Dedication

To our families

To the
Department of Anesthesiology at Northwestern University Feinberg School of Medicine,
Johns Hopkins University School of Medicine,
Virginia Mason Clinic,
and the University of California, Davis School of Medicine.

Contents

Contributors

Burak Alptekin, MD
Medical Doctor; Fellow, Clinical and Research Pain; Fellow, Clinical and Research Critical Care, Critical Care and Pain Medicine, Department of Anesthesiology, Beth Israel Deaconess Medical Center, Harvard Medical School, Boston, Massachusetts.
Classification of Headache

Michael L. Ault, MD
Assistant Professor, Associate Chief, Section of Critical Care Medicine, Department of Anesthesiology, Northwestern University Fienberg School of Medicine; Attending Physician, Northwestern Memorial Hospital; Consulting Physician, Rehabilitation Institute of Chicago, Chicago, Illinois.
Pain Control in the Critically Ill Patient

Zahid H. Bajwa, MD
Assistant Professor of Anesthesiology (Neurology), Harvard Medical School; Director, Education and Clinical Pain Research, Beth Israel Deaconess Medical Center, Boston, Massachusetts.
Classification of Headache

Bernard R. Bendok, MD
Assistant Professor of Neurological Surgery and Radiology, Northwestern University Feinberg School of Medicine; Attending Physician, Northwestern Memorial Hospital, Chicago, Illinois.
Osteoporosis and Percutaneous Vertebroplasty

Honorio T. Benzon, MD
Professor of Anesthesiology; Senior Associate Chair, Academic Affairs; Chief, Division of Pain Medicine; Director, Pain Medicine Fellowship Program, Northwestern University Feinberg School of Medicine, Northwestern Memorial Hospital, Chicago, Illinois.
Taxonomy: Definition of Pain Terms and Chronic Pain Syndromes; Physical Examination of the Pain Patient; Membrane Stabilizers; Drugs for the Interventional Physician: Botulinum Toxin, Steroids, Radiopaque Dye; Patient-Controlled Analgesia; Intraarticular and Intraperitoneal Opioids for Postoperative Pain; Postdural Puncture Headache and Spontaneous Intracranial Hypotension; Cervicogenic Headache and Orofacial Pain; Overview of Low Back Pain Disorders; Interlaminar Epidural Steroid Injections for Lumbosacral Radiculopathy; Selective Nerve Root Blocks and Transforaminal Epidural Steroid Injection for Back Pain and Sciatica; Facet Syndrome: Facet Joint Injections and Facet Nerve Block; Pain Originating from the Buttock: Sacroiliac Joint Dysfunction and Piriformis Syndrome; Phantom Pain; Geriatric Pain; Lumbar Discography; Fluoroscopy and Radiation Safety; Lumbar Plexus, Femoral, Lateral Femoral Cutaneous, Obturator, Saphenous, and Fascia Iliaca Blocks; Sciatic Nerve Block; Issues in Peripheral Nerve Blocks: Use of Nerve Stimulators, Multiple- Versus Single-Injection Techniques, and Use of Adjuvants; Peripheral Sympathetic Blocks; Anticoagulants and Neuraxial Anesthesia

Patrick K. Birmingham, MD, FAAP
Associate Professor of Anesthesiology, Northwestern University Feinberg School of Medicine; Director, Pain Management Services; Attending Physician, Children's Memorial Medical Center, Chicago, Illinois.
Pediatric Postoperative Pain

E. Richard Blonsky, MD
Professor of Clinical Neurology, Northwestern University Feinberg School of Medicine; Attending

Physician, Northwestern Memorial Hospital;
Medical Director, The Pain & Rehabilitation Clinic of
Chicago, Chicago, Illinois.
Determination of Disability

Allen W. Burton, MD
Associate Professor; Section Chief of Pain Management,
Department of Anesthesiology, University of Texas M.D.
Anderson Cancer Center, Houston, Texas.
Spinal Cord Stimulation

Kenneth D. Candido, MD
Associate Professor of Anesthesiology; Chief, Section of
Acute Pain Medicine, Northwestern Memorial
Hospital, Northwestern University Feinberg
School of Medicine, Chicago, Illinois.
*Diagnostic Nerve Blocks; Intraarticular and
Intraperitoneal Opioids for Postoperative Pain; Caudal
Anesthesia; Brachial Plexus Block: Techniques Above the
Clavicle; Brachial Plexus Block: Techniques Below the
Clavicle; Lumbar Plexus, Femoral, Lateral Femoral
Cutaneous, Obturator, Saphenous, and Fascia Iliaca
Blocks; Issues in Peripheral Nerve Blocks: Use of Nerve
Stimulators, Multiple- Versus Single-Injection Techniques,
and Use of Adjuvants*

Zenobia Casey, MD
Assistant Professor, Department of Anesthesiology and
Critical Care Medicine, Johns Hopkins Medical
Institutions, Baltimore, Maryland.
Epidural Opioids for Postoperative Pain

Yuan Chen, MD
Medical Director of Pain Management, Rush-Copley
Medical Center, Aurora, Illinois.
Pharmacology for the Interventional Physician

Michael R. Clark, MD, MPH
Associate Professor and Director, Chronic Pain
Treatment Programs, Department of Psychiatry and
Behavioral Sciences, Johns Hopkins Medical
Institutions, Baltimore, Maryland.
Substance Use Disorders and Detoxification

Christopher M. Criscuolo, MD
Associate Professor of Anesthesiology and
Orthopaedic Surgery; Director, Division of
Pain Medicine, Department of Anesthesiology,
University of Nebraska College of Medicine,
Omaha, Nebraska.
Acupuncture

Lowell Davis, DO
Fellow, Division of Pain Medicine, Department of
Anesthesiology, Northwestern University Feinberg
School of Medicine, Northwestern Memorial Hospital,
Chicago, Illinois.
Geriatric Pain

Oscar A. de Leon-Casasola, MD
Director, Pain Fellowship Program; Vice-chair for
Clinical Affairs, Department of Anesthesiology,
University at Buffalo, School of Medicine; Chief, Pain
Medicine, Roswell Park Cancer Institute, Buffalo,
New York.
Neurolytic Visceral Sympathetic Blocks

Robert Doty, Jr., MD
Assistant Professor, Department of Anesthesiology,
Northwestern University Feinberg School of Medicine;
Attending Anesthesiologist, Northwestern Memorial
Hospital, Chicago, Illinois.
Ankle Block

Patrick M. Dougherty, PhD
Associate Professor, Department of Anesthesiology,
Division of Anesthesiology and Critical Care Medicine,
The University of Texas M.D. Anderson Cancer Center,
Houston, Texas.
*Anatomy and Physiology of Somatosensory and Pain
Processing; Neurochemistry of Somatosensory and
Pain Processing*

Robert H. Dworkin, PhD
Professor of Anesthesiology, Neurology, Oncology, and
Psychiatry, University of Rochester School of Medicine
and Dentistry; Director, Anesthesiology Clinical
Research Center, Strong Memorial Hospital, Rochester,
New York.
Herpes Zoster and Postherpetic Neuralgia

Robert R. Edwards, PhD
Assistant Professor, Department of Psychiatry and
Behavioral Sciences, Johns Hopkins University School
of Medicine, Baltimore, Maryland.
Pain Assessment

Frank D. Ferris, MD
Medical Director, Palliative Care Standards/Outcome
Measures, San Diego Hospice and Palliative Care;
Clinical Professor, Voluntary, Department of Family &
Preventative Medicine, University of California,
San Diego, School of Medicine, San Diego, California;
Assistant Professor, Adjunct, Department of Family and

Community Medicine, University of Toronto, ON, Canada; Affiliate, Buehler Center on Aging, Northwestern University Feinberg School of Medicine, Chicago, Illinois.
Approach to the Management of Cancer Pain

Scott M. Fishman, MD
Professor of Anesthesiology; Chief, Division of Pain Medicine, Department of Anesthesiology and Pain Medicine, University of California, Davis School of Medicine, Sacramento, California.
Opioid Receptors; Major Opioids in Pain Management; Minor and Short-Acting Opioids; Opioid Therapy: Adverse Effects Including Addiction; Drugs for the Interventional Physician: Botulinum Toxin, Steroids, Radiopaque Dye

Mikhail Fukshansky, MD
Fellow in Cancer Pain Medicine, Department of Anesthesiology, University of Texas M.D. Anderson Cancer Center, Houston, Texas.
Spinal Cord Stimulation

Rollin M. Gallagher, MD, MPH
Director, Pain Management Service, Philadelphia VA Medical Center; Professor of Psychiatry and Anesthesiology, Department of Psychiatry and Anesthesiology, University of Pennsylvania School of Medicine; Editor in Chief of *Pain Medicine*.
Psychopharmacology for Pain Medicine

Robert Gould, MD
Assistant Professor, Northwestern University Feinberg School of Medicine; Medical Director, Simulator Center; Consulting Physician, Rehabilitation Institute of Chicago; Attending Physician, Northwestern Memorial Hospital, Chicago, Illinois.
Pain Control in the Critically Ill Patient

Theodore S. Grabow, MD
Assistant Professor, Department of Anesthesiology and Critical Care Medicine, Division of Pain Medicine, Johns Hopkins University School of Medicine; Active Staff, Department of Anesthesiology, St Joseph Medical Center, Baltimore, Maryland.
Complex Regional Pain Syndrome: Terminology and Pathophysiology; Complex Regional Pain Syndrome: Diagnosis and Treatment

Anthony H. Guarino, MD
Director of Pain Management, Barnes-Jewish West County Hospital; Faculty, Washington University Medical School, St. Louis, Missouri.

Complex Regional Pain Syndrome: Terminology and Pathophysiology; Complex Regional Pain Syndrome: Diagnosis and Treatment

Jennifer A. Haythornthwaite, PhD
Associate Professor, Department of Psychiatry and Behavioral Sciences, Johns Hopkins Medical Institutions, Baltimore, Maryland.
Psychological Evaluation and Testing; Psychological Interventions for Chronic Pain

James R. Hebl, MD
Staff Consultant, Department of Anesthesiology, Mayo Clinic College of Medicine, Rochester, Minnesota.
Complications After Peripheral Nerve Block

Ursula Heck, MS, MD
Fellow, Pain Medicine, Department of Anesthesiology, Georgetown University Hospital, Washington, DC.
Preemptive Analgesia: Physiology and Clinical Studies

Leslie J. Heinberg, PhD
Associate Professor, Department of Psychiatry, Division of Child and Adolescent Psychiatry, Case Western Reserve University School of Medicine, Cleveland, Ohio.
Psychological Evaluation and Testing; Psychological Interventions for Chronic Pain

Matthew D. Hepler, MD
Assistant Professor, Department of Orthopaedic Surgery, Northwestern University Feinberg School of Medicine, Chicago, Illinois.
Overview of Low Back Pain Disorders

Mark Holtsman, Pharm.D.
Co-Director, Acute Pain Service; Associate Clinical Professor, Department of Anesthesiology and Pain Medicine, University of California, Davis School of Medicine, Sacramento, California.
Opioid Receptors

Rasha Snan Jabri, MD
Fellow, Pain Medicine, Department of Anesthesiology, Northwestern University Feinberg School of Medicine, Northwestern Memorial Hospital, Chicago, Illinois.
Overview of Low Back Pain Disorders

Jeffrey A. Katz, MD
Associate Professor of Anesthesiology, Northwestern University Feinberg School of Medicine; Associate Director, Section of Pain Medicine; Staff Member,

Department of Anesthesiology, Northwestern Memorial Hospital, Chicago, Illinois.
NSAIDs and COX-2-Selective Inhibitors; Diabetic and Other Peripheral Neuropathies; Issues in Peripheral Nerve Blocks: Use of Nerve Stimulators, Multiple- Versus Single-Injection Techniques, and Use of Adjuvants

Mark J. Lema, MD, PhD
Professor and Chair, Department of Anesthesiology, State University of New York at Buffalo, School of Medicine and Biomedical Sciences; Chairman of Anesthesiology and Pain Medicine, Roswell Park Cancer Institute, Buffalo, New York.
Neurolytic Visceral Sympathetic Blocks

Robert M. Levy, MD, PhD
Professor of Neurological Surgery; Associate Professor of Physiology, Departments of Neurosurgery and Physiology, Northwestern Comprehensive Pain Clinic, Northwestern University Institute for Neuroscience, Northwestern University Feinberg School of Medicine; Attending Physician, Northwestern Memorial Hospital, Chicago, Illinois.
Neurosurgical Procedures for Treatment of Intractable Pain; Implanted Drug Delivery Systems for Control of Chronic Pain

Henry M. Liu, MD
Vice Chair, Department of Anesthesiology, Lake Forest Hospital, Lake Forest, Illinois.
Acupuncture

John C. Liu, MD
Assistant Professor, Department of Neurosurgery, Northwestern University Feinberg School of Medicine; Attending Physician, Northwestern Memorial Hospital, Chicago, Illinois.
Osteoporosis and Percutaneous Vertebroplasty

Spencer S. Liu, MD
Staff Anesthesiologist, Virginia Mason Medical Center; Clinical Professor of Anesthesiology, University of Washington School of Medicine, Seattle, Washington.
Local Anesthetics: Clinical Aspects

Gagan Mahajan, MD
Assistant Professor; Director, Fellowship in Pain Medicine, Department of Anesthesiology and Pain and Medicine, University of California, Davis School of Medicine, Sacramento, California.

Major Opioids in Pain Management; Opioid Therapy: Adverse Effects Including Addiction

Atif B. Malik, MD
Arnold Pain Center, Department of Anesthesia, Beth Israel Deaconess Medical Center, Boston, Massachusetts.
Classification of Headache

James J. Mathews, MD
Professor of Clinical Medicine, Northwestern University Feinberg School of Medicine; Senior Attending Staff, Northwestern Memorial Hospital, Chicago, Illinois.
Pain Management in the Emergency Department

Susan B. McDonald, MD
Staff Anesthesiologist, Virginia Mason Medical Center, Seattle, Washington.
Combined Spinal–Epidural Technique

Onur Melen, MD
Assistant Professor of Neurology and Ophthalmology, Northwestern University Feinberg School of Medicine, Chicago, Illinois.
Muscle Relaxants

Michael M. Minieka, MD
Assistant Professor of Clinical Neurology, Department of Neurology, Northwestern University Feinberg School of Medicine; Attending Neurologist, Northwestern Memorial Hospital, Chicago, Illinois.
Neurophysiologic Testing for Pain; Entrapment Neuropathies

Veronica Mitchell, MD
Director of Pain Medicine Services, Department of Anesthesiology, Georgetown University Hospital, Washington, DC.
Preemptive Analgesia: Physiology and Clinical Studies

Robert E. Molloy, MD
Assistant Professor of Anesthesiology; Director, Residency Program, Northwestern University Feinberg School of Medicine, Chicago, Illinois.
Membrane Stabilizers; Diagnostic Nerve Blocks; Interlaminar Epidural Steroid Injections for Lumbosacral Radiculopathy; Myofascial Pain Syndrome; Fibromyalgia; Sickle Cell Anemia; Geriatric Pain; Neurolytic Visceral Sympathetic Blocks; Intrathecal and Epidural Neurolysis; Head and Neck Blocks; Truncal Blocks: Intercostal, Paravertebral, Interpleural, Suprascapular, Ilioinguinal and Iliohypogastric Nerve Blocks

John D. Moore, MD
Fellow, Pain Medicine, Department of
Anesthesiology, Northwestern University Feinberg
School of Medicine, Northwestern Memorial Hospital,
Chicago, Illinois.
*Physical Examination of the Pain Patient; Postdural
Puncture Headache and Spontaneous Intracranial
Hypotension*

Kenji Muro, MD
Resident Physician, Department of Neurologicalsurgery,
Northwestern University Feinberg School of Medicine,
Chicago, Illinois.
*Implanted Drug Delivery Systems for Control of
Chronic Pain*

Antoun Nader, MD
Assistant Professor of Anesthesiology, Northwestern
University Feinberg School of Medicine, Chicago,
Illinois.
*Intraarticular and Intraperitoneal Opioids for
Postoperative Pain; Caudal Anesthesia; Peripheral
Sympathetic Blocks*

Joseph M. Neal, MD
Staff Anesthesiologist, Virginia Mason Medical Center;
Clinical Professor of Anesthesiology, University of
Washington, Seattle, Washington.
Complications After Peripheral Nerve Block

Takashi Nishida, MD
Assistant Professor of Clinical Neurology,
Department of Neurology, Northwestern University
Feinberg School of Medicine, Chicago, Illinois.
*Neurophysiologic Testing for Pain; Entrapment
Neuropathies*

Umeshraya T. Pai, MD
Professor of Clinical Anesthesia; Adjunct Professor of
Anatomy, University of Cincinnati Medical Center,
Cincinnati, Ohio.
Head and Neck Blocks

Judith Paice, RN, PhD
Director, Cancer Pain Program, Division of
Hematology-Oncology; Research Professor of Medicine,
Northwestern University Feinberg School of Medicine,
Robert H. Lurie Comprehensive Cancer Center,
Chicago, Illinois.
Management of Pain at End of Life

Sunil J. Panchal, MD
Director, Interventional Pain Medicine, H. Lee Moffitt
Cancer Center and Research Institute; Associate
Professor of Oncology and Anesthesiology, University
of South Florida College of Medicine, Tampa, Florida.
Pelvic Pain

James C. Phero, DMD
Professor of Clinical Anesthesia, Pediatrics and Surgery;
Faculty, Pain Control Center, College of Medicine,
University of Cincinnati, Cincinnati, Ohio.
Cervicogenic Headache and Orofacial Pain

Heidi Prather, DO
Assistant Professor; Chief of Section, Physical Medicine
and Rehabilitation, Department of Orthopaedic
Surgery, Washington University School of Medicine,
St. Louis, Missouri.
*Physical Medicine and Rehabilitation Approaches to Pain
Management*

Joel M. Press, MD
Assistant Professor, Department of Physical Medicine
and Rehabilitation, Northwestern University Feinberg
School of Medicine, Chicago, Illinois.
*Physical Medicine and Rehabilitation Approaches to
Pain Management*

Srinivasa N. Raja, MD
Professor of Anesthesiology and Critical Care; Director
of Pain Research, Division of Pain Medicine; Interim
Director, Division of Pain Medicine, Johns Hopkins
University School of Medicine, Baltimore, Maryland.
*Anatomy and Physiology of Somatosensory and Pain
Processing; Neurochemistry of Somatosensory and Pain
Processing; Complex Regional Pain Syndrome:
Terminology and Pathophysiology; Complex Regional Pain
Syndrome: Diagnosis and Treatment; Phantom Pain;
Central Pain States*

Rebecca Rallo Clemans, MD
Fellow, Pain Medicine, Department of Anesthesiology,
Northwestern University Feinberg School of Medicine,
Northwestern Memorial Hospital, Chicago, Illinois.
*Pharmacology for the Interventional Physician;
Facet Syndrome: Facet Joint Injections and Facet
Nerve Blocks*

Maunak V. Rana, MD
Interventional Pain Physician, The Illinois Pain
Treatment Institute, Elgin, Illinois.

Physical Examination of the Pain Patient; Membrane Stabilizers

James P. Rathmell, MD
Professor of Anesthesiology, University of Vermont College of Medicine; Director, Center for Pain Medicine, Fletcher Allen Health Care, Burlington, Vermont.
Diabetic and Other Peripheral Neuropathies

Jeffrey M. Richman, MD
Assistant Professor of Anesthesiology, Department of Anesthesiology and Critical Care Medicine, Johns Hopkins Medical Institutions, Baltimore, Maryland.
Intrathecal Opioid Injections for Postoperative Pain

Jack M. Rozental, MD, PhD, MBA
Vice Chair, Davee Department of Neurology, Northwestern University Feinberg School of Medicine; Chief, Neurology Service, Jesse Brown VA Medical Center, Chicago, Illinois.
Migraine Headache and Cluster Headache; Tension-Type Headache, Chronic Tension-Type Headache, and other Chronic Headache Types

Eric J. Russell, MD
Professor and Chairman, Department of Radiology; Professor of Neurosurgery and Otolaryngology, Northwestern University Feinberg School of Medicine, Chicago, Illinois.
Anatomy, Imaging, and Common Pain-Generating Degenerative Pathologies of the Spine

Francis V. Salinas, MD
Clinical Assistant Professor of Anesthesiology, University of Washington School of Medicine; Staff Anesthesiologist, Virginia Mason Medical Center, Seattle, Washington.
Spinal Anesthesia

Kenneth E. Schmader, MD
Associate Professor of Medicine, The Center for the Study of Aging and Human Development, Duke University Medical Center; Vice-Chief, Division of Geriatrics, Geriatric Research, Education and Clinical Center, Durham VA Medical Center, Durham, North Carolina.
Herpes Zoster and Postherpetic Neuralgia

Ali Shaibani, MD
Assistant Professor of Radiology and Neurosurgery, Northwestern University Feinberg School of Medicine;

Co-director, Neuroendovascular Program, Interventional Neuroradiology, Northwestern Memorial Hospital, Chicago, Illinois.
Lumbar Discography

Nigel E. Sharrock, MD, ChB
Attending Anesthesiologist; Senior Scientist, Department of Anesthesiology, Hospital for Special Surgery, New York, New York.
Epidural Anesthesia

Edward R. Sherwood, MD, PhD
Associate Professor; James F. Arens Endowed Chair, Department of Anesthesiology, The University of Texas Medical Branch, Shriners Hospital for Children, Galveston, Texas.
Patient-Controlled Analgesia

B. Todd Sitzman, MD, MPH
Director, The Center for Pain Medicine, Wesley Medical Center, Hattiesburg, Mississippi.
Pharmacology for the Interventional Pain Physician

Eric M. Spitzer, MD
Clinical Instructor, Northwestern University Feinberg School of Medicine, Fellow in Neuroradiology, Northwestern Memorial Hospital, Chicago, Illinois.
Anatomy, Imaging, and Common Pain Generating Degenerative Pathologies of the Spine

Steven P. Stanos, DO
Instructor, Department of Physical Medicine and Rehabilitation, Northwestern University Feinberg School of Medicine; Medical Director, Chronic Pain Care Center, Rehabilitation Institute of Chicago, Chicago, Illinois.
Physical Medicine and Rehabilitation Approaches to Pain Management

Rom A. Stevens, MD
Captain, Medical Corps U.S. Naval Reserve; Adjunct Associate Professor, Department of Anesthesiology, Uniformed Services University of the Health Sciences, Bethesda, Maryland.
Epidural Anesthesia

Lila A. Sueda, MD
Staff Anesthesiologist, Virginia Mason Medical Center, Seattle, Washington.
Complications After Neuraxial Blockade

Radha Sukhani, MD
Associate Professor of Anesthesiology; Director,
Regional Anesthesia Service, Northwestern University
Feinberg School of Medicine, Chicago, Illinois.
Sciatic Nerve Block; Ankle Block

Santhanam Suresh, MD, FAAP
Associate Professor of Anesthesiology, Northwestern
University Feinberg School of Medicine; Co-Director,
Pain Management Services, Children's Memorial
Hospital, Chicago, Illinois.
Chronic Pain Management in Children

Jay R. Thomas, MD, PhD
Clinical Medical Director, San Diego Hospice and
Palliative Care; Assistant Clinical Professor of Medicine,
University of California, San Diego, School of
Medicine, San Diego, California.
Approach to the Management of Cancer Pain

Muthukumar Vaidyaraman, MBBS
Post-Doctoral Clinical Fellow, Division of Pain
Medicine, Department of Anesthesiology and Critical
Care Medicine, Johns Hopkins Medical Institutions,
Baltimore, Maryland.
Central Pain States

Murugusundaram Veeramani, MD
Clinical Instructor, Northwestern University Feinberg
School of Medicine; Fellow in Neuroradiology,
Northwestern Memorial Hospital, Chicago, Illinois.
*Anatomy, Imaging, and Common Pain Generating
Degenerative Pathologies of the Spine*

Charles F. von Gunten, MD, PhD, FACP
Medical Director, Center for Palliative Studies,
San Diego Hospice and Palliative Care; Editor-in-Chief,
Journal of Palliative Medicine; Associate Clinical
Professor of Medicine, University of California,
San Diego, School of Medicine, San Diego,
California.
Approach to the Management of Cancer Pain

David R. Walega, MD
Assistant Professor of Anesthesiology, Northwestern
University Feinberg School of Medicine; Director,
Anesthesiology Pain Medicine Center, Northwestern
Memorial Hospital, Chicago, Illinois.
*Intradiscal Techniques: Intradiscal Electrothermal
Therapy and Nucleoplasty*

Matthew T. Walker, MD
Chief, Neuroradiology; Assistant Professor, Northwestern
University Feinberg School of Medicine Chicago,
Illinois.
*Anatomy, Imaging, and Common Pain-Generating
Degenerative Pathologies of the Spine*

Ajay D. Wasan, MD, MSc
Instructor in Pain Medicine, Department of
Anesthesiology, Perioperative, and Pain Medicine,
Department of Psychiatry, Brigham and Women's
Hospital, Harvard Medical School, Boston,
Massachusetts.
Psychopharmacology for Pain Medicine

Barth L. Wilsey, MD
Associate Clinical Professor of Anesthesiology and
Pain Medicine; Director, Residency Program in
Pain Medicine, University of California,
Davis School of Medicine, Sacramento,
California.
*Minor and Short-Acting Opioids; Opioid Therapy:
Adverse Effects Including Addiction*

Cynthia A. Wong, MD
Associate Professor of Anesthesiology; Director of
Obstetric Anesthesiology; Medical Director, Labor and
Delivery, Northwestern University Feinberg School of
Medicine, Chicago, Illinois.
Pain Management During Pregnancy and Lactation

Christopher L. Wu, MD
Associate Professor of Anesthesiology, Department of
Anesthesiology and Critical Care Medicine,
Johns Hopkins Medical Institutions, Baltimore,
Maryland.
*Intrathecal Opioid Injections for Postoperative Pain;
Epidural Opioids for Postoperative Pain*

Edward Yaghmour, MD
Instructor in Anesthesiology, Northwestern University
Feinberg School of Medicine, Chicago, Illinois.
Brachial Plexus Block: Techniques Below the Clavicle

Jeffrey L. Young, MD, MA
Director, Musculoskeletal Health Program, Hudson
Valley Physical Medicine and Rehabilitation, Sleepy
Hollow, New York.
*Physical Medicine and Rehabilitation Approaches to
Pain Management*

Preface

The first edition of our book provided a quick reference and easy reading. It was ideal for residents who were looking for short and precise discussions of a subject. It was not adequate for the fellows who were reviewing for their pain medicine boards or for the researcher looking for a comprehensive treatise on a topic. The short format constrained us from satisfying readers looking for more detailed information.

We made several changes in this second edition. We expanded each chapter to make it more authoritative and comprehensive in depth and in its references. Several important topics on pharmacology, back pain and the other pain syndromes, and interventional procedures were added to be more representative of the complex nature of pain management and to incorporate the recent advances in the field. The chapters on regional anesthesia were increased, expanded, and updated. We added key points at the end of most chapters to highlight the important contents of the chapter. However, we maintained one format of the first edition: the discussion of each topic in a separate chapter. Readers who voiced their opinions to us appreciated this unique feature of the book. Readers also informed us that they prefer a hard cover for the book, as the soft cover nature of the first edition did not lend itself to repeated usage.

An endeavor of this kind cannot be completed without the help of many people. Our contributors took time off from their busy schedules to write their chapters. Our secretaries, especially Robb Rabito and Sandra Taylor, performed numerous tasks to bring this book into fruition. Our editors, Katie Miller and Melissa Fisch, showed diplomacy in waiting for the manuscripts and patience in correcting our mistakes. To all of you, thank you.

This second edition of our book shows maturity. We hope the readers like it.

Honorio T. Benzon, M.D.
Srinivasa N. Raja, M.D.
Robert E. Molloy, M.D.
Spencer S. Liu, M.D.
Scott M. Fishman, M.D.
EDITORS

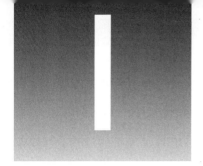

Anatomy and Physiology of Somatosensory and Pain Processing

Srinivasa N. Raja, M.D., and
Patrick M. Dougherty, Ph.D.

Pain is a physiological consequence of impending or actual tissue injury that serves a vital protective function. For example, clinical observations in patients with congenital insensitivity to pain and in patients with leprosy have clearly demonstrated that the absence of pain results in chronic disabilities. However, pain can become a disease itself when it occurs or persists in the absence of tissue damage or following appropriate healing of injured tissues. Chronic pain becomes tremendously disabling and has considerable negative impact on quality of life.

The International Association for the Study of Pain defines pain as "an unpleasant sensory and emotional experience associated with actual or potential tissue damage, or described in terms of such damage."[1] The definition acknowledges that pain is not only a sensory experience, but may be associated with affective and cognitive responses. The definition also recognizes that the relationship between pain and tissue damage is not constant. Thus, an understanding of the anatomical substrates and physiological mechanisms by which noxious and non-noxious stimuli are perceived provide the essential background to understand the mechanisms of both acute and chronic pain.

SOMATOSENSATION, NOCICEPTION, AND PAIN

Somatosensation is the physiological process by which neural substrates are activated by physical stimuli resulting in the perception of what we describe as touch, pressure, pain, etc. *Nociception* is the physiological process of activation of neural pathways by stimuli that are potentially or actually damaging to tissue. In experimental situations a stimulus is considered nociceptive based on a behavioral avoidance or escape response of an animal or by studying the activity evoked by the stimulus in specialized groups of afferent fibers. Clinically, the degree of

nociception is inferred by overt evidence of tissue damage. *Pain*, in contrast to nociception, is a conscious experience, and while the stimulus-induced activation of afferent neural pathways may play an important role, other factors may influence the overall perception of pain. These factors include the alterations in somatic sensory processing following injury to tissues and/or nerves as well as psychosocial factors. The experience of pain, particularly chronic pain, often results in suffering. Suffering results from a multitude of factors that includes loss of physical function, social isolation, family distress, and a sense of inadequacy or spiritual loss. This chapter briefly reviews the basic anatomy and physiology of the neural pathways that respond to somatosensory stimuli, especially nociceptive stimuli, and emphasizes the plasticity in this system following an injury. This knowledge is fundamental in the evaluation and subsequent management of patients with painful disorders.

The sequence of events by which a stimulus is perceived involves four processes: (1) transduction, (2) transmission, (3) modulation, and (4) perception. *Transduction* occurs in the peripheral terminals of primary afferent neurons where different forms of energy, e.g., mechanical, heat, or cold, are converted to electrical activity (action potentials). *Transmission* is the process by which electrical activity induced by a stimulus is conducted through the nervous system. There are three major components of the transmission system. The peripheral sensory cells in the dorsal root ganglia transmit impulses from the site of transduction at their peripheral terminal to the spinal cord where the central terminals synapse with second-order neurons. The spinal neurons are the second component in the transmission network. These cells send projections to various brain stem and diencephalic structures. Finally, neurons of the brainstem and diencephalon form the third component of the transmission network as they project to various cortical sites.

Modulation is the process whereby neural activity may be altered along the pain transmission pathway. The dorsal horn of the spinal cord is one major site where modulation occurs involving a multitude of neurotransmitter systems. Activation of pain modulation systems usually results in less activity in the pain transmission pathway following a noxious stimulus. Examples of activation of this process include stress-induced analgesia. However, in some circumstances modulation can also result in an enhancement of pain signaling. *Perception* is the final stage of the pain-signaling process by which neural activity in the somatosensory transmission pathway results in a subjective sensation of pain. It is presumed that this process results from the concerted activation of primary and secondary somatosensory and limbic cortices.

PERIPHERAL MECHANISMS

Primary afferent fibers are part of the peripheral nervous system with their cell bodies located in the dorsal root ganglia. Primary afferent fibers are initially classified based on their conduction velocity and the cutaneous stimuli by which they are activated. Information on the intensity of a given stimulus is coded by the frequency of impulses in a population of primary afferents with a generally monotonic relationship between the stimulus intensity and the number of impulses generated by afferent fibers in reply. There are three classes of primary afferent fibers in skin based on conduction velocity that may be activated by a given cutaneous stimulus.[2,3] The fastest conducting fibers are the large-diameter myelinated A-beta (Aβ) fibers. These fibers when activated do not normally transmit the sensation of pain, but rather of light touch, pressure, or hair movement. The axons of the nociceptive neurons are generally unmyelinated C fibers or thinly myelinated A-delta (Aδ) fibers. Nociceptors have the capacity to respond to intense heat, cold, mechanical, and chemical stimuli. The functional role of the Aδ and C fiber nociceptors may be different. The C fibers (0.3 to 3.0 μM) conduct at velocities of less than 2 m/second and are the predominant (>75%) type of afferent fiber in peripheral nerves. Recordings from C fibers in humans suggest that C fiber activity is associated with a prolonged burning sensation. In contrast, activation of faster conducting (5 to 20 m/second) Aδ fibers evokes a sharp, intense, tingling sensation. The combined activation of these two groups of afferents, such as by an intense brief heat stimulus, results in a dual pain sensation.[4] Aδ fibers convey the rapid-onset first sensation of pricking pain while C fibers mediate the slower-onset second burning pain sensation that follows brief intense heat stimulation to the skin. Combined, Aδ and C fiber nociceptors encode and transmit information to the central nervous system concerning the intensity, location, and duration of noxious stimuli.

Nociceptive afferents are further subclassified based on the molecules expressed on their cell surface (e.g., receptors, glycoconjugates), based on the molecules they store and release (e.g., peptides), and based on the enzymes they contain. While none of these cell markers is completely specific for the peripheral target tissue innervated, nevertheless the percentage of dorsal root ganglion cells positive for a given marker differs significantly among target tissues. For example, almost all visceral afferents are peptidergic, but only about half of the afferents projecting to the skin are,[5] and only a small percentage of the non-peptidergic afferents, characterized by binding the plant lectin IB4 from *Griffonia simplicifolia*,[6] project to muscle.[7,8] Similarly, the central projection areas of peptidergic and non-peptidergic afferents differ with peptidergic fibers mainly projecting to lamina I and lamina II outer, and IB4 binding (non-peptidergic) afferents projecting preferably to lamina II inner (e.g., Silverman and Kruger,[6] but see also Woodbury et al.[9]). Most peptidergic neurons express the tyrosine kinase receptor A (trk A), suggesting that they depend on nerve growth factor (NGF) for survival.[10] In contrast, most IB4 positive dorsal root ganglion cells do not express trk A[11] (see also Kashiba et al.[12]) but express one of the GDNF family receptors (GDNFRα1–4) together with receptor tyrosine kinase Ret.[13,14] Peptidergic and non-peptidergic neurons also express different patterns of receptors involved in signal transduction, and they may therefore display different sensitivities to a given stimulus. Thus the P2X$_3$ receptor, which mediates nociceptor excitation by ATP, is primarily expressed in IB4 positive neurons.[15] In contrast, the vanilloid receptor 1 (VR1/TRPV1), which mediates responses to heat, capsaicin, and protons, is expressed in only a minority of IB4 positive cells in mice,[16] and IB4 positive neurons are less responsive to these stimuli than their IB4 negative counterparts.[17,18]

SPINAL MECHANISMS

The first synapse in somatosensory processing of information from the body surface occurs at either the spinal dorsal horn or in the dorsal column nuclei at the spinal cord–brainstem junction.[19] Somatosensory processing for information from the face is similarly processed either in the spinal trigeminal nucleus (pain and temperature) or in the chief sensory nucleus of the trigeminal nerve located in the midpons region of the brainstem. Both nociceptive and non-nociceptive fibers provide inputs to both of these initial targets. However, under normal circumstances the dorsal column nuclei and the chief sensory nucleus can be considered to process selectively inputs from the large myelinated Aβ fiber classes related to light touch while the spinal dorsal horn and spinal trigeminal nucleus processes inputs of the nociceptive Aδ and C fibers. This separation of modalities in the somatosensory system is the basis for the localization of neural lesions based on quantitative sensory examination.

Nociceptive primary afferent fibers terminate in a highly ordered way in the spinal dorsal horn on the same side of the body of their origin.[20,21] The dorsal horn is anatomically organized in the form of layers or laminae as first recognized by Rexed in the cat[22] (Fig. 1-1). The unmyelinated C fibers terminate primarily in the most superficial lamina (I and II outer), while the thinly myelinated Aδ fibers end in lamina I, and in laminae III to V. Collaterals of the large myelinated fibers (Aβ) terminate laminae III to V of the dorsal horn.

Two predominant types of second-order nociceptive spinal and spinal trigeminal projection neurons have been identified: wide dynamic range neurons (WDR) and nociceptive specific (NS) neurons.[19] WDR cells are especially concentrated in the deeper laminae of the dorsal horn (III to V) where they receive input from both low-threshold Aβ and nociceptive Aδ and C fibers and hence are activated by both innocuous and noxious stimuli. However, the responses of WDR cells to these stimuli are graded so that the noxious stimuli evoke a greater response than non-noxious stimuli. WDR spinal projection neurons in monkeys have an average spontaneous discharge rate of

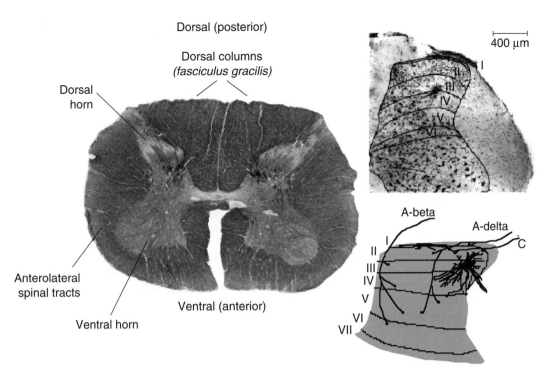

FIGURE 1-1. Histological sections and schematic diagrams of the spinal dorsal horn. The histological section at left from human lumbar spinal cord is labeled to show the relationship between the major spinal somatosensory structures. The histological section at right is from rat spinal cord. The outer heavy lines show the boundary of the spinal gray matter while the inner heavy lines show the boundaries of Rexed's laminae. These boundaries are established by the histological characteristics of each zone, and the layers are identified by the numerals at the right of the dorsal horn boundary. Finally, the schematic at the bottom illustrates the pattern of primary afferent innervation to the non-human primate spinal dorsal horn. The large myelinated (A-beta) fibers segregate to the dorsal aspect of an entering rootlet and then course medially in the dorsal horn and terminate in layers III to V. The small myelinated (A-delta) fibers and C fibers which carry nociceptive information segregate ventrally in the entering roots, course laterally in the dorsal horn, and then largely terminate in the more superficial layers (I and II) of the dorsal horn. The cell profiles inserted in laminae I and II to IV are representative of superficial and deep classes of spinothalamic neurons.

approximately 11 Hz, average responses to innocuous cutaneous stimulation by a soft camel hair brush of approximately 25 Hz, and average responses to noxious mechanical stimulation by a small arterial clip applied to the skin of approximately 50 Hz (Fig. 1-2).

In contrast to WDR cells, NS projection cells respond only to noxious stimuli under physiological conditions. The majority of NS cells are found in the superficial laminae of the dorsal horn (I and outer II). These cells have a lower rate of spontaneous activity than WDR cells averaging about 3 to 5 Hz. The discharge rates to the noxious stimuli of NS cells are comparable to those of WDR cells averaging about 50 Hz (Fig. 1-3).

The axons of both the WDR and NS second-order neurons cross the midline near the level of the cell body, gather into bundles of ascending fibers in the contralateral anterolateral spinal region, and then ascend toward targets in the brainstem and diencephalon (Fig. 1-4). The conduction velocity of the WDR cells is usually faster than that of the NS cells (approximately 30 m/second versus 12 m/second). Additionally, the axons of the NS cells that largely arise from laminae I of the dorsal horn and those of the WDR cells arising primarily from laminae III to V tend to run in slightly different positions in the anterolateral spinal funiculus. In the anterolateral spinal column the NS cell axons are found in the dorsal medial region while axons of WDR cells are more concentrated in the ventral lateral region.

SPINAL MODULATION

The concept of modulation of noxious inputs at spinal levels was highlighted by the gate control theory of Melzack and Wall.[23] This theory suggested that input along low-threshold (Aβ) fibers inhibits the responses of WDR cells to nociceptive input. The theory was offered as an explanation for the efficacy of transcutaneous electrical stimulation for pain relief. Subsequent studies have identified intrinsic spinal neurons that release several different neurotransmitters in the spinal cord that play a role in the modulation of nociceptive impulses. Furthermore, a number of inputs to the dorsal horn from various brainstem sites have been shown to also modulate peripheral inputs as well as outputs of intrinsic cells.[24,25] Both types of modulation, that arising in the local network of cells at the spinal levels as well as that from the descending inputs, can result in either augmented or inhibited output from spinal cord pain signaling neurons. It is the combined effects of spinal excitatory and inhibitory systems that determine what messages are delivered to the higher levels of the central nervous system (CNS).

A special type of spinal modulation that is observed under certain circumstances is known as *central sensitization*.[26] In this phenomenon the capacity for transmission in the nociceptive system is changed or shows *neuronal plasticity*. The result of this plasticity is that following a noxious stimulus of sufficient intensity and duration, such as a surgical incision, the coding

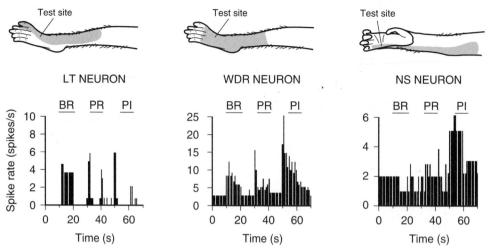

FIGURE 1-2. The rate histograms show responses of primate spinothalamic tract neurons representative of low threshold (LT), wide dynamic range (WDR), and nociceptive specific (NS) classes. The responses of these cells were evoked by application of a series of mechanical stimuli of graded intensity to multiple sites across the receptive field for each cell. The times and sites of each stimulus application are indicated by the lines and labels at the top of each histogram. The brush stimulus (BR) was provided by a soft camel hair brush while a large arterial clip was used to produce innocuous pressure (PR) and a small arterial clip was used to produce a noxious pinch (PI) sensation. The WDR cell in the center shows responses that are graded with the intensity of the stimuli. The NS neuron at the right shows no significant responses to any stimuli but the most intense, while the LT neuron on the left responds to innocuous brushing of the skin alone (the transient responses with the application and removal of the arterial clips are due to the touch stimuli provided at contact). The diagrams of the hindlimbs show the receptive field locations of each neuron (shaded region) and the site on skin where each of the mechanical stimuli were applied (spots).

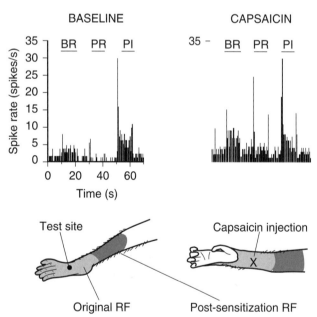

FIGURE 1-3. The rate histograms show the background activity and responses of a representative wide dynamic range spinothalamic tract neuron to mechanical stimulation of the hindlimb before and following sensitization by an intradermal injection of capsaicin. The baseline responses to the mechanical stimuli are shown on the left, while the matching records after capsaicin are shown on the right. The mechanical stimuli were applied to the spot shown on the drawing of the leg at the bottom. The "X" shows the site at which capsaicin was delivered. The light gray area shows the receptive field during the baseline recordings while the dark gray area shows the expansion in receptive field induced by capsaicin.

of pain-signaling neurons for a given stimulus may be increased. One example of central plasticity is the phenomenon of *windup* whereby repeated stimulation of C fibers at intervals of 0.5 to 1 Hz results in a progressive increase in the number of discharges evoked by each volley.[27] In addition to an increase in discharges evoked by a given stimulus, sensitized spinal neurons also show an expansion of receptive field size and an increase in spontaneous discharge rate. WDR cells tend to become sensitized more readily than do NS cells. However, in those circumstances where NS cells do show sensitization they often acquire novel responsiveness to innocuous stimuli and hence could be recategorized as WDR neurons. Our increase in the understanding of the pharmacology of this and other types of plasticity will have profound consequences in the development of new analgesic pharmacotherapies.

SUPRASPINAL MECHANISMS

Supraspinal structures involved in somatosensory processing include brainstem, diencephalic, and cortical sites.[28] There are two sets of somatosensory inputs to the brainstem and diencephalon. First, many axons and axon collaterals of the spinal projection neurons that ascend in the anterolateral spinal quadrant depart this ascending tract to terminate in a number of nuclei of the brainstem and midbrain. These target sites include brainstem autonomic regulatory sites that influence cardiovascular and respiratory functions, while in the midbrain there are multiple inputs to centers from which both descending as well as ascending (e.g., to thalamus) modulation of somatosensory processing is evoked. The remainder of the so-called anterolateral system fibers continues through the brainstem and midbrain to terminate in diencephalic structures, including the hypothalamus and posterior, lateral, and medial regions of the thalamus (see Fig. 1-4).

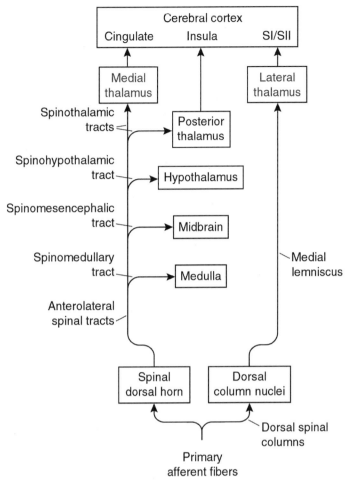

FIGURE 1-4. Schematic diagram summarizing the central nociceptive pathways. Each box represents the discrete anatomical locations at which noxious stimuli are processed and/or registered. The lines indicate the neural pathways which interconnect each of the anatomical locations.

The second set of somatosensory inputs to the brain stem includes those primary afferent fibers that ascend in the dorsal (posterior) columns of the spinal cord to form their first synapse at the dorsal column nuclei. These inputs are organized so that the fibers from the lower extremities synapse most medially in the nucleus gracilis and inputs from the upper extremities synapse laterally in the nucleus cuneatus. The trunk is represented in regions of both nuclei. Comparative inputs from the face are processed in the chief sensory nucleus of the trigeminal nerve located at the site of origin of cranial nerve five in the midpons of the brainstem. The axons of the second-order cells in the dorsal column nuclei cross the midline and form the medial lemniscus on the contralateral side of the brainstem. These fibers then ascend through the brainstem and midbrain acquiring the functionally related fibers from the trigeminal nerve as pass and continue on to provide the second somatosensory input to the diencephalon as they terminate in the ventral posterior lateral (VPL) nucleus (inputs from the body) and ventral posterior medial (VPM) nucleus (inputs from the face) of the thalamus.

The somatosensory inputs to the cortex include the third-order projections from thalamic somatosensory relay neurons of VPL and VPM as well as third- (and higher-) order neurons projecting from brainstem and midbrain relay neurons.[29,30] Some of these projections are highly organized and quite specific. For example, the cells in the core of VPL that receive inputs from the dorsal column–medial lemniscus fibers project to cortical areas SI and SII. The neurons in the posterior region of the lateral thalamus receiving inputs from the anterolateral system project to SII and the retro-insular areas of cortex, while medial thalamic nuclei ultimately project to the anterior cingulate cortex. Similarly, somatosensory relay neurons of the midbrain parabrachial nucleus project specifically to the amygdaloid nucleus of the neocortex. On the other hand, other third-order projections into cortex are quite diffuse. Outputs from cells of the brainstem reticular activating system that receive somatosensory inputs from the spinoreticular tract, for example, project throughout the neocortex.

SUPRASPINAL MODULATION OF NOCICEPTION

Several lines of research have clearly indicated that plasticity and modulation of somatosensory signaling occur at brainstem, midbrain, and diencephalic levels. Examples of plasticity of responses of dorsal column neurons following intradermal injection of the irritant capsaicin have been documented in the rat and monkey. Similarly, with the development of acute inflammation and following deafferentation, neurons of the thalamus alter their patterns of spontaneous discharge so that a large increase in bursting of these cells is observed. Ascending modulation from the brainstem dorsal raphe nucleus also influences signaling of thalamic neurons. However, unlike at spinal levels, our understanding of these processes at these higher levels of the somatosensory system is not as fully developed.

KEY POINTS

- The processes resulting in a noxious stimulus-inducing pain are transduction, transmission, modulation, and perception.
- Nociceptors in the periphery respond to intense heat, cold, mechanical, or chemical stimuli and encode the intensity, location, and duration of noxious stimuli.
- The dorsal horn is anatomically organized in laminae. Unmyelinated C fibers terminate in Rexed's laminae I and II, and large myelinated fibers terminate in the laminae III to V.
- Two types of second-order nociceptive spinal and spinal trigeminal projection neurons are wide dynamic range (WDR) and nociceptive specific (NS). WDR cells receive input from both Aβ and nociceptive (C and Aδ) fibers.
- The somatosensory system is composed of two main signaling channels.
- The anterolateral system is the primary pain signaling channel.
- In contrast the dorsal column–medial lemniscal system is primarily a high-speed, very discrete signaling channel for innocuous stimuli.
- The two sensory channels project to both unique as well as overlapping brain regions.
- Derangements can occur in both these signaling systems at any and all levels that result in the generation of chronic pain.

REFERENCES

1. Merskey H: Pain terms: A supplementary note. Pain 14:205–206, 1982.
2. Besson JM, Chaouch A: Peripheral and spinal mechanisms of nociception. Physiol Rev 67:67–186, 1987.
3. Burgess PR, Perl ER: Myelinated afferent fibres responding specifically to noxious stimulation of the skin. J Physiol 190:541–562, 1967.
4. Meyer RA, Campbell JN: Myelinated nociceptive afferents account for the hyperalgesia that follows a burn to the hand. Science 213:1527–1529, 1981.
5. Perry MJ, Lawson SN: Differences in expression of oligosaccharides, neuropeptides, carbonic anhydrase, and neurofilament in rat primary afferent neurons retrogradely labelled via skin, muscle or visceral nerves. Neuroscience 85:293–310, 1998.
6. Silverman JD, Kruger L: Lectin and neuropeptide labeling of separate populations of dorsal root ganglion neurons and associated "nociceptor" thin axons in rat testis and cornea whole-mount preparations. Somatosens Res 5:259–267, 1988.
7. Ambalavanar R, Moritani M, Haines A, et al: Chemical phenotypes of muscle and cutaneous afferent neurons in the rat trigeminal ganglion. J Comp Neurol 460:179, 2003.
8. Plenderleith MB, Snow PJ: The plant lectin Bandeiraea simplicifolia I-B4 identifies a subpopulation of small diameter primary sensory neurons which innervate the skin in the rat. Neurosci Lett 159:17–20, 2003.
9. Woodbury CJ, Ritter AM, Koerber HR: On the problem of lamination in the superficial dorsal horn of mammals: a reappraisal of the substantia gelatinosa in postnatal life. J Comp Neurol 417:88–102, 2000.
10. Averill S, McMahon SB, Clary DO, et al: Immunocytochemical localization of trkA receptors in chemically identified subgroups of adult rat sensory neurons. Eur J Neurosci 7:1484–1494, 1995.
11. Molliver DC, Radeke MJ, Feinstein SC, Snider WD: Presence or absence of TrkA protein distinguishes subsets of small sensory neurons with unique cytochemical characteristics and dorsal horn projections. J Comp Neurol 361:404–416, 1995.
12. Kashiba H, Uchida Y, Senba E: Difference in binding by isolectin B4 to trkA and c-ret mRNA-expressing neurons in rat sensory ganglia. Brain Res Mol Brain Res 95:18–26, 2001.
13. Bennett DL, Michael GJ, Ramachandran N, et al: A distinct subgroup of small DRG cells express GDNF receptor components and GDNF is protective for these neurons after nerve injury. J Neurosci 18:3059–3072, 1998.
14. Orozco OE, Walus L, Sah DW, et al: GFRalpha3 is expressed predominantly in nociceptive sensory neurons. Eur J Neurosci 13:2177–2182, 2001.
15. Vulchanova L, Riedl MS, Shuster SJ, et al: P2X3 is expressed by DRG neurons that terminate in inner lamina II. Eur J Neurosci 10:3470–3478, 1998.
16. Zwick M, Davis BM, Woodbury CJ, et al: Glial cell line-derived neurotrophic factor is a survival factor for isolectin B4-positive, but not vanilloid receptor 1-posirive, neurons in the mouse. J Neurosci 22:4057–4065, 2002.
17. Dirajlal S, Pauers LE, Stucky CL: Differential response properties of IB(4)-positive and -negative unmyelinated sensory neurons to protons and capsaicin. J Neurophysiol 89:513–524, 2003.
18. Stucky CL, Lewin GR: Isolectin B(4)-positive and -negative nociceptors are functionally distinct. J Neurosci 19:6497–6505, 1999.
19. Willis WD: The Pain System. The Neural Basis of Nociceptive Transmission in the Mammalian Nervous System. Karger, Basel, 1985.
20. Light AR, Perl ER: Differential termination of large-diameter and small-diameter primary afferent fibers in the spinal dorsal gray matter as indicated by labeling with horseradish peroxidase. Neurosci Lett 6:59–63, 1977.
21. Woolf CJ, Fitzgerald M: Somatotopic organization of cutaneous afferent terminals and dorsal horn neuronal receptive fields in the superficial and deep lamine of the rat lumbar spinal cord. J Comp Neurol 251:517–531, 1986.
22. Rexed B: The cytoarchitectonic organization of the spinal cord in the cat. J Comp Neurol 96:415–466, 1952.
23. Melzack R, Wall PD: Pain mechanisms: A new theory. Science 150:971–979, 1965.
24. Basbaum AI, Fields HL: Endogenous pain control mechanisms: review and hypothesis. Ann Neurol 4;451–462, 1978.
25. Besson JM, Guilbaud G, LeBars D: Descending inhibitory influences exerted by the brain stem upon the activities of dorsal horn lamina V cells induced by intra-arterial injection of bradykinin into the lilmbs. J Physiol 248:725-739, 1975.
26. Woolf CJ: Evidence for a central component of post-injury pain hypersensitivity. Nature 306:686–688, 1983.
27. Mendell LM, Wall PD: Responses of single dorsal cord cells to peripheral cutaneous unmyelinated fibres. Nature 206:97–99, 1965.
28. Albe-Fessard D, Berkley KJ, Kruger L, et al: Diencephalic mechanisms of pain sensation. Brain Res Rev 9:217–296, 1985.
29. Casey KL, Minoshima S, Berger KL, et al: Positron emission tomographic analysis of cerebral structures activated specifically by repetitive noxious heat stimuli. J Neurophysiol 71:802–807, 1994.
30. Sweet WH: Cerebral localization of pain. In Thompson RA, Green JR (eds): New Perspectives in Cerebral Localization. Raven Press, New York, 1982, pp 205–242.

Neurochemistry of Somatosensory and Pain Processing

**Patrick M. Dougherty, Ph.D., and
Srinivasa N. Raja, M.D.**

The neurochemistry of somatosensory processing provides the clinician with two general levels of intervention: modification of pain transduction at the level of nociceptors in skin; and modification of pain transmission through the central nervous system.

NEUROCHEMISTRY OF PAIN TRANSDUCTION

Tissue injury results in the local release of numerous chemicals which either directly induce pain transduction by activating nociceptors or facilitate pain transduction by increasing the excitability of nociceptors. The list of mediators is extensive as one can see quickly in the graphical summary presented in Fig. 2-1, and as such is frequently referred to simply as an "inflammatory soup."

Inflammatory Soup: Several of the key "ingredients" of this soup include the following components.

Bradykinin plays a critical role in inflammatory pain and hyperalgesia (see Dray[1] and Couture et al.[2] for reviews). Bradykinin produces acute pain in humans by activation of unmyelinated and myelinated nociceptors.[3] Bradykinin also produces transient heat hyperalgesia in humans by sensitization of nociceptors through activation of phospholipase C (PLC), protein kinase C (PKC), the production of eicosanoids, and modulation of the TRPV1 (VR1) channel (see below).

Low pH (excess free H+) levels found in inflamed tissues also contribute to the pain and hyperalgesia associated with inflammation, as this selectively causes activation and sensitization of nociceptors to mechanical stimuli. Recent studies suggest that the effects of pH are mediated by the opening of a dorsal root ganglion neuron specific acid-sensing ion channel (DRASIC/ASIC-3, see Waldmann[4] for a review). Excitation of nociceptors

by protons does not undergo tachyphylaxis or adaptation, and a synergistic excitatory effect of protons and a combination of inflammatory mediators has been reported.[5,6]

Serotonin, released from platelets in response to platelet-activating factor derived from mast cell degranulation, causes pain when applied to a human blister base[7] by activation of nociceptors.[8] Serotonin also potentiates bradykinin-induced pain and nociceptor activation.

Histamine, released from mast cells by *substance P* derived from axon reflexes in activated nociceptors, produces a variety of responses including vasodilation and edema. Exogenous histamine applied to the skin produces itch and not pain,[9] but histamine excites polymodal visceral nociceptors and potentiates the responses of nociceptors to bradykinin and heat.[10]

Eicosanoids are a large family of arachidonic acid metabolites that include the *prostaglandins*, *thromboxanes*, and *leukotrienes*. Eicosanoids directly activate articular afferents and sensitize these, as well as those in skin and viscera, to natural stimuli and other endogenous chemicals (for reviews see Cunha and Ferreira[11] and Schaible et al.[12]). Prostaglandins, synthesized by the constitutive enzyme COX-1, and by COX-2, induced in peripheral tissues by inflammation,[13] reduce the activation threshold of tetrodotoxin-resistant Na+ currents in nociceptors, increase intracellular cAMP levels, and increase the excitability of sensory neurons. Leukotrienes, metabolites of the lipoxygenase pathway, contribute to hyperalgesia and sensitization to mechanical stimuli.

Adenosine and its mono- and polyphosphate derivates (AMP, ADP, ATP) are released or leaked into the extracellular space with tissue injury and inflammation where they contribute to pain and hyperalgesia (for reviews see Hamilton and McNahon[14] and Ralevic and Burnstock[15]). Adenosine induces pain in humans by direct activation of nociceptors. ATP also

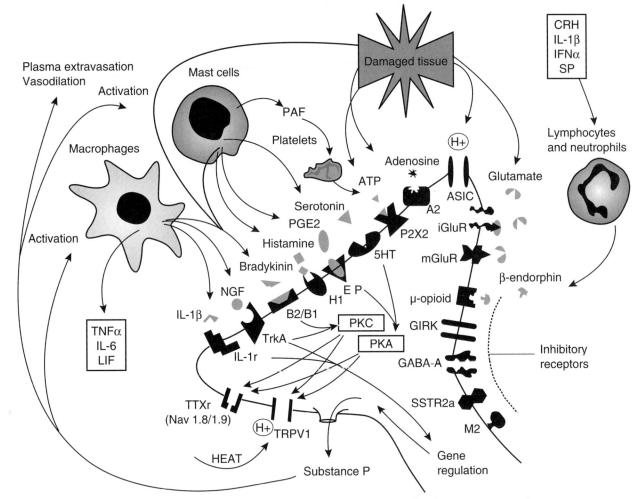

FIGURE 2-1. Schematic of the neurochemistry of somatosensory processing at peripheral sensory nerve endings.

induces pain in humans and activates C nociceptors in healthy human skin, but does not sensitize C fibers to mechanical or heat stimuli. ATP presumably activates nociceptive neurons in normal skin via the $P2X_3$ and the heteromeric $P2X_2/P2X_3$ receptor.[16]

Cytokines (e.g., interleukin-1β (IL-1β), tumor necrosis factor α (TNFα), interleukin-6 (IL-6)) are released by a variety of cells (e.g., macrophages, astrocytes, Schwann cells) to regulate inflammatory cell responses (see Cunha and Ferreira[11] for a review). However, cytokines also promote pain signaling. Both IL-1β and TNFα directly excite and sensitize nociceptive afferent fibers to thermal and mechanical stimuli. IL-6 in combination with its soluble IL-6 receptor also sensitizes nociceptors to heat. Clinical studies show that TNFα levels are increased in synovial fluid of painful joints, and treatment with antibodies against TNFα improves symptoms accompanying rheumatoid arthritis, including pain.[17]

Excitatory amino acid (EAA) receptors are present on dorsal root ganglion cells and the presynaptic terminals of primary afferents and play a role in the modulation of nociceptive impulses.[18] Peripheral application of glutamate activates nociceptors through binding to both ligand-gated ion channels (ionotropic glutamate receptors, iGlu) and G-protein-coupled metabotropic (mGlu) type 1 and type 5 (mGluR1, mGluR5)

receptors on unmyelinated axons in the skin and enhance pain behavior. Neurons in the DRG labeled for mGluR5 also express VR1 receptors characteristic of nociceptive neurons.[19]

Nerve growth factor (NGF) may contribute to inflammatory pain via direct and indirect mechanisms. Inflammatory mediators, such as cytokines, increase NGF production in inflamed tissues.[20] NGF stimulates mast cells to release histamine and serotonin and induces heat hyperalgesia by acting directly on the peripheral terminals of primary afferent fibers.[21] NGF sensitizes nociceptors and may alter the distribution of Aδ fibers such that a greater proportion of fibers have nociceptor properties.[22] NGF is implicated in the inflammation-induced changes in nociceptor response properties, such as an increase in incidence of ongoing activity, increase in maximum fiber following frequency, and changes in the configuration of the action potential of DRG neurons. NGF-induced hyperalgesia may be mediated via its actions on the TTXr sodium channel, Nav 1.8, and by potentiation of the responses of the VR1 receptor.[21]

Peripheral Anti-hyperalgesic Mechanisms: In addition to the pain-enhancing mediators listed above, there are also numerous mediators that may act to limit or modulate pain transmission. Some of these components are discussed here.

Opioids are another component of inflammatory soup that, unlike the other constituents listed above, may produce analgesia in inflamed tissues by a peripheral mechanism (see Machelska and Stein[23] for a review). Opioid receptors are preset on peripheral terminals of afferent fibers, and axonal transport of these receptors is enhanced during inflammation. Increased amounts of endogenous opioids are found in inflamed tissues likely arising from inflammatory cells such as macrophages, monocytes, and lymphocytes induced by IL-1β and corticotropin-releasing hormone (CRH) originating from the inflamed tissue.

An alternate mechanism for the activation of peripheral endogenous opioid analgesia is via endothelin-1 (ET-1), a potent vasoactive peptide, synthesized and released by epithelia after tissue injury.[24] Although ET-1 can trigger pain by activating ET_A receptors on nociceptors, it also has an analgesic effect through its actions on ET_B receptors. Activation of ET_B receptors on keratinocytes by ET-1 results in release of β-endorphins and analgesia that are mediated via peripheral μ- and κ-opioid receptors, which are linked to G-protein-coupled inward rectifying potassium channels (GIRKs).

Acetylcholine acting on peripheral cholinergic receptors after release from non-neuronal sources may have a modulatory role on nociception. Nicotine has a weak excitatory effect on C nociceptors and induces a mild sensitization to heat, but no alterations in mechanical responsiveness. In contrast, muscarine desensitizes C nociceptors to mechanical and heat stimuli.[25] Studies in mice with targeted deletions of the M2 receptor gene suggest that M2 receptors on cutaneous nerve endings depress the responsiveness of nociceptive fibers to noxious stimuli (see Wess[26] for a review).

Gamma-aminobutyric acid (GABA) may have a peripheral role in modulation of pain transmission similar to acetylcholine. $GABA_A$ receptors have been found in DRG cells and on their central terminals in the dorsal horn.

Somatostatin (SST) type 2a receptors (SSTR2a) are present in about 10% of unmyelinated primary afferent fibers innervating the glabrous skin of rat.[27] The intraplantar administration of the SST receptor agonist octreotide reduces the phase II response after formalin injection. In addition, octreotide reduces the response of CMHs to heat stimuli and attenuates the thermal responses of nociceptors sensitized by bradykinin. The peripheral effects of SST agonists may be mediated by a direct effect on primary afferents, or by its anti-inflammatory effects.

Peripheral Second Messenger Pathways: As described above, inflammation is associated with the release of a host of chemical mediators. While some of these agents may directly activate nociceptors, most of the inflammatory mediators lead to changes in the sensory neuron rather than directly activating it. These changes in sensory neurons include early post-translational changes, such as phophorylation of transducer molecules (e.g., VR1 receptor) and voltage-gated ion channels (e.g., sodium channels) in the peripheral terminals of nociceptors (peripheral sensitization) as well as longer-lasting transcription-dependent changes in effector genes in DRG cells.[28,29] The *vanilloid receptor* TRPV1 (also known as VR1) present on a subpopulation of primary afferent fibers that are activated by capsaicin, heat, and protons is subject to both short- and long-term changes in function. Inflammatory mediators, such as bradykinin and NGF, lower the threshold of TRPV1-mediated heat-induced currents in DRG neurons and increase the proportion of DRG cells that respond to capsaicin[30,31] by PLC-dependent phosphorylation by PKC, by phosphorylation by protein kinase A (PKA),[32,33] and by hydrolysis of the membrane phospholipid phosphatidylinosital-4-5-biphophate (PIP_2).[21] PKA and PKC also induce a short-term sensitization of nociceptors to heat by modulating the activity of tetrodotoxin-resistant sodium currents.[34,35] Longer-term changes in TRPV1 following inflammation in primary afferent fibers are associated with increases in the activity of the various transcription factors including cAMP-responsive element-binding protein (CREB)[36] and the mitogen-activated protein kinases (MAPK), most especially the extracellular signal-regulated kinases (ERK), the c-Jun amino-terminal kinases (JNK), and the p38 enzymes.[37–39]

NEUROCHEMISTRY OF PAIN TRANSMISSION

As reviewed in Chapter 1, the pain transmission pathways through the central nervous system (CNS) can be broadly divided into the anterolateral and dorsal column–medial lemnsical pathways based on differences in both anatomy and physiology of constituent neurons. The neurochemistry, unlike the anatomy and physiology, of somatosensory processing in both the anterolateral and dorsal column–medial lemniscal systems is very similar. Both systems involve three classes of transmitter compounds, excitatory neurotransmitters, inhibitory neurotransmitters, and neuropeptides, that are found in three anatomical compartments, sensory afferent terminals, local circuit terminals, and descending (or ascending) modulatory circuit terminals (Fig. 2-2).

Excitatory Neurotransmitters: The main excitatory neurotransmitters in the somatosensory system are the amino acids glutamate and aspartate. These excitatory amino acids mediate transmission at each of the afferent connections in the somatosensory system, including the synaptic connection between primary afferent fibers and spinal neurons,[40] from spinal neurons to thalamic neurons,[41] etc. There are four receptor types for glutamate and aspartate in the somatosensory system. These receptors are named for the synthetic agonists by which they are best activated. Thus, one class of receptors best activated by *N*-methyl-D-aspartate (NMDA) is termed the NMDA glutamate receptor.[42] A second class of receptors not activated by NMDA (non-NMDA receptors) includes three subtypes: a kainate receptor, an AMPA ((R,S)-α-amino-3-hydroxy-5-methylisoxazole-4-propionic acid) receptor, and the metabotropic receptor.[43] The AMPA and kainate receptors are linked to sodium channels and are considered to mediate the majority of the fast synaptic afferent signaling in this system for all modalities and intensities of stimuli. The NMDA receptor is usually considered as recruited only by intense and/or prolonged somatosensory stimuli. This characteristic is due to the NMDA receptor's well-known magnesium block that is only relieved by prolonged depolarization of the cell membrane. The NMDA receptor is linked to a calcium ionophore that when activated results in many long-term changes in excitability of sensory neurons (*sensitization*). The AMPA/kainate and NMDA receptors are also frequently considered to mediate mono- and polysynaptic contacts of primary afferent fibers to dorsal horn neurons. Finally, the metabotropic glutamate receptors (mGluR) are actually

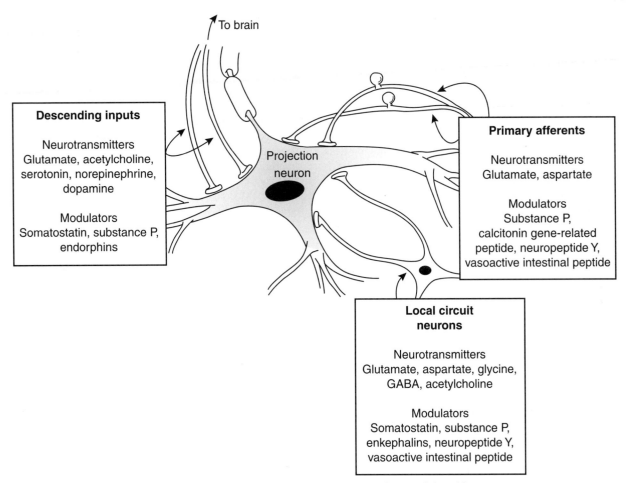

FIGURE 2-2. Schematic of the neurochemistry of somatosensory processing in the spinal dorsal horn.

a family of G-protein-linked sites. The group I mGluRs when activated are coupled to $G_{q/11}$ that activates phospholipase C liberating inositol phosphate, which in turn results in the release of cytosolic calcium and activation of protein kinase C. The group II and III metabotropic receptors are negatively coupled by G_i/G_o to adenyl cyclase and so reduce intracellular cyclic AMP and protein kinase A activity. Given the complexity of these receptor transduction mechanisms, it should come as no surprise that activation of mGluRs can result in the modulation of multiple cellular kinases, receptors, ion channels, and transcription factors and so have complex and sometimes variable effects on somatosensory and pain processing. However, as a general rule the group I mGluRs have cooperative effects with NMDA receptors in promoting cellular excitability and pain signaling, while the group II and III mGluRs most often have inhibitory effects on pain transmission.

A second type of excitatory substance that may have a transmitter role in the somatosensory system is adenosine triphosphate (ATP). ATP modulates somatosensory transmission by activation of the P2X family of receptors that is composed of seven subunits expressed in six homomeric and at least four heteromeric subtypes.[44] P2X receptors are present on the central terminals of primary afferent fibers innervating neurons in laminae V and II of the dorsal horn where they function to increase the release of the glutamate.

Inhibitory Neurotransmitters: The primary inhibitory neurotransmitters of the somatosensory system include the amino acids glycine and GABA. *Glycine* is particularly important at spinal levels while GABA is the chief inhibitory transmitter at higher levels. Glycine has two receptor sites: a chloride-linked strychnine-sensitive inhibitory receptor as well as a strychnine-insensitive modulatory site on the NMDA glutamate receptor complex. GABA is an inhibitory amino acid neurotransmitter found in local circuit neurons of spinal laminae I, II, and III of the dorsal horn. Three types of GABA receptors have been identified. The $GABA_A$ receptor is linked to a chloride channel and modulated by barbiturates, benzodiazepines, and alcohol. Selective $GABA_A$ agonists include muscimol and selective antagonists include gabazine. The $GABA_B$ receptor has been associated with both a potassium ionophore and with a G-protein-linked complex. Baclofen is a selective $GABA_B$ receptor agonist and phaclofen is a selective antagonist. Finally the newly described $GABA_C$ receptor has also been described as associated with a potassium channel ionophore. CACA is a selective agonist for this site, but there is no selective antagonist for $GABA_C$ receptors at present. $GABA_C$ receptors do not appear to have any role in the modulation of somatosensory information.

Alterations in the functions of the inhibitory neurotransmitters may be particularly important with the induction of hyperalgesia and following the development of neuropathic pain.

For example, a GABA$_A$-mediated link between large myelinated fibers and C fiber nociceptors has been proposed as a mechanism for the development of allodynia following intradermal injection of the irritant capsaicin.[45] Additionally, a selective loss of inhibitory interneurons at both spinal and thalamic levels has been suggested as contributing to some neuropathic pain conditions.[46]

Norepinephrine is an important inhibitory neurotransmitter in descending brainstem projections to the dorsal horn.[47,48] The adrenergic receptors include two broad classes termed the alpha and beta receptors each of which in turn have several subtypes. The alpha 2 adrenergic receptor is the primary form found in the spinal dorsal horn that has an inhibitory role in the processing of sensory information. However, it should be noted that the function of norepinephrine following injury to the nervous systems might become reversed from an inhibitory, analgesic role into one of promoting and/or sustaining an on-going chronic pain state.

Serotonin has historically been considered as one of the major inhibitory transmitters in pathways descending to the spinal dorsal horn from the midbrain raphe nuclei.[47,49] There are multiple serotonin receptor subtypes, including 5HT-1, -2, and -3 receptors. Each of these major types also has several subtypes. Controversy has arisen in recent years concerning which of these subtypes mediate the analgesic properties of serotonin, which has in turn cooled the interest in serotonin as a clinically useful target for the treatment of pain. In part, this controversy may be due to the fact that some serotonin receptor subtypes, in fact, promote nociception, while others are inhibitory. If more selective tools are developed with which to dissect this pharmacology, serotonin may regain its former status as potentially useful clinical target.

Another important inhibitory neurotransmitter at spinal levels is the purine *adenosine*.[50] There are at least two types of adenosine receptors termed the A1 and A2 sites. Occupation of these sites by adenosine results in G-protein-mediated alterations of cyclic AMP levels in target cells. However, elevations, as well as decreases, in cAMP formation have been reported in various conditions. Adenosine may mediate a portion of the analgesia produced by brainstem norepinephrine projections to the spinal cord and appears to have especially robust analgesic properties in neuropathic pain conditions.

Finally, *acetylcholine* is yet another neurotransmitter that mediates antinociception at the level of the spinal dorsal horn.[51] This transmitter likely mediates the inhibition of pain transmission that is observed on stimulation of the vagus nerve and may also contribute to the analgesia produced by the alpha-2 adrenergic receptor agonist clonidine. The antinociceptive effects of acetylcholine appear mediated by the muscarinic and not by the nicotinic acetylcholine receptor subtypes.

Neuropeptides: There are multiple neuropeptides that contribute to signaling of somatosensory information. Some of these could be classified as excitatory compounds and others as inhibitory. However, instead of considering these compounds together with the excitatory and inhibitory neurotransmitters above, we have separated these into a section of their own because of the distinct profile of action of these compounds as opposed to the neurotransmitters. Unlike the very rapid onset and termination of action of the transmitters, neuropeptides tend to have more gradual onset of effects as well as much more prolonged duration of action once released.

The excitatory neuropeptides in the somatosensory system include *substance P* and *neurokinin A*.[52,53] These peptides are especially concentrated in primary afferent fibers but also may be present in intrinsic neurons of the spinal dorsal horn and thalamus. The receptors for these peptides include the neurokinin 1 and 2 sites, each of which has been associated with elevation of intracellular calcium levels, perhaps through liberation of inositol phosphate. At the spinal level these peptides are only released following application of noxious stimuli that are sufficient to produce sustained discharges in C nociceptors, although some small myelinated (Aδ) fibers may also contain substance P. These peptides do not appear to signal as synaptic transmitters, but rather as trans-synaptic transmitters. Thus, once released, the peptides are not confined to a site of action on the immediate postsynaptic membrane, but instead tend to spread throughout the dorsal horn potentially acting on multiple synapses at some distance from their point of release. It has been suggested that stimuli of particular modalities (e.g., mechanical versus thermal) are associated with selective release of one peptide versus another; however, this suggestion has not been corroborated. Activation of neurokinin 1 and/or 2 receptors by substance P and/or neurokinin A are considered key steps needed for the induction of sensitization and hence the expression of hyperalgesia following cutaneous injury. It has been further proposed that the mechanism of neurokinin receptor involvement in the expression of sensitization is through facilitation of the synaptic actions of the excitatory amino acid neurotransmitters.

The inhibitory neuropeptides at spinal levels include somatostatin, the enkephalins, and possibly dynorphin. These peptides are contained in both intrinsic neurons of the dorsal horn and in the fibers descending to the dorsal horn from various brainstem nuclei. At thalamic levels the inhibitory neuropeptides also include the endorphins which are contained in ascending antinociceptive pathways. The receptor types for the opioid peptides include the μ-, δ-, and κ-receptor subtypes at all levels of the somatosensory system. These receptors are associated with modulation of both intracellular cAMP and potassium levels. There is also an important cooperative functional link between mu-opioid and alpha$_2$-adrenergic receptors that has yet to be fully exploited for clinical applications.

Finally, a number of neuropeptides are present in the somatosensory system whose functions have yet to be clearly identified and, for now, should be considered as a third category. These peptides include calcitonin gene-related peptide (CGRP), vasoactive intestinal peptide (VIP), neuropeptide Y (NPY), and cholecystokinin (CCK), among others. Future studies will no doubt have more to say about the role of these peptides in the neurochemistry of synaptic transmission in the somatosensory system.

Central Signal Propagation and Second Messenger Systems: Propagation of bioelectric signals in the CNS is fundamentally dependent on the movement of various ions and the activity of cellular enzymes and metabolites. The proteins that form ion channels and function as second messenger enzymes can be blocked by a number of agents and many of these have been studied as putative analgesics. However, since ion channels and second messengers are found in all neural elements, the effects of compounds acting at these sites are not specific to pain circuitry. Side effects are therefore often encountered with these drugs that limit their usefulness. There are four ion channels involved in pain signal propagation in the CNS, those for sodium, calcium, potassium, and chloride.

The opening of *sodium channels* is the primary event underlying the depolarization of nerve membranes and so is the key to propagation of neural impulses throughout the nervous system. Sodium currents in dorsal horn neurons are mediated by at least three types of tetrodotoxin-sensitive channels and these are inactivated by local anesthetics such as lidocaine and bupivacaine. Prolonged infusions of local anesthetics for postoperative pain in humans became widespread in the 1990s,[54–56] and cancer and chronic nonmalignant pain are treated with continuous infusions of intrathecal local anesthetics outside of the hospital.[57,58] Side effects are, however, common[57–60] and include delayed urinary retention, paresthesia, paresis/gait impairment, periods of orthostatic hypotension, bradypnea, and dyspnea.

Calcium ions are essential for regulation of neuronal excitability and for the release of neurotransmitter with synaptic depolarization.[61] At least four different types of calcium channels, the L-, N-, T-, and P-types, have been identified in dorsal horn neurons. There are numerous chemical antagonists of L-type calcium channels,[61] whereas N-type calcium channels are blocked using toxins of *Conus magnus*.[62] P-channels are especially prevalent in Purkinje cells and are sensitive to venom toxins of the funnel web spider (*Agelenopsis aperta*).[61] T-channels are involved in the regulation of neuronal excitability and pacemaker activity[63] and are blocked by some omega conotoxins. Antinociceptive effects have been shown for N-, L-, and P-type calcium channels in animals[62–66] and for L- and N-type channels in humans.[67]

Potassium is the second main cation of the neuronal action potential. There are two large families of potassium channels, the voltage-gated channels and the inwardly rectifying channels.[68] The voltage-gated channels include the "A" fast transient conductances sensitive to 4-aminopyridine, barium, and cobalt; and the calcium-activated potassium channels sensitive to cobalt, manganese, and cadmium. Opening of voltage-gated potassium channels allows outward positive current flow from neurons, such as during repolarization following an action potential. Blockade of these channels initially prolongs generation of action potentials. Continued application, however, prevents repolarization and so ultimately produces a failure to generate action potentials. The inwardly rectifying channels establish and regulate neuronal excitability. Potassium channel agonists/antagonists are not likely to be soon used for the treatment of pain.

Three major classes of *chloride channels* have been identified.[69] The first class identified was the ligand-gated chloride channels, including those of the GABA type A (GABAA) and glycine receptors. The ligand-gated chloride channels are common dorsal horn neurons. The second class, also likely common at spinal levels, is the voltage-gated chloride channels. The final chloride channel class is activated by cyclic adenosine monophosphate and may include only the cystic fibrosis transmembrane regulator. Activation of chloride currents usually produces inward movement of chloride to cells that hyperpolarize neurons; facilitation of these hyperpolarizing currents underlies the mechanisms of many depressant drugs. An important exception at spinal levels, however, is that GABAA receptors on primary afferent terminals gate a chloride channel that allows efflux of chloride with a net effect therefore of depolarizing primary afferent terminals. Chloride channel antagonists, such as bicuculline and strychnine, have not been given to relieve pain, but instead to produce an experimental pain state characterized by a pronounced opiate-refractory allodynia.[46,70,71] These compounds were also used to exacerbate the anatomical consequences of nerve constriction injury.[72]

The role of *second messenger systems* in pain sensitivity has been examined in a number of studies. Levels of membrane-bound protein kinase C increase following both nerve injury and intraplantar injection of formalin.[73,74] Spinal infusion of phorbol esters to activate protein kinase C increases the behavioral response to intraplantar formalin and increases the spontaneous and evoked activity of primate spinothalamic tract neurons. In contrast, antagonists for protein kinase C decrease pain behavior following nerve injury,[75] intraplantar formalin,[76] intraspinal N-methyl-D-aspartate, and intradermal capsaicin. Similarly, inhibition of phospholipase C[75] or phospholipase A[76] (needed for release of cofactors to protein kinase C) reduce hyperalgesia following intraplantar formalin and zymosan, respectively. Finally, animals engineered with defects in protein kinase C had less pain following nerve injury,[77] while those engineered with defects in protein kinase A had decreased responses to formalin, capsaicin, and hindpaw inflammation.[78]

In summary, many second messenger systems could become targets for clinical pain treatment. At present, however, the role of these systems in pain management is indirect through the action of various drugs that interact with surface receptors linked to G-proteins. Receptors linked to G_s (receptors associated with $\beta\gamma\alpha$ S subunits) include the β1-adrenergic, dopaminergic type 1, and adenosine type 2 receptors. Those that activate $G_{q,12}$ ($\beta\gamma\alpha$ q,12) include the serotonin 2c, α_1-adrenergic, histamine, thromboxane A2, metabotropic glutamate, and the muscarinic type 1, 3, and 5 receptors. Finally, G_i ($\beta\gamma\alpha$ i)-linked receptors include the adenosine 1, serotonin 1B, GABA type B, muscarinic 2, μ-, δ-, and κ-opioid receptors.[79] Neurotransmitter receptors linked to G_s and $G_{q,12}$ generally increase pain transmission while G_i-linked receptors inhibit pain signaling.[79–82]

KEY POINTS

- The excitatory amino acids glutamate and aspartate are the key excitatory neurotransmitters in the somatosensory system.
- The four types of excitatory amino acid receptors are the NMDA, AMPA, kainite, and metabotropic receptors.
- GABA and glycine are the key inhibitory neurotransmitters.
- Substance P is the key excitatory neuropeptide in the somatosensory system.
- The enkephalins and somatostatin are the key inhibitory neuropeptides in the somatosensory system.

REFERENCES

1. Dray A: Kinins and their receptors in hyperalgesia. Can J Physiol Pharmacol 75:704–712, 1997.
2. Couture R, Harrisson M, Vianna RM, Cloutier F: Kinin receptors in pain and inflammation. Eur J Pharmacol 429:161–176, 2001.
3. Beck PW, Handwerker HO: Bradykinin and serotonin effects on various types of cutaneous nerve fibres. Pflugers Arch Physiol 347: 209–222, 1974.
4. Waldmann R: Proton-gated cation channels – Neuronal acid sensors in the central and peripheral nervous system. Adv Exp Med Biol 502:293–304, 2001.

5. Steen KH, Steen AE, Kreysel HW, Reeh PW: Inflammatory mediators potentiate pain induced by experimental tissue acidosis. Pain 66:163–170, 1996.

6. Steen KH, Steen AE, Reeh PW: A dominant role of acid pH in inflammatory excitation and sensitization of nociceptors in rat skin, in vitro. J Neurosci 15:3982–3989, 1995.

7. Richardson BP, Engel G: The pharmacology and function of 5-HT3 receptors. Trends Neurosci 9:424–427, 1986.

8. Lang E, Novak A, Reeh PW, Handwerker HO: Chemosensitivity of fine afferents from rat skin in vitro. J Neurophysiol 63:887–901, 1990.

9. Simone DA, Alreja M, LaMotte RH: Psychophysical studies of the itch sensation and itchy skin ("allokinesis") produced by intracutaneous injection of histamine. Somatosens Mot Res 8:271–279, 1991.

10. Mizumura K, Minagawa M, Koda H, Kumazawa T: Influence of histamine on the bradykinin response of canine testicular polymodal receptors in vitro. Inflamm Res 44:376–378, 1995.

11. Cunha FQ, Ferreira SH: Peripheral hyperalgesic cytokines. Adv Exp Med Biol 521: 22–39, 2003.

12. Schaible HG, Ebersberger A, Von Banchet GS: Mechanisms of pain in arthritis. Ann NY Acad Sci 966:343–354, 2002.

13. Ballou LR, Botting RM, Goorha S, et al: Nociception in cyclooxygenase isozyme-deficient mice. Proc Natl Acad Sci USA 97:10272–10276, 2000.

14. Hamilton SG, McMahon SB: ATP as a peripheral mediator of pain. J Auton Nerv Syst 81:187–194, 2000.

15. Ralevic V, Burnstock G: Receptors for purines and pyrimidines. Pharmacol Rev 50:413–492, 1998.

16. Chen CC, Akopian AN, Sivilotti L, et al: A P2X purinoceptor expressed by a subset of sensory neurons. Nature 377:428–431, 1995.

17. Elliott MJ, Maini RN, Feldmann M, et al: Randomised double-blind comparison of chimeric monoclonal antibody to tumour necrosis factor alpha (cA2) versus placebo in rheumatoid arthritis. Lancet 344:1105–1110, 1994.

18. Carlton SM: Peripheral excitatory amino acids. Curr Opin Pharmacol 1:52–56, 2001.

19. Walker K, Bowes M, Panesar M, et al: Metabotropic glutamate receptor subtype 5 (mGlu5) and nociceptive function. I. Selective blockade of mGlu5 receptors in models of acute, persistent and chronic pain. Neuropharmacology 40:1–9, 2001.

20. McMahon SB: NGF as a mediator of inflammatory pain. Philos Trans R Soc Lond B Biol Sci 351:431–440, 1996.

21. Chuang HH, Prescott ED, Kong H, et al: Bradykinin and nerve growth factor release the capsaicin receptor from PtdIns(4,5)P2-mediated inhibition. Nature 411:957–962, 2001.

22. Stucky CL, Koltzenburg M, Schneider M, et al: Overexpression of nerve growth factor in skin selectively affects the survival and functional properties of nociceptors. J Neurosci 19:8509–8516, 1999.

23. Machelska H, Stein C: Pain control by immune-derived opioids. Clin Exp Pharmacol Physiol 27:533–536, 2000.

24. Khodorova A, Navarro B, Jouaville LS, et al: Endothelin-B receptor activation triggers an endogenous analgesic cascade at sites of peripheral injury. Nat Med 9:1055–1061, 2003.

25. Bernardini N, Roza C, Sauer SK, et al: Muscarinic M2 receptors on peripheral nerve endings: A molecular target of antinociception. J Neurosci 22:1–5, 2002.

26. Wess J: Novel insights into muscarinic acetylcholine receptor function using gene targeting technology. Trends Pharmacol Sci 24:414–420, 2003.

27. Carlton SM, Du J, Davidson E, et al: Somatostatin receptors on peripheral primary afferent terminals: inhibition of sensitized nociceptors. Pain 90:233–244, 2001.

28. Kidd BL, Urban LA: Mechanisms of inflammatory pain. Br J Anaesth 87:3–11, 2001.

29. Woolf CJ, Costigan M: Transcriptional and posttranslational plasticity and the generation of inflammatory pain. Proc Natl Acad Sci USA 96:7723–7730, 1999.

30. Stucky CL, Abrahams LG, Seybold VS: Bradykinin increases the proportion of neonatal rat dorsal root ganglion neurons that respond to capsaicin and protons. Neuroscience 84:1257–1265, 1998.

31. Sugiura T, Tominaga M, Katsuya H, Mizumura K: Bradykinin lowers the threshold temperature for heat activation of vanilloid receptor 1. J Neurophysiol 88:544–548, 2002.

32. Distler C, Rathee PK, Lips KS, et al: Fast Ca^{2+}-induced potentiation of heat-activated ionic currents requires cAMP/PKA signaling and functional AKAP anchoring. J Neurophysiol 89:2499–2505, 2003.

33. Rathee PK, Distler C, Obreja O, et al: PKA/AKAP/VR-1 module: a common link of G_s-mediated signaling to thermal hyperalgesia. J Neurosci 22:4740–4745, 2002.

34. Gold MS, Levine JD, Correa AM: Modulation of $TTX-RI_{Na}$ by PKC and PKA and their role in PGE_2-induced sensitization of rat sensory neurons in vitro. J Neurosci 18:10345–10355, 1998.

35. Khasar SG, Lin YH, Martin A, et al: A novel nociceptor signaling pathway revealed in protein kinase C epsilon mutant mice. Neuron 24:253–260, 1999.

36. Ji RR, Rupp F: Phosphorylation of transcription factor CREB in rat spinal cord after formalin-induced hyperalgesia: relationship to c-fos induction. J Neurosci 17:1776–1785, 1997.

37. Dai Y, Iwata K, Fukuoka T, et al: Phosphorylation of extracellular signal-regulated kinase in primary afferent neurons by noxious stimuli and its involvement in peripheral sensitization. J Neurosci 22:7737–7745, 2002.

38. Ji RR, Befort K, Brenner GJ, Woolf CJ: ERK MAP kinase activation in superficial spinal cord neurons induces prodynorphin and NK-1 upregulation and contributes to persistent inflammatory pain hypersensitivity. J Neurosci 22:478–485, 2002.

39. Ji RR, Samad TA, Jin SX, et al: p38 MAPK activation by NGF in primary sensory neurons after inflammation increases TRPV1 levels and maintains heat hyperalgesia. Neuron 36:57–68, 2002.

40. Dougherty PM, Palecek J, Paleckova V, et al: The role of NMDA and non-NMDA excitatory amino acid receptors in the excitation of primate spinothalamic tract neurons by mechanical, thermal, chemical, and electrical stimuli. J Neurosci 12:3025–3041, 1992.

41. Dougherty PM, Li YJ, Lenz FA, et al: Evidence that excitatory amino acids mediate afferent input to the primate somatosensory thalamus. Brain Res 278:267–273, 1997.

42. Cotman CW, Iversen LL: Excitatory amino acids in the brain – Focus on NMDA receptors. Trends Neurosci 10:263–302, 1987.

43. Asztely F, Gustafsson B: Ionotropic glutamate receptors. Their possible role in the expression of hippocampal synaptic plasticity. Mol Neurobiol 12:1–11, 1996.

44. Li J, Perl ER: ATP modulation of synaptic transmission in the spinal substantia gelatinosa. J Neurosci 15:3357–3365, 1995.

45. Cervero F, Laird JMA: Mechanisms of touch-evoked pain (allodynia): A new model. Pain 68:13–23, 1996.

46. Sivilotti L, Woolf CJ: The contribution of GABAA and glycine receptors to central sensitization: Disinhibition and touch-evoked allodynia in the spinal cord. J Neurophysiol 72:169–179, 1994.

47. Basbaum AI, Fields HL: Endogenous pain control mechanisms: Review and hypothesis. Ann Neurol 4:451–462, 1978.

48. Jones SL: Descending noradrenergic influences on pain. Prog Brain Res 88:381–394, 1991.

49. Yaksh TL, Wilson PR: Spinal serotonin terminal system mediates antinociception. J Pharmacol Exp Therap 208:446–453, 1979.

50. Sawynok J: Adenosine receptor activation and nociception. Eur J Pharmacol 347:1–11, 1998.

51. Iwamoto ET, Marion L: Characterization of the antinociception produced by intrathecally administered muscarinic agonists in rats. J Pharmacol Exp Therap 266:329–338, 1993.

52. Carter MS, Krause JE: Structure, expression, and some regulatory mechanisms of the rat preprotachykinin gene encoding substance p, neurokinin a, neuropeptide k, and neuropeptide y. J Neurosci 10:2203–2221, 1990.

53. Nakanishi S: Substance P precursor and kininogen: Their structures, gene organizations and regulation. Physiol Rev 67:1117–1142, 1987.

54. Dahm P, Nitescu P, Appelgren L, Curelaru I: Efficacy and technical complications of long-term continuous intraspinal infusions of opioid and/or bupivicaine in refractory nonmalignant pain: A comparison between the epidural and the intrathecal approach with externalized or implanted catheters and infusion pumps. Clin J Pain 14:4–16, 1998.

55. Lubenow TR, Faber LP, McCarthy RJ, et al: Postthoracotomy pain management using continuous epidural analgesia in 1,324 patients. Ann Thoracic Surg 58:924–930, 1994.

56. Shafer AL, Donnelly AJ: Management of postoperative pain by continuous epidural infusion of analgesics [published erratum appears in Clin Pharmacol 10:824, 1991]. Clin Pharmacol 10:745–764, 1991.

57. Berde CB, Sethna NF, Conrad LS, et al: Subarachnoid bupivicaine analgesia for seven months for a patient with a spinal cord tumor. Anesthesiology 72:1094–1096, 1990.

58. Sjoberg M, Appelgren L, Einarsson S, et al: Long-term intrathecal morphine and bupivicaine in refractory cancer pain: I. Results from the first series of 52 patients. Acta Anaesth Scand 35:30–43, 1991.

59. Appelgren L, Janson M, Nitescu P, Curelaru I: Continuous intracisternal and high cervical intrathecal bupivicaine analgesia in refractory head and neck pain. Anesthesiology 84:256–272, 1996.

60. Hardy PAJ, Wells JCD: Continuous intrathecal lignocaine infusion analgesia: A case report of a nine-week trial. Palliat Med 3:23–25, 1989.

61. Lynch C, Pancrazio JJ: Snails, spiders, and stereospecificity – Is there a role for calcium channels in anesthetic mechanisms? Anesthesiology 81:1–5, 1994.

62. Bowersox SS, Gadbois T, Singh T, et al: Selective N-type neuronal voltage-sensitive calcium channel blocker, SNX-111, produces spinal antinocicepion in rat models of acute, persistent and neuropathic pain. J Pharm Exp Ther 279:1243–1249, 1996.

63. Omote K, Kawamata M, Satoh O, et al: Spinal antinociceptive action of an N-type voltage-dependent calcium channel blocker and the synergistic interaction with morphine. Anesthesiology 84:636–643, 1996.

64. Hara K, Saito Y, Kirihara Y, et al: Antinociceptive effects of intrathecal L-type calcium channel blockers on visceral and somatic stimuli in the rat. Anesth Analg 87:382–387, 1998.

65. Malmberg AB, Yaksh TL: Voltage-sensitive calcium channels in spinal nociceptive processing: Blockade of N- and P-type channels inhibits formalin-induced nociception. J Neurosci 14:4882–4890, 1994.

66. Sluka KA: Blockade of calcium channels can prevent the onset of secondary hyperalgesia and allodynia induced by intradermal injection of capsaicin in rats. Pain 71:157–164, 1997.

67. Brose WG, Cherukuri S, Longton WC, et al: Safety and efficacy of intrathecal SNX-111, a novel analgesic, in the management of intractable neuropathic and nociceptive pain in humans: preliminary results. APS Abstracts A-116, 1995.

68. Jan LY, Jan YN: Structural elements involved in specific K^+ channel functions. Ann Rev Physiol 54:537–555, 1992.

69. Jentsch TJ, Gunther W: Chloride channels: An emerging molecular picture. BioEssays 19:117–126, 1997.

70. Sherman SE, Loomis CW: Morphine insensitive allodynia is produced by intrathecal strychnine in the lightly anesthetized rat. Pain 56:17–29, 1994.

71. Yaksh TL: Behavioral and autonomic correlates of the tactile evoked allodynia produced by spinal glycine inhibition: Effects of modulatory receptor systems and excitatory amino acid antagonists. Pain 37:111–123, 1989.

72. Sugimoto T, Bennett GJ, Kajander KC: Transsynaptic degeneration in the superficial dorsal horn after sciatic nerve injury: effects of a chronic constriction injury, transection, and strychnine. Pain 42:205–213, 1990.

73. Mayer DJ, Mao J, Price DD: The association of neuropathic pain, morphine tolerance and dependence, and the translocation of protein kinase C. NIDA Res Monogr 147:269–298, 1995.

74. Yashpal K, Pitcher GM, Parent A, et al: Noxious thermal and chemical stimulation induce increases in 3H-phorbol 12,13-dibutyrate binding in spinal cord dorsal horn as well as persistent pain and hyperalgesia, which is reduced by inhibition of protein kinase C. J Neurosci 15:3263–3272, 1995.

75. Coderre TJ: Contribution of protein kinase C to central sensitization and persistent pain following tissue injury. Neurosci Lett 140:181–184, 1998.

76. Meller ST: Thermal and mechanical hyperalgesia. A distinct role for different excitatory amino acid receptors and signal transduction pathways? APS J 3:215–231, 1998.

77. Malmberg AB, Chen C, Tonegawa S, Basbaum AI: Preserved acute pain and reduced neuropathic pain in mice lacking PKC gamma. Science 278:279–283, 1997.

78. Malmberg AB, Brandon EP, Idzera RL, et al: Diminished inflammation and nociceptive pain with preservation of neuropathic pain in mice with a targeted mutation of the type I regulatory subunit of cAMP-dependent protein kinase. J Neurosci 17:7462–7470, 1997.

79. Linden J, Auchampach JA, Jin X, Figler RA: The structure and function of A_1 and A_{2B} adenosine receptors. Life Sci 62:1519–1524, 1998.

80. Duggan AW, Griersmith BT: Methyl xanthines, adenosine 3′,5′-cyclic monophosphate and the spinal transmission of nociceptive information. Brit J Pharm 67:51–57, 1979.

81. Manji HK, Potter WZ, Lenox RH: Signal transduction pathways. Molecular targets for lithium's actions. Arch Gen Psychiat 52:531–543, 1995.

82. Pacheco MA, Jope RS: Phosphoinositide signaling in human brain. Prog Neurobiol 50:255–273, 1996.

Taxonomy: Definitions of Pain Terms and Chronic Pain Syndromes

Honorio T. Benzon, M.D.

Analgesia — Absence of pain in response to a stimulus that is normally painful.

Anesthesia — Absence of all sensory modalities.

Anesthesia dolorosa — Pain in an area or region that is anesthetic.

Carpal tunnel syndrome — Pain in the hand, usually occurring at night, due to entrapment of the median nerve in the carpal tunnel. The quality of the pain is a pins-and-needles sensation, stinging, burning, or aching. There may be decreased sensation on the tips of the first to third fingers, positive Tinel's sign, and, rarely, atrophy of the thenar muscles. A nerve conduction study shows delayed conduction across the carpal tunnel. The syndrome is caused by compression of the median nerve in the wrist between the carpal bones and the flexor retinaculum (transverse carpal ligament).

Central pain — Regional pain caused by a primary lesion or dysfunction in the central nervous system, usually associated with abnormal sensibility to temperature and to noxious stimulation.

Complex regional pain syndrome (CRPS) — A term describing a variety of painful conditions following injury that appear regionally, having a distal predominance of abnormal findings, exceeding in both magnitude and duration the expected clinical course of the inciting event, often resulting in significant impairment of motor function, and showing variable progression over time. CRPS is a new term for disorders previously called reflex sympathetic dystrophy (RSD).

CRPS type I (RSD)

1. Type I is a syndrome that develops after an initiating noxious event.
2. Spontaneous pain or allodynia/hyperalgesia occurs, is not limited to the territory of a single peripheral nerve, and is disproportionate to the inciting event.

3. There is or has been evidence of edema, skin blood flow abnormality, or abnormal sudomotor activity in the region of the pain since the inciting event.
4. This diagnosis is excluded by the existence of conditions that would otherwise account for the degree of pain and dysfunction.

CRPS type II (causalgia)

1. Type II is a syndrome that develops after a nerve injury. Spontaneous pain or allodynia/hyperalgesia occurs and is not necessarily limited to the territory of the injured nerve.
2. There is or has been evidence of edema, skin blood flow abnormality, or abnormal sudomotor activity in the region of the pain since the inciting event.
3. This diagnosis is excluded by the existence of conditions that would otherwise account for the degree of pain and dysfunction.

Chronic pain — Pain that persists beyond the course of an acute disease or a reasonable time for an injury to heal or that is associated with a chronic pathologic process that causes continuous pain, or the pain recurs at intervals of months or years. Some investigators use a pain duration of ≥6 months to designate a pain as chronic.

Cubital tunnel syndrome — Entrapment of the ulnar nerve in a fibro-osseous tunnel formed by the trochlear groove between the olecranon process and the medial epicondyle of the humerus. A myofascial covering converts the groove to a tunnel causing the nerve entrapment. There is pain, numbness, and paresthesia in the distribution of the ulnar nerve and, sometimes, weakness and atrophy in the same distribution. Tinel's sign is positive at the elbow. Nerve conduction velocity shows slowing of conduction in the ulnar nerve across the elbow. The intrinsic muscles of the hand may show signs of denervation. Surgery may be required to decompress the entrapment or to transpose the ulnar nerve.

Deafferentation pain — Pain due to loss of sensory input into the central nervous system. This may occur with lesions of peripheral nerves such as avulsion of the brachial plexus or due to pathology of the central nervous system.

Dysesthesia — An unpleasant abnormal evoked sensation, whether spontaneous or evoked.

Fibromyalgia — Diffuse musculoskeletal aching and pain with multiple predictable tender points. There is pain on digital palpation in at least 11 of 18 tender sites:

- Occiput: bilateral, at the suboccipital muscle insertions.
- Low cervical: bilateral, at the anterior aspects of the inter-transverse process at C5–C7.
- Trapezius: bilateral, at the midpoint of the upper border.
- Supraspinatus: bilateral, at the origins above the scapula spine near the medial border.
- Second rib: bilateral, at the second costochondral junctions, just lateral to the junctions on upper surfaces.
- Lateral epicondyle: bilateral, 2 cm distal to the epicondyles.
- Gluteal: bilateral, in upper outer quadrants of buttocks in anterior fold of muscle.
- Greater trochanter: bilateral, posterior to the trochanteric prominence.
- Knees: bilateral, at the medial fat pad proximal to the joint line.

Hyperalgesia — An increased response to a stimulus that is normally painful.

Hyperesthesia — Increased sensitivity to stimulation; this excludes the special senses.

Hyperpathia — A painful syndrome, characterized by increased reaction to a stimulus, especially a repetitive stimulus, as well as increased threshold.

Hypoalgesia — Diminished sensitivity to noxious stimulation.

Hypoesthesia — Diminished sensitivity to stimulation; this excludes the special senses.

Lateral epicondylitis (tennis elbow) — Pain in the lateral epicondylar region of the elbow due to strain or partial tear of the extensor tendon of the wrist. The pain may radiate to the lateral forearm or to the upper arm. There is pain in the elbow during grasping and supination of the wrist and on repeated wrist dorsiflexion. Physical examination shows tenderness of the wrist extensor tendon approximately 5 cm distal to the epicondyle.

Neuralgia — Pain in the distribution of a nerve or nerves.

Neuritis — Inflammation of a nerve or nerves. (Not to be used unless inflammation is thought to be present.)

Neurogenic pain — Pain initiated or caused by a primary lesion, dysfunction, or transitory perturbation in the peripheral or central nervous system.

Neuropathic pain — Pain initiated or caused by a primary lesion or dysfunction in the peripheral or central nervous systems.

Central neuropathic pain: a lesion in the central nervous system causing pain. These include thalamic pain syndrome, poststroke pain, and postspinal cord injury pain.

Peripheral neuropathic pain: pain caused by a lesion or dysfunction of the central nervous system. Examples are postherpetic neuralgia (PHN), painful diabetic neuropathy (PDN), and complex regional pain syndrome (CRPS).

Neuropathy — A disturbance of function or pathologic change in a nerve. This may involve one nerve (mononeuropathy), several nerves (mononeuropathy multiplex), or it may be bilateral or symmetrical (polyneuropathy).

Nociceptive pain — Pain caused by activation of nociceptive afferent fibers. This type of pain satisfies the criteria for pain transmission, i.e., transmission to the spinal cord, thalamus then to the cerebral cortex.

Somatic pain — Pain carried along the sensory fibers; this pain is usually discrete and intense.

Visceral pain — Pain carried by the sympathetic fibers; this pain is diffuse and poorly localized.

Nociceptor — A receptor preferentially sensitive to a noxious stimulus or to a stimulus that would become noxious if prolonged.

Noxious stimulus — A stimulus that is actually or potentially damaging to body tissue.

Pain — An unpleasant sensory and emotional experience associated with actual or potential tissue damage, or described in terms of damage.

Pain threshold — The least experience of pain that a subject can recognize.

Pain tolerance level — The greatest level of pain that a subject is prepared to tolerate.

Pain of psychological origin:

Delusional or hallucinatory: pain of psychological origin and attributed by the patient to a specific delusional cause.

Hysterical, conversion, or hypochondriacal: pain specifically attributable to the thought process, emotional state, or personality of the patient in the absence of an organic or delusional cause or tension mechanism.

Pain associated with depression: pain occurring in the course of a depressive illness, not preceding the depression and not attributable to any other cause.

Paresthesia — An abnormal sensation, whether spontaneous or evoked. (Note. Paresthesia is an abnormal sensation that is not unpleasant while dysesthesia is an abnormal sensation that is considered unpleasant. Dysesthesia does not include all abnormal sensations, but only those that are unpleasant.)

Peripheral neuropathy — Constant or intermittent burning, aching, or lancinating limb pain due to generalized or focal diseases of peripheral nerves.

Phantom pain — Pain referred to a surgically removed limb or portion thereof.

Piriformis syndrome — Pain in the buttock and posterior thigh due to myofascial injury of the piriformis muscle itself or dysfunction of the sacroiliac joint or pain in the posterior leg and foot, groin, and perineum due to entrapment of the sciatic or other nerves by the piriformis muscle within the greater sciatic foramen, or a combination of these causes.

Post-thoracotomy pain syndrome — Pain along a thoracotomy scar persisting at least two months after a thoracotomy. There is aching sensation in the distribution of the surgical incision. Sensory loss and tenderness may be present along the thoracotomy scar. A trigger point may be present, secondary to a neuroma, that responds to a trigger point injection.

Radicular pain — Pain perceived as arising in a limb or the trunk wall caused by ectopic activation of nociceptive afferent fibers in a spinal nerve or its roots or other neuropathic mechanisms. The pain is usually lancinating and travels in a narrow band. Etiologic causes include anatomic lesions affecting the spinal nerve and dorsal root ganglion including herniated intervertebral disc and spinal stenosis.

Radiculopathy — Objective loss of sensory and/or motor function as a result of conduction block in axons of a spinal nerve or its roots. Symptoms include numbness and weakness in the distribution of the affected nerve. Neurologic examination and diagnostic tests confirm the neurologic abnormality. (Note. Radicular pain and radiculopathy are not synonymous. The former is a symptom caused by ectopic impulse generation. The latter relates to objective neurological signs due to conduction block. The two conditions may coexist and may be caused by the same lesion.)

Raynaud's disease — Episodic attacks of aching, burning pain associated with vasoconstriction of the arteries of the extremities in response to cold or emotional stimuli.

Raynaud's phenomenon — Attacks like those of Raynaud's disease but related to one or more other disease processes. Systemic and vascular diseases such as collagen disease, arteriosclerosis obliterans, nerve injuries, and occupational trauma may all contribute to the development of Raynaud's phenomenon.

Referred pain — Pain perceived as occurring in a region of the body topographically distinct from the region in which the actual source of pain is located.

Somatic — Derived from the Greek word for "body." Although somatosensory input refers to sensory signals from all tissues of the body including skin, viscera, muscles, and joints, it usually signifies input from body tissue other than the viscera.

Stump pain — Pain at the site of an extremity amputation.

Suffering — A state of severe distress associated with events that threaten the intactness of the person; it may or may not be associated with pain.

Stylohyoid process syndrome (Eagle's syndrome) — Pain following trauma in the region of a calcified stylohyoid ligament.

Thoracic outlet syndrome — Pain in the root of the neck, head, shoulder, radiating down the arm into the hand due to compression of the brachial plexus by hypertrophied muscle, congenital bands, post-traumatic fibrosis, cervical rib or band, or malformed first thoracic rib.

BIBLIOGRAPHY

Bonica JJ: The Management of Pain, ed 2. Lea & Febiger, Philadelphia, 1990, pp 18–27.

Derasari MD. Taxonomy of pain syndromes: Classification of chronic pain syndromes. *In* Raj PP (ed): Practical Management of Pain, ed 3. Mosby, St. Louis, 2000, pp 10–16.

Mersky H, Bogduk N: International Association for the Study of Pain (IASP) Classification of Chronic Pain, ed 2. IASP Press, Seattle, 1994.

Stanton-Hicks M, Janig W, Hassenbuch S, et al: Reflex sympathetic dystrophy: Changing concepts and taxonomy. Pain 63:127–133, 1995.

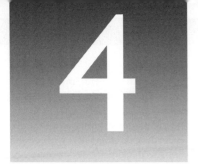

Physical Examination of the Pain Patient

John D. Moore, M.D.,
Honorio T. Benzon, M.D., and
Maunak Rana, M.D.

The physical examination of a patient with pain is the most significant diagnostic tool, only surpassed in importance by the pain history. The goals of the physical examination are multiple and include developing the patient's trust, gaining insight into the impact of pain on the patient's level of functioning, and ultimately identifying potential pain generators and other neurological derangements. Due to the obvious importance of a thorough and complete physical examination, methodical templates that are easily reproducible, efficient, and targeted toward a specific region should be developed. A comprehensive physical examination must be based on anatomical and physiological principles and an examination that fulfills this criterion is an invaluable diagnostic tool.

A review of the physical examination must include a review of the anatomical and physiological basis that explains the significance of physical findings. The physical examination of the pain patient is largely based on a comprehensive neurological examination which can be divided into four main categories: sensation, motor, reflexes, and coordination.

SENSATION AND SENSORY EXAMINATION

The physiological basis of the sensory examination is the differentiation of nerve fiber sensation. From a pain perspective the foundations of the sensory system are peripheral nociceptors. There are three main types of nociceptors which are differentiated based on the type of damaging stimuli they detect: *mechanical nociceptors* respond to pinch and pin-prick, *heat nociceptors* respond to a temperature greater than 45°C, and *polymodal nociceptors* respond equally to mechanical, heat, and chemical noxious stimuli. All nociceptors are connected to the central nervous system (CNS) and transmit information via the A-delta and C fibers. Based on the transmitting fibers, pain can be sensed as fast or slow pain. *Fast pain* is transmitted by

well-localized myelinated A-delta fibers and is characterized as sharp, shooting pain. *Slow pain* is transmitted by unmyelinated C fibers and is characterized as dull, poorly localized burning pain. Although all examination findings should be described with specific established terms reviewed in Chapter 3, there are certain terms unique to the sensory examination which must be understood and agreed upon. *Hyperesthesia* is a broad general description of a sensation out of proportion to the stimuli applied. From a pain perspective hyperesthesia is further divided into hyperalgesia and allodynia. *Hyperalgesia* is severe pain in response to mild noxious stimuli, for example pinprick. *Allodynia* is severe pain in response to non-noxious stimuli, for example light touch or a light breeze on the skin. Allodynia is an important indicator of neuropathic pain and its distribution, frequently nondermatomal, should be documented.[1]

An initial gross sensory examination will direct a more in-depth investigation of an affected region. The more detailed examination is generally based on physiological differentiation of sensory nerve fibers and often uses the contralateral side as a control. *C fibers* are tested using both pain stimulus (pinprick) and temperature. These are readily accomplished with the sharp edge of a broken tongue blade and a cold tuning fork or glove filled with ice. *A-delta fibers* are tested with pinprick and light touch stimulus. Light touch is tested with a cotton wisp or tissue. Although A-delta and C fibers transmit painful stimuli which are tested with pinprick, there are cases of sensory dissociation. Sensory dissociation presents as a patient reporting a sharp sensation to pinprick in an area without pain or temperature sensation. This can occur in lesions that interrupt fibers crossing the spinal cord. An example of such lesion is a syrinx which is a progressive myelopathy that presents as a central high cervical cord syndrome with a sensory deficit in a cape or shawl distribution, and neck, shoulder, and arm

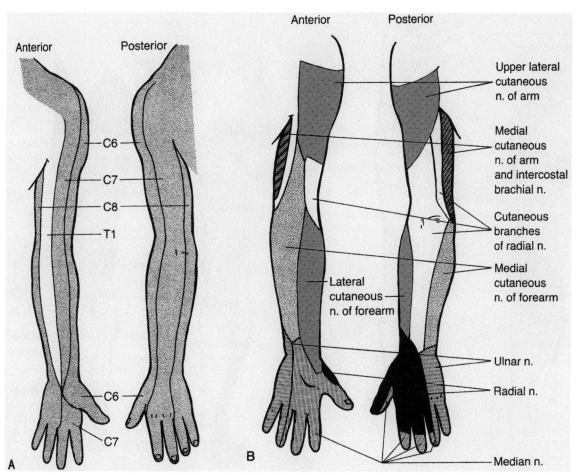

FIGURE 4-1. *A*, Cutaneous distribution of the cervical roots. *B*, Cutaneous distribution of the peripheral nerves of the upper extremity. (From Wedel DJ: Nerve blocks. *In* Miller RD (ed): Anesthesia, ed 4. Churchill Livingstone, New York, 1994, p 1537.)

muscle wasting. *A-beta fibers* are examined through light touch, vibration, and joint position. Vibration is tested with a 128 Hz tuning fork and has increased value when combined with joint position testing. Isolated decreased vibratory sense is an early sign of large-fiber neuropathy and if combined with position sense deficit indicates posterior column disease or peripheral nerve involvement. Posterior column disease is also indicated by the loss of graphesthesia or the ability to interpret a number outlined on the patient's palm or calf. Isolated joint position sense deficit is an indication of parietal lobe dysfunction or peripheral nerve lesion.[1,2]

The anatomical significance of sensory changes is represented in the classic dermatome and peripheral cutaneous nerve maps (Figs. 4-1 and 4-2). Through careful differentiation and mapping of sensory changes and comparison with established maps it is possible to pinpoint the anatomical location of a lesion (Table 4-1). Anatomically, lesions can be divided into central, spinal nerve root (dermatomal), and peripheral nerve lesions.[3]

MOTOR EXAMINATION

Although more limited than the sensory examination, an examination of motor function can indicate the level of a

lesion and knowledge of muscle innervation is essential. The motor examination begins with inspection. Detailed inspection can identify signs of hypertrophy, atrophy, and fasciculations among other pathologies. Following inspection palpation is a valuable tool to identify pain generators, specifically myofascial trigger points. Tone, the sensation of resistance felt as one manipulates a joint through its expected range of motion with the patient relaxed, is described in terms of hypotonia and hypertonia. *Hypotonia*, a decrease in the normal expected muscular resistance to passive manipulation, is believed due to a depression of alpha or gamma motor unit activity. Hypotonia is seen in extrapyramidal or cerebellar motor disorders, polyneuropathy, myopathy, and spinal cord lesions. *Hypertonia*, a greater than expected normal resistance to passive joint manipulation, is divided into spasticity and rigidity. *Spasticity*, a velocity-dependent increase in tone with joint movement, is due to increased excitation at the spinal reflex arc level or from loss of descending inhibitory control in the reticulospinal or rubrospinal tracts. Spasticity is commonly seen after brain and spinal cord injury, stroke, and in multiple sclerosis. *Rigidity*, a generalized increase in muscle tone, is characteristic of extrapyramidal diseases and is due to lesions in the nigrostriatal system. Finally, isolated voluntary muscle strength is tested and graded from 0 to 5 (normal strength).

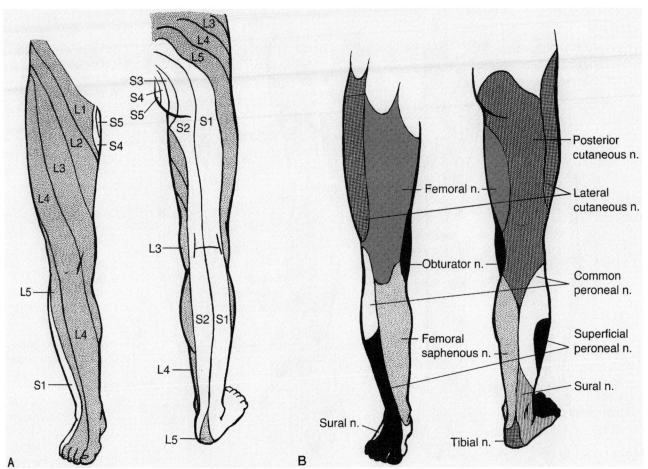

FIGURE 4-2. *A,* Cutaneous distribution of the lumbosacral nerves. *B,* Cutaneous distribution of the peripheral nerves of the lower extremity. (From Wedel DJ: Nerve blocks. *In* Miller RD (ed): Anesthesia, ed 4. Churchill Livingstone, New York, 1994, p 1547.)

TABLE 4-1. **SENSORY INNERVATION LANDMARKS BY DERMATOME**

Dermatome	Landmark	Dermatome	Landmark
C4	Shoulder	L1	Half way between T12 and L2
C5	Lateral aspect of the elbow	L2	Mid-anterior thigh
C6	Thumb	L3	Medial femoral condyle
C7	Middle finger	L4	Medial malleolus
C8	Little finger	L5	Dorsum of foot
T1	Medial aspect of the elbow	S1	Lateral heel
T2	Axilla	S2	Popliteal fossa at midline
T3–T11	Corresponding intercostal space; T4, nipple line; T10, umbilicus	S3	Ischial tuberosity
T12	Inguinal ligament at midline	S4–S5	Perianal area

TABLE 4-2. **STANDARD MUSCLE GRADING SYSTEM**

Grade	Description
0	No movement
1	Trace movement, no joint movement
2	Full range of motion with gravity eliminated
3	Full range of motion against gravity
4	Full range of motion against gravity and partial resistance
5 (normal)	Full range of motion against gravity and full resistance

Table 4-2 describes the standard muscle strength grading system. Greater proximal muscle weakness, in contrast to distal muscle weakness, indicates a myopathy. Greater distal muscle weakness, compared to proximal muscle weakness, indicates a polyneuropathy. Single innervation muscle weakness indicates a peripheral nerve lesion.[1,4]

REFLEXES AND COORDINATION

In coordination with the sensory and motor examinations deep tendon reflexes (muscle stretch reflexes) serve as a valuable guide to the anatomical localization of a lesion. Similar to motor and sensory tests, reflexes are indicative of specific spinal levels. The most commonly tested reflexes are listed in Table 4-3. A standardized grading system for deep tendon reflexes from 0 to 4 is presented in Table 4-4. In cases of hypoactive reflexes, *Jendrassik's maneuver*, which is the facilitation of underactive reflexes by voluntary contraction of other muscles, can provide a more accurate assessment of the reflex. *Clonus*, a grade four reflex, is characterized by rhythmic, uniphasic muscle contractions in response to sudden sustained muscle stretch. Clonus is typical of upper motor neuron disease.

TABLE 4-3. **COMMON REFLEXES NERVE ROOT LEVEL TESTED**

Nerve Root Level	Reflex
S1–S2	Achilles reflex
L3–L4	Patellar reflex
C5–C6	Biceps reflex
C7–C8	Triceps reflex

TABLE 4-4. **DEEP TENDON REFLEX GRADING SYSTEM**

Grade	Description
0	No response
1+	Reduced, less than expected
2+	Normal
3+	Greater than expected, moderately hyperactive
4+	Hyperactive with clonus

A positive plantar or *Babinski's reflex*, wherein the great toe moves upward and the toes fan outward in response to a key scratch along the lateral aspect and metatarsal heads on the plantar surface of the foot, further indicates upper motor neuron disease. Ultimately the confidence level in the localization of a lesion is quite high when confirmed by sensory, motor, and a reflex derangement.[1,5]

Coordination and gait testing is a sensitive indicator of cerebellar function and equilibrium. Cerebellar function is tested by traditional finger-nose-finger and heel-knee-shin tests. Equilibrium is assessed by observation of normal gait, heel and toe walk, and tandem gait testing. Tandem gait instructs a patient to walk heel to toe along an imaginary line and observes the results. Equilibrium is further tested by Romberg's test.[6]

DIRECTED PAIN EXAMINATION TEMPLATE

In addition to structuring the physical examination based on physiological principles, the examination should be standardized and reproducible with regards to the observations and tests performed on an examined region and the descriptive terminology used. The development of a standardized approach promotes thoroughness and consistency. A descriptive template should include inspection, palpation, percussion, range of motion, motor examination, sensory examination, reflexes, and additional indicated regional provocative tests. Table 4-5 lists a sample template. Although there are multiple standardized descriptive terms to describe the physical findings, the most important for a pain examination is whether the pain elicited during a portion of the examination is concordant or discordant. *Concordant* pain is the same pain in location, nature, or intensity with the patient presented. *Disconcordant* pain is painful, however different from the pain with which the patient presented.

The examination should begin with inspection and description of the affected region with attention to symmetry and the cutaneous landmarks. Particular vigilance for signs of infection or rash, surgical or traumatic scars, sudomotor alterations, congenital cutaneous discoloration, and abnormal hair growth should be maintained. Subcutaneous alterations such as edema, muscular atrophy or hypertrophy, and masses should

TABLE 4-5. **DIRECTED PAIN EXAMINATION TEMPLATE**

Examination	Observation
Inspection	Cutaneous landmarks, symmetry, temperature
Palpation	Gross sensory changes, masses, trigger points, pulses
Percussion	Tinel's sign, fractures
Range of motion	Described in degrees, reason for limitation
Motor examination	Graded 0–5, correlated with innervation
Sensory examination	Dermatomal distribution of changes, description of affected fibers
Reflexes	Graded 0–4
Provocative tests	Description of concordant vs. disconcordant pain, appropriate for region

also be documented. In addition to visual inspection, the cutaneous temperature should be measured in suspected cases of sympathetically maintained pain and compared to the contralateral side. The initial temperature measurement is a guide to effectiveness of subsequent therapy.

Palpation of the affected region provides both insight into alterations observed on inspection and contributes to the sensory examination. Palpation is dependent on the patient tolerating touch. Patients with allodynia, dysesthesia, hyperesthesia, or other sensory derangements often are unable to tolerate palpation. When tolerated, palpation should be performed in a systematic, comprehensive manner from the least to most painful area. This permits an appreciation of the normal tissues against which to compare the painful region. The objectives of palpation are to identify and delineate subcutaneous masses, edema, muscle contractures, assess pulses, and to localize trigger points and tender points. Palpation can also identify painful bony or neural structures indicating potential pain generators.

Similar to palpation, percussion is dependent on the patient tolerating touch. Pain on percussion of bony structures can indicate a fracture, abscess, or infection. Pain on percussion over a sensory nerve, or *Tinel's sign*, can indicate nerve entrapment or the presence of a neuroma. Although the force of percussion is limited, all provoked pain should be specified as concordant or disconcordant.

Range of motion is limited to articulated areas. Range of motion is an active test limited by the patient's effort and report of limitation. There are six possible movements depending on the joint: flexion, extension, right lateral flexion, left lateral flexion, and right and left rotation. The range of motion for each possible movement is described in terms of maximum degrees of movement the patient performed and the reported reason for any limitation. All reported induced pain should be described as concordant or disconcordant. Each joint has generally agreed upon normal limits of motion.

Motor and sensory examinations of a region are based upon the physiological principles reviewed and are standard. The descriptions obviously must specify the dermatomes or muscles tested and any alterations. Similarly reflexes are graded and reported in the established manner presented. An in-depth knowledge and understanding of the examined region is vital in order to integrate the results of the sensory, motor, and reflex examinations and come to a meaningful conclusion about the localization and nature of the lesion.

In addition to the universal descriptive examinations reviewed, each region has specific unique tests for the structures of that area. The most specific and unique are the tests for cranial nerve function. All regionally directed pain examinations have evolved specific provocative pain tests for many of the potential pain generating structures. Since these maneuvers are unique to each area a detailed knowledge of the anatomy and function of the local structures is essential. All provoked pain should be described in terms of concordant versus disconcordant pain.[7]

GENERAL OBSERVATIONS

The physical examination should begin as early as possible through careful observation of the patient's mannerisms, coordination, interpersonal interactions, and gait. These are frequently observed starting in the waiting room and provide insight into the patient's mental, emotional, and physical status. Early observations in a less obvious setting provide a basis against which to measure pain behaviors and gait abnormalities and can indicate signs of emotional and mental disturbance that will be more formally tested later. Since obtaining a history precedes the physical examination this provides an opportunity to develop the patient's trust and provides indications of the patient's mental status and whether a more detailed mental examination is warranted.[8] By establishing the nature of the patient's complaint during the history, the physical examination can be efficiently directed toward the affected region and can also explore possible causes of the chief complaint. A structured plan of examination ensures a comprehensive evaluation. The degree of disrobement should be a balance between adequate exposure for a thorough examination and respect for patient privacy and comfort.

Following the above preparations the directed physical examination should begin with a general assessment of the patient's global physical status and by obtaining vital signs. The vital signs are an objective indication of the patient's general health status and provide a baseline against which to compare the patient's condition following any procedures. Additionally the patient's hydration and nutritional status should be documented.

MENTAL EXAMINATION

Based on observations made while obtaining the history, a mental examination can be performed and documented as an

TABLE 4-6. BRIEF MENTAL EXAMINATION

Orientation to person and place, date repetition

Ability to name objects (e.g., pen, watch)

Memory immediate at 1 minute, and at 5 minutes, repeat the names of three objects

Ability to calculate serial 7s or if patient refuses have them spell "world" backward

Signs of cognitive deficits, aphasia

indicator of general health status. A basic mental examination is described in Table 4-6. Descriptors of the general mental status include the patient's level of consciousness, alertness, orientation to person place and time, and demeanor toward the examiner.[9] Signs of mental deterioration should correlate with the patient's history or initiate a search for an underlying pathology. The examiner should be especially vigilant for signs of undiagnosed depression frequently associated with chronic pain. Documentation and description of specific pain behaviors during the examination are particularly important to gauge the response to possible therapies.

GAIT

Another general indicator of health status is the patient's gait. In general terms gait is divided into two main phases, the swing and the stance phases, which are further divided into several components. Although there are numerous detailed descriptions of normal and pathological gaits and their analysis, for a directed pain physical examination it suffices to describe the gait as normal, antalgic, or abnormal. An antalgic gait is characterized by the avoidance of bearing weight on an affected limb or joint secondary to pain. An abnormal non-antalgic gait is a broad category that includes balance, neurological, and musculoskeletal disorders. Since an abnormal gait is an indicator of pathology, an adequate explanation for this should be obtained and documented in the history or a more thorough investigation should be directed toward detecting the cause of the gait abnormality.[6]

EXAMINATION OF THE DIFFERENT REGIONS OF THE BODY

By definition the directed pain physical examination concentrates on a specific painful region of the body identified by the history that is unified by location, innervation, and function. Based on these criteria the physical examination is broadly divided into the face, cervical region, thoracic region, and lumbosacral region. Obviously with such broad definitions overlap occurs and the examination should be tailored to the patient's signs and symptoms. Equally a more limited examination can be indicated and performed based upon the presenting pathology.

FACE

A directed examination of the face is largely based on an examination of the cranial nerves. Table 4-7 provides a description

of a detailed strategy. Although a comprehensive cranial nerve examination covers the facial innervation, a standard examination of the face should be performed and can provide valuable clues as to the origin of the patient's pain. Inspection of the face begins by observing the cutaneous landmarks for signs of infection, herpetic lesions, sudomotor changes, and scarring both traumatic and postherpetic. Oral inspection is indicated since intraoral lesions frequently refer pain to distant facial regions. It is also crucial to observe the symmetry of the face; signs of asymmetry should be investigated. Facial palpation is important to identify masses, sensory changes, and tenderness over the sinuses. Percussion can confirm sinus tenderness and distal neurological derangements. The most common facial percussive test is Chvostek's test. Facial range of motion largely refers to temporomandibular joint function. A facial examination is indicated in headache patients secondary to referred pain patterns.[5,10]

CERVICAL AND THORACIC AREAS AND UPPER EXTREMITIES

A directed cervical examination including the upper thorax, shoulders, and upper extremities is indicated by complaints of pain in the examined areas and by headaches. Inspection should focus on symmetry, muscle condition, scarring, and head, shoulder, and upper extremity position at rest. Additionally the upper extremities should be examined for sudomotor changes and cutaneous temperature when indicated. Palpation in the cervical and trunk region should be vigilant for muscle spasms, myofascial trigger points, tender points, occipital nerve entrapment, and pain over the bony structures that can indicate facet arthropathy. Upper extremity palpation should identify gross sensory changes and pulse symmetry.

The normal cervical ranges of motion (ROM) are flexion, $0°$ to $60°$; extension, $0°$ to $25°$; bilateral lateral flexion, $0°$ to $25°$; and bilateral lateral rotation, $0°$ to $80°$. Any reduction in the patient controlled active range of motion should be documented with the reported reason for limitation. Pain should be documented as concordant or disconcordant and the exact distribution of the reported pain noted. Pain in a dermatomal pattern often indicates a spinal cord or nerve root lesion.[5,10]

The remainder of the examination of the cervical region is based on dermatomal and large peripheral nerve function that can be corroborated by motor, sensory, and reflex test results. In consideration of this the cervical region motor, sensory, and reflex examinations are best reviewed in an integrated manner. Table 4-8 lists appropriate tests for the C4–T1 nerve roots.[1]

PROVOCATIVE TESTS

There are provocative maneuvers in the cervical area and the upper extremities. The *distraction test* is a maneuver that evaluates the effect of cervical traction on a patient's pain perception. The patient's head is slightly elevated superiorly, offloading the cervical spine. This motion allows widening of the neural foramina relieving compression caused by neural foraminal stenosis. In contrast, the cervical *compression test* involves downward pressure on the head causing compression

TABLE 4-7. **CRANIAL NERVE EXAMINATION**
Summary of Cranial Nerve Functions and Tests

Cranial Nerve	Function	Test
I. Olfactory	Smell	Use coffee, mint, etc., held to each nostril separately; consider basal frontal tumor in unilateral dysfunction
II. Optic	Vision	Assess optic disc, visual acuity; name number of fingers in central and peripheral quadrants; direct and consensual pupil reflex; note Marcus–Gunn pupil (paradoxically dilating pupil)
III, IV, and VI. Oculomotor, trochlear, and abducens	Extraocular muscles	Pupil size; visually track objects in 8 cardinal directions, note diplopia (greatest on side of lesion); accommodation; note Horner's pupil (miosis, ptosis, anhydrosis)
V. Trigeminal: motor, sensory	Facial sensation, muscles of mastication	Cotton-tipped swab/pinprick to all 3 branches; recall bilateral forehead innervation (peripheral lesion spares forehead, central lesion affects forehead); note atrophy, jaw deviation to side of lesion
VII. Facial	Muscles of facial expression	Wrinkle forehead, close eyes tightly, smile, purse lips, puff cheeks; corneal reflex
VIII. Vestibulocochlear (acoustic)	Hearing, equilibrium	Use timing fork, compare side–side; Rinne's test for air vs. bone conduction, (BC > AC); Weber's test for sensorineural hearing
IX. Glossopharyngeal	Palate elevation, taste to posterior third of tongue, sensation to posterior tongue, pharynx, middle ear, and dura	Palate elevates away from the lesion; check gag reflex
X. Vagus	Muscles of pharynx, larynx	Check for vocal cord paralysis, hoarse or nasal voice
XI. Accessory	Muscles of larynx, sternocleidomastoid, trapezius	Shoulder shrug, sternocleidomastoid strength
XII. Hypoglossal	Intrinsic tongue muscles	Protrusion of tongue; deviates toward lesion

TABLE 4-8. **CERVICAL REGION NERVE ROOT TESTING**

Root Level	Nerve	Muscle(s) Tested	Position	Action	Sensory	Reflex
C4	Dorsal scapular	Levator scapulae	Sitting	Shoulder shrug	Shoulders	None
C5	Musculotaneous (C5–6)	Biceps	Forearm fully supinated, elbow flexed 90°	Patient attempts further flexion against resistance	Lateral arm	Biceps
C6	Radial (C5–6)	Extensor carpi, radialis, longus, and brevis	Elbow flexed at 45°, wrist extended	Maintain extension against resistance	Lateral forearm, first and second finger	Brachioradialis
C7	Radial (C6–8)	Triceps	Shoulder slightly abducted, elbow slightly flexed	Extend forearm against gravity	Middle finger	Triceps
C8	Anterior interosseous (median) (C7–8)	Flexor digitorum profundus		Finger flexion of middle finger	Fourth, fifth finger medial forearm	None
T1	Ulnar, deep branch (C8–T1)	Dorsal interossei	Patient extends and spreads all fingers	Examiner pushes patient's fingers together, patient resists	Medial arm	None

of the cervical spine and narrowing of the foramina. The exacerbation of symptoms indicates foraminal stenosis. A *Valsalva maneuver* may also be helpful in delineating pathology in the cervical spine. An increase in intrathecal pressure develops with this maneuver and increased pain may be secondary to compression of the disc material or tumor.

The presence of a rotator cuff derangement can cause pain in the shoulder. The *drop arm test* may help identify the presence of tear in the rotator cuff. In this test the patient with rotator cuff dysfunction will not be able to retain their arm in an abducted position. The *Yergason test* examines the integrity of the biceps tendon in its bony groove in the humerus. In this maneuver the patient flexes his elbow. The examiner grasps the elbow and wrist of the patient and attempts to rotate the arm externally while the patient resists the maneuver. Instability of the tendon is manifested by the presence of pain in the area of the tendon. Patients with lateral epicondylitis pain can have their symptoms reproduced by the *tennis elbow test*. The test involves wrist extension by the patient as the lateral forearm is stabilized by the examiner. An attempt to flex the wrist is made while the patient resists. In the presence of lateral epicondylitis the patient will notice tenderness in the area.

Tinel's sign is a maneuver that is designed to elicit pain in the distribution of the ulnar nerve by tapping over the groove between the olecranon and the medial epicondyle. The eponym for tapping the median nerve at the wrist is also known as Tinel's sign, a test utilized for the diagnosis of carpal tunnel syndrome. Similarly, *Phalen's sign* also tests for the presence of carpal tunnel syndrome; tingling of the fingers by flexing the patient's wrist to dorsal surfaces and holding for a minute may indicate median nerve pathology.

THORACIC REGION

Examination of the thoracic region is indicated by pain in the thorax, abdomen, and back. Inspection should focus on the cutaneous landmarks, especially surgical or traumatic scars, herpetic lesions, ecchymotic lesions, and masses. Detection of thoracic kyphosis or scoliosis is an important indicator of thoracic alignment and possible neural and intrathoracic compression. Palpation can indicate cutaneous sensory deficits, delineate masses, and confirm bony integrity of the thorax. Palpation of the abdominal wall may differentiate between superficial and deep pain generators. Deep palpation can detect pulsatile masses consistent with an abdominal aortic aneurysm that can present as low thoracic back pain. A comprehensive sensory examination is often necessary to delineate the extent of a sensory lesion, specify the type of fibers involved, and the affected dermatomes. This is especially true in postherpetic neuralgia and postsurgical lesions. The evaluation of the range of motion and motor and reflex examinations of the thoracic area is limited because of its location.

LUMBOSACRAL REGION

The lumbosacral region is the most common location of pain complaints and contains the most potential pain-generating structures. Similar to the other regional examinations a structured evaluation begins with inspection. A global inspection of the patient's gait and posture at rest reveals signs of asymmetry and the degree of spinal curvature. A detailed analysis of an antalgic gait provides valuable information concerning potential pain-generating structures. Lumbar scoliosis, kyphosis, and excess lordosis also provide direction in the search for pain generators. A detailed inspection of the cutaneous landmarks should emphasize signs of infection, rash, cutaneous discoloration, subcutaneous masses, and postsurgical scars. The orientations of surgical scars are important indicators of postsurgical anatomical changes. Lower extremity inspection includes vigilance for sudomotor changes and temperature measurement.[5]

Palpation in the lumbar spine begins with identification of the bony landmarks, specifically the iliac crests. The horizontal line connecting the iliac crests traverses the lumbar spine at L4–L5. Identification of this landmark provides a reference point against which to orient any further observations. Common bony structure pain generators in the lumbar region include the facet joints, sacroiliac joints, and the coccyx. Soft tissue palpation is important to evaluate paraspinous muscle tone, the localization of trigger points and the presence of masses such as lipomas. Pain on palpation over the iliac crest can indicate cluneal nerve entrapment.[11]

The normal lumbar spine ranges of motion (ROM) are flexion, 0° to 90°; extension, 0° to 30°; bilateral lateral flexion, 0° to 25°; and bilateral lateral rotation, 0° to 60°.[5] Chapter 39 on low back pain provides a review of the possible causes of limitation of ROM and pain. However, general guidelines are that pain on flexion can indicate a disc lesion, and pain on extension can indicate a facet arthropathy or muscular pain generator.

Similar to the cervical region the confidence in lumbosacral lesions localized by confirmatory muscle, sensory and reflex test results is extremely high. Table 4-9 provides an integrated sensory, motor, reflex test outline for L2–S1. In addition to specific nerve root tests, two complimentary tests are heel walk, which tests L4–L5 function, and toe walk, which tests S1–S2 integrity.

There are multiple provocative tests described for the lumbar region which are presented in Chapter 39. The majority of tests are directed toward pathology in the disc and nerve roots, facet joints, sacroiliac joint, hip, and piriformis muscle. The most frequently performed test for nerve root irritation is back flexion (range of movement and presence of pain) and straight leg raise, both sitting and standing. Tests for facet pathology include back extension, lateral flexion, and lateral rotation. *Faber Patrick test*, *Gaenslen's test*, *Yeoman's test*, and *posterior shear test* are tests for sacroiliac joint dysfunction.[11] It is hard to distinguish normal from abnormal sacroiliac joint response with the *Gillet test*. Tests for piriformis syndrome include the *Pace, Laseque,* and *Freiberg signs*. All of these are described in Chapter 43. General tests for intrathecal lesions include the Kernig test for meningeal irritation, and the Valsalva, and Milgram test for intrathecal pathology. In the *Kernig test* a supine patient flexes the chin onto the chest. A positive sign is when the patient complains of pain in the spine. The *Milgram* test involves a supine patient raising the leg a few inches off the examination table. The inability of the patient to hold this position for thirty seconds may indicate an intrathecal lesion.[1,12]

In addition to the standard provocative tests, which rely on patient cooperation, there have been developed confirmatory tests used to grade patient participation and pain behaviors. These tests include the Hoover test and Waddell's signs. The *Hoover test* may be used to confirm the presence of malingering with regards to paralysis of the legs. In this test the patient is supine and the examiner raises one leg of the patient while the other hand of the examiner is underneath the patient's other (supine) leg. The tendency is for the patient to press down on the supine leg (the downward movement of the heel of the foot is felt by the examiner's hands), the absence of movement of the supine leg indicates true leg paralysis.[12] Although controversial, *Waddell's signs* are a measurement of patient pain behaviors and provide indications of a nonorganic source for the patient's pain. There are five potential Waddell's signs, the presence of three or more positive signs is a strong indication of a nonorganic source for the patient's pain. The five signs or tests are tenderness, simulation testing, distraction testing, regional disturbances, and overreaction. *Tenderness* is deep tenderness or a diffuse nondermatomal report of pain to a superficial stimulus most often a light skin roll or pinch. *Simulation testing* is a report of pain in the lumbar region to axial loading of the head or to body rotation with the shoulders and pelvis in line. *Distraction testing* is repetition and comparison of the results of a provocative test in an obvious and less obvious nonstandard fashion; the most common is sitting versus supine straight leg raises. If the results are contrary this is considered positive. *Regional disturbances* are primarily motor and sensory deficits that do not follow an anatomical distribution. They can be nondermatomal distribution of sensory changes, for example glove and stocking distribution or complete limb weakness. Finally *overreaction* in the context of cultural variation includes disproportionate verbal and facial expressions, unconventional anatomical movements and postures, and inappropriate responses to the examination. These examinations do not indicate an anatomical source for the patient's pain but place the results of the physical examination in the context of the patient's effort and can provide support for the results.[5,11]

TABLE 4-9. **LUMBAR REGION NERVE ROOT TESTING**

Root Level	Nerve	Muscle(s) Tested	Position	Action	Sensory	Reflex
L2	Femoral (L2–4)	Psoas, iliacus	Hip and knee flexed at 90°	Flex hip further against resistance	Anterior upper thigh	Patellar
L3	Femoral (L2–4)	Quadriceps femoris	Supine, hip flexed, knee flexed at 90°	Extend knee against resistance	Anterior lower thigh	Patellar
L4	Deep peroneal (L4–5)	Tibialis anterior	Ankle dorsiflexed, heel walk	Maintain dorsiflexion against resistance	Anterior knee	Patellar*
L5	Deep peroneal (L4–5)	Extensor hallucis longus	Great toe extended	Maintain extension against resistance	Lateral calf, web between big and second toe	Medial hamstring
	Superficial peroneal	Peroneus longus and brevis	Foot everted	Maintain eversion against resistance	Dorsum of foot	
S1	Sciatic (L5–S2)	Hamstrings	Prone, knee flexed, toe walk	Maintain flexion against resistance	Foot (except medial aspect)	Achilles

* Patellar reflex is mainly secondary to L4.

CONCLUSION

The physical examination is secondary in importance only to the pain history. In addition to developing the patient's trust a complementary physical examination should explore the complaints raised in the history and provide physical information that confirms or rejects the proposed explanations for the symptoms. In order to gain a meaningful understanding of the patient's symptoms the physical examination should be based on anatomical and physiological principles. Following a brief global assessment of the patient's health, the pain examination should be focused toward the affected region and consistently performed in a structured pattern. Diagnosis supported by confirmatory physical examination findings and appropriate provocative test results instill high degrees of confidence. Ultimately a physical examination that fulfills these criteria is an invaluable component in establishing the diagnosis in a pain patient.

REFERENCES

1. Ho J, DeLuca KG: Neurologic assessment of the pain patient. *In* Benzon HT, Raja SN, Borsook D, et al (eds): Essentials of Pain Medicine and Regional Anesthesia. Churchill Livingstone, New York, 1999, pp 14–19.
2. Fuller G: Sensation: General. *In* Fuller G (ed): Neurological Examination Made Easy, ed 2. Churchill Livingstone, London, 1999, pp 151–161.
3. Fuller G: Sensation: What you find and what it means. *In* Fuller G (ed): Neurological Examination Made Easy, ed 2. Churchill Livingstone, London, 1999, 163–168.
4. Fuller G: Motor system: What you find and what it means. *In* Fuller G (ed): Neurological Examination Made Easy, ed 2. Churchill Livingstone, London, 1999, pp 145–150.
5. Simon SM: Physical examination of the patient in pain. *In* Raj PP, Abrams BM, Benzon HT, et al (eds): Practical Management of Pain, ed 3. Mosby, St. Louis, 2000, pp 339–359.
6. Hoppenfeld S, Hutton R: Examination of gait. *In* Hoppenfeld S, Hutton R (eds): Physical Examination of the Spine and Extremities. Appleton & Lange, Connecticut, 1976, pp 133–142.
7. Haldeman S: Differential diagnosis of low back pain. In Kirkaldy-Willis WH, Bernard TN (eds): Managing Low Back Pain, ed 4. Churchill Livingstone, New York, 1999, pp 227–249.
8. Donohoe CD: Targeted history and physical examination. *In* Waldman SD (ed): Interventional Pain Management, ed 2. W B Saunders, Philadelphia, 2001, pp 83–94.

9. Fuller G: Mental state and higher function. *In* Fuller G (ed): Neurological Examination Made Easy, ed 2. Churchill Livingston, London, 1999, pp 19–34.

10. Hoppenfeld S, Hutton R: Physical examination of the cervical spine and temporomandibular joint. *In* Hoppenfeld S, Hutton R (eds): Physical Examination of the Spine and Extremities. Appleton & Lange, Connecticut, 1976, pp 105–132.

11. Quon JA, Bernard TN, Burton CV, et al: The site and nature of the lesion. *In* Kirkaldy-Willis WH, Bernard TN (eds): Managing Low Back Pain, ed 4. Churchill Livingstone, New York, 1999, pp 122–152.

12. Hoppenfeld S, Hutton R: Physical examination of the lumbar spine. *In* Hoppenfeld S, Hutton R (eds): Physical Examination of the Spine and Extremities. Appleton & Lange, Connecticut, 1976, pp. 237-263.

Pain Assessment

Robert R. Edwards, Ph.D.

By its very definition, pain is an internal, subjective experience that cannot be directly observed by others or by the use of physiological markers or bioassays. The assessment of pain, therefore, relies largely upon the use of self-report. Although the self-report of pain or any other construct is subject to a number of biases, a good deal of effort has been invested in testing and refining self-report methodology within the field of human pain research. The purpose of this chapter is to provide an overview of this research, to critically evaluate pain assessment tools, and to assist clinicians and researchers in selecting the pain assessment methods best suited to serve their purposes.

CHALLENGES OF PAIN MEASUREMENT

Assessing pain requires measurement tools that are valid and reliable, as well as an ability to communicate (using language, movements, etc.). However, even when these basic requirements are met, additional challenges abound. For example, over what time frame is pain to be measured? Many ratings scales query current pain, or pain over the past week, but longer time frames are often used and these may introduce additional memory biases.[1] In addition, pain is a multidimensional experience incorporating sensory and affective components which are correlated but which may be assessed separately.[2] Generally, most self-report pain assessment tools described below focus on pain intensity ratings over a relatively brief and recent period of time (e.g., the past week).

TYPES OF SELF-REPORT PAIN SCALES

The three most commonly utilized methods to quantify the pain experience (pain intensity, usually) are verbal rating scales, numeric rating scales, and visual analogue scales.

Verbal Rating Scales (VRSs): A VRS generally consists of a series of adjectives (or phrases), ordered from least intense (or unpleasant) to most intense (or unpleasant). An adequate VRS should span a maximum possible range of the pain experience (e.g., from "no pain" to "extremely intense pain"). Patients are asked to select the adjective or phrase that best characterizes their level of pain. Dozens of VRSs have been described and validated; one of the more common examples appears in Table 5-1.[3]

In general, a VRS is scored by assigning each adjective or phrase a number according to its rank (e.g., 0–4 in the example in Table 5-1). The strengths of the VRS include simplicity, ease of administration and scoring, as well as face validity (i.e., they appear to measure directly exactly what they purport to measure—for example, the intensity of pain). In addition, because they are so easy to comprehend, compliance rates for the VRS can be superior to the rates obtained with other scales, especially within certain populations such as the elderly.[4] The VRS has demonstrated good reliability (e.g., consistency over short periods of time) in a number of studies. The validity of the VRS has also been repeatedly established; these scales correlate positively with other self-report measures of pain intensity and with pain behaviors.[5]

Despite their substantial strengths, the VRSs also exhibit a number of weaknesses, based on which other pain researchers have hesitated to recommend these scales. First, the scoring method for a VRS assumes equal intervals between adjectives. That is, the change in pain from "none" to "mild" is quantified identically with the change in pain from "moderate" to "severe." This assumption is rarely tested, and is likely often violated. This property of the VRS poses difficulties in both the interpretation and analysis of VRS-derived data. Second, in order to use VRS properly a patient must both be familiar with all of the words used on the scale and must be able to find one that accurately describes his or her pain. A recent review indicated that the VRS is being used less often in pain outcome research than has been the case in the past.[6]

Numerical Rating Scales (NRSs): An NRS typically consists of a series of numbers with verbal anchors representing the entire possible range of pain intensity. Generally, patients rate their pain from 0 to 10, from 0 to 20, or from 0 to 100. Zero represents "no pain" while the 10, 20, or 100 represents the opposite end of the pain continuum (e.g., "the most intense pain imaginable," "pain as intense as it could be,"

TABLE 5-1. VERBAL RATING SCALE (VRS) FOR PAIN INTENSITY

Five-point VRS
None
Mild
Moderate
Severe
Very severe

"maximum pain"); see Fig. 5-1 for an example. Like VRSs, the NRSs have well documented validity; they correlate positively with other measures of pain and show sensitivity to treatments that are expected to affect pain.[6,7] The NRS can be administered verbally or in a written format, is simple and easily understood, and is easily administered and scored. The principal weakness of the NRS is that, statistically, it does not have ratio qualities.[8]

Visual Analogue Scales (VASs): A VAS consists of a line, often 10 cm long, with verbal anchors at either end, similar to an NRS (e.g., "no pain" on the far left and "the most intense pain imaginable" on the far right). The patient places a mark at a point on the line corresponding to the patient's rating of pain intensity. The line may be depicted with a horizontal or vertical orientation, though a horizontal line is generally preferred (see Fig. 5-2). Recent versions include the mechanical VAS, which uses a sliding marker superimposed on a horizontal VAS drawn on a ruler[8] and is easily scored from the back, which includes numbers for each marker placement. The VAS has often been recommended as the measure of choice for assessment of pain intensity. Substantial evidence supports its validity, and the VAS is sensitive to treatment effects. Although most studies suggest minimal differences in sensitivity among rating scales, significant differences that do emerge generally favor a VAS over a VRS or an NRS. In addition, VAS scores correlate with pain behaviors and do show ratio-level scoring properties.

The VAS does possess some limitations, however. It can be difficult to administer to patients with perceptual-motor problems, which are rather common in the context of chronically painful conditions. In addition, a VAS is generally scored using a ruler (the score is the number of centimeters or millimeters from the end of the line), making scoring more time-consuming and adding additional possible sources of bias or error. Finally, relative to other rating scales, use of a VAS produces higher

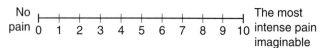

FIGURE 5-1. Sample numerical rating scale (NRS) for pain intensity.

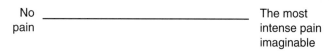

FIGURE 5-2. Sample visual analogue scale (VAS) for pain intensity.

non-completion rates among certain populations, primarily among those with cognitive limitations and among elderly samples (see below).

McGill Pain Questionnaire (MPQ): The MPQ,[9] or its brief analogue the short-form MPQ,[10] are among the most widely utilized measures of pain. In general, the MPQ is considered to be a multidimensional measure of pain quality; however, it also yields numerical indices of several dimensions of the pain experience. Researchers[11] have proposed three dimensions of the experience of pain: sensory-discriminative, affective-motivational, and cognitive-evaluative. The MPQ was created to assess these multiple aspects of pain. It consists of 20 sets of verbal descriptors, ordered in intensity from lowest to highest. These sets of descriptors are divided into those assessing the sensory (10 sets), affective (5 sets), evaluative (1 set), and miscellaneous (4 sets) dimensions of pain. Patients select the words that describe their pain, and their word selections are converted into a pain rating index, based on the sum of all of the words after they are assigned a rank value, as well as the total number of words chosen. In addition, the MPQ contains a present pain intensity VRS (i.e., the PPI), ordered from "mild" to "excruciating."

The more frequently utilized short form of the MPQ consists of 15 representative words from the sensory (11 items) and affective (4 items) categories of the original MPQ. Each descriptor is ranked on a 0 ("none") to 3 ("severe") intensity scale. The PPI, along with a VAS, is also included (see Fig. 5-3). The short form correlates highly with the original scale, can discriminate among different pain conditions, and may be easier than the original scale for geriatric patients to use.[4]

Pain Relief: Studies of interventions designed to reduce pain often include a post-treatment assessment of pain relief in addition to measures of pain intensity obtained at both baseline and post-treatment. Pain relief is often measured using a VAS, a VRS with gradations of relief (e.g., "none," "slight," "moderate," "complete"), or an NRS assessing the percentage of relief. While conceptually attractive, measures of pain relief have demonstrated problems with validity. For example, a significant minority of patients report at least moderate relief on these scales when an analysis of sequential pain ratings (i.e., pretreatment compared to post-treatment) reveals *increases* in reported pain intensity. In one recent trial, while average pain ratings increased by 28% early in the study, approximately 90% of patients reported some degree of relief on a VAS.[12] This phenomenon (i.e., the apparent over-reporting of relief) seems to be due in part to a memory for past pain as being substantially greater than previous ratings would indicate.[1]

BEHAVIORAL OBSERVATION

Although pain is by definition a private and subjective experience, its manifestations are often apparent to others. People in

	None	Mild	Moderate	Severe
Throbbing	0)_____	1)_____	2)_____	3)_____
Shooting	0)_____	1)_____	2)_____	3)_____
Stabbing	0)_____	1)_____	2)_____	3)_____
Sharp	0)_____	1)_____	2)_____	3)_____
Cramping	0)_____	1)_____	2)_____	3)_____
Gnawing	0)_____	1)_____	2)_____	3)_____
Hot-burning	0)_____	1)_____	2)_____	3)_____
Aching	0)_____	1)_____	2)_____	3)_____
Heavy	0)_____	1)_____	2)_____	3)_____
Tender	0)_____	1)_____	2)_____	3)_____
Splitting	0)_____	1)_____	2)_____	3)_____
Tiring-exhausting	0)_____	1)_____	2)_____	3)_____
Sickening	0)_____	1)_____	2)_____	3)_____
Fearful	0)_____	1)_____	2)_____	3)_____
Punishing-cruel	0)_____	1)_____	2)_____	3)_____

Rate the intensity of your pain on the two scales below. Make a mark on the line to indicate where your pain falls between *No pain* and *Worst possible pain* and then circle the appropriate number on the second scale.

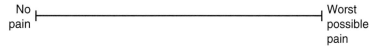

No
pain   Worst
                                                 possible
                                                 pain

Circle the one of the following words that best describes your current pain:

    0 No pain
    1 Mild
    2 Discomforting
    3 Distressing
    4 Excruciating

FIGURE 5-3. Short form MPQ. (Reprinted from Pain, Volume 30: Melzack R, The Short Form McGill Pain Questionnaire, pp 191–7. Copyright (1987), with permission from International Association for the Study of Pain.)

pain may communicate their discomfort by vocalizations, facial expressions, body postures, and actions. These verbal and non-verbal behaviors have been termed pain behaviors, and they have emerged as an important component of behavioral models of pain. Numerous pain behavior coding systems have been developed, although many of them are specific to particular pain conditions. For example, the osteoarthritis (OA) pain behavior coding system[13] assesses the position, movement, and specific pain behaviors (e.g., guarding, rubbing, flexing) observed in OA patients during standardized tasks. Assessment of pain behaviors can be valuable in establishing a patient's level of physical functioning (e.g., the amount of activity engaged in), in analyzing the factors that may reinforce displays of pain (e.g., solicitous responses from others), or in assessing pain in nonverbal individuals. A recent review concluded that while pain behaviors and self-report of pain are moderately related, these measures are not interchangeable.[14] Interestingly, correspondence between pain report and pain behavior was lower in the context of chronic pain than acute pain and, not surprisingly, was highest when observation and verbal report of pain were recorded at the same time.

EXPERIMENTAL PAIN ASSESSMENT

Administration of standardized noxious stimulation under controlled conditions constitutes an important subdiscipline within the field of pain.[15] Several modalities of noxious stimulation are commonly used to induce pain (e.g., thermal, mechanical, electrical, chemical, ischemic, etc.); typical parameters that are measured include pain threshold, pain tolerance, and ratings of suprathreshold noxious stimuli using an NRS, a VAS, or a VRS. The clinical relevance of experimental pain assessment is gradually being established; quantitative sensory testing can be used to subtype patients with chronically painful conditions,[16] to identify mechanisms of chronic pain,[17] and to predict prospectively postoperative pain.[18]

PSYCHOPHYSIOLOGICAL ASSESSMENT

Psychophysiological data serve a number of important functions in the assessment of acute and chronic pain. First, they are a prerequisite for performing biofeedback or related procedures in which patients are taught to bring physiological processes under some degree of voluntary control. Second, psychophysiological measures can help to elucidate some of the concomitants of pain not easily measured by self-report (e.g., arousal, central processing of information related to noxious stimulation). It should be noted that none of the following measures constitute "objective" measures of pain, which is by definition dependent on self-report, and none can substitute for some type of patient rating of their experience of pain.

Surface electromyography (EMG) is often used to record levels of local muscle tension in the context of musculoskeletal pain syndromes, such as low back pain or tension headache, in which heightened muscle tension is thought to contribute to the experience of pain.[19] Electroencephalography (EEG) has been used in a number of studies to assess brain responses to noxious stimulation. While the spatial resolution of EEG is rather limited, its temporal resolution is quite good; several studies have now shown that EEG-measured cortical responses to standardized noxious stimuli are enhanced in patients with chronic pain relative to healthy controls.[20] Heart rate and blood pressure are frequently assessed in the context of experimental pain administration. However, while resting blood pressure and pain responses are inversely correlated,[21] no consistent relationships between cardiovascular reactivity and pain responses have been observed. Collectively, psychophysiological measures can provide unique information about pain responses; they cannot, however, serve as proxy measures for the experience of pain.

SPECIAL POPULATIONS

Children: The assessment of pain in children obviously presents a number of challenges to the healthcare professional. Many providers may (inaccurately) assume that children cannot reliably provide information about their pain. In fact, many pain assessment tools for use specifically in children have been developed and validated, and factors similar to those that influence pain in adults (e.g., the presence and magnitude of tissue damage, affective state, social responses, etc.) have been shown to relate in similar ways to children's pain.[22]

Over a dozen behavioral pain rating scales for infants have been developed. While demonstration of the validity of these scales is often difficult, many have been shown to be consistently reliable. As an example, one of the more commonly used measures is the Neonatal Infant Pain Scale (NIPS),[23] which codes the presence and intensity of six pain-related behaviors: facial expressions, crying, breathing, arm movement, leg movement, and arousal state. Among older children who can more readily self-report sensory and affective experiences, researchers have suggested that direct questioning (e.g., "How is your pain today?"), while clinically useful, is particularly susceptible to bias and demand characteristics. Standardized pain assessment scales have been developed for children of various ages, some of them specific to particular ethnic groups. For example, among these are the Faces scale and the Oucher scale[24] which do not require language and are used for younger children (see Fig. 5-4). Pain thermometers, consisting of a vertical NRS superimposed on a VAS shaped to resemble a thermometer, have also been widely used, while for children over 6 years, a standard VAS is a valid and reliable measure of pain.[25]

The Elderly: The past decade has witnessed a steady increase in research related to pain in the elderly. Most pain assessment tools that have been validated in middle-aged adults have also been psychometrically examined in older subjects. In general, this body of research indicates that increasing age is associated with a higher frequency of incomplete or non-scorable responses on a VAS, but not on a VRS or NRS. Across studies, VAS failure rates in cognitively intact elderly samples range from 7% to 30% of respondents, with the percentages increasing substantially (up to 73%) in cognitively impaired samples.[4] Studies of preferences indicate that, in general, a VAS is rated as one of the least preferred measures among the elderly while a VRS often receives the highest preference scores.

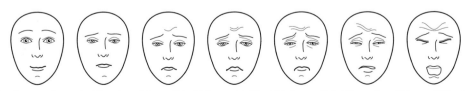

FIGURE 5-4. The Faces pain scale. (Reprinted from Pain, Volume 41: Bieri D, Reeve RA, Champion GD, et al. The Faces Pain Scale for the self-assessment of the severity of pain experienced by children, pp 139–150. Copyright (1990), with permission from International Association for the Study of Pain.

In addition, it has been suggested that the MPQ (long form) is inappropriate for use in elderly samples due to its complexity and time requirements. Although research does not support the contention that the elderly make more errors on the MPQ, several studies have now shown that older adults report less pain on the MPQ (i.e., choose fewer words) even when NRS- or VRS-rated pain does not differ.[26,27] These findings may suggest that the MPQ assesses the construct of pain differently across age groups, and caution may be warranted before using this instrument with older samples.

Collectively, recent findings suggest that a VRS produces the fewest "failure" responses among samples of cognitively intact and cognitively impaired elderly subjects while a VAS produces the largest number. It is therefore recommended that studies of pain in the elderly utilize, at minimum, a VRS to assess pain intensity.

BIASES IN PAIN MEASUREMENT

Inaccurate assessments of pain have a number of substantive consequences; underestimation of pain can lead to improper management, unnecessary suffering, and delay in recovery, while overestimation of pain can lead to over-treatment and potentially to adverse iatrogenic consequences. A number of studies have examined the congruence, or lack thereof, between patient reports of pain and healthcare providers' assessments of patients' pain. In general, findings from this body of research suggest that a good deal of caution is warranted when medical professionals attempt to estimate patients' levels of pain.

The majority of studies examining the congruence between health professional and patient ratings of pain have used samples of nurses. One study found that 43% of nurses underestimated the pain experienced by burn patients during a therapeutic procedure and nurses also overestimated the amount of pain relief following administration of analgesic medication.[28] Similar findings have also emerged from a number of other studies.[29] In one study[30] agreement scores (i.e., kappa statistics) between nurses and postsurgical pain patients ranged from 0.01 to 0.12, which indicates no significant correlation between nurse and patient ratings of pain. In a study of cancer patients and their providers no correlations between patients' VAS pain ratings and ratings of patient pain made by nurses, house officers, or oncology fellows were significant.[31] Finally, in addition to findings relating to the inaccuracy or systematic underestimation of patients' pain, there is little evidence for the validity of expert judgments regarding the prognosis of patients in pain. For example, among back pain patients followed longitudinally, no relationship was observed between providers' estimates of patients' rehabilitation potential and actual rehabilitation outcomes.[32]

SUMMARY AND RECOMMENDATIONS

Although pain is a private and subjective experience, a wide array of valid and reliable measurement tools is available. Any study of pain should include at least one self-report measure, and it is often beneficial to use either multiple measures or a multidimensional measure of pain (e.g., the short form of the MPQ, which includes both verbal descriptors and a VAS). A recent review of the cancer pain literature indicated that single-item VAS, VRS, and NRS all showed good validity and reliability, and it was concluded that no one of these measures was consistently superior.[5] However, we can advise that in studies of elderly or cognitively compromised subjects, use of a VRS or NRS is strongly preferable to use of a VAS. Pain relief should be measured using sequential ratings (i.e., changes from pre- to post-treatment) rather than a retrospective impression. Behavioral observation, experimental pain assessment, and psychophysiological assessment are all useful and potentially informative adjunctive measures of pain responses, but none can substitute for self-report of the pain experience. The one exception to this standard is infants, in whom coding of behavioral or facial responses is the current gold standard for pain assessment. For slightly older children, a pictorial scale such as the Faces or Oucher scale may be utilized, while in children who are 6 years or older a standard VAS may be the optimal choice. Finally, substantial research suggests that healthcare professionals, no matter how expert or experienced, are not reliable judges of patients' report of pain. Their estimates are both inaccurate and systematically biased in the direction of underestimating patients' experiences of pain.

The assessment of pain is vitally important to both clinicians and researchers. Self-report is the most direct manner of assessing pain and a variety of self-report measurement options exist. In this chapter we have attempted to provide those with an interest in treating or studying pain with some of the requisite information on which to base choices regarding pain assessment. Measures should be selected with as complete a knowledge as possible of their properties, strengths, and limitations.

KEY POINTS

- Although pain is a subjective experience, standardized assessment of pain using validated self-report measures is essential.
- Any study of pain should include at least one of the following measures: a numeric rating scale, a visual analogue scale, a verbal rating scale, or a multidimensional measure such as the McGill pain questionnaire.
- In studies of elderly or cognitively compromised subjects investigators should strongly consider using a verbal or numeric rating scale, while in studies of infants the use of a standardized coding system for facial and behavioral responses is recommended.
- Behavioral observation, experimental pain assessment, and psychophysiological assessment are informative adjunctive measures of pain responses, but none can substitute for self-report of the pain experience (except in infants, as noted above).
- In treatment outcome studies pain relief should be measured using sequential ratings (i.e., changes from pre- to post-treatment) rather than a retrospective rating of the degree or percentage of relief.
- Healthcare professionals, no matter how experienced, are generally not reliable judges of patients' reports of their pain. The estimates of physicians, nurses, and other providers are both inaccurate and systematically biased in the direction of underestimating patients' experiences of pain. Only in rare and extreme circumstances should a healthcare professional's judgment be substituted for a patient's self-report of his or her pain.

REFERENCES

1. Haythornthwaite JA, Fauerbach JA: Assessment of pain, pain relief, and patient satisfaction. *In* Turk DC, Melzack R (eds): Handbook of Pain Assessment. Guilford, New York, 2001, pp 417–430.
2. Melzack R: Pain — An overview. Acta Anaesthesiol Scand 43:880–884, 1999.
3. Frank AJ, Moll JM, Hort JF: A comparison of three ways of measuring pain. Rheumatol Rehabil 21:211–217, 1982.
4. Gagliese L, Melzack R: The assessment of pain in the elderly. *In* Ostofsky D, Lomranz J (eds): Handbook of Pain and Aging. Plenum Press, New York, 1997.
5. Jensen MP: The validity and reliability of pain measures in adults with cancer. J Pain 4:2–21, 2003.
6. Jensen MP, Karoly P: Self-report scales and procedures for assessing pain in adults. *In* Turk DC, Melzack R (eds): Handbook of Pain Assessment. Guilford, New York, 2001, pp 15–34.
7. Jensen MP, Karoly P, Braver S: The measurement of clinical pain intensity; a comparison of six methods. Pain 27:117–126, 1986.
8. Price DD, Bush FM, Long S, Harkins SW: A comparison of pain measurement characteristics of mechanical visual analogue and simple numerical rating scales. Pain 56:217–226, 1994.
9. Melzack R: The McGill Pain Questionnaire: Major properties and scoring methods. Pain 1:277–299, 1975.
10. Melzack R. The short-form McGill Pain Questionnaire. Pain 30:191–197, 1987.
11. Melzack R, Casey KL: Sensory, motivational, and central control determinants of pain: A new conceptual model. *In* Kenshalo D (ed): The Skin Senses. CC Thomas, Springfield, IL, 1968, pp 423–443.
12. Feine JS, Lavigne GJ, Dao TT, et al: Memories of chronic pain and perceptions of relief. Pain 77:137–141, 1998.
13. Keefe FJ, Caldwell DS, Queen K, et al: Osteoarthritic knee pain: A behavioral analysis. Pain 28:309–321, 1987.
14. Labus JS, Keefe FJ, Jensen MP: Self-reports of pain intensity and direct observations of pain behavior: When are they correlated? Pain 102:109–124, 2003.
15. Gracely R. Studies of pain in human subjects. *In* Wall P, Melzack R (eds): Textbook of Pain. Churchill Livingstone, New York, 1999, pp 385–407.
16. Pappagallo M, Oaklander AL, Quatrano-Piacentini AL, et al: Heterogenous patterns of sensory dysfunction in postherpetic neuralgia suggest multiple pathophysiologic mechanisms. Anesthesiology 92:691–698, 2000.
17. Sarlani E, Greenspan JD: Evidence for generalized hyperalgesia in temporomandibular disorders patients. Pain 102:221–226, 2003.
18. Granot M, Lowenstein L, Yarnitsky D, et al: Postcesarean section pain prediction by preoperative experimental pain assessment. Anesthesiology 98:1422–1426, 2003.
19. Jensen R, Olesen J: Initiating mechanisms of experimentally induced tension-type headache. Cephalalgia 16:175–182; discussion 138–139, 1996.
20. Flor H: Cortical reorganisation and chronic pain: Implications for rehabilitation. J Rehabil Med 66–72, 2003.
21. Ghione S: Hypertension-associated hypalgesia. Evidence in experimental animals and humans, pathophysiological mechanisms, and potential clinical consequences. Hypertension 28:494–504, 1996.
22. McGrath PA: Pain in the pediatric patient: Practical aspects of assessment. Pediatr Ann 24:126–128, 1995.
23. Lawrence J, Alcock D, McGrath P, et al: The development of a tool to assess neonatal pain. Neonatal Netw 12:59–66, 1993.
24. Luffy R, Grove SK: Examining the validity, reliability, and preference of three pediatric pain measurement tools in African-American children. Pediatr Nurs 29:54–59, 2003.
25. McGrath PA, Gillespie J: Pain assessment in children and adolescents. *In* Turk DMR (ed): Handbook of Pain Assessment. Guilford Press, New York, 2001, pp 97–118.
26. Gagliese L, Melzack R: Age-related differences in the qualities but not the intensity of chronic pain. Pain 104:597–608, 2003.
27. Gagliese L, Katz J: Age differences in postoperative pain are scale dependent: A comparison of measures of pain intensity and quality in younger and older surgical patients. Pain 103:11–20, 2003.
28. Choiniere M, Melzack R, Girard N, et al: Comparisons between patients' and nurses' assessment of pain and medication efficacy in severe burn injuries. Pain 40:143–152, 1990.
29. Stephenson NL: A comparison of nurse and patient: Perceptions of postsurgical pain. J Intraven Nurs 17:235–239, 1994.
30. Thomas T, Robinson C, Champion D, et al: Prediction and assessment of the severity of post-operative pain and of satisfaction with management. Pain 75:177–185, 1998.
31. Grossman SA, Sheidler VR, Swedeen K, et al: Correlation of patient and caregiver ratings of cancer pain. J Pain Symptom Manage 6:53–57, 1991.
32. Jensen IB, Bodin L, Ljungqvist T, et al: Assessing the needs of patients in pain: A matter of opinion? Spine 25:2816–2823, 2000.

Psychological Evaluation and Testing

**Leslie J. Heinberg, Ph.D., and
Jennifer A. Haythornthwaite, Ph.D.**

The experience of pain is a private, subjective phenomenon. There is no simple instrument, such as a thermometer, that can accurately assess an individual's pain experience. As a result, numerous instruments have been offered to measure multiple domains of pain (Table 6-1). Voluminous research has demonstrated that a psychological perspective is helpful in conceptualizing, evaluating, and treating chronic pain. This chapter focuses on the psychological evaluation and assessment of chronic pain. The components of a psychological evaluation for chronic pain are reviewed and the psychological assessment of pain is examined in the domains of disability/impairment, negative affect, and coping. Multidimensional instruments and measures of more global psychopathology are outlined followed by a brief discussion of specialized assessment.

PSYCHOLOGICAL EVALUATION

A comprehensive evaluation of individuals with chronic pain must include assessment of psychological, social, and behavioral factors associated with their experience of pain. This is best accomplished by combining interview techniques with the administration of one or more standardized questionnaires. Psychological evaluation should not only include an examination of psychological aspects of the pain experience but also a more comprehensive psychiatric interview to diagnose current or past psychiatric disorders, particularly depression.

Although structured clinical interviews for pain have been developed, the majority of practitioners choose to conduct semi-structured interviews. Because patients with chronic pain complaints may be reticent to undergo psychological evaluation, it is recommended that a history of the pain complaint be taken first. This assessment will focus upon the intensity, frequency, and affective and sensory quality of pain, as well as the efficacy of previous treatment interventions. It is important to identify events that act as precipitants to pain exacerbations; assess daily activities, disability, and perceived interference,

evaluate familial/social factors; and identify any psychiatric disorders. Because of the high coprevalence of chronic pain and major depression, it is recommended that all depressive symptoms be carefully assessed. In addition, practitioners generally assess symptoms of anxiety disorders, alcohol and substance abuse and dependence, personality disorders, and any relevant family psychiatric history.

PSYCHOLOGICAL ASSESSMENT/TESTING

Disability/Impairment: Individuals with chronic pain describe significant variability in the degree of interference, impairment, and disability due to their pain complaints. As a result, a number of measures have been offered to assess perceived disability. The *Brief Pain Inventory* (BPI; see Figure 6.1) was originally developed by the Pain Research Group of the WHO Collaborating Center for Symptom Evaluation in Cancer Care[1] to measure pain severity and pain-related interference in patients with cancer in many different countries. Recently its use has been extended to non-cancer pain assessment, including heterogeneous pain conditions,[2] osteoarthritis,[3] neuropathic pain[4] including HIV/AIDS,[5] and cerebral palsy.[6] The most widely used version of the pain interference scale uses 11-point numeric rating scales (0 = no interference to 10 = interferes completely) to assess pain-related interference in seven areas: general activity, mood, walking ability, normal work including outside the home and housework, relations with other people, enjoyment of life, and sleep.[1] The time frame for assessment can vary from "the past week"[1] to "the past 24 hours."[7] Factor analyses of the pain intensity and pain interference scales support a two-factor structure that is robust across cultures.[1] The BPI has been used to demonstrate the efficacy of pain medication in a variety of chronic painful conditions[3] and appears to be sensitive to change due to treatment.

An alternative scale that is quite similar to the BPI is the *Pain Disability Index* (PDI) that measures perceived disability

TABLE 6-1. **SUMMARY OF MEASURES**

Domain/Scale	Estimated Time to Complete	Comments
Disability/impairment		
Brief Pain Inventory	<5 min	2 primary domains: pain severity and interference
Sickness Impact Profile	15 min	
Roland–Morris Disability Scale	5 min	3 primary domains: psychosocial function, physical function, other; used primarily in the assessment of low back pain
Negative affect		
Beck Depression Inventory	15 min	Includes an item assessing suicide
CES-D	10 min	Available on the Internet
Coping		
Coping Strategies Questionnaire	15 min	6 cognitive and 2 behavioral pain coping strategies
Pain Catastrophizing Scale	5 min	3 dimensions of pain catastrophizing
Chronic Pain Coping Inventory	10 min	12 primarily behavioral pain coping strategies
Multidimensional scales		
Multidimensional Pain Inventory	15 min	Comprehensive scale that includes social responses to pain
SF-36	10 min	Captures general health-related function
Psychopathology		
MMPI-2	120 min	Available only through licensed professionals, 9 dimensions
SCL-90-R	15 min	of psychological disturbance and 3 global distress scales

due to pain. It consists of seven questions assessing disability due to pain in the following domains: family/home, recreation, social activities, occupation, sexual behavior, self-care, and life support activities. Each item is rated on an 11-point scale (0 = no disability to 10 = total disability) and the responses are summed. Although early analyses suggested these seven domains assessed two factors,[8] more recent analyses with a large group of patients suggest a single factor[9] that does not include the life-support activity item.[10] The PDI is also sensitive to change following pain treatment, as treatment with controlled-release codeine led to an improvement in each area of role functioning, except life-support activities.[11]

Although widely used, the *Sickness Impact Profile* (SIP)[12] is complicated by length (136 items) and a complex scoring algorithm. The SIP has been comprehensively tested and revised and has been normed on a number of medical populations including individuals with chronic pain. The 136 items of the SIP are separated into 12 scales: sleep and rest, eating, work, home management, recreation and pastimes, ambulation, mobility, body care and movement, social interaction, alertness behavior, emotional behavior, and communication. Respondents mark only those statements that describe the respondent "today" and are related to health, and its instructions are typically changed from "your state of health" to "your pain." Each statement is weighted and percentage scores for three areas are computed as weighted sums: physical function (personal care, mobility, and walking), psychosocial function

(emotions, cognitive function, social interactions, and communication), and other function (sleep/rest, household, work, recreation, and eating). A total score is calculated as a weighted sum of these three scales. The distribution of SIP scores can be quite skewed, necessitating transformations to normalize the distribution prior to conducting parametric analyses.[13]

Early in its application, 24 of the original SIP items were developed as a measure of function in back pain by adding the stem to each statement "because of my back pain"—the *Roland–Morris Disability Scale*.[14,15] Items were selected based on the likely impact back pain would have on the physical function; however, not all items are from the SIP Physical Function scale. Items include assessment of irritability, appetite, and housework. This measure has become one of a select group of standard outcome measures in the back pain literature.[16,17] Although primarily used for the assessment of function in low back pain, some investigators have used this shorter scale to assess function in heterogeneous groups of patients seen through multidisciplinary programs. A later analysis identified 20 items that were most sensitive to change in patients with low back pain, only seven of which were included in the Roland–Morris scale.[18,19]

Negative Affect: Because depression and other types of negative affect often result from chronic pain and unduly influence its experience, it is important to determine whether the patient has experienced any change in mood or affect.[20]

FIGURE 6-1. **BRIEF PAIN INVENTORY**

Please rate your pain by circling the one number that best describes your pain DURING THE PAST WEEK:

Please rate your pain at its *worst* during the past week

       0   1   2   3   4   5   6   7   8   9   10

No pain   Pain as bad as you can imagine

Please rate your pain at its *least* during the past week

       0   1   2   3   4   5   6   7   8   9   10

No pain   Pain as bad as you can imagine

Please rate your pain on the *average* during the past week

       0   1   2   3   4   5   6   7   8   9   10

No pain   Pain as bad as you can imagine

Please rate how much pain you have *right now*

       0   1   2   3   4   5   6   7   8   9   10

No pain   Pain as bad as you can imagine

Circle the one number that describes how, DURING THE PAST WEEK, pain has interfered with your:

General activity

       0   1   2   3   4   5   6   7   8   9   10

Does not interfere   Completely interferes

Mood

       0   1   2   3   4   5   6   7   8   9   10

Does not interfere   Completely interferes

Walking ability

       0   1   2   3   4   5   6   7   8   9   10

Does not interfere   Completely interferes

Normal work (includes both work outside the home and housework)

       0   1   2   3   4   5   6   7   8   9   10

Does not interfere   Completely interferes

Relations with other people

       0   1   2   3   4   5   6   7   8   9   10

Does not interfere   Completely interferes

Sleep

       0   1   2   3   4   5   6   7   8   9   10

Does not interfere   Completely interferes

Enjoyment of life

       0   1   2   3   4   5   6   7   8   9   10

Does not interfere   Completely interferes

Modified from Cleeland CS, Ryan KM: Pain assessment: Global use of the Brief Pain Inventory. Ann Acad Med Singapore 23:129–138, 1994.

One of the most frequently utilized measures is the *Beck Depression Inventory* (BDI).[21] The BDI is a 21-item, multiple choice measure that requires individuals to endorse one of a series of four statements which best describes his or her subjective experience. The four statements reflect progressively more severe symptomatology. The BDI was developed to measure symptoms of depression or distress as operationally defined by: alterations in mood, a negative self-concept associated with self-devaluation and self-blame, self-punitive wishes, vegetative symptoms, and alterations in activity level. The BDI is frequently used in psychiatric and general medical populations. Although brief and easy to score and interpret, the BDI may overestimate the degree of depression among chronic pain patients because of its focus on a number of somatic and vegetative symptoms.

Another frequently used measure of depression is the *Center for Epidemiological Studies Depression Scale* (CES-D).[22] The CES-D was originally developed for use in large epidemiologic studies involving the general population, has been shown to be quite reliable and valid, and copies and reviews of this instrument are widely available on the worldwide web. Respondents are asked to report the frequency with which they have experienced each of 20 symptoms during the past week on a 4-point scale. Like the BDI, the CES-D is brief and has excellent psychometric properties. However, because of the overlap between somatic symptoms of depression and symptoms of chronic pain, it also has been criticized for possibly overestimating the prevalence and severity of depression among pain populations. Comparative analysis suggests that the CES-D and BDI are relatively comparable, with the CES-D demonstrating greater sensitivity and the BDI exhibiting better specificity.[23]

Coping: Coping is a term that encompasses the many techniques that people utilize to attempt to control or tolerate stressors, including the experience of pain. The use of some pain-specific coping strategies differentially relate to outcome among chronic pain patients[24] and many psychosocial interventions aim to increase these more effective strategies. Because of the interest in enhancing pain-coping techniques, a number of measures of coping in chronic pain patients have been developed. The *Coping Strategies Questionnaire*[25] is a 50-item measure assessing 6 cognitive and 2 behavioral coping strategies including (1) diverting attention, (2) reinterpreting pain sensations, (3) coping self-statements, (4) ignoring pain sensations, (5) praying and hoping, (6) catastrophizing, (7) increasing behavioral activity, and (8) increasing pain behaviors. Catastrophizing (e.g., "I feel I can't stand it anymore") has been consistently identified as a maladaptive coping strategy[26] and the *Pain Catastrophizing Scale*—a scale measuring three dimensions of catastrophizing—is available.[27] Despite the inclusion of cognitive strategies in psychological interventions for pain management (e.g., coping self-statements), these strategies have not been consistently demonstrated to be adaptive.[24]

More recently, a more behavioral measure of coping in chronic pain patients has been developed with the *Chronic Pain Coping Inventory*.[28] The scale was designed to include strategies that are encouraged, as well as discouraged, in multidisciplinary pain treatment that have not been assessed with other measures of coping. This 65-item scale has 12 subscales including guarding, resting, asking for assistance, relaxation, task persistence, exercise/stretch, seeking social support, coping self-statements, and medication use. Guarding, resting, asking for assistance, and task persistence are closely associated with measures of functioning.

Multidimensional Instruments: Rather than administering patients large batteries of assessments in order to measure the various domains of interest, multidimensional instruments have been developed. One of the most frequently used, and widely studied, is the *Multidimensional Pain Inventory* (MPI).[29] This 56-item measure is comprised of three sections and examines multiple pain domains including pain severity; interference of pain with daily activities; work; family relationships and social activities; pain-specific support from spouse or partner; perceived life control; and negative affect. Patients' responses may be compared against normative data from other chronic pain patients. In addition, validity studies[30] demonstrate that MPI profile patterns, labeled "dysfunctional," "interpersonally distressed," and "adaptive coper," can be readily identified and interpreted. This measure is valuable in its ability to assess multiple dimensions of pain, its comprehensive focus on psychological, behavioral, and social factors, its relative brevity, and its demonstrated sensitivity to treatment.

The *Short Form 36 Health Survey* (SF-36)[31] is a 36-item self-report measure of health-related quality of life yielding 8 subscales. The scale was developed for diverse applications, and factor analysis yields two major factors: physical health and mental health. Although not specific to pain, an advantage of the SF-36 is the opportunity to compare scores for different diagnostic groups, since this instrument has been widely used.

Measures of Psychopathology: In addition to assessing the presence of psychopathology during a psychiatric interview, psychologists often administer self-report instruments of psychopathology to patients with chronic pain. Unlike interview data, these measures provide standardized, reliable, and valid assessments of psychopathology that may influence the experience of pain. The *Minnesota Multiphasic Personality Inventory* (MMPI) is the psychological instrument most commonly used to evaluate the psychological status of patients with chronic pain. A revised version, the MMPI-2,[32] has been introduced which, like the original MMPI, includes ten clinical scales which assess psychopathology and three validity scales. The MMPI has been shown to differentiate samples of rheumatoid arthritis and low back pain. However, it has been criticized due to its length (566 items), frequency of items relating to physical symptoms, and lack of predictive validity among populations with chronic pain.[33]

Shorter inventories, such as the 90-item *Symptom Checklist-90-Revised* (SCL-90-R),[34] have been utilized to assess psychopathology among chronic pain patients. The SCL-90-R assesses 9 different types of psychological disturbance and yields 3 global measures of distress. Although often favored for its briefer length and, because of its focus on symptoms, less patient resistance, it also has not demonstrated predictive validity with regard to treatment outcome.

SPECIALIZED ASSESSMENT

Invasive Therapies: Because psychosocial factors are involved in the maintenance and exacerbation of pain and disability, as well as influencing recovery from some spine surgeries, psychological evaluation is often recommended prior to pursuing invasive therapies. Such evaluations have numerous goals, including screening for major psychopathology, retardation, dementia or delirium, which could impede the patient's ability to provide informed consent. In addition, it has been suggested that active psychosis, suicidality/homicidality, or active alcohol or drug dependency are psychosocial "red flags" for pursuing invasive therapy, at least until these clinical conditions are successfully managed. For most patients, this evaluation will focus upon screening for, and potentially intervening upon, psychosocial factors that may impede optimal outcome (e.g., a high degree of disability), help educate the patient as part of preparation for informed consent, and guide both the patient and physician in identifying the individual's strengths and weaknesses. These evaluations generally include psychological testing, a psychiatric interview, and an educational component. Such evaluations are often recommended prior to the implantation of an intrathecal pump or a spinal cord stimulator or more extensive orthopedic and/or neurological surgery. It is important to note that both physical and psychological criteria for patient selection for surgery are somewhat imprecise and the predictive ability of psychological measures is relatively mixed. Excellent detailed discussions of these procedures are available elsewhere.[35-38]

Chronic Opioid Therapy: Patients are often referred for psychological evaluation as part of considering or continuing chronic opioid therapy. When done prior to beginning therapy, this evaluation provides a baseline assessment of the patient's pain intensity, affective state, disability, and quality of life. In addition, potential behavioral and/or psychological contraindications for chronic opioid use can be identified such as current alcohol abuse or dependence, illicit or prescription drug abuse or dependence, severe major depression, or antisocial or borderline personality disorder. Other psychological factors that may require closer supervision by the physician or referral for psychiatric care can also be assessed. Unfortunately, little work has focused on developing screening tools that successfully predict problematic use of prescription opioids,[39] although patients classified as addicted to prescription opioids were more likely to respond positively to three screening items: patient believes he/she is addicted; increases in opioid dose or frequency have occurred; and patient prefers one route of administration.[40]

Psychological evaluation can be helpful for patients who are concerned about the effects of opioid treatment on cognitive functioning, particularly if they continue to work. Brief screening of intellectual functioning, memory, psychomotor speed, and attention prior to initiation of chronic opioids and again following titration to therapeutic doses can demonstrate to patients (and often employers) the lack of significant cognitive effects of opioid medications. If such an evaluation is considered, it is important that the baseline testing occurs when the patient has not taken any opioid therapy for at least one week and is not taking other medications (e.g., benzodiazepines) that may impair cognitive functioning. Psychological evaluation may be helpful for patients who exhibit problematic behavior while using chronic opioid therapy (e.g., early prescription refills or excessive telephone interactions with clinic staff), although the goal for these evaluations needs to be carefully outlined for patients and providers.

SUMMARY

Assessment of chronic pain requires careful multidisciplinary assessment to arrive at an optimally helpful treatment plan. A physical examination is generally not sufficient to capture the number of psychological, behavioral, and social factors that should be considered. Psychological assessment and clinical interviewing can be helpful adjuncts to physicians' evaluations. However, it is important that the assessment be multidimensional and utilize instruments that are reliable and valid. The preceding discussion of instruments should provide a starting place for the selection of appropriate instruments.

KEY POINTS

- Psychological evaluations for pain and disability typically include psychological testing and an interview.
- Key domains for assessment include pain-related disability, negative affect, and pain coping strategies; multidimensional instruments also offer an assessment of social/familial factors.
- When the presence of psychopathology is a particular concern, personality assessment—often using the MMPI-2—is indicated.
- When invasive therapy is being considered in the patient with chronic pain, it is often advisable to obtain a specialized psychological consultation that includes evaluation, screening, and education.
- Psychological evaluation as part of chronic opioid therapy can provide reassurance and valuable information about the patient's response to therapy.

REFERENCES

1. Cleeland CS, Ryan KM: Pain assessment: global use of the Brief Pain Inventory. Ann Acad Med Singapore 23:129–138, 1994.
2. Palangio M, Northfelt DW, Portenoy RK, et al: Dose conversion and titration with a novel, once-daily, OROS osmotic technology, extended-release hydromorphone formulation in the treatment of chronic malignant or nonmalignant pain. J Pain Symptom Manage 23:355–368, 2002.
3. Roth SH, Fleischmann RM, Burch FX, et al: Around-the-clock, controlled-release oxycodone therapy for osteoarthritis-related pain: Placebo-controlled trial and long-term evaluation. Arch Intern Med 160:853–860, 2000.
4. Jensen MP, Ehde DM, Hoffman AJ, et al: Cognitions, coping and social environment predict adjustment to phantom limb pain. Pain 95:133–142, 2002.
5. Breitbart W, Rosenfeld B, Passik S, et al: A comparison of pain report and adequacy of analgesic therapy in ambulatory AIDS patients with and without a history of substance abuse. Pain 72:235–243, 1997.
6. Tyler EJ, Jensen MP, Engel JM, Schwartz L: The reliability and validity of pain interference measures in persons with cerebral palsy. Arch Phys Med Rehabil 83:236–239, 2002.
7. Anderson KO, Syrjala KL, Cleeland CS: How to assess cancer pain. In Turk DC, Melzack R (eds): Handbook of Pain Assessment, ed 2. Guilford Press, New York, 2001, pp 579–600.
8. Tait RC, Pollard CA, Margolis RB, et al: The Pain Disability Index: Psychometric and validity data. Arch Phys Med Rehabil 68:438–441, 1987.
9. Chibnall JT, Tait RC: The Pain Disability Index: Factor structure and normative data. Arch Phys Med Rehabil 75:1082–1086, 1994.

10. Tait RC, Chibnall JT: Attitude profiles and clinical status in patients with chronic pain. Pain 78:49–57, 1998.
11. Arkinstall W, Sandler W, Goughnour B, et al: Efficacy of controlled-release codeine in chronic non-malignant pain: A randomized, placebo-controlled clinical trial. Pain 62:169–178, 1995.
12. Pollard WE, Bobitt RA, Bergner M, et al: The sickness impact profile: Reliability of a health status measure. Medical Care 14:146–155, 1976.
13. Romano JM, Turner JA, Jensen MP: The Chronic Illness Problem Inventory as a measure of dysfunction in chronic pain patients. Pain 49:71–75, 1992.
14. Roland M, Morris R: A study of the natural history of back pain: I. Development of a reliable and sensitive measure of disability in low-back pain. Spine 8:141-144, 1983.
15. Roland M, Fairbank J: The Roland–Morris Disability Questionnaire and the Oswestry Disability Questionnaire. Spine 25:3115–3124, 2000.
16. Deyo RA: Comparative validity of the sickness impact profile and shorter scales for functional assessment in low-back pain. Spine 11:951–954, 1986.
17. Deyo RA, Battie M, Beurskens AJ, et al: Outcome measures for low back pain research. A proposal for standardized use. Spine 23:2003–2013, 1998.
18. Stratford P, Solomon P, Binkley J, et al: Sensitivity of Sickness Impact Profile items to measure change over time in a low-back pain patient group. Spine 18:1723–1727, 1993.
19. Linton SJ, Hellsing AL, Larsson I: Bridging the gap: Support groups do not enhance long-term outcome in chronic back pain. Clin J Pain 13:221–228, 1997.
20. Fishbain DA, Cutler R, Rosomoff HL, Rosomoff RS: Chronic pain-associated depression: Antecedent or consequence of chronic pain? A review. Clin J Pain 13:116–137, 1997.
21. Beck A, Rush AJ, Shaw BF, Emery G: Cognitive Therapy of Depression. Guilford Press, New York, 1979.
22. Radloff LS: The CES-D scale: A self report depression scale for research in the general population. Appl Psychol Measures 1:385–401, 1977.
23. Geisser ME, Roth RS, Robinson ME: Assessing depression among persons with chronic pain using the Center for Epidemiological Studies-Depression Scale and the Beck Depression Inventory: A comparative analysis. Clin J Pain 13:163–170, 1997.
24. Jensen MP, Turner JA, Romano JM, Karoly P: Coping with chronic pain: A critical review of the literature. Pain 47:249–283, 1991.
25. Rosenstiel AK, Keefe FJ: The use of coping strategies in chronic low back pain patients: Relationship to patient characteristics and current adjustment. Pain; 3:1–8, 1983.
26. Sullivan MJ, Thorn B, Haythornthwaite JA, et al: Theoretical perspectives on the relation between catastrophizing and pain. Clin J Pain 17:52–64, 2001.
27. Sullivan MJ, Bishop SR, Pivik J: The Pain Catastrophizing Scale: Development and validation. Psychol Assessm 7:524–532, 1995.
28. Jensen MP, Turner JA, Romano JM, Strom SE: The Chronic Pain Coping Inventory: Development and preliminary validation. Pain 60:203–216, 1995.
29. Kerns R, Turk D, Rudy T: The West Haven-Yale Multidimensional Pain Inventory (WHYMPI). Pain 23:345–356, 1985.
30. Turk DC, Rudy TE: The robustness of an empirically derived taxonomy of chronic pain patients. Pain 43:27–35, 1990.
31. Ware JE, Snow KK, Kosinski M, et al: SF-36 Health Survey: Manual and Interpretation Guide. Nimrod Press, Boston, 1993.
32. Hathaway SR, McKinley JC, Butcher JN, et al: Minnesota Multiphasic Personality Inventory-2: Manual for Administration. University of Minnesota Press, Minneapolis, 1989.
33. Bradley LA, McKendree-Smith NL: Assessment of psychological status using interviews and self-report instruments. In Turk DC, Melzack R (eds): Handbook of Pain Assessment, ed 2. Guilford Press, New York, 2001, pp 292–319.
34. Derogatis L: The SCL-90R: Administration, Scoring, and Procedures Manual, ed 2. Clinical Psychometric Research, Towson, 1983.
35. Block AR: Presurgical Psychological Screening in Chronic Pain Syndromes. Lawrence Erlbaum, Mahwah, NJ, 1996.
36. Epker J, Block AR: Presurgical psychological screening in back pain patients: A review. Clin J Pain 17:200–205, 2001.
37. Prager J, Jacobs M: Evaluation of patients for implantable pain modalities: Medical and behavioral assessment. Clin J Pain 17:206–214, 2001.
38. Carragee EJ: Psychological screening in the surgical treatment of lumbar disc herniation. Clin J Pain 17:215–219, 2001.
39. Robinson RC, Gatchel RJ, Polatin P, et al: Screening for problematic prescription opioid use. Clin J Pain 17:220–228, 2001.
40. Compton P, Darakjian J, Miotto K: Screening for addiction in patients with chronic pain and "problematic" substance use: Evaluation of a pilot assessment tool. J Pain Symptom Manage 16:355–363, 1998.

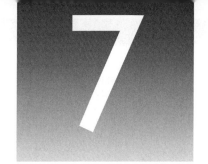

Neurophysiologic Testing for Pain

Takashi Nishida, M.D., and
Michael M. Minieka, M.D.

Electrophysiologic testing when properly applied is a useful tool for the evaluation of patients with pain. Understanding the indications and limitations of each test is absolutely essential for appropriate diagnosis and subsequent treatment.

Electrophysiologic studies are a very sensitive indicator of central and peripheral nervous system involvement but do not indicate underlying disease. For example, testing can diagnose radiculopathy but cannot determine if it is caused by osteophytes, a herniated disc, or diabetes. This chapter describes conventional electrophysiologic tests such as electromyography (EMG) and short latency somatosensory evoked potentials (SSEPs), as well as newer techniques including quantitative sensory testing (QST), and laser evoked potentials (LEPs). Invasive testing such as microneurography is not discussed here.

The role of the sympathetic nervous system in the production of pain is complex and controversial; nonetheless, testing of the autonomic function is also important for the evaluation of pain complaints because it gives an objective measure of autonomic nervous system involvement as well as evidence of the therapeutic interventions such as sympathetic nerve blocks. The most frequent referrals to the autonomic laboratory are patients with painful peripheral neuropathy such as diabetic polyneuropathy and so-called complex regional pain syndrome/reflex sympathetic dystrophy (CRPS/RSD). Based on accuracy, reproducibility, and easiness to perform, two quantitative methods, sympathetic skin response (SSR) and quantitative sudomotor axon reflex test (QSART), are discussed here.

ELECTROMYOGRAPHY (EMG)

When strictly defined, EMG indicates only a needle examination of muscles. However, EMG is often used to include both needle studies and nerve conduction studies. Nerve conduction studies are often referred to by the letters NCV, with "V" standing for velocity, although nerve conduction studies measure more than velocity. For clarity, we use EMG/NCV to indicate the combination of needle electromyography and nerve conduction studies.[1]

EMG/NCV is extremely useful in the evaluation of the peripheral nervous system. Indeed, the three most common diagnoses in EMG laboratories—peripheral neuropathy, carpal tunnel syndrome, and lumbosacral radiculopathy—all cause pain. EMG/NCV can identify the anatomic site of injury (anterior horn cell, spinal root, plexus, nerve, neuromuscular junction, or muscle), the type of neurons or fibers involved (motor, sensory, or autonomic), the nature of pathologic alteration (demyelination or axonal degeneration), time course (acute, subacute, or chronic), and severity of injury.

By stimulating peripheral nerve with supramaximal intensity, compound muscle action potential (CMAP) for motor nerve and sensory nerve action potential (SNAP) for sensory nerve are recorded. Amplitude of action potentials as well as the time from stimulation to response is recorded. Latency is the interval between the onset of a stimulus and the onset of a response, expressed in milliseconds. Conduction velocity is obtained by dividing the distance between two stimulation points (mm) of the same nerve by the difference between proximal and distal latencies (ms). This calculated velocity, expressed in meters per second (m/s) represents the conduction velocity of the fastest nerve fibers between two points of stimulation. It is important to note that studies may be normal if a disorder is limited to small nerve fibers such as $A\delta$ and C fibers.

The amplitude of CMAP is measured from baseline to negative peak in millivolts, and the amplitude of SNAP is measured from the first positive peak to negative peak in microvolts. Most laboratories have their own normal values for major motor and sensory nerves with minor differences occurring among laboratories. A lower temperature will prolong distal latencies, reduce conduction velocities, and increase the amplitude of CMAP and SNAP. Age also affects NCVs. Adult values are not attained until 4 years of age, and they decline after age 60 years at a rate of 1 to 2 m/s per decade. Waveform analysis of CMAP and SNAP helps estimate normal vs. abnormal nerve function (Fig. 7-1). The amplitude of a response should be similar when the same nerve is stimulated proximally and distally.

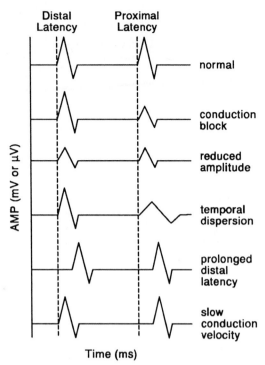

FIGURE 7-1. Schematic representation of normal and pathological findings obtained from a NCV study.

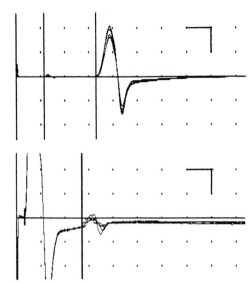

FIGURE 7-2. H reflex with tibial nerve stimulation (top); time marker 10 ms; amplitude marker 5 mV. F response with median nerve stimulation (bottom); time marker 10 ms; amplitude marker 1 mV.

A greater than 20% to 50% reduction between distal and proximal stimulation of a motor nerve suggests an abnormal block in conduction between two stimulation points. Many laboratories are now computerized and the area under an action potential curve can be calculated. Greater than 20% to 40% reduction in area also suggests conduction block. A significant reduction in amplitude from proximal to distal stimulation sites without a reduction in area under the response curve, and a significant increase in duration (>15%) suggest temporal dispersion resulting from a relative desynchronization of the components of an action potential which is due to different rates of conduction of each nerve fiber. This also suggests nerve pathology between the proximal and distal stimulation sites.

The H reflex is the electrophysiological equivalent of a muscle stretch reflex. A sensory nerve is stimulated with submaximal intensity, and a late motor response is recorded owing to reflex activation of motor neurons. In adults, H reflexes are easily obtained from soleus muscle and less easily from flexor carpi radialis muscle following the stimulation of tibial and median nerves, respectively. The tibial H reflex is useful in identifying S1 radiculopathy.

F waves are late responses recorded from muscle after supramaximal stimulation of a motor nerve. F waves represent a response to a stimulus that travels first to and then from the cord via motor pathways. Thus F waves are useful in studying the proximal portion of motor nerves (Fig. 7-2). Unfortunately there is no consensus as to methodology for obtaining responses, and to the patterns of abnormality to be identified.

Repetitive nerve stimulation (RNS) studies are used primarily for evaluation of neuromuscular junction disorders like myasthenia gravis. As such they are not usually useful in the evaluation of pain and therefore will not be discussed further.

The electrical activity in a muscle can be measured using disposable needle electrodes. Needle examination is performed in proper steps. An examiner observes activity on insertion of a needle (insertion activity), activity when the needle is maintained in a relaxed muscle (spontaneous activity), and activity during varying degrees of voluntary muscle contraction. The electrical activity is evaluated by sight and sound, as specific activities have specific waveforms and characteristic sounds. Observations are made by the electromyographer during the study; therefore, the results of a needle examination are dependent on the experience of the examiner.

Insertion activity, also referred to as injury potential, is caused by movement of the needle electrode, resulting in mechanical damage to the muscle fibers. Increased insertion activity consists of unsustained fibrillation potentials and positive sharp waves. A muscle at rest should be electrically silent. Spontaneous activity in a resting muscle usually suggests a pathologic condition. The type and significance of various spontaneous activities are summarized in Table 7-1, and some examples are shown in Fig. 7-3.

As a muscle contracts motor unit action potentials (MUAPs) are observed. MUAP represents the summation of muscle fiber action potentials of a given motor unit. With increasing voluntary muscle contraction, individual motor units fire more frequently, and more motor units are recruited to fire. The term onset frequency is used to describe the firing rate of a single MUAP maintained at the lowest voluntary muscle contraction (normally less than 10 Hz). Recruitment frequency is defined as the frequency of first MUAP when second MUAP is recruited (normally less than 15 Hz). Reduced number of MUAP (high recruitment frequency) can be seen in neuropathic processes. Increased number of MUAP (low recruitment frequency), however, can be seen in myopathic disorder or defect of neuromuscular junction. During maximum contraction, a full interference pattern consisting of overlapping motor units is seen. MUAPs are analyzed in terms of amplitude, duration, number of phases, and stability. The morphology of the MUAPs is affected by the type of needle

TABLE 7-1. **POTENTIALS RECORDED IN THE MUSCLE AT REST**

Spontaneous Activity	Firing Pattern	Frequency	Waveform	Amplitude	Duration	Significance
Complex repetitive discharge	Regular, abrupt onset and cessation, "motor cycle idling"	5–100 Hz	Polyphasic or serrated, MFAP	100 μV–1 mV		Neurogenic (chronic), myopathic (dystrophy)
Cramp discharge	Increase and subside gradually	(1) <150 Hz; (2) 4–15 Hz	MUAP			(1) Ischemic, ↑Na, (2) ↓Ca, ↓Mg, ↑K
End plate noise	Dense and steady, "sea shell hissing"	>150 Hz	Monophasic (negative), MEPP	10–20 μV	0.5–1 ms	Normal
End plate spike	Irregular short burst, "sputtering fat in a frying pan"	50–100 Hz	Biphasic (negative–positive), MFAP	100–300 μV	2–4 ms	Decrease in denervated muscle, increase in reinnervated muscle
Fasciculation potential	Spontaneous, sporadic, "typing on cardboard"	0.1–10 Hz	MUAP			Normal, neurogenic (motor neuronopathy), myopathic
Fibrillation potential	Regular, "rain on a tin roof", "ticking of clock"	1–50 Hz	Biphasic (positive–negative), MFAP	<1 mV	<5 ms	Neurogenic, NMJ defect, myopathic
Myokymic discharge	Semi-regular, "marching soldiers"	(1) 2–60 Hz brief; (2) 1–5 Hz continuous	MUAP			Neurogenic (chronic, radiation), face (MS, brainstem tumor, Bell's palsy)
Myotonic discharge	Wax and wane, "dive bomber"	20–80 Hz	(1) Biphasic (positive–negative); (2) positive	(1) <1 mV; (2) <1 mV	(1) <5 ms; (2) 5–20 ms	Myopathic (myotonic syndromes)
Neuromyotonic discharge	Start and stop abruptly, wane, "pinging"	150–300 Hz	MUAP			Isaac's syndrome, stiff-man syndrome, tetany
Positive sharp wave	Regular	1–50 Hz	Biphasic (positive–negative), MFAP	<1 mV	10–100 ms	Same as fibrillation

MFAP, muscle fiber action potential; MUAP, motor unit action potential; MEPP, miniature endplate potential; NMJ, neuromuscular junction.

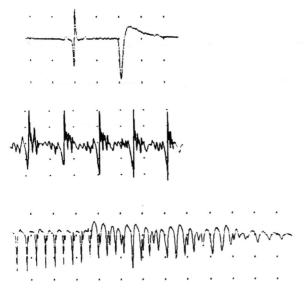

FIGURE 7-3. Spontaneous activities. Fibrillation potential and positive wave (top), and complex repetitive discharges (middle); time marker 10 ms, amplitude marker 100 μV. Myotonic discharges (bottom); time marker 20 ms, amplitude marker 200 μV.

electrode used, location of the needle within the motor unit territory, age, temperature, and specific muscle being examined. Large, long-duration polyphasic units suggest denervation and re-innervation. Short-duration, small polyphasic units can be seen in myopathic processes. EMG findings in neuropathic and myopathic disorder are summarized in Table 7-2.

While performing an EMG/NCV study several questions must be answered by the examiner,[2] as discussed in the following.

Where is the Lesion? (Localization): EMG/NCV is very useful in localizing the specific anatomical site of a lesion that is causing pain. For example, a complaint of burning feet can be caused by a diffuse peripheral neuropathy (as in diabetes), by a plexus injury after surgery, or by a lumbosacral radiculopathy due to spinal stenosis. Each of these has different

findings and can be localized by EMG/NCV. In general, changes in conduction, either a prolonged distal latency or a slow velocity, suggest a pathologic lesion between the site of stimulation and the recording site. Abnormally small amplitude, however, can occur from an injury anywhere distal to the motor or sensory neuron. A sampling on needle examination of muscles representing different nerves and roots can further localize the site of injury. Using the example of burning feet, let us examine the differential diagnosis and its EMG/NCV findings. In radiculopathy, motor conduction velocity would be normal, and CMAP amplitude would be reduced if there were axonal degeneration from nerve root compromise. SNAP would be normal because the lesion is proximal to the dorsal root ganglion. (Note that most radiculopathies occur within the spinal canal. The dorsal root ganglion is located in the neuroforamina distal to most radicular pathologic lesions. The dorsal root ganglion is a bipolar neuron with one axon extending distally to limb and one extending proximally to the spinal cord.) EMG abnormalities first appear in appropriate paraspinal muscles, because of their proximity to the injury site. Abnormalities are next seen in the proximal and then distal muscles within the specific myotomal distribution of the injured nerve root. In a plexus injury both CMAP and SNAP amplitudes would be decreased if axons were injured. NCV is usually normal unless stimulation is applied proximal to the lesion. Paraspinal muscles are spared because posterior rami innervate these muscles while the plexus is in the anterior rami distribution. Combined motor and sensory NCV abnormalities are characteristic of most peripheral neuropathies. Needle findings would depend on the severity of motor nerve involvement, and these are usually normal unless the neuropathy is severe. Anatomic localization based on EMG/NCV is summarized in Table 7-3.

Is the Lesion Axonal or Demyelinating? (Pathophysiology): Based on the EMG/NCV findings, the distinction can be made with relative ease. If an injury occurs at the cell body or axon, axonal degeneration results. If an injury is directed against the myelin, demyelination ensues. In the majority of peripheral neuropathy both demyelination and axonal injury will occur; however, characterizing the primary

TABLE 7-2. EMG FINDINGS IN NEUROGENIC AND MYOPATHIC DISORDERS

EMG	Normal	Neurogenic (axonal)	NMJ Defect	Myopathic
Insertional activity	N	↑	↑	↑
Spontaneous activity	–	+	+	+
MUAP amplitude	0.1–5 mV	↑	↓	↓
Duration	3–15 ms	↑	↓	↓
Phase	<5	↑	↑	↑
Stability	N	N	Variable	N
Recruitment	N	↓	N	↑

MUAP, motor unit action potential; NMJ, neuromuscular junction; N, normal.

TABLE 7-3. **ANATOMICAL LOCALIZATION BASED ON THE EMG AND NCV STUDIES**

Lesion	Motor Nerve Conduction	Sensory Nerve Conduction	RNS	EMG
Dorsal root ganglia (sensory neuronopathy)	N	N, ↓ amp	N	N
Anterior horn cell (motor neuronopathy)	N, ↓ amp	N	N/Abn	Abn
Root (radiculopathy)	N, ↓ amp	N	N	Abn
Plexus (plexopathy)	N, ↓ amp	N, ↓ amp	N	Abn
Nerve (neuropathy)	Abn	Abn	N	Abn
NMJ defect	N, ↓ amp	N	Abn	Abn
Muscle (myopathy)	N, ↓ amp	N	N/Abn	Abn

RNS, repetitive nerve stimulation; NMJ, neuromuscular junction; N, normal; Abn, abnormal.

pathological process is important to establish an etiology and to assess the extent of injury. Demyelinating neuropathies can be further divided into segmental (acquired) and uniform (hereditary) types. In the former nonuniform slowing in individual myelinated nerve fibers results in conduction block and temporal dispersion. In the latter prolonged latency and slowing of conduction predominate as a result of uniform involvement of all myelinated fibers. Table 7-4 summarizes the EMG/NCV characteristics of demyelinating and axonal injuries.

Is the Lesion Motor, Sensory, or Autonomic? (Fiber Type Specificity): NCV tests motor and sensory components separately. Many peripheral nervous system diseases affect both motor and sensory nerves. In a case of distal sensory or motor neuropathies amplitudes as well as velocities are abnormal. With a dorsal root ganglia lesion or anterior horn cell disease, NCV studies show small-amplitude SNAP or CMAP, respectively, and as a rule normal velocity. Routine EMG/NCV studies do not test the integrity of the autonomic nervous system. Autonomic tests are discussed separately.

Is the Lesion Focal, Multifocal, or Diffuse? (Distribution): By determining the distribution of abnormalities, neuropathy, for example, can be further divided into mononeuropathy, multifocal neuropathy, and polyneuropathy. A focal lesion such as carpal tunnel syndrome will result in abnormalities limited to the distal segment of a median nerve. If the same nerve is affected disproportionately in the opposite

TABLE 7-4. **NCV AND EMG CHARACTERISTICS OF THE DEMYELINATING AND AXONAL INJURIES**

	NCV	EMG
Demyelination	1. Prolonged latency, more than 13% of normal 2. Slow NCV, less than 70% of normal 3 Conduction block 4. Temporal dispersion	1. Normal insertional activity, no spontaneous activity 2. Reduced recruitment with conduction block 3. Normal MUAP morphology
Axonal injury	1. Normal latency 2. Slow NCV, more than 70% of normal 3. Small CMAP/SNAP amplitude	1. Increased insertional activity, spontaneous activity 2. Reduced recruitment 3. Large amplitude, long-duration polyphasics with reinnervation 4. Satellite potentials

CMAP, compound muscle action potential; SNAP, sensory nerve action potential; MUAP, motor unit action potential.

TABLE 7-5. CHRONOLOGY OF THE NCV AND EMG FINDINGS FOLLOWING AXONAL INJURY

	NCV	EMG
0–1 week	↓ amp, proximal	↓ recruitment
1–2 weeks	↓ amp, proximal and distal	↓ recruitment, ↑insertional activity
2–3 weeks	↓ amp, proximal and distal	↓ recruitment, ↑ fibrillation potentials
1–3 months	↑ amp	↓ fibrillation potentials, ↓ amp, ↑ duration, ↑ phase
3–6 months	↑ amp	↑ recruitment, ↑ amp, ↑ duration, ↑ phase

limb or one nerve is affected more than the other in the same limb, a multifocal disorder is suggested. In a fully developed polyneuropathy motor and sensory nerves in both upper and lower extremities are affected in equal and symmetrical fashion; in milder cases, however, the abnormalities will be more significant in distal sensory nerves of the lower extremities.

How Old is the Injury? (Chronicity): Following an axonal injury, the nerve distal to the lesion undergoes wallerian degeneration. For the first 2 to 3 days motor conductions distal to a lesion will be normal. Then CMAP amplitude drops progressively, reaching a nadir at about 7 days. SNAP amplitudes distal to a lesion are unaffected for 5 to 6 days but by day 10 to 11 the nadir is reached. After an axonal motor nerve injury, EMG findings will change slowly. Initially, insertional activity is increased. Positive sharp waves and fibrillation potentials may not occur for 2 to 3 weeks following a nerve injury, depending on the length between site of nerve injury and corresponding muscles. The abnormal spontaneous activity can resolve in 3 to 6 months. Therefore, needle studies performed less than 2 to 3 weeks after injury, or later than 3 to 6 months after injury, may be normal. Large-amplitude, long-duration polyphasic MUAPs seen in denervation and re-innervation develop 3 to 6 months after an injury. Table 7-5 summarizes the chronology of EMG/NCV findings after axonal injury.

How Bad is the Injury? (Severity and Prognosis): The severity of an injury can be determined if EMG/NCV is done in a timely manner. The amplitude difference between the same nerve on affected and unaffected sides gives an idea of extent of injury and potential recovery if they are determined sequentially. A paucity of spontaneous activity in affected muscles 3 weeks after injury indicates an excellent outcome for the return of muscle function. Markedly reduced recruitment of MUAPs indicates severe lesion except for neurapraxia. In general, axonal injury has a worse prognosis than demyelinating disorders.

QUANTITATIVE SENSORY TESTING (QST)

The test provides a quantitative measure to detect large and small fiber dysfunction. Various stimuli at varying intensities are applied to the skin and a patient is asked to indicate when he or she begins to feel the stimulus. A consensus report defines "sensory detection threshold" as "the smallest stimulus that can be detected at least 50% of the time."[3] By increasing and decreasing stimulus intensity from the predetermined level, "appearance" and "disappearance" thresholds can be determined. Sensory modalities commonly used are vibration and thermal senses: warm, cold, heat pain, and cold pain (Fig. 7-4). Vibration threshold measures large myelinated fiber function, whereas warm, heat pain, and cold pain thresholds reflect the function of unmyelinated C-fibers. Cold threshold measures small myelinated Aδ fiber function.

QST measures not only peripheral nerve fiber function but also central pathway function. Vibratory sense is carried by the dorsal columns and thermal senses via the spinothalamic tract. Normal values depend on methodology, sensory modality tested, and site of test. Sensory detection threshold increases with age; therefore results should be compared with the age-matched reference values.

QST can be used to detect subtle sensory changes that may be missed by NCV study. Increased or decreased thermal detection threshold (hypoesthesia or hyperesthesia) and thermal pain threshold (hypoalgesia or hyperalgesia) have been reported in many painful neuropathies. Cold or heat hyperalgesia is

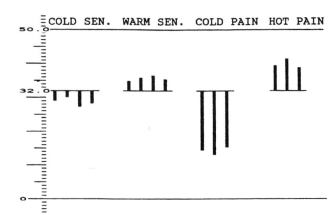

FIGURE 7-4. Example of a thermal QST in a normal subject. Temperature, in degrees centigrade, on vertical scale. Solid bar represents each trial. Sen, sensation.

a feature of reflex sympathetic dystrophy. Heat hyperalgesia is common in erythromeralgia, and angry backfiring C nociceptor (or ABC) syndrome. Cold hypoesthesia, cold hyperalgesia, and cold limb are features of the CCC syndrome, whereas thermal hypoesthesia and hyperalgesia (anesthesia dolorosa) are typical manifestations of postherpetic neuralgia.

QST allows early detection of disease. Sequential testing can be used to monitor disease progression and therapeutic efficacy. However QST is not objective and relies on patient cooperation. QST does not localize a lesion, as it tests the integrity of the entire sensory pathway from nerve ending to cortex.

SHORT LATENCY SOMATOSENSOSRY EVOKED POTENTIALS (SSEPS)

Conventional sensory NCV studies assess a lesion distal to the dorsal root ganglion. SSEPs provide a quantitative measure to study the entire sensory pathway. Typically, a mixed nerve, such as median nerve at the wrist or tibial nerve at the ankle, is repeatedly stimulated and responses are recorded along the sensory pathway. Those responses are averaged to improve signal-to-noise ratio.[4] Stimulations of the skin within a dermatome or cutaneous nerve, such as superficial radial or sural nerve, have more limited value because of the low-amplitude response. Submaximal intensity and longer duration of stimulus are required to elicit an optimal response.

Stimulations are mediated by group Ia and II sensory afferents, dorsal root ganglion (neuron I), dorsal columns, gracilis and cuneatus nuclei (neuron II), contralateral medial lemniscus, ventroposterolateral nucleus of the thalamus (neuron III), and sensory cortex. Clinically, touch–pressure, position–movement senses are affected with the injury to the dorsal column pathway in both the central and peripheral nervous system. Each identifiable component is labeled according to its polarity (negative or positive) and its mean peak latency (in milliseconds) following stimulation. Useful obligate potentials after median nerve

stimulation include EP (Erb's point), N13 (dorsal column of the cervical cord), P14 (caudal medial lemniscus), N18 (thalamus), and N20 (sensory cortex). Identifiable potentials after tibial nerve stimulation are PF (popliteal fossa), LP (lumbar potential), P31 (caudal medial lemniscus), N34 (thalamus), and P37 (sensory cortex) (Fig. 7-5). Knowledge of the generator source of these peaks allows one to localize lesions to parts of the pathway. Age, temperature, limb length, medications, level of attention, and sleep may alter latency and amplitude. Therefore, every laboratory has its own normal values. Adult norms are reached at about 8 years of age. Criteria for abnormality include absence of any obligate waves and prolongation of interpeak intervals. For example, absence of N18 and N20 or a prolonged P14–N20 interval suggests a lesion between the medulla and sensory cortex. Table 7-6 summarizes some typical SSEP findings and resulting localization. Absolute latency is a less reliable indicator of abnormality because it varies with limb length. A side-to-side amplitude ratio less than half is considered abnormal by some. Application of SSEPs for a patient with pain is limited to the identification of a potential structural or compressive lesion involving peripheral or central sensory pathway.

LASER EVOKED POTENTIALS (LEPS)

A carbon dioxide laser can be used to generate pain-related cerebral potentials.[5] Laser stimulation produces heat quickly and activates $A\delta$ and C fibers. Late component, which occurs at approximately 500 ms following stimulation of the hand, corresponds to $A\delta$ fiber conduction, and ultra-late component at 1500 ms corresponds to C fiber; both components are maximum in amplitude at the vertex (CZ). LEP is a noninvasive test and no tissue damage has been reported. LEPs provide an objective measure to assess the function of pain pathway in patients with neuropathic pain. LEP is not yet available in most electrophysiology laboratories.

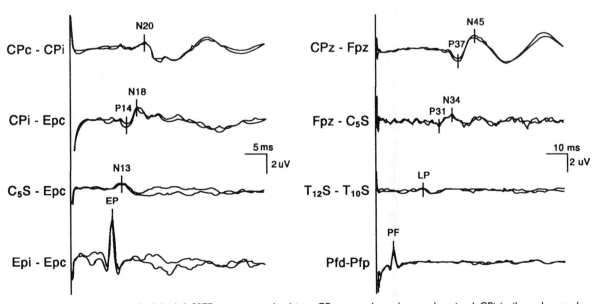

FIGURE 7-5. Median (left) and tibial (right) SSEPs in a normal subject. CPc, contralateral central-parietal; CPi, ipsilateral central-parietal; EPc, contralateral Erb's point; EPi, ipsilateral Erb's point; CS, cervical spine; CPz, midline central-parietal; Fpz, midline frontopolar; TS, thoracic spine; Pfd, popliteal fossa, distal; Pfp, popliteal fossa, proximal; EP, Erb's potential; LP, lumbar potential; PF, popliteal fossa.

TABLE 7-6. TYPICAL SSEP FINDINGS AND RESULTING LOCALIZATION

SSEPs	Abnormality	Lesion
Median nerve	1. Absent EP, P14, N20 2. Prolonged EP–P14, P14–N20	Median nerve–brachial plexus; above plexus; above medulla Brachial plexus–medulla; medulla–sensory cortex
Tibial nerve	1. Absent LP, P37 2. Prolonged LP–P37	Tibial nerve–cauda equina; above lumbar spinal cord Spinal cord–sensory cortex

EP, Erb's potential; LP, lumbar potential.

SYMPATHETIC SKIN RESPONSE (SSR)

The first report of the galvanic skin response appeared in 1890. Since then various terminologies have been introduced on the basis of different stimulating and recording methods (e.g., electrodermal activity, sympathetic skin response, peripheral autonomic surface potential, and psychogalvanic reflex). A standard method of obtaining SSR is to place a recording electrode on the palmar and plantar surface, because these recording sites yield higher amplitudes. A stimulator is placed on either the median or the tibial nerve of the opposite limb, and the stimulus is given randomly at a rate of less than one per minute, and with a stimulus intensity that is sufficient to cause mild pain. A minimum of 5 to 10 responses should be recorded, and SSR responses are obtainable 60% to 100% of the time in normal subjects. Waveforms are usually triphasic, with an initial small negativity followed by a large positive wave, and a subsequent prolonged negative wave (Fig. 7-6). Waveforms can also be monophasic or diphasic with an initial negative or positive peak. Maximal peak-to-peak amplitudes and mean latencies are measured. Amplitude and latency variability can be minimized by reducing stimulus frequency, increasing stimulus intensity, and/or changing stimulus site or mode.

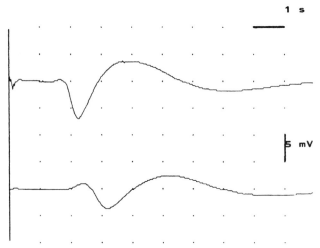

FIGURE 7-6. Normal sympathetic skin response (SSR) recorded simultaneously from the palm of the hand (top) and sole of the foot (bottom) by electrical stimulation.

Low skin temperature, low level of attention, medication (especially anticholinergics), age, and habituation will also attenuate the response. Normal amplitude is more than 1 mV for hand, and more than 0.2 mV for foot. Mean palmar latency is 1.4 ± 0.1 seconds and plantar latency is 1.9 ± 0.1 seconds. SSR measures change of epidermal resistance due to sweat gland activity. The somatic afferent limb depends on the stimulus type (electrical shock, loud noise, visual threat, deep breathing); with the electrical stimulation, the afferent limb occurs via large myelinated fibers. The efferent limb is a sympathetic pathway, originating in the posterior hypothalamus, descending through the spinal cord to the intermediolateral cell column (T1 to L2), and paravertebral ganglia and then to the sweat gland via small unmyelinated fibers. Therefore, it is important to note that neuropathy affecting large myelinated fibers exhibits abnormal SSR when electrical stimulation is used.

Low-amplitude or absent response indicates abnormal sympathetic reflex arc, and the lesion can be central or peripheral, preganglionic or postganglionic. A side-to-side amplitude difference of more than 50% is considered to be abnormal by some. In studies of diabetic, uremic, and amyloid neuropathies the results of SSR correlated well with autonomic symptoms. As a rule, SSR is abnormal in axonal neuropathies. An exception is the demyelinating neuropathy with prominent autonomic features, such as Guillain–Barré syndrome. Some studies have reported abnormal SSR test results in patients with CRPS/RSD and others have not.[6] Immediately following the sympathetic nerve block or sympathectomy, SSR is absent or reduced in amplitude. The SSR is usually normal in entrapment neuropathy and radiculopathy. SSR evoked by magnetic stimulation in the neck bypasses the afferent limb and directly stimulates postganglionic fibers. This method has less of a propensity to habituate and therefore less fluctuation of amplitude and latency occurs .[7]

QUANTITATIVE SUDOMOTOR AXON REFLEX TEST (QSART) AND RESTING SWEAT OUTPUT (RSO) TEST

This is a sensitive, reproducible, and quantitative method to test sudomotor function. A multicompartment plastic "sweat cell" is tightly secured to the skin. The outer compartment is filled with acetylcholine solution, and nitrogen gas flows constantly to an inner compartment through an instrument that measures the change of humidity (sudorometer). A direct current is applied

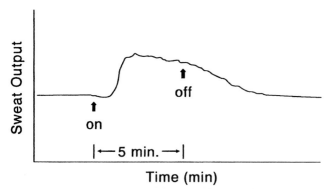

FIGURE 7-7. Example of a normal quantitative sudomotor axon reflex test (QSART). On, off, stimulator on and off.

and the water content in the inner compartment is continuously measured before, during, and after the stimulus. The basis of the test is that the axon terminal of the sweat gland under the outer compartment is activated by acetylcholine iontophoresis; the impulse travels centripetally to a branch point and then distally to the axon terminal under the inner compartment where acetylcholine is released and a sweating response results. Use of the term "axon reflex" should be discouraged because only the postganglionic sympathetic sudomotor axon is considered to be involved in this setup. With a latency of 1 to 2 minutes after the induction of the stimulus, sweat output increases rapidly while stimulation continues; then the stimulator is turned off, and sweat output returns to its prestimulus baseline within 5 minutes (Fig. 7-7). The area under the curve represents the total amount of sweat output expressed in microliters per square centimeter, and the normal value varies depending on the site of testing, gender, and age of the subject. Distal limbs and male and younger subjects tend to sweat more. Reduced or absent response indicates postganglionic disorder. Normal response does not rule out preganglionic involvement. Excessive and persistent sweating is also considered abnormal. Comparison is made between the two limbs, and an asymmetry of more than 25% is considered to be abnormal.

RSO test is basically similar to the QSART; a capsule with one chamber is attached to the skin, and the rate of water evaporation is continuously recorded for 5 minutes. The presence of RSO indicates that the sweat gland is spontaneously activated by the sympathetic fibers.

In a patient with painful diabetic neuropathy RSO studies show the presence of increased sweat activity and QSART exhibits short latency, excessive, and persistent sweat patterns, which is evidence of sympathetic overactivity.[8] A recent study seems to indicate that sweat test abnormalities correlate well with the symptoms of CRPS/RSD-related pain,[9] for which the pathophysiologic mechanism of those is uncertain; perhaps a lower firing threshold, or an increased firing frequency due to denervation hypersensitivity of the sudomotor axons may produce excitation of the sweat glands. Recently, an FDA-approved Q-Sweat device became available. This device uses dry air instead of nitrogen gas to measure water content.

KEY POINTS

- Electrophysiological studies are a very sensitive indicator of central and peripheral nervous system involvement but do not indicate underlying disease.
- EMG/NCV studies can identify the anatomic site of injury, the type of neurons or fibers involved, the nature of the pathologic alteration, and severity of injury.
- In QST cold threshold measures Aδ fiber function, whereas warm, heat pain, and cold pain thresholds reflect the function of C fibers.
- SSEPs provide a quantitative measure to study the entire sensory pathway, mediated by Ia and II sensory afferents.
- LEPs, by using a carbon dioxide laser, measure the function of Aδ and C fibers.
- SSR and QSART have a limited role but useful for the evaluation of painful diabetic neuropathy or CRPS/RSD.

REFERENCES

1. AAEE glossary of terms in electrodiagnostic medicine. Muscle Nerve 10(Suppl):S1–S50, 2001.
2. Guidelines in electrodiagnostic medicine. Muscle Nerve 22(Suppl):S1–S300, 1999.
3. Quantitative sensory testing: A consensus report from the Peripheral Neuropathy Association. Neurology 43:1050–1052, 1993.
4. Guidelines on evoked potentials. J Clin Neurophysiol 11:40–73, 1994.
5. Kakigi R, Shibasaki H, Ikeda A: Pain-related somatosensory evoked potentials following CO_2 laser stimulation in man. Electroencephalogr Clin Neurophysiol 74:139–146, 1989.
6. Rommel O, Tegenthoff M, Peru U, et al: Sympathetic skin response in patients with reflex sympathetic dystrophy. Clin Auton Res 5:205–210, 1995.
7. Uozumi T, Nakano S, Matsunaga K, et al: Sudomotor potential evoked by magnetic stimulation of the neck. Neurology 43:1397–1400, 1993.
8. Low PA (ed): Laboratory evaluation of autonomic failure. *In* Clinical Autonomic Disorders: Evaluation and Management. Little Brown, Boston, 1992.
9. Chelimsky TC, Low PA, Naessens JM, et al: Value of autonomic testing in reflex sympathetic dystrophy. Mayo Clin Proc 70:1029–1040, 1995.

Anatomy, Imaging, and Common Pain-Generating Degenerative Pathologies of the Spine

Matthew T. Walker, M.D.,

Eric Spitzer, M.D.,

Murugusundaram Veeramani, M.D., and

Eric J. Russell, M.D.

ANATOMY

Osseous Spinal Column: The spinal column is comprised of 7 cervical, 12 thoracic, 5 lumbar, and 5 fused sacral segments. The terminal portion of the osseous spinal column, the coccygeal segments, varies in number, but typically 4 segments can be visualized. The morphology of the individual vertebrae is quite consistent throughout, with the exception of the first two cervical segments (C1 and C2) and the sacrococcygeal levels.

The C1 level, commonly referred to as the atlas, is comprised of an anterior arch, posterior arch, and paired lateral masses (Fig. 8-1A). The lateral masses articulate with the occipital condyles superiorly and the body of C2 inferiorly (Fig. 8-1B). C1 does not have a vertebral body nor is it separated from adjacent levels by an intervertebral disc. The C2 vertebra, commonly referred to as the axis, has some of the typical features of the remainder of the vertebral segments but is unique in having a superior extension of bone from the vertebral body which articulates with the dorsal margin of the anterior arch of C1: this bony projection is called the odontoid process or dens and allows for head rotation (Fig. 8-1B). Unique to the segments from C3 through C7 are the uncinate processes that arise from the dorsolateral margins of the superior endplates of the vertebral bodies and articulate with the level above (Fig. 8-2).[1]

The typical cervical, thoracic, and lumbar vertebrae consist of an anterior body, paired pedicles, articular pillars and laminae, and a single dorsal midline spinous process (Fig. 8-3). The pedicles attach the body to the posterior neural elements. The articular pillars are comprised of the pars interarticularis and the superior and inferior articular processes. Each level from C3 to L5 has superior and inferior articular processes that serve as the main posterior contact between adjacent levels. The surface of the superior articular process is the inferior facet of the associated zygapophyseal joint, and the surface of the inferior articular process is the superior facet of the joint. The "superior processes" at C1 and C2 and the "inferior process" at C1 are more descriptively referred to as articular surfaces as they do not have a true morphological extension away from the vertebral segments. The two laminae extend dorsomedially and connect to form the root of the spinous process. The spinous process projects dorsally and serves as an attachment point for the posterior ligamentous structures. The pedicles, articular pillars, and lamina serve to enclose and protect the spinal canal and contents particularly the spinal cord and nerve roots. Transverse processes vary in size from short in the cervical spine to long in the lumbar spine. In the mid-cervical spine the transverse processes help to enclose and form the osseous transverse foramina which transmit the vertebral artery and contents.

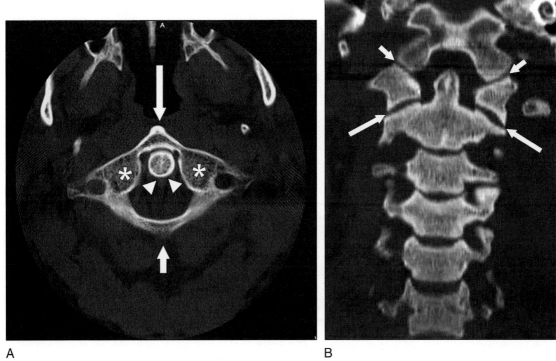

A   B

FIGURE 8-1. (A) Axial CT image through the atlas shows the anterior arch (long arrow), posterior arch (short arrow) and paired lateral masses (asterisks). The tip of the odontoid process (arrowheads) articulates with the anterior arch of C1. (B) Coronal CT reconstruction through the cervical spine demonstrates the articulations between the occipital condyles and the lateral masses of C1 (atlanto-occipital joints, small arrows). Also note the atlantoaxial joints (long arrows) between the lateral masses of C1 and the body of C2.

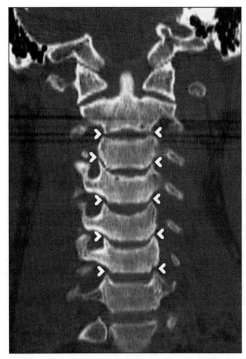

FIGURE 8-2. Coronal CT reconstruction through the cervical spine profiles the uncinate processes and uncovertebral joints (arrowheads).

In the thoracic and lumbar spine the transverse processes serve as anchoring points for the muscles that help to stabilize and protect the spinal column and its contents.

Joints: Six specific types of synovial joints exist from the skull base to the lumbosacral junction including the atlanto-occipital, atlantoaxial, uncovertebral, costovertebral, costotransverse, and zygoapophyseal (facet) joints.[2] The atlanto-occipital joint is formed by the bilateral superiorly convex occipital condyles and the bilateral concave superior articular surfaces of the C1 lateral masses (Fig. 8-1B). The main atlantoaxial joint is formed by the inferior articular surfaces of C1 and the superior articular surfaces of C2 (Fig. 8-1B). A true synovial-lined joint also exists between the ventral dens and the dorsal surface of the C1 anterior arch, and the dorsal aspect of the dens and the posterior ligamentous structures. The uncovertebral joints (joints of Luschka) exist only in the cervical spine below C2. The osseous uncinate processes arise from the dorsolateral margin of the superior endplates of the C3–C7 vertebral bodies and articulate with the level above: uncovertebral joints therefore exist from C2–3 to C6–7 (Fig. 8-2). The joints of Luschka have features of both cartilaginous and synovial joints and when degenerated can result in foraminal stenosis and even central stenosis.[1,3] As their names imply, the costovertebral and costotransverse joints are articulations between the ribs (costo-) and the vertbral bodies or transverse processes of the thoracic spine (Fig. 8-4).

The facet joints are the most prevalent joint in the spinal column and are formed by the inferior and superior articular

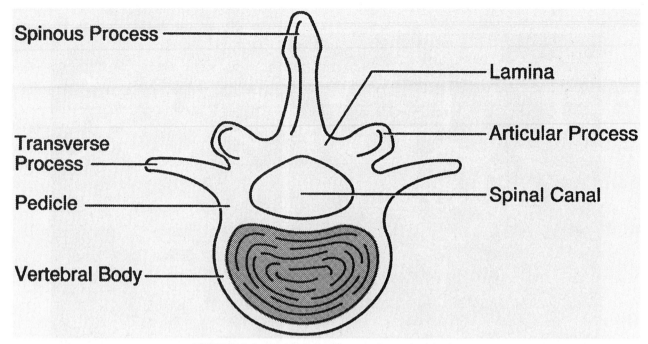

FIGURE 8-3. Axial diagram of a typical vertebral body.

processes of adjacent vertebral bodies. The facet surfaces (named relative to the joint space as described below) are covered with articular cartilage which allows for bending motion and offers some protection to shearing forces. The joints are encapsulated by a true synovial lining and loose capsular ligaments.[4] In the cervical spine, there is a thick fibrous capsule laterally under which a small synovial recess may protrude. In the lumbar spine, a thick fibrous capsule is present along the posterior margin of the facet joint. The inferior synovial recess occurs at the caudal extent of this capsule and is the common location for access to the joint space.[5,6] A complete discussion of the innervation of the facet joints is beyond the scope of this chapter. Generally speaking, the facet joints are dually innervated from paired medial branches of the dorsal primary rami.[7,8] This dual innervation explains why complete denervation of a symptomatic facet joint requires treatment of both medial branches. Knowledge of the different facet joint orientations is important when planning facet joint interventions. The cervical facet joints are obliquely oriented from superior to posterior with a ventral to dorsal angle when viewed in the sagittal plane (Fig. 8-5A). The thoracic facet joints are oriented in the coronal plane limiting access for percutaneous procedures (Fig. 8-5B). The lumbar facet joints have a lunate configuration with the posterior margin oriented in the oblique sagittal plane and the anterior margin oriented in the oblique coronal plane (Fig. 8-5C). Access to the joint under fluoroscopy is accomplished from a shallow oblique sagittal projection.[9]

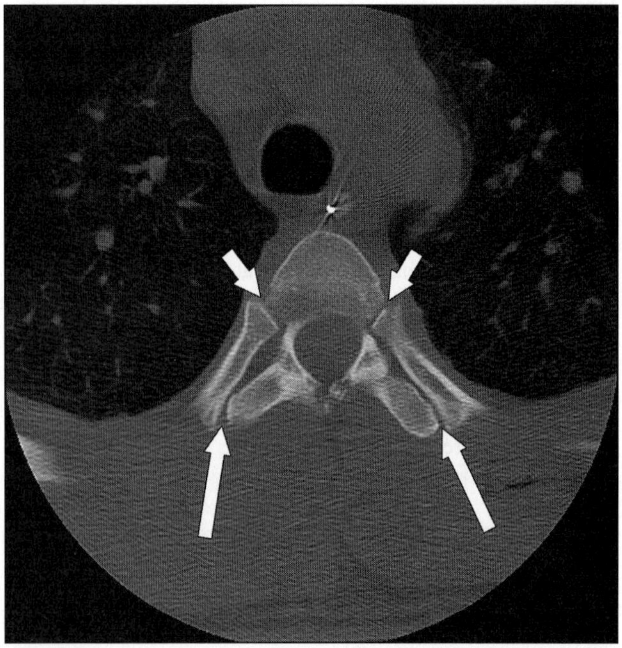

Transverse Foramen, Intervertebral Foramen, and Nerve Roots: The transverse foramen, also known as the vertebral foramen or foramen transversarium, occurs in the cervical spine from C1 to C7. The transverse foramina develop when the neural processes posteriorly fuse with the vestigial costal element anteriorly.[10,11] The contents of the transverse foramina include the vertebral artery, vertebral venous plexus, fibers of the sympathetic chain, and fat. Typically round or oval, these foramina vary in size and shape and often reflect the underlying size of the traversing vertebral artery.[12] The vertebral artery typically enters the foramen at C6, but can enter as high as C3. In the sagittal projection, the vertebral artery is a few millimeters ventral to the adjacent exiting nerve root (Fig. 8-6).

In the cervical spine, the intervertebral foramen runs obliquely anterolaterally. It is bounded by the pedicles, uncinate

FIGURE 8-4. Axial CT image through the mid-thoracic spine identifies the costotransverse (long arrows) and costovertebral joints (short arrows).

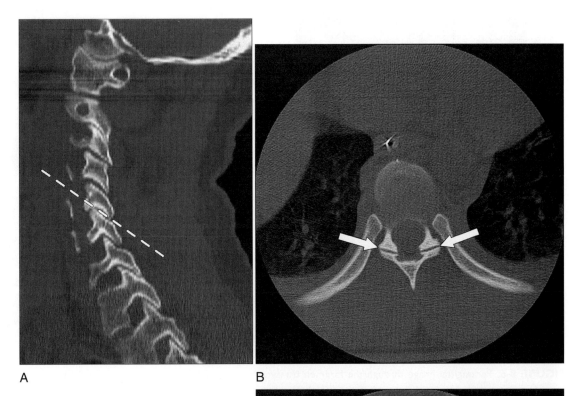

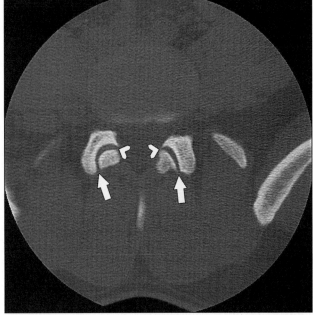

FIGURE 8-5. (A) Sagittal CT reconstruction of the cervical spine. Note the oblique orientation of the cervical facet joints (dashed line). There are several approaches to the cervical facets including anterolateral, direct lateral, and posterolateral obliquities. (B) Axial CT image through the mid-thoracic spine. The facet joints (short arrows) are oriented in the oblique coronal plane. Safe and reliable access to these joints is best achieved under CT guidance. (C) Axial CT image through the mid-lumbar spine. Note the lunate configuration of these facet joints. With the patient in the prone position, a shallow oblique projection will profile the dorsal margin (arrows) of the joint space thus allowing safe access to the joint. A steeper oblique projection will profile the ventral component (arrowheads) of the joint space but access to the joint will be impeded by the intervening articular process.

process, vertebral body, and superior articular facet. The exiting cervical nerves are positioned posteroinferiorly in the intervertebral foramina (Fig. 8-6). Small veins connecting the epidural venous plexus and the anterior longitudinal intraspinal venous channel with the perivertebral venous plexus within the transverse foramina traverse the intervertebral foramen (Fig. 8-7).[13] There are eight paired cervical nerve roots, the first exiting the spinal canal between the skull base and C1. Therefore, in the cervical spine, the number of the nerve root passing through the foramen is one greater than the number of the pedicle that it passes beneath. For example, the nerve root passing through the intervertebral foramen at C3–4 is the C4 nerve root.

The thoracic spine intervertebral foramina are rather constant bounded by the pedicles, vertebral body, disc, and superior articular process of the vertebra below. The thoracic spinal nerves are more closely associated with the superiorly positioned articular process compared to the cervical spine. Small veins run through the intervertebral foramina as in the cervical spine. The exiting nerve roots are designated by the pedicle under which they immediately course. For example, at the T8–9 level, the T8 spinal nerve root exits.

Much like the thoracic spine, the lumbar spine intervertebral foramina are bounded by the pedicles, vertebral body, disc, and superior articular process. The spinal nerve roots exit

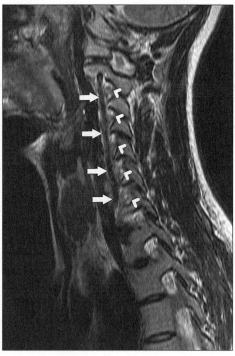

FIGURE 8-6. Parasagittal image through the foramen transversaria. The linear dark flow void (arrows) is the vertebral artery. Note the position of the vertebral artery immediately ventral to the exiting spinal nerve roots (arrowheads).

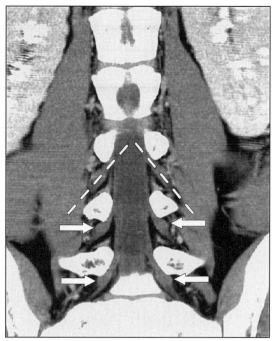

FIGURE 8-8. Coronal CT reconstruction after contrast administration. Note the orientation of the exiting lumbar nerve roots (dashed lines) relative to the spinal canal and intervertebral foramina. Enhancement of the dorsal root ganglia (arrows) is evident.

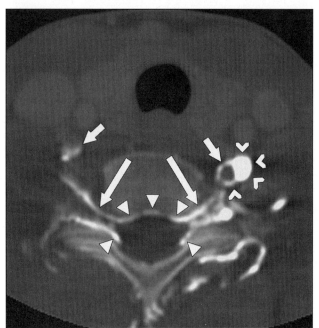

FIGURE 8-7. Axial CT image through the lower cervical spine. Contrast was administered for a neck CT but, as commonly occurs, some contrast filled the venous system in a retrograde fashion. The venous connection between the epidural space (closed arrowheads) and the perivertebral venous plexus (open arrowheads) via branches through the intervertebral foramina (long arrows) are well seen. The vertebral arteries (short arrows), not yet within the vertebral foramina, are encircled with venous opacification particularly on the left.

at a 45° angle inferolaterally and are closely associated with the medial and inferior margins of the pedicle under which they exit (Fig. 8-8). The spinal nerve roots are numbered as in the thoracic spine; the numbered root exits below the same numbered pedicle. For example, at the L4–5 level, the L4 spinal nerve exits.

Throughout the spine, the exiting nerve roots are comprised of a smaller, ventral motor root and a larger, dorsal sensory root. The dorsal root contains a ganglion which can range in size from 5 to 15 mm.[14] This dorsal root ganglion (DRG) occurs in the intervertebral foramen and is most apparent in the lumbar and sacral spine. Small arterial branches from the lumbar arteries supply the DRG and have a fenestrated capillary endothelium. This anatomic configuration results in normal enhancement of the DRG on contrast examinations (Figs. 8-8 and 8-9).[15]

When contemplating a transforaminal or periganglionic intervention in the thoracolumbar region, one must consider the potential complication resulting from damage to the artery of the lumbar enlargement (artery of Adamkiewicz). This artery is the primary supply to the lower two-thirds of the spinal cord and enters the spinal canal via an intervertebral foramen. Although it typically enters on the left from T9–L1, the artery of Adamkiewicz can enter on either side from T5–L4. The artery usually runs in the more superior and ventral aspect of the foramen (Fig. 8-10).[16]

Intervertebral Discs: Intervertebral discs separate the vertebral bodies and contribute a significant proportion (20% to 35%) of the height to the spinal column. The discs are thicker in the cervical and lumbar regions and thicker anteriorly than posteriorly contributing to the lordotic curvatures of the spine

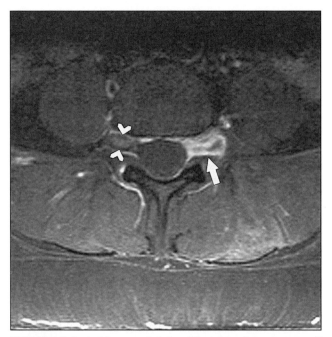

FIGURE 8-9. Axial postgadolinium T1-weighted fat-suppressed MR image. In the left foramen, the oval peripherally enhancing lesion (arrow) is a sequestered disc fragment. In the right foramen, normal enhancement of the dorsal root ganglion (arrowheads) is identified.

in these regions. The primary function of the disc is to absorb the impact of daily axial loading and confer some flexibility. Discs are composed of three main components: the nucleus pulposus, annulus fibrosis, and the cartilaginous endplate.[17,18] The nucleus pulposus contains type II collagen, hyaluronic acid, and glycosaminoglycans. This composition confers excellent compressive resistance and, when hydrated, has characteristic imaging findings on magnetic resonance imaging (MRI). The annulus fibrosis consists of an outer dense circumferential fibrous band and an inner fibrocartilagenous layer. The outer layer fibers, also known as Sharpey's fibers, insert into the ring apophyses. The cartilaginous endplate is composed of hyaline cartilage which tightly adheres to the vertebral endplate. Vascular supply to the disc is primarily via small nutrient channels through this cartilaginous endplate.[19,20]

Ligaments: Ligaments of the spine provide stability while allowing flexion, extension, and rotation. There are five main ligamentous structures seen throughout the spinal column: anterior longitudinal ligament (ALL), posterior longitudinal ligament (PLL), ligamentum flavum, interspinous ligaments, and the supraspinous ligament. The ALL and PLL run along the anterior and posterior margins of the vertebral bodies, respectively (Fig. 8-11).[21] The ALL adheres to the vertebral body and intervertebral discs. The PLL adheres to the annulus fibrosis of the disc but does not contact the posterior vertebral margin to any significant degree. The ligamentum flavum runs along the length of the spinal canal extending between adjacent laminar segments and defining the dorsolateral margins of the spinal canal. The interspinous ligaments run between adjacent spinous processes whereas the supraspinous ligament runs along the tips of the spinous processes.

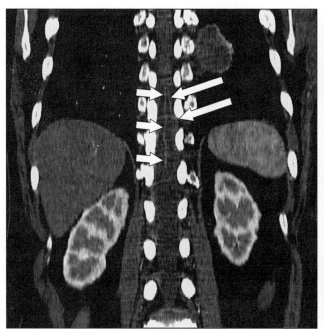

A

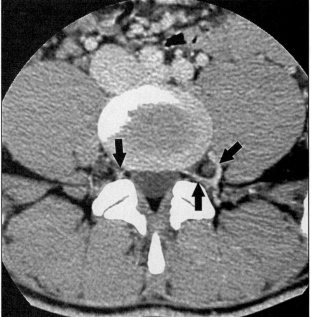

B

FIGURE 8-10. (A) Coronal CT reconstruction of a contrast-enhanced aorta study. The high-density linear structure on the surface of the spinal cord is the anterior spinal artery (short arrow). The artery of Adamkiewicz (long arrows) enters the spinal canal through the left T10–11 intervertebral foramen. (B) Axial CT image postcontrast through the mid-lumbar spine demonstrates typical venous structures (arrows) within and lateral to the intervertebral foramen.

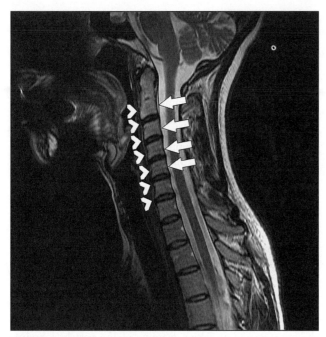

FIGURE 8-11. Sagittal T2-weighted image through the cervical spine. The thin linear hypointense signal paralleling the ventral margins of the vertebral bodies and discs represents the ALL (arrowheads). The PLL (arrows) has a similar appearance but runs along the dorsal margin of the intervertebral discs.

Specialized ligaments are present at the craniocervical junction including the atlanto-occipital ligament, apical ligament, tectorial membrane, and the cruciate ligaments which form the transverse ligament.[22] These ligaments provide stability and flexibility at the craniocervical junction. Further discussion of these ligaments is beyond the scope of this chapter.

IMAGING OVERVIEW

Conventional Radiographs (X-Rays): Conventional or plain radiographs record differential attenuation of the X-ray beam by tissues based on their differential densities. For example, cortical bone is very dense and completely attenuates the beam. The heart is soft tissue and partially attenuates the beam and the lung is mostly air thus attenuating very little of the beam. Conventional radiographs are quick, inexpensive, easy to perform, and have excellent spatial resolution. Important information about the spine can be obtained with conventional radiographs including alignment, structure, and mineralization. Dynamic, weightbearing upright flexion and extension views can reveal a stable or unstable spine in chronic and acute scenarios. This is the only modality to date that routinely achieves that type of stress-related imaging. Osseous foraminal stenosis and spondylolysis can be diagnosed with oblique projections. Vertebral fractures and joint dislocations can be detected although acuity can be difficult to discern. Although conventional radiographs are less optimal than computed tomography (CT) for soft tissue evaluation, degenerative changes of the disc can be identified such as disc dehydration (air in disc) and disc collapse.

Standard frontal (including odontoid view when imaging the cervical spine) and lateral projections are the minimum required for adequate evaluation (Figs. 8-12A–C, 13A,B, 14A–C). In the cervical and lumbar regions, oblique projections are helpful in evaluating the facet joints, articular processes, and intervertebral foramina (Figs. 8-12D,E, 14D,E). When spondylolisthesis or spondylolysis is present, flexion and extension views aid in demonstration of abnormal motion. Flexion and extension views may be supplemented by direct real-time observation using flouroscopy.

Plain films can detect changes related to systemic diseases such as ankylosing spondylitis and diffuse sclerotic/lytic states (Fig. 8-15). Also, there is no good substitute for plain radiographs to evaluate overall alignment abnormalities in patients with extensive kyphoscoliotic deformities.

Conventional radiography is the easiest and most cost-effective method of assessing alignment and structure of the spine in both traumatic and nontraumatic conditions. On lateral projection, three longitudinal curves may be used to evaluate alignment of the vertebrae (Fig. 8-16). The anterior and posterior spinal lines trace the course of the anterior and posterior longitudinal ligaments, respectively. The spinolaminar line traces the course of the ligamentum flavum along the deep surface of the laminae. On frontal projection, a vertical line drawn through the tips of the spinous processes serves as a reference for evaluation of lateral curvature (Fig. 8-17). The relationship of this line and the pedicles will demonstrate rotational malalignment.

Plain radiographs can easily depict hardware failure such as fractures. Even known hardware fractures can be difficult to detect with CT due to beam-hardening artifact which can obscure large portions of the images.

Myelography and Postmyelography CT Scan: Myelography is the radiographic technique utilized to evaluate the contents of the spinal canal by the introduction of a nonionic, water-soluble, radiographically dense iodinated contrast material into the spinal subarachnoid space. This contrast material outlines the spinal cord and nerve roots, which appear as filling defects in the radiodense contrast column on conventional radiographs. Extradural indentations into the contrast column are observed and generally represent disc abnormalities, ligament thickening, or hypertrophic facet degenerative changes. Spinal stenosis can be diagnosed and nerve root impingement can be detected. Redundant thickened nerve roots and arachnoiditis can also be demonstrated (Fig. 8-18). Myelography should always be followed by a postmyelography CT scan to provide better definition of anatomic relationships of the contents of the spinal canal to the surrounding structures.

The use of myelography has decreased significantly due to the invasive nature of the procedure and the availability of other noninvasive imaging tools including CT and MRI which provide excellent spatial and contrast resolution. The risks of myelography are directly related to the lumbar puncture (LP) and injection including positional headache, contrast-related seizure, and infection. The most common of these complications is the post-LP positional headache.[23] If this headache does not respond to conservative therapy, an epidural blood patch can be performed for more definitive treatment.[24] Seizures related to intrathecal contrast administration are uncommon but the seizure threshold does decrease with certain medications including numerous anti-depressants.[25] In general, patients should be screened for specific medications and rescheduled if they are found to be on any seizure threshold-reducing medications. Myelography is now used mainly as

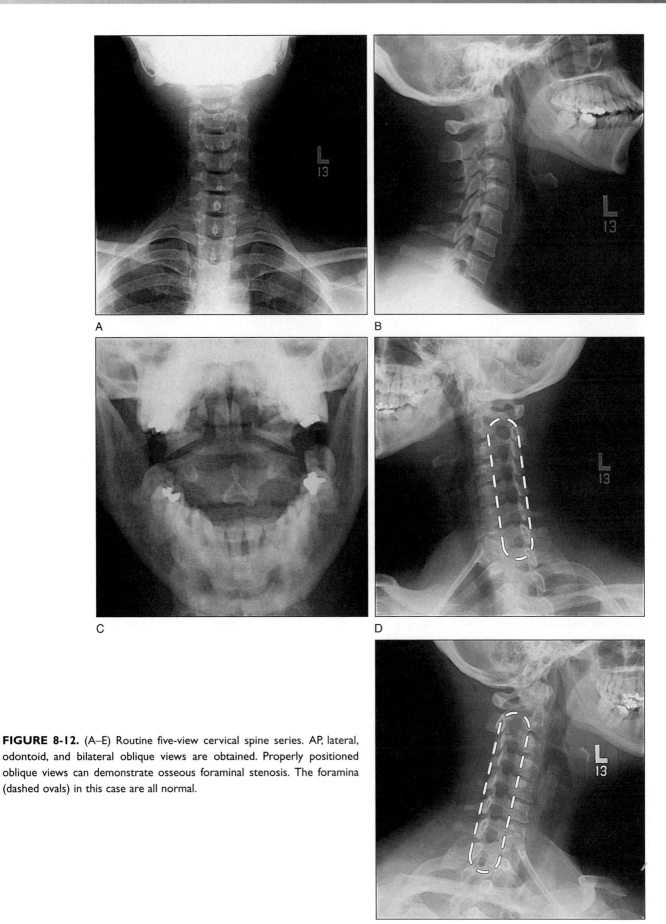

FIGURE 8-12. (A–E) Routine five-view cervical spine series. AP, lateral, odontoid, and bilateral oblique views are obtained. Properly positioned oblique views can demonstrate osseous foraminal stenosis. The foramina (dashed ovals) in this case are all normal.

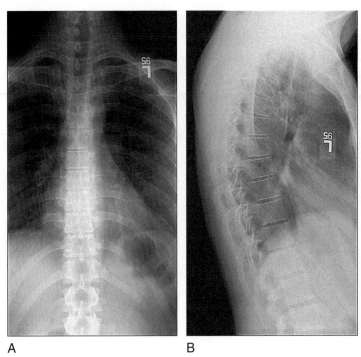

FIGURE 8-13. (A, B) Standard images of the thoracic spine include an AP and lateral view.

a problem-solving tool when CT or MRI examination cannot be performed due to contraindications, are equivocal, or are limited due to artifacts from surgical hardware.

Computer-Assisted Tomography (CAT or CT Scan): CT is an X-ray technique that is considerably more sensitive to the differential attenuation of the X-ray beam than plain film radiography. CT provides the best possible definition of osseous structures and has excellent spatial resolution. The newest generation of CT scanners employ slip-ring technology (helical acquisition), multidetector systems, high-speed rotation, and dynamic table translation to image optimally the spine. Dose-reduction software now changes the patient dose "on the fly": the current (mA) and therefore the dose changes in response to the thickness of the individual patient at each slice. Overlapping data sets can be acquired which allow for multiplanar reformatting and three-dimensional data sets can be acquired for volumetric analysis or volume rendering applications.

As with conventional radiographs, CT imaging is based upon differential attenuation of the X-ray beam but can differentiate not only bone from soft tissue but also between different densities of bone and soft tissue structures. Differences in radiographic density of ligament, disc material, and cerebrospinal fluid (CSF) make identification of disc herniations and ligamentous disorders possible using CT (Fig. 8-19). Subtle areas of bone sclerosis or lysis can easily be displayed with CT. Windowing techniques used in the display of CT images allow optimal viewing of image data, depending on the tissue type of interest. The administration of intravenous iodinated contrast material may be valuable in certain circumstances to highlight vascular structures, such as the epidural venous plexus or adjacent arteries.

Artifacts from metallic surgical implants, such as spinal rods, transpedicular screws, laminar wires/hooks, and intervertebral/vertebral body cages can severely limit the diagnostic value of CT images. In these cases, conventional radiographs and myelography may prove to be the best diagnostic imaging modalities. Even this limitation will improve as CT scanners evolve from 4 slices to 16 slices and beyond. The radiation dose from CT can be several times that of plain radiography depending on technique and protocols. Hence appropriate care should be exercised in using it in the more sensitive populations including children, pregnant females, and other young adults.

Magnetic Resonance Imaging (MRI): MRI uses gradient fields and radiofrequency waves to localize and characterize tissues based on the amount and state of the ubiquitously present hydrogen atoms (protons). There is no ionizing radiation employed with MRI, but there are risks including those related to electrical and metal implants and an unknown/unquantified risk to the fetus.[26–30] The very good soft tissue contrast resolution afforded by MRI combined with its multiplanar tomographic capability make it the most versatile and useful diagnostic imaging modality for spinal disorders. It provides a wide field of view with excellent definition of tissue types, such as bone marrow, muscle, ligament, disc material, and nerve roots. MRI allows precise definition of extradural, intradural extramedullary, and intramedullary pathology. Evaluation of medullary bone with MRI is excellent, and many osseous conditions resulting in marrow edema or marrow replacement (e.g., metastatic disease) are well demonstrated. However, demonstration of dense cortical bone, sclerotic lesions, and osteophytes is less precise than by CT.

Standard MRI protocols usually include sagittal and axial images with T1- and T2-weighted sequences. T1 weighting provides excellent anatomical delineation. Generally speaking, high signal intensity on T1 represents fat (such as in fatty bone marrow, subcutaneous fat) whereas low signal intensity represents fluid (such as CSF, bone marrow edema, normal nucleus

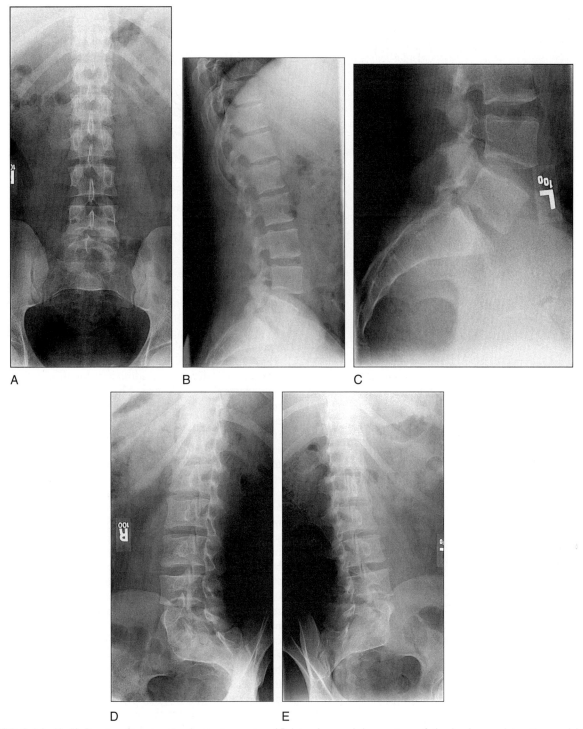

A   B   C

D   E

FIGURE 8-14. (A–E) Routine five-view lumbar spine series. AP, lateral, coned-down view of the lumbosacral junction and bilateral oblique views.

pulposus) (Fig. 8-20A). T2 weighting makes fat-containing structures less bright than on T1 and makes fluid-containing structures hyperintense (bright) (Fig. 8-20B). Soft tissue structures such as muscles and spinal cord have intermediate signal intensities on T1 and T2 sequences. The STIR (short-tau inversion recovery) sequence is a fat suppressed, T2-weighted sequence that is extremely sensitive to minute amounts of fluid (Fig. 8-20C). This sequence is particularly useful in detecting edema as can be seen with traumatic injury, malignancy, and infection.[31] Gradient recalled echo (GRE) T2-weighted imaging is exquisitely sensitive to blood products and calcium and is particularly useful in the setting of spine trauma for evaluating the spinal cord (Fig. 8-20D).[32,33] When evaluating scoliosis, coronal T1- or T2-weighted imaging may be added to better assess the extent of curvature (Fig. 20E).

In the cervical spine, thin-section axial two- or three-dimensional GRE T2 images are utilized to further evaluate central canal and intervertebral foraminal stenosis. The degree

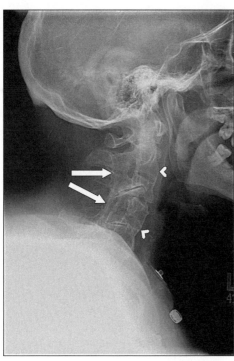

FIGURE 8-15. In this single lateral cervical spine film, the findings consistent with ankylosing spondylitis are easily identified including facet joint ankylosis (arrows) and vertebral body fusion (arrowheads).

of stenosis produced by osteophytes may be exaggerated on the GRE T2 sequence because of the sensitivity to susceptibility artifacts. Proton density (intermediate T2) and T2-weighted axial images are utilized in the lumbar region. Whether using a GRE T2 axial image in the cervical spine or a spin echo

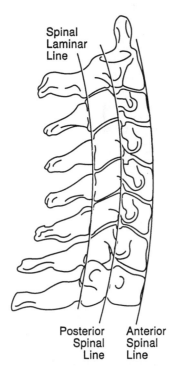

FIGURE 8-16. Lateral diagram of the cervical spine demonstrating the spinal laminar, posterior spinal, and anterior spinal lines.

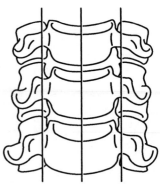

FIGURE 8-17. Frontal diagram of the cervical spine showing normal alignment of the spinous processes.

T2-weighted axial image in the thoracic or lumbar spine, the effect is the same: a "myelographic" effect is produced with hyperintense CSF within the thecal sac surrounding the intermediate signal intensity of the spinal cord and nerve roots (Fig. 8-21).

When evaluating for infection, multiple sclerosis, intramedullary neoplasm, metastatic disease, or postoperative scarring, sagittal and axial T1-weighted images prior to and following the intravenous administration of gadolinium contrast material are indicated. The addition of fat-suppression techniques can further highlight areas of pathological enhancement especially in the bone marrow. The combination of contrast administration and fat suppression will increase diagnostic sensitivity in cases of osteomyelitis/discitis, epidural abscess or tumor, meningitis, leptomeningeal carcinomatosis, and perineural scarring (Fig. 8-22).

Unfortunately, some patients cannot be examined using MRI. The most common problem encountered is claustrophobia. This is often overcome by light/moderate sedation but sometimes requires the services of the anesthesiology department. Another alternative is the "open-magnet" MRI systems but the trade-off is lower field strength and therefore poorer spatial resolution, less signal-to-noise, and fewer sequence options.[34] Strict contraindications for MRI relate to the very strong magnetic field required for imaging. Patients with cardiac pacemakers, metallic foreign bodies, and specific metallic surgical implants cannot be evaluated using MRI. Cardiac pacemakers may be disabled or reprogrammed or their leads repositioned by the magnetic field. Metallic foreign bodies or surgical implants, such as cerebral aneurysm clips and heart valves, may be displaced by the magnetic field with catastrophic outcomes. Comprehensive references are available to determine which implants are safe to be placed into the magnetic field.[35] Metallic implants may also create severe artifact and distort the images significantly, rendering them nondiagnostic.

DEGENERATIVE DISC DISEASE

Overview: Discogenic pain refers to back pain arising from the disc itself. Degenerative disc disease is a pathologic process, not entirely related to aging, of uncertain etiology that may cause acute or chronic low back pain.[36,37] The conventional radiographic findings in degenerative disc disease include disc space narrowing, vacuum disc, endplate sclerosis, and osteophyte formation (Fig. 8-23A).[38,39] CT scans will identify these same changes but earlier in the course of degeneration (Fig. 8-23B). Due to its excellent soft tissue contrast and multi-planar capabilities, MRI is the modality of choice to evaluate disc degeneration and much effort has been placed into correlating MRI findings with potentially symptomatic levels. In the right hands, a provocative test, discography, can be used to correlate clinical symptoms with the MRI appearance. Although each finding of degenerative disc disease will be discussed separately, the imaging findings are most often seen together when degenerative disc disease is present.

Disc Dehydration and Narrowing: With T1 weighting, the distinction between hydrated and nonhydrated disc is unapparent and therefore the disc appears homogeneous (Fig. 8-24A). The water content of the intervertebral disc is responsible for the bright signal on T2-weighted MRI (Fig. 8-24B).[40] The tightly packed annular fibers represent the dark T2 signal surrounding the centrally bright nucleus pulposus. Disc hydration and therefore T2 disc signal normally decreases with age but should remain brighter than the signal of bone marrow on T2-weighted sequences. The pathologic process of degenerative

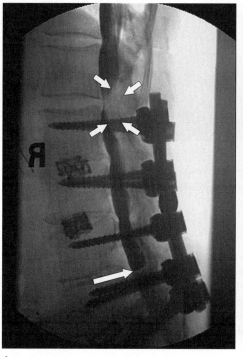

A

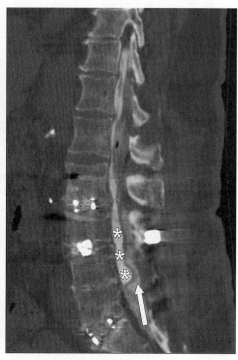

B

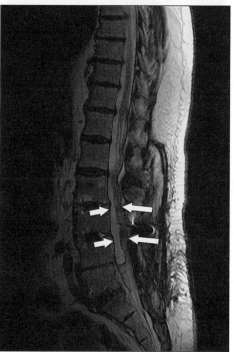

C

FIGURE 8-18. (A) This lateral lumbar spine film was obtained after routine myelography. The patient has undergone posterolateral fusion from L2–S1. A waist of contrast column attenuation (short arrows) is seen at L1–2 indicating ligamentum flavum thickening. At the L4–5 level, the intrathecal contrast is compartmentalized (long arrow) suggesting arachnoiditis. (B) Sagittal CT reconstruction demonstrates a dense ventral subarachnoid collection of contrast (asterisks) and a less dense collection dorsally (arrow). This appearance is consistent with arachnoiditis. (C) Sagittal T2-weighted MRI identifies the dorsal position of the nerve roots (long arrows) in the thecal sac and the compartmentalization of the CSF spaces (short arrows).

(Continued)

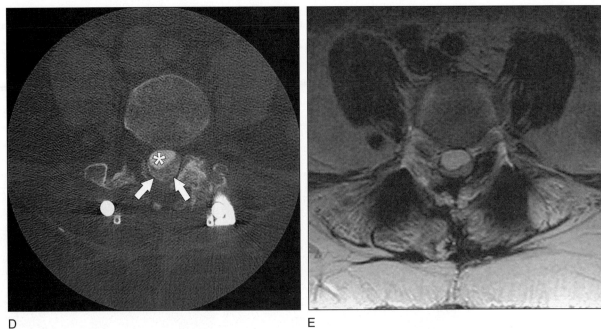

D   E

FIGURE 8-18. *cont'd* (D) This axial CT myelographic image shows clumping and peripheral displacement of the spinal nerve roots (arrows) with ventral accumulation of contrast (asterisk). (E) Axial T2-weighted MRI was obtained at the same level as the CT image and demonstrates the same findings.

disease results in accelerated disc desiccation, which results in a more significant decrease in disc signal, the most severe end of the spectrum of which is complete loss of the signal (Fig. 8-23B–D). Degenerated discs occasionally demonstrate an accumulation of intradiscal gas (nitrogen) which can be detected on plain film, CT, and MRI.[41] On MRI, this "vacuum

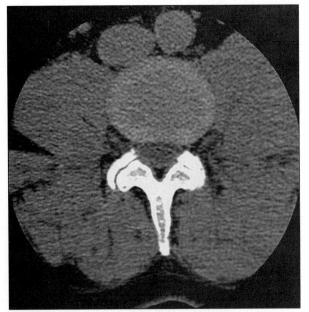

FIGURE 8-19. CT images represent differential attenuation of the x-ray beam by the bones and soft tissues. Fat is low density and is hypodense on CT. CSF is less dense than the ligamentum flavum which are similar in density to the disc and muscles. Cortical bone is generally the densest endogenous structure.

disc phenomenon" is typically hypointense on T1- and T2-weighted sequences due to lack of protons. Inexplicably, vacuum discs occasionally fill with fluid and can demonstrate high signal intensity on T2-weighted sequences.

Disc height is interpreted relative to other intervertebral levels in the same patient. Individual disc heights can be categorized as either normal or as mildly, moderately, or severely diminished based on percentage loss of disc height compared to a normal level. In a study comparing the disc heights of young versus middle-aged males, it was found that young, healthy males had narrower disc heights compared with middle-aged men.[42] Taken alone, therefore, disc height is not used as an indicator of disc degeneration. The main importance of loss of disc space height is the concomitant decrease in size of the intervertebral foramina and the related potential for nerve root compression.

Annular Fissure/Tears: In 1992 Aprill and Bogduk reported a high intensity zone within the midline posterior annulus, discontinuous with the central high signal nucleus pulposus, as a strong predictor of positive discography in patients with low back pain.[43] The linear hyperintense signal on T2-weighted images in the posterior or posterolateral disc represents radial and concentric fissuring of the annular fibers extending from the nucleus to the outer one-third of the annulus.[44] An element of inflammation (granulation tissue) is also thought to contribute to the high intensity zone based on enhancement on postcontrast T1-weighted images. Annular degeneration can be divided into three types including concentric fissuring, transverse tears, and radial tears.[45] Concentric fissuring occurs due to collagen fiber delamination of the annulus fibrosis with deposition of mucoid material.[45,46] This fissuring is high-signal intensity on T2-weighted sequences and parallels

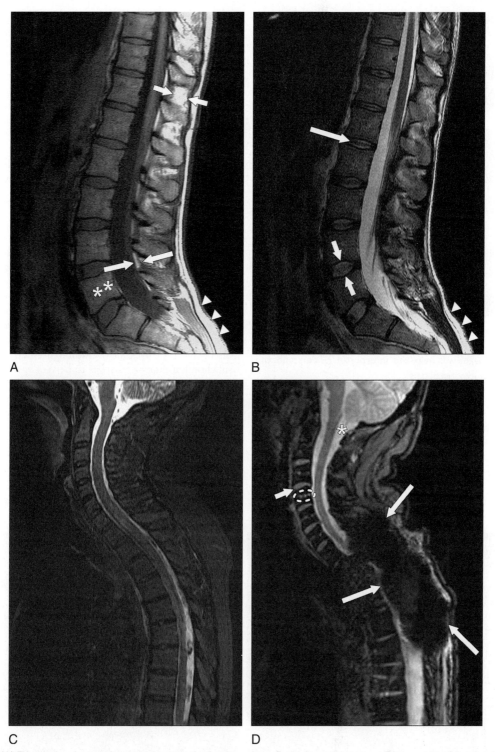

FIGURE 8-20. (A) T1-weighted sagittal image through the lumbar spine. Fat is hyperintense on T1 images and is seen in the subcutaneous soft tissues (arrowheads), interspinous regions (short arrows), epidural space (long arrows), and bone marrow (asterisks). The intervertebral discs are mildly hypointense relative to the vertebral marrow. The CSF is hypointense relative to all but cortical bone. (B) T2-weighted sagittal image. In this sequence, the CSF is the most hyperintense (white) structure. Fat remains hyperintense (arrowheads) but is less bright than on the T1-weighted sequence. Note the high signal intensity within the intervertebral discs indicating normal disc hydration (short arrows). A small, normal hypointense intranuclear cleft is visible in many discs including at L1–2. (C) The STIR sequence is a T2-weighted sequence with a fat-suppression technique. The CSF remains hyperintense but the fat has "dropped out" and is now hypointense. Edema is easily depicted in the vertebral bodies or soft tissues using this sequence. (D) The GRE sequence is a fast T2-weighted sequence that is particularly susceptible to inhomogenities in the magnetic field as are produced by blood, calcium, and metal. In this image the discs (short arrow), CSF (asterisk), and basivertebral plexi (dashed oval) are hyperintense whereas the bone and fascial planes are hypointense. Blooming (long arrows) is seen dorsal to C7–T5 due to metallic surgical hardware.   *(Continued)*

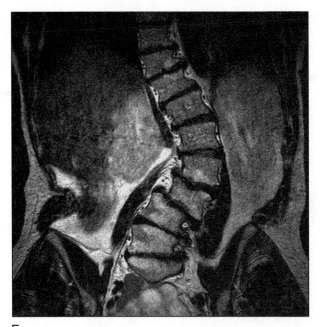

E

FIGURE 8-20. cont'd (E) Any coronal acquisition, in this case a T2-weighted image, will help the interpreter understand the curves involved in kyphoscoliosis.

the margins of the disc (Fig. 8-25). Transverse tears are small foci of T2 hyperintensity at the junction of Sharpey's fibers with the vertebral body ring apophyses.[45,46] Both concentric fissuring and transverse tears may imply disc degeneration but are not generally symptomatic. Radial tears are full-thickness disruptions of the annulus and represent primary failure of the annulus (Fig. 8-26).[46] The lateral and posterior margins of the

outer third of the annulus fibrosis and the PLL are richly innervated by nociceptive nerve endings and therefore disruption is felt to be a source of discogenic back pain.[47] It is this particular feature that supports the notion that radial tears can produce pain whereas transverse tears and concentric fissures should not.

Subchondral Marrow Changes: Degenerative disease in the vertebral end plates, referred to as Modic-type changes, are classified into three types based on signal characteristics of T1- and T2-weighted signal characteristics.[48] Type I changes refer to low signal in the vertebral end plates on T1- and increased signal on T2-weighted images, representing vascularized marrow (Fig. 8-27A,B). Enhancement of Modic changes, particularly type 1, is not uncommon (Fig. 8-27C).

Type II changes show increased signal intensity on T1- and increased signal or isointensity on T2-weighted images, representing fatty replacement of the bone marrow (Fig. 8-28). Type III changes consist of low signal on both T1- and T2-weighted sequences due to subchondral sclerosis (Fig. 8-29).

It has been suggested that subchondral marrow changes represent chemical inflammation in the vertebral end plates that is a reaction to the diffusion of toxic substances from a degenerated disc.[49,50] Modic changes, therefore, could be a secondary sign of discogenic low back pain. Although Braithwaite et al found subchondral marrow changes to be very specific, low sensitivity limits the value of Modic changes in detecting the source of a patient's low back pain.[51] One investigator found no relationship between Modic changes and provocative discography.[52]

DISC HERNIATION

Overview: In an attempt to standardize the reporting of normal and pathologic conditions of the lumbar spine, the North American Spine Society (NASS), the American Society of

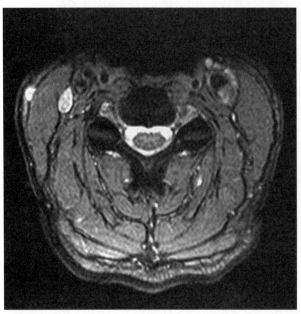

A

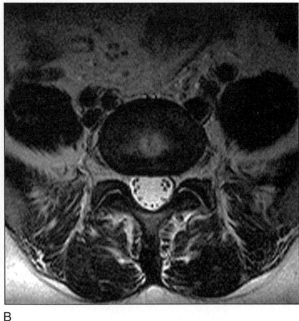

B

FIGURE 8-21. (A) In the cervical spine, the "myelographic effect" is achieved with a T2-weighted GRE sequence. This sequence is less susceptible to pulsation artifact but very sensitive to susceptibility artifact. The latter property can lead to overestimation of foraminal or canal stenosis from osteophytes. (B) In the lumbar spine, CSF pulsation is dampened and typically not an issue. A conventional or fast spin echo T2-weighted technique is utilized to achieve the "myelographic effect."

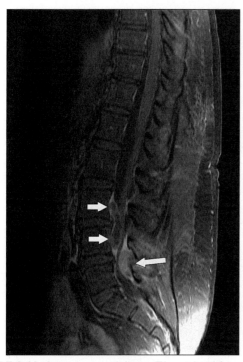

FIGURE 8-22. Sagittal postgadolinium T1-weighted fat saturated image. Inflammatory processes are easily identified such as the large ventral (short arrows) and dorsal (long arrow) epidural abscess seen here.

Neuroradiology (ASNR), and the American Society of Spine Radiology (ASSR) put their efforts together and created recommendations that provide a common nomenclature to promote uniform descriptions of pathological processes affecting the discs.[53]

Due to its superior soft tissue resolution, MRI is the imaging modality of choice to evaluate disc herniations. CT is also useful, but is typically relegated to use as a secondary study either to better delineate bony abnormalities or for patients who cannot undergo or tolerate an MRI examination. Myelography can be added when contraindications preclude the use of MRI and plain CT is inadequate to define the clinical problem.

Disc Contour: Disc herniation has been defined as a localized displacement of disc material beyond the limits of the intervertebral disc space. A "circumferential bulge" describes disc material bulging out beyond 50% to 100% of the edges of the vertebral body's ring apophysis and is not considered a disc herniation. Localized herniated disc material, i.e., disc extending beyond the endplate margin less than 50% of the disc circumference, can be termed "focal" (less than 25%) or "broad-based" (25% to 50%). A focal disc herniation can also occur into adjacent vertebral endplates, commonly referred to as a Schmorl's node (Fig. 8-30).

The terms protrusion and extrusion describe disc herniations based on the shape of the herniated disc fragment and its relationship to the parent disc margin. A protrusion describes a localized disc herniation that has its base wider than the furthest extent of the apex of herniated disc material (Fig. 8-31A). An extruded disc is defined by the presence of a herniated disc fragment which is larger in diameter at any point away from

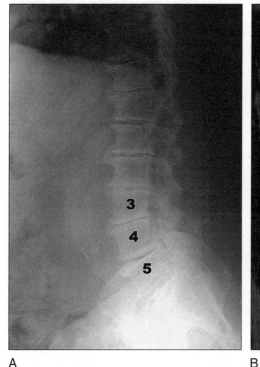

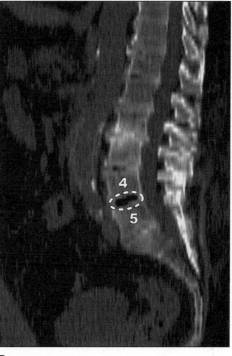

A   B

FIGURE 8-23. (A) The conventional radiographic findings of disc degenerative changes are seen here including loss of disc space height, vacuum disc phenomenon, end plate sclerosis, and osteophyte formation. (B) This sagittal reconstruction from an abdominal CT scan easily depicts the same changes. A vacuum disc is particularly well seen at L4–5 (dashed oval).

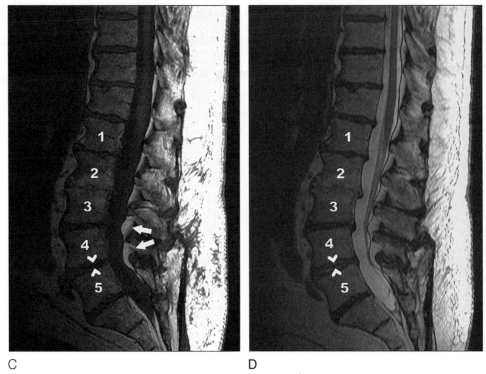

FIGURE 8-23. *cont'd* (C) Sagittal T1-weighted image in the same patient shows classic degenerative changes. The vacuum disc at L4–5 is hypointense (arrowheads). The dorsal epidural space (short arrows) behind L3–4 and L4–5 is large and would be an easy target for epidural steroid injections. (D) This T2-weighted image shows diffuse disc dessication and complete loss of disc space height at L2–3. Multiple disc bulges are seen indenting the ventral subarachnoid space at all levels except L5–S1. The linear hypointense signal representing the vacuum disc (arrowheads) at L4–5 is smaller than would be predicted by the CT image.

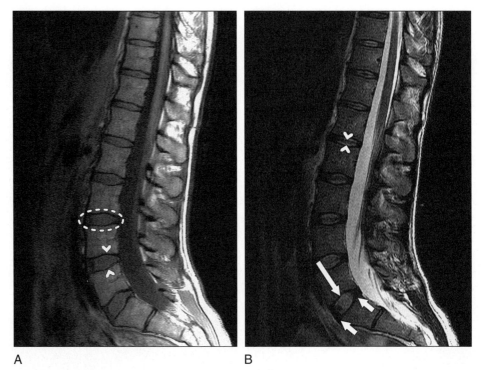

FIGURE 8-24. (A) On T1-weighted images, the normal intervertebral disc is homogeneously isointense (dashed oval). The black signal outlining the superior and inferior margins of the disc (arrowheads) represents the cortex of the adjacent vertebral bodies. (B) In this T2-weighted image, the tightly packed annular fibers are hypointense (short arrows). The hydrated nucleus (long arrow) is hyperintense except for the central linear intranuclear cleft (arrowheads). This intranuclear cleft is a normal finding and should not be misinterpreted as focal desiccation.

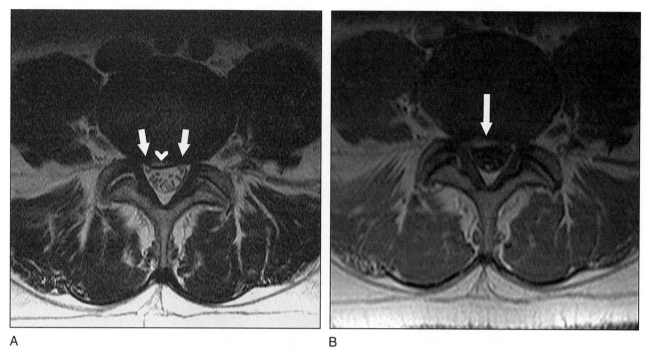

FIGURE 8-25. (A) Axial T2-weighted image through the L4–5 level. There is a right paracentral protrusion (short arrows) which indents the ventral thecal sac. Linear hyperintense signal in the central dorsal annulus (arrowhead) parallels the disc margin and represents mucoid deposition within a concentric fissure or tear. (B) On postgadolinium T1-weighted imaging, annular tears of any type can enhance (arrow) as in this case. Enhancement implies nothing other than the likely presence of a reparative process such as granulation tissue.

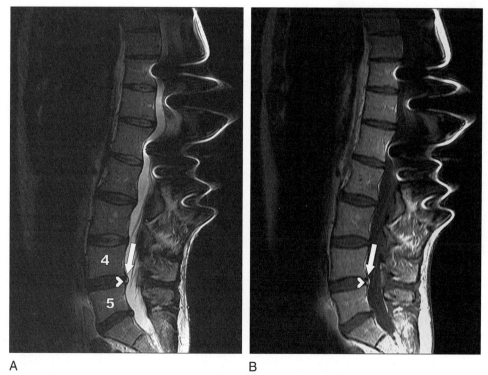

FIGURE 8-26. (A, B) At the L4–5 level, a dorsal concentric annular fissure/tear (arrow) and a radial tear (arrowhead) are identified. Both of these tears enhance on the postgadolinium T1-weighted sagittal image.

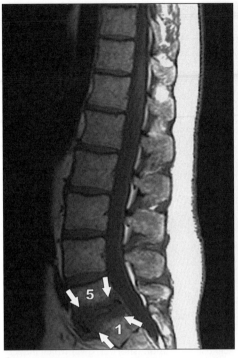

A

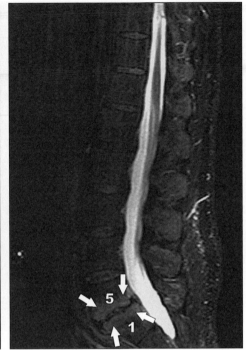

B

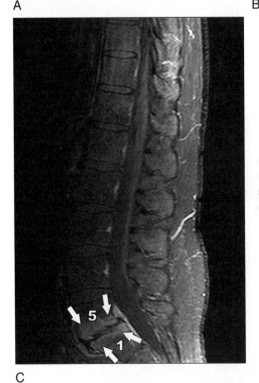

C

FIGURE 8-27. Sagittal (A) T1, (B) STIR, and (C) postgadolinium T1-weighted fat saturation images show the typical Modic type 1 subchondral marrow changes (arrows) at L5–S1. The signal and enhancement resemble that which is seen with early osteomyelitis.

the base at the annular margin, than is the width of the fragment at the base (Fig. 8-31B). A sequestered or free-fragment disc herniation is disc material that has completely separated from the parent disc. Describing disc herniations using these terms is not meant to imply any significance regarding symptom production or the best method of treatment.

Disc migration in the cranial or caudal directions is best evaluated in the sagittal plane. A posterior disc extrusion may be contained by the posterior longitudinal ligament and migrate inferiorly or less commonly, superiorly. Such extrusions

may appear on axial imaging as a protrusion but are easily identified as a migrated extrusion on sagittal imaging. Measurements are taken from the posterior margin of the superior or inferior end plate of the intervertebral body, to describe the extent of migration for the surgeon. Migrated fragments are usually paramedian, since the posterior longitudinal ligament at midline tends to direct the fragment unilaterally.

Disc Herniation Position: Using anatomic landmarks to describe the location of a disc herniation provides a precise and

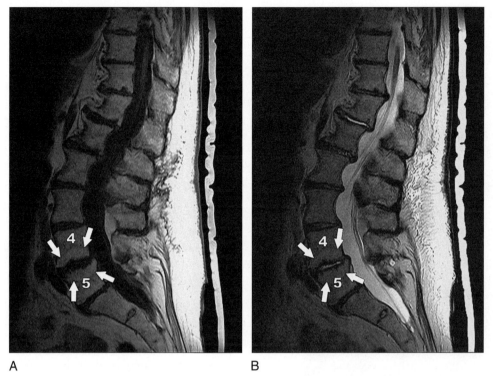

FIGURE 8-28. Sagittal (A) T1- and (B) T2-weighted images show classic Modic type 2 changes at L4–5. The hyperintense endplate signal (arrows) on both sequences represents focal fatty replacement of bone marrow.

consistent classification.[54] An axial image at the level of the disc has four "zones" based on arbitrary sagittal and parasagittal lines drawn through specific anatomic landmarks. The term "central" means the posterior midline aspect of the disc, between the medial aspects of the articular facets. Right and

left paracentral/paramedian descriptors can be added if the disc favors one side or the other. The "subarticular" zone is between the medial aspect of the articular process and the medial aspect of the ipsilateral pedicle. The "foraminal" zone is between the parasagittal planes defined by the medial and

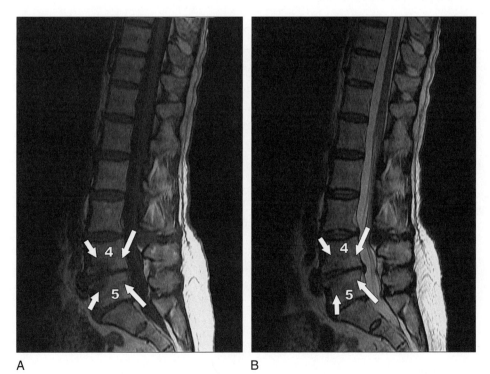

FIGURE 8-29. Sagittal (A) T1- and (B) T2-weighted images show Modic type 3 changes (short arrows) along the ventral half of the L4–5 endplates. Interestingly, Modic type 2 changes (long arrows) are present at the same level along the dorsal margin of the endplates.

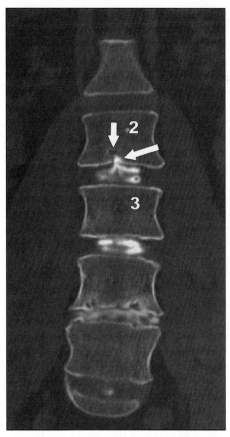

FIGURE 8-30. CT coronal reconstruction after lumbar discography from L2 to L5. There is a Schmorls node extending through the inferior endplate of L2. A sclerotic margin (short arrow) is present. Contrast (long arrow) from the L2–3 discogram is seen extending into the Schmorls node (intervertebral disc herniation).

lateral aspects of the pedicle. Finally, the extraforaminal zone is beyond the parasagittal line of the lateral aspect of the pedicle.

Of note, the term lateral recess describes the area along the medial border of the pedicle, below the level of the disc and the superior vertebral endplate, and is a part of but does not describe the entire subarticular zone (Fig. 8-32). Disc herniations can reach the lateral recess, but the anatomic term lateral recess should not be used in a description of a disc herniation at the level of the disc.

On sagittal images, the position of a herniated disc in the craniocaudal direction can be separated into levels based on anatomic landmarks. The suprapedicular level extends from just above the pedicle to the superior end plate. The pedicle level is defined by the superior and inferior edges of the pedicle. The infrapedicular level extends from below the inferior edge of the pedicle to the inferior end plate.

Depending on the position of a herniated disc, it can potentially compress adjacent nerve roots. In the cervical spine, a central or paramedian disc herniation will affect the descending nerve roots and not the exiting nerve root at that level. For instance, a right paramedian small disc extrusion at C3–4 will most likely compress the descending right C5 nerve root. A foraminal disc abnormality will affect the exiting nerve root at that level. For instance, a right foraminal disc extrusion at C3–4 will likely compress the right C4 nerve root. In the thoracic and lumbar spine, the nerve roots are numbered differently (exiting root is associated with superior level). A right paramedian disc extrusion at T3–4 or L3–4 would likely affect the descending right T4 or right L4 nerve roots, respectively. A right foraminal disc extrusion at T3–4 or L3–4 would compress the exiting right T3 or L4 nerve roots.

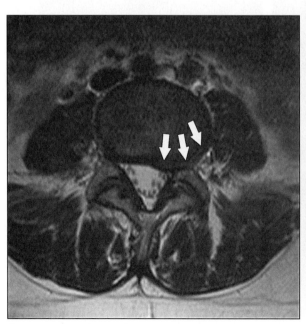

A

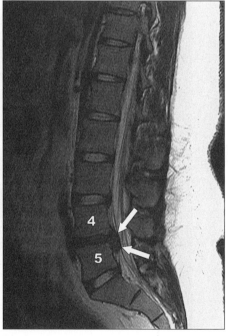

B

FIGURE 8-31. (A) Axial T2-weighted MRI demonstrating a broad-based left parasagittal, foraminal, and far lateral herniation (arrows). This morphology is consistent with a disc protrusion. (B) Parasagittal T2-weighted MRI shows a large disc extrusion (arrows) at the L4–5 level. Disc material elevates the PLL and has migrated 6 mm caudal to the parent disc.

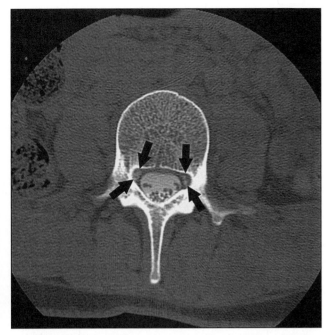

FIGURE 8-32. Axial CT myelogram image in the mid-lumbar spine. The lateral recesses (arrows) reside just medial to the medial margin of each pedicle and contain the exiting nerve roots. In this image, the exiting nerve root sleeves are opacified with contrast.

The degree of neural compression can be graded based on the change in the normal round or oval configuration of the spinal cord, nerve root, or root ganglion produced by the herniated disc. Mild compression is defined as 75% to 99% of the normal diameter of the structure being maintained. Similarly, moderate and severe compression is described as 50% to 74% and <50% of the normal diameter, respectively.

FACET JOINT

Overview: The facet joint is another potential source of low back pain. Considering the numerous potential causes of low back pain, it can be difficult to isolate the facet joint clinically or by imaging as the primary cause of a patient's pain. Facet joint syndrome is a controversial diagnosis referring to focal or referred pain arising from or anatomically correlating with a degenerated facet joint.[55,56]

Imaging: Facet joint arthropathy includes hypertrophic osteophytic overgrowth, subchondral sclerosis, bone marrow edema, joint space narrowing/widening, joint effusions, and periarticular soft tissue edema.[57] Osteophytosis and subchondral sclerosis are hypointense on T1- and T2-weighted imaging. Bone marrow and periarticular soft tissue edema are hypointense on T1- but hyperintense on T2-weighted sequences (Fig. 8-33A,B). A fat-suppressed T2-weighted sequence is particularly sensitive at detecting marrow or soft tissue edema. The joint space can narrow or, if instability and abnormal motion occur, widen. A small amount of synovial fluid exists in the joint space but effusions are commonly seen, particularly in widened facet joints (Fig. 8-33C). Facet joint arthropathy can result in pain secondary to the intrinsic abnormalities of the bone and joint or can result in extrinsic compression of descending nerve roots in the lateral recess or exiting nerve roots in the intervertebral foramen. Facet joint osteoarthritis can be accurately diagnosed by CT scanning although the ability to detect bone marrow or periarticular edema is limited. In the cervical spine, subtle sclerotic changes and osteophytes are easily detected on CT whereas on MRI the

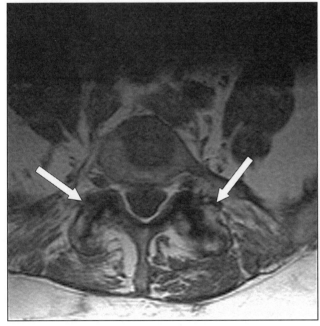

A

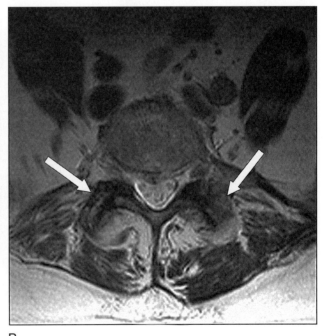

B

FIGURE 8-33. Axial (A) T1-weighted and (B) T2-weighted MRI through the L5–S1 level demonstrate facet degenerative changes (arrows) including loss of the joint space, osteophyte overgrowth, and subchondral sclerosis.

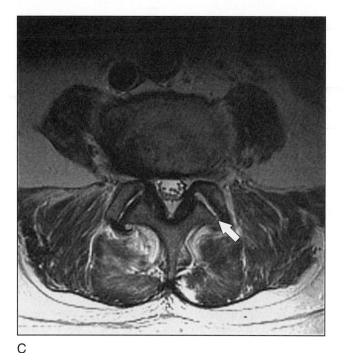

C

FIGURE 8-33. cont'd (C) Axial T2-weighted MRI shows a typical facet joint effusion (arrow).

changes are either more difficult to detect or are overestimated, particularly on the GRE sequence images. Plain films can detect some facet degenerative changes including sclerosis and hypertrophic overgrowth but are generally the least sensitive modality.

INTRASPINAL FACET CYSTS

Overview: Intraspinal facet cysts are fluid-filled, rounded structures with a smooth border that originate from the facet joint. Facet joint arthritic changes and spinal instability is thought to lead to protrusion of articular tissue forming an adjacent cyst.[58,59] The lining of a cyst may contain synovial epithelial cells (synovial cyst) or a fibrous wall surrounding myxoid material (ganglion cyst).[60] Radiologically, both types of cysts appear identical. Treatment and prognosis of synovial and ganglion cysts are the same (decompression) and distinguishing between them is not clinically important. It has been postulated that ganglion cysts represent synovial cysts that have undergone degeneration and lost their communication with the facet joint.[61] For simplicity, the following discussion will refer to all facet-related cysts as synovial cysts.

Synovial cysts are almost invariably discovered adjacent to a degenerated facet joint. They can arise off the dorsal surface of the joint, protruding into the soft tissues but not compressing

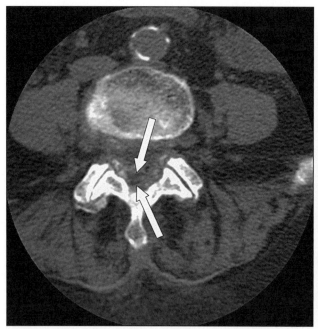

A

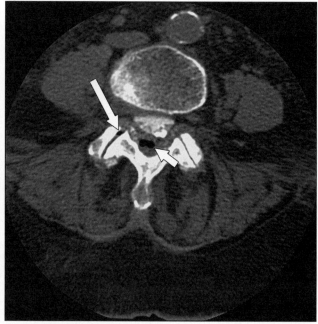

B

FIGURE 8-34. (A, B) CT imaging of a synovial cyst. The axial noncontrast CT image (A) shows facet degenerative changes particularly on the patient's right. Ligamentum thickening and calcification are also present. Just deep to the right lamina and partially within the ligamentum flavum, the hypodense synovial cyst (arrows) is identified. The patient underwent myelography followed by percutaneous aspiration and steroid injection of the cyst. The postprocedure axial CT image (B) shows persistent mass effect by the partially calcified cyst. Note the presence of air in the cyst (short arrow) and the joint (long arrow) which was introduced through the injection and confirms communication between the degenerated facet and the synovial cyst.

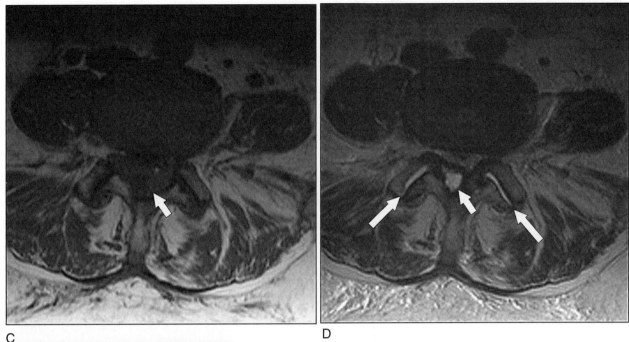

C   D

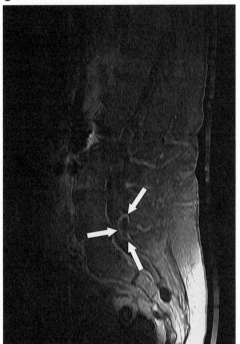

FIGURE 8-34. *cont'd* (C–E) MRI imaging of a synovial cyst. On T1-weighted imaging (E), the cyst (arrow) is almost indistinguishable from ligamentum flavum thickening. The T2-weighted image (D) identifies hyperintense fluid within the synovial cyst (short arrow) and the joint spaces (long arrows) which is consistent with synovial fluid. Peripheral enhancement (arrows) of the synovial cyst wall is common as is demonstrated in the parasagittal postgadolinium T1-weighted fat saturation image (E).

E

any neural structures. These cysts can also arise off the ventral surface and protrude into the intervertebral foramen, lateral recess, or lateral spinal canal. Depending upon the location, a synovial cyst can compress an exiting nerve root (in the foramen) or a descending nerve root (in the lateral recess or lateral spinal canal). Synovial cysts can also be intrinsically painful because they are often lined with a nociceptive synovial lining.

Imaging: On CT scan, an uncomplicated synovial cyst is isodense to CSF, located next to a degenerated facet joint and occasionally has a calcified wall (Fig. 8-34A,B).[62] Proteinaceous material or blood within the cyst may be isodense to the adjacent muscle or ligament. CT can also clearly demonstrate gas located within a juxta-articular cystic structure which, when present, almost always represents a synovial cyst. CT myelography may better demonstrate the degree of mass effect or stenosis related to an intraspinal or foraminal synovial cyst, by better defining the spinal subarachnoid space with contrast.

Typical MRI findings for synovial cysts include T1- and T2-prolongation and therefore generally follow CSF signal

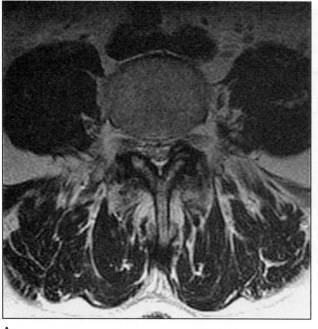

A

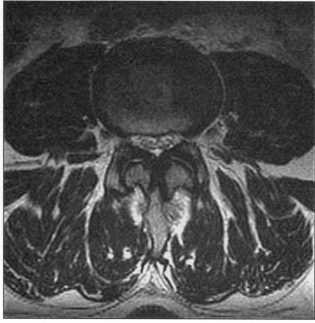

B

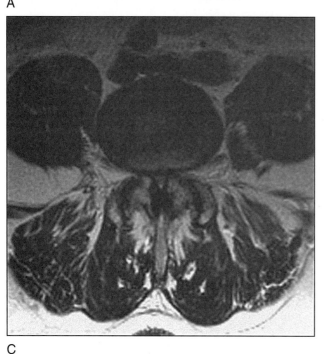

C

FIGURE 8-35. Axial T2-weighted images in the same patient showing (A) mild, (B) moderate, and (C) severe spinal stenosis. In this patient, mild stenosis is produced by subtle facet degenerative changes. Moderate stenosis is produced by the "trifecta" of disc bulging, ligament thickening, and facet degenerative changes. In severe stenosis, the trifecta is again responsible and result in severe compression of the lumbar nerve roots.

(Fig. 8-34C,D).[63] Some synovial cysts contain proteinaceous or hemorrhagic material and can also demonstrate T1 hyperintensity. Acute hemorrhage can cause a rapid increase in the size of the cyst and result in acute pain or radiculopathy. The wall of a synovial cyst is typically composed of tough fibrous material and it may be partially or completely calcified. The degree of calcification is anecdotally predictive of the potential success of percutaneous decompression. Peripheral enhancement of a synovial cyst is common and should not be mistaken as an aggressive feature (Fig. 8-34E).

An important consideration in the differential diagnosis of a juxta-articular cyst is an extruded disc fragment. Recognizing that the lesion is juxta-articular, and is related to a degenerated facet joint is the key to making the correct diagnosis. Alternatively, a short-term follow-up MRI might show resolution of a disc fragment, but no change in the case of a synovial cyst. Treatment options include conservative management, percutaneous decompression, or surgical removal. Successful outcomes have been reported with all approaches.[64,65]

SPINAL STENOSIS

Overview: CT effectively evaluates spinal stenosis caused by bony abnormalities of the vertebral column and can show a contributing component of a bulging or herniated disc. CT myelography requires a lumbar puncture, but has the added benefit of outlining nerve roots and the contour of the thecal sac particularly as it relates to disc abnormalities and hypertrophic ligaments.

MRI, using axial GRE T2 images in the cervical spine and conventional or fast spin echo T2-weighted images in the thoracic and lumbar spine, provides a noninvasive technique to evaluate the central canal and intervertebral foramen without significant artifact from CSF flow within the canal.

If surgical hardware is present, conventional T2-weighted images are used to minimize susceptibility artifact. In some circumstances, axial T1-weighted sequences can be helpful.

Grading Spinal Stenosis: Although there are various methods to grade spinal stenosis, no one technique has proved reliable in predicting symptoms or favorable surgical outcome. Also, the reliability of grading the severity of lumbar spinal stenosis has been challenged.[66] Consequently, it is difficult to interpret studies examining the efficacy of treatment if there is disagreement on the grading of stenosis.

One grading scheme used by Renfrew and colleagues in a large spinal imaging practice compares the AP dimension of an abnormal level to an adjacent normal level of the spinal canal in the same patient.[67] The inherent spinal canal diameter is also evaluated to take into account the possibility of a developmentally narrow canal.

Mild, moderate, and severe stenoses are assigned relative to the degree of narrowing (Fig. 8-35). Mild stenosis is defined as 75% to 99% maintenance of the AP dimension of the normal level, while moderate and severe are 50% to 74% and <50%, respectively. Using the AP dimension is not absolute, and stenosis can be up- or downgraded depending on the developmental size of the canal and the amount of space surrounding the nerve roots.

In a similar manner, the subarticular recess and foramen can be graded. The intervertebral foramen is evaluated in the AP and craniocaudad dimension. Stenosis in the foramen can be described as craniocaudal, AP, or combined depending on the site of narrowing. Mild foraminal stenosis usually reflects some narrowing of the inferior part of the foramen by a disc bulge or hypertrophic superior articular process. Moderate narrowing implies loss of fat along a portion of the nerve root and some nerve root displacement. Severe foraminal stenosis is used when little to no fat is visible in the foramen and the nerve root is clearly displaced and/or compressed. These changes are most sensitively detected on a sagittal T1-weighted MRI sequence (Fig. 8-36).

SPONDYLOLYSIS AND SPONDYLOLISTHESIS

Overview: Spondylolysis refers to a discontinuity in the pars intra-articularis of the articular pillar. The etiology is uncertain but felt to be related to chronic microtrauma leading to a

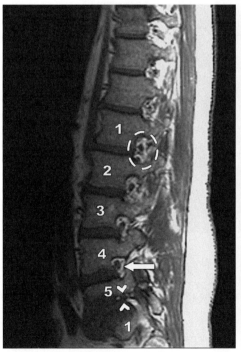
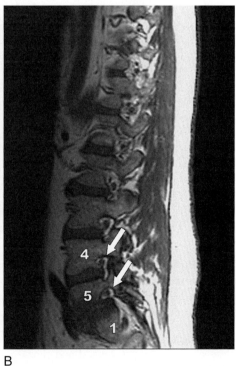

A   B

FIGURE 8-36. Parasagittal T1-weighted images show (A) mild and severe and (B) moderate foraminal stenosis. In (A) mild stenosis is identified at L4–5 (arrow) and severe stenosis at L5–S1. The severe stenosis is due to loss of disc space height, disc bulging, and osteophyte formation off the vertebral body and superior articular process and results in compression of the exiting nerve root (arrowheads). Note the normal appearance on the foramen at L1–2 (dashed oval). In (B) moderate stenosis is identified at L4–5 and L5–S1 secondary to similar degenerative changes (arrows). Note early encroachment on the exiting L4 nerve root at L4–5.

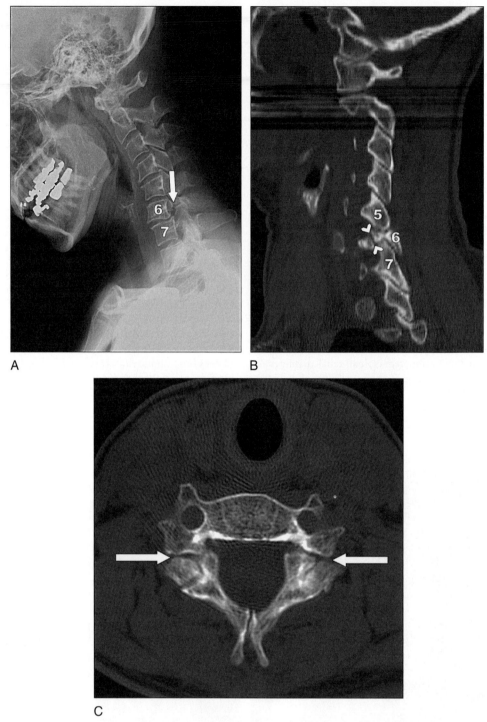

FIGURE 8-37. Developmental cervical spondylolysis on (A) lateral plain film, (B) sagittal CT reconstruction, and (C) axial CT imaging. The plain film reveals a reversed lordosis and anterior subluxation of C6 on C7. Pars deficiencies are suggested (arrow). One of the pars fractures is well profiled on the sagittal CT reconstruction (arrowheads). The axial CT image demonstrates bilateral pars intra-articularis fractures (arrows). The sclerotic margins support a chronic process.

stress-type reaction or fracture, particularly in the lumbar spine.[68] Spondylolysis can occur in the cervical and thoracic spine, albeit rarely, and may be more related to a developmental abnormality as opposed to trauma in these locations (Fig. 8-37). When bilateral pars fractures are present, the vertebral body can slip forward. This is most apparent in the lumbar spine where axial loading and incompetent pars result in spondylolisthesis. Mild and moderate slips generally do not narrow,

but paradoxically enlarge, the central canal. Severe spondylolisthesis elongates the spinal canal in the AP direction and narrows the spinal canal in the sagittal plane. All degrees of listhesis tend to result in foraminal stenosis and nerve root compression.

Imaging: The test of choice to diagnose spondylolysis is CT. Sclerosis and fractures of the pars can be optimally depicted in any plane and the degree of osseous canal or foraminal

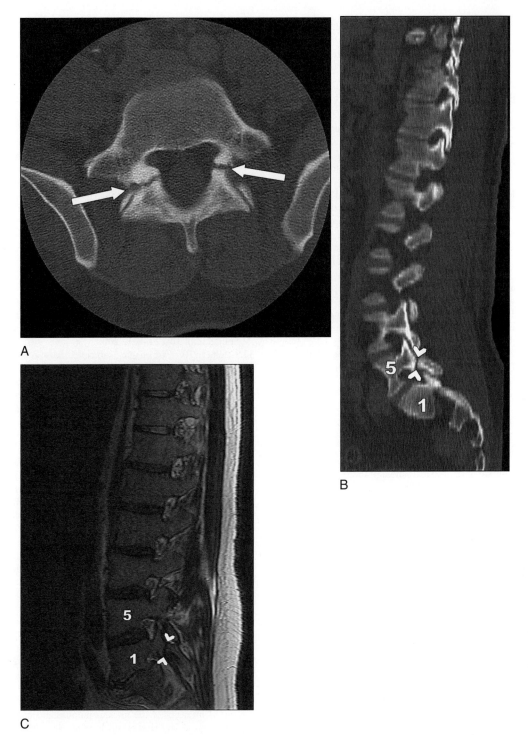

FIGURE 8-38. Developmental lumbar spondylolysis on (A) axial CT, (B) sagittal CT reconstruction, and (C) sagittal T2-weighted MRI. The axial CT image shows the deficient pars intra-articularis (arrows) and associated sclerosis. One of the pars defects is easily confirmed on the sagittal CT reconstruction (arrowheads) and is identifiable but more subtle on sagittal MRI (arrowheads).

narrowing can be assessed. MRI can show similar findings although the actual fracture can sometimes be elusive (Fig. 8-38A,B). MRI exquisitely demonstrates the foraminal stenosis and nerve root compression that are invariably present with spondylolysis and spondylolisthesis (Fig. 8-38C). MRI also demonstrates cartilaginous overgrowth in the area of the pars

fracture that may also contribute to canal and foraminal stenosis. Plain films can easily depict the spondylolisthesis and can demonstrate the pars defect, particularly with an oblique projection. Plain films can be effectively employed to correlate bone detail with an MRI examination although most imagers prefer CT.

ACKNOWLEDGMENT

The authors would like to thank Ms. Rita Jarmon and Mr. David Botos for help in preparing this chapter.

REFERENCES

1. Ebraheim NA, Lu J, Biyani A, et al: Anatomic considerations for uncovertebral involvement in cervical spondylosis. Clin Orthop 334:200–206, 1997.
2. Osborn A: Normal anatomy and congenital anomalies of the spine and spinal cord. In Osborn A (ed): Diagnostic Neuroradiology. Mosby, St Louis, 1994, pp 783–819.
3. Hayashi K, Yabuki T: Origin of the uncus and of the Luschka's joint in the cervical spine. J Bone Joint Surg North Am 67A: 788–791, 1985.
4. Tournade A, Patay Z, Krupa A, et al: A comparative study of the anatomical, radiological, and therapeutic features of the lumbar facet joints. Neuroradiol 34:257–261, 1992.
5. Xu GL, Haughton VM, Carrera GF: Lumbar facet joint capsule: appearance at MR imaging and CT. Radiol 177:415–420, 1990.
6. Yamashita T, Minaki Y, Ozaktay AC, et al: A morphological study of the fibrous capsule of the human lumbar facet joint. Spine 21:538–543, 1996.
7. Ashton IK, Ashton BA, Gibson SJ, et al: Morphological basis for back pain. The demonstration of nerve fibers and neuropeptides in the lumbar facet joint capsule but not in the ligamentum flavum. J Orthop Res 10:72–78, 1992.
8. Hogan QH, Abram SE: Diagnostic and prognostic neural blockade. In Cousins MJ (ed): Neural Blockade in Clinical Anesthesia and Management of Pain, ed 3. Lippincott-Raven, Philadelphia, 1998, pp 837–877.
9. Carrera GF. Lumbar facet joint injection in low back pain and sciatica: Description of technique. Radiology 137:661–664, 1980.
10. Osborn A: The vertebrobasilar system. In Osborn A (ed): Diagnostic Cerebral Angiography, ed 2. Lippincott Williams and Wilkins, Philadelphia, 1999, pp 173–193.
11. Morris P: Embryology of the cranial circulation. In Morris P (ed): Practical Neuroangiography. Lippincott Williams and Wilkins, Philadelphia, 1997, pp 89–98.
12. Erbil KM, Sargon MF, Celik HH, et al: A study of variations of transverse foramens of cervical vertebras in humans: Accessory foramina in shape and number. Morphologie 85:23–24, 2001.
13. Flannigan BD, Lufkin RB, McGlade C, et al: MR imaging of the cervical spine: Neurovascular anatomy. AJNR Am J Neuroradiol 8:27–32, 1987.
14. Cohen MS, Wall EG, Brown RA, et al: Cauda equina anatomy II: Extrathecal nerve roots and dorsal root ganglia. Spine 15: 1248–1251, 1990.
15. Czervionke LF, Haughton VM: Degenerative disease of the spine. In Atlas SW (ed): Magnetic Resonance Imaging of the Brain and Spine, ed 3, vol II. Lippincott Williams and Wilkins, Philadelphia, 2002, pp 1633–1650.
16. Alleyne CH Jr, Cawley CM, Shengelaia GG, et al: Microsurgical anatomy of the artery of Adamkiewicz and its segmental artery. J Neurosurg 89:791–795, 1998.
17. Peacock A: Observations on the postnatal structure of the intervertebral disk in man. J Anat 86:162–179, 1952.
18. Rabischong P, Louis R, Vignaud J, et al: The intervertebral disk. Anat Clin 1:55–64, 1978.
19. Ibrahim MA, Jesmanowicz A, Hyde JS, et al: Contrast enhancement in normal intervertebral disks: Time and dose dependence. AJNR Am J Neuroradiol 15:419–423, 1994.
20. Urban JPG, McMullen JF: Fifth international congress on biorheology symposium: Some biorheological aspects of joint diseases. Biorheology 22:145–157, 1985.
21. Grenier N, Greselle J-F, Vital J-M, et al: Normal and disrupted lumbar longitudinal ligaments. Radiology 171:197–205, 1989.
22. Harris JH Jr: How I do it; the cervicocranium: Its radiographic assessment. Radiology 218:337–351, 2001.
23. Hess JH: Postdural puncture headache: A literature review. J Am Assoc Nurse Anes 59:549–555, 1991.
24. Bart AJ, Wheeler S: Comparison of epidural saline placement and epidural blood placement in the treatment of post-lumbar-puncture headache. Anesthesiology 48:221–223, 1978.
25. Fedutes BA, Ansani NT: Seizure potential of concomitant medications and radiographic contrast media agents. Ann Pharmacother 37:1506–1510, 2003.
26. Kanal E, Shellock FG: Burns associated with clinical MR examinations. Radiology 175:585, 1990.
27. Schenk JF: Safety of strong, static magnetic fields. J Magn Reson Imaging 12:2–19, 2000.
28. Schaefer DJ, Bourland JD, Nyenhuis JA: Review of patient safety in time-varying gradient fields. J Magn Reson Imaging 12:20–29, 2000.
29. Shellock FG: Radiofrequency energy-induced heating during MR procedures. J Magn Reson Imaging 12:30–36, 2000.
30. McJury M, Shellock FG: Auditory noise associated with MR procedures. J Magn Reson Imaging 12:37–45, 2000.
31. Vanel D, Dromain C, Tardivon A: MRI of bone marrow disorders. Eur Radiol 10:224–229, 2000.
32. Mulkern RV: Fast imaging principles. In Atlas SW (ed): Magnetic Resonance Imaging of the Brain and Spine, ed 3, vol I. Lippincott Williams and Wilkins, Philadelphia, 2002, pp 127–196.
33. Czervionke LF, Daniels DL: Cervical spine anatomy and pathologic processes. Radiol Clin North Am 26:921–947, 1988.
34. Marti-Bonmati L, Kormano M: MR equipment acquisition strategies: Low-field or high-field scanners. Eur Radiol. 7(Suppl 5):263–268, 1997.
35. Shellock, FG: Reference Manual for Magnetic Resonance Safety: 2003 Edition. WB Saunders, Philadelphia, 2003.
36. Pritzker KPH: Aging and degeneration in the lumbar intervertebral disk. Orthop Clin North Am 8:65–77, 1977.
37. Twomey LT, Taylor JR: Age changes in lumbar vertebrae and intervertebral disks. Clin Orthop Rel Res 224:97–104, 1987.
38. Hirsch C, Schajowicz F: Studies on structural changes in the lumbar annulus fibrosus. Acta Orthop Scand 22:184–231, 1952.
39. Yu S, Haughton VM, Sether LA, et al: Criteria for classifying normal and degenerated lumbar intervertebral disks. Radiology 170:523–526, 1989.
40. Yu S, Haughton VM, Lynch KL, et al: Fibrous structure in the intervertebral disk: Correlation of MR appearance with anatomic sections. AJNR Am J Neuroradiol 10:1105–1110, 1989.
41. Grenier N, Grossman RI, Schiebler ML, et al: Degenerative lumbar disk disease: Pitfalls and usefulness of MR imaging in detection of vacuum phenomenon. Radiology 164:861–865, 1987.
42. Luoma K, Vehmas T, Riihimaki H, Raininko R: Disc height and signal intensity of the nucleus pulposus on magnetic resonance imaging as indicators of lumbar disc degeneration. Spine 26:680–686, 2001.
43. Aprill C, Bogduk N: High-intensity zone: A diagnostic sign of painful lumbar disc on magnetic resonance imaging. Br J Radiol 65:361–369, 1992.
44. Yu S, Haughton VM, Sether LA, Wagner M: Comparison of MR and discography in detecting radial tears of the annulus: A postmortem study. AJNR Am J Neuroradiol 10:1077–1081, 1989.
45. Yu S, Haughton VM, Sether LA, et al: Criteria for classifying normal and degenerated intervertebral disks. Radiol 170:523–526, 1989.
46. Yu S, Sether LA, Ho PSP, et al: Tears of the annulus fibrosus: Correlation between MR and pathologic findings in cadavers. AJNR Am J Neuroradiol 9:367–370, 1988.

47. Rabischong P, Louis R, Vignaud J, et al. The intervertebral disk. Anat Clin 1:55–64, 1978.
48. Modic MT, Steinberg PM, Ross JS, et al: Degenerative disk disease: assessment of changes in vertebral body marrow with MR imaging. Radiology 166:193–199, 1988.
49. Crock HV: A reappraisal of intervertebral disc lesions. Med J Aust 1:983–989, 1970.
50. Crock HV: Internal disc disruption. A challenge to disc prolapse fifty years on. Spine 11:650–653, 1986.
51. Braithwaite I, White J, Saifuddin A, et al: Vertebral end-plate (Modic) changes on lumbar spine MRI: Correlation with pain reproduction at lumbar discography. Eur Spine J 7:363–368, 1998.
52. Sandhu HS, Sanchez-Caso LP, Parvataneni HK, et al: Association between findings of provocative discography and vertebral endplate signal changes as seen on MRI. J Spinal Disord 12:438–443, 2000.
53. Fardon DF, Milette PC: Nomenclature and classification of lumbar disc pathology: Recommendations of the Combined Task Forces of the North American Spine Society, American Society of Spine Radiology, and the American Society of Neuroradiology. Spine 26:E93–E113, 2001.
54. Wiltse LL, Berger PE, McCulloch JA: A system for reporting the size and location of lesions in the spine. Spine 22:1534–1537, 1997.
55. Jackson RP: The Facet syndrome. Myth or reality? Clin Orthop 279:110–121, 1992.
56. Schwarzer AC, Aprill CN, Derby R, et al: Clinical features of patients with pain stemming from the lumbar zygapophysial joints. Spine 19:1132–1137, 1994.
57. Resnick D: Degenerative diseases of the vertebral column. Radiology 156:3–14, 1985.
58. Fujiwara A, Tamai K, An HS, et al: The relationship between disc degeneration, facet joint osteoarthritis and stability of the degenerative lumbar spine. J Spinal Disord 13:444–450, 2000.
59. Fujiwara A, Lim T, An HS, et al: The effect of disc degeneration and facet joint osteoarthritis on the segmental flexibility of the lumbar spine. Spine 25:3036–3044, 2000.
60. Hsu KY, Zucherman JF, Shea WJ, Jeffrey RA: Lumbar intraspinal synovial and ganglion cysts (facet cysts). Spine 20:80–89, 1995.
61. Yuh WTC, Drew JM, Weinstein JN, et al: Intraspinal synovial cysts: Magnetic resonance evaluation. Spine 16:740–745, 1991.
62. Farrokh D: Lumbar intraspinal synovial cysts of different etiologies: Diagnosis by CT and MR imaging. J Belge Radiol 81:275–278, 1998.
63. Apostolaki E, Davies AM, Evans N, et al: MR imaging of lumbar facet joint synovial cysts. Eur Radiol 10:615–623, 2000.
64. Howington JU, Connolly ES, Voorhies RM: Intraspinal synovial cysts: 10 year experience at the Ochsner Clinic. J Neurosurg 91(Suppl 2):193–199, 1999.
65. Sabo RA, Tracy PT, Weinger JM: A series of 60 juxtafacet cysts: Clinical presentation, the role of spinal instability, and treatment. J Neurosurg 85:560–565, 1996.
66. Drew B, Bhandari M, Kulkarni AV, et al: Reliability in grading severity of lumbar spinal stenosis. J Spinal Disord 13:253–258, 2000.
67. Renfrew DL: Degenerative disease. In Atlas of Spine Imaging. Elsevier Science, Saunders, Philadelphia, 2003, pp 11–129.
68. Wiltzer LL, Widell EH, Jackson DW. Fatigue fracture: the basic lesion in isthmic spondylolisthesis. J Bone Joint Surg Am 57:17–22, 1975.

Determination of Disability

E. Richard Blonsky, M.D.

Disability is defined as the inability of an individual to perform various activities of daily living based on the physical and/or cognitive requirements of the tasks relevant to the individual's impairments. Impairment is an alteration of an individual's health status and includes the loss of, or loss of use of, a physical, cognitive, or psychological part or function. Physicians are trained to determine impairment, but the majority does not evaluate patients from a functional perspective unless specifically requested to do so. The goal of most physicians is to establish a diagnosis and determine a course of treatment as quickly and accurately as possible. Acute disorders are most easily dealt with. Chronic illness and impairment are more difficult matters because of the demands made on the physician to look beyond the medical model. This is especially true when pain is an issue.

The American Medical Association's *Guides to Evaluation of Permanent Impairment*[1] enables the examiner to assess an individual and to accurately establish the nature and degree of each impairment displayed. Every organ system is considered in this book, as are chapters on psychiatric disturbances and pain. All but two chapters assign a value for a particular impairment (e.g., loss of the part due to injury or disease; loss of use due to immobility (ankylosis), injury, or disease; diminished function of a part or system). The decision of disability is administrative, not medical, although the question is regularly asked of treating and examining physicians. To establish disability status it is necessary (1) to identify fully all pertinent impairments attributed to an individual, (2) to determine what restrictions are imposed on performance by the impairments, (3) to understand the complete requirements of the tasks or job to be completed, and (4) to be aware of possible accommodations that would enable the impaired individual to perform the requisite tasks.

DISABILITY PROGRAMS

The determination of disability is critical for the claimant in various societal and legal settings. Federally mandated disability programs include Title II—Social Security Disability (individuals who work and have paid taxes into the Social Security system) and Title XVI—Supplemental Security Disability Income (individuals who have not worked or do not qualify for regular Social Security benefits); Workers' compensation

programs; and individual and group short- and long-term disability policies. A brief discussion of each will allow the reader to become familiar with the similarities and differences between them. The Social Security Act defines disability as an "inability to engage in any substantial gainful activity by reason of a medically determinable physical or mental impairment which can be expected to result in death or has lasted or can be expected to last for a continuous period of not less than 12 months."[2] Disability is entirely based on vocational rather than medical issues, although the medical justification is essential. The adjudicator utilizes a Listing of Impairments to determine the severity of the problem, and if a single impairment is inadequate a combination of impairments might suffice to justify a disability determination.

The treating physician is requested to provide information as to the claimant's condition. Lack of this documentation may lead to the conclusion that the impairment is not severe, and disability may be denied. Specific forms are provided, although narrative documentation and office records are often sufficient. The approved claimant will not receive benefits until a year has elapsed. The Act allows an injured worker to attempt to return successfully to work for 9 months before benefits are rescinded. If a worker is determined to be unemployable benefits continue for his or her lifetime.

Workers' compensation programs are administered by each state and territory and, while the principles are similar in each jurisdiction, the practices vary widely from state to state. In many states the employer/insurance company determines the provider of medical care to the injured worker. In other venues, the worker has the choice, and, in Illinois, can choose a second provider if he or she is dissatisfied with the first. Direct referral to consultants also is allowed, often leading to several treaters involved in the claimant's case. The stated purpose of these programs is to provide the injured worker prompt and appropriate treatment in order to restore the worker to his or her pre-injury state and enable the worker to return to work. The worker also is provided monetary benefits to compensate for lost wages, but usually at a tax-free rate of 66% of the *base* wage (not considering overtime).

The hearing officers who decide these cases are medically uneducated, and may not even be attorneys. The medical records and testimony they have to consider must be clear enough to be understandable and comprehensive enough to establish the nature and degree of impairment suffered by the worker and why this prevents the worker from working. Four categories of disability are possible: 1. *Temporary partial*; 2. *Temporary total*; 3. *Permanent partial*; 4. *Permanent total*. The duration and extent of benefits are determined by the category into which the claimant falls. Statistics suggest that approximately 85% of workers' compensation cases are handled routinely in a "no fault" fashion. The worker receives wage benefits while being treated, recovers, returns to work, and may receive a small settlement for the injury. The other 15% represent cases that are contested because either the circumstances of injury, the degree of injury, or the extent of treatment is questionable or the alleged permanent disability is disputed. The treating physician is called upon to prepare detailed reports regarding the injuries sustained by the claimant (petitioner) and the treatment provided. Records are required and may be obtained by subpoena. In contested cases, the employer (respondent) may obtain an independent examination by a chosen expert to provide an assessment of the facts in the case. Examination of the claimant is usual, as is detailed scrutiny of the treater's records. Scrupulous attention to detail and documentation of findings is essential to the claimant's case.

Short-term disability policies supplement sick day allowances in many organizations. If an employee's illness/injury prevents him or her from working the benefits pay a fixed percentage of salary. An individual must be temporarily totally disabled to qualify, and these benefits are paid for a fixed period (usually 3 or 6 months). Unlike workers' compensation plans, short-term disability does not provide medical payments. Medical payments derive from the individual's health coverage. Persons receiving workers' compensation benefits are not eligible for short-term disability. The administrators of short-term disability plans closely monitor the medical treatment received and anticipated recovery times for each illness. Unnecessarily prolonged care is questioned and claims may be terminated without valid medical documentation of ongoing disability. Long-term disability plans may be independent or an extension of short-term plans. Many professionals purchase individual policies to cover unexpected illness or injury. The definition of disability refers to the inability to perform either the majority of activities required of a specific occupation (the claimant's own occupation) or any occupation. A surgeon who loses an arm cannot perform his or her occupation but could teach, read radiographs, etc., and would be considered totally disabled under an "own occupation" policy. High benefit policies frequently are challenged by insurance companies when obvious catastrophic impairments are not evident. Pain-related claims require detailed documentation by the treating physician in order to substantiate them. Group policies may pay only for two years while individual policies often pay benefits until age 65 or 70. Some may provide coverage as long as the claimant is gainfully employed in his or her occupation.

TREATING PHYSICIAN vs. EXPERT EXAMINATIONS

In all the scenarios described, the treating physician's records and opinions hold the greatest weight with examiners and judges. A detailed history from the claimant, and, possibly, family and friends, regarding onset of the problem, course of treatment, outcome, and present state, is essential. A careful, comprehensive examination with documentation of all positive findings will prevent claims of physician carelessness and provide the factual basis for opinions. Physical findings should be discoverable by other examiners and symptoms should be consistent with recognized anatomic pathways or physiologic functions. The treater must justify the credibility attributed to his or her statements.

An expert retained by either party provides important medical information and opinions that either confirm or refute the statements of the treating physician. The expert acts as an agent of that party. The opinions, of necessity, are "biased" in favor of the party for whom the expert works, but must be based on careful examination of the patient and/or review of the medical records. The expert's "employer" expects a report that will be beneficial, but the expert must retain objectivity and credibility and avoid flawed and unsubstantiated opinions. There are occasions when the two sides in an adversarial situation agree on an individual to examine a claimant and provide an independent opinion. An adjudicating body (a court, industrial commission, etc.) may request an unbiased evaluation by an expert in the medical condition in question. These represent truly "independent" examinations.

When pain is an issue in the disability determination process, it is important that the examiner documents the nature of the physical changes that are responsible for it or result from it. Observed restriction of movement, spontaneous pain behaviors, and limitations in activities of daily living resulting from the pain are important factors when supporting a disability status. Conversely, inappropriate pain behaviors, evidence of symptom exaggeration and malingering, and symptoms that are anatomically and physiologically impossible should be documented when acting for the insurance company.

In every situation it is obligatory that the "expert" act professionally and honestly, providing opinions based on actual findings in the case. A reputable attorney wants to know the truth about his case. Pursuing a noncredible case is expensive and an unfavorable decision provides no financial benefits. Similarly, defense firms need to know the real medical condition in order to inform their (insurance company) clients about necessary reserves and the monetary potential of an adverse verdict. Many physicians find the role as an expert to be mentally challenging and economically rewarding and enjoy the give-and-take of the legal setting. Many more, however, are terrified of the process. Treating physicians often feel threatened when their judgment is questioned, and become defensive. It is for this reason that detailed documentation of the patient's complaints, physical findings, results of diagnostic testing, and rational justification for treatment rendered, especially invasive anesthetic and surgical procedures, is essential. While there may be differences in opinions between physicians as to a particular course of treatment if the facts are present the treater can securely defend his or her decisions.

DETERMINATION OF IMPAIRMENT

The *Guides to Evaluation of Permanent Impairment* integrate the effects of injury, disease, and disuse in an evaluation process that assesses disturbance in functional use of the affected part or system. The first two chapters of the fourth edition provide the philosophy and methodology of the work. Inherent in the impairment ratings are associated phenomena such as pain and sensory changes. For example, a surgically treated disc lesion with residual medically documented pain receives a higher rating than a similar lesion with no residual symptoms. This is a well-recognized situation, and an additional rating for pain is not warranted. Each affected part, organ, or system must be individually evaluated and documented. Impairment, however, affects the whole person, and the *Guides to Evaluation of Permanent Impairment* are structured according to this principle. Impairment of a finger relates to a percentage of the hand, which is a proportion of the upper extremity, which is a percentage of the whole person (Tables 9-1 and 9-2). If multiple parts and/or systems are affected, each impairment percentage is determined and the cumulative impairment is established, based on the grid located at the end of the book that facilitates this process.

The concept behind use of the *Guides to Evaluation of Permanent Impairment* is that any competent physician who utilizes the methods described should arrive at a determination of impairment consistently comparable to that determined by another evaluator. Another essential concept is that the condition being evaluated is stable and permanent. No attempt to determine impairment should be made until complete resolution has occurred. If additional treatment can be expected to improve function, it should be recommended; if the treatment is carried out, re-evaluation should be performed subsequently. The chapter on pain discusses how residual pain interferes with performance of activities of daily living. It utilizes a grid arrangement (Table 9-3) whereby an individual's symptoms are classified in terms of intensity vs. frequency, and an impairment rating is assigned on the basis of the examiner's perception of the problem. There is no way to objectify pain. This assessment is entirely dependent on the patient's statements regarding pain characteristics (location and distribution, quality, intensity, duration, frequency of occurrence, and precipitating and relieving factors) and on the examiner's experience with similar conditions (either personally or through training), his or her belief in the patient's description, and personal bias.

Impairment for psychiatric reasons is based on an individual's inability to perform in society because of his or her mental and emotional disturbances. The chapter "Mental and Behavioral Disorders" requires determination of a diagnosis based on specific criteria as set forth in the fourth edition of the *Diagnostic and Statistical Manual of Mental Disorders* (DSM-IV).[3] This mandates obtaining a detailed history from the patient regarding onset, precipitating causes, duration, periodicity, and interference in functional state caused by the disorder. A person with a mental disorder is often least qualified to provide an accurate statement concerning these matters. Other observers (e.g., family, friends, previous treaters) need to be interviewed or their records and/or reports reviewed to determine the chronologic and longitudinal aspects of a mental disorder; this is a time-consuming process that is rarely carried out. A clever, tutored person could easily recite the appropriate statements to establish the presence of a major emotional disturbance if he or she were trying to gain a disability rating.

Unlike physical impairments, those relating to pain and psychiatric issues are almost entirely dependent on the clinician's judgment. There are projective tests (e.g., Rorschach test, Thematic Apperception Test) that provide some measurable data regarding mental impairment and thought disorders and are useful in confirming such a diagnosis. The Minnesota Multiphasic Personality Interview (Revised Version) (MMPI-2)[4] is a well-established means of determining a person's affective and attitudinal self-perception and likely behavioral response in various situations. The validity measures built in to this instrument can be utilized effectively to determine whether responses meet criteria for credibility or represent the subjects' attempts to make themselves appear more or less impaired than they are.

DETERMINATION OF RESTRICTIONS

The limitations imposed on a person based on a specific set of impairments are usually related to the training and experience of the evaluator. A student adopts principles and practices espoused by a respected mentor, but, hopefully, modifies them on the basis of subsequent experience. Lifting, carrying, walking, sitting—all the varied activities of daily living—may be restricted in an injured subject because of the nature of the original problem, the effects of surgical and other treatments employed to correct it, and potential future problems if restrictions are not imposed. Examiner bias often also plays a role. When setting limits for a personal patient the physician tends to be more lenient regarding duration of recovery time and restrictions following return to work or other activities. When evaluating a person as a retained medical examiner the physician tends to be more rigorous and demanding of higher levels of performance. Realistically, financial issues (keeping the patient in the practice) or legal considerations (concern about legal action if the person is judged to be fit and claims re-injury on return to work) may cloud the objectivity of the evaluation process.

In an attempt to objectify this process, many physicians and insurance companies rely on the findings of a functional capacity evaluation (FCE) and/or work capacity evaluation (WCE). Several standardized protocols have been established, but all require that a person perform a set number of different tasks over a measured period of time in various positions. Validity measures are built in, and some incorporate the Waddell criteria[5] as measures of symptom magnification. Because all of these protocols allow the person to discontinue an activity on the basis of pain or fatigue, for example, similar activities presented in a different format (for distraction) allow the evaluator to confirm the disparity or reproducibility of performance. Motivation on the part of the examinee also is crucial. A person who makes no attempt to perform at maximal effort will, predictably, have a poor outcome, and the performance will be unreliable as an indicator of the person's physical activity potential.

An FCE assesses the maximum physical performance of a person and determines limits that should allow for regular, consistent performance. If the maximum lift is 50 lb, the person would not be expected to perform at that level continuously. Reducing the lift by 20% permits a 40 lb lift occasionally, and reducing it by 30% justifies a 35 lb lift on a regular basis. Tolerances for sitting, standing, walking, and climbing, for example, can be determined in a similar fashion, by direct observation during a given timed session and extrapolation for longer periods. For this reason, an FCE should be carried out for at least 5 to 6 hours, preferably over a span of 2 days to establish a confident analysis.

A WCE gauges an individual's ability to carry out all of the numerous physical tasks required in the performance of

TABLE 9-1. **RELATIONSHIP OF IMPAIRMENT OF THE DIGITS TO IMPAIRMENT OF THE HAND***

% Impairment					
Thumb	**Hand**	**Index or Middle Finger**	**Hand**	**Ring or Little Finger**	**Hand**
0–1	= 0	0–2	= 0	0–4	= 0
2–3	= 1	3–7	= 1	5–14	= 1
4–6	= 2	8–12	= 2	15–24	= 2
7–8	= 3	13–17	= 3	25–34	= 3
9–11	= 4	18–22	= 4	35–44	= 4
12–13	= 5	23–27	= 5	45–54	= 5
⋮	⋮ ⋮	⋮	⋮ ⋮	55–64	= 6
49–51	= 20	73–77	= 15	65–74	= 7
52–53	= 21	78–82	= 16	75–84	= 8
54–56	= 22	83–87	= 17	85–94	= 9
57–58	= 23	88–92	= 18	95–100	= 10
59–61	= 24	93–97	= 19		
62–63	= 25	98–100	= 20		
64–66	= 26				
⋮	⋮ ⋮				
87–88	= 35				
89–91	= 36				
92–93	= 37				
94–96	= 38				
97–98	= 39				
99–100	= 40				

* The table is illustrative only. Material has been deliberately deleted for brevity. Deletions indicated by dotted lines.
Modified from Guides to the Evaluation of Permanent Impairment, ed 4. American Medical Association, Chicago, 1993.

a specific job. Availability of heavy tools, special equipment, and mock-up vehicles, for example, are necessary for this evaluation, and only specialized centers are equipped to properly perform these assessments. Sedentary and light-level jobs can be simulated more easily, and a determination of ability to perform them can be made in the regular physical and occupational therapy department settings. It is acceptable for a physician to rely on the results of such testing to specify restrictions for an individual only if the results are valid and are based on maximal effort and motivation; less effort on the part of the

TABLE 9-2. **RELATIONSHIP OF IMPAIRMENT OF THE HAND TO IMPAIRMENT OF THE UPPER EXTREMITY***

% Impairment					
Hand	Upper extremity	Hand	Upper extremity	Hand	Upper extremity
0	= 0	17	= 15	68	= 61
1	= 1	⋮	⋮ ⋮	69	= 62
2	= 2	53	= 48	⋮	⋮ ⋮
3	= 3	54	= 49	88	= 79
4	= 4	55	= 50	89	= 80
5	= 5	56	= 50	90	= 81
6	= 5	57	= 51	91	= 82
7	= 6	58	= 52	92	= 83
8	= 7	59	= 53	93	= 84
9	= 8	60	= 54	94	= 85
10	= 9	61	= 55	95	= 86
11	= 10	62	= 56	96	= 86
12	= 11	63	= 57	97	= 87
13	= 12	64	= 58	98	= 88
14	= 13	65	= 59	99	= 89
15	= 14	66	= 59	100	= 90
16	= 14	67	= 60		

*The table is illustrative only. Material has been deliberately deleted for brevity. Deletions indicated by dotted lines.
Modified from Guides to the Evaluation of Permanent Impairment, ed 4. American Medical Association, Chicago, 1993.

subject produces a flawed outcome and the results would be unreliable.

JOB REQUIREMENTS

In order to determine a claimant's ability to return to work the physician must be provided with an accurate and complete job description for the individual in question. This must include not only the purpose of the job (what should be accomplished as a result of its performance) but also its physical and cognitive requirements. It is not enough to rely on a written job description provided by the claimant's company if it is several years old, particularly when it is at great variance with the description given by the claimant. This information can be obtained from a case manager or vocational specialist if involved in the case. In other circumstances the human relations department of the employer often will provide this information.

With regard to the physical requirements, the physician must be made aware of how much actual time is spent performing various tasks. Sitting, standing, walking, climbing, lifting, and carrying, etc., must be known. Other factors include the weights of items lifted, carried, pushed, or pulled; how

TABLE 9-3. **PAIN INTENSITY–FREQUENCY GRID**

Intensity	Frequency			
	Intermittent	Occasional	Frequent	Constant
Minimal				
Slight				
Moderate				
Marked				

Modified from Guides to the Evaluation of Permanent Impairment, ed 4. American Medical Association, Chicago, 1993.

often the task is performed in an hour or a day; what positions are required of the neck, upper limbs, trunk, and legs; and how often various movements are performed by the components of the upper limbs, for example. If the physical demands exceed the claimant's capabilities an alternative job must be considered.

From a cognitive perspective, the physician must understand the amount of decision-making required by the patient as compared to performance of simple repetitive activities. Other affective considerations include the amount of required interaction with co-workers, supervisors, and outsiders, and the level of stress induced by production quotas. Knowledge of these and other issues is essential for the physician to provide a realistic and reasonable statement regarding the claimant's potential to return successfully to work.

ACCOMMODATIONS

It is reasonable to suggest simple accommodations or modification at work to enable an impaired, handicapped worker to perform his or her job, or another job, as mandated by the Americans With Disabilities Act.[6] The vast majority of accommodations or work-site modifications cost less than $300. These recommendations may emanate from the evaluator's own clinical experience with other patients with similar problems or may reflect observations and statements contained in the FCE/WCE reports. The optimal vocational outcome would be for the injured person to return to his or her previous job for the previous employer. An uncooperative employer creates major problems in returning an injured person to work, and alternative jobs must be identified and located.

SUMMARY

The treating physician should use his or her best judgment in providing care for the injured person. Neither over- nor under-treatment is appropriate, no matter who pays the medical bills. The overriding goal should be to return the claimant to normal activity, including work. Creating an invalid does not benefit the claimant and does not enhance the value of the claim. Iatrogenic impairment due to unnecessary treatment or over-medication may prevent the patient from performing requisite activities of daily living and engaging in social and recreational activities that add quality to life. The evaluating expert physician has obligations to the injured person, the party that retained him or her, and society to perform a scrupulous examination of the claimant and to provide as honest and appropriate a report as possible.

Although reasonable minds might differ to some extent regarding physical capability, if FCE/WCE results are available those differences should be slight. There should be no disagreement between examiners about the nature or degree of impairment if both utilize the AMA *Guides to the Evaluation of Permanent Impairment*. For those reasons, a claims examiner, Social Security adjudicator, Industrial Commission arbitrator, or other insurance administrator realistically should be able to determine disability on the basis of the information provided by the physician.

REFERENCES

1. Guides to the Evaluation of Permanent Impairment, ed 4. American Medical Association, Chicago, 1993.
2. US Department of Health and Human Services, Social Security Administration, Office of Operational Policy and Procedures: Social Security Regulations: Rules for Determining Disability and Blindness, 4.04, 1505. SSA Publication No. 64-014. US Government Printing Office, Washington, DC, 1981.
3. Diagnostic and Statistical Manual of Mental Disorders: DSM-IV ed 4. American Psychiatric Association, Washington, DC, 1994.
4. Butcher JN, Dahlstrom WG, Graham J, et al: Minnesota Multiphasic Personality Inventory-2 (MMPI-2): Manual for Administration and Scoring. University of Minnesota Press, Minneapolis, 1989.
5. Waddell G, McCullock JA, Kummel E, et al: Nonorganic physical signs in low-back pain. Spine 5:117, 1980.
6. US Department of Justice: The Americans with Disabilities Act [brochure]. US Government Printing Office, Washington, DC, 1991.

FURTHER READING

Dusik LA, Menard MR, Cooke C, et al: Concurrent validity of the ERGOS work simulator versus conventional functional capacity evaluation techniques in a workers' compensation population. J Occup Med 35:759, 1993.

Isernhagen SJ: Role of functional capacities assessment after rehabilitation. *In* Bullock MI (ed): Ergonomics: The Physiotherapist in the Workplace. Churchill Livingstone, New York, 1990, p 259.

Matheson LN: Functional capacity evaluation. *In* Demeter SL, Andersson GBJ, Smith GM (eds): Disability Evaluation. Mosby-Year Book, St. Louis, 1996, p 168.

Nadolsky JM: Social Security: In need of rehabilitation. J Rehabil 50:6, 1984.

Turk DC, Rudy TE, Stieg RL: The disability determination dilemma: Toward a multiaxial solution. Pain 34:217, 1988.

Ziporyn T: Disability evaluation: A fledgling science? JAMA 250:873, 1983.

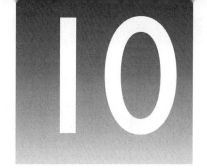

Opioid Receptors

Mark Holtsman, Pharm.D., and
Scott M. Fishman, M.D.

Research over the past 25 years has dramatically increased our knowledge of the sites where opioids take effect and their mechanisms of action.[1] Opiates had been used for their pain releving effects for thousands of years before researchers discovered opioid receptors in the brain in 1973. Later endogenous opioid peptides were discovered in 1975.[2–5] Opioid receptors and endogenous opioid peptides combine to form a complex neurotransmitter system known as the endogenous opioid system.[6]

OPIOID RECEPTOR PHARMACOLOGY

Opioid Pharmacodynamics: Analgesia from opioids varies greatly between individuals because of unique differences in each opioid system. For example, in a study looking at morphine doses required to produce adequate analgesia after C sections, researchers found that women using morphine via patient-controlled analgesia (PCA) pumps required from 0.6 to 5.2 mg/hour of intravenous morphine to achieve the same level of pain relief.[7,8] These variations are due to the differences in morphology and physiology of opioid systems between individuals.

The opioid system consists of at least three distinct opioid receptors: mu, kappa, and delta. These receptors are widely distributed in the brain, spinal cord, and peripheral nociceptors. At one time a fourth opioid receptor designated sigma was proposed, but research has since proven this receptor to be an NMDA subtype of the glutamate receptor. The recent discovery of a sensory neuron-specific G-protein-coupled receptor, which binds proenkephalin A with high affinity, raises the possibility that more distinct opioid receptors may be defined in the future.[9]

Opioid receptors are found at the pre and postsynaptic sites of the ascending pain transmission system in the dorsal horn of the spinal cord, the brain stem, thalamus, and the cortex. Opioid receptors are also found in the midbrain periaqueductal gray, the nucleus raphe magnus, and the rostral ventral medulla, that comprise the descending inhibitory system modulating spinal pain transmission.[10] Opioid receptors bind to three major groups of endogenous opioid peptides including enkephalins, endorphins, and dynorphins (Table 10-1).

Opioid receptors are activated by exogenous opiates (such as morphine) or endogenous peptides (such as beta-endorphin) modulating nociception, the reward pathways, and responses to stress. Recent studies that used mice to target single and combinatorial opioid receptors support the existence of an antinociceptive opioid tone. Mu receptors influence responses to mechanical, chemical, and thermal nociception at a supraspinal level. Kappa receptors appear to modulate spinally mediated thermal nociception and chemical visceral pain. Delta receptors may modulate mechanical nociception and inflammatory pain. Thus, endogenous opioid peptides bind to opioid receptors to modulate nociceptive information and control pain sensitivity.[11] Opioid receptors have extracellular, transmembrane regions that provide receptor specificity and intracellular regions that link to G proteins. Activation of the opioid receptor sends a signal via potassium ion channels and protein kinase C enzyme systems located in the cytosol and cell membrane resulting in reduction of both action potential duration and neurotransmitter release (Fig. 10-1).[12]

Opioid Agonists: Opioid agonist analgesics bind predominantly to the mu receptor and can be grouped into three distinct chemical classes: phenanthrene opioid agonists, phenylpiperidine opioid agonists, or the diphenylhepatane opioid agonists. The first class includes morphine, hydromorphone, codeine, oxycodone, oxymorphone, and hydrocodone. The second class includes meperidine, fentanyl, sufentanil, alfentanil, and remifentanyl. The third class contains methadone and propoxyphene.

Mu receptor activation generates desired effects such as analgesia and adverse effects such as constipation. Research with mice using gene targeting (knockout) technology to disrupt the codes for each of the three opioid receptors has confirmed the central role of the mu receptor in mediating both analgesia and adverse effects. Mice lacking the mu receptor did not respond to morphine with any responses of analgesia, respiratory depression, constipation, physical dependence, or reward behaviors.[13]

Opioid Agonist–Antagonist Analgesics: Opioid agonist–antagonist analgesics bind to one opioid receptor activating agonist activity that goes on to bind to another opioid

TABLE 10-1. **OPIOID RECEPTOR TYPES**[1,46,74–77]

Receptor Type	Ligand		
	Endogenous Agonist	Exogenous Agonist	Exogenous Antagonist
μ	β-endorphin	Morphine	Naloxone
δ	Enkephalin	TAN-67	Naltrindole
κ	Dynorphin	TRK-820	Norbinaltorphimine

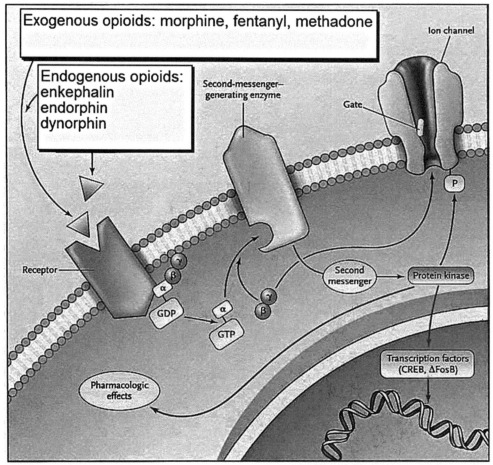

FIGURE 10-1. Metabotropic (G-protein-coupled) receptors mediate slow synaptic transmission. G proteins are trimeric structures composed of two functional units: an α subunit that catalyzes GTPase activity (converting guanosine triphosphate (GTP) to guanosine diphosphate (GDP)) and a β–γ dimer that interacts with the α subunit when bound to GDP (inactive state). The binding of the agonist activates a nearby G protein. The α subunit bound to GTP subsequently dissociates from its β and γ subunits. Both can activate or inhibit enzymes (adenylyl cyclase or phospholipase C) that synthesize second messengers such as cyclic adenosine monophosphate (cAMP), cyclic guanosine monophosphate, inositol triphosphate, and diacylglycerol. In addition, the β and γ subunits directly regulate calcium-, sodium-, and potassium-ion channels. Second messengers also regulate ion channels by activating protein kinases, which phosphorylate (P) such channels. Protein kinases induce pharmacologic effects and produce changes in transcription factors such as cAMP-responsive element-binding protein (CREB) and ΔfosB. Opioids bind to opioid receptors (which reduce cAMP levels). (Modified with permission from Cami J, Farree M: N Engl J Med 349:975–986, 2003.)

receptor producing no or low receptor activation (antagonist activity). Commercially available examples of opioid agonist–antagonist analgesics include butorphanol, nalbuphine, and pentazocine. These agents are agonists at the kappa receptor and antagonists at the mu receptor. If given to a patient with a history of chronic opiate use and physical dependence to opiates, the opioid agonist–antagonist analgesics can precipitate opioid withdrawal symptoms.

Opioid Partial-Agonist Analgesics: Opioid partial-agonist analgesics bind to an opioid receptor producing a fraction of the full agonist response.[14] Buprenorphine is an example of a partial agonist at the mu receptor. Buprenorphine is gaining interest for use in patients with addiction histories. The use of a partial agonist agent can offer some analgesia which may have a ceiling effect. Later administration of full agonists can result in partial antagonism effects.

Opioid Antagonists: Opioid antagonists bind to opioid receptors producing no or low antagonist activity that may reverse or inhibit the effects of opioid agonists by preventing receptor access. Naloxone, naltrexone, and nalmefene are commercially available opioid antagonists. Naloxone and nalmefene are useful for reversing opioid-induced sedation and respiratory depression. Naltrexone is used in the treatment of both opiate and alcohol addiction.[15]

Opioid Phamacokinetics: Opioid analgesics have significant interindividual variability in both absorption into and clearance from the body. This variability requires that each patient receive a dose titrated to produce the desired response with a chosen opioid agent. To illustrate, consider hydromorphone, a useful opioid analgesic for the treatment of moderate to severe pain. Hydromorphone has an oral bioavailability of approximately 51%, but ranges from 10% to 65% as the medication undergoes extensive presystemic liver elimination (first pass hepatic metabolism).[16,17] The elimination half-life of hydromorphone varies from 1 to 4 hours after oral administration. As a result, patients may experience analgesic effects within 30 minutes after administration of a dose and continue to have pain relief for 2 to 4 hours afterward.[18]

Opioids such as hydromorphone and morphine are metabolized in the liver via uridine diphosphate glucuronosyl transferase (UGT) enzymes. Adding a glucuronic acid moiety to the drugs produces the metabolites hydromorphone-3-glucuronide, morphine-6-glucuronide, and morphine-3-glucuronide. Each of these metabolites is then excreted renally and may potentially produce both desirable and undesirable effects especially in patients with significant renal dysfunction.[19] The widely used opioids fentanyl and methadone are metabolized primarily by cytochrome P450 enzymes, designated CYP3A4, to inactive the metabolites norfentanyl, EDDP, and the N-demethylated methadone.[20] As a result, both fentanyl and methadone can interact with drugs that affect the CYP3A4 isoenzymes. Some drugs, such as macrolide antibiotics (erythromycin), inhibit CYP3A4 enzymes resulting in the possible decreased clearance of fentanyl and methadone. Other drugs like the anticonvulsant phenytoin cause CYP3A4 enzyme induction that results in increased clearance of fentanyl and methadone.[21,22] As most opioid analgesics are metabolized by the liver to active or inactive metabolites, patient hepatic function, renal function, and potential drug interactions must be assessed and the opioid analgesic regimen tailored to the individual patient's analgesic requirements.

RECEPTOR ACTIVITY INVOLVED IN OPIOID ADVERSE EFFECTS

Common Side Effects

CONSTIPATION: Constipation is the most common opioid side effect and can cause patients to experience abdominal pain, bloating, nausea and vomiting, and urinary retention.[23] Endogenous opioid peptides and opioid receptors are located in the digestive tract with high concentrations in the gastric antrum and proximal duodenum.[24] While it is thought that opioids may produce constipation via several mechanisms, the most significant is the decrease in intestinal motility which results in increased colonic transit time.[25]

Opioid analgesics and their active metabolites have differing actions on opioid receptors which subsequently may have differing effects on the gastrointestinal tract. For example, the active metabolite of morphine, morphine-6-glucuronide, is also a potent mu receptor agonist capable of inhibiting gastrointestinal transport. There is currently little data available to indicate that particular opioids at equianalgesic dosages produce different levels of constipation. Recent comparative trials of transdermal fentanyl vs. sustained-release morphine showed a trend towards less constipation in the fentanyl group but the trials were not well controlled. Opioid antagonists such as naloxone given orally have been studied in patients with opioid-induced constipation with mixed results. While some patients had bowel evacuation within 1 to 4 hours after a naloxone dose others experienced withdrawal symptoms.[26–28]

Opioid-induced constipation can be treated with laxatives but there is no research demonstrating a clear advantage of one laxative over another. Treatment with a stool softener such as docusate and a stimulant laxative such as senna, lactulose, and/or bisacodyl on a regular prophylactic basis often allows patients on opioid analgesics to have regular bowel movements and avoid the symptoms associated with constipation.[29,30]

NAUSEA AND VOMITING: Nausea and vomiting are common opioid side effects. These side effects can be so severe that patients choose to suffer with significant pain rather than endure the nausea associated with taking an opioid dose. Fortunately, these patients usually develop rapid tolerance to opioid-induced nausea. Opioid-induced nausea and vomiting is mediated by opioid receptors in the chemoreceptor trigger zone. Animal studies show these side effects can be prevented by pretreatment with naloxone and blocked by methylnaltrexone, a quaternary opioid antagonist with peripherally restricted action. This suggests opioid-induced emesis is produced by opioid receptors outside the blood–brain barrier. The chemoreceptor trigger zone, known as the area postrema, has an incomplete blood–brain barrier and is available to interact with peripheral opioid antagonists.[31,32]

Opioids can cause nausea and vomiting via several mechanisms including stimulating the vestibular apparatus, chemoreceptor trigger zone, and, as mentioned previously, constipation. As a result, clinicians need to assess the patient's complaints of nausea to determine when the patient last had a bowel movement, whether or not the nausea gets worse with movement, and if there is a temporal relationship between opioid dose administration and onset of nausea. Nausea secondary to stimulation of the vestibular apparatus usually decreases when treated with meclizine, promethazine, or scopolamine. Nausea associated with stimulation of the chemoreceptor trigger zone is often controlled with droperidol, prochlorperazine, ondansetron, or hydroxyzine. In some patients multiple mechanisms may be involved at the onset of nausea and vomiting. These patients may require two or more antiemetic agents simultaneously in order to control their nausea.[33,34]

SEDATION: Opioids can produce sedation and drowsiness, especially in opioid-naive patients or in patients undergoing chronic opioid therapy following opioid dose escalation. The presence of pain may antagonize the sedating effects of opioids. Once the patients are on stable doses of opioids for an extended period of time, tolerance to the sedating effects of opioids usually develops. Most patients on stable doses of opioids for at least seven days have no psychomotor impairment.[35–37] This observation is very important as some clinicians routinely counsel their patients to never drive while on opioids. As more cancer and noncancer patients have lived for years with moderate to severe pain requiring opioid therapy, evidence has accumulated showing that patients on long-term opioid therapy are alert enough to drive safely.[38,39] Some patients may continue to experience intolerable sedation with chronic opioid therapy. Usually, these patients have contributing factors including additive drug interactions between central nervous system (CNS) depressant medications (e.g., antiemetics), renal and/or hepatic dysfunction, neuropathic pain, disease-related fatigue, or intracerebral metastases.[40] Minimizing other CNS depressant medications, lowering the opioid dose in comfortable patients, utilizing nonopioid adjuvant analgesics, switching opioids, and/or starting psychostimulants such as methylphenidate can help alleviate sedation in the patient requiring chronic opioid therapy.

ITCHING: Generalized itching is a common side effect of opioids and is found more frequently in patients receiving neuraxial opioids than in those utilizing opioids given by the oral or parenteral route. Usually this side effect is mild and does not require treatment. Some opioid agonists such as morphine can produce histamine release and may stimulate itching by activating (H1) receptors on itch-specific C fibers. Other opioids such as fentanyl do not produce clinically significant histamine release but cause itching via another mechanism. Proposed opioid-induced itching mechanisms include involvement of serotonergic receptors and/or mu and kappa receptors. Recent studies have shown ondansetron, a 5HT3-receptor antagonist, decreases itch caused by intrathecal morphine as well as intrathecal fentanyl but not the combination of intrathecal morphine and sufentanil.[41–43] Nalbuphine, a mu receptor antagonist and kappa receptor agonist, works effectively to reduce itching in patients receiving epidural or intrathecal morphine without reversing analgesia.[44,45] A recent animal study provides evidence suggesting stimulation of kappa receptors by a kappa opioid receptor-selective agonist (TRK-820) inhibits itching induced by histamine and substance P.[46]

Less Common Side Effects
RESPIRATORY DEPRESSION: Respiratory depression is rare in patients whose opioid dose is carefully titrated to the desired analgesic effect. When respiratory depression is seen, it is usually in opioid-naive patients following acute administration of an opioid. This is usually heralded by increasing sedation and decreased respiratory rate. Opioid agonists activate mu receptors in the brainstem respiratory centers decreasing both hypoxic and hypercapnic respiratory drive, resulting in respiratory depression.[47–50]

Pain is a physiological antagonist of the respiratory depressant effects of opioids. As a result, opioid dose reductions should be anticipated and initiated in patients whenever sudden pain relief may occur. Patients that may experience sudden pain relief include those treated with effective neurolytic procedures, radiation therapy, adjuvant analgesics (e.g., corticosteroids), surgical procedures, or those with disease progression compromising pain pathways.[51,52]

When the adult patient cannot be aroused and opioid overdose is strongly suspected, 0.4 mg of naloxone can be diluted in 10 cm³ of normal saline and administered in 0.5 cm³ boluses every 2 minutes. Children and adults weighing less than 40 kg should be given 0.5 µg/kg IV naloxone every 2 minutes. The naloxone dose should be titrated to avoid precipitation of profound withdrawal, seizures, and severe pain, especially in patients on opioid analgesics for greater than one week. The patient should then be closely observed as naloxone has a shorter duration of action than most opioid agonist analgesics.[53]

COGNITIVE DYSFUNCTION: When opioid-naive patients are started on opioid analgesics, a decrease in speed of reaction with minimal or no reduction in accuracy is seen in studies examining the psychomotor and cognitive effects of opioids. As a result, clinicians should warn their patients that cognitive impairment could occur with the initiation of opioid therapy and with dose increases of at least 30%. Tolerance usually develops to this side effect over several days of continuous opioid therapy. Patients should be counseled not to drive for 7 days after initiation of opioid therapy or opioid dose escalation in patients on chronic opioid therapy. After 7 days of continuous opioid therapy, patients may choose to drive but should not drive if they ever feel sedated, unsteady, or cognitively impaired. In addition, they should not utilize alcohol, cannabinoids, or other medications known to produce sedation such as benzodiazepines or over-the-counter antihistamines.[54]

DELIRIUM: Opioid-induced delirium is uncommon in patients treated with opioids for noncancer-related pain. In patients with cancer-related pain the incidence of opioid-induced delirium is greater especially in the terminally ill cancer patient. Opioids have been reported to be the chief cause of delirium in 27% of cancer patients consulting a specialized pain service with refractory pain.[55] Opioid metabolites may contribute to delirium especially in patients with decreased renal function. Work by several investigators has implicated higher plasma levels of morphine-6-glucuronide and morphine-3-glucuronide as being associated with development of delirium in cancer patients. Normeperidine, the toxic metabolite of meperidine, has also been implicated in the development of delirium. Each of these metabolites requires clearance by the kidneys thus putting patients with decreased renal function at greater risk for development of delirium when using morphine or meperidine.[56,57] Patients with significant risk factors for development of delirium or those showing signs of cognitive impairment after being on chronic stable opioid doses often benefit by switching to an alternative opioid analgesic without active metabolites cleared by the kidneys such as fentanyl and methadone, or with less active metabolites such as oxycodone and hydromorphone.[58,59]

MYOCLONUS: At high doses, all of the opioid analgesics can cause multifocal myoclonus. This side effect is most commonly seen with patients on higher doses of morphine and meperidine that have decreased renal function as the metabolites morphine-3-glucuronide and normeperidine accumulate in these patients. Normeperidine, with its elimination half-life of 14 to 21 hours, can precipitate myoclonus and occasionally seizures in patients with normal renal function when meperidine is repeatedly given.[60]

FUTURE DIRECTIONS IN OPIOID ANALGESIA

Opioid Agonist–Antagonist Combinations: Evidence suggests opioid antagonists at ultra-low doses may potentiate the analgesic effects of opioid agonists and decrease development of opioid tolerance. This may occur through inhibition of an opioid-mediated excitatory effect (prolongation of the action potential) believed to be involved with the activation of $Gs\alpha$ protein as a second messenger. Animal studies provide evidence that naltrexone, in ultra-low doses, enhances morphine analgesia and inhibits or reverses tolerance. A recently published case report demonstrated ultra-low doses of naltrexone (1 μg orally twice a day) administered to a patient decreased his opioid-induced side effects and increased his sensitivity to methadone.[61–63] In a study investigating the effects of low-dose naloxone infusions on morphine PCA use, a group of patients receiving 0.25 μg/kg/hour IV naloxone used less morphine to control their pain and had a lower incidence of opioid-induced side effects such as nausea and itching.[64] Other investigators utilizing combinations of naloxone and morphine administered via PCA machines have not been able to duplicate these results.[65,66] At least one phase III clinical trial is underway comparing the analgesic efficacy of a combination product containing oxycodone and naltrexone with oxycodone and placebo. The naltrexone has been added in combination to oxycodone with the goal of enhancing analgesia and attenuating tolerance, physical dependence, and addiction.

Peripheral Opioid Agonists: Efforts to find analgesics that treat specific types of pain such as visceral pain without dose-limiting opioid-induced side effects have led to studies of peripheral kappa receptor agonists such as ADL 10-0101 that minimally penetrate the brain producing no central side effects at doses less than 300 μg/kg. Investigators administered ADL 10-0101 at 10 μg/kg/minute over 30 minutes to a small number of patients with chronic pancreatitis pain and observed reductions in pain scores ranging from 14% to 100%. No severe side effects were observed in any patient. Early study results suggest that opioids that target specific opioid receptors or subreceptors within a receptor class may offer greater analgesia with reduced side-effect profiles. These novel, targeted opioids may treat pain states that presently have poor responses to conventional opioids.[67,68]

Opioid Neuropeptide Gene Regulator Analgesics and Gene Therapy: Research on genetic expression of endogenous opioid neuropeptides suggests that there are targets for medications that may allow a patient to increase his or her own production of endogenous opioids. Proteins that regulate dynorphin production have been identified. Modification of these proteins through deleting a key transcription factor called downstream regulatory element antagonistic modulator (DREAM) can increase production of dynorphin in the spinal cord. If a medication can be designed to inhibit DREAM activity, then possibly a patient can take a DREAM inhibitor and experience analgesia resulting from increased endogenous dynorphin levels. Other investigators have used a gene gun to deliver genetic material capable of producing endogenous opioid peptides to targeted sites and decrease pain at those sites. Pro-opiomelanocortin (POMC), a precursor molecule for endogenous opioid peptides, can be produced utilizing genetic engineering technology. Human POMC cDNA has been cloned into a modified pCMV plasmid and delivered via a gene gun into the bladder wall of adult female rats. The rats that received POMC gene gun treatments had a decreased nociceptive response to intravesical instillation of acetic acid that could be reversed with naloxone. Increased endorphin immunoreactivity with antiendorphin antibodies was observed in the bladder of gene gun-treated animals.[69–71]

Peripheral Opioid Antagonists: As the mechanisms of opioid-induced side effects become more clearly defined, medications targeting receptors responsible for these side effects are being developed. Methylnaltrexone and Alvimopan are two peripheral opioid antagonists in clinical trials that may become available in the near future. Both medications block opioid receptors in the gut and area postrema but cannot penetrate the blood–brain barrier. As a result, these drugs do not block opioid receptors in the CNS and produce no reversal of analgesia in patients as they decrease constipation and nausea.[72,73]

KEY POINTS

- Opioid analgesics provide clinicians with powerful tools to manage many types of moderate to severe pain.
- Each patient requires careful dose titration of their opioid analgesic to ensure adequate analgesia because of significant variability in opioid pharmacokinetics and pharmacodynamics between patients.
- Opioid analgesics commonly produce side effects such as constipation, nausea, and sedation. Patients rapidly develop tolerance to nausea and sedation from opioids. Constipation can be prevented with stool softeners and stimulant laxatives. In the future, peripheral opioid antagonists may be used to prevent constipation.

REFERENCES

1. Snyder S, Pasternak G: Historical review: Opioid receptors. Trends Pharmacol Sci 24:198–205, 2003.
2. Pert CB, Snyder SH: Opiate receptor: Demonstration in nervous tissue. Science 179:1011–1014, 1973
3. Simon EJ, Hiller JM, Edelman I: Stereospecific binding of the potent narcotic analgesic [3H] etorphine to rat brain homogenate. Proc Natl Acad Sci 70:1947–1949, 1973.
4. Simantov R, Snyder SH: Morphine-like peptides in mammalian brain: Isolation, structure elucidation, and interactions with the opioid receptor. Proc Natl Acad Sci 73:2515–2519, 1976.
5. Hughes J, Kosterlitz HW, et al: Identification of two related pentapeptides from the brain with potent opiate agonist activity. Nature 258:577–579, 1975.
6. Gaveriaux-Ruff C, Kieffer BL: Opioid receptor genes inactivated in mice: The highlights. Neuropeptides 36:62–71, 2002.
7. Eisenach JC, Grice SC, Dewan DM: Patient-controlled analgesia following caesarian section: A comparison with epidural and intramuscular narcotics. Anesthesiology 68:444–448, 1988.

8. Foster DJR, Somogyi AA, Bochner F: Methadone N-demethylation in human liver microsomes: Lack of stereoselectivity and involvement of CYP3A4. Br J Clin Pharmacol 47:403–412, 1999.

9. Lembo PM, et al: Proenkephalin A gene products activate a new family of sensory neuron-specific GPCRs. Nat Neurosci 5:201–209, 2002.

10. Terman G, Bonica JJ: Spinal mechanisms and their modulation. *In* Loeser JD, Butler SD, Chapman CR, et al (eds): Bonica's Management of Pain, ed 3. Lippincott Williams and Wilkins, 2001, pp 73–152.

11. Martin M, Matifas A, Maldonado R, et al: Acute antinociceptive responses in single and combinatorial opioid receptor knockout mice: Distinct mu, delta and kappa tones. Eur J Neurosci 24:198–205, 2003.

12. Suresh S, Anand KJS: Opioid tolerance in neonates: Mechanisms, diagnosis, assessment, and management. Semin Perinatol 22:425–433, 1998.

13. Kieffer BL: Opioids: First lessons from knockout mice. Trends Pharmacol Sci 20:19–26, 1999.

14. Traynor JR, Clark MJ, Remmers AE: Relationship between rate and extent of G protein activation: Comparison between full and partial opioid agonists. J Pharmacol Exp Ther 300:157–161, 2002.

15. Ferrante FM: Principles of opioid pharmacotherapy: Practical implications of basic mechanisms. J Pain Symptom Manage 11:265–273, 1996.

16. Parab PV, Ritschel WA, Coyle DE, et al: Pharmacokinetics of hydromorphone after intravenous, peroral, and rectal administration to human subjects. Biopharm Drug Dispos 9:187–199, 1988.

17. Vallner JJ, Stewart JT, Kotzan JA, et al: Pharmacokinetics and bioavailability of hydromorphone following intravenous and oral administration to human subjects. J Clin Pharmacol 21:152–156, 1981.

18. Sarhill N, Walsh D, Nelson KA: Hydromorphone: Pharmacology and clinical applications in cancer patients. Support Care Cancer 9:84–96, 2001.

19. Armstrong SC, Cozza KL: Pharmacokinetic drug interactions of morphine, codeine, and their derivatives: Theory and clinical reality: I. Psychosomatics 44:167–171, 2003.

20. Labroo RB, Paine MF, Thummel KE, et al: Fentanyl metabolism by human hepatic and intestinal cytochrome P4503A4: Implications for interindividual variability in disposition, efficacy, and drug interactions. Drug Metab Dispos 25:1072–1080, 1997.

21. Davis MP, Walsh D: Methadone for relief of cancer pain: a review of pharmacokinetics, pharmacodynamics, drug interactions and protocols of administration. Support Care Cancer 9:73–83, 2001.

22. Tempelhoff R, Modica PA, Spitznagel EL: Anticonvulsant therapy increases fentanyl requirements during anaesthesia for craniotomy. Can J Anaesth 37:327–332, 1990.

23. Bruera E, Suarez-Almazor M, Velasco A, et al: The assessment of constipation in terminal cancer patients admitted to a palliative care unit: A retrospective review. J Pain Symptom Manage 9:515–519, 1994.

24. Polack JM, Bloom SR: Neuropeptides of the gut: A newly discovered control mechanism. World J Surg 3:393, 1979.

25. DeLuca A, Coupar IM: Insights into opioid action in the intestinal tract. Pharmacol Ther 69:103–115, 1996.

26. Choi YS, Billings JA: Opioid antagonists: A review of their role in palliative care, focusing on use in opioid-related constipation. J Pain Symptom Manage 24:71–90, 2002.

27. Radbruch L, Sabatowski R, Loick G, et al: Constipation and the use of laxatives: A comparison between transdermal fentanyl and oral morphine. Pall Med 14:111–119, 2000.

28. Ahmedzai S, Brooks D: Transdermal fentanyl versus sustained-release oral morphine in cancer pain: Preference, efficacy, and quality of life. J Pain Symptom Manage 13:254–261, 1997.

29. Agra Y, Sacristan A, Gonzalez M, et al: Efficacy of senna versus lactulose in terminal cancer patients treated with opioids. J Pain Symptom Manage 15:1–7, 1998.

30. Inturrisi CE: Clinical pharmacology of opioids for pain. Clin J Pain 18:S3–S13, 2002.

31. Simoneau II, Hamza MS, Mata HP, et al: The cannabonoid agonist WIN55,212–2 suppresses opioid induced emesis in ferrets. Anesthesiology 94:882–887, 2001.

32. Foss JF, Bass AS, Goldberg LI: Dose-related antagonism of the emetic effect of morphine by methylnaltrexone in dogs. J Clin Pharmacol 33:747–751, 1993.

33. Frederich ME: Nonpain symptom management. Prim Care 28:299–316. 2001.

34. Cherny NI, Portenoy RK: The management of cancer pain. CA Cancer J Clin 44:262–303, 1994.

35. Zacny JP: Should people taking opioids for medical reasons be allowed to work and drive? Addiction 91:1581–1584, 1996.

36. Zacny JP: A review of the effects of opiates on psychomotor and cognitive functioning in humans. Exper Clin Psychopharm 3:432–466, 1995.

37. Bruera E, Macmillan K, Hanson J, et al: The cognitive effects of the administration of narcotic analgesics in patients with cancer pain. Pain 39:13–16, 1989.

38. Sabatowski R, Schwalen S, Rettig K, et al: Driving ability under long-term treatment with transdermal fentanyl. J Pain Symptom Manage 25:38–47, 2003.

39. Fishbain, DA, Cutler, RB, Rosomoff HL, et al: Are opioid-dependent/tolerant patients impaired in driving-related skills? A structured evidence-based review. J Pain Symptom Manage 25:559–577, 2003.

40. Lawlor PG: The panorama of opioid-related cognitive dysfunction in patients with cancer. Cancer 94:1836–1853, 2002.

41. Yeh HM, Chen LK, Lin CJ, et al: Prophylactic intravenous ondansetron reduces the incidence of intrathecal morphine induced pruritis in patients undergoing cesarean delivery. Anesth Analg 91:172–175, 2000.

42. Yavuz G, Toker K: Prophylactic ondansetron reduces the incidence of intrathecal fentanyl-induced pruritus. Anesth Analg 95:1763–1766, 2002.

43. Yazigi A, Chalhoub V, Madi-Jebara S, et al: Prophylactic ondansetron is effective in the treatment of nausea and vomiting but not on pruritus after cesarean delivery with intrathecal sufentanil-morphine. J Clin Anesth 14:183–186, 2002.

44. Charuluxananan S, Kyokong O, Somboonviboon W, et al: Nalbuphine versus propofol for treatment of intrathecal morphine-induced pruritus after cesarean delivery. Anesth Analg 93:162–165, 2001.

45. Charuluxananan S, Kyokong O, Somboonviboon W, et al: Nalbuphine versus ondansetron for prevention of intrathecal morphine-induced pruritus after cesarean delivery. Anesth Analg 96:1789–1793, 2003.

46. Togashi Y, Umeuchi H, Okano K, et al: Antipruritic activity of the kappa-opioid receptor agonist, TRK-820. Eur J Pharmacol 435:259–264, 2002.

47. Leino K, Mild L, Lertola K, et al: Time course of changes in breathing pattern in morphine- and oxycodone-induced respiratory depression. Anaesth 54:835–840, 1999.

48. Weil JV, McCulloough RE, Kline JS, et al: Diminished ventilatory response to hypoxia and hypercapnia after morphine in normal man. N Eng J Med 292:1103–1106, 1975.

49. May CN, Dashwood MR, Whitehead CJ, et al: Differential cardiovascular and respiratory responses to central administration of selective opioid agonists in conscious rabbits: Correlation with receptor distribution. Br J Pharmacol 98:903–913, 1989.

50. Dahan A, Sarton E, Teppema L, et al: Anesthetic potency and influence of morphine and sevoflurane on respiration in mu-opioid receptor knockout mice. Anesthesiology 94:824–832, 2001.

51. Hanks GC, Twycross RG, Lloyd JM: Unexpected complication of successful nerve block (morphine-induced respiratory depression precipitated by removal of severe pain). Anaesth 36:37–39, 1981.

52. Quevedo F, Walsh D: Morphine-induced ventilatory failure after spinal cord compression. J Pain Symptom Manage 18:140–142, 1999.

53. Manfredi PL, Ribeiro S, Chandler SW, et al: Inappropriate use of naloxone in cancer patients with pain. J Pain Symptom Manage 11:131–134, 1996.

54. Fishbain DA, Cutler RB, Rosomoff HL, et al: Are opioid-dependent/tolerant patients impaired in driving-related skills? A structured evidence-based review. J Pain Symptom Manage 25:559–577, 2003.

55. Caraceni A, Nanni O, Maltoni C, et al: Impact of delirium on the short term prognosis of advanced cancer patients. Cancer 1;89(5):1145–1149, 2000.

56. Morita T, You T, Tsunoda J, et al: Increased plasma morphine metabolites in terminally ill cancer patients with delirium: An intra-individual comparison. J Pain Symptom Manage 23:107–113, 2002.

57. Eisendrath SJ, Goldman B, Douglas J, et al: Meperidine-induced delirium. Am J Psychiat 144:1062–1065, 1987.

58. de Stoutz ND, Bruera E, Suarez-Almazor M: Opioid rotation for toxicity reduction in terminal cancer patients. J Pain Symptom Manage 10:378–384, 1995.

59. Indelicato RA, Portenoy RK: Opioid roation in the management of refractory cancer pain. J Clin Oncol 20:348–352, 2002.

60. Inturrisi CE. Clinical pharmacology of opioids for pain. Clin J Pain 18:S3–S13, 2002.

61. Crain SM, Shen K-F: Antagonists of excitatory opioid receptor functions enhance morphine's analgesic potency and attenuate opioid tolerance/dependence liability. Pain 84:121–131, 2000.

62. Powell KJ, Abul-Husn NS, Jhamandas A, et al: Paradoxical effects of the opioid antagonist naltrexone on morphine analgesia, tolerance, and reward in rats. J Pharmacol Exp Ther 300:588–596, 2002.

63. Cruciani RA, Lussier D, Arbuck DM, et al: Ultra-low dose oral naltrexone decreases side effects and potentiates the effect of methadone. J Pain Symptom Manage 25:491–494, 2003.

64. Gan TJ, Ginsberg B, Glass PSA, et al: Opioid-sparing effects of a low-dose infusion of naloxone in patient-administered morphine sulfate. Anesthesiology 87:1075–1081, 1997.

65. Cepeda MS, Africano JM, Manrique AM, et al: The combination of low dose of naloxone and morphine in PCA does not decrease opioid requirements in the postoperative period. Pain 96:73–79, 2002.

66. Sartain JB, Barry JJ, Richardson CA, et al: Effect of combining naloxone and morphine for intravenous patient-controlled analgesia. Anesthesiology 99:148–151, 2003.

67. DeHaven-Hudkins DL, Gauntner EK, Gottshall SL, et al: Peripheral restrictions of kappa opioid receptor agonists as defined by pharmacokinetic parameters correlates with behavioral indices of sedation in the rat. Soc Neurosci 26:915, 2000.

68. Eisenach JC, Carpenter R, Curry R: Analgesia from a peripherally active kappa-opioid receptor agonist in patients with chronic pancreatitis. Pain 101:89–95, 2003.

69. Vogt BA: Knocking out the DREAM to study pain. N Engl J Med 347:362–364, 2002.

70. Cheng H-YM, Pitcher GM, Laviolette SR, et al: DREAM is a critical transcriptional repressor for pain modulation. Cell 108:31–43, 2002.

71. Chuang YC, Chou AK, Wu PC, et al: Gene therapy for bladder pain with gene gun particle encoding pro-opiomelanocortin cDNA. J Urol 170:2044–2048, 2003.

72. Choi YS, Billings JA: Opioid antagonists: A review of their role in palliative care, focusing on use in opioid-related constipation. J Pain Symptom Manage 24:71–90, 2002.

73. Friedman JD, Dello Buono FA: Opioid antagonists in the treatment of opioid-induced constipation and pruritus. Ann Pharmacother 35:85–91, 2001.

74. Nagase H, Hayakawa J, Kawamura K, et al: Discovery of a structurally novel opioid κ-agonist derived from 4,5-epoxymorphinan. Chem Pharm Bull 46:366–369, 1998.

75. Ferrante FM: Principles of opioid pharmacotherapy: Practical implications of basic mechanisms. J Pain Symptom Manage 11:265–273, 1996.

76. Tseng LF, Narita M, Mizoguchi H, et al: δ1 opioid receptor-mediated antinociceptive properties of a non-peptidic δ opioid receptor agonist, (–)TAN-67, in the mouse spinal cord. J Pharmacol Exp Ther 280:600–605, 1997.

77. Drower EJ, Stapelfeld A, Rafferty MF, et al: Selective antagonism by naltrindole of the antinociceptive effects of the δ opioid agonist cyclic[D-penicillamine2-D-penicillamine5]-enkephalin in the rat. J Pharmacol Exp Ther 259:725–731, 1991.

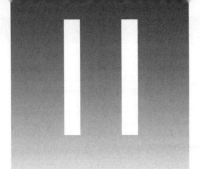

Major Opioids in Pain Management

Gagan Mahajan, M.D., and
Scott M. Fishman, M.D.

While analgesic options are growing each year, opioids continue to remain the "gold standard." The use of opioids has become more widespread and yet remains controversial, with polarized arguments on either side of the debate over their effectiveness in chronic pain. The debate over opioid use in terminally ill patients is less encumbered by social, legal, and professional taboos. Extensive documented experience in treating cancer pain with opioids has broadened the understanding of this important drug therapy that has long been used with apprehension and reluctance. However, opioid use in chronic nonmalignant pain (CNMP) remains controversial.[1–3] Resistance to opioids for CNMP predominantly stems from old or inaccurate understandings of appropriate prescribing and the associated risks of abuse and side effects. This issue is further complicated by societal attitudes and beliefs related to addiction, and the attendant concerns about efficacy, toxicity, abuse potential, physical dependence, and tolerance when using opioids for CNMP. Because the CNMP population varies between those utilizing relatively small and stable doses to those frequently escalating their dosage due to a self-perceived lack of adequate analgesia, rational opioid prescribing should be predicated upon definitive and observable treatment endpoints and management of adverse effects.[4,5] Even in patients with a history of substance abuse and whose acute or chronic pain (malignant or nonmalignant) has not responded to nonopioid regimens (medications, interventional procedures, physical therapy, or behavioral therapy), their abuse history represents a relative contraindication to opioid therapy.

Florence Nightingale first resorted to opium injections to treat her chronic back pain over a century ago.[6] While the decision to implement opioids for the management of acute or chronic pain of malignant origin is far less challenged than ever before, there remains a lack of compelling scientific data to argue convincingly for or against long-term opioid therapy in patients with CNMP. The scarcity of evidence for opioid prescribing with no validated endpoints of analgesic therapy makes its role in clinical practice formidable. Since pain and pain relief are both impossible to prove or refute, clinicians have turned toward improvements in function and quality of life as outcomes that potentially offer observable endpoints of therapy. Nonetheless, measuring the positive and negative impact of treatment with opioids on the patient's quality of life can be time consuming and challenging. This chapter reviews these issues and discusses the principles of opioid selection and usage, including the determination of functional endpoints of opioid therapy in pain of malignant and nonmalignant origin.

RATIONALE

Opioids produce reliable analgesia and their adverse effects (e.g., constipation, nausea and vomiting, sedation, and respiratory suppression) often can be preempted, treated, or reversed. Opioid therapy can be an integral part of a multidisciplinary approach to acute and chronic pain management. An attempt to optimize a patient's pain management may include concurrently combining opioids with nonopioid adjuvant analgesics (nonsteroidal anti-inflammatory drugs (NSAIDs), acetaminophen, antidepressants, anticonvulsants, etc.), physical therapy, psychological therapy, and/or interventional procedures. Much of the debate concerning the role of opioid therapy in CNMP management, however, has centered on whether opioids should be used as a first-line treatment or whether they should be used at all on a chronic basis. Whether or not physicians should withhold opioid therapy until other nonopioid treatment options have failed remains controversial. Although a consensus opinion on this important issue is lacking, health care professionals tend to utilize opioid therapy as a second-line treatment for CNMP for the following reasons: (1) nonopioid medications, such as NSAIDs and anticonvulsants or tricyclic antidepressants, can be efficacious in treating CNMP secondary to arthritic pain[7] and neuropathic pain,[8] respectively; (2) injection therapies can be more effective in certain types of CNMP (e.g., sympathetically maintained pain secondary to complex regional pain syndrome, types I or II) than chronic drug management; and (3) considering the noteworthy side effects and liability profiles of opioid treatment (see below), the risk–benefit ratio often demands that alternative treatments be implemented before instituting opioid therapy.

Although the effectiveness of opioid therapy in certain types of CNMP remains controversial, no evidence suggests an absolute contraindication to opioid therapy under circumstances in which it is not necessarily the first choice. Animal studies have shown a rightward shift of the opioid dose–response curve in experimental models of pain related to nervous system injury,[9,10] suggesting that higher opioid doses may be required for patients primarily suffering from neuropathic pain or other forms of chronic severe pain. The limiting factor for opioid therapy in neuropathic pain treatment may be related to the development of significant side effects associated with the requirement of high opioid dosages rather than to the inherent tolerance found in these pain states. In instances where tolerance is suspected, methadone may offer extra benefits in treating neuropathic pain because of its N-methyl-D-aspartate (NMDA) receptor blocking action that may reduce tolerance to opioids as well as provide analgesia. While these potential benefits of methadone remain intriguing, they have yet to be clinically proven.

In summary, an opioid trial should be considered when alternative analgesics, interventional pain procedures, and physical and psychological therapies have been inadequate, contraindicated, or otherwise exhausted. While nonopioid drugs may appear to be better and/or safer choices for patients with CNMP, long-term use of such agents may have deleterious or life-threatening effects. Furthermore, drugs such as antidepressants and anticonvulsants have been shown to provide only 50% pain relief for one out of three patients.[11] Ultimately, rational opioid prescribing mandates a comprehensive treatment program that includes consideration of alternative therapies that carry relatively less risk, observable treatment endpoints, and ongoing patient follow-up for recognizing and correcting potential adverse effects related to the treatment plan.

GUIDELINES

Since opioids are controlled substances with potential for abuse, they are often associated with stigma as well as regulation by federal and state agencies. One of the major concerns of opioid prescribers is the potential of diversion through fraud, theft, forged prescriptions, or illegal activities of unprincipled health professionals. Several national organizations, including the American Pain Society and the American Academy of Pain Medicine, have developed guidelines for rational approaches to prescribing opioids and avoiding potential adverse effects.[12] In 1998 the House of Delegates of the Federation of State Medical Boards of the United States established and adopted the *Model Guidelines for the Use of Controlled Substances for the Treatment of Pain*, which offers clear practice standards for opioid prescribers (Table 11-1).[13] These guidelines emphasize the importance of an evaluation, physical examination, and follow-up to monitor and evaluate for therapeutic efficacy, which includes the patient's functional status.

TABLE 11-1. **MODEL GUIDELINES FOR THE USE OF CONTROLLED SUBSTANCES FOR THE TREATMENT OF PAIN**
The Federation of State Medical Boards of the United States, Inc.

(Adopted 2 May 1998)

Section I: Preamble

The [name of board] recognizes that principles of quality medical practice dictate that the people of the State of [name of state] have access to appropriate and effective pain relief. The appropriate application of up-to-date knowledge and treatment modalities can serve to improve the quality of life for those patients who suffer from pain as well as to reduce the morbidity and costs associated with untreated or inappropriately treated pain. The Board encourages physicians to view effective pain management as a part of quality medical practice for all patients with pain, acute or chronic, and it is especially important for patients who experience pain as a result of terminal illness. All physicians should become knowledgeable about effective methods of pain treatment as well as statutory requirements for prescribing controlled substances.

Inadequate pain control may result from physicians' lack of knowledge about pain management or an inadequate understanding of addiction. Fears of investigation or sanction by federal, state, and local regulatory agencies may also result in inappropriate or inadequate treatment of chronic pain patients. Accordingly, these guidelines have been developed to clarify the Board's position on pain control, specifically as related to the use of controlled substances, to alleviate physician uncertainty, and to encourage better pain management. The Board recognizes that controlled substances, including opioid analgesics, may be essential in the treatment of acute pain due to trauma or surgery and chronic pain, whether due to cancer or non-cancer origins. Physicians are referred to the US Agency for Health Care and Research Clinical Practice Guidelines for a sound approach to the management of acute* and cancer-related pain.†

* Acute Pain Management Guideline Panel: Acute pain management: Operative or medical procedures and trauma. Clinical Practice Guideline. AHCPR Publication No. 92-0032. Agency for Health Care Policy and Research, Rockville, MD, US Department of Health and Human Resources, Public Health Service, February 1992.
† Jacox A, Carr DB, Payne R, et al: Management of cancer pain. Clinical Practice Guideline No. 9. AHCPR Publication No. 94-0592. Agency for Health Care Policy and Research, Rockville, MD, US Department of Health and Human Resources, Public Health Service, March 1994.

Continued

TABLE 11-1. MODEL GUIDELINES FOR THE USE OF CONTROLLED SUBSTANCES FOR THE TREATMENT OF PAIN—CONT'D
The Federation of State Medical Boards of the United States, Inc.

The medical management of pain should be based upon current knowledge and research and includes the use of both pharmacologic and nonpharmacologic modalities. Pain should be assessed and treated promptly and the quantity and frequency of doses should be adjusted according to the intensity and duration of the pain. Physicians should recognize that tolerance and physical dependence are normal consequences of sustained use of opioid analgesics and are not synonymous with addiction.

The [state medical board] is obligated under the laws of the State of [name of state] to protect the public health and safety. The Board recognizes that inappropriate prescribing of controlled substances, including opioid analgesics, may lead to drug diversion and abuse by individuals who seek them for other than legitimate medical use. Physicians should be diligent in preventing the diversion of drugs for illegitimate purposes.

Physicians should not fear disciplinary action from the Board or other state regulatory or enforcement agency for prescribing, dispensing, or administering controlled substances, including opioid analgesics, for a legitimate medical purpose and in the usual course of professional practice. The Board will consider prescribing, ordering, administering, or dispensing controlled substances for pain to be for a legitimate medical purpose if based on accepted scientific knowledge of the treatment of pain or if based on sound clinical grounds. All such prescribing must be based on clear documentation of unrelieved pain and in compliance with applicable state or federal law.

Each case of prescribing for pain will be evaluated on an individual basis. The board will not take disciplinary action against a physician for failing to adhere strictly to the provisions of these guidelines, if good cause is shown for such deviation. The physician's conduct will be evaluated to a great extent by the treatment outcome, taking into account whether the drug used is medically and/or pharmacologically recognized to be appropriate for the diagnosis, the patient's individual needs including any improvement in functioning, and recognizing that some types of pain cannot be completely relieved.

The Board will judge the validity of prescribing based on the physician's treatment of the patient and on available documentation, rather than on the quantity and chronicity of prescribing. The goal is to control the patient's pain for its duration while effectively addressing other aspects of the patient's functioning, including physical, psychological, social, and work-related factors. The following guidelines are not intended to define complete or best practice, but rather to communicate what the Board considers to be within the boundaries of professional practice.

Section II: Guidelines
The Board has adopted the following guidelines when evaluating the use of controlled substances for pain control:
1. Evaluation of the Patient
   A complete medical history and physical examination must be conducted and documented in the medical record. The medical record should document the nature and intensity of the pain, current and past treatments for pain, underlying or coexisting diseases or conditions, the effect of the pain on physical and psychological function, and history of substance abuse. The medical record should also document the presence of one or more recognized medical indications for the use of a controlled substance.
2. Treatment Plan
   The written treatment plan should state objectives that will be used to determine treatment success, such as pain relief and improved physical and psychosocial function, and should indicate if any further diagnostic evaluations or other treatments are planned. After treatment begins, the physician should adjust drug therapy to the individual medical needs of each patient. Other treatment modalities or a rehabilitation program may be necessary depending on the etiology of the pain and the extent to which the pain is associated with physical and psychosocial impairment.
3. Informed Consent and Agreement for Treatment
   The physician should discuss the risks and benefits of the use of controlled substances with the patient, persons designated by the patient, or with the patient's surrogate or guardian if the patient is incompetent. The patient should receive prescriptions from one physician and one pharmacy where possible. If the patient is determined to be at high risk for medication abuse or have a history of substance abuse, the physician may employ the use of a written agreement between physician and patient outlining patient responsibilities including (1) urine/serum medication levels screening when requested, (2) number and frequency of all prescription refills, and (3) reasons for which drug therapy may be discontinued (i.e., violation of agreement).
4. Periodic Review
   At reasonable intervals based upon the individual circumstance of the patient, the physician should review the course of treatment and any new information about the etiology of the pain. Continuation or modification of therapy should depend on the physician's evaluation of progress toward stated treatment objectives such as improvement in patient's pain intensity and improved physical and/or psychosocial function, such as ability to work, need of health care resources, activities of daily living,

Continued

TABLE 11-1. MODEL GUIDELINES FOR THE USE OF CONTROLLED SUBSTANCES FOR THE TREATMENT OF PAIN—CONT'D
The Federation of State Medical Boards of the United States, Inc.

and quality of social life. If treatment goals are not being achieved, despite medication adjustments, the physician should re-evaluate the appropriateness of continued treatment. The physician should monitor patient compliance in medication usage and related treatment plans.

5. Consultation

The physician should be willing to refer the patient as necessary for additional evaluation and treatment in order to achieve treatment objectives. Special attention should be given to those pain patients who are at risk for misusing their medications and those whose living arrangements pose a risk for medication misuse or diversion. The management of pain in patients with a history of substance abuse or with a comorbid psychiatric disorder may require extra care, monitoring, documentation, and consultation with or referral to an expert in the management of such patients.

6. Medical Records

The physician should keep accurate and complete records to include (1) the medical history and physical examination, (2) diagnostic, therapeutic, and laboratory results, (3) evaluations and consultations, (4) treatment objectives, (5) discussion of risks and benefits, (6) treatments, (7) medications (including date, type, dosage, and quantity prescribed), (8) instructions and agreements, and (9) periodic reviews. Records should remain current and be maintained in an accessible manner and readily available for review.

7. Compliance with Controlled Substances Laws and Regulations

To prescribe, dispense, or administer controlled substances, the physician must be licensed in the state, and comply with applicable federal and state regulations. Physicians are referred to the Physicians Manual of the US Drug Enforcement Administration and [any relevant documents issued by the state medical board] for specific rules governing controlled substances as well as applicable state regulations.

Section III: Definitions

For the purposes of these guidelines, the following terms are defined as follows:

Acute pain: Acute pain is the normal, predicted physiological response to an adverse chemical, thermal, or mechanical stimulus and is associated with surgery, trauma, and acute illness. It is generally time limited and is responsive to opioid therapy, among other therapies.

Addiction: Addiction is a neurobehavioral syndrome with genetic and environmental influences that results in psychological dependence on the use of substances for their psychic effects and is characterized by compulsive use despite harm. Addiction may also be referred to by terms such as "drug dependence" and "psychological dependence." Physical dependence and tolerance are normal physiological consequences of extended opioid therapy for pain and should not be considered addiction.

Analgesic Tolerance: Analgesic tolerance is the need to increase the dose of opioid to achieve the same level of analgesia. Analgesic tolerance may or may not be evident during opioid treatment and does not equate with addiction.

Chronic Pain: A pain state that is persistent and in which the cause of the pain cannot be removed or otherwise treated. Chronic pain may be associated with a long-term incurable or intractable medical condition or disease.

Pain: An unpleasant sensory and emotional experience associated with actual or potential tissue damage or described in terms of such damage.

Physical Dependence: Physical dependence on a controlled substance is a physiologic state of neuroadaptation which is characterized by the emergence of a withdrawal syndrome if drug use is stopped or decreased abruptly, or if an antagonist is administered. Physical dependence is an expected result of opioid use. Physical dependence, by itself, does not equate with addiction.

Pseudoaddiction: Pattern of drug-seeking behavior of pain patients who are receiving inadequate pain management that can be mistaken for addiction.

Substance Abuse: Substance abuse is the use of any substance(s) for nontherapeutic purposes; or use of medication for purposes other than those for which it is prescribed.

Tolerance: Tolerance is a physiologic state resulting from regular use of a drug in which an increased dosage is needed to produce the same effect or a reduced effect is observed with a constant dose.

The guidelines also recommend the use of specialty consultations and additional referrals when patients present with complex histories, troubling adverse effects, or lack of progress towards analgesia or improved function.

ADMINISTRATION

The usual goal of opioid administration for treatment of chronic pain is to achieve sustained analgesia over regular intervals.[14] Use of short-acting opioids in this setting can produce a "roller coaster" effect whereby patients have pain, take analgesics, experience brief periods of relief, followed by repetition of this cycle when the pain returns. Typical chronic opioid therapy aims to avoid perpetuation of this phenomenon by producing stable analgesia that is targeted less at total abolition of pain and more towards augmentation of the patient's function at a tolerable level of pain.

Prescribing opioids for long-term therapy necessitates the consideration of multiple factors. For instance, changing from one opioid to another requires knowledge of equianalgesic dosages. Since cross-tolerance between opioids may be incomplete, a patient who has become tolerant to one opioid can respond with effective analgesia to another opioid of less than equianalgesic dose. Management of pain in tolerant patients can be a challenge because typical dosages for the opioid-naive patient do not apply. In such cases, opioids are slowly and incrementally increased until analgesia with tolerable side effects is reached. The occurrence of analgesia only in conjunction with intolerable side effects indicates that the particular opioid is suboptimal, and there may be a need to change to a different opioid. Analgesia that occurs only in combination with sedation after an individual trial of most or all opioids suggests opioid-insensitive pain. Additionally, analgesia may also have more to do with the effects related to sedation rather than direct antinociceptive properties of the drug. As one would expect, side effects without analgesia indicate failure for that particular opioid. In such cases, another opioid may be worth trying, as it may not share this same profile.

Chronic opioid treatment strategy has recently tended towards using fixed dosing as a superior treatment option to "as needed" (PRN, pro re nata) dosing, with each strategy offering possible advantages for different reasons. Fixed dosing permits consistent delivery for reaching steady state and avoids the peak-and-trough effect associated with on-demand dosing. Such fixed dose schedules with long-acting opioids (LAOs) and sustained-release opioids (SROs) are thought to have less reward-associated reinforcement of potentially dysfunctional cycles where pain and pain medication become a conditioned part of the patient's life. However, such benefits of LAO therapy have not been conclusively proven in the scientific literature. Nonetheless, the use of fixed dosing may prevent delays in delivery that can occur with on-demand schedules.

Due to their longer half-life or sustained delivery, LAOs and SROs may accumulate in fixed doses. This feature may make it more difficult to titrate than shorter-acting opioids (SAOs) upon initiation or change of an LAO or SRO regimen. Patients who are opioid naive may require test dosing that is most safely given on demand. For example, morphine and hydromorphone may take less than 24 hours to reach steady state, whereas levorphanol or methadone can take up to a week. While some clinicians advocate the use of only LAOs or SROs for chronic opioid therapy, employing conservative fixed dosing combined with PRN breakthrough dosing can also be effective in the management of chronic pain, particularly when there is a need to assess a patient's analgesic threshold. However, consensus in this area of pharmacotherapy is elusive at present.

Achievement of safe, effective steady-state levels with regard to fixed dosing intervals is the major benefit of using SROs and LAOs.[15] Various SROs are now available, including morphine (MS-Contin, Oramorph, Kadian, Avinza), oxycodone (Oxycontin), and fentanyl (Duragesic Patch). LAOs, e.g., methadone and levorphanol, are not formulated for sustained release but have intrinsically longer plasma half-lives than other typical opioids such as codeine (Tylenol 2, 3, and 4), propoxyphene (Darvon, Darvocet-N, Darvocent-N 100), hydrocodone (Vicodin, Vicoprofen, Lortab, Lorcet, Norco, Hydrocet, and Zydone), oxycodone (Percocet, Percodan, Endocet, Endodan, Roxicet, Roxicodone, and Tylox), hydromorphone (Dilaudid), or morphine.

The convenience of orally administered opioids has made this the preferred route of delivery. Many patients with cancer or acute postoperative pain, however, are unable to tolerate oral ingestion or temporarily are not permitted oral ingestion. Therefore, having multiple means of administering opioids is advantageous.[16] An intravenous (IV) or subcutaneous (SQ) infusion is commonly used in cancer patients, often with around-the-clock dosing for constant effect. Both routes avoid the first-pass effect and can be supplemented by PRN doses for breakthrough pain. The SQ route has several advantages, including faster onset of analgesia compared with most oral preparations (although slower than IV), uncomplicated access in patients with poor venous access, and safer administration compared with the intramuscular route in patients with bleeding disorders or reduced muscle mass.

A variant of the above is patient-controlled analgesia (PCA), most commonly using morphine, hydromorphone, or fentanyl. Widely used for treating postoperative pain, PCA is rapidly finding broader use in also treating cancer pain. PCA immediately delivers a preprogrammed IV or SQ dosage of an opioid when the patient activates a button, thereby permitting rapid analgesia without having to wait for a nurse to deliver an IV PRN dose. By placing a maximum limit on the dose and frequency of opioid administered, the physician helps the patient titrate his/her opioid requirement. Because the PCA machine records the patient's individual dosing and frequency parameters, useful information can be obtained about the patient's analgesic requirements, which also simplifies subsequent conversion to a non-PCA opioid regimen.

Alternatives for patients unable to use parenteral or oral preparations include rectal (suppositories are available containing morphine, hydromorphone, and oxymorphone), sublingual, buccal, intranasal, transdermal, epidural, and intrathecal routes of administration. Epidural and intrathecal opioids, commonly used in the perioperative, postoperative, obstetrical, and cancer population, make opioids directly available to the opiate receptor-rich neuraxis. These two forms of selective analgesia have the advantage of requiring relatively small quantities of opioids, thereby reducing the risk of central and autonomic complications. Patient-controlled epidural analgesia (PCEA), a new variant of patient-controlled drug delivery systems, administers epidural dosages of opioid, and potentially other drugs, via a similar mechanism as IV PCA.

TREATMENT ENDPOINTS AND OPIOID SELECTION

Since pain is an untestable hypothesis that can neither be proved nor disproved, using pain relief as the endpoint of opioid therapy is also untestable and subjective. The most feared adverse effect from chronic opioid therapy is drug addiction, which manifests as a compulsive use of a drug that causes dysfunction, and the continued use despite the harm related to that dysfunction. Thus, clinicians are advised to focus on functional improvement as an objective endpoint for analgesia that also offers evidence of opioid efficacy that exists in contrast to addiction. The challenge, however, is to develop outcome measures for chronic opioid therapy beyond a lower pain score that distinguish function from dysfunction, and that emphasize therapy expectations, goal setting, goal monitoring, and collaboration with the patient's entire treatment team. The two critical issues related to treatment endpoints in chronic opioid therapy include defining what outcomes should be expected and followed to demonstrate an effective and safe trial of opioids, and determining when and how opioid therapy should be discontinued (or tapered) if the treatment is either effective or ineffective. Clinical studies in this area are limited.

Markers of opioid benefit in patients treated for CNMP include subjective pain reduction and evidence of improved functional status and quality of life. Determining functional improvement can be accomplished with standardized instruments (SF-36, TOPS, Oswestry, etc.) or through a simple process of ascertaining limitations in function and quality of life prior to treatment and following these endpoints through the course of opioid therapy. The ideal functional assessment model should be simple, brief, individualized, and comprehensive, something which most formalized scales fail to accomplish.

Implementation of chronic opioid therapy should encourage the patient to become the responsible party for demonstrating his/her own functional gain(s). In turn, clinicians must provide an environment that is conducive to facilitating and reinforcing functional improvement. The detection of dysfunction is as important as identifying signs of functional improvement, as the former suggests that adversity may be related to the therapeutic trial. Assessment should consider encompassing the biopsychosocial aspects of a patient's life, including social activities related to family, support networks, and work, as well as areas where rehabilitation is necessary, such as participation and progress in physical or occupational therapies, weight reduction, psychological counseling, and group educational and support programs. Demonstration of function should be in more than one single domain, recognizing that no one functional achievement is solely indicative of efficacy, just as one indication of dysfunction may not be proof of therapeutic failure. Typically, collateral sources (e.g., family members, friends, physical therapist, psychologist, or other healthcare professionals) are necessary to help document functional gains. Patients may be required to collect and document participation and progress in structured programs such as a gym or other therapeutic activities.

The foundation of a functional clinic environment is a well-planned and detailed program with sufficient patient education to support patients in their quest for improved function. Prior to beginning an opioid trial, the healthcare provider must be committed to documenting and tracking function once the therapy is started. Documenting functional improvement is a critical component of safe and comprehensive opioid management and can go a long way towards mitigating concerns about addiction. As noted above, vigilant recognition of decreased function is equally important, as this may be a sign of treatment failure or even addiction.

Psychological and social factors, as well as coexistent diseases that may influence pain perception and suffering, can affect the overall assessment of pain.[17–19] Initiation of opioid therapy is unlikely to offer concomitant and proportional improvement in all of these areas. If the psychological amplifiers of pain perception have not been adequately addressed, opioid-induced analgesia may not be maximally effective. Likewise, analgesia and functional improvement resulting from opioid therapy may be discordant with achievements occurring from psychological treatment. Many possible variations in efficacy and functional gain may dictate flexibility in ascertaining treatment endpoints.

Because pain reduction is subjective, it can only serve as a single aspect of adequate chronic opioid therapy. Consider, for example, the patient who has a constant pain rated "6 out of 10" ("0" being no pain and "10" being severe pain) with significantly associated disability. While opioid therapy may only decrease the patient's pain from a "6" to a "5" a successful outcome has been achieved if the patient demonstrates improvements in activities of daily living (ADL), ability to participate in physical rehabilitation, and/or ability to return to work. Conversely, an opioid trial can be considered counterproductive if the patient reports increased pain relief without observable functional gains, and possibly even signs of functional loss (daytime sedation, impaired cognition, voluntary unemployment, dysfunctional interpersonal or family relationships, diminished physical activity, or legal difficulties). In situations of functional decline, it is imperative to assess the possible contribution of opioid side effects or simply persistent pain related to opioid ineffectiveness. Signs of dysfunction should raise the suspicion of addiction but do not always conform to this. Unlike the addict, whose functional status is impaired by substance use, the chronic pain patient's functional status should improve with appropriate opioid therapy.

While effectiveness of opioid therapy is a primary concern, an equally important part of opioid management relates to deciding when to discontinue opioid therapy if the treatment is deemed to be unsatisfactory. Determination of a treatment failure requires consideration of multiple contributing factors, including (1) underdosing, (2) inappropriate dosing schedule, (3) improper drug delivery route, (4) potentially diminished opioid responsiveness relating to the nature of the pain generator (e.g., neuropathic pain), (5) involvement of unresolved contributors to pain, such as physical, psychological, and social disability, and (6) development of side effects that limit dose escalation. In the face of apparent opioid ineffectiveness from a single agent, opioids as a class may not be problematic as patients can appear resistant to one opioid yet sensitive to another.[20]

The duration of opioid therapy remains a question with no clear consensus amongst practitioners and minimal science to guide the debate. Pharmacological tolerance to opioids can develop during treatment, and may require either escalating the dose to maintain the same level of analgesia or switching to a different opioid. The need to rotate to another opioid is expected to occur in less than 2% to 3% of cases.[21] Although some clinical studies have suggested stabilization of opioid dose requirement following an initial dose increase, it is possible that periodic increases may be warranted during chronic opioid therapy. Clearly, determining the duration of effective opioid therapy must be individualized based on treatment efficacy balanced with side effects and progression or regression of the underlying disease process. Ultimately, it may be impossible to know how much pain would be present without opioid therapy unless the medication is tapered.

A benefit as well as a pitfall of (single-agent) opioid therapy is its lack of an absolute upper limit to dosing necessary to control a patient's pain. Other analgesics such as NSAIDs, acetaminophen, or aspirin have ceiling effects whereby either analgesia is not increased above a certain dose or toxicity can manifest. Thus, opioids compounded with NSAIDs, acetaminophen, or aspirin present a problem of commingling a drug with no known ceiling effect that can cause tolerance with another drug that has a ceiling effect but no accrual of tolerance. In a setting of suboptimal analgesia increased dosages of a combination agent (Darvocet, Vicodin, Lortab, Norco, Percocet, etc.) may be required to maximize the opioid portion, which may simultaneously raise the nonopioid component above its ceiling dose and into the toxicity range.

While selection of any SAO or LAO largely appears to be empirical, a rational approach to prescribing can be aided by a careful review of the patient's medical history. Patients with moderate to severe acute and/or chronic pain who have not improved with nonopioid therapies are potential candidates for opioid analgesics. Whether or not a patient is opioid naive can help determine if he/she should be started on an SAO or LAO/SRO. Patients with minimal to no recent opioid exposure should be given a titration trial with a low-dose SAO to establish their opioid requirement. The brief half-life of an SAO should minimize its toxic accumulation, and thereby minimize risk of side effects. The severity and frequency of the patient's pain should determine whether PRN versus "around-the-clock" dosing is necessary. For example, in those with acute pain secondary to an injury or surgery, PRN dosing may be sufficient if the anticipated healing process is rapid and short. Conversely, in those with either a slow and prolonged recovery process or persistent chronic pain SAOs may be best delivered at fixed dosing intervals, just as with an LAO or SRO. Such a strategy avoids both the reinforcement of pain complaints and behaviors with additional analgesics as well as the precipitation of anxiety. If a patient responds to the SAO and tolerates its side effects, chronic opioid therapy may be best delivered by converting to an equianalgesic LAO or SRO if dosing permits.

SELECTED OPIOIDS

Meperidine: While meperidine (Demerol) is a common analgesic, particularly by the intramuscular (IM) route, its primary use in the pain management setting has steadily declined due to potential for neurotoxicity. Meperidine was developed in Nazi Germany as a synthetic opioid with relatively weak μ-opioid receptor agonist properties. Compared to morphine, it is one-tenth as potent and has a slightly more rapid onset and shorter duration of action.[22] At equianalgesic doses meperidine produces less sedation and pruritis and may be more effective in neuropathic pain.[22] However, it possesses significant cardiac (orthostatic hypotension, and direct myocardial depression),[22] anticholinergic, and local anesthetic properties, which decrease its therapeutic window.[23]

Unlike other opioids, epidural or spinal administration of meperidine can produce sensory, motor, and sympathetic blockade.[22] Meperidine does have a beneficial use in the operative setting for treatment of postanesthetic shivering.

While meperidine has a relatively short half-life of 3 hours,[23] prolonged administration (greater than 3 days) is problematic due to the potential for accumulation of its neurotoxic metabolite, normeperidine. Meperidine is demethylated in the liver to normeperidine, which has a half-life of 12 to 16 hours and is well documented to produce central nervous system (CNS) hyperactivity and, ultimately, seizures.[24] Since normeperidine is excreted by the kidneys, its adverse effects are most commonly, although not exclusively, seen in patients with renal impairment. Normeperidine toxicity initially manifests as subtle mood alteration and may progress to potentially naloxone-irreversible tremors, myoclonus, and seizures.[24] Because the hyperexcitability of normeperidine can also occur in patients with normal renal function, chronic administration of meperidine is not recommended. Finally, for patients on monoamine oxidase inhibitors, coadministration of meperidine can have potentially fatal outcomes. Caution may be prudent in coadministering meperidine and any other serotonergic drugs such as selective serotonin reuptake inhibitors (SSRIs), tramadol, or methadone.

Morphine: Morphine is the prototypical μ-opioid receptor agonist against which all other opioids are compared for equianalgesic potency. It can be given via IV, epidural, or intrathecal routes for perioperative and postoperative pain management. Orally, it is available in sustained-release (SR) or immediate-release (IR) formulations for the management of chronic pain and breakthrough pain, respectively. As an SRO, its dosing frequency ranges from every 8 to 24 hours (MS Contin, Oramorph, Kadian, and Avinza). With an oral bioavailability of 35% to 75%, morphine's relative hydrophilicity is less than ideal as an analgesic. Because of the delay in transport across the blood–brain barrier, morphine has a slower onset of action compared to other opioids. Conversely, morphine has a relatively longer analgesic effect of 4 to 5 hours relative to its plasma half-life (2 to 3.5 hours), thereby minimizing its accumulation and contributing to its safety.[24] The disproportional duration of analgesia versus plasma half-life is due in part to its low solubility and slower elimination from the brain compartment relative to the plasma concentration.[23]

Although morphine's pharmacological activity is primarily due to the parent compound, morphine's efficacious and toxic effects can also be mitigated or perpetuated by two of its major metabolites: morphine 3-glucuronide (M3G) and morphine 6-glucuronide (M6G). M3G lacks any μ- and δ-opioid receptor activity and accounts for approximately 50% of morphine's metabolites. It has been shown in animals to cause generalized hyperalgesia, CNS irritability, seizure, myoclonus, and development of tolerance.[25] Whether this explains why neuroexcitatory side effects occur in humans exposed to chronic dosing of morphine has yet to be conclusively proven. Although M3G is devoid of opioid receptor activity, its true mechanism of action remains unknown. Conversely, M6G is a μ- and δ-opioid receptor agonist and accounts for approximately 5% to 15% of morphine's metabolites. M6G has intrinsic opioid agonism and sustains analgesia in addition to side effects. The route of morphine administration may account for variations in concentration of both glucuronide metabolites. Because the intravenous[26] and rectal[27] routes of administration avoid hepatic biotransformation, their glucuronide concentrations are less than with oral administration. Chronic use of oral morphine ultimately results in higher circulating concentrations of the glucuronides (mean ratios of M3G:M6G range from 10:1 to 5:1) than the parent compound.[23] Patients experiencing side effects attributable to M3G and/or M6G may be candidates for rotation to an alternative opioid.

Since morphine's elimination is dependent upon hepatic mechanisms, it should be used with caution in cirrhotic patients. However, enterohepatic cycling and extrahepatic metabolism of morphine have also been reported to occur in the gastric and intestinal epithelia.[23] The glucuronides can also undergo deconjugation back to morphine by colonic flora and subsequently reabsorbed.[23] Because morphine metabolites are excreted through the kidneys, the dose should be adjusted in those with renal impairment in order to minimize the risk of adverse side effects associated with the accumulation of glucuronide metabolites. Smith reported that while respiratory depression, sedation, and vomiting due to relatively high concentrations of M6G can be reversed by naloxone, the most concerning adverse affect in patients with compromised renal function is encephalopathy and myoclonus.[25] Peterson et al. found the ratio of M6G to morphine correlated with increased blood urea nitrogen or creatinine levels.[27] Ultimately, morphine's analgesic effects and side effects are likely related to complex interactions between the parent compound and its glucuronide metabolites. Exactly how specific diseases, polypharmacy, and patient age influence ratios of the individual glucuronide metabolites to morphine remains unclear.[23]

Oxycodone: Oxycodone is a semisynthetic congener of morphine that has been used as an analgesic for over 80 years.[28] As an SAO, it is available in IR preparations as a single agent (OxyIR or Roxicodone) or compounded with acetaminophen (Percocet, Endocet, or Roxicet®) or aspirin (Percodan or Endodan). Oxycodone is also available in SR formulation (OxyContin) with the advantage of decreased dosing frequency. IR oxycodone has been shown to deliver equivalent analgesia as the SR version.[29]

SR oxycodone possesses many of the characteristics of an ideal opioid including no ceiling dose, minimal side effects, absence or minimal active metabolite, easy titration, rapid onset of action, short half-life, long duration of action, and predictable pharmacokinetics.[30] In comparison to SR morphine, it has a prolonged pharmacokinetic profile, which theoretically allows it to be solely administered on an every 12-hour dosing schedule. This, however, reflects a characteristic of the drug delivery system rather than a property of the drug itself. Oxycodone's narrower oral bioavailability (50% or more) than morphine's (15% to 64%)[28] can account for variations in dose conversion ratios between the two drugs. Milligram-to-milligram, oxycodone is more potent than morphine and has a shorter onset of analgesia with less plasma variation. Accordingly, oxycodone is associated with fewer side effects (hallucinations, dizziness, and pruritis) than morphine.

While it possesses some intrinsic analgesic properties via activation of the κ-opioid receptors, oxycodone is predominantly a prodrug. It undergoes hepatic metabolism via the cytochrome P450 2D6 enzyme where it is converted into oxymorphone, an active metabolite with μ-opioid agonist properties, and noroxycodone, an inactive metabolite. While the role

of oxymorphone is not well known, Kaiko et al. reported that it is often produced in undetectable amounts and is 14 times as potent as the parent compound.[31] Currently, oxymorphone is available as a prescribed analgesic in limited formulations as a suppository or intravenously, although efforts are underway to develop an SR formulation.[24]

In the approximately 10% of the population with genetically low levels of the cytochrome P450 2D6 enzyme, lower concentrations of oxymorphone may account for the fact that higher than usual doses of oxycodone may be necessary to obtain pain relief. Analgesic efficacy may also be decreased in those concurrently taking medications that competitively inhibit the P450 2D6 enzyme. Whether the relationship between impaired hepatic metabolism and decreased analgesia has anything to do with lower levels of oxymorphone remains uncertain. Therefore, careful dose titration must be made in those concurrently taking medications with potential interaction such as SSRIs, tricyclic antidepressants (TCAs), or neuroleptics. Finally, because the kidneys excrete oxycodone, the dose should be adjusted in renal dysfunction.

Hydromorphone: Hydromorphone (Dilaudid) is a hydrogenated ketone analogue of morphine that can be formed by N-demethylation of hydrocodone. It can be given via IV, epidural, or intrathecal routes for perioperative and postoperative pain management. As an oral medication, it is available only in the IR formulation in the USA, limiting its use as an SAO. In other countries, however, it is available in an oral SR formulation, affording every 12-hour dosing for chronic pain management. Various randomized, double-blinded cross-over trials on patients with stable cancer pain have demonstrated equivalent analgesic efficacy and safety of SR hydromorphone when compared to IR hydromorphone given every 4 hours or SR oxycodone.[21]

Like morphine, hydromorphone is hydrophilic, possesses strong μ-opioid receptor agonist activity, and has a similar duration of analgesic effect (3 to 4 hours). However, side effects of pruritis, sedation, and nausea and vomiting occur less frequently with hydromorphone.[21] Depending on whether it is administered orally or parenterally, hydromorphone's milligram-to-milligram potency is estimated to be 5 to 7 times that of morphine, respectively. Onset of analgesic effect occurs within 30 minutes when administered orally and 5 minutes when administered parenterally.[21] Peak analgesic effect of parenteral hydromorphone occurs within 8 to 20 minutes, most likely because its hydrophilicity impairs its ability to cross the blood–brain barrier.[32] Although it is hydrophilic, it is 10 times as lipid soluble as morphine.[21] This feature, plus its greater milligram-to-milligram potency than morphine, allows equianalgesic doses to be infused subcutaneously but in smaller volumes (10 or 20 mg/mL). Possessing 78% of the bioavailability of IV hydromorphone,[21] SQ administration offers a safe alternative in hospice patients with impaired gastrointestinal (GI) function and requires less maintenance than with an IV site.

Hydromorphone undergoes hepatic biotransformation into its primary metabolite, hydromorphone-3-glucuronide (H3G), with both the parent compound and metabolite being renally excreted. Similar to morphine's M3G metabolite, H3G is an active metabolite that lacks analgesic efficacy but possesses potent neuroexcitatory properties which are 10 times stronger than the parent compound and have been shown to produce neuroexcitation (allodynia, myoclonus, and seizures) when administered directly into the lateral ventricle of rat brains.[23] Because H3G is produced in such small quantities, its effects are negligible except in cases of renal insufficiency where it may accumulate. In those with renal insufficiency hydromorphone is not preferable to morphine. Concentrations of H3G are dose dependent and clear with time once hydromorphone is discontinued.

Methadone: According to the American Heritage Dictionary, the name "methadone" is a derivative merging of the words that describe its chemical structure, 6-di**meth**ylamino-4,4-**d**iphenyl-3-heptan**one**.[33] Methadone has recently received increased attention and use due to its many attractive features as an analgesic medication: low cost (wholesale price is approximately 1/15th to 1/20th that of the more expensive proprietary SROs), high bioavailability with absorption and activity within 30 minutes, multiple receptor affinities, and lack of known metabolites that produce neurotoxicity. Methadone has an oral bioavailability (approximately 80%; range 40% to 99%)[34,35] that is approximately three-fold that of morphine. Methadone's absence of neurotoxic metabolites theoretically positions it as a second-line opioid for those requiring high doses of opioids which may otherwise subject them to the potential accumulation of opioid metabolites that produce sedation, confusion, hallucinations, and myoclonus. Unfortunately, the pharmacokinetics and pharmacodynamics of methadone, exemplified by unpredictable bioavailability and high interindividual variability in steady-state serum levels, can make it a challenge to determine precisely appropriate dosages, thereby increasing the potential for delayed neurotoxicity.

Methadone, which is structurally unrelated to other opium-derived alkaloids, is available as a hydrochloride powder that can be reconstituted for oral, rectal, or parenteral administration. It is lipophilic, basic (pK_a = 9.2), and usually exists as a racemic mixture of its two isomers, d-methadone (S-met) and l-methadone (R-Met), both of which have separate modes of action. The d-isomer antagonizes the NMDA receptor and inhibits 5-hydroxytryptamine and norepinephrine reuptake, while the l-isomer (R-met) possesses the opioid receptor agonist properties. Among opioid receptor subtypes, methadone demonstrates variable affinity. Animal models demonstrate that it has a lower affinity than morphine for the μ-opioid receptor, which may explain why methadone may have fewer μ-opioid receptor-related side effects.[36] Conversely, methadone has a greater affinity than morphine for the δ-opioid receptor.[37] While δ-opioid receptor activity is felt to be crucial to the development of morphine-induced tolerance and dependence, methadone's δ-opioid receptor agonism leads to its desensitization. This feature may partially account for methadone's ability to counteract opioid-induced tolerance and dependence.[38] Aside from acting as an opioid receptor agonist, methadone also acts as an NMDA receptor antagonist.[39–42] Numerous studies have demonstrated the involvement of the NMDA receptor mechanisms in the development of opioid tolerance[41] and neuropathic pain.[42] Hypothetically, methadone's ability to mitigate opioid-induced tolerance and treat neuropathic pain remains an intriguing concept.

Methadone's lipophilicity most likely accounts for its extensive tissue distribution (mean 6.7 mL/kg) and slow elimination (mean half-life = 26.8 hours).[35,43] Its delayed clearance (mean 3.1 mL/minute/kg) provides the basis for dosing it once per day for methadone maintenance therapy, thereby preventing the onset of opioid withdrawal syndrome for 24 hours or more.[43] Unfortunately, the same does not hold true for analgesia. Furthermore, there is extensive interindividual variation in the relationship between changes in plasma methadone concentration and analgesia.[44] The ability to use methadone for either opioid detoxification or analgesia can be explained by methadone's biphasic elimination phase. The α-elimination phase, which lasts 8 to 12 hours, equates to the period of analgesia that typically does not exceed 6 to 8 hours. Consequently, initial dosing for analgesia may need to be frequent because steady-state kinetics is required for reaching the biphasic profile. The β-elimination phase, which ranges from 30 to 60 hours, may be sufficient for preventing withdrawal symptoms but is insufficient for providing analgesia. This provides the rationale for prescribing methadone every 24 hours for opioid maintenance therapy and every 4 to 8 hours for analgesia.

Unlike other opioids whose breakdown products contribute to potential neurotoxicity, methadone has no known active metabolites. It undergoes hepatic metabolism by the cytochrome P450 family of enzymes. Thus, there are multiple potential drug interactions with respect to the different isoenzymes that metabolize methadone compared with other opioids. Methadone's drug interactions are largely attributed to inducers or inhibitors of the cytochrome P450 enzymes, especially the CYP3A4 subtype.[45] Even in the absence of other drugs, CYP3A4 is an autoinducible enzyme. Thus, methadone can bring about its own metabolism, increasing its clearance over time.[36]

In addition to the possibility of drug interactions, gastric pH can affect methadone's degree of absorption. For example, patients who are also taking omeprazole will absorb more methadone. While changes in urinary pH can also influence renal excretion of methadone, it does not accumulate in renal failure and does not appreciably filter during hemodialysis.[46] Thus, the possibility of methadone toxicity is increased in the setting of polypharmacy and/or changes in either gastric or urinary pH. Finally, variability in protein binding, excretion, and equianalgesic potency can further contribute to methadone's potential instability by provoking either overdose or withdrawal symptoms. While signs of toxicity are often clear, signs of decreased analgesia or withdrawal symptoms due to involuntary decreases in free circulating methadone may not be as apparent. Such patients may be erroneously characterized as drug seeking because they display signs and symptoms of pseudoaddiction, requiring higher doses of methadone.

Methadone's duration of effect is inherently long acting, as opposed to having SR properties. This is especially beneficial for those with impaired GI absorption secondary to "short-gut syndrome" or "dumping syndrome." Unlike the SROs, methadone tablets can be broken in half or chewed. Methadone is also available in an elixir formulation (1 mg/mL or 10 mg/mL), which is advantageous for those with a gastrostomy feeding tube, thus minimizing the risk of clogging the tube by not having to crush a tablet. In addition, the low-concentration elixir theoretically allows for a relatively more careful and precise titration of methadone, which can potentially minimize the risk of delayed-onset toxicity. Ultimately, methadone's pharmacodynamic property as an LAO makes it beneficial for those with impaired GI absorption secondary to "short-gut syndrome" or "dumping syndrome." It is also ideal for those with renal impairment, as it does not accumulate in renal failure and is insignificantly removed during dialysis.

The many attractive features of methadone relate to its pharmacological complexity. The latter, however, can increase the risk of side effects, especially in those with a concomitant illness or those on multiple medications. Furthermore, uncertainty remains regarding methadone's equianalgesic dosing conversion. Contrary to logic as it relates to tolerance, methadone appears to have greater potency (milligram-per-milligram) in patients rotating from high dosages of other opioids. In the opioid-tolerant patient the exact equianalgesic dose for methadone as a conversion from morphine equivalents is uncertain. Older equianalgesic tables are usually based on studies that included normal controls or opioid-naive patients and, therefore, do not take into account chronic opioid exposure. This tends to lead to excessive dosages. Therefore, methadone presents the inexperienced clinician with the challenge of predicting effects, not only in the face of unreliable equianalgesic dosing ratios that may be nondirectional, but also due to fluctuations related to altered hepatic metabolism that can be influenced by drug–drug interactions, protein binding changes, and altered renal clearance.

Fentanyl: Originally formulated as part of a balanced anesthetic for use during surgical procedures, fentanyl continues to be used parenterally, epidurally, and intrathecally for perioperative and postoperative pain management. Because fentanyl is highly lipophilic, this can present advantages or disadvantages, depending on the desired effect, due to its limited spread along the neuraxis when used epidurally or intrathecally. Fentanyl possesses predominantly μ-opioid receptor agonist properties. Compared to morphine, it has an inherently faster onset of action and is 75 to 125 times as potent.[22,24] Its greater degree of potency compared to other opioids allows for the delivery of smaller quantities of the drug measured in micrograms per hour. Although considered short acting, its lipophilicity allows for transdermal and transmucosal applications for the management of chronic pain and breakthrough pain, respectively.

Transdermal fentanyl (Duragesic Patch) is recommended for use only in patients with chronic or cancer pain based on several studies reporting a 20% incidence of hypoventilation when it was used in acute postoperative pain management.[47] In addition to a peel strip that protects the adhesive, the patch consists of four layers: (1) the polyester backing layer is impermeable to drug loss or moisture penetration; (2) the drug reservoir contains fentanyl gelled with hydroxyethyl cellulose and ethanol, the latter of which enhances transdermal absorption of fentanyl; (3) the rate-controlling membrane helps control the rate of drug absorption, whereby 50% of the absorption rate is controlled by the membrane and 50% by the inherent resistance of the skin;[48] and (4) the silicone adhesive layer keeps the patch in place when affixed to the skin. The patch should be placed on the upper body on a hairless (clipped, not shaved), flat surface of skin free of defects. Once applied to the skin, sustained levels of analgesia can be achieved via fentanyl's continuous transdermal absorption.

Transdermal fentanyl permits 3-day dosing with avoidance of the first-pass effect of the liver, where fentanyl is metabolized primarily by the cytochrome P450 family of enzymes. Because transdermal fentanyl does not pass through the GI tract, it theoretically causes less constipation than oral opioids. Furthermore, not having to depend on the GI tract provides the rationale for prescribing it in those with an inability to tolerate oral medications secondary to chronic nausea and vomiting, in those with impaired GI absorption secondary to "short-gut syndrome" or "dumping syndrome," and in those who are noncompliant with taking oral medications.

Unlike the oral LAOs, dose titration of the patch can sometimes be difficult due to individual variations in transdermal rate absorption, adherence of the patch to the skin due to perspiration (~10%),[48] skin temperature, fat stores, and muscle bulk.[23] Because of the slow and variable rate of absorption after initial patch application or increase in patch dose, it can take 1 to 30 hours (mean value of 13 hours) before therapeutic serum levels are achieved.[49] Therefore, during the first 12 hours patients should be prescribed an SAO or IV PCA to address breakthrough pain and to minimize withdrawal symptoms if rotation is from another opioid, especially since it can take as long as 6 days before steady state is achieved.[23] The amount of SAO required after steady state is achieved may also determine if the patch dose needs to be changed, although caution is recommended in making rapid dose adjustments. Conversely, because it takes at least 16 hours before serum fentanyl concentrations drop by 50% after the patch is removed, one would also expect a delay in resolution of analgesia or side effects upon removing the patch. Patients should be advised to avoid submerging the patch in hot water, placing a heating pad over the patch, or placing the patch over broken skin, as all of these can influence the rate of drug absorption and attendant side effects. The most common side effects of the transdermal delivery system (<1%) are adhesive related and include erythema, itching, and occasional pustule formation.[48]

Unlike transdermal fentanyl, oral transmucosal fentanyl citrate (OTFC; brand name Actiq) has a rapid onset of analgesia (5 to 10 minutes) and short duration of action. Buccal absorption avoids the first-pass hepatic metabolism and yields peak serum concentrations within 22 minutes of starting a 15-minute application.[50] In a study comparing OTFC to IV morphine in acute postoperative pain both demonstrated a similar onset of analgesia.[51] Rapid absorption and short duration of effect make OTFC an ideal analgesic for breakthrough pain, especially in patients with an impaired swallow or GI tract. Finally, fentanyl is also widely used as an epidural and intrathecal analgesic. Since its lipophilic properties limit its spread along the neuraxis, this can present advantages or disadvantages depending on the desired effect.

Sufentanil: Used primarily in the operative setting as an IV or neuraxial analgesic, sufentanil (Sufenta) is a thiamyl analogue of fentanyl. Both are lipophilic, are predominantly hepatically metabolized by the CYP3A4 isoenzyme, and have a rapid onset with short duration of effect. While the pharmacokinetics and pharmacodynamics of these two drugs are similar, sufentanil has a smaller volume of distribution, greater analgesic potency (IV, 5 to 7 times; epidural or intrathecal, 2 to 5 times), shorter half-life (2.7 hours versus 3.1 to 7.9 hours), and more rapid onset of analgesia (IV, 1 to 3 minutes; epidural or intrathecal, 4 to 10 minutes) with a shorter duration of effect (IV, 20 to 45 minutes; epidural or intrathecal, 2 to 4 hours).[22,23] Sufentanil may also produce dose-related skeletal muscle rigidity.

Alfentanil: Also used primarily in the operative setting as an IV or neuraxial analgesic, alfentanil (Alfenta) is less lipophilic compared to fentanyl and sufentanil. Its lower lipid solubility means it has a smaller volume of distribution (~25% of that of fentanyl and sufentanil). This, coupled with its short elimination half-life (70 to 111 minutes) and rapid onset of analgesia (IV, 1 to 2 minutes; epidural, 5 to 15 minutes) with a short duration of effect (IV, 10 to 15 minutes; epidural 4 to 8 hours), makes it ideal in an operative setting due to the lower probability of accumulation with repeated dosing or continuous infusion and its ease of rapid titration.[22,23] Like fentanyl and sufentanil, alfentanil is extensively metabolized in the liver by the CYP3A4 isoenzyme.

Remifentanil: The most potent μ-opioid receptor agonist of the opioids discussed above, remifentanil (Ultiva) is administered IV for the induction and maintenance of anesthesia.[23] More lipophilic than fentanyl, sufentanil, and alfentanil, remifentanil also has a larger volume of distribution, a more rapid distribution and metabolism, a shorter elimination half-life (3 to 10 minutes), and a more rapid analgesic onset (1 minute) with shorter duration of effect (5 to 10 minutes).[23] Unlike fentanyl, sufentanil, and alfentanil, remifentanil is not metabolized to any appreciable degree by the liver. Instead, its ester side-chain linkage subjects it to rapid degradation by tissue and plasma esterases into an inactive carboxylic acid metabolite that is renally excreted.[23] This confers unique pharmacokinetic and pharmacodynamic parameters that makes remifentanil's actions brief and unaffected by renal or hepatic insufficiency. Brisk clearance and lack of accumulation with repeated dosing are advantageous features in an operative setting, but discontinuation of the infusion results in a rapid loss of analgesia.

SUMMARY

With an informed and cautious approach, opioids are safe and effective for treating moderate to severe pain of both malignant and nonmalignant origin. Clinicians who choose to offer chronic opioid therapies must formulate rational and individualized regimens according to strategies such as those described above. Safe opioid therapy requires a program for continuous and close observation of analgesia and possible side effects. Furthermore, subjective reports of pain relief should be corroborated by documentation of objective signs of success, such as improvement in function. Experience dictates that improvements in functionality are more frequently encountered when a multidisciplinary treatment plan is employed.

REFERENCES

1. Portenoy RK: Opioid therapy for chronic nonmalignant pain: A review of the critical issues. J Pain Symptom Manage 11:203–217, 1996.
2. Robinson RC, Gatchel RJ, Polatin P, et al: Screening for problematic prescription opioid use. Clin J Pain 17:220–228, 2001.
3. Pappagallo M, Heinberg LJ: Ethical issues in the management of chronic nonmalignant pain. Semin Neurol 17:203–211, 1997.
4. Barkin RL, Barkin D: Pharmacologic management of acute and chronic pain: Focus on drug interactions and patient-specific pharmacotherapeutic selection. South Med J 94:756–770, 2001.
5. Society AP: Principles of analgesic use in the treatment of acute pain and chronic cancer pain. Clini Pharmacy 9:601–611, 1990.
6. Prest VQAJ: Dear Miss Nightingale: A selection of Benjamin Jowett's letters to Florence 1860–1893. Oxford University Press, New York, 1987.
7. Bertin P: Current use of analgesics for rheumatological pain. Eur J Pain 4:9–13, 2000.
8. Watson CP: The treatment of neuropathic pain: Antidepressants and opioids. Clin J Pain 16:S49–S55, 2000.
9. Ossipov MH, Lopez Y, Nichols ML, et al: Inhibition by spinal morphine of the tail-flick response is attenuated in rats with nerve ligation injury. Neurosci Lett 199:83–86, 1995.
10. Mao J, Price DD, Mayer DJ: Experimental mononeuropathy reduces the antinociceptive effects of morphine: Implications for common intracellular mechanisms involved in morphine tolerance and neuropathic pain. Pain 61:353–364, 1995.
11. McQuay H, Moore R: An Evidence-based Resource for Pain Relief. Oxford University Press, Oxford, 1998.
12. http://www.ampainsoc.org/advocacy/opioids.htm.
13. http://www.fsmb.org/. Model Guidelines for the Use of Controlled Substances for the Treatment of Pain, 1998.
14. Portenoy RK: Current pharmacotherapy of chronic pain. J Pain Symptom Manage 19:S16–S20, 2000.
15. Reder RF: Opioid formulations: Tailoring to the needs in chronic pain. Eur J Pain 5:109–111, 2001.
16. Mercadante S, Fulfaro F: Alternatives to oral opioids for cancer pain. Oncology (Huntingt) 13:215–220, 225, discussion 226–229, 1999.
17. Dworkin RH, Hetzel RD, Banks SM: Toward a model of the pathogenesis of chronic pain. Semin Clin Neuropsychiatry 4:176–185, 1999.
18. Vlaeyen JW, Crombez G: Fear of movement/(re)injury, avoidance and pain disability in chronic low back pain patients. Man Ther 4:187–195, 1999.
19. Feldman SI, Downey G, Schaffer-Neitz R: Pain, negative mood, and perceived support in chronic pain patients: A daily diary study of people with reflex sympathetic dystrophy syndrome. J Consult Clin Psychol 67:776–785, 1999.
20. Quang-Cantagrel ND, Wallace MS, Magnuson SK: Opioid substitution to improve the effectiveness of chronic noncancer pain control: A chart review. Anesth Analg 90:933–937, 2000.
21. Sarhill N, Walsh D, Nelson KA: Hydromorphone: Pharmacology and clinical applications in cancer patients. Support Care Cancer 9:84–96, 2001.
22. Omoigui S: Sota Omoigui's Pain Drugs Handbook. Blackwell Science, Oxford, 1999, p 816.
23. Janicki PK, Parris WC: Clinical pharmacology of opioids. In Smith HS (ed): Drugs for Pain. Hanley & Belfus, Philadelphia, 2003, pp 97–118.
24. Inturrisi CE: Clinical pharmacology of opioids for pain. Clin J Pain 18:S3–S13, 2002.
25. Smith MT: Neuroexcitatory effects of morphine and hydromorphone: Evidence implicating the 3-glucuronide metabolites. Clin Exp Pharmacol Physiol 27:524–528, 2000.
26. Osborne R, Joel S, Trew D, Slevin M: Morphine and metabolite behavior after different routes of morphine administration: Demonstration of the importance of the active metabolite morphine-6-glucuronide. Clin Pharmacol Ther 47:12–19, 1990.
27. Peterson GM, Randall CT, Paterson J: Plasma levels of morphine and morphine glucuronides in the treatment of cancer pain: Relationship to renal function and route of administration. Eur J Pharmacol 38:121–124, 1990.
28. Anderson R, Saiers JH, Abram S, Schlicht C: Accuracy in equianalgesic dosing. Conversion dilemmas. J Pain Symptom Manage 21:397–406, 2001.
29. Kaplan R, Parris WC, Citron ML, et al: Comparison of controlled-release and immediate-release oxycodone tablets in patients with cancer pain. J Clin Oncol 16:3230–3237, 1998.
30. Levy MH: Advancement of opioid analgesia with controlled-release oxycodone. Eur J Pain 5:113–116, 2001.
31. Kaiko RF, Benziger DP, Fitzmartin RD, et al: Pharmacokinetic–pharmacodynamic relationships of controlled-release oxycodone. Clin Pharmacol Ther 59:52–61, 1996.

32. Coda B, Tanaka A, Jacobson RC, et al: Hydromorphone analgesia after intravenous bolus administration. Pain 71:41–48, 1997.

33. The American Heritage Stedman's Medical Dictionary, vol xxxiii. Houghton Mifflin, Boston, 2002, p 923.

34. Kristensen K, Blemmer T, Angelo HR, et al: Stereoselective pharmacokinetics of methadone in chronic pain patients. Ther Drug Monit 18:221–227, 1996.

35. Rostami-Hodjegan A, Wolff K, Hay AW, et al: Population pharmacokinetics of methadone in opiate users: Characterization of time-dependent changes. Br J Clin Pharmacol 48:43–52, 1999.

36. Fishman SM, Wilsey B, Mahajan G, Molina P: Methadone reincarnated: Novel clinical applications with related concerns. Pain Medicine 3:339–348, 2002.

37. Davis MP, Walsh D: Methadone for relief of cancer pain: A review of pharmacokinetics, pharmacodynamics, drug interactions, and protocols of administration. Support Care Cancer 9:73–83, 2001.

38. Liu JG, Liao XP, Gong ZH, Qin BY: The difference between methadone and morphine in regulation of delta-opioid receptors underlies the antagonistic effect of methadone on morphine-mediated cellular actions. Eur J Pharmacol 373:233–239, 1999.

39. Gagnon B, Bruera E: Differences in the ratios of morphine to methadone in patients with neuropathic pain versus non-neuropathic pain. J Pain Symptom Manage 18:120–125, 1999.

40. Sang CN: NMDA-receptor antagonists in neuropathic pain: Experimental methods to clinical trials. J Pain Symptom Manage 19:S21–S25, 2000.

41. Price DD, Mayer DJ, Mao J, Caruso FS: NMDA-receptor antagonists and opioid receptor interactions as related to analgesia and tolerance. J Pain Symptom Manage 19:S7–S11, 2000.

42. Parsons CG: NMDA receptors as targets for drug action in neuropathic pain. Eur J Pharmacol 429:71–78, 2001.

43. Wolff K, Hay AW, Raistrick D, Calvert R: Steady-state pharmacokinetics of methadone in opioid addicts. Eur J Clin Pharmacol 44:189–194, 1993.

44. Inturrisi CE, Colburn WA, Kaiko RF, et al: Pharmacokinetics and pharmacodynamics of methadone in patients with chronic pain. Clin Pharmacol Ther 41:392–401, 1987.

45. Garrido MJ, Troconiz IF: Methadone: A review of its pharmacokinetic/pharmacodynamic properties. J Pharmacol Toxicol Methods 42:61–66, 1999.

46. Fainsinger R, Schoeller T, Bruera E: Methadone in the management of cancer pain: A review. Pain 52:137–147, 1993.

47. Sandler A: Transdermal fentanyl: Acute analgesic clinical studies. J Pain Symptom Manage 7:S27–S35, 1992.

48. Gourlay GK: Treatment of cancer pain with transdermal fentanyl. Lancet Oncol 2:165–172, 2001.

49. Gourlay GK, Kowalski SR, Plummer JL, et al: The transdermal administration of fentanyl in the treatment of postoperative pain: Pharmacokinetics and pharmacodynamic effects. Pain 37:193–202, 1989.

50. Coluzzi PH, Schwartzberg L, Conroy JD, et al: Breakthrough cancer pain: A randomized trial comparing oral transmucosal fentanyl citrate (OTFC) and morphine sulfate immediate release (MSIR). Pain 91:123–130, 2001.

51. Lichtor JL, Sevarino FB, Joshi GP, et al: The relative potency of oral transmucosal fentanyl citrate compared with intravenous morphine in the treatment of moderate to severe postoperative pain. Anesth Analg 89:732–738, 1999.

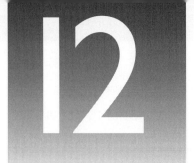

Minor and Short-Acting Opioids

Barth L. Wilsey, M.D., and
Scott M. Fishman, M.D.

Opioids have a long history of being the standard analgesic used for the management of pain, by which other medications in this category are measured. They come in two varieties: long- and short-acting preparations. Long-acting opioids are believed to be preferable for chronic pain because they provide less variation in analgesic blood levels and possibly promote less adverse pain related behavior. This is thought to result in a lower tendency for the development of tolerance and abusive behaviors. However, there is no definitive data regarding these attributes and the entire issue of preference for long-acting opioids in chronic pain patients remains in the realm of speculation. Nonetheless, its validity is suggested by finding a preponderance of diverted street opioids to be of the short-acting variety.

Short-acting opioids are generally employed for acute or breakthrough pain but do have some role in the treatment of chronic pain. When used for acute pain, short-acting opioids tend to be employed in combination with adjuvant analgesics such as acetaminophen, aspirin, or nonsteroidal anti-inflammatory medications in an effort to provide increased analgesia. The combination therapy may also offer drug sparing effects since a lower dose of each medication is used, thus avoiding side effects associated with higher doses. A potential problem is created by combining a drug like an opioid, which can produce tolerance and that has no dose ceiling, with acetaminophen or a nonsteroidal anti-inflammatory drug (NSAID), which causes toxicity beyond a certain dosage. Patients and clinicians are often very concerned about the opioid portion of these combination preparations but are unaware that their patients may have incurred potential renal or hepatic toxicity from the nonopioid component. The newer COX-2 anti-inflammatory medications have also undergone direct comparisons with short-acting opioids that are compounded with acetaminophen. These newer agents may prove to have the advantage of a superior side-effect profile, but only time will tell if they replace the short-acting opioids as first choice agents for treating mild to moderate postoperative pain.

Combinations of short-acting opioids and other nonopioid analgesics are also employed in chronic pain where the titration of drugs requires not only monitoring of pain relief and adverse effects but also other endpoints like improvement in function, Opioids such as oxycodone, hydrocodone, codeine, tramadol, and propoxyphene have pain-relieving properties by virtue of their ability to stimulate endogenous opioid receptors as well as other receptor complexes. This is exemplified by tramadol's agonism at noradrenergic and serotinergic reuptake sites or antagonism of N-methyl-D-aspartate (NMDA) receptors by methadone or propoxyphene.

When opioids are administered with aspirin, acetaminophen, or ibuprofen these medications are referred to as "weak opioids." This misnomer refers only to the limit to which they can be prescribed in any single patient due to the restrictive dosing of the acetaminophen, aspirin, or nonsteroidal anti-inflammatory component. When administered alone, opioid analgesics can be as potent as morphine. Table 12-1 compares dosages of other opioids to standard, morphine 10 mg IV. However, combination therapy has been widely shown to be beneficial and subsequently widely employed. Efficacy in these opioid medications has been seen in combination with acetaminophen, aspirin, and NSAIDs. A recent randomized, controlled trial compared the analgesic efficacy and safety of the oxycodone 10 mg/acetaminophen 325 mg formulation to a 20 mg dose of controlled-release (CR) oxycodone for the treatment of acute pain following oral surgery.[1] The combination treatment of oxycodone/acetaminophen was superior to CR oxycodone in outcome measures of pain intensity and pain relief. The combination treatment also provided a faster onset and 24% reduction in the number of patients reporting treatment-related adverse events. Thus, the "opioid-sparing" effect was significant and resulted in fewer side effects leading to better compliance.[2] A similar scenario exists for codeine in combination with acetaminophen and hydrocodone with ibuprofen added.[3] Additive effects with aspirin combinations have not been clearly demonstrated.

TABLE 12-1. **EQUIANALGESIC (MORPHINE 10 mg IV OR 30 mg PO) VALUES OF SHORT-ACTING OPIOIDS**

Generic Name	Equianalgesic Amount	Comments
Codeine	200 mg	Most widely employed naturally occurring opioid; has strong antitussive effects
Hydrocodone	30 mg	Many products combining hydrocodone and nonopioid analgesics available; has strong antitussive effects
Oxycodone	20–30 mg	High abuse potential; many products combining oxycodone and nonopioid analgesics available
Propoxyphene	130 mg	Not more effective than APAP alone; neurotoxic metabolite
Tramadol	120 mg	Avoid in patients at risk for seizures; avoid in patients taking SSRIs

The Federal Controlled Substances Act (CSA) of 1970 regulates the production and distribution of controlled substances. The CSA is "the legal foundation of the government's fight against the abuse of drugs and other substances." The CSA devised the current classification system that classifies drugs as schedule I through V. The difference between the classification levels is based on the individual medication's abuse potential and medical utility. Schedule I controlled substances include drugs with high abuse potential and no medical use while schedule V controlled substances include those with low abuse potential (Table 12-2). Short-acting opioids belong to either schedule II or schedule III. Both categories contain medications that have accepted medical use in treatment in the USA and are recognized as having the potential to be associated

TABLE 12-2. **FEDERAL CONTROLLED SUBSTANCE SCHEDULES**

	Description of Criteria	Examples
Schedule I C-I	High potential for abuse Lack of accepted safety No current accepted medical use	Heroin, lysergic acid, marijuana, mescaline, methaqualone
Schedule II C-II	High potential for abuse Severe psychological or physical dependence liability Current accepted medical use	Morphine, hydromorphone, methadone, oxycodone, cocaine, amphetamine, methylphenidate
Schedule III C-III	Less abuse potential than I or II Moderate or low physical dependence or high psychological dependence Current accepted medical use	Opioids combined w/non-narcotic drugs (e.g., hydrocodone/acetaminophen, codeine comb), dronabinol, anabolic steroids, benzphetamine
Schedule IV C-IV	Less potential for abuse than CI–CIII Limited physical or psychological dependence Current accepted medical use	Benzodiazepines, chloral hydrate, dextropropoxyphene, phenobarbital, fenfluramine
Schedule V C-V	Low abuse potential Limited physical dependence or psychological dependence relative to CI–IV Current accepted medical use	Dephenoxylate in combination w/atropine (antidiarrheals), antitussives w/limited amounts of narcotics (e.g., codeine)

Modified from Fujimoto D: Regulatory issues in pain management. Clin Geriat Med 17:537–551, 2001.

with physical dependence, addiction, or drug abuse. Individual state regulatory agencies determine the guidelines by which these medications are prescribed. In general, they have acted to make the more abusable schedule II medications undergo greater barriers to diversion by using multiple copy prescriptions and/or limitations on refills. This chapter reviews the use of short-acting opioids and provides the reader with a practical approach to employing these medications in both acute and chronic pain conditions.

SPECIFIC SHORT-ACTING OPIOIDS

Oxycodone: Oxycodone is a semisynthetic opioid processed from thebaine, an organic chemical found in opium. It is one of the most popular opioids in the USA. A study conducted to determine the frequency of opioid prescriptions used by primary care physicians showed the most frequently prescribed oral opioids were oxycodone/acetaminophen (31%), morphine (19%), Tylenol #3 (15%), and hydrocodone/acetaminophen (14%).[1] These results are in some part due to its suitability for oral administration due to high bioavailability (60%). As a result of this property, oxycodone is twice as potent as morphine, a medication that is only 33% bioavailable. When provided orally, oxycodone reaches peak serum concentrations within 1 to 2 hours and exhibits half-lives of 2.5 to 4.0 hours. It may be given by alternative routes, such as intramuscularly, intravenously, subcutaneously, and rectally, but these routes of administration are rarely employed. Postoperative pain is the usual model for analyzing analgesics for acute pain. Oxycodone has been evaluated recurrently since, when combined with acetaminophen, it makes an excellent choice for mild to moderate acute pain after dental procedures. Oxycodone has also been shown to be effective in chronic low back pain.[4,5]

Oxycodone abuse has an infamous history. The first report that oxycodone, sold under the brand name Eukodal, produced a "striking euphoria" and addiction was published in Germany in the 1920s. Oxycodone is equipotent to morphine in relieving abstinence symptoms from heroin administration. Consequently, street users of heroin or methadone may use it to alleviate or prevent the onset of opiate withdrawal. In the 1960s the Addiction Research Center in Lexington, Kentucky, found that the subjective and physiological effects of oxycodone were greater than an equivalent dose of morphine in opiate substance abusers.[6] More recently, oxycodone was noted to produce pleasant and unpleasant subjective effects similar to those of morphine. One study reported no distinguishable euphoric effect between oxycodone and morphine in normal volunteers.[7] Perhaps details of the genomic influence will provide an explanation of why an addict has a different subjective response to oxycodone than the naive subject. Unlike morphine, oxycodone is known to be active at the kappa receptor. As of now, there is no supporting evidence that this binding has a known role in abuse or addiction.

Although oxycodone has been placed in the more restricted schedule II category, oxycodone abuse has been a continuing problem in the USA. The abuse of the sustained-release formulation of oxycodone, known as Oxycontin®, has brought about a renewed interest in the abuse potential of oxycodone. Abusers crushed the long-acting preparation, Oxycontin®, and either inhaled the powder or injected a solution into their veins. Mortality from the use of this product was usually associated with comorbid polysubstance abuse.[8] As a consequence of the popularity of abusing Oxycontin®, the number of Emergency Department visits related to oxycodone abuse more than tripled in recent years: 3,190 episodes in 1996 to 10,825 in 2000.[9]

Hydrocodone: Hydrocodone bitartrate occurs as fine white crystals or as a crystalline powder. Like oxycodone, it reaches peak serum concentrations within 1 to 2 hours and exhibits a half-life of 2.5 to 4.0 hours. Unlike oxycodone, this opium derivative is a schedule III medication. Rumor has it that objections were raised concerning the classification of hydrocodone and codeine as schedule II medications because this would have restricted the use of these drugs as antitussive medications. Hydrocodone abuse potential is similar to that seen with the schedule II classified oxycodone. In a recent study using urine toxicology screening products containing hydrocodone were found to be most frequently misused (20.3%), followed closely by oxycodone products (19.7%).[10] Low doses of hydrocodone have been found to be effective and safe to treat cough in advanced cancer. A starting dose of only 10 mg per day in divided doses seems effective.[11] Initial comparisons concluded that hydrocodone and morphine were equipotent for pain control in humans. However, more recent equianalgesic studies suggest that a dose of 15 mg (1/4 gr) of hydrocodone is equivalent to 10 mg (1/6 gr) of morphine. Hydrocodone combined with ibuprofen has been studied in moderate to severe postoperative pain from abdominal or gynecologic surgery. These studies found analgesia from the combination provided an additive effect.[12] In contrast to oxycodone, in which analgesia was comparable to the opioid plus an anti-inflammatory, COX-2 inhibitors have demonstrated simultaneous enhanced analgesia and tolerability compared with hydrocodone and acetaminophen combinations under settings of mild to moderate postoperative pain after ambulatory orthopedic surgery.[13]

Codeine: Codeine is the most widely employed naturally occurring opioid in developed countries. This alkaloid is found in opium in concentrations ranging from 0.7% to 2.5%. Rather than rely upon this source, most codeine used in this country is produced from morphine. Codeine is readily absorbed from the gastrointestinal tract. The plasma concentration does not correlate with brain concentration or relief of pain. Urinary excretion products include codeine (about 70%), norcodeine (about 10%), morphine (about 10%), normorphine (4%), and hydrocodone (1%). Codeine is prepared in both oral and parenteral preparations. It is frequently administered in combination with acetaminophen, butalbital, and caffeine intended for the treatment of tension headache. It is also commonly employed as an antitussive. Several years ago a clinical trial demonstrated temporary efficacy of codeine in nonmalignant pain.[6] Similar studies evaluating short-acting opioids in chronic pain are not available.

Tramadol: Tramadol has several mechanisms of activity including agonist activity at the mu opioid receptor as well as inhibition of the reuptake of norepinephrine and serotonin. Tramadol is metabolized in the liver to its active metabolite, O-demethyl tramadol, which is excreted by the kidneys. Tramadol has an elimination half-life of approximately 5 hours. It was initially thought to lack abuse potential as substantiated by postmarketing surveillance data. More recently, abuse potential of tramadol has been noted in several patients. Still an unscheduled drug, it has been studied in moderate to severe pain associated with osteoarthritis,[14] fibromyalgia,[15] low back pain,[16] and diabetic neuropathy.[17–19] Although useful in these conditions, the analgesia produced is often less than optimal. Like therapy with other opioids in nonmalignant pain, the treatment of these conditions requires rational polypharmacy with combinations of coanalgesics and alternative physical and psychological therapies. Like hydrocodone and codeine, tramadol may be useful in the pediatric population. Tramadol 1 to 2 mg/kg has been found to be an effective oral agent in postoperative children ready to be transitioned from patient-controlled analgesia.[20] Commonly reported adverse events with tramadol included nausea, dizziness, somnolence, and headache. More problematic has been the association of seizure activity, albeit in less than 1% of users. The risk of seizure activity is increased by a history of alcohol abuse, stroke, head injury, or renal compromise. Patients receiving serotonin selective reuptake inhibitors should avoid taking tramadol due to the risk of producing the serotonin syndrome.

Propoxyphene: Propoxyphene hydrochloride is an odorless, white crystalline powder with a bitter taste. It is freely soluble in water. Chemically, it is alpha (+)-4-(dimethylamino)-3-methyl-1,2-diphenyl-2-butanol propionate hydrochloride. Peak plasma concentrations of propoxyphene are reached in 2 to 2½ hours. Propoxyphene is metabolized by the liver to norpropoxyphene, an active metabolite with a propensity to accumulate. The most frequently reported adverse effects are dizziness, sedation, nausea, and vomiting. However, there are more serious potential problems including seizures, cardiac dysrhythmias, and even heart block if propoxyphene is purposefully or accidentally taken in excessive amounts. Patients who are depressed and suicidal are at risk for the purposeful ingestion of this medication. Concomitant use of alcohol, sedatives, tranquilizers, muscle relaxants, antidepressants, or other central nervous system (CNS)-depressant drug places patients in jeopardy of the additive depressant effects of propoxyphene. In fact, accidental ingestion of quantities of propoxyphene in excess of that prescribed has been fatal in several instances. Unfortunately, several studies have demonstrated inappropriate prescribing of propoxyphene, particularly in the elderly.[21–23] Although propoxyphene is no stronger than aspirin, it remains a relatively popular analgesic. The combination of propoxyphene with a mixture of aspirin and caffeine is thought to produce additive analgesia and is utilized frequently for patients with headaches. This combination also poses the potential of producing rebound headaches if taken on a daily basis. For this reason, the combination of propoxyphene, aspirin, and caffeine is best provided in limited quantities. Increased interest in propoxyphene has been spurred by finding that d-isomer, dextropropoxyphene, is a non-competitive NMDA receptor antagonist.[24] Thus, it may have extra-opioid effects with some potential benefit in cases of neuropathic pain.

SPECIAL CONSIDERATIONS

World Health Organization Analgesic Ladder: The general treatment strategy for cancer pain developed by the World Health Organization (WHO) program involves three steps in the analgesic ladder (see Fig. 12-1). Mild pain is usually treated with over-the-counter (OTC) analgesics such as aspirin, ibuprofen, or acetaminophen. These agents exert their analgesic effect by acting upon the algogenic soup that follows tissue injury. For mild to moderate pain, the WHO analgesic ladder advocates the use of short-acting opioids either alone or in conjunction with OTC analgesics. Opioids such as oxycodone, hydrocodone, and codeine are usually employed for this type of cancer pain. In addition, adjunctive therapy such as acupuncture, transcutaneous electrical nerve stimulation, and/or psychotherapy may be brought into play at this step of the analgesic ladder. The third step of the WHO ladder entails the use of strong opioids, used either alone or with adjunctive therapy to achieve relief of moderate to severe pain. At this point, it may be necessary to prescribe strong opioids such as morphine, hydromorphone, or fentanyl, or long-acting opioids such as sustained-release (SR) morphine, SR oxycodone, transdermal fentanyl, or methadone for cancer pain that is not responsive to the so called "weak opioids." However, even strong opioids may or may not be effective for some forms of pain and there are steps beyond the analgesic ladder that include other analgesics such anticonvulsants, antidepressants, or interventional pain procedures. Thus, the astute clinician will see that weak opioids can become strong opioids with increased dosing and strong opioids may only offer side effects in pain that is not responsive to opioid analgesia.

NSAIDs versus Short-Acting Opioids for Acute and Postoperative Pain: Recent studies have pointed to the efficacy of the newer COX-2 inhibitors for mild to moderate pain following minor surgery. NSAIDs should be considered possible first-line agents for most acute injuries and minor surgical procedures. Since the COX-2 inhibitors have not been shown to have greater analgesic potency than standard NSAIDs, the specific NSAID should be chosen on the basis of cost, availability, and individual risk for potential side effects. On the basis of increased risk of anti-inflammatory medications, there are several scenarios in which opioids may be preferable. As much as NSAIDs cause platelet dysfunction, use

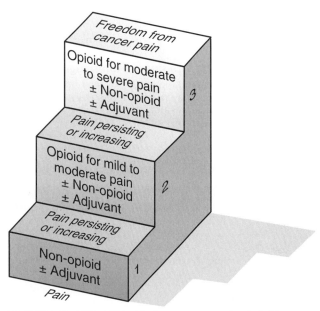

FIGURE 12-1. World Health Organization analgesic ladder.

in a patient with a low platelet count is relatively contra-indicated. Likewise, the patient with a low threshold for bronchospasm may do better perioperatively with an opioid. Women may want to avoid NSAIDs during pregnancy as these medications may increase the risk of miscarriage. This association is stronger if the initial NSAID is used around the time of conception or if the NSAID usage lasts more than a week. NSAIDs as a group tend to exacerbate reflux esophagitis, esophageal strictures, nonulcer dyspepsia, and peptic ulcer. Individuals prone to these conditions may be better off with opioids. Although rare, fatal outcomes from liver necrosis have been reported with almost all NSAIDs. Opioids are probably preferable in patients with liver disease although caution should also be exercised with medication combinations containing acetaminophen by limiting the dosage to less than 2 g per day. In susceptible patients suppression of compensatory prostaglandin production may result in acute reduction in renal blood flow and glomerular filtration. At risk are patients with congestive heart failure, intrinsic renal disease, liver failure with ascites, and those receiving diuretics. Opioid analgesics might be advantageous in these scenarios although they too must be used with caution because most are excreted by the kidneys and metabolized by the liver. Even without comorbid conditions, opioid analgesics should be substituted or supplemented for more severe pain that does not respond to the use of an NSAID.

The use of various analgesic medications in the pediatric population for acute and postoperative pain follows a stepwise approach similar to the WHO's analgesic ladder. When analgesia is poorly controlled with acetaminophen, salicylates, or an NSAID, a weak opioid (e.g., codeine, oxycodone, tramadol, or hydrocodone) can be added to bring about additional pain relief. There are special elixirs of these medications that make them more palatable in this age group (see Table 12-3). There are special precautions that are necessary in this age group because of the propensity to produce excessive sedation and respiratory depression. These problems are extremely uncommon except with excessive dosing or the presence of an underlying medical condition, which predisposes the pediatric patient to the central respiratory depressant effects of opioids. This is particularly true in younger infants. Hepatic and renal dysfunction makes opioids potentially hazardous as do a history of apnea and the use of concomitant sedative medications.

Use of Short-Acting Opioids in Nonmalignant Pain:
It is logical that short-acting opioids, with their fast onset and high serum peak levels, are better suited than long-acting opioids for inducing psychoactive nonanalgesic effects.

Theoretically, at least, this euphoric effect of short-acting preparations (e.g., oxycodone, hydrocodone, codeine, etc.) might then be more prone to abuse and addiction. The use of long-acting opioids (e.g., levorphanol, sustained release preparations of morphine and oxycodone, transdermal fentanyl) have been championed because of their gradual onset and reduced chance that a euphoric effect may occur. Therefore, to reduce the incidence of prescription opioid abuse, it can be argued that all patients who are on persistent continuous dosages of opioids for nonmalignant pain receive long-acting opioids.

There probably is a role for short-acting opioids as both an initial and titrating agent. For instance, short-acting opioids might be valuable in acclimation of dose-related side effects. Starting with a low dose of a short-acting agent and then titrating upward might increase patient compliance with opioid medications as many instances of nonadherence are related to adverse events. Likewise, such dosing titration strategies help establish the opioid requirement of a patient prior to committing to a longer half-life compound. Once accustomed to the short-acting opioids, a patient may be rotated to a long-acting agent. Theoretically, rotation from short- to long-acting opioids would tend to establish stable analgesia, minimize withdrawal symptoms, and, thus, the risk of tolerance and addiction.

In addition to titration, there are several situations in which it is necessary to continue short-acting opioids in the treatment of nonmalignant pain. For instance, some patients who receive SR opioids may be provided with an immediate-release opioid to treat pain that may break through the around-the-clock scheduled medication. As stated above, this is particularly important when initiating long-acting opioids, since there may be an end of dose failure, a situation in which there is decreasing blood levels of the analgesic before the next regularly scheduled dose. It ordinarily would be preferable to shorten the interval or increase the dose of the long-acting agent to negate the necessity to continue prescribing short-acting opioids. It may be necessary to maintain a person on short-acting opioids for breakthrough pain in some instances. Take the example of the elderly patient whose incidental pain is related to weight bearing or another activity that compromises their daily activity. In order to prevent cognitive impairment from larger doses of long-acting opioids, it might be preferable to provide this patient with short-acting opioids to be taken prior to any planned activity. It might also be prudent to treat an elderly patient with spontaneous breakthrough pain from a neuropathic pain syndrome (postherpetic neuralgia, diabetic neuropathy, spinal cord injury pain, or poststroke pain) with short-acting opioids for the same reason. Finally, the

TABLE 12-3. COMBINATIONS OF WEAK OPIOIDS AND ACETAMINOPHEN ELIXIRS

Generic Name	Brand Name	Formulation	Dose
Codeine	Tylenol with Codeine #3	Elixir (120 mg acetaminophen/12 mg per 5 mL)	0.8–1.0 mg/kg every 4 hours by mouth based on codeine
Hydrocodone	Lortab	Elixir (167 mg acetaminophen/2.5 mg per 5 mL)	Start at 0.1 mg/kg every 3 or 4 hours based upon hydrocodone

patient with sleep apnea deserves similar consideration but for another reason: the respiratory depressant effect of opioids. It may be justifiable to allow patients with sleep apnea to use short-acting opioids for their chronic pain to forestall the development of excessive sedation and respiratory depression during periods when they might be experiencing hypercapnea. In addition to maintaining them on short-acting opioids, it is also advisable to ensure that they are using their continuous positive airway pressure (CPAP) device if they are regular users of nasal CPAP therapy to minimize upper airway obstruction. Both the elderly patient and the patient with sleep apnea require frequent reassessment of their analgesic regimen to curtail cognitive impairment in the former and excessive sedation and respiratory depression in the latter.

Addiction Issues: The rationale of the federal government in regulating opioid analgesics through the CSA of 1970 was to ensure appropriate utilization of these agents when medically indicated and minimizing abuse. While theoretically sound, there is evidence to suggest that these medications are still being diverted.[25] In 1998 an estimated 1.6 million Americans used prescription pain relievers for nonmedical purposes for the first time. This was a significant change from the 1980s, when there were fewer than 500,000 first-time users per year. In 1999 an estimated 2.6 million people used pain relievers nonmedically in the month prior to taking a national survey. The nonmedical use of pain relievers such as oxycodone with aspirin (Percodan) and hydrocodone (Vicodin) is on the rise. The 1999 Drug Abuse Warning Network (DAWN), which collects data on drug-related episodes in metropolitan hospital emergency departments, reported that incidents involving hydrocodone as a cause for visiting an emergency room increased by 37% from 1997 to 1999. Opiate-containing medications are now being offered for sale without a prescription on-line.[26] Many of these organized drug rings are willing to sell opioids as well as other abusable medications including barbiturates, stimulants, benzodiazepines, and "date rape" drugs. A majority of these commercial opiate sites are registered to owners outside the USA.

With attestation of diversion and nonmedical use abundant, it is important to reaffirm the intent of the CSA to ensure appropriate utilization of these agents when medically indicated. Physicians should continue to treat all patients in need of opioid medications without fear of regulatory scrutiny. To do so, special attention needs to be given to documenting the need for the medication (history, physical examination, and diagnostic test/laboratory results, consultations) and the treatment objectives with attention to functional outcome as discussed in a separate chapter. One may also want to focus on rational use of short- versus long-acting opioids depending on the acute or chronic nature of the case. If done in this manner, there is little likelihood of a physician being involved in defending the practice of writing prescriptions for opioids. The problematic issue of diversion will require continued vigilance by legal authorities but should not present an obstacle to the appropriate treatment of acute and chronic pain.

CONCLUSIONS

There is a definite role for the use of short-acting opioids in the management of mild to moderate pain in acute and cancer pain.

Whether or not long-acting opioids would be better suited for chronic pain purposes is a matter of opinion and awaits evaluation of future data regarding the comparative development of tolerance and addictive behavior. Anti-inflammatory medications are being touted as an alternative to short-acting opioids in acute pain conditions including pain states following surgery. There are many variables that go into the decision of whether or not to use an anti-inflammatory medication. It is not clear if short-acting opioids will retain their pre-eminence for the treatment of mild to moderate acute pain. There are also individual issues among the short-acting opioids that mandate comparisons and warrant individualization of therapy in many instances. The use of the WHO analgesic ladder provides a basis upon which to model therapy for all types of painful conditions.

REFERENCES

1. Adams NJ, Plane MB, Fleming MF, et al: Opioids and the treatment of chronic pain in a primary care sample. J Pain Symptom Manage 22:791–796, 2001.
2. Gammaitoni AR, Galer BS, Bulloch S, et al: Randomized, double-blind, placebo-controlled comparison of the analgesic efficacy of oxycodone 10 mg/acetaminophen 325 mg versus controlled-release oxycodone 20 mg in postsurgical pain. J Clin Pharmacol 43:296–304, 2003.
3. Palangio M, Wideman GL, Keffer M, et al: Combination hydrocodone and ibuprofen versus combination oxycodone and acetaminophen in the treatment of postoperative obstetric or gynecologic pain. Clin Ther 22:600–612, 2000.
4. Jamison RN, Raymond SA, Slawsby EA, et al: Opioid therapy for chronic noncancer back pain. A randomized prospective study. Spine 23:2591–2600, 1998.
5. Gammaitoni AR, Galer BS, Lacouture P, et al: Effectiveness and safety of new oxycodone/acetaminophen formulations with reduced acetaminophen for the treatment of low back pain. Pain Med. 4:21–30, 2003.
6. Arkinstall W, Sandler A, Goughnour B, et al: Efficacy of controlled-release codeine in chronic non-malignant pain: A randomized, placebo-controlled clinical trial. Pain 62:169–178, 1995.
7. Zacny JP, Gutierrez S. Characterizing the subjective, psychomotor, and physiological effects of oral oxycodone in non-drug-abusing volunteers. Psychopharmacology (Berl) 170:242–254, 2003.
8. Davis MP, Varga J, Dickerson D, et al: Normal-release and controlled-release oxycodone: Pharmacokinetics, pharmacodynamics, and controversy. Support Care Cancer 11:84–92, 2003.
9. Intelligence Production Unit ID, DEA Headquarters. Drug Intelligence Brief: Oxycontin Pharmaceutical Diversion: DEA, March 2002.
10. Vaglienti RM, Huber SJ, Noel KR, Johnstone RE: Misuse of prescribed controlled substances defined by urinalysis. W V Med J 99:67–70, 2003.
11. Homsi J, Walsh D, Nelson KA, et al: A phase II study of hydrocodone for cough in advanced cancer. Am J Hosp Palliat Care 19:49–56, 2002.
12. Wideman GL, Keffer M, Morris E, et al: Analgesic efficacy of a combination of hydrocodone with ibuprofen in postoperative pain. Clin Pharmacol Ther 65:66–76, 1999.
13. Gimbel JS, Brugger A, Zhao W, et al: Efficacy and tolerability of celecoxib versus hydrocodone/acetaminophen in the treatment of pain after ambulatory orthopedic surgery in adults. Clin Ther 23:228–241, 2001.
14. Silverfield JC, Kamin M, Wu SC, Rosenthal N: Tramadol/acetaminophen combination tablets for the treatment of

osteoarthritis flare pain: A multicenter, outpatient, randomized, double-blind, placebo-controlled, parallel-group, add-on study. Clin Ther 24:282–297, 2002.

15. Bennett RM, Kamin M, Karim R, Rosenthal N: Tramadol and acetaminophen combination tablets in the treatment of fibromyalgia pain: A double-blind, randomized, placebo-controlled study. Am J Med 114:537–545, 2003.

16. Ruoff GE, Rosenthal N, Jordan D, et al: Tramadol/acetaminophen combination tablets for the treatment of chronic lower back pain: A multicenter, randomized, double-blind, placebo-controlled outpatient study. Clin Ther 25:1123–1141, 2003.

17. Harati Y, Gooch C, Swenson M, et al: Double-blind randomized trial of tramadol for the treatment of the pain of diabetic neuropathy. Neurology 50:1842–1846, 1998.

18. Moulin D. Tramadol for the treatment of the pain of diabetic neuropathy. Neurology 52:1301, 1999.

19. Harati Y, Gooch C, Swenson M, et al: Maintenance of the long-term effectiveness of tramadol in treatment of the pain of diabetic neuropathy. J Diabetes Complications 14:65–70, 2000.

20. Finkel JC, Rose JB, Schmitz ML, et al: An evaluation of the efficacy and tolerability of oral tramadol hydrochloride tablets for the treatment of postsurgical pain in children. Anesth Analg. 94:1469–1473, table of contents, 2002.

21. Aparasu RR, Fliginger SE: Inappropriate medication prescribing for the elderly by office-based physicians. Ann Pharmacother 31:823–829, 1997.

22. Piecoro LT, Browning SR, Prince TS, et al: A database analysis of potentially inappropriate drug use in an elderly medicaid population. Pharmacotherapy 20:221–228, 2000.

23. Kamal-Bahl SJ, Doshi JA, Stuart BC, Briesacher BA: Propoxyphene use by community-dwelling and institutionalized elderly medicare beneficiaries. J Am Geriatr Soc 51:1099–1104, 2003.

24. Ebert B, Thorkildsen C, Andersen S, et al: Opioid analgesics as noncompetitive N-methyl-D-aspartate (NMDA) antagonists. Biochem Pharmacol 56:553–559, 1998.

25. Trends in Prescription Drug Abuse: US National Institute on Drug Abuse, April 2001.

26. Allen GJ, Hartl TL, Duffany S, et al: Cognitive and motor function after administration of hydrocodone bitartrate plus ibuprofen, ibuprofen alone, or placebo in healthy subjects with exercise-induced muscle damage: A randomized, repeated-dose, placebo-controlled study. Psychopharmacology (Berl) 166:228–233, 2003.

FURTHER READING

Barkin RL: Pharmacotherapy for nonmalignant pain. Am Fam Physician 63:848, 2001.

Cramer GW: A drug use evaluation of selected opioid and nonopioid analgesics in the nursing facility setting. J Am Geriatr Soc 48:398–404, 2000.

Schecter WP: Pain control in outpatient surgery. J Am Coll Surg 195:95–104, 2002.

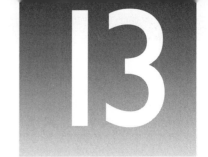

Opioid Therapy: Adverse Effects Including Addiction

Gagan Mahajan, M.D.,
Barth Wilsey, M.D., and
Scott M. Fishman, M.D.

Opioids represent a special class of medications that can be extremely helpful in improving the quality of life for those suffering from acute or chronic pain of either malignant or nonmalignant origin. When used for chronic pain, they are usually reserved for analgesia when other forms of treatment have proven to be insufficient. Since complaints of pain are entirely subjective and impossible to verify, opioid therapy can present challenges to both the prescriber and patient. Although they are excellent pain relievers, opioids can themselves be a source of suffering which may inherently limit the ability to maximize the medication's full analgesic potential. An opioid's ability to relieve pain as well as contribute to side effects is a function of interactions with various opioid and potentially other nonopioid receptor systems. The major opioid receptor classes are mu, kappa, and delta, which are located throughout the central nervous system (CNS) and periphery. Mu-opioid receptors mediate analgesia, respiratory depression, euphoria, sedation, and gastrointestinal (GI) dismotility. Kappa-opioid receptors mediate analgesia, dysphoria, diuresis, and psychotomimetic effects. Delta-opioid receptors mediate analgesia and possibly other effects which are not yet known.[1] While the mu-opioid receptor is the primary target for opioid-induced analgesia, escalating doses may lead to stimulation of the other receptor subtypes along with concomitant side effects. In a 1998 survey of patients receiving opioids for chronic pain 82% reported opioid-related side effects.[1] For some individuals these side effects can be so overwhelming that they would rather cope with the pain. Since it is virtually impossible to anticipate which patients will have side effects and which opioids will cause them, it is easier to assume side effects will occur and to implement preventative measures whenever and wherever possible.

This chapter also reviews the issues of addiction in prescribing opioids for chronic pain and some of the inherent difficulties in treating patients who have pain coupled with addiction. We review some of the issues surrounding the problem of prescription drug abuse found in some chronic pain patients, with emphasis on the broad range of aberrant behaviors that can indicate confusion or lack of education or addiction, pseudoaddiction, psychopathology, criminal intent, or a combination of these.

OPIOID ADVERSE EFFECTS

Constipation: Approximately one-third of the population of Western industrial countries suffers from constipation at one time or another, with a higher prevalence in women and increasing incidence as people age.[2] While there are multiple etiologies of constipation, each can be broadly categorized as either somatopathic (gastroenteric, oncologic, endocrinologic, neurologic, or metabolic) or functional (medications, prolonged GI transit time, inadequate fluid or dietary fiber intake, or immobility) in nature.[2] Opioid-induced constipation occurs as a result of interaction with opioid receptors located in the gut and CNS. Within the longitudinal muscle layer of the small and large intestine, opioids inhibit acetylcholine release, thereby decreasing propulsive effects. As a result of the increased transit time, retained fecal material absorbs more water. Constipation is further exacerbated by impaired defecation flex and decreased intestinal, gastric, biliary, and pancreatic secretions.[2] Among the various medications with potential for causing constipation, opioids are the most notorious. Furthermore, lack of constipation in a patient with normal GI function may, in part, suggest that the opioid dose is too low or even that the medication is being diverted.

Constipation is the most common dose-dependent side effect of opioids. Because minimal to no tolerance develops to opioid-induced constipation, it should be anticipated during the course of opioid therapy, irrespective of the route of administration (oral, intravenous, epidural, or intrathecal). Prophylactic treatment with cathartics (senna tablet Qd or BID, cascara 4–12 mL Qhs, bisacodyl 5 mg PO Qhs or bisacodyl 10 mg suppository Qhs) and adequate oral or intravenous fluid hydration (1.5–2.0 L/day)[2] should be instituted upon initiation and continuation of opioid therapy. Opioid-related constipation results from increased tone and decreased gut motility. Stool softeners and bulking agents such as bran or psyllium derivatives alone will be inadequate for constipation relief. The addition of a laxative is required.

Pharmacologically, laxatives soften hard stool by affecting water and electrolyte transfer within the small and large intestine. While it is beyond the scope of this chapter to discuss each type of laxative, it is important to understand that each is categorized based on its mechanism of action: bulk-forming, osmotic, stimulating, or other. Bulk-forming agents are minimally absorbed and promote water retention, thereby softening the stool, increasing the intestinal wall diameter, and augmenting peristalsis. Without adequate fluid hydration, bulk-forming agents can worsen constipation. Similar to bulk-forming agents, osmotic laxatives (e.g., lactulose and polyethylene glycol) are minimally absorbed. Lactulose causes both a pH- and volume-induced increase in stool propulsion, but has common side effects of flatulence, abdominal cramping, and bloating.[2] Unlike lactulose, polyethylene glycol's affects only depend on orally consumed fluids and do not affect intraluminal water. It is also better tolerated and has a lower incidence of side effects than lactulose. Stimulating laxatives (e.g., senna, bisacodyl, and castor oil) work directly on the myenteric plexus and also increase intestinal fluid content both by preventing fluid resorption and by promoting an influx of electrolytes into the intestine. Abdominal cramping tends to be a common side effect. Rectal laxatives (suppositories and enemas) should be used if the goal is to trigger the defecation reflex in order to empty the rectal vault.[2]

Besides anti-constipation medications, other options are available. For example, there is some evidence that suggests that transdermal fentanyl may be less likely to cause constipation than oral opioids because it bypasses the gut.[3] Such findings still require confirmation, and it remains to be seen if this applies to other new opioid delivery systems, such as the transmucosal fentanyl system.[4] Nonetheless, all opioids produce constipation no matter that some may produce less potent effects than others.

One could also consider a drug whose side effect profile includes diarrhea. Misoprostol (Cytotec), which is commonly prescribed to protect the gastric mucosa from the irritating effects of nonsteroidal anti-inflammatory drugs (NSAIDs), is often associated with diarrhea. Therefore, it can potentially serve a dual purpose in those patients taking both opioids and NSAIDs. However, misoprostol must be avoided in pregnant patients and should be used with extreme caution in women of child-bearing capacity due to its potential abortifacient property via stimulation of uterine contraction.

Finally, an opioid antagonist such as naloxone may be considered. Typically given intravenously for reversal of opioid-induced overdose or respiratory depression, naloxone is a competitive mu-opioid receptor antagonist that has a rapid onset of effect (within 2 minutes) and a short serum half-life of 1 to 1.5 hours.[1,5] While it exerts its primary effects on central opioid receptors, naloxone also works on peripheral receptors. By taking naloxone orally, it primarily antagonizes the opioid receptors in the gut. The enteral route also allows one to take advantage of naloxone's limited potential for systemic bioavailability (less than 3%) due to its extensive first-pass

hepatic metabolism (greater than 97%).[5,6] At the same time, one must remain cognizant of the possibility of reversing opioid analgesia and/or precipitating withdrawal symptoms since oral naloxone is lipid-soluble and crosses the blood–brain barrier. Studies evaluating the efficacy of using naloxone to reverse constipation have been mixed with some showing benefit, no benefit, side effects of partially or completely reversing analgesia, or precipitation of withdrawal symptoms.[7–10] While the exact dosing regimen of oral naloxone for constipation is uncertain, the initial dose could be as low as 0.8 mg BID but should not exceed 5 mg per day with gradual titration up to 12 mg per day.[5] In our institution we usually start with 1.2–2.4 mg PO (3–6 small ampules) every 4 hours until the first bowel movement, or for 5 doses. If ineffective, another series with a higher dose (3–5 mg per dose) may be tried. It should be realized that naloxone doses will likely have to be at least 20% of the daily oral morphine or morphine-equivalent dose in most patients before efficacy is noted. Dosing ranges have varied extensively from 0.5% to 60%.[5]

Similar in structure to naloxone, naltrexone and nalmefene have a prolonged duration of effect due to their longer elimination half-life (4 and 8.5 to 10.8 hours, respectively). Both have limited efficacy in reversing constipation due to their intended advantage of oral absorption with the tendency to concomitantly reverse analgesia or precipitate a withdrawal syndrome. Alternatively, opioid antagonists that cannot cross the blood–brain barrier due to poor lipid solubility have the greatest chance of reducing peripherally mediated opioid side effects without reversing analgesia or inducing withdrawal. Thus far, clinical trials on oral formulations of methylnaltrexone and the investigational drug ADL 8-2698 (Adolor Corporation, Malverin, PA) look promising in this regard.[1,5,11] It is critically important to realize these poorly lipid-soluble antagonists cannot treat any concomitant centrally mediated side effects, i.e., sedation and respiratory depression. Since nonopioid medications (e.g., anticholinergics, antispasmodics, antiepileptics, and antacids), metabolic and endocrinologic disorders (e.g., hypercalcemia and diabetic autonomic neuropathy), and other disease states (e.g., spinal cord injury and Parkinson's) can contribute to constipation, it is crucial to remember that oral opioid antagonists only work when the constipation is solely or primarily opioid-related.

When constipation occurs, it is important to differentiate whether or not it is due in part or completely to GI obstruction.[2] In the presence of a complete obstruction laxatives should be avoided and a surgical consultation obtained. With a partial obstruction, laxatives may be tried. In the absence of obstruction, a rectal examination should be performed to assess for stool presence and consistency. If the stool is soft, treat with both a stimulating suppository and oral laxative. If the stool is hard, treat with both a stool softening suppository and oral laxative. If no stool is detected in the rectum, obstruction must be ruled out. If stool is detected in the colon, an enema should be prescribed in addition to laxatives and stimulants.

Nausea and Vomiting: Opioid-induced nausea and vomiting is primarily a centrally mediated effect on the brainstem medulla and secondarily a peripherally mediated effect on the GI tract.[5,11] While nausea and vomiting may occur with the initiation of opioid therapy, cases of severe, protracted nausea and vomiting are seldom due to opioids alone. In the majority of cases the nausea and vomiting is mild and can be treated with antiemetics. Since most patients develop tolerance to the nausea and vomiting within two to three days, decreasing the opioid dose may be sufficient to decrease symptoms prior to resuming upward titration. Alternatively, changing the route of administration may also alleviate the symptoms (e.g., IV to PR, etc.). If these simple measures fail, substituting an equianalgesic dose of a different opioid analgesic should be considered. It remains unclear why opioids should have differential emetic side effects in an individual patient, or why opioid rotation reduces or eliminates these side effects. Avoiding a known offending opioid or premedication with an antiemetic should be considered in those with a history of opioid-induced severe nausea and vomiting.

Stimulation of various receptors in the brainstem's medullary chemoreceptor trigger zone is felt to be the primary mechanism of opioid-induced nausea and vomiting. Effective antiemetic agents include the antihistamines H-1 blockers such as hydroxyzine, serotonin antagonists 5HT-3 blockers such as ondansetron, dopamine antagonists such as droperidol, haloperidol, and metoclopramide, anticholinergics such as scopolamine, and cholinergics such as low-dose metoclopramide. Benzodiazepines such as lorazepam may also possess antiemetic properties, but it is not known whether this is due to direct effects on receptors found in the CTZ or indirect treatment of anxiety and conditioning. Since it is unclear which of these drug classes is most effective for opioid-induced nausea and vomiting, selection is often empirical but should theoretically be guided by the antiemetic's potential secondary ability to treat GI dismotility, sedation, pruritus, anxiety, or psychosis. For example, opioid-related nausea may be associated with orthostasis, thereby implicating vestibular dysfunction which may best respond to antiemetics that are antihistamines and anticholinergics. Scopolamine is especially advantageous because of its transdermal patch administration.

If side effects of nausea and vomiting persist, consider administering the antiemetic on a scheduled basis. Some antiemetics can cause additive side effects of sedation; therefore patients should be forewarned and carefully monitored. Addition of an opioid antagonist such as intravenous naloxone or oral methylnaltrexone may also be helpful in reversing direct GI side effects,[12,13] and they do not cause sedation.

Of course, nonopioid-related mediators of nausea and vomiting also must be considered. These include chemotherapy (particularly cisplatin), radiation therapy, brain or GI metastases, elevated intracranial pressure, peptic ulcer disease, esophagitis, gastritis, electrolyte and acid-base imbalance, uremia, liver disease, infection, pregnancy, and fear and/or anxiety.

Sedation: Opioid-induced sedation is a common side effect with opioid therapy and can often times be the rate-limiting step for further dose escalations. In opioid-naive patients the sedation usually resolves over time as tolerance develops. Conversely, for those who are opioid-tolerant and require dose escalation due to worsening pain, accommodation to the sedative side effects may be only partial. While the mechanism of opioid-induced sedation has not been well characterized, clinical and laboratory evidence strongly implicates the involvement of acetylcholine.[14]

In those with persistent sedation strategies for management include decreasing the opioid dose to the smallest amount necessary for adequate analgesia and ruling out other causes of sedation such as other drugs or even nighttime insomnia.

It is important to evaluate whether concurrent medications may be contributing to the symptoms and determine if adjuvant nonmedication therapies (nerve blocks, neuromodulation therapy, or radiation therapy) may be helpful and opioid sparing.[14] Initial attempts can include decreasing the dose or decreasing the dosing frequency, while maintaining the same overall daily dose. This strategy should decrease the peak serum and CNS concentrations of the opioid.[15] If accumulation of the opioid is suspected, either increase the dose interval or change to a shorter-acting agent. For unremitting sedation, stimulants such as dextroamphetamine or methylphenidate can be used. Additional benefits of such stimulants include potentiation of analgesia, improvement in cognitive function, and treating depression. However, these medications are not without their disadvantages. It is not uncommon for patients with underlying cardiovascular disease, agitation, or anxiety to experience an exacerbation of these symptoms.[16] Tolerance can also develop to amphetamines. Furthermore, their abuse potential and, therefore, classification as schedule II controlled substances implies greater risk and vigilance on the part of the prescriber.

Modafinil (Provigil®), a novel wake-promoting drug that is a schedule IV controlled substance, may be an appealing alternative. Its inability to produce psychoactive or euphoric effects is due to its weak increase in dopamine levels in the nucleus accumbuns, unlike amphetamines and methylphenidate.[17,18] Furthermore, modafinil's lower abuse potential is attributed to its (1) insolubility in water, which makes it noninjectable; (2) degradation when heated, which makes it impossible to smoke; and (3) long duration of effect, thereby not requiring more than three times per day dosing.[19,20] While modafinil's exact mechanism of action remains unknown, its wake-promoting effect is thought to be due to inhibition of gamma-aminobutyric acid (GABA) transmission in the anterior hypothalamus. In various studies, it has been shown to improve fatigue associated with multiple sclerosis and fibromyalgia and to augment treatment of depression.[18] In a retrospective chart review of patients receiving modafinil for opioid-induced sedation Webster et al found subjective improvements in levels of alertness, wakefulness, and fatigue.[18]

The states of arousal, attention, and respiratory regulation are, in part, mediated by central cholinergic activity. Opioids have been shown to inhibit this pathway.[14] Furthermore, animal models suggest acetylcholine can affect nociception.[14] Donepezil (Aricept®), an oral selective acetylcholinesterase inhibitor, approved for the treatment of cognitive dysfunction in Alzheimer's disease, may be an intriguing option. In addition to having long-acting properties, donepezil exhibits linear pharmacokinetics, does not have any significant drug interactions, and appears to be well tolerated by most patients (common side effects may include fatigue, diarrhea, nausea, vomiting, and muscle cramps).[14,21] Nonetheless, it should be used with caution as other acetylcholinesterase-inhibiting agents have been associated with weight loss and bradycardia.[14] While only reporting on a case series of six cancer patients taking greater than 200 mg of oral morphine equivalents per day, Slatkin et al described successful results in treating sedation and improving daily function in most when given donepezil.[14] Similarly, a one-week open prospective pilot study by Bruera et al using donepezil 5 mg every morning in cancer patients on high doses of opioids (median oral morphine equivalent was 180 mg/day) showed improvements in sedation, fatigue, sensation of well-being, anxiety, and constipation.[21] Donepezil's potentially beneficial side effect of diarrhea may also be a welcoming benefit for those suffering from constipation.

Sedation in the setting of respiratory slowing is managed differently, and occurs most commonly with opioids that have long plasma half-lives. Withholding one or two doses and then decreasing the overall dose to 25% of the original dose until symptom resolution is usually sufficient and will usually avoid withdrawl.[15]

Respiratory Depression: Respiratory depression is a potentially serious complication of opioid therapy. This side effect is mediated centrally in the medulla, whereby opioid-induced respiratory depression leads to both an increase in PCO_2 and a decrease in the medulla's sensitivity to carbon dioxide concentrations, which further decreases the respiratory rate.[5] Clinically apparent signs of irregular breathing indicate severe respiratory depression.[22] Fortunately, tolerance occurs early with chronic opioid administration. Combining oral or intravenous opioids with epidural or intrathecal opioids has long been considered to potentially lead to additive depressant effects on respiration. Evidence for this widely held conclusion is lacking. When administered neuraxially, the greatest risk of respiratory depression occurs within 4 to 8 hours and is more likely to occur with hydrophilic versus lipophilic opioids.[23]

When respiratory depression occurs, naloxone should be administered. While its onset of action may be rapid, its duration of action is brief. Therefore, naloxone may need to be administered more often than once or even continuously. Since fully therapeutic doses of naloxone can precipitate withdrawal in physically dependent patients,[1] careful dosing is advised (0.4 mg diluted in 10 mL of normal saline, administered in 0.5 mL [0.02 mg] IV boluses every minute until resolution of the respiratory depression; or a continuous infusion of 0.8 mg mixed with 250 mL of normal saline).[15] Reversal of sedation to the point of alertness is usually not the goal, as this will more than likely be associated with reversal of analgesia and precipitation of withdrawal symptoms. In certain situations antagonization of opioid actions can promote pulmonary edema. This effect is likely the result of reversal of opioid-induced pulmonary vascular smooth muscle relaxation. This is usually of minimal concern unless the patient is predisposed toward pulmonary edema (e.g., congestive heart failure, adult respiratory distress syndrome).

Pruritus: Pruritus is an uncommon side effect with oral opioids. Parenteral opioids typically produce mild pruritus, although it can be moderate to severe in a minority of patients. Pruritus tends to occur most commonly when opioids are administered neuraxially. The incidence of opioid-induced pruritus varies from 30% to 100% and occurs most commonly with intrathecal morphine[24] and in parturients.[25] The reported incidence of pruritus after administration of intrathecal morphine, fentanyl, and sufentanil is 62% to 85%, 67% to 100%, and 80%, respectively.[26] The incidence after epidural administration of the same three drugs is 65% to 70%, 67%, and 55%, respectively. With neuraxially administered opioids, symptoms typically occur within 2 to 5 hours and are dose related.[27] Fortunately, tolerance to this side effect develops rapidly, with resolution occurring within one to two days for those receiving spinal opioids.[5]

Opioid-related pruritus is usually localized to the face or less often the perineum and can also become generalized. The mechanism of oral or parenteral opioid-induced pruritus is not well understood, although morphine and some related opioids can cause mast cells to release histamine.[5] Mu-opioid receptors may also be involved, as administration of an opioid antagonist can reverse pruritus. Conversely, spinal opioid-induced pruritus is felt to be a centrally mediated phenomenon (presence of an "itch center" in the CNS, excitation of medullary dorsal horn neurons, central migration of spinal opioids to the brainstem, and antagonism of inhibitory transmitters), as histamine release is not always seen.[4,5,25] Prostaglandin release can lead to histamine release and potentiate histamine-induced pruritus.[25] Serotonergic pathways may also be involved. In patients with pruritus associated with cholestatic jaundice evidence suggests a link between the release of endogenous opioids and the serotonin system. Furthermore, administration of ondansetron (Zofran®), a 5-HT$_3$-receptor antagonist, in this patient population reduced pruritus.[24,28] Interestingly, morphine's effect is partially mediated by serotonin release.[29] The 5-HT$_3$-receptors are located in the dorsal part of the spinal cord and the spinal nucleus of the trigeminal nerve, the latter of which probably explains why itching occurs on the nose and upper face after administering an intrathecal opioid.[24,25] Finally, opioid antagonism of the inhibitory neurotransmitters GABA and glycine may also contribute to pruritus. Intrathecal administration of a glycine antagonist in cats produced the same side effects as intrathecal morphine.[25]

Since pruritus may be an idiosyncratic response to a particular opioid, opioid rotation may be a sufficient treatment. When this is insufficient, medications to treat the symptoms should be considered. Naloxone is currently the most effective therapy and is useful for opioid-related pruritus from any route of administration. An intravenous naloxone infusion (0.25 µg/kg/hour)[5] can treat intravenous morphine-induced pruritus without reversing analgesia, although this may not be the case if the infusion exceeds 2 µg/kg/hour.[5,25] Besides naloxone, other antagonists (oral naltrexone [6–9 mg], methylnaltrexone, nalmefene) and agonist–antagonists (butorphanol and nalbuphine) can be used.[5,25] While effective, dosing must be done cautiously to prevent reversal of analgesia.

Antihistamines may be more effective when pruritus is related to systemic rather than neuraxial opioids. Since antihistamines can potentiate opioid analgesia, a decrease in opioid dose might further reduce pruritus. The antipruritic efficacy of antihistamine therapy may, in part, be related to sedation since nonsedating antihistamines are less effective than sedating antihistamines.[4] If an antihistamine is given but does not adequately treat the pruritus, remember that sedative effects of antihistamines and opioids will be additive, and that administration of an opioid antagonist may decrease analgesia.

Due to morphine-associated serotonin release and the high density of 5-HT$_3$ receptors located in the dorsal part of the spinal cord and the spinal nucleus of the trigeminal nerve, a 5-HT$_3$-receptor antagonist might be a reasonable option. Epidural administration of droperidol, a weak 5-HT$_3$-receptor antagonist to parturients receiving epidural anesthesia with 0.5% bupivacaine with 1:200,000 epinephrine and morphine 2 mg demonstrated a dose-dependent decrease in pruritus, but at the risk of increased side effects of sedation.[30] Intravenous ondansetron has also demonstrated efficacy in reducing the incidence of pruritus. Kyriakides et al. randomized surgical patients receiving alfentanil 10 mg/kg IV into two groups: ondansetron 4 mg IV vs. 0.9% saline IV (placebo).[24] The authors showed a statistically significant reduction in scratching with the ondansetron (42.5%) vs. placebo (70%) group and a statistically insignificant reduction in itching (30% vs. 42.5%, respectively). In parturients receiving intrathecal morphine, Yeh et al. found that the incidence of pruritus was 25%, 80%, and 85% in the IV ondansetron, diphenhydramine, and placebo groups, respectively.[31] Based on ondansetron's dose-related efficacy in treating opioid-induced nausea and vomiting, the same might hold true in the treatment of pruritus.[24]

Recently, Torn et al. demonstrated that even small doses of propofol IV (10 mg bolus followed by 30 mg/24 hour infusion) prevented intrathecal opioid-induced pruritus, most likely by inhibiting posterior horn transmission in the spinal cord.[32] While adverse effects from low-dose propofol are minimal, administration of this sedative hypnotic should be limited to a monitored setting.

Finally, one could consider the use of an NSAID as a prophylaxis against pruritus in addition to using it as an adjuvant analgesic. In patients receiving epidural fentanyl or intrathecal morphine, Colbert et al. demonstrated a reduced incidence of pruritus when patients were also given intravenous tenoxicam[33] or rectal diclofenac,[34] respectively.[33]

While agents from multiple drug classes can be tried, it is not clear how they compare against each other in terms of efficacy. Ultimately, ondansetron may be the ideal medication for treating pruritus because it produces minimal sedation while addressing any postoperative nausea and vomiting without reversing analgesia.

ADDICTION AND OPIOIDS

Predicting and detecting addiction in patients on chronic opioids can be a limiting step in treating chronic pain. Patients with legitimate needs for opioid analgesics are often denied appropriate treatment because of their previous history of addiction or due to fear of potential addiction in individuals with no prior history. Although it may appear clear-cut to distinguish abusers from non-abusers, this is not necessarily always feasible. Aberrant behaviors may or may not be indicative of compulsive use or abuse of medications. Nonetheless, therapy with opioids is often avoided or abandoned because of misunderstood concepts of addiction, tolerance, and/or physical dependence.

Chronic pain and addiction are clinical disorders that frequently occur together. The prevalence of drug abuse, dependence, or addiction in chronic pain patients has been stated to range from 3% to 19%.[35] Diagnosis of chronic pain and addiction are complicated medical problems in their own right, but treatment is made even more difficult when both are treated concurrently in the same patient. Twenty-three percent of pain patients in an inpatient rehabilitation facility were found to meet the criteria for addiction.[36] Likewise, chronic severe pain is believed to be prevalent in outpatient substance abuse treatment, especially those in methadone maintenance programs. Thirty seven percent of patients on methadone for heroin addiction reported having a significant pain complaint.[37] Even when chronic pain presents without the complexities of a dual diagnosis, residual attitudinal barriers related to the stigma of addiction can lead to inadequate care. The mere threat of the mishandling of medications or the potential

for addiction often impedes appropriate opioid prescribing. While 6% to 15% of the population suffering from chronic pain were found to have an addiction problem, the other 85% to 94% received less than optimal treatment due to the association between misuse and opioid prescribing.[38]

Despite indications that addiction is a concern in the pain clinic setting, rational opioid prescribing has not been linked with stimulating addiction. A recent study by Joranson et al evaluated the trend in opioid use and abuse.[39] These authors performed an analysis of the national use of five opioid analgesics used to treat severe pain along with a retrospective chart review of emergency room visits associated with abusive behaviors. From 1990 to 1996 there were increases in medical use of morphine (59%; 2.2 to 3.5 million g), fentanyl (1168%; 3263 to 41,371 g), oxycodone (23%; 1.6 to 2.0 million g), and hydromorphone (19%; 118,455 to 141,325 g), and a decrease in the medical use of meperidine (35%; 5.2 to 3.4 million g). During this same interval, the total number of drug abuse cases per year due to opioid analgesics increased only 6.6%, from 32,430 to 34,563. Although somewhat alarming, this increase was not due to more instances of opioid abuse. On the contrary, the proportion of reported opioid abuse relative to total drug abuse decreased from 5.1% to 3.8%. Reports of abuse decreased for meperidine (39%; 1335 to 806), oxycodone (29%; 4526 to 3190), fentanyl (59%; 59 to 24), and hydromorphone (15%; 718 to 609), and increased for morphine (3%; 838 to 865). The authors concluded that the trend of increasing medical use of opioid analgesics to treat pain does not appear to contribute to increases in opioid analgesic abuse.

Stigma is not the only reason that patients with chronic pain have difficulty obtaining opioids. Fear of physical dependence and the development of tolerance are other obstacles that impede the use of these agents. Tolerance and physical dependence are often confused for addiction in patients receiving opioid treatment. These entities are completely separate phenomena that coincidently may occur when patients are treated with opioid analgesics for their chronic pain.[35] Conflicting definitions of addiction, tolerance, and physical dependence cloud the literature. The American Pain Society (APS), the American Academy of Pain Medicine (AAPM), and the American Society of Addiction Medicine (ASAM) convened a consensus conference to reduce the misunderstanding that has been caused by the use of these terms in reference to patients who are receiving opioids for pain.[40] It was hoped that these misunderstandings among regulators and health care providers would promote appropriate treatment of pain. The three organizations unanimously approved the following definitions in 2001:

- **Addiction** is a primary, chronic, neurobiological disease, with genetic, psychosocial, and environmental factors influencing its development and manifestations. It is characterized by behaviors that include one or more of the following: impaired control over drug use, compulsive use, continued use despite harm, and craving.
- **Physical dependence** is a state of adaptation that is manifested by a drug class-specific withdrawal syndrome that can be produced by abrupt cessation, rapid dose reduction, decreasing blood level of the drug, and/or administration of an antagonist.
- **Tolerance** is a state of adaptation in which exposure to a drug induces changes that result in a diminution of one or more of the drug's effects over time.

Legal Barriers to the Treatment of Chronic Pain in Patients with an Addiction: There is a bewildering array of laws and regulations that govern the areas of chronic pain and addiction.[41] The legality of prescribing controlled substances to patients with prior histories of addiction is often misunderstood, even amongst lawyers and regulators. Although most addiction specialists would discourage prescribing controlled substances to practicing addicts because of the significant risk of enabling dysfunctional behavior and further harm, the undertreatment of pain in patients with prior histories of addiction may trigger aberrant behavior and relapse. While it is lawful under federal policy to prescribe, administer, and dispense controlled substances to people with addictive diseases, many practitioners have incorrectly assumed that this is not the case.

There is legal precedent in case law that is deferential to physicians who treat chronic pain in patients with addiction. In 1993 the administrator of the Drug Enforcement Administration (DEA) investigated an Ohio physician who prescribed opioids to a drug abuser for treatment of non-malignant pain.[42] The DEA sought to penalize the physician under the jurisdiction of federal law. During the administrative hearing, the DEA contended that the physician had prescribed a variety of controlled substances to his patients over extended periods of time and that one of his patients had a serious substance abuse problem. Ruling against the DEA, it was ruled that the physician could legitimately use these medications in the treatment of chronic pain syndrome, indicating that there was no evidence that the controlled substances had been prescribed for illegitimate purposes. In subsequent cases the DEA has recognized that a physician's prescribing of controlled substances to treat pain is a legitimate medical practice, even for patients who may be drug abusers.

It remains illegal under federal law for a practitioner to prescribe controlled substances solely for maintenance therapy unless specifically authorized to do so as part of a narcotic treatment program. Physicians may treat pain in a patient who is simultaneously enrolled in one of these narcotic treatment programs. The law does not have difficulty differentiating the nuances of a patient receiving medication from a narcotic treatment program and from a physician for treating pain as long as a physician fully documents that the medication being provided is solely for pain. It would be wise for a practitioner to be very clear in his/her documentation regarding the treatment plan of opioid prescribed for pain, especially when a history of narcotic addiction is a factor.

State regulations regarding opioid prescribing are now undergoing evolutionary changes from a very restrictive climate to one in which practitioners are being allowed to treat chronic pain patients without interference. There have been numerous intractable pain treatment acts (IPTA) passed in the last decade stating that a physician may not be disciplined for treating chronic pain with appropriate controlled substances. Unfortunately, several of these legislative mandates contain confusing language. For instance, there are several states in which an addict is defined as someone with a physical dependence. Additional prohibitions in the language of several states IPTA (Texas, North Dakota, and Tennessee) limit a physician from treating a patient with opioids if they are known to be addicts.[41]

As of 2001, federal laws regarding narcotic treatment programs were revised, adopting the new name Opioid Treatment Programs.[43] One of the major thrusts for modifying federal laws was to alter admission criteria as defined by the Diagnostic and Statistical Manual for Mental Disorders and the International Classification of Disorders.[44] The policy change will restrict the criteria to individuals with active addictive disorders and refrain from encompassing individuals who previously sought opioid medications for pain treatment.[41]

Treatment of Pain in Patients with a History of Addiction: Many providers have trepidation when confronted with a substance abuser in need of pain medication. Even when the physicians are aware of the legitimate use of opioids in the aftermath of an acute injury or surgery, they are often still not willing to prescribe the appropriate amount of analgesics to control pain. For example, trauma and postoperative states occur in patients with substance abuse issues, yet in these circumstances analgesia is often suboptimal. Lack of knowledge regarding opioid requirements in this setting may be a factor. Undertreatment of pain is problematic amongst patients in methadone maintenance programs.[45] Since aberrant drug-related behaviors are part of the repertoire of these individuals, it is not surprising that they do not receive the appropriate care even in the setting of acute injury and pain. Ironically, it may be through desperation that they exhibit drug-seeking behavior that appears to be mistaken for manipulation.

The term pseudoaddiction has been given to the false conclusions from behaviors that suggest drug abuse rather than the legitimate need for additional medications.[46] The manipulation or drug-seeking behavior resolves once the pain is alleviated, usually via additional opioids. This differs from addiction where dysfunctional behavior continues unabated regardless of the dosage increase. There are some expert guidelines that can be followed in the setting of addiction, opioid maintenance therapy, and acute pain, such as following surgery or trauma.[45,47] First, if maintenance dosing is already in place, it is recommended that the dosage of methadone for opioid addiction maintenance be continued. This can be administered intravenously, if the patient is NPO. Under federal law, any physician with a standard DEA license may prescribe maintenance methadone to a patient who is hospitalized. Obviously, the intent is to prevent withdrawal and relapse during limited periods of high stress such as those accompanying medical illness, trauma, and/or surgery. Second, a short-acting opioid for the acute painful condition for which the patient has been hospitalized may be used. The route of administration may initially be parenteral and patient-controlled analgesia may be necessary and optimal. If the patient is opioid tolerant, higher than usual doses for nontolerant patients may be required. Optimal agents include morphine 1 mg per mL, dilaudid 0.2 mg per mL or fentanyl 10 mL/cm^3. Initial dosing would depend upon the amount of methadone maintenance but are usually at least 2–3 mL per bolus. Subsequent escalations of the bolus are based on titration to the patient's response. If the patient is NPO, it may be necessary to add a continuous infusion of one of these agents. Supplemental intravenous analgesic medication in the form of injections by the nursing staff may be administered early on in the course of therapy while the patient's requirements are being assessed. If supplemental injections are necessary, it would be best to have the continuous opioid infusion increased. Once the patient resumes oral intake, they can be converted back to their standard dose of methadone with the addition of a short-acting opioid (dilaudid, oxycodone, hydrocodone, or codeine) for continuing breakthrough pain.

The use of this breakthrough pain medication may be continued for a maximum of 4 to 6 weeks as consistent with the course and resolution of the acute painful condition. Should the pain persist, it will be necessary to proceed as if it were a chronic pain problem with special considerations that are discussed below.

There is sparse literature on maladaptive behaviors seen in the addicted population during treatment for pain with opioids. Dunbar and Katz examined 20 patients with a history of substance abuse and were treated with opioids for their nonmalignant pain.[48] The retrospective study looked at the predictive factors associated with prescription abuse. They found that those who did not abuse their opioid prescriptions were more likely to either (1) have a history of isolated alcohol abuse as opposed to abusing multiple substances or (2) have a remote history of polysubstance abuse. In addition, they were found more likely to be active members of Alcoholics Anonymous and to have a stable support system (e.g., family). The group that abused opioids tended to escalate medications and request early refills soon after initiating their opioids. A recent history of polysubstance abuse or simply a prior history of oxycodone abuse was a predictive risk factors for prescription drug abuse.[48] Individuals who are actively abusing opioids are best managed in a drug treatment facility where they receive their medication for pain as well as treatment for addiction in a controlled setting. Studies suggest that 30% to 80% of substance abusers suffer from coexisting psychiatric disorders.[49] Psychiatric evaluation and treatment should be implemented at the beginning of therapy.

Patients in methadone maintenance programs have been successfully treated for pain in a substance abuse recovery program by a physician knowledgeable in prescribing opioids for both purposes. Patients on methadone maintenance may have decreased pain thresholds and/or increased tolerance to opioids. This may be why they often require higher doses of pain medications and suggests that one should allow them to titrate their medication during brief periods in which they are experiencing acute pain. These patients can receive daily methadone maintenance and see a physician for prescribing additional opioids for their pain with close and frequent monitoring. These office visits initially occur every few days with the goal of progressive lengthening of the interval between visits as mutual trust develops. The physician develops trust by demonstrating empathy while at the same time establishing clear behavioral boundaries. These behavioral boundaries are often supported with an opioid agreement or contract and objective screening. During this opioid trial, the patient must demonstrate compliance with all aspects of the treatment regimen, including demonstration of functional improvement. This delicate period usually involves pill counts, periodic and frequent urine toxicology screens to exclude illicit drug use, questions regarding functionality and percentage of pain relief, and family or other care giver corroboration. Enrollment in a support group and/or professional counseling for substance abusers is usually mandatory. The type of organized meeting or counselor varies and is usually left to the discretion of the treater and patient. For instance, some prefer narcotics anonymous while others utilize group psychotherapy. The importance of this type of support activity cannot be overemphasized.

The percentage of pain relief provides one measure of improvement, while functional assessments provide another.

Patients are informed at the onset of their treatment with opioids that it will not be possible to eliminate their pain entirely. A treatment plan is prearranged whereby only a percentage of pain relief will be sought. Implementing a clear, rational, and mutually agreed upon course helps lead to reduction of drug-seeking behavior normally encountered in this setting. Pain relief is not as important as improved function since dysfunction is the hallmark of addiction.

Prescription Drug Abuse: There are multiple sources by which prescription drugs can be obtained. Addiction specialists have long maintained lists of bizarre and illegal behaviors that are encountered in their practices (Table 13-1). Due to the potential role in illicit trafficking, physicians have a reasonable fear of being deceived by drug-abusing patients. This potential risk can lead physicians to assume that a patient is drug abusing rather than simply requesting additional medications for undertreated pain. Conversely, when confronted with a hostile and suspicious physician, patients often feel stigmatized.[50] The paucity of data into the predictive and mitigating factors for prescription drug abuse remains a significant factor in the contentious nature of the debate over the appropriate use of opioids to treat patients with chronic pain. Concerns regarding efficacy and drug abuse abound.[51–54] It appears difficult to distinguish abusers from non-abusers based upon behavior alone. One study demonstrated that 21% of chronic pain patients being prescribed opioids for chronic pain with no behavioral issues were actually abusing prescription medications or illicit drugs as evidenced by "dirty" urine tox screens.[55] Clinicians must be aware of the potential for prescription abuse while simultaneously recognizing that, in practice, there are rarely absolutely confirming behaviors of abuse. Most are relative indicators that warrant suspicion without warranting a firm conclusion.

There are several types of aberrant behaviors that may be suggestive of, but not conclusive for, prescription drug abuse.

TABLE 13-1. ILLEGAL DRUG-RELATED BEHAVIORS

Selling prescription drugs
Forging prescriptions
Stealing or "borrowing" drugs from another person
Injecting oral preparations
Obtaining prescription drugs from nonmedical sources
Ongoing use of illicit drugs
Multiple unsanctioned dose escalations
Repeated episodes of lost prescriptions

Modified from Jaffe: Opiates: Clinical aspects. In Lowinson JRP, Mullman R (eds): Substance Abuse: A Comprehensive Text. Williams and Wilkins, Baltimore, 1992, pp 186–194.

Prescription drug abuse is differentiated from the more classic form of opioid addiction whereby an abuser consumes illicit substances obtained from the street. Prescription drug abusers usually are unable to take medications according to an agreed upon schedule and may take multiple doses together: so called self-escalation of opioids. To cover up their self-escalation when they run out of medication, they often report their prescriptions lost or stolen. Such reports take the form of excuses that can range from comical to disturbing. Alternatively, patients may find multiple prescribers to avoid the consequences of reporting self-escalation. While some patients may openly consider this acceptable practice, it is usually contrary to the mutually agreed upon treatment plan for opioid prescribing. Insurance companies are quick to point out this type of activity, as do pharmacists involved in tracking prescriptions on computer databases for state agencies. There are many other behaviors that may raise suspicion of abusive behavior. The use of opioids for nonintended symptoms, i.e., sedation at bedtime, anxiolysis, or for the psychomimetic effect from a short-acting opioid, is to be viewed with apprehension by the prescribing physician. There are obviously more optimal treatments for sleep and/or anxiety and depression. The use of opioids for their psychomimetic effects may be avoided by relying primarily on long-acting opioids which tend to be slow in onset (and slow in offset) thus avoiding any sense of a "rush." Such practices are strongly advised since, at present, there is no accepted screening questionnaire available to determine who would be at greatest risk of developing prescription drug abuse.

Without a rapid screening examination, it behooves practicing physicians to assess periodically for the presence of prescription drug abuse to limit their liability and regulatory scrutiny. Many practitioners rely on their impression of the patient's "drug-seeking behavior" to provide them with a rationale to refuse prescribing opioids. The meaning of "drug-seeking behavior" is controversial as the term is often used pejoratively and signs of these behaviors can easily be based upon incorrect impressions that lead to false conclusions.

Repeated prescription loss, multiple prescribers, and requests for early refills may simply be manifestations of inadequate analgesia by a patient who is attempting self-medication to alleviate pain. The psychiatric and addiction literature has, until recently, been a source of confusion regarding addiction in the patient with chronic pain. To diagnose addictive disease, the DSM-IV Diagnostic Criteria for Substance Dependence requires evidence of certain drug-seeking behaviors whereby "important social, occupational, or recreational activities were given up or reduced because of substance use." Classic evidence of compulsive opioid use may be missing in pain patients because opioid medication is being prescribed and, thus, readily available. In addition, pain patients usually do not have to compromise their lifestyle nor run the risk of endangering their lives to obtain the prescribed opioid. Likewise, an illicit life style (i.e., involvement in criminal activity, drug diversion) is generally not seen in the chronic pain population. The form of addiction seen in the pain patient is different from the type seen in the street addict. The subtle signs of prescription drug abuse (Table 13-2) are deciphered from multiple observations and encounters.

A number of opioids and opioid preparations are available for clinical use. The types of vehicles for drug administration are expanding as basic scientists and pharmaceutical companies recognize the need for different method of drug delivery and the need for sustained-release medications that are slow in onset to reduce reinforcing psychomimetic effects. Evidence that short-acting opioids are responsible for escalating tolerance and addiction is incomplete. Reinforcing euphoric effects from a short-acting opioid would be more likely than from a long-acting opioid because of the rapid uptake of the former. For instance, while nicotine may be the most addictive drug to be commonly abused in our society, the transdermal nicotine patch is not abused. Heroin addicts are well known to derive much less euphoria from oral methadone maintenance than from intravenous heroin.

Physicians tend to use short-acting schedule III opioids to avoid stigma or burdensome paperwork such as monthly prescriptions that are required for schedule II opioids in some states. Physicians thus avoid prescribing long-acting schedule II opioids (e.g., sustained-release morphine, transdermal fentanyl, sustained-release oxycodone, or methadone) for chronic non-malignant pain. A study of 300 patients on opioids for nonmalignant pain found that the majority were prescribed the short-acting variety by their primary care physicians.[56] Some of these physicians may have considered more potent opioids to be problematic from the standpoint of a "slippery slope" that could lead them to undesirable consequences. Concerns about physical dependence, tolerance, and addiction provide other obstacles that are not easily overcome.[57] Whether or not the use of long-acting opioids offers less risk of stimulating addiction has not been well studied; it is suggested by many and supported by finding a preponderance of diverted street opioids to be of the short-acting variety.[39,58,59] Since short-acting opioids have fast onset and high serum peak levels, they may be better suited than long-acting opioids for inducing psychoactive nonanalgesic effects which might then foster addiction. A collaborative case study demonstrated successful prescribing of long-acting opioids in patients with a history of prescription opioid addiction, although not all patients were successfully able to maintain compliance.[60]

TABLE 13-2. PRESCRIPTION ABUSE CHECKLIST

A focus on opioid issues during clinic visits impeding progress with other treatment issues and persisting beyond the third appointment
A pattern of early refills or escalating drug use in the absence of any clinical change
Multiple telephone calls or visits about opiate prescriptions
A pattern of prescription problems (e.g., lost, spilled, stolen)
Supplemental sources of opioids

Modified from Chabal C, Erjavec MK, Jacobson L, et al: Prescription opiate abuse in chronic pain patients: Clinical criteria, incidence, and predictors. Clin J Pain 13:150–155, 1997.

Contracts are often employed in the chronic administration of opioids and are intended to improve adherence to a treatment regimen. In addition to enhancement of compliance, contracts provide education and documentation. Fishman et al compared 39 opioid contracts from major academic programs finding wide variability of content.[61] However, there was also a core group of themes found consistently amongst the contracts reviewed. The "opioid contract" often included clear descriptions of what constitutes medication use and abuse, terms for random drug screening, consequences of contract violations, and measures for opioid discontinuation should this become required. Some instances of minor deviations of the contract are often tolerated before resorting to severing of the contract on the part of the physician. However, unlawful activities such as forging prescriptions, selling drugs, and/or resumption of alcohol or illicit drug intake or abuse are grounds for immediate tapering and discharge. If there is evidence of emotional distress accompanying prescription drug abuse, visitation to a mental health provider, if not already in progress, should be encouraged to evaluate psychosocial issues. In cases of comorbid addiction and chronic pain requiring opioid therapy, it may be most prudent to coordinate care with both a pain and an addiction specialist.

Differentiating Substance Abuse, Dependence, and Prescription Drug Abuse: Unfortunately, the DSM-IV definitions of abuse and dependence imply that long-term opioid therapy (with or without prescription drug abuse) may be synonymous with the DSM-IV characterization of substance abuse and dependence. Substance abuse is defined by DSM-IV as "a maladaptive pattern of substance use manifested by recurrent and significant adverse consequences related to the repeated use of substances." There may be repeated failure to fulfill major role obligations (i.e., at school, home, or at work), repeated use in situations in which it is physically hazardous (i.e., driving a car), multiple legal problems such as arrests for driving under the influence, and recurrent social and interpersonal problems (i.e., fights). Substance dependence is regarded as a more serious offense defined as "a cluster of cognitive, behavioral, and physiological symptoms indicated by the individual's continued use of the substance despite significant substance related problems." The problems referred to in this definition are tolerance, withdrawal, escalation of dose, unsuccessful taper, spending a great deal of time and energy to obtain the drug, missing important social functions because of substance use, and continued use of the substance despite knowing that it might be harmful. The DSM-IV criteria have been considered inappropriate for use in the chronic pain patient taking long-term opioids.[62] Patients using chronic opioids normally become physically dependent and may become tolerant. Self-escalation of dosage is central to the diagnosis of prescription drug abuse as it leads all of the other excuses seen when this type of abusive behavior develops, like repeated prescription loss or unscheduled visits to the doctor's office. Globally equating opioid self-escalation with addiction is overly simplistic and may miss the pseudoaddict or the patient with other needs or even psychopathology.

In the patient with chronic pain who uses chronic opioids, physical dependence and tolerance in and of themselves should not raise concerns of abuse. Refusing to prescribe opioids solely because someone has evidence of physical dependence or tolerance is medically inappropriate. On the other hand, repeated failure to fulfill major role obligations, multiple legal problems

including drug diversion, and recurrent social and interpersonal problems are not anticipated in this population and should raise suspicions. Opioid tapering would be warranted should these events occur regardless of the patient prior history. Rather than denying a pain management tool that has shown itself to be effective, barring the presence of obvious red flags, a prescribing physician should assume that the patient has legitimate pain and proceed accordingly. Monitoring to detect aberrant behavior and drug abuse should be part of any opioid treatment plan. As noted previously, aberrant behaviors most often begin early in therapy. According to Sees and Clark, "improvement in functioning should be the primary treatment goal for the chronic pain patient. Unlike the chemically dependent patient whose level of function is impaired by substance use, the chronic pain patient's level of function may improve with adequate, judicious use of medications, which may include opioids."[62] Thus, it is incumbent upon the clinician who is prescribing opioids to inquire about functionality at every visit to insure that opioids are improving performance in key activities.

CONCLUSIONS

In treating patients with acute or chronic pain of malignant or nonmalignant origin, opioid therapy can often ameliorate the suffering associated with pain. Unfortunately, utilization of opioid therapy is sometimes limited by the patient's tolerance of centrally and/or peripherally mediated side effects. When opioid dose adjustments or opioid rotation unsuccessfully minimizes the side effects, clinicians must look towards symptom management with medications. While at times selection of the most appropriate agent may seem haphazard, rational prescribing should be based upon a careful assessment of the patient's symptoms. If possible, one should consider using an agent that can possibly address multiple side effects without reversing analgesia.

Although addiction is a major public health crisis that reaches into the pain management arena, rational opioid therapy does not necessarily lead to addictive sequelae. On the contrary, as drug addiction hinges on dysfunctional use that produces harm, effective analgesia hinges on increased function that improves quality of life. Nonetheless, addiction looms as one of the many outcomes to opioid therapy, and just as in the case of a myelosuppressive drug that requires regular white blood cell count studies, chronic opioid therapy requires vigilant observation of function, and particularly any dysfunction that will warn of addictive effects. Doctor shopping, multiple prescribers, prescription loss, visiting without a prescription, frequent telephone calls to the clinic, multiple drug intolerances or "allergies" and frequent dose escalations are common manifestations of misuse in the pain population. There is rarely a single behavior or event that confirms the diagnosis of addiction. Making this diagnosis requires careful consideration of diverse information and firm conclusions cannot always be supported. The decision to alter or discontinue opioid therapy is often based on evidence of dysfunction or misuse but may be more securely based on the finding of insufficient gains in function from the therapeutic trial of opioids. There are many tools and strategies that can make chronic opioid therapies less risky for clinicians and more efficacious for patients. At the heart of rational chronic opioid therapy is the recognition of function as the main outcome measure and lack of functional improvement or dysfunction as a sign of treatment failure that may or may not involve addiction.

REFERENCES

1. Friedman JD, Dello Buono FA: Opioid antagonists in the treatment of opioid-induced constipation and pruritus. Ann Pharmacother 35:85–91, 2001.
2. Klaschik E, Nauck F, Ostgathe C: Constipation – Modern laxative therapy. Support Care Cancer 11:679–685, 2003.
3. Allan L, Hays H, Jensen NH, et al: Randomised crossover trial of transdermal fentanyl and sustained release oral morphine for treating chronic non-cancer pain. BMJ 322:1154–1158, 2001.
4. Wilsey BL, Mahajan G, Fishman SM: Opioid therapy in chronic non-malignant pain. *In* Smith HS (ed): Drugs for Pain. Hanley & Belfus, Philadelphia, 2003, pp 119–132.
5. Choi YS, Billings JA: Opioid antagonists: A review of their role in palliative care, focusing on use in opioid-related constipation. J Pain Symptom Manage 24:71–90, 2002.
6. De Ponti F: Methylnaltrexone progenics. Curr Opin Investig Drugs 3:614–620, 2002.
7. Sykes NP: Oral naloxone in opioid-associated constipation. Lancet 337:1475, 1991.
8. Robinson BA, Johansson L, Shaw J: Oral naloxone in opioid-associated constipation. Lancet 338:581–582, 1991.
9. Culpepper-Morgan JA, Inturrisi CE, Portenoy RK, et al: Treatment of opioid-induced constipation with oral naloxone: A pilot study. Clin Pharmacol Ther 52:90–95, 1992.
10. Latasch L, Zimmermann M, Eberhardt B, Jurna I: [Treatment of morphine-induced constipation with oral naloxone]. Anaesthesist 46:191–194, 1997.
11. Murphy DB, Sutton JA, Prescott LF, Murphy MB: Opioid-induced delay in gastric emptying: A peripheral mechanism in humans. Anesthesiology 87:765–770, 1997.
12. Gan TJ, Ginsberg B, Glass PS, et al: Opioid-sparing effects of a low-dose infusion of naloxone in patient-administered morphine sulfate. Anesthesiology 87:1075–1081, 1997.
13. Yuan CS, Foss JF, O'Connor M, et al: Efficacy of orally administered methylnaltrexone in decreasing subjective effects after intravenous morphine. Drug Alcohol Depend 52:161–165, 1998.
14. Slatkin NE, Rhiner M, Bolton TM: Donepezil in the treatment of opioid-induced sedation: Report of six cases. J Pain Symptom Manage 21:425–438, 2001.
15. Pharmacologic Management. Clinical Practice Guideline for the Management of Cancer Pain, vol 9. Agency for Health Care Policy and Research, 1994, pp 61–64.
16. Rozans M, Dreisbach A, Lertora JJ, Kahn MJ: Palliative uses of methylphenidate in patients with cancer: A review. J Clin Oncol 20:335–339, 2002.
17. Ferraro L, Antonelli T, O'Connor WT, et al: Modafinil: An anti-narcoleptic drug with a different neurochemical profile to d-amphetamine and dopamine uptake blockers. Biol Psychiatry 42:1181–1183, 1997.
18. Webster L, Andrews M, Stoddard G: Modafinil treatment of opioid-induced sedation. Pain Med 4:135–140, 2003.
19. Jasinski DR: An evaluation of the abuse potential of modafinil using methylphenidate as a reference. J Psychopharmacol 14:53–60, 2000.
20. Jasinski DR, Kovacevic-Ristanovic R: Evaluation of the abuse liability of modafinil and other drugs for excessive daytime sleepiness associated with narcolepsy. Clin Neuropharmacol 23:149–156, 2000.
21. Bruera E, Strasser F, Shen L, et al: The effect of donepezil on sedation and other symptoms in patients receiving opioids for cancer pain: A pilot study. J Pain Symptom Manage 26:1049–1054, 2003.
22. Bouillon T, Bruhn J, Roepcke H, Hoeft A: Opioid-induced respiratory depression is associated with increased tidal volume variability. Eur J Anaesthesiol 20:127–133, 2003.
23. Anwari JS, Iqbal S: Antihistamines and potentiation of opioid induced sedation and respiratory depression. Anaesthesia 58:494–495, 2003.
24. Kyriakides K, Hussain SK, Hobbs GJ: Management of opioid-induced pruritus: A role for 5-HT3 antagonists? Br J Anaesth 82:439–441, 1999.
25. Szarvas S, Harmon D, Murphy D: Neuraxial opioid-induced pruritus: A review. J Clin Anesth 15:234–239, 2003.
26. Kjellberg F, Tramer MR: Pharmacological control of opioid-induced pruritus: A quantitative systematic review of randomized trials. Eur J Anaesthesiol 18:346–357, 2001.
27. Larijani GE, Goldberg ME, Rogers KH: Treatment of opioid-induced pruritus with ondansetron: Report of four patients. Pharmacotherapy 16:958–960, 1996.
28. Raderer M, Muller C, Scheithauer W: Ondansetron for pruritus due to cholestasis. N Engl J Med 330:1540, 1994.
29. Krajnik M, Zylicz Z: Understanding pruritus in systemic disease. J Pain Symptom Manage 21:151–168, 2001.
30. Horta ML, Ramos L, Goncalves ZR: The inhibition of epidural morphine-induced pruritus by epidural droperidol. Anesth Analg 90:638–641, 2000.
31. Yeh HM, Chen LK, Lin CJ, et al: Prophylactic intravenous ondansetron reduces the incidence of intrathecal morphine-induced pruritus in patients undergoing cesarean delivery. Anesth Analg 91:172–175, 2000.
32. Torn K, Tuominen M, Tarkkila P, Lindgren L: Effects of sub-hypnotic doses of propofol on the side effects of intrathecal morphine. Br J Anaesth 73:411–412, 1994.
33. Colbert S, O'Hanlon DM, Chambers F, Moriarty DC: The effect of intravenous tenoxicam on pruritus in patients receiving epidural fentanyl. Anaesthesia 54:76–80, 1999.
34. Colbert S, O'Hanlon DM, Galvin S, et al: The effect of rectal diclofenac on pruritus in patients receiving intrathecal morphine. Anaesthesia 54:948–952, 1999.
35. Fishbain DA, Rosomoff HL, Rosomoff RS: Drug abuse, dependence, and addiction in chronic pain patients. Clin J Pain 8:77–85, 1992.
36. Hoffmann NG, Olofsson O, Salen B, Wickstrom L: Prevalence of abuse and dependency in chronic pain patients. Int J Addict 30:919–927, 1995.
37. Rosenblum A, Joseph H, Fong C, et al: Prevalence and characteristics of chronic pain among chemically dependent patients in methadone maintenance and residential treatment facilities. JAMA 289:2370–2378, 2003.
38. Passik SD: Responding rationally to recent report of abuse/diversion of Oxycontin. J Pain Symptom Manage 21:359, 2001.
39. Joranson DE, Ryan KM, Gilson AM, Dahl JL: Trends in medical use and abuse of opioid analgesics. JAMA 283:1710–1714, 2000.
40. Addiction LCoPa. Definitions related to the use of opioids for the treatment of chronic pain. A consensus document from the American Academy of Pain Medicine, the American Pain Society, and the American Society of Addiction Medicine, 2001. www.ampainsoc.org.
41. Gilson AM, Joranson DE: US policies relevant to the prescribing of opioid analgesics for the treatment of pain in patients with addictive disease. Clin J Pain 18:S91–98, 2002.
42. Code of Federal Regulations 58FR 37507–37508 July 12, 1993.
43. Code of Federal Regulations 42 Section 8.12. October 1, 2002.
44. American Psychiatric Association: Diagnostic aand Statistical Manual of Mental Disorders: DSM-IV, 4th ed. American Psychiatric Publishing Inc., Arlington, 1994.
45. Portenoy RK, Dole V, Joseph H, et al: Pain management and chemical dependency. Evolving perspectives. JAMA 278:592–593, 1997.
46. Weissman DE, Haddox JD: Opioid pseudoaddiction – An iatrogenic syndrome. Pain 36:363–366, 1989.
47. Scimeca MM, Savage SR, Portenoy R, Lowinson J: Treatment of pain in methadone-maintained patients. Mt Sinai J Med 67:412–422, 2000.

48. Dunbar SA, Katz NP: Chronic opioid therapy for nonmalignant pain in patients with a history of substance abuse: Report of 20 cases. J Pain Symptom Manage 11:163–171, 1996.

49. Savage S: Management of acute pain, chronic pain and cancer pain in the addicted patient. *In* Miller N (ed): Principles of Addiction Medicine, vol sec VIII. American Society of Addiction Medicine (ASAM), Chevy Chase, MD, 1994, p 4.

50. Merrill JO, Rhodes LA, Deyo RA, et al: Mutual mistrust in the medical care of drug users: The keys to the "narc" cabinet. J Gen Intern Med 17:327–333, 2002.

51. Mendelson D: Legal liability for pain management involving opioid medication: An American perspective. J Law Med 10:145–154, 2002.

52. Fleischman J, Galler D: Prescription for addiction? Adv Nurse Pract 9:27, 2001.

53. Zacny J, Bigelow G, Compton P, et al: College on Problems of Drug Dependence taskforce on prescription opioid non-medical use and abuse: Position statement. Drug Alcohol Depend 69:215–232. 2003.

54. Wasserman S: States respond to growing abuse of painkiller. State Legis 27:33–34, 2001.

55. Katz NP, Sherburne S, Beach M, et al: Behavioral monitoring and urine toxicology testing in patients receiving long-term opioid therapy. Anesth Analg 97:1097–1102, table of contents, 2003.

56. Clark JD: Chronic pain prevalence and analgesic prescribing in a general medical population. J Pain Symptom Manage 23:131–137, 2002.

57. Potter M, Schafer S, Gonzalez-Mendez E, et al: Opioids for chronic nonmalignant pain. Attitudes and practices of primary care physicians in the UCSF/Stanford Collaborative Research Network. University of California, San Francisco. J Fam Pract 50:145–151, 2001.

58. McCarberg BH, Barkin RL: Long-acting opioids for chronic pain: Pharmacotherapeutic opportunities to enhance compliance, quality of life, and analgesia. Am J Ther 8:181–186, 2001.

59. Heit HA: The truth about pain management: The difference between a pain patient and an addicted patient. Eur J Pain 5(Suppl A):27–29, 2001.

60. Mahoney ND, Devine JE, Angres D: Multidisciplinary treatment of benign chronic pain syndrome in substance abusing patients. Curr Rev Pain 3:321–331, 1999.

61. Fishman SM, Bandman TB, Edwards A, Borsook D: The opioid contract in the management of chronic pain. J Pain Symptom Manage 18:27–37, 1999.

62. Sees KL, Clark HW: Opioid use in the treatment of chronic pain: Assessment of addiction. J Pain Symptom Manage 8:257–264, 1993.

14

Psychopharmacology for Pain Medicine

**Ajay D. Wasan, M.D., M.Sc., M.A., and
Rollin M. Gallagher, M.D., M.P.H.**

A large percentage of patients with chronic pain disorders have coexisting, or comorbid, psychiatric conditions, which are the most prevalent comorbidities in patients with chronic pain. Compared to patients with little or no psychiatric comorbidity, these patients have a worse pain and disability outcome, regardless of treatment, be it medications, nerve blocks, or physical therapy.[1–3] These patients are commonly referred to pain medicine clinics and frequently present on psychoactive medications. Many of these medications, such as antidepressants and anticonvulsants, also have analgesic properties, and are a mainstay of the drug armamentarium of the pain physician. Consequently, it behoves the astute pain practitioner to be familiar with the psychiatric comorbidities of patients with chronic pain and to understand how to use psychoactive medications to treat both pain and/or psychopathology. Psychotherapeutic modalities, such as cognitive behavioral therapy, relaxation training, or biofeedback, play an important role in the treatment of both psychiatric and chronic painful illness, and in some cases are the preferred method of treatment. However, this chapter focuses on the use of medications as they pertain to treating patients with pain and psychiatric comorbidity. As with many of the medications used in pain medicine, psychoactive medications with reported analgesic properties do not always have an FDA indication for this purpose, but can legally be prescribed for off-label use.

EPIDEMIOLOGY

Over two decades of studies of US pain clinic populations have shown that 60% to 80% of these patients have psychiatric illnesses by DSM criteria.[4–6] Estimates are lower in persons with pain in primary care, institutional, and community settings, but regardless of setting, given the prevalence of persistent pain in adults, estimated at 20% to 45%, pain–psychiatric comorbidity constitutes an important public health problem.[7,8] Patients with psychiatric illness report greater pain intensity, more pain-related disability, and a larger affective component to their pain.[3,9,10]

The majority of patients with psychiatric comorbidity developed their psychiatric illness after the onset of chronic pain. Major depression alone affects 30% to 50% of all pain clinic patients, followed by anxiety disorders, personality disorders, somatoform disorders, and substance use disorders.[4,11,12] Virtually all psychiatric conditions are treatable, and the majority of patients provided with appropriate treatment significantly improve. Of the disorders that most frequently affect patients with chronic pain, major depression and anxiety disorders are the most common and have the best response to medications, and so their treatment is the focus of this chapter. Regardless of the specific psychopathology, improvement in psychiatric illness results in: diminished pain levels, greater acceptance of the chronicity of pain, improved functionality, and an improved quality of life. Although this chapter focuses on psychopharmacological treatment, it is important to note that, in general, combined pharmacological and psychotherapeutic treatments are more effective in treating depression and anxiety than pharmacologic treatment alone. Psychotherapeutic treatments (e.g., cognitive behavioral therapies, relaxation and biofeedback, interpersonal therapies, group therapies, etc.) are covered in other chapters in this book.

PSYCHIATRIC NOSOLOGY

Mental health practitioners utilize the *Diagnostic and Statistical Manual of Mental Disorders IV* (DSM-IV) or the tenth revision of the *International Statistical Classification of Diseases and Related Health Problems* (ICD-10) as an aid in making psychiatric diagnoses.[13] While these manuals elegantly outline the suggested criteria for psychiatric diagnosis, they are not very good at highlighting which symptoms are more or less important in making a diagnosis. While the criteria have high reliability, i.e., two psychiatrists applying the criteria to the assessment of the same patient will very often come up with the same diagnosis, the criteria do not all have equally high validity. That is, there is no universal agreement that the symptoms listed under diagnostic criteria for a particular condition are the best description of that illness.[14] In this light, and in an attempt to demystify psychiatric diagnosis for the pain physician, the following descriptions of psychopathology will emphasize the hallmark features of each illness.

MAJOR DEPRESSION AND SUBTHRESHOLD DEPRESSION

Symptoms: As the most prevalent of the psychiatric comorbidities, major depression can be distinguished from situational depression (also termed demoralization or an adjustment disorder with depressed mood) by the triad of persistently low mood, self-attitude changes, and changes in vital sense, all lasting at least two weeks.[14] Low mood manifests itself by emotions of "feeling blue," down, or depressed. Anhedonia, or the inability to experience pleasure, is a key reflection of low mood. A diminished self-attitude is seen in thoughts of guilt or thinking that one is a bad person. Changes in vital sense refer to changes in sleep, appetite, or energy levels. Patients with major depression often feel that their thinking is slow or fuzzy and have difficulty concentrating. Depressed patients may feel anxious, have panic attacks, or PTSD symptoms, which if they occur in the presence of significant depression symptoms are consistent with a major depressive disorder, not a separate anxiety disorder. Depressive symptoms may present as Beck's triad, with patients feeling hopeless, hapless, and helpless. They see the future as bleak, they feel they cannot help themselves, and no one can help them.[15] Suicidal thoughts reflect the severity of depressive symptoms. Untreated or undertreated major depression has a lifetime risk of death through completion of suicide of 10% to 15%.[16] Major depression is a serious complication of persistent pain, and if not treated effectively it will reduce the effectiveness of all pain treatments. Even low levels of depression ("sub-threshold depression") may worsen the physical impairment associated with chronic pain conditions and should also be treated.[9]

Treatment: All antidepressants take 2 to 4 weeks to see a clinical improvement after a typical dose is reached. Patients should remain on them for 6 to 12 months for the treatment of an initial depressive episode, and five years for the treatment of a recurrent depressive episode. Regardless of the medication chosen, approximately 60% of patients will respond (have at least a 50% improvement) to the initial antidepressant prescribed. At least 80% of patients will respond to at least one medication, either with or without an augmentation agent, such as lithium, an anticonvulsant, or another antidepressant.[17] There is some evidence that pain patients with major depression have increased treatment resistance, particularly when their pain is not effectively managed.[7] Older adults tend to respond at lower doses of antidepressants, and dose titration should occur more slowly in this group because of their heightened sensitivity to side effects and toxicity.[18] A good rule of thumb in starting antidepressants in any age group is to begin with 1/4 to 1/2 of the standard initial treatment dose for a week, and then advance gradually over the next 2 to 3 weeks to the treatment dose. This minimizes side effects and increases treatment compliance. Often, patients with chronic pain are on multiple medications that can potentiate the side effects of antidepressants, e.g., headache, nausea, constipation, or sedation, so "starting low and going slow," is even more important in this population. Typically, in the initial treating period re-evaluations are done every 2 to 4 weeks, with dose adjustments if indicated. Monoamine oxidase inhibitors

(MAOIs), such as phenelzine, which are rarely prescribed anymore, should not be prescribed with other antidepressants concurrently. Because of the inherent risks of these medications, they should be used only by experienced psychopharmacologists.[19]

Cognitive behavioral therapy (CBT) in conjunction with antidepressant therapy is the most efficacious treatment for major depression. Cognitive behavioral therapy examines negative and destructive thoughts that arise in conjunction with low moods, helping patients to see the unrealistic and maladaptive qualities of thoughts and behaviors.[20]

SELECTIVE SEROTONIN REUPTAKE INHIBITORS (SSRIs): Since the introduction of fluoxetine (Prozac) in 1987, many SSRIs have been introduced. They have an immediate effect on the blockade of the presynaptic serotonin reuptake pump in the central nervous system (CNS), which has been shown in animals to increase the duration of serotonin in the synaptic cleft, increasing the effects of neurotransmission.[21] The antidepressant efficacy of SSRIs and their low side effect profiles have made them the most widely prescribed class of antidepressants.

However, the SSRIs have few independent pain properties. Pain patients whose depression responds to an SSRI may have diminished pain that is attributable to improvements in the affective components of their pain, but there is little evidence supporting independent analgesic activity of SSRIs. While a few case reports have shown improvements in diabetic neuropathic pain on SSRIs, double-blind, placebo-controlled clinical trials that exclude patients with depression have not consistently demonstrated analgesic benefit.[22–26]

In deciding to prescribe an SSRI there are no absolute contraindications except in patients on MAOIs. No additional laboratory workup is required, and dose titration is based on clinical response and side effects. Fluoxetine tends to be more activating and is prescribed in the morning, while paroxetine with its anticholinergic effect of activating muscarinic receptors, is more sedating and has greater anxiolytic properties. Sertraline and citalopram tend to be less sedating than paroxetine and are generally prescribed in the morning.[19]

Patients should begin on one-half of the usual dose for a week (see Table 14-1) and then to the standard dose, to minimize the side effects of nausea, diarrhea, tremor, and headache. Some patients can experience sedation or overstimulation. Approximately 15% of patients on SSRIs experience sexual side effects, such as decreased libido, impotence, ejaculatory disturbances, or anorgasmia. Rare side effects include dystonia, akathesia, palpitations, a lowered seizure threshold, serotonin syndrome, or syndrome of inappropriate antidiuretic hormone (SIADH).[27]

SSRIs are metabolized by hepatic oxidation, and their use may alter the serum levels of other hepatically metabolized drugs. SSRIs induce and/or inhibit various cytochrome P450 enzymes. Most significantly, they can increase levels of tricyclic antidepressants and benzodiazepines.[28] They may also affect levels of carbamezepine, lithium, antipsychotics, and a commonly used analgesic, methadone.[29] If taken in an overdose, SSRIs are rarely, if ever, lethal. In discontinuing SSRIs, they should be tapered down slowly to avoid a withdrawal syndrome, which has the same symptoms as initiation of SSRIs (headache, nausea, diarrhea, or myalgias).

TRICYCLIC ANTIDEPRESSANTS (TCAs): TCAs are one of the oldest classes of antidepressants and they act by inhibiting both serotonergic and noradrenergic reuptake. This lengthens the

TABLE 14-1. **SELECTIVE SEROTONIN REUPTAKE INHIBITORS (SSRIs)**

Drug	Usual Start Dose	Average Dose	Maximum Dose
Citalopram (Celexa)	10 mg qd	20–40 mg qd	60 mg/day
Fluoxetine (Prozac)	10 mg qd	20–40 mg qd	80 mg/day
Fluvoxamine (Luvox)	25 mg qd	50–100 mg bid	300 mg/day
Paroxetine (Paxil)	5–10 mg qd	20–40 mg qd	60 mg/day
Sertraline (Zoloft)	25 mg qd	50–150 mg qd	200 mg/day

time serotonin and norepinephrine remain in the synaptic cleft, enhancing their neurotransmission.[30] The analgesic properties of TCAs independent of their treatment effects on depression make them a good choice for treating depression in the patient with chronic pain, particularly if cost is a factor.

All TCAs are equally effective for the treatment of depression, and the choice of a particular one is determined by side effects. The magnitude of anticholinergic and antihistaminic effects is the largest determinant. Amitriptyline and imipramine are more sedating, with more weight gain and orthostatic hypotension. Other anticholinergic side effects include dry mouth, constipation, blurred vision, urinary retention, sexual side effects, excessive sweating, and confusion or delirium. TCAs also decrease the seizure threshold. Desipramine and nortriptyline have fewer anticholinergic side effects, and of all of the TCAs, nortriptyline has the fewest anticholinergic side effects. Serum plasma levels can be monitored for TCAs, and this is particularly important for amitriptyline and nortriptyline, which have the best correlation of blood levels to therapeutic antidepressant response.[18]

Prior to initiating treatment patients should have laboratory screening of electrolytes, BUN, creatinine, and LFTs. TCAs also have quinidine-like properties, are potentially proarythmic, and can prolong the QTC interval. All patients over 40 years or with any history of cardiac disease should have a baseline EKG, with particular attention to the QTC interval, checking that it is less than 450 milliseconds.[30] TCAs are strongly protein-bound (85% to 95%) and undergo first-pass hepatic metabolism. Subsequent stages involve demethylation, oxidation, and glucuronide conjugation. Amitriptyline is demethylated to nortriptyline, and imipramine is demethylated to desipramine. Hepatic clearance involves the P450 enzyme system, and so drugs such as SSRIs, cimetidine, and methylphenidate increase TCA plasma levels. SSRIs and TCAs should not be prescribed at the same time unless plasma levels are carefully monitored. Phenobarbital, carbamazepine, and cigarette smoking induce the P450 enzyme system, and thus decrease serum TCA levels.[28]

As with SSRIs, to minimize side effects and increase adherence initiation of TCAs should begin at lower doses (usually 25 mg for a week) than the target doses for antidepressant effect (typically 75 to 150 mg, see Table 14-2). The elderly are more sensitive to their side effects, and many psychiatrists begin at doses of

TABLE 14-2. **TRICYCLIC ANTIDEPRESSANTS (TCAs)**

Drug	Usual Start Dose	Average Dose	Maximum Dose
Amitriptyline (Elavil)	10–25 mg qd	75–150 mg qd	300 mg/day
Amoxapine (Asendin)	25 mg bid	75–200 mg bid	600 mg/day
Clomipramine (Anafranil)	25 mg qd	150–250 mg qd	250 mg/day
Desipramine (Norpramin)	10–25 mg qd	75–150 mg qd	300 mg qd
Doxepin (Sinequan)	10–25 mg qd	75–150 mg qd	300 mg qd
Nortriptyline (Pamelor)	10–25 mg qd	75–150 mg qd	200 mg qd
Protriptyline (Vivactil)	5 mg qd	10 mg tid	60 mg/day

10 to 20 mg in this age group.[18] With diminished or altered metabolism of TCAs, as well as the multiple medications older patients are frequently taking, they are more prone to develop toxic serum levels, and monitoring should be more frequent. There is a withdrawal syndrome with abrupt discontinuation of TCAs, characterized by fever, sweating, headaches, nausea, dizziness, or akathisia. Unlike the SSRIs, overdose can be lethal. TCA overdose is a leading cause of drug-related overdose and death. Three to five times the therapeutic dose is potentially lethal, so this narrow therapeutic range must be respected, and blood levels serially done. Toxicity results from anticholinergic and proarythmic effects, such as seizures, coma, and QTC widening.[31]

Also unlike the SSRIs, TCAs have independent pain properties. A series of studies by Max and others have illustrated the analgesic properties of TCAs, which are independent of its effects on improving depression.[32,33] TCAs have been shown to be effective for diabetic neuropathy pain, chronic regional pain syndrome, chronic headache, poststroke pain, and radicular pain.[17,32–36]. Additionally, TCAs are useful as preemptive analgesics, being opioid-sparing in the postoperative period.[37] While the initial studies were done with amitriptyline and desipramine, subsequent studies have confirmed that the other TCAs have equivalent analgesic properties. Of note, the typical doses for the analgesic benefit of TCAs (25 to 75 mg) are lower than the typical doses for antidepressant effect (75 to 150 mg). Many patients are referred to the pain specialist after a failed trial of TCAs at lower doses. And yet there is a dose–response relationship for analgesia. So even if one is using a TCA solely for pain relief, patients may benefit with a dose in the antidepressant range, in conjunction with blood level monitoring.

SEROTONIN–NOREPINEPHRINE REUPTAKE INHIBITORS (SNRIs):

The nontricyclic SNRIs are a newer group of antidepressants which, like the TCAs, act by inhibiting serotonin and norepinephrine reuptake. This appears to be one of the mechanisms accounting both for the higher rates of depression remission and the analgesic efficacy associated with TCAs and SNRIs as compared with SSRIs.[26,38] Venlafaxine and duloxetine are the main drugs in this category and have no alpha-1,

cholinergic, or histamine inhibition. This results in fewer side effects than the tricyclics, with equivalent antidepressant and potentially equal analgesic benefits. Placebo-controlled studies have demonstrated efficacy in neuropathic pain for both venlafaxine[38,39] and duloxetine.[40] A numbers-needed-to-treat analysis suggested superior analgesic properties of TCAs which may be due their properties of NMDA antagonism and sodium channel blockade, in addition to their combined serotonin and norepinephrine reuptake inhibition.[38]

Venlafaxine is given in two or three divided daily doses (even with extended-release formulations), beginning at 37.5 mg per day for a week and then slowly increased to as high as 375 mg per day (Table 14-3). A typical dose is 150 to 225 mg/day. Generally, patients are escalated over a month to 75 mg/day, and then dependent on clinical response, the dose is adjusted.

Prior to starting venlafaxine no laboratory studies are needed, and caution should be taken in patients with hypertension. Particularly at doses over 150 mg/day, venlafaxine may increase systolic blood pressure by 10 mm or more. This is likely due to the onset of norepinephrine reuptake inhibition, which occurs at higher doses of venlafaxine[38] that appear to be needed for analgesic efficacy in neuropathic pain, unlike tricyclics that may be effective at lower than antidepressant doses. Other side effects include nausea, somnolence, dry mouth, dizziness, nervousness, constipation, anorexia, or sexual dysfunction. Venlafaxine may affect hepatic metabolism of other medications.

Structurally, venlafaxine is similar to tramadol, and in mice venlafaxine demonstrates opioid-mediated analgesia that is reversed by naloxone. Both controlled studies and case reports indicate that venlafaxine has analgesic properties independent of its antidepressant effects in a variety of neuropathic conditions.[41–44] Many patients are unable to tolerate the side effects of tricyclics, so both venlafaxine and duloxetine are promising agents in patients with major depression and chronic pain.

OTHER ANTIDEPRESSANTS:

Buproprion is a noradrenergic and dopaminergic reuptake pump inhibitor, prolonging the time norepinephrine and dopamine remain in the synaptic cleft.[21] Unlike many of the other antidepressants it has significant

TABLE 14-3. MISCELLANEOUS ANTIDEPRESSANTS

Drug	Usual Start Dose	Average Dose	Maximum Dose
Buproprion (Wellbutrin)	75 mg bid	100–150 mg bid	600 mg qd
Duloxetine (Cymbalta)*	40 mg qd	40–60 mg bid	?
Mirtazepine (Remuron)	15 mg qhs	30–45 mg qd	60 mg qd
Nefazodone (Serozone)	100 mg bid	150–300 mg bid	600 mg/day
Trazadone (Desyrel)	50 mg qhs	150–250 mg bid	600 mg/day
Venlafaxine (Effexor)	37.5 mg qd	75–112.5 mg bid	375 mg/day

* At the time of writing Duloxetine had not yet been officially released by Eli Lilly.

psychostimulant properties. It is used in the treatment of depression, ADHD, and smoking cessation, at doses up to 600 mg per day (Table 14-3). Two recent studies have shown that bupropion has independent analgesic effects in a variety of neuropathic conditions.[45] Anecdotal reports have also indicated that bupropion is effective in alleviating the sedative effects of opioids. Consequently, bupropion will have an emerging use in pain medicine.

Treatment should start at 75 to 100 mg in the morning to avoid insomnia which may occur if the drug is starting at night. After 5 days this dose is advanced to the average treatment dose of 100 to 150 mg bid, even for sustained-release preparations. At these doses there is a very slight decrease in seizure threshold. Doses from 450 to 600 mg per day may cause seizures in 4% of patients, so these doses should be avoided.[46] Buproprion should not be prescribed to patients with seizures, eating disorders, or those taking MAOIs. Side effects include nervousness, headache, irritability, and insomnia.

Mirtazapine is a newer antidepressant with antagonism of serotonin and central presynaptic alpha2-adrenergic receptors, stimulating serotonin and norepinephrine release. This serves to potentiate serotonergic and noradrenergic transmission, while having no anticholinergic effects.[28] It is thought to preferentially augment serotonergic transmission and have an antihistaminic effect at lower doses, 15 to 30 mg/day. At higher doses, 45 to 60 mg/day, it augments more noradrenergic transmission (Table 14-3). As a result, at lower doses it is more sedating and has antianxiety effects, with the side effect of weight gain. At higher doses it is more activating and can provoke anxiety symptoms. Agranulocytosis and neurotropenia can rarely occur with this medication, at an incidence of 0.3%.[19] One case report and an open-label study indicate that there may be analgesic benefits to mirtazapine, but improvements in depression were not adequately controlled.[47,48] Theoretically and yet to be reported, with its central alpha2 *antagonism* properties, mirtazapine may counteract the analgesic benefits of muscle relaxants such as tizanidine, which act through central alpha2 *agonism* mechanisms.

Trazodone and nefazodone are serotonin-2 antagonist/reuptake inhibitors (SARIs) and are used for major depression and insomnia. The sedative qualities of trazodone are so great that few patients are able to get to high enough of a dose to be in the effective antidepressant range. Trazodone is most often prescribed for insomnia that accompanies depressive, anxious, or pain symptoms and is the preferred treatment for insomnia for many pain physicians.[17] Typical dosing for sleep is 25 to 100 mg at bedtime (Table 14-3). For depression, dosing for trazodone and nefazodone is 50 to 600 mg/day in 2 divided doses. A rare but serious side effect of trazodone is priapism, occurring in 1 in 1,000 to 1 in 10,000 cases.[49] Side effects common to both medications are sedation, dizziness, dry mouth, orthostatic hypotension, constipation, and headache. Studies have shown that trazodone has few analgesic properties. No such studies have been done with nefazodone, but one would not expect a different result.

ANXIETY DISORDERS

Symptoms: Anxiety disorders are a broad spectrum of disorders, including generalized anxiety disorder, panic disorder, obsessive compulsive disorder, and post-traumatic stress disorder (PTSD). There is high prevalence rate of anxiety disorders in chronic pain clinic populations, with 30% to 60% of patients having anxiety

at pathological levels.[2,5,7] Generalized anxiety disorder is the most frequent anxiety disorder affecting pain patients.

Anxiety is a broad concept with many dimensions. Anxiety can be an enduring personality trait that at times becomes excessive. It can be a symptom among a constellation of symptoms as part of another disorder, such as major depression. Or, it may be an episodic disorder, provoked by stressful and taxing challenges, such as chronic pain. Anxiety also has a biological component and is responsive to medications.[4] It is difficult to determine when anxiety is pathological, but one guideline is when anxiety interferes with normal functioning. There is both trait anxiety and situational anxiety. Trait anxiety is excessive worry and concern, often about routine matters. The amount of worry and anxiety is out of proportion to the likelihood of the negative consequences occurring, and the patient has great difficulty controlling worry.

In pain patients situational anxiety is often anxiety about pain and its negative consequences. Patients may be conditioned to be excessively fearful that activities will cause uncontrollable pain, causing avoidance of those activities, which in some patients can be extreme, almost phobic. Also, pain may activate thoughts that patients are seriously ill.[50] Anxiety amplifies pain perception and pain complaints through several biopsychosocial mechanisms, including sympathetic arousal with noradrenergically mediated lowering of nociceptive threshold, increased firing of ectopically active pain neurons, excessive cognitive focus on pain symptoms, and poor coping skills. Patients with pathological anxiety are often restless, fatigued, irritable, and have poor concentration. They may have muscle tension and sleep disturbances. Their mood is often low, but not at the severity level found in major depressive disorder.[17]

Treatment: Overall, cognitive behavioral therapy demonstrates the best treatment outcomes for anxiety disorders. Significant improvements are further obtained with relaxation therapy, meditation, and biofeedback.[51] Antidepressants are effective, but generally at higher doses than what is typically prescribed for depression. Anxiolytics, such as benzodiazepines and buspirone, are most useful in the initial treatment stages to stabilize a disorder. However, the side effects and physiologic dependency associated with benzodiazepines in particular make them a poor choice for long-term treatment.

ANTIDEPRESSANTS: As in depression treatment, it may take 2 to 4 weeks after the patient is on the target dose to see improvement. To improve compliance, escalation of doses must be done very slowly, because anxious patients are poorly tolerant of side effects. Antidepressants are useful to diminish the overall level of anxiety and to prevent anxiety or panic attacks, but they have no role in treating acute anxiety. The SSRIs are the most effective agents among antidepressants. Paroxetine tends to have greater antianxiety effects, but all of the SSRIs have good anxiolytic properties.[52] Effective doses are higher than those for depression, typically 60 to 80 mg/day.[53]

Of the TCAs, clomipramine is the most effective, with particular usefulness in obsessive compulsive disorder. Nefazadone has antianxiety effects, as does venlafaxine at higher doses. Mirtazapine has anxiolytic properties at the lower, more sedating doses, and higher doses of 45 to 60 mg can worsen anxiety with its activating qualities.[54] Similarly, while there are reports that buproprion is effective in depressions with anxious features, its stimulating effects make it less attractive as a primary antianxiety agent.

SNRIs, specifically venlafaxine, have also demonstrated efficacy in generalized anxiety.[64]

BENZODIAZEPINES (BZDs) AND BUSPIRONE: These medications are useful for acute anxiety, panic attacks, and to stabilize generalized anxiety. Occasionally, anxiety cannot be stabilized with antidepressants and patients remain on BZDs in the long term. Benzodiazepines bind to the benzodiazepine component of the gamma-aminobutyric acid (GABA) receptor, an inhibitory neurotransmitter. They depress the CNS at the levels of the limbic system, brainstem reticular formation, and cortex.[21] While they are widely prescribed by pain practitioners, studies indicate that they have few independent pain properties.

Acute anxiety or panic attacks can be treated with short-acting BZDs, such as lorezepam 0.5 to 2 mg q6hr, prn, which has a rapid onset of action (10 to 15 minutes) and a half-life of 10 to 20 hours.[28] Table 14-4 lists these features of many BZDs. Caution should be taken in prescribing short-half-life drugs, such as alprazolam. While it has a rapid onset of action, it typically lasts only 2 to 3 hours and many patients have significant rebound anxiety, resulting in a roller coaster of peaks and valleys of anxiety during the day.

Buspirone is also an effective acute anxiolytic. It acts as a serotonin agonist. It is especially useful in treating patients with a history of substance abuse who may abuse BZDs. It has no addictive properties, and does not impair psychomotor or cognitive functions. It is started at 5 mg tid and can be advanced as high as 10 mg tid.[30] Unlike the short-acting BZDs that deliver anxiolysis with the first dose, buspirone requires 1 to 4 weeks of administration for antianxiety benefits to appear. Patients can experience headache, dizziness, fatigue, paresthesias, and GI upset.

Clonazepam 0.25 to 2 mg tid, a long-acting BZD, is often used in conjunction with a short-acting agent or an antidepressant to stabilize persistent anxiety or prevent acute anxiety attacks. Diazepam, which also has psychoactive metabolites lasting several days, and flurazepam are other agents with long half-lives.

The side effects of BZDs limit their use as long-term agents. Acutely, all of the BZDs can cause profound sedation, confusion, or respiratory depression, and can be fatal in overdose. Caution is taken in prescribing these medications concurrently with opioids, which can compound the risk of these side effects. Rarely but with more frequency in the elderly, BZDs can be disinhibiting agents, in which patients can become agitated on them. All of the BZDs have addiction potential. All of them can cause physical and psychological dependence, and often require long tapering schedules from 1 to 3 months to minimize withdrawal symptoms.[17] Abrupt discontinuation of BZDs can cause insomnia, anxiety, delirium, psychosis, or seizures. Recent evidence indicates that long-term prescription of BZDs adversely affects short- and long-term memory, as well as learning abilities.[55] Furthermore, given that CBT with coping skills training is one of the most effective treatments for anxiety disorders, anxiolytics can undermine this treatment

TABLE 14-4. BENZODIAZEPINES (BZDs)

Drug	Onset	Half-life (hours)
Alprazolam (Xanax)	intermediate	6–20
Chlordiazepoxide (Librium)	intermediate	30–100
Clonazepam (Klonopin)	intermediate	18–50
Clorazepate (Tranxene)	rapid	30–100
Diazepam (Valium)	rapid	30–100
Estazolam (ProSom)	intermediate	10–24
Flurazepam (Dalmane)	rapid-intermediate	50–160
Lorazepam (Ativan)	intermediate	10–20
Midazolam (Versed)	rapid	2–3
Oxazepam (Serax)	intermediate-slow	8–12
Temazepam (Restoril)	intermediate	8–20
Triazolam (Halcion)	intermediate	1.5–5

because it may reinforce the notion that only a pill can solve a patient's anxiety problems, decreasing their self-efficacy for anxiety control.

MOOD STABILIZERS

Mood stabilizers are agents that possess both antimanic and antidepressant properties. In psychiatry, they are most frequently prescribed for bipolar disorder. There is no evidence that bipolar disorder occurs at a higher frequency in patients with chronic pain.[2] There are two medications in this class, lithium and valproic acid (Depakote is the longer-acting brand name formulation). While many of the other anticonvulsants have antimanic properties if prescribed either as a sole agent or in combination with other agents, they have little, if any, antidepressant effects of their own, and thus are not true mood stabilizers. The other anticonvulsants are useful as secondary or tertiary agents in bipolar disorder, or as augmentation agents in the treatment of major depression. The anticonvulsants are frequently prescribed in pain medicine and are documented analgesics for a variety of conditions. Their use is covered in more detail in other chapters of this text.

Lithium: Lithium is the most commonly prescribed mood stabilizer for bipolar disorder and is the only one demonstrating a clear decrease in suicide attempts for those taking it.[56] It is also used as an augmentation agent for major depressive disorder, administered in conjunction with antidepressants to which a patient has had a partial response. With mixed results, lithium has been used as prophylaxis for chronic daily headaches and cluster headaches. Lithium has a narrow therapeutic range for both benefit and toxicity, thus obtaining serum levels is important. Lethal overdoses can involve as little ingestion of 4 to 5 times the daily dose. Lithium has effects on the thyroid and kidney, and their function must be monitored. These difficulties in using lithium and its sparse analgesic benefits make it less useful to the pain practitioner. Typically, patients with chronic pain on lithium are followed by a psychiatrist.

Valproic Acid: Depakote is the brand name of long-acting valproic acid, with a duration of action of 8 to 12 hours. It has both antimanic and antidepressant effects, although with less antidepressant effect than lithium. It is also useful as an augmentation agent in depression. Valproic acid has an established use in migraine prophylaxis, and neurologists have extensive experience with it in seizure treatment. Starting dose is 250 mg/day and a typical dose used in pain medicine is 250 mg tid, while doses used in treatment of bipolar disorder are higher, 500 to 1,000 mg tid.[28] Serum levels are monitored for therapeutic and toxicity ranges. Prior to initiating treatment, CBC and liver function tests are done. Anemia and neurotropenia are rare side effects of valproic acid, but thrombocytopenia is more common. Platelet levels should be checked at least two weeks after the start of treatment and two weeks after reaching a therapeutic dose. Fortunately, platelet levels quickly rise after discontinuation of valproic acid. Sedation, dizziness, and hepatitis are other side effects.

NEUROLEPTICS

Also termed antipsychotics, neuroleptics have been available for almost 50 years. They are used to treat any psychotic process, the hallmark illness being schizophrenia, and psychotic symptoms in depression, mania, or delirium are also indications for their use. Both the typical and newer-generation atypical neuroleptics have independent pain properties, and are effective analgesics for nociceptive and neuropathic conditions.[57] Yet their serious side effects of Parkinsonism and tardive dyskinesia have limited their use in pain medicine. More often, neuroleptics are used in inpatient settings where other analgesic agents have produced delirium.

Typical Neuroleptics: Typical neuroleptics (Table 14-5) act as antipsychotics through their antagonism of dopamine receptors, particularly the D2 receptors. They also have actions on histaminic, cholinergic, and alpha-1 adrenergic receptors. Haloperidol is the prototypical agent in this class, with a molecular structure similar to morphine. All of the typical

TABLE 14-5. SELECTED TYPICAL NEUROLEPTICS

Drug	Usual Dose	Maximum Dose
Fluphenazine (Prolixin)	5–10 mg bid-tid	40 mg/day
Haloperidol (Haldol)	2–5 mg bid-tid	100 mg/day
Perphenazine (Trilafon)	8–16 mg bid-tid	64 mg/day
Thiothixene (Navane)	5–10 mg tid	60 mg/day
Trifluoperazine (Stelazine)	5–10 mg bid	40 mg/day
Loxapine (Loxitane)	20–50 mg bid-tid	250 mg/day
Chlorpromazine (Thorazine)	10–50 mg bid-qid	2000 mg/day
Thioridazine (Mellaril)	100–200 mg bid-qid	800 mg/day

TABLE 14-6. **ATYPICAL NEUROLEPTICS**

Drug	Usual Dose	Maximum Dose
Clozapine (Clozaril)	100–300 mg qd-bid	900 mg/day
Olanzapine (Zyprexa)	5–15 mg qd	20 mg/day
Quetiapine (Seroquel)	50–150 mg bid-tid	800 mg/day
Risperidone (Risperdal)	2–4 mg qd-bid	16 mg/day
Ziprasidone (Geodon)	20–40 mg bid	160 mg/day

neuroleptics have varying degrees of anticholinergic side effects: dry mouth, dizziness, sedation, weight gain, constipation, or blurred vision. They are also plagued by varying degrees of extrapyramidal effects: tremor, dystonia, akathesia, and, most seriously, tardive dyskinesia which is permanent. All of these agents very slightly lower the seizure threshold and may elevate serum glucose levels. Cardiovascular effects include hypotension, tachycardia, nonspecific EKG changes (including 'Torsades de Pointes'), and, exceedingly rare, sudden cardiac death.[28]

Atypical Neuroleptics: The first atypical neuroleptic was clozapine, which is used in treatment-refractory schizophrenia. Subsequently, several other agents have been released in this class: risperidone, olanzapine, quetiapine, and ziprasidone (Table 14-6). The atypicals have a lesser degree of dopamine D2 receptor antagonism and a greater degree of D4 receptor antagonism than the typical neuroleptics.[46] Additionally, they have some degree of serotonin-2 receptor blocking. This mixed receptor profile results in far fewer extrapyramidal, anticholinergic, and cardiac side effects. However, virtually all the side effects of the typical agents can occur with atypicals. Caution should be used in prescribing this class for patients with diabetes. Emerging evidence indicates that the atypicals, particularly olanzapine, lower glucose tolerance and can elevate serum glucose levels.[58] Overall, since the atypicals are better tolerated than typical neuroleptics, they are quickly becoming the first-line treatment for psychotic symptoms. Both classes are equally as effective for the "positive symptoms" of psychosis: hallucinations and delusions. However, the atypicals are more effective for the "negative symptoms" flat affect, poor motivation, and social withdrawal. Additionally, these agents are increasingly used as augmentation agents for treatment-resistant depression or anxiety, and may be very useful in helping patients disabled by pain and comorbid agitated depression control their anger.[17,59]

The use of atypical neuroleptics in pain medicine will grow. Case reports and retrospective studies indicate that they may be effective as a secondary or tertiary agents for migraine and chronic daily headache prophylaxis.[60,61] They have been effective as abortive agents for cluster headache.[60] A small study showed analgesic benefit in those with cancer pain.[62] In mice, studies of risperidone demonstrate an opioid-mediated analgesia to thermal pain.[63] The dosage range for the analgesic benefit of atypicals is yet unclear.

Whether an atypical or typical is prescribed, in starting a neuroleptic patients *must* be warned about the side effects, especially the risks of tardive dyskinesia which is permanent, if it occurs. In prescribing a neuroleptic for a nonpsychotic patient, initial dose should be very low with a slow escalation, since these patients are neuroleptic-naive and are very prone to its side effects.

CONCLUSIONS

Some 60% to 80% of patients with chronic pain attending pain clinics have significant psychiatric pathology. This comorbidity worsens their pain and disability, and this mental distress is an independent source of suffering, further reducing quality of life. The boom in psychotherapeutic medications over the past 15 years, combined with more effective psychotherapies, has resulted in significantly improved treatment. Many of these medications have analgesic benefits independent of their treatment effects on depression, anxiety, or psychosis. The antidepressants, anticonvulsants, and antipsychotics are the most notable for their pain properties. The improved treatment results for psychopathology and the emergence of additional analgesics is a boon to pain medicine practice.

REFERENCES

1. Fishbain D: Approaches to treatment decisions for pychiatric comorbidity in the management of the chronic pain patient. Med Clin North Am 83:737–759, 1999.
2. Koenig T, and Clark M: Advances in comprehensive pain management. Psych Clin North Am 19: 589–611, 1996.
3. Evers AW, Kraaimaat FW, van Reil PL, Bijlsma JW: Cognitive, behavioral and physiological reactivity to pain as a predictor of long-term pain in rheumatoid arthritis patients. Pain 9:139–146, 2001.
4. Clark MR, Cox TS: Refractory chronic pain. Psych Clin North Am 25:71–88, 2002.
5. Katon W, Egan K, Miller D: Chronic pain: Lifetime psychiatric diagnoses and family history. Am J Psychiatry 142:1156–1160, 1985.
6. Fishbain D, Goldberg M, Meagher BR, et al: Male and female chronic pain patients characterized by DSM-III psychiatric diagnostic criteria. Pain 26:181–197, 1986.
7. Gallagher RM, Verma S: Managing pain and co-morbid depression: A public health challenge. Semin Clin Neuropsych 4:203–220, 1999.
8. Gallagher, R: Primary care and pain medicine: A community solution to the public health problem of chronic pain. Med Clin North Am 83:555–583, 1999.
9. Mossey J, Gallagher RM, Tirumalasetti F: The effects of pain and depression on physical functioning in elderly residents of a continuing care retirement community. Pain Med 1:340–350, 2000.

10. Harkins SW, Price DD, Braith J: Effects of extraversion and neuroticism on experimental pain, clinical pain, and illness behavior. Pain 36:209–218, 1989.

11. Fishbain D, Cutler R, Rosomoff H, et al: Chronic pain associated depression: Antecedent or consequence of chronic pain? A review. Clin J Pain 13:116–137, 1997.

12. Dersh J, et al: Prevalence of psychiatric disorders in patients with chronic work-related musculoskeletal pain disability. J Occupat Environm Med 44:459–468, 2002.

13. Diagnostic and Statistical Manual of Mental Disorders, ed 4. American Psychiatric Association Press, Washington, DC, 1994.

14. McHugh PM, Slavney P: The Perspectives of Psychiatry. Johns Hopkins University Press, 1998.

15. Alford BA, Lester JM, Patel RJ, et al: Hopelessness predicts future depressive symptoms: A prospective analysis of cognitive vulnerability and cognitive content specificity. J Clin Psychol 51:331–339, 1995.

16. Janicak PG, Davis JM, Preskorn SH, Ayd FJ: Indications for antidepressants. In Principles and Practice of Psychopharmacotherapy. Lippincott-Williams, 2001, pp 193–214.

17. Verma S, Gallagher RM: The psychopharmacologic treatment of depression and anxiety in the context of chronic pain. Curr Pain Headache Rep 6:30–39, 2002.

18. Clark M: Pain. In Coffey C, Cummings J (eds): The American Psychiatric Textbook of Geriatric Neuropsychiatry. American Psychiatric Press, 1999.

19. Janicak PG, Davis JM, Preskorn SH, Ayd FJ: Treatment with antidepressants. In Principles and Practice of Psychopharmacotherapy. Lippincott Williams, 2001, pp 215–326.

20. Sonawalla SB, Fava M: Severe depression: Is there a best approach? CNS Drugs 15:765–776, 2001.

21. Stahl SM. Essential Psychopharmacology. Neuroscientific Basis and Clinical Applications. Cambridge University Press, 1996.

22. Max M: Antidepressants as analgesics. In Progress in Pain Research and Management, vol 1. IASP Press, Seattle, 1994.

23. Max MB, Lynch SA, Muir J, et al: Effects of desipramine, amitriptyline and fluoxetine on pain in diabetic neuropathy. N Engl J Med 326:1250–1256, 1992.

24. Lynch ME: Antidepressants as analgesics: A review of randomized controlled trials. J Psychiatry Neurosci 26:30–36, 2001.

25. Sindrup SH, Jensen TS: Pharmacologic treatment of pain in polyneuropathy. Neurology 55:915–920, 2000.

26. Fishbain DA, Cutler R, Rosomoff HL, Rosomoff RS: Evidence-based data from animal and human experimental studies on pain relief with antidepressants: A structured review. Pain Med 1:310–316, 2000.

27. Ener RA, Meglathery SB, Van Decker WA, Gallagher RM: Serotonin syndrome and other serotonergic disorders. Pain Med 4:63–74, 2003.

28. Fishman SM, Dougherty D: Psychopharmacology for the pain specialist. Curr Rev Clin Anesth 18:17–28, 1997.

29. Fishman SM, Wilsey B, Mahajan G, et al: Methadone reincarnated: Novel clinical applications with related concerns. Pain Med 3:339–348, 2002.

30. Bezchlibnyk-Butler KZ, Jefferies JJ, Martin BA: Clinical Handbook of Psychotropic Drugs, ed 4. Hogrefe and Huber, Seattle, 1994.

31. Guze B, Richeimer S, Szuba M: The Psychiatric Drug Handbook. Mosby Year Book, Boston, 1995.

32. Max MB, Culnane M, Schafer SC, et al: Amitriptyline relieves diabetic neuropathy pain in patients with normal or depressed mood. Neurology 37:589–596, 1987.

33. Onghena P, Van Houdenhove B: Antidepressant-induced analgesia in chronic non-malignant pain: A meta-analysis of 39 placebo controlled studies. Pain 49:205–209, 1992.

34. Leijon G, Boivie J: Central post-stroke pain: Controlled trial of amitriptyline and carbamezepine. Pain 36:27–36, 1989.

35. Panerai AE, Monza G, Movilla P, et al: A randomized, within patient, crossover, placebo-conrolled trail on the efficacy and

36. Watson CP, Vernich L, Chipman M, Reed K: Nortriptyline versus amitriptyline in postherpetic neuralgia: A randomized trial. Neurology 51:1166–1167, 1998.

37. Levine JD, Gordon NC, Smith R, et al: Desipramine enhances opiate postoperative analgesia. Pain 27:45–49, 1986.

38. Thase ME, Entsuah AR, Rudolph RL: Remission rates during treatment with venlafaxine or selective serotonin reuptake inhibitors. Br J Psychiatry 178:234–241, 2001.

39. Sindrup SH, Bach FW, Madsen C, et al: Venlafaxine versus imipramine in painful neuropathy: A randomized, controlled trial. Neurology 60:1284–1289, 2003.

40. Goldstein DJ, et al: Duloxetine in the treatment of pain associated with diabetic neuropathy. 156th American Psychiatric Association Meeting, San Francisco, 17–22 May 2003.

41. Davis JL, Smith RL: Painful peripheral diabetic neuropathy treated with venlafaxine HCl extended release capsules. Diabetes Care 22:1909–1910, 1999.

42. Pernia A: Venlafaxine for the treatment of neuropathic pain. J Pain Symptom Manage 19:408–410, 2000.

43. Tasmuth T, Hartel B, Kalso E: Venlafaxine in neuropathic pain following treatment of breast cancer. Eur J Pain 6:17–24, 2002.

44. Songer, DA, Schulte H: Venlafaxine for the treatment of chronic pain. Am J Psychiatry 153:737, 1996.

45. Semenchuk MR, Sherman S, Davis B: Double-blind, randomized trial of bupropion SR for the treatment of neuropathic pain. Neurology 57:1583–1588, 2001.

46. Hyman SE, Arana GW, Rosenbaum JF: Handbook of Psychiatric Drug Therapy, ed 3. Little, Brown, Boston, 1995.

47. Brannon GE, Stone KD: The use of mirtazapine in a patient with chronic pain. J Pain Symptom Manage 18:382–385, 1999.

48. Theobald DE, Kirsh KL, Holtsclaw E, et al: An open-label, crossover trial of mirtazapine (15 and 30 mg) in cancer patients with pain and other distressing symptoms. J Pain Symptom Manage 23:442–447, 2002.

49. Tarascon Pocket Pharmacopoeia. Tarascon, Loma Linda, CA, 2003.

50. McCracken LM, Gross RT, Aikens J, Carnrike CL: The assessment of anxiety and fear in persons with chronic pain: A comparison of instruments. Behav Res Ther 34:927–933, 1996.

51. Borkovec TD, Ruscio AM: Psychotherapy for generalized anxiety disorder. J Clin Psychiatry 62(Suppl 11):37–42; discussion 43–45, 2001.

52. Rocca P, Fonzo V, Scotta M, et al: Paroxetine efficacy in the treatment of generalized anxiety disorder. Acta Psychiatr Scand 95:444–450, 1997.

53. Rickels K, Rynn M: Pharmacotherapy of generalized anxiety disorder. J Clin Psychiatry 63(Suppl 14):9–16, 2002.

54. Bienvenu OJ, Cannistraro PA: The significance of the concept of obsessive-compulsive spectrum disorder to the treatment of chronic nonmalignant pain. Curr Pain Headache Rep 6:40–43, 2002.

55. Janicak PG, Davis JM, Preskorn SH, Ayd FJ: Treatment with anti-anxiety and sedative-hypnotic agents. In Principles and Practice of Psychopharmacotherapy. Lippincott-Williams, 2001, pp 471–522.

55. Rickels K, Pollack MH, Sheehan DV, Haskins JT: Efficacy of extended-release venlafaxine in nondepressed outpatients with generalized anxiety disorder. Am J Psychiatry 157:968–974, 2000.

56. Goodwin FK, Fireman B, Simon GE, et al: Suicide risk in bipolar disorder during treatment with lithium and divalproex. JAMA 290:1467–1473, 2003.

57. Zitman FG, Linssen AC, Edelbroek PM, Van Kempen GM: Clinical effectiveness of antidepressants and antipsychotics in chronic benign pain. Clin Neuropharmacol 15(Suppl 1): 377A–378A, 1992.

58. Lindenmayer JP, Nathan AM, Smith RC: Hyperglycemia associated with the use of atypical antipsychotics. J Clin Psychiatry 62(Suppl 23):30–38, 2001.

59. Fe-Bornstein M, Watt SD, Gitlin MC: Improvement in the level of psychosocial functioning in chronic pain patients with the use of risperidone. Pain Med 3:128–131, 2002.

60. Rozen TD: New treatments in cluster headache. Curr Neurol Neurosci Rep 2:114–121, 2002.

61. Silberstein SD, Peres MF, Hopkins MM, et al: Olanzapine in the treatment of refractory migraine and chronic daily headache. Headache 42:515–518, 2002.

62. Khojainova N, Santiago-Palma J, Kornick C, et al: Olanzapine in the management of cancer pain. J Pain Symptom Manage 23:346–350, 2002.

63. Schreiber S, Backer MM, Weizman R, Pick CG: Augmentation of opioid induced antinociception by the atypical antipsychotic drug risperidone in mice. Neurosci Lett 228:25–28, 1997.

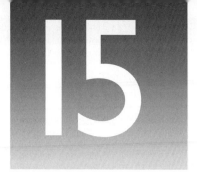

Membrane Stabilizers

Maunak Rana, M.D.,
Honorio T. Benzon, M.D., and
Robert E. Molloy, M.D.

There are many sources of pathology for the development of pain problems in an acute setting. Continued derangement to the normal structure and function of peripheral sensory neurons[1] can lead to the chronic persistence of pain sensation. Plasticity or alterations in the way that nerve fibers respond to and send subsequent input to the central nervous system (CNS) follows, leading to the development of a concept called *central sensitization.*[2]

Changes occur to the way that the nervous system responds to stimuli. Tissue injuries affect the A-delta and C fibers, decreasing their threshold to activation. As a result, prior nonnoxious stimuli can cause activation leading to the perception of pain.[3] This is termed *allodynia.*

Neuronal membrane excitability increases with an increase in various ion channels being present at the site of pathology.[4] The presence of the excess channels can lead to the production of ectopic, abnormal impulses.[5] These aberrant signals are sensed as signals of painful transmission by patients.

Situations that lead to the development of the abnormal pain signals as a result of nervous system remodeling lead to a state of pain characterized as *neuropathic.* A significant number of patients suffer from these remodeled maladies with figures ranging from 10% of all low back pain patients to as many as 1.5% of the US population suffering from some form of neuropathic pain.[5] The causes of neuropathic pain encountered by a pain provider include, but are not limited to, trigeminal neuralgia, intercostal neuralgia, HIV-associated polyneuropathy, diabetic neuropathy, complex regional pain syndrome (CRPS), and central poststroke pain.

Research into pharmacologic management of the source of neuropathic pain led to the study of sodium and calcium channels as a source of the ectopic signals. As a result of this, researchers have focused on attempting to inhibit these sources of aberrant signals by blocking the sodium and calcium channels.[3,5] The pathology leading to epilepsy was extrapolated and studied as a possible source for the development of neuropathic pain in patients. Membrane stabilizers are those agents that have typically been used for the treatment of epileptic foci in the brain. As a result of this logic, these agents have been tried in patients with neuropathic pain states.

Multiple classes of medications are grouped under the heading "membrane stabilizers," including sodium channel blocking agents (antiepileptics and local anesthetics, and antiarrhythmics) and calcium channel blocking agents (gabapentin, w-conopeptides, and calcium channel blockers). Devor showed that lidocaine, via a sodium channel blocker mechanism, was effective in decreasing ectopic firing from the dorsal root ganglia and neuromas in a rodent model.[2,5] Table 15-1 shows the mechanisms of action and side effects of the commonly used membrane stabilizers.

SODIUM CHANNEL BLOCKERS

These agents include the anticonvulsants, local anesthetics, and antiarrhythmics. They as a whole block the development and propagation of ectopic discharges. The primary agents utilized for neuropathic pain are the anticonvulsants. Gabapentin,[6] also an anticonvulsant, is considered separately under calcium channel antagonists, as the mechanism of action of this agent is different from that of the other agents that are typically used for epilepsy and convulsions.

This class of drug is the primary therapy or adjunctive treatment for such processes as trigeminal neuralgia, CRPS, diabetic neuropathy, and postherpetic neuralgia. When utilizing these agents, as with all membrane stabilizers, it is crucial to be aware of dosages, toxicities, and effect of coadministration of

TABLE 15-1. COMMONLY USED MEMBRANE STABILIZERS: THEIR MECHANISMS OF ACTION AND COMMON SIDE EFFECTS

Membrane Stabilizer	Mechanism	Side Effects
Carbamazepine (Tegretol)	Na channel blockade	Sedation, dizziness, gait abnormalities, hematologic changes
Oxcarbazepine	Na channel blockade	Hyponatremia, somnolence, dizziness
Phenytoin	Na channel blockade	Sedation, motor disturbances
Lamotrigine (Lamictal)	Stabilize slow Na channel; suppress release of glutamate from presynaptic neurons	Rash, dizziness, somnolence
Gabapentin	Binds to alpha-2-delta subunit of GABA; increased GABA	Dizziness, sedation
Valproic acid (Valproate)	Na channel blockade; increase GABA	Somnolence, dizziness, gastrointestinal upset
Topiramate (Topamax)	Na channel blockade; potentiate GABA inhibition	Sedation, kidney stones, glaucoma

other drugs. As a general rule, the dose should be titrated to patient comfort within safety standards.

ANTICONVULSANTS

Phenytoin (Dilantin): The initial dosage of phenytoin is 100 mg BID-TID. Major uses include the treatment of diabetic neuropathy. Phenytoin provides pain relief by blocking sodium channels, preventing the release of excitatory glutamate, and inhibiting ectopic discharges.

Studies have been performed looking at the trial of phenytoin for diabetic neuropathy with conflicting results on the efficacy of this therapy.[7] As a result, this agent would not be considered first-line therapy for neuropathic pain. IV phenytoin has been studied in the pain management setting. Doses of this agent at 15 mg/kg have provided relief of acute pain when administered over a short-term two-hour period. The exact role of phenytoin in the treatment of neuropathic pain is yet to be fully elucidated. Side effects include slowing of mentation, somnolence, and giddiness. Nystagmus and ataxia may also be seen in some patients. Unique to phenytoin, among the antiepileptics, is the development of facial alterations including gum hyperplasia and a coarsening of the features.

Phenytoin activates the P450 enzyme system in the liver, and therefore careful assessment of cotherapy is warranted. For example, phenytoin decreases the efficacy of meperidine, mexilitine, haloperidol, lamotrigine, and carbamazepine. As a result, dosages of these medications need to be adjusted accordingly. Coadministration with antidepressants and valproic acid could lead to increased blood concentration of phenytoin, lowering the subsequent doses required for effect in patients.

Carbamazepine (Tegretol): The initial dosage of carbamazepine is 100 mg BID, titrated to effect, with typical dose ranges of 300 to 1,000 mg/day, administered in divided dosages. The chemical structure of this compound is similar to that of the tricyclic antidepressants. This agent is thought to inhibit pain via peripheral and central mechanisms. Carbamazepine selectively blocks active fibers, having no effect on normally functioning C and A-delta nociceptive fibers. Major uses of the drug include primary therapy for trigeminal neuralgia (tic doloreux), thalamic-mediated poststroke pain, postherpetic neuralgia, and diabetic neuropathy. Nausea and vomiting and sedation are common side effects.

Carbamazepine is considered to be the pharmacologic treatment of choice for trigeminal neuralgia, a sharp severe facial pain in the areas supplied by the trigeminal nerve.[7–9] Patients often describe their symptoms as "stabbing or lancinating." While the pathology of this process has not fully been elucidated it is believed that the compression of the trigeminal nerve at the pontine origin of the nerve by the superior cerebellar artery is developmental in the disease.

Prior studies have highlighted the usefulness of carbamazepine therapy for trigeminal neuralgia.[9] One study highlighted the effect of carbamazepine in 70 patients with trigeminal neuralgia, with a 68% decrease in pain episodes and a 58% decrease in the severity of pain. Research from other studies showed a verbal response by patients of "excellent" or "good" upon initiation of therapy for two weeks.[7,10] Additionally, the positive effect of carbamazepine on trigeminal neuralgias has been tested by crossover, placebo, controlled double-blinded studies.[9] Still, even with these positive results, trigeminal neuralgia is a difficult disease process to treat fully in many patients, often requiring multiple agents utilized by the pain physician.

Carbamazepine has also been studied for use in pain states caused by diabetic neuropathy. Carbamazepine showed a decrease in the hyperalgesia to various stimuli in the study animals. The agent has been shown to be more beneficial than placebo in the human diabetic patient population.[7] Carbamazepine therapy was found to be equally effective, with less side effects, when compared with nortriptyline/fluphenazine combination in patients with painful diabetic neuropathy.[7]

Patients on carbamazepine therapy should have blood tests every 2 to 4 months, as there is an increased risk of developing agranulocytosis and aplastic anemia with this agent. Other notable side effects include gait alterations and sedation.

Oxcarbazepine: Oxcarbazepine, the keto-analogue of carbamazepine, is less likely to cause CNS side effects such as dizziness or hematological abnormalities such as leukopenia. A major advantage of oxcarbazepine is that monitoring of drug plasma levels and hematological profiles is generally not necessary. Similar to carbamazepine, oxcarbazepine blocks sodium channels; it does not affect gamma-aminobutyric acid (GABA) receptors.

Significant hyponatremia (sodium < 125 mmol/L) may develop during treatment with oxcarbazepine. This typically occurs during the first 3 months and normalization of sodium levels usually occurs within a few days of discontinuing the drug. Monitoring of sodium levels should be performed when instituting oxcarbazepine therapy. The frequently reported adverse effects of oxcarbazepine include dizziness and somnolence.

The better side-effect profile of oxcarbazepine compared to carbamazepine has led to its increased use. In several countries oxcarbazepine is now the drug of choice in trigeminal neuralgia. While case series reported its efficacy in the treatment of neuropathic pain, prospective randomized controlled studies are lacking at this time.

Valproic Acid: This drug acts at the GABA A receptor. There are conflicting reports in the literature as to the efficacy of this agent in neuropathic pain, although studies have demonstrated the efficacy of this agent in migraine therapy with dosages of 800 mg/day for a period of 8 weeks.[9] Side effects include gastrointestinal upset, somnolence, and dizziness. The exact role of this agent in the armamentarium of the pain practitioner is yet to be elucidated.[11]

Lamotrigine (Lamictal): The initial dosage is 20 to 50 mg at bedtime, increased to 300 to 500 mg per day given in divided doses BID, with a slow increase in dosage over the first month of therapy. Drug administration can be slowly tapered over a 2 week time period safely. As with previously discussed agents, lamotrigine is an agent that blocks sodium channels in actively firing nerves. The agent has no effect on sensation in the native, normally functioning nervous system. Unique to lamotrigine is the fact that in addition to acting as a sodium channel blocker the drug prevents release of an excitatory transmitter involved in pain propagation, glutamate.

A major use for lamotrigine is in trigeminal neuralgia. It also has an indication for cold-induced pain.[7] Studies have analyzed this particular scenario. Volunteers were subjected to a warm water bath (37°C) in which they placed their hands for a few minutes, with subsequent immediate transfer of their hands to a cold bath (2°C). The volunteers were surveyed for their responses ranging from a state of none/minimal pain to maximum pain. The efficacy of lamotrigine, phenytoin, and opioid therapy was tested, with lamotrigine therapy and the opioid therapy providing the best relief in the shortest time

period. This improvement in cold-induced pain could be of benefit in the setting of trauma, peripheral vascular disease, and other temperature-induced pain states.

While carbamazepine has been advocated as the first-line therapy for trigeminal neuralgia, it is not always effective in these patients. Lamotrigine has been studied in this patient model as a co-drug and also as a substitute for carbamazepine.[12,13] A study involving 21 patients being treated for trigeminal neuralgia with no benefit from carbamazepine therapy were treated with lamotrigine.[7] The population of 7 men and 14 women had 14 of the patients noting significant to complete relief of their symptoms after the institution of lamotrigine therapy. The remaining 7 patients did not have benefit from the lamotrigine treatment. The use of lamotrigine may therefore be indicated in carbamazepine-resistant trigeminal neuralgia.

Lamotrigine has also been studied via a double-blinded placebo-controlled trial with positive results on patients who are being treated for trigeminal neuralgia.[12] Fourteen patients were randomized to receive lamotrigine or placebo for a period of two weeks, with a crossover period. Patients who were on lamotrigine noted a significant improvement over their co-subjects treated with placebo. Additionally, patients who were initially on lamotrigine and who were then switched to placebo on crossover continued to have improvement in their symptoms. By the termination of the study, 64% of patients decided to continue their lamotrigine therapy because of beneficial outcome results.

This positive result has also been seen in follow-up with a group of 15 patients with trigeminal neuralgia receiving lamotrigine therapy.[7,13] Seventy-three percent of patients were free of their painful symptoms at the conclusion of the study. Subsequent interval follow-up revealed a continued positive result with no change in pain scores provided by patients. As a result of these studies, lamotrigine may have a role in prevention of trigeminal neuralgia in susceptible patients.

Lamotrigine has also been evaluated in the diabetic neuropathy population. It has been studied in the above mentioned streptozotocin animal-induced hyperalgesic state, decreasing the hyperalgesic state in the diabetic neuropathy models. Patients suffering from diabetic neuropathy may receive benefit from lamotrigine therapy.[11] A group of 15 patients with diabetes (type I and II combined in the study) induced peripheral neuropathy were treated in an open study. Patients were tested with brush and cold stimuli for allodynia, and pinprick for hyperalgesia. Patients developed improvement in pain in all settings tested on completion of the study and persisted in their relief as noted during subsequent 6-month interval follow up.

Lamotrigine can also be considered as therapy for patients suffering from HIV-associated polyneuropathy.[7,13] HIV-associated neuropathy is believed to be on the rise with an increase in the number of patients who become diagnosed with the virus. Patients with distal sensory peripheral neuropathy associated with HIV infection were subjected to a placebo-controlled randomized double-blind study to identify the benefit of lamotrigine therapy. While both placebo-treated patients and patients receiving lamotrigine had a decrease in pain, the rate of decrease was quicker in the lamotrigine group. Patients who were on antiretrovirals and lamotrigine, however, were noted to have slower pain relief than patients who were maintained on lamotrigine without the antiretroviral agents. It is not readily apparent why cotherapy patients have a decreased potency of lamotrigine.

A rash is the most common side effect seen in patients. This rash is more likely to develop in pediatric patients, especially when lamotrigine is combined with valproic acid. The development of a rash is also seen with a rapid titration in the dose of the drug. Prescribing physicians should also be aware that the efficacy of lamotrigine may be diminished with coadministration of phenytoin and carbamazepine.

Topiramate (Topamax): The initial dose is 50 mg at bedtime, increasing upward to an upper limit of 200 mg BID. Studies have shown that pain relief begins to occur at doses of 200 mg/day. In addition to affecting sodium channels and calcium channels, topiramate enhances the action of the GABA (inhibitory) neurotransmitter, and inhibits the AMPA-type glutamate (excitatory) receptor.

Topiramate has been studied in patients with diabetic neuropathy. A 14-week double-blinded study showed that topiramate therapy had more efficacy than placebo in relieving the pain sensed by patients with diabetic neuropathy.[7] Other double-blinded studies have not corroborated these results, however. This agent should therefore be utilized as an adjunct for pain management with other membrane stabilizer agents. Case reports in the literature have also highlighted the use of this agent for additional forms of neuropathic pain including postherpetic neuralgia, intercostal neuralgia, and CRPS.[7]

The primary side effect seen with topiramate is sedation. Other unique occurrences include the potential for development of kidney stones and ocular glaucoma, as topiramate is an inhibitor of the enzyme carbonic anhydrase.[9]

Levetiracetam (Keppra): This agent is a relatively new antiepileptic. The mechanism of its action is yet to be elucidated. Starting dose for this medicine is 500 mg po BID to a goal of 1500 mg BID. At the time of writing there were no double-blinded studies looking at the efficacy of this agent in neuropathic pain states via a MEDLINE search. Side effects to be noted include rash, hives, itching, and dizziness.

LOCAL ANESTHETICS

Local anesthetics are utilized in neuropathic pain states to block the aberrant firing of the abnormal nerves; they do not block normally conducting nerves. As a group they are effective agents in the treatment of postherpetic neuralgia, trigeminal neuralgia, radiculopathies, and peripheral neuropathies.

Lidocaine: The usual dose is 1 to 5 mg/kg IV. Side effects of the CNS include dizziness, blurred vision, and seizure, present when the plasma level is 10 μg/mL.[9] As lidocaine is an antiarrhythmic, bradycardia and cardiac depression (present at 20 to 25 μg/mL plasma concentration) is a potential risk of this agent; therefore, obtaining electrocardiography studies is indicated for the long-term use of lidocaine. A formulation of 5% lidocaine is available in transdermal application, which has been of benefit to patients with various types of neuropathic pain, including postherpetic neuralgia, post-thoracotomy pain, intercostal neuralgia, and meralgia parasthetica.[14]

The eutetic mixture of local anesthetics (EMLA)—comprised of prilocaine and lidocaine—has also been advocated for use as a topical local anesthetic. This agent is sometimes utilized as an adjunct for venipuncture in the pediatric population; care must be taken with the amount of EMLA cream given to patients to avoid toxicity. Prilocaine is readily metabolized to o-toluidine, which can lead to methemoglobinemia. Clinical methemoglobinemia is less likely to develop if dosages of prilocaine are kept below 600 mg.

Mexilitene: The usual dose is 150 mg/day up to a goal of 300 to 450 mg/day. This agent is an antiarrhythmic, and for pain purposes can be considered to be an oral analogue of lidocaine. Pain physicians may provide IV lidocaine for pain management and monitor dose and effect. On obtaining a dose of intravenously administered drug, this may be readily converted to oral mexilitine.

Mexilitine can be used for diabetic neuropathy, thalamic stroke pain, spasticity, and myotonia. Side effects include somnolence, irritability, blurred vision, and nausea. Patients are also at risk for developing blood dyscrasias and should have blood tests on a regular basis. Prescribing physicians should be aware that mexilitene administered with theophylline will increase the levels of the latter, necessitating a decrease in dosage of the mexilitine.

CALCIUM CHANNEL BLOCKERS

Blockade of calcium channels also has a role in pain management. There are six different calcium channel current types found in nervous tissue: L, N, P, Q, R, T.[15] Knowledge of the channel type allows investigators to design specific drugs for precise indications.[16] L-type blockers, for example, have historically been utilized for the treatment of cardiovascular disease.

Gabapentin: Gabapentin binds at the alpha-2-delta subunit of the L-type calcium channel, stabilizing the membrane as its major mechanism of action. Gabapentin, while similar to GABA structurally, does not bind to nor does it have activity at this receptor. It also has no effect on uptake or metabolism of GABA. Also, gabapentin does not change the thresholds for nociception in animal models.[6] In fact, in animals with an intact nervous system, gabapentin may increase the response of dorsal horn neurons to A-delta and C fiber input.[7] As a result, in non-neuropathic native states, gabapentin may enhance pain.

The selective role of gabapentin in pain is seen in its inability to block the sodium channel-mediated potentials in intact neurons. In animals that are placed in a neuropathic state, gabapentin decreases the dorsal horn responses to C fibers.

The usual initial dose is 100 to 300 mg at bedtime, increasing the dose gradually to a maximum of 4,800 mg a day in TID divided doses. If necessary, gabapentin may be continued with a gradual tapering of the agent. Introduced in 1994, the agent has uses for patients suffering from multiple pain conditions. Studies have been performed on patients being treated for CRPS, postherpetic neuralgia, and other forms of neuropathic pain.[6,17–21] When considering the descriptive quality of pain, patients with allodynic, burning, and lancinating pain are more likely to get positive benefit from gabapentin therapy as opposed to patients with hyperalgesic dull and achy pain.[6]

Concerning the effect of gabapentin on postherpetic neuralgia pain, double-blinded studies have been performed testing for benefit in this patient population.[20] Patients with postherpetic neuralgia being maintained on opioids and/or TCA were identified. Patients were divided into two groups, 113 patients receiving gabapentin and 116 receiving placebo therapy, in addition to their current background pain regimen. For a period of 8 weeks patients were maintained on their respective therapies with increased titration of the drug to a maximum goal dose of 3,600 mg/day, achieved in 4 weeks. Results indicated that the gapabentin patients had a decrease in their visual analogue score (VAS) for pain of nearly 2 points, compared to a decrease of only 0.5 in the placebo-treated patients. Along with a decrease in pain, patients also reported improvement in their SF-36 (quality of life) scores as they noted improved functionality, feeling better and more restful sleep at night.

The effect of gapapentin on the neuropathic pain of diabetes has also been evaluated.[19] A randomized, double-blinded, placebo-controlled trial pooling patients from multiple centers showed a decrease of 2.5 on the VAS for patients receiving gabapentin up to 3,600 mg/day vs. a decrease of 1.4 for the patients in the control group.[19] As with the postherpetic neuralgia study, patients also had an increase in their SF-36 scores, more restful sleep at night, and an overall improvement in functioning.

In a double blind, randomized, placebo-controlled 8-week trial gabapentin reduced pain and improved some quality of life measures in patients with a variety of neuropathic pain syndromes.[21] In this study, gabapentin was initially started at 900 mg/day for three days then increased to a maximum of 2,400 mg/day at the end of week five. The patients studied suffered from complex regional pain syndrome, postherpetic neuralgia, radiculopathy, postlaminectomy syndrome, poststroke syndrome, phantom limb pain, and other neuropathic pain syndromes.[21] Gabapentin has also been found to be effective in reducing the pain associated with multiple sclerosis, specifically the paroxysmal pain with throbbing, pricking, and cramping quality rather than the dull, aching pain in multiple sclerosis patients.[17] Finally, gabapentin appears to improve the analgesic efficacy of opioids in patients with neuropathic cancer pain.[17]

Gabapentin has a favorable side-effect profile. Also, with higher doses (greater than 1,800 mg/day) the agent is tolerated better than when doses administered are less than 1,800 mg/day.[17] The efficacy of gabapentin may also be reduced with low doses of the agent. The side effects seen include fatigue, somnolence, and dizziness and may increase with rapid increase in dosage of the drug.

Zonisamide (Zonegran): The initial dose is 100 mg QD for two weeks, increasing by 200 mg/week for a goal of 600 mg/day. This agent functions by blocking the T-type calcium channels, and sodium channels; it also acts to increase GABA release. It has uses in various types of neuropathic pain. An open label dose titration study[7] showed minimal change in VAS scores after 8 weeks of therapy. Side effects to be noted for include ataxia, decreased appetite, rash, and renal calculi (due to the carbonic anhydrase inhibitor effect).

In children there is an increased risk of oligohydrosis and susceptibility to hyperthermia. The exact role of zonisamide in the management of patients with neuropathic pain is therefore yet to be elucidated, and further research studies need to be performed.

ω-conopeptides: These agents are administered intrathecally given the peptidic structure of these drugs, of which

Ziconotide (previously knows as SNX-111) is an example. These agents (CVID, GVIA, and MVIIA are analogues of SNX-111) are derived from the venom of a marine snail (genus *Conus*).[22] W-conopeptides have action at the N-type calcium channels that are present in the dorsal horn laminae of the spinal cord.[18] Intrathecal doses in humans range from 0.3 to 1 ng/kg/hour.[22] Studies have been performed utilizing this agent in an animal setting with intrathecal administration of the agent to cause antinociception in rats to formalin and hot-plate set-ups.[23]

These agents have also been studied in the HIV and cancer populations as a modality for pain relief in opioid-resistant pain. Additionally, case reports have appeared in the literature for the novel use of SNX-111 in intractable pain secondary to brachial plexus avulsion injury.[22] A double-blinded study has shown decreased morphine requirements for patients receiving ziconotide in a perioperative setting.[24] As a result, this agent may be a possible agent for future use in an acute postperioperative setting as well as in a chronic setting as an agent utilized in intrathecal pump therapy. The major side effects of these agents include hypotension, histamine release, sedation, nystagmus, and a tremor.

Nifedipine, Verapamil, Diltiazem, Nimodipine: These agents are mentioned[25] briefly as they are calcium channel blockers, used in a cardiovascular setting classically. As with other agents in this class, these drugs have a role in decreasing central sensitization.[15] Nimodipine has been shown to decrease dose of morphine in cancer pain in 9 of 14 patients.[16] In a colorectal surgery population, concomitant calcium channel blocker therapy does not decrease opioid requirements. L- and N-type calcium channel antagonists may have an adjunctive role with opioids in this category of patient; they do not have a role as monotherapy, however.[16,25]

Magnesium: Research has recently been performed evaluating the antagonists of the *N*-methyl-D-aspartate (NMDA) receptor, including the membrane stabilizing effect of magnesium. In a study of 7 patients with postherpetic neuralgia the intravenous infusion of 30 mg/kg of magnesium sulfate over 30 minutes was found to be more effective in relieving the pain when compared to an intravenous infusion of saline.[26]

NUMBERS NEEDED TO TREAT (NNT)

"Numbers needed to treat" is the number of patients treated with a certain drug in order to obtain one patient with a defined degree of relief. The NNT of drugs permit a comparison between different drugs and diseases to better judge the efficacy of an agent more precisely.[11,27] Usually, the NNT > 50% pain relief is utilized because it is easily understood and seems to be related to relevant clinical effect.[27] The NNT of the different membrane stabilizers in the treatment of neuropathic pain is seen in Table 15-2. The NNTs of the antidepressants and other drugs are included for comparison of their efficacy with the membrane stabilizers. The "numbers needed to harm" (NNH) is the number needed to treat with a certain drug before a patient experience a significant side effect. The NNH of several drugs for pain management is not yet known. The drugs with a low NNT/NNH ratio are superior to the drugs with high NNT/NNH ratio.

TABLE 15-2. NUMBERS NEEDED TO TREAT (NNT) 50% OF SOME THE COMMONLY USED DRUGS FOR NEUROPATHIC PAIN

Drug/Class of Drug	PHN	PDN
Carbamazepine	ND	3.3
Gabapentin	3.2	3.7
Mexilitine	ND	10
TCAs	2.3	3.0
TCA serotonin/noradrenaline	2.4	2.0
TCA noradrenaline	1.9	3.4
SSRI	ND	6.7
Tramadol	ND	3.4
Oxycodone	2.5*	ND

Adapted from Sindrup SH, Jensen TS: Efficacy of pharmacological treatments of neuropathic pain and effect related to mechanism of drug action. Pain 83:389–400, 1999; Jensen TS: Anticonvulsants in neuropathic pain: Rationale and clinical evidence. Eur J Pain 6S:61–68, 2002.

* Add-on therapy to carbamazepine or phenytoin.

PHN, postherpetic neuralgia; PDN, painful diabetic neuropathy; TCA, tricyclic antidepressant; SSRI, specific serotonin reuptake inhibitor; ND, no study done; NNT, number of patients needed to treat with a certain drug to obtain one with a defined degree of pain relief; NNT 50%, numbers needed to obtain one patient with >50% pain relief.

KEY POINTS

- In neuropathic pain there are altered processing and changes in central modulation. These include pathologic activity in injured nerves (resulting in hyperexcitability, spontaneous and evoked pain), loss of C fibers and sprouting of the large fibers in the outer laminas of the dorsal horn where the nociceptive-specific neurons are located (resulting in allodynia), and increased activity in the sympathetic nervous system.
- Some of the molecular changes in neuropathic pain include the accumulation and novel expression of sodium channels in peripheral nerves, increased activity of glutamate receptor subpopulations especially the NMDA receptor, reduction of GABA inhibition, and changes in the penetration of calcium into the cells.
- The mechanisms of action of the membrane stabilizers include blockade of the sodium channel, suppression of the release of glutamate or blockade of glutamate activity, increase in the GABA content, and binding to the alpha-2-delta subunit of GABA (see Table 15-1).

- The most common side effect of lamotrigine is the development of a rash. This is usually seen in pediatric patients and when the dose of the drug is rapidly titrated.
- The most common side effect of oxcarbazepine is hyponatremia.
- Gabapentin is an effective drug in neuropathic pain, specifically postherpetic neuralgia and painful diabetic neuropathy. It is well tolerated. Its common side effects include dizziness and sedation.

REFERENCES

1. Baron R: Peripheral neuropathic pain: From mechanisms to symptoms. Clin J Pain 16:S12–20, 2000.
2. Devor M, Wall PD, Catalan N: Systemic lidocaine silences neuroma and DRG discharge without blocking nerve conduction. Pain 48:261–268, 1992.
3. Nicholson B: Gabapentin use in neuropathic pain syndromes. Acta Neurol Scand 101:359–371, 2000.
4. England JD, Happel LT, Kline DG, et al: Sodium channel accumulation in humans with painful neuromas. Neurology 47:272–276, 1996.
5. Devor M, Setlzer Z: Pathophysiology of damaged nerves in relation to chronic pain. In Wall P, Melzack R (eds): Textbook of Pain, ed 4. Churchill-Livingstone, Edinburgh, 1999, pp 129–165.
6. Mellegers MA, Furlan AD, Mailis A: Gabapentin for neuropathic pain: Systematic review of controlled and uncontrolled literature. Clin J Pain 17:284–295, 2001.
7. Backonja MM: Anticonvulsants (antineuropathics) for neuropathic pain syndromes. Clin J Pain 16:S67–72, 2000.
8. Munglani R, Hill RG: Other drugs including sympathetic blockers. In Wall P, Melzack R (eds): Textbook of Pain, ed 4. Churchill-Livingstone, Edinburgh, 1999, pp 1233–1251.
9. Tremont-Lukats IW, Megeff C, Backjona MM: Anticonvulsants for neuropathic pain syndromes: mechanisms and place in therapy. Drugs 60:1029–1052, 2000.
10. Ross EL: The evolving role of antiepileptic drugs in treating neuropathic pain. Neurology 55:S41–46, 2000.
11. Sindrup SH, Jensen TS: Efficacy of pharmacological treatments of neuropathic pain and effect related to mechanism of drug action. Pain 83:389–400, 1999.
12. Zakrzewska JM, Chaudry Z, Nurmikko TJ, et al: Lamotrigine in refractory trigeminal neuralgia: Results from a double-blinded placebo-controlled crossover trial. Pain 73:223–230, 1997.
13. McCleane GJ: Lamotrigine in the management of neuropathic pain: A review of the literature. Clin J Pain 16:321–326, 2000.
14. Argoff CE: New analgesics for neuropathic pain: The Lidoderm patch. Clin J Pain 16:S62–66, 2000.
15. McGuire D, Bowersox S, Fellmann JD, et al: Sympatholysis after neuron-specific, N-type, voltage-sensitive calcium channel blockade: First demonstration of N-channel function in humans. J Cardiovasc Pharm 30:400–403, 1997.
16. Wallace MS: Calcium and sodium channel antagonists for the treatment of pain. Clin J Pain 16:S80–85, 2000.
17. Mao J, Chen L: Gabapentin in pain management. Anesth Analg 91:680–687, 2000.
18. Fields H, Baron R, Rowbotham M: Peripheral neuropathic pain: An approach to management. In Wall P, Melzack R (eds): Textbook of Pain, ed 4. Churchill-Livingstone, Edinburgh, 1999, pp 1523–1535.
19. Backonja MM, Beydoun A, Edwards KR, et al: Gabapentin monotherapy for the treatment of painful neuropathy: A multicenter, double-blind, placebo-controlled trial in patients with diabetes mellitus. JAMA 280:1831–1836, 1998.

20. Rowbotham M, Harden N, Stacey P, et al: Gabapentin for the treatment of post-herpetic neuralgia: A multi-center, double-blind, placebo-controlled study. JAMA 280:1837–1842, 1998.

21. Serpell MG, and Neuropathic Pain Study Group: Gabapentin in neuropathic pain syndromes: A randomised, double-blind, placebo-controlled trial. Pain 99:557–566, 2002.

22. Browse W: Use of intrathecal SNX-111, a novel, N-type, voltage-sensitive, calcium channel blocker, in the management of intractable brachial plexus avulsion pain. Clin J Pain 13:256–259, 1997.

23. Malmberg AB, Yaksh TL: Effect of continuous intrathecal infusion of omega-conopeptide N-type calcium-channel blockers, on behavior and antinociception formalin and hot plate tests in rats. Pain 60:83–90, 1995.

24. Atanassoff PG, Hartmannsgruber MWB, Thrasher J, et al: Ziconotide, a new N-type calcium channel blocker, administered intrathecally for acute postoperative pain. Reg Anesth Pain Med 25:274–278, 2000.

25. Smutch TP, Sutton KG, Zamponi GW: Voltage-dependent calcium channels – Beyond dihydropyridine antagonists. Curr Opinion Pharmacol 1:11–16, 2000.

26. Brill S, Sedgwick PM, Hamann W, et. al. Efficacy of intravenous magnesium in neuropathic pain. Br J Anesth 2002; 89(5) 711–714.

27. Jensen TS: Anticonvulsants in neuropathic pain: Rationale and clinical evidence. Eur J Pain 6S:61–68, 2002.

NSAIDs and COX-2-Selective Inhibitors

Jeffrey A. Katz, M.D.

HISTORY AND BACKGROUND

The nonopioid analgesics most often used are the nonsteroidal anti-inflammatory drugs (NSAIDs)—in 1984 one estimate noted that 1 in 7 Americans were treated with an NSAID.[1] In 1991, 70 million prescriptions for NSAIDs were given (excluding aspirin), and this does not even account for the increasing availability of over-the-counter NSAIDs. Those prescriptions resulted in a retail cost of $2.2 billion, with the worldwide market exceeding $6 billion per year.[2,3] This cost does not even cover the expense of using medications to treat dyspepsia, which can occur in up to 15% of NSAID users.[4] Another estimate suggests that more than 30 million people use NSAIDs on a daily basis worldwide, with 25% of all adverse drug effects coming from this class of drug.[5]

The glycoside salicin was first extracted from the bark of the willow tree (*Salix alba*) and was documented for use in fever since at least 1827. The first published report of the use of salicylic acid was by Stone in 1763, when he treated 50 rheumatic patients with willow bark.[7] Both acetylsalicylic acid (aspirin) as well as sodium salicylate were both synthesized in 1899 by Felix Hoffman as part of Bayer Corporation, with salicylate being used for rheumatologic disorders since 1927.[6,7] The first of the newer NSAIDs was phenylbutazone, which was synthesized in 1946. In 1971 it was discovered that aspirin acts as an inhibitor of cyclooxygenase (COX), preventing the formation of prostaglandins from arachidonic acid.[8]

The NSAID class of drug contains compounds that are often chemically unrelated and which are grouped together based on their therapeutic actions.[9] Figure 16-1 shows just how chemically unrelated many of these compounds actually are. All NSAIDs have analgesic, anti-inflammatory, and antipyretic properties, despite formal claims that some are indicated only for various diagnoses such as arthritis or dysmenorrhea.[10] Unlike the opioids, the NSAIDs do not demonstrate

tolerance, and they often are more effective at controlling certain pain conditions with fewer side effects than the opioids.[11] They have even demonstrated clear clinical utility in such severe pain states as metastatic spread of cancer to bone, usually supplementing rather than replacing the role of opioids.[12]

In 1998 the NSAID class was expanded to include a new sub-class, the COX-2-selective inhibitors. Although some consider this subclass to be separate from the NSAIDs based on their clinical profile (see below), as their mechanism of action still involves inhibition of COX (and since the US Food and Drug Administration language classifies them as NSAIDs), the COX-2-specific inhibitors will be assumed to be included when the term 'NSAID' is used.[13]

For the purposes of this chapter, acetaminophen is not discussed. It is, however, considered by many to be an NSAID despite its lack of peripheral anti-inflammatory effect. Its mechanism of analgesia, which is primarily in the central nervous system (CNS), remains unclear. Nonetheless it is a popular analgesic option due to its lack of platelet, gastric, bone, and renal effects. However, its hepatotoxicity when taken in overdose is profound and must be recognized as a significant clinical risk in selected patients.

One must be cautious reviewing the literature on NSAIDs since the majority of studies involves responsiveness of patients treated for rheumatic or other arthritic conditions. In those studies inflammation of the joints rather than analgesia is often emphasized as the measured variable. While such data are useful in predicting the ability of an NSAID to control inflammatory changes of joint structures, they have little bearing on NSAID efficacy for other analgesic purposes, since there is a clearly documented lack of association between analgesia and anti-inflammatory effect of NSAIDs.[14]

The difference between the arthritis and pain usage of NSAIDs is also reflected in dosage requirements. The dosing for acute pain for NSAIDs is typically higher than that used

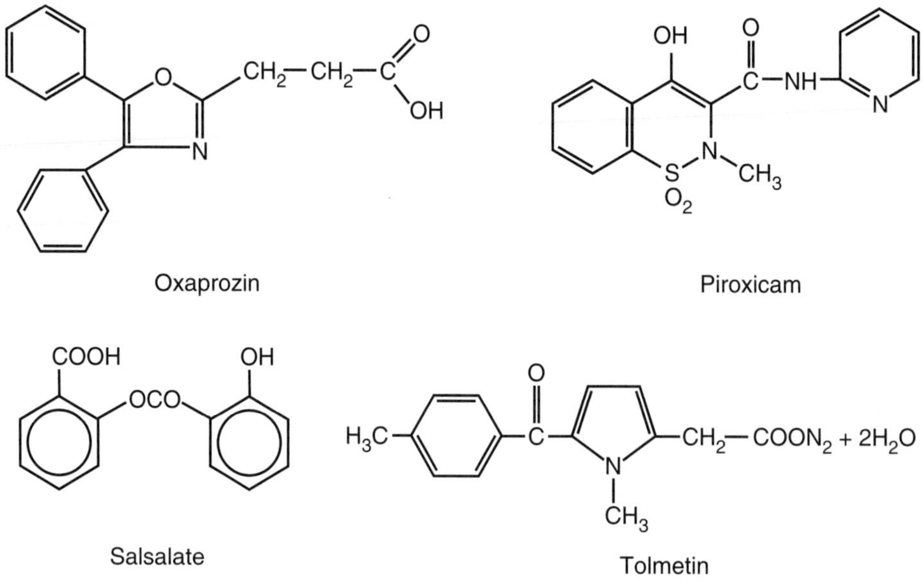

FIGURE 16–1. Structures of several different NSAIDs, revealing the wide variation in chemical structure of these compounds that are grouped into this one therapeutic class.

for either rheumatoid or osteoarthritis, reflecting differences in the pain model used (Table 16-1). Further, even within the arthritis pain model there may be differences: rheumatoid arthritis pain has a clear inflammatory component that osteoarthritis pain may not necessarily share. Acute postoperative pain shares several types of pain, including visceral, inflammatory, neuropathic, as well as nociceptive and hence arthritis data may not predict efficacy in perioperative pain management.

Similarly, most toxicity studies of NSAIDs have been performed in elderly patients with concomitant medical conditions—there is not as much toxicity data specifically in healthier patients using the NSAIDs solely for pain. Toxicity is also related to duration of usage—the longer an NSAID is used, the greater the likelihood that toxicity will develop over time. Again, there is limited data (short of endoscopic studies) on the clinically relevant toxicity of NSAIDs in short-term (days to weeks) usage.

Lastly, the NSAIDs are actually not analgesics. Rather, they function as antihyperalgesics. Fentanyl and other opioids are capable of raising the threshold of tolerance to the nociception of an acute injury, such as a surgical incision; the NSAIDs, however, do not. Rather, these drugs demonstrate a significant

ability to reduce the hyperalgesia and allodynia following injury, often performing better in this manner than opioids but more often providing a major synergism to opioid analgesia.[15]

MECHANISM OF ACTION

Svensson aptly stated that "the circle is now complete" when referring to our beliefs regarding the mechanism of analgesia of the NSAIDs. Although Woodbury in the third edition of Goodman and Gilman's textbook of pharmacology noted that the salicylates provide analgesia by a "selective depressant effect on the CNS," a change occurred in belief in the 1980 sixth edition that noted, "aspirin works peripherally."[15] Currently, however, there is ample evidence that prostaglandins play a key role in the CNS in pain modulation especially following inflammation and the NSAIDs probably exert some, if not most, of their analgesic effect on the CNS.

Prostaglandin Physiology: Traditional teaching indicates that the NSAIDs provide analgesia primarily through actions outside the CNS by inhibiting the formation of prostaglandins (PG).[16] When cell membranes are damaged, a class of substance called the eicosanoids (which includes arachidonic acid)

TABLE 16-1. RECOMMENDED DOSAGES FOR ACUTE vs. CHRONIC PAIN STATES IN VARIOUS NSAIDs[13]

Drug	Dose for Osteoarthritis/ Rheumatoid Arthritis	Dose for Acute Pain/ Dysmenorrhea
Celecoxib	100–200 mg bid	400 mg load, 200 mg bid prn
Rofecoxib	12.5–25 mg/day	50 mg/day up to 5 days
Valdecoxib	10–20 mg/day	20 mg bid prn

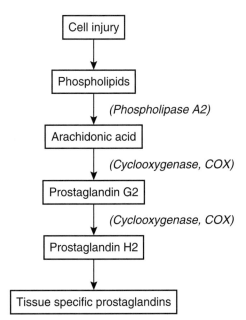

FIGURE 16–2. Pathway for formation of prostaglandins.

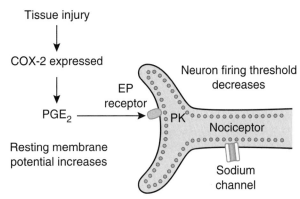

FIGURE 16–3. Mechanism of peripheral nociceptor sensitization by prostaglandins. Tissue injury results in increased expression of COX-2 that in turn increases production of PGE_2. PGE_2 binds to the EP receptor causing intracellular phosphokinases to alter sodium channels in the nociceptor to increase sodium permeability. The net effect is a reduction in firing threshold. PK, phosphokinases; EP, prostaglandin E receptor.

is formed by the action of phospholipases (phospholipase A_2 and C and diglyceride lipase) on membrane phospholipids. Arachidonic acid in turn is broken down by the lipooxygenase system or the COX (also called prostaglandin G/H synthetase, PGHS) enzyme system (Fig. 16-2).

The COX system converts arachidonic acid to cyclic endoperoxide prostaglandin G2 (PGG_2) that is subsequently acted on by hydroperoxidase to form the endoperoxide PGH_2. This endoperoxide is then converted to different prostaglandins by tissue-specific prostaglandin synthases as determined by the cell type. For example, platelets will convert the endoperoxide to thromboxane A_2, whereas vascular endothelium will convert it to prostacyclin (PGI_2).

Arachidonic acid is also acted on by lipooxygenase to form leukotrienes. Some of the leukotrienes are involved in affecting pain transmission: leukotriene B4, for example, produces thermal hyperalgesia in humans.[17] Although leukotrienes are relevant to the manner in which aspirin-induced asthma (AIA) may be triggered by NSAIDs (but not necessarily by selective COX-2 inhibitors, see below) their role in pain and hyperalgesia is not well elucidated at present. While all NSAIDs inhibit COX, some (such as ketoprofen) also inhibit lipooxygenase to varying degrees, although whether there is any advantage to this activity has yet to be demonstrated.

Prostaglandins and Pain: Peripheral Actions: By themselves, the prostaglandins such as PGE_1 or PGE_2 are not important mediators of pain transmission, but they contribute to hyperalgesia peripherally by sensitizing nociceptive sensory nerve endings to other mediators (such as histamine and bradykinin) and by sensitizing nociceptors to respond to nonnociceptive stimuli (e.g., touch).[10,18] Prostaglandin E_2 binds to EP (prostaglandin E) receptors on nociceptive nerve endings, triggering the action of phosphokinases intracellularly to increase sodium channel permeability. The result is an elevation of the resting membrane potential and a reduction in the firing threshold. Hence, low-intensity stimuli may cause the

nociceptor to fire (i.e., touch and movement cause pain) as well as hyperalgesia[19] (Fig. 16-3).

Prostaglandins and Pain: Central Actions: Prostaglandins are recognized to have direct actions at the level of the spinal cord to enhance nociception, notably at the terminals of sensory neurons in the dorsal horn.[20] Minute amounts of prostaglandins are capable of enhancing pain transmission by a number of mechanisms: (1) increasing release of neurotransmitters such as substance P and glutamate from primary nociceptive afferents where they terminate in the dorsal horn, (2) increasing the sensitivity of second-order neurons responsible for nociceptive transmission, and (3) inhibiting the release of descending inhibitory neurotransmitters.[21–23]

While both COX-1 and COX-2 (see below in the section on COX isoforms) are present in the CNS, studies using selective inhibitors of these enzymes applied intrathecally confirm that inhibition of COX-2 and not COX-1 reduces hyperalgesia.[15] COX-2 is upregulated significantly following inflammatory injury, and while direct neural input can trigger this production, humoral factors also play a major role. In the presence of inflammation, inflammatory proteins, cytokines, are released into the circulation. At present, evidence suggests that interleukin 6 (IL-6) triggers the formation of IL-1beta in the CNS, which in turn causes increased production of COX-2 and PGE_2, producing hyperalgesia.[24] Blockade of the nerves carrying the pain from the affected site do not prevent this upregulation since it is a humoral response. Further, it is a systemic response, causing upregulation of COX-2 not only in the segment of the spinal cord corresponding to the injured area, but throughout the CNS including the thalamus and cerebral cortex ipsi- and contralaterally.[24] COX-2 is formed in several cells types including both neurons and glial cells.[25]

COX Isoforms: In the late 1980s evidence accumulated indicating that there was more than one form of COX. This discovery that mammalian cells contain two related but unique COX isoenzymes led to further research to clarify the different roles of the two forms. The two forms are about 60% identical in terms of molecular structure, but the significant difference is in terms of their expression and functions.[26] Type I COX (COX-1) is a constitutively expressed enzyme which is present in variable amounts in most cells, including vascular endothelium, platelets, and renal tubules.[27] COX-1 levels remain fairly stable although hormonal stimuli can cause increases. Type II COX (COX-2) is almost undetectable in most tissues under normal physiologic conditions, but during inflammation COX-2 expression significantly increases, by as much as 10 to 80 fold.[26,28] COX-2 is known to be present, however, under basal conditions in the brain and renal cortex.[29]

COX-1 is the primary form of the enzyme expressed in platelets, kidney, stomach, and vascular smooth muscle, apparently serving an important function in cellular homeostasis.[26]

As discussed later, prostaglandins formed by COX-1 are important in protecting the gastric mucosa, in ensuring proper platelet function, and in maintaining renal function.

COX-2 appears to be key in the production of hyperalgesia following injury. Although some studies suggest that COX-1 plays a role in spinal transmission of pain,[30] a much greater body of evidence is available supporting the concept that it is almost entirely COX-2 that is responsible for forming the prostaglandins involved in hyperalgesia both in the periphery as well as in the CNS. Compounds specific for blocking COX-1 repeatedly fail to reduce hyperalgesia whereas COX-2 and mixed COX-1/COX-2 inhibitors are antihyperalgesic.[15]

It is not surprising, then, that interest in developing pure COX-2 inhibitors has increased, with the goal being to prevent formation of prostaglandins associated with pain and hyperalgesia while leaving unaffected the formation of prostaglandins needed to preserve normal function in the gastrointestinal (GI) mucosa, kidney, and vasculature. Table 16-2 shows the selectivity of various NSAIDs for COX-2 vs. COX-1; however, any such data must be interpreted cautiously. Inhibition of COX can vary by species and by experimental model; for example, a model done in the absence of protein will fail to account for the high protein binding of NSAIDs that occurs in vivo. There is no clear evidence that once a clinically relevant level of COX-2 selectivity has been achieved (as evidenced by lack of platelet effect in supratherapeutic doses, for example) that greater selectivity confers any further benefit.

There has been some evidence to suggest the existence of a third COX isoenzyme, COX-3. COX-3 is essentially a genetic modification of the COX-1 enzyme, and has been shown to be present in the brain of dogs and rats. However, although some have suggested that COX-3 may play a role in CNS pain processing (and might explain the analgesic action of acetaminophen), there is minimal evidence at present to support the contention.[31–33]

NSAID Analgesic Actions: NSAIDs are characterized by their ability to inhibit COX. It should be noted, though, that other drugs (e.g., tricyclic antidepressants) might also be inhibitors of this enzyme.[34] The apparent mechanism of preventing sensitization of peripheral nociceptors by diminishing prostaglandin formation (and thereby preventing peripheral nociceptor sensitization) is the most commonly stated mechanism of action of NSAID analgesia. Furthermore, there is evidence that NSAIDs have peripheral cellular effects unrelated to the synthesis of prostaglandins, such as inhibiting the release of inflammatory mediators from neutrophils and macrophages.[35] Nonetheless, the recognized dissociation between the anti-inflammatory potency of various NSAIDs and their respective analgesic actions supports evidence that the NSAIDs produce analgesia also through mechanisms in the central nervous system.[36–41]

There are many potential sites of action for NSAIDs in the CNS. NSAIDs have been shown in animals to reduce apparent hyperalgesia evoked by spinal action of substance P and N-methyl-D-aspartate (NMDA).[42] Central mechanisms for NSAID analgesia may also involve reversing the inhibition by prostaglandins of the descending opioid-mediated noradrenergic pathways involved in pain inhibition.[39,43,44] Demonstrated sites of actions of the NSAIDs in animals models have included the hypothalamus, thalamus, and periaqueductal gray.[45–47] Additionally, there is evidence that NSAIDs may exert some actions through central opioid mechanisms, as evidenced by the ability of naloxone to inhibit early diclofenac analgesia and the finding that diclofenac can counteract the withdrawal symptoms of heroin addicts.[10,48] Evidence also exists suggesting important roles of serotonin and nitric oxide in the production of analgesia by NSAIDs.[10]

NSAIDs are known to cross the blood–brain barrier to enter the CNS, sometimes (but not always) in proportion to plasma concentrations.[49,50] More recent studies have focused on the COX-2-selective inhibitors, which also demonstrate the ability to enter the CNS.[51] Perhaps the simplest evidence of the central action of the NSAIDs would be in their antipyretic action, which is based on their action on the hypothalamus.[52]

There is evidence to indicate that the analgesic response to a particular NSAID will vary depending on the individual. That is, while the mean response of a population is the same for all NSAIDs, the individual response can be highly variable, reflected in the clinical situation of some patients being better responders to some NSAIDs and not responsive to others.[53,54] Some studies have stated that due to the interpatient variability in side effects, efficacy, and pharmacokinetics, 10 to 15 different NSAIDs are necessary to provide a reasonable range of

TABLE 16-2. **SELECTIVITY OF VARIOUS NSAIDs FOR COX-1 vs. COX-2**[7]

Drug	Ratio of IC50* for COX-2/COX-1
Aspirin	166
Indomethacin	60
Ibuprofen	15
Diclofenac	0.7
Naproxen	0.6
Nabumetone	0.2
Etodolac	0.1

*The IC50 ratio is the mean inhibitory concentration of the drug needed to inhibit COX-2 vs. COX-1 by 50%. A higher value implies greater selectivity of inhibition of COX-2. Note that all values are derived from in vitro studies and may not reflect the clinical situation.

alternative therapy.[55] The wide variety of possible mechanisms of analgesia and the array of chemical structures in this therapeutic class of drug may account for the large interindividual response to various NSAIDs and COX-2 inhibitors.

COX-2 Selectivity of NSAIDs: One classification scheme of NSAIDs based on COX selectivity divides the NSAIDs into four classes. Aspirin comprises the first class, causing irreversible inhibition of both COX-1 and COX-2. Ibuprofen is in the second class, which causes reversible competitive inhibition of both isoforms. The third proposed class causes a slower, time-dependent inhibition of both isoforms; flurbiprofen and indomethacin are in this class. The fourth class consists of those compounds that are largely COX-2 selective, and celecoxib, rofecoxib, valdecoxib, etoricoxib, parecoxib, and lumericoxib are in this class. This last class is comprised of weak competitive inhibitors of COX-1 (for all clinical purposes, there is no COX-1 inhibition) but inhibit COX-2 in a slower, more time-dependent process.[56]

One additional area of interest relating to COX-2 is in the pathogenesis of colon cancer and possibly other malignancies. Previous epidemiologic studies have shown a reduced risk of colon cancer in people using NSAIDs, and this concept has been supported in animal models. COX-2 expression is increased notably in colorectal carcinomas and adenomas, and it may be that COX-2 expression could be a major contributor to the dysfunctions seen in malignant cells.[8,57]

Enantiomer Activity: Evaluation of the activities of the enantiomers of NSAIDs reveals that most of the COX inhibitory activity lies with the S form, although for the enantiomers studied no selectivity between COX-1 or COX-2 inhibition has been shown for ketoprofen, ketorolac, or ibuprofen.[58] In studies of flurbiprofen both enantiomers when given systemically produced reduced neural response in the animal model of an inflamed knee joint, but only the S form produced such effect when given at the site of inflammation. Such information implies that while peripheral analgesia is only mediated by the S form, both the R and S forms may mediate central analgesia produced by flurbiprofen.[59] Similar data exist for ketoprofen, which also has most of its peripheral anti-inflammatory activity in the S(+) enantiomer (dexketoprofen). Furthermore, as with flurbiprofen, conversion from the R(–) enantiomer to the S(+) form can occur in vivo, but the reverse process does not occur. Of greatest interest was the finding in rats that dexketoprofen showed significantly less ulcerogenic tendencies than the racemic form.[60]

PHARMACOKINETICS

Basic pharmacokinetic data of most NSAIDs are summarized in Table 16-3. Reviews of the clinical pharmacokinetics of NSAIDs have been previously published.[61] The NSAIDs overall have similar pharmacokinetic characteristics: they are rapidly and extensively absorbed after oral administration, tissue distribution is very limited (due to high protein binding), they are metabolized extensively in the liver with little dependence on renal elimination, and they have low clearances.[62] Of particular clinical relevance is the observation that toxicity of many NSAIDs may be related to their plasma half-lives—the longer the elimination half-life, the greater the risk of toxicity.[63] However, this information regarding the half-life relationship

to toxicity is based on epidemiologic retrospective data; it may be that improved compliance with once daily dosing led to more consistent use of the long-half-life NSAIDs with resulting increases in apparent toxicity.

The high protein binding ($\geq$90%) of the NSAIDs has particular relevance in the elderly population. The elderly tend to have decreased concentrations of serum albumin, resulting in higher free fractions of NSAIDs in the blood. While such elevated free fractions may enhance efficacy, they can also increase toxicity.[64] Another area of concern with the high protein binding would be with the NSAIDs interaction with warfarin, which when combined with the platelet-inhibiting effect of nonselective NSAIDs could cause a significant risk of bleeding.

Despite the overall similarity between NSAIDs in their pharmacokinetic profiles, there are subclasses of the drugs with unique features. The most studied NSAIDs are the salicylates, which demonstrate increasing half-life with increasing dose (Michaelis–Menton kinetics). It takes about 2 days to achieve steady-state blood concentrations when 1.5 g/day of aspirin is given to adults, while more than 1 week may be needed to achieve steady-state concentrations when the dose is 3 g/day.[65] Salicylates also displace other NSAIDs such as naproxen and phenylbutazone from plasma binding sites, increasing the free concentrations of those drugs and increasing the risk of toxicity.[66] Other clinically relevant pharmacokinetic characteristics are described in the sections dealing with individual agents.

Differences in efficacy between NSAIDs may be more related to the relative doses of the drugs being compared rather than the properties of the medications. For example, one paper comparing diclofenac, indomethacin, and piroxicam noted wide differences in bioavailability and elimination between patients, and suggested these pharmacokinetic differences as a contributor to the phenomena of interpatient differences in drug responsiveness.[67] Such data must be interpreted relative to the data mentioned previously regarding individual variability in pharmacodynamic response to NSAIDs.

TOXICITY

Although they do not demonstrate tolerance or physical dependence like the opioids, NSAIDs present a toxicity profile that is very significant. For example, it was estimated using 1981–1983 Medicaid data that treating GI side effects added 45% to the cost of treating arthritis patients.[68] While the use of NSAIDs increased more than 100% between 1973 and 1983, more recently the prescription rate has been stable, most likely due to physician awareness of the significance of the complications of NSAIDs.[69] Nonetheless, recent studies regarding informed consent prior to institution of NSAID therapy revealed that while epigastric discomfort was discussed 72% of the time, other side effects were mentioned less than 15% of the time.[70] Such statistics are disconcerting, given the rather severe reactions to NSAIDs possible in significant numbers of patients. Several reviews document that the complications from NSAIDs result in an increased mortality in elderly arthritic patients who use NSAIDs vs. those who do not.[71,72] Also, the risk of toxicity from NSAIDs for any organ system is greater with increasing age.[73] The three most common adverse drug reactions to NSAIDs are GI, dermatological, and neuropsychiatric, the last one oddly not being age related.[74] However, most clinically significant complications involve the GI, renal, hematologic, and hepatic organ systems.

TABLE 16-3. **PHARMACOKINETIC DATA OF NSAIDs**

Drug (Generic)	Drug (Brand)	T1/2β (hour)	Vd (L/kg)	Cl (L/kg/hour)
Acetaminophen		2.8	1.0	0.25
Aspirin		0.25	0.2	0.55
Celecoxib	Celebrex	11.2		
Diclofenac	Voltaren	1–2	0.12	0.04–0.08
Diflunisal	Dolobid	5–20	0.1	0.007
Etodolac	Lodine	7	0.36	0.047
Fenoprofen	Nalfon	2–3	0.1	0.02–0.04
Flurbiprofen	Ansaid	3–4	0.1	0.03–0.04
Ibuprofen	Motrin, Nuprin	2–2.5	0.14	0.04–0.05
Indomethacin	Indocin	6	0.12	0.014
Ketoprofen	Orudis	1.5	0.11	0.07
Ketorolac	Toradol	5.5	0.28	0.035
CMT	Trilisate, Trisalicylate	7	0.11	0.01
Meloxicam	Mobic	20.1		
Nabumetone	Relafen	26	0.68	0.018
Naproxen	Naprosyn, Anaprox	12–15	0.10	0.005–0.006
Oxaprozin	Daypro	40–60	0.15	0.002
Piroxicam	Feldene	48.5	0.1	0.002
Rofecoxib	Vioxx	17		
Salsalate	Mono-Gesic	3.8		0.21
Sulindac	Clinoril	1.5	0.52	0.21
Tolmetin	Tolectin	1	0.09	0.07
Valdecoxib	Bextra	8.11		

Modified from Denson D, Katz J: Nonsteroidal antiinflammatory agents. *In* Raj P (ed): *Practical Management of Pain.* Mosby Year Book, St Louis, 1992, p 607.

One question repeatedly brought up particularly by pharmaceutical manufacturers is whether one NSAID is more toxic than another. One review of 2,747 rheumatoid arthritis patients, even controlling for patient factors, found more problems with indomethacin, tolmetin, and meclofenamate. The least toxic were coated or buffered aspirin, salsalate, and ibuprofen. The most toxic drugs were those usually taken in the lowest doses.[75]

Gastrointestinal Toxicity: NSAIDs affect the GI tract with symptoms of gastric distress alone and through actual damage with ulceration. Dyspepsia (upper abdominal pain in the absence of documented gastric mucosal damage) has been shown to have an annual prevalence with NSAID use of about 15%. One study demonstrated that over 12 weeks of use, 2% to 5% of patients stopped NSAID use because of dyspepsia.[76] In another study comparing five NSAIDs, gains in pain control were generally at a cost in quality of life due to GI complaints.[77] Hence, even in the absence of serious ulceration, GI side effects can be frequent and severe enough to warrant their discontinuation.

GI bleeding and perforation are the most frequently reported significant complication of NSAID use. One review estimated 7,000 deaths and 70,000 hospitalizations per year in the USA among NSAID users. Among rheumatoid arthritis patients, an estimated 20,000 hospitalizations and 2,600 deaths per year are related to NSAID GI toxicity.[78] Costs for the evaluation and treatment of GI symptoms (not even those associated with hospitalization) have been estimated by some to account for more than one-half of the expenditures for NSAID-related GI disease.[79] This has been confirmed with more recent data suggesting that 16,500 deaths per year can be attributed to NSAID use alone, exceeding the number of deaths per year of cervical cancer, asthma, and malignant melanoma.[80]

The earliest evidence of a link between aspirin and stomach damage was reported in 1938, and in the 1950s and 1960s further reports and case series associated with aspirin use began to appear. More evidence of the association between NSAIDs and gastropathy accrued in the 1970s with the increased use of gastroscopy and the introduction of several new NSAIDs.[7] It should be noted, however, that while endoscopic studies demonstrating ulcer formation with NSAID usage appear on the surface to reflect the risk of clinically significant ulcer formation, no such connection has been clearly made, and some question the validity of using endoscopic ulcer observation as a marker for gastric toxicity of NSAIDs.[80] On the other hand, it is often said that one "can't bleed from an ulcer that isn't there." Interpretation of endoscopic studies should be done with care.

NSAID use is associated with many potential alterations in GI function. In the stomach NSAIDs affect mucus and bicarbonate secretion, blood flow, epithelial cell turnover and repair, and mucosal immunocyte function. One of the more common effects seen is hemorrhagic gastric erosion, typically found in the corpus. These lesions are the result of topical irritation by acidic NSAIDs, and they heal quickly in a few days with the cessation of NSAID use. This topical irritation, however, contributes little to the formation of gastric or duodenal ulcers, which seem to be primarily the result of COX inhibition. Interestingly, the topical gastric irritation effect occurs less often as NSAID use is continued. This is the result of an adaptation of the gastric mucosa to the acidic irritant over time, although the mechanism of this adaptation is not understood.[7]

The ulcerogenic aspects of NSAID injury to the GI system seem to predominantly be the result of inhibition of prostaglandin synthesis, and these injuries usually involve antral and prepyloric gastric lesions. Despite the frequency of dyspepsia, silent ulceration is still common, necessitating vigilance on the part of the prescribing physician.[81,82] One endoscopic study screening for ulcers associated with NSAID use found that there was a lack of symptoms in 70% of patients with documented NSAID-related ulcers.[4] The relative risk of inducing ulceration with NSAIDs is not entirely clear, although some prevalence studies show that in arthritics gastric ulcers will be present in 13% of those on NSAIDs (11% will have duodenal ulcers) vs. a 0.3% incidence (1.4% for duodenal) in the normal population.[83]

Several factors that increase the risk of NSAID gastropathy and development of gastroduodenal ulcers have been identified. Proposed risk factors for NSAID gastropathy include age over 60 years, prior history of peptic ulcer disease, steroid use, alcohol use, multiple NSAID use, and possibly the first 3 months of use of the NSAID.[84] However, some studies challenge whether steroid use adds significant risk of ulceration with concomitant NSAID use.[76] Furthermore, while original thinking led many to believe that the risk of ulceration was highest in the first few months of NSAID use before gastric adaptation had occurred, more recent data suggest that the risks in fact do not decrease with continued drug exposure.[83] Recent studies have implicated the bacteria *H. pylori* in the pathogenesis of peptic ulcer disease; however, prevalence of the bacteria is not affected by NSAID use.[85] Again, other data challenge this contention, showing that *H. pylori* neither increases the risk of gastric injury among long-term NSAID users nor does NSAID use affect the dynamics of *H. pylori* infection.[76]

The role of NSAIDs in producing small intestine and colonic lesions has not been well characterized. Exacerbation of colitis has been observed with NSAIDs, but not all NSAIDs have been shown to produce intestinal lesions.[7] A condition called NSAID enteropathy has been described, reflecting the impact of the NSAIDs in the small intestine.[86] Due to the lack of technology to evaluate for erosions in the small intestine, data are limited. However, changes in permeability and protein wasting are characteristics of this syndrome, which may be prevented by use of misoprostol.[87] There is also animal evidence to suggest that the COX-2-selective inhibitors may also protect the small intestine, as evidenced by reduced changes in permeability and no mitochondrial uncoupling as seen with indomethacin.[88]

In terms of prevention of NSAID gastropathy, antacids and enteric coating of the NSAIDs have had limited success: one study found that the use of Maalox instead of placebo in combination with naproxen actually resulted in an increased incidence of gastric lesions.[89] Cimetidine and ranitidine are effective in treating gastric ulcers caused by NSAID use, but most data indicate they are not effective in preventing such ulcers, although some studies claim otherwise.[90–93]

Another drug used to prevent NSAID gastropathy is sucralfate. Sucralfate is a basic aluminum salt of sucrose octasulfate that aids in the healing of gastric and duodenal ulcers by several mechanisms: (1) forming a complex with proteins at an ulcer base thereby protecting it from further erosion, (2) stimulating prostaglandin synthesis in gastric mucosa, and (3) promoting gastric mucus secretion by a prostaglandin-independent mechanism. Its major advantage is a low side-effect profile, but it has not been demonstrated to be very effective in preventing

NSAID gastropathy.[94] However, a study of a gel formulation of sucralfate showed promise in reducing both side effects and significantly reducing the incidence of gastroduodenal ulcers.[95]

A more successful drug available in preventing NSAID gastropathy is misoprostol. It is a synthetic analogue of prostaglandin E_1. In a study comparing it to placebo and sucralfate, misoprostol 200 μg taken qid resulted in far fewer gastric lesions in patients taking NSAIDs.[94] However, diarrhea can occur in up to 50% of patients using 200 μg qid, and in 25% of patients using 100 μg qid. It is also relatively expensive, so it is probably best to restrict use of the drug to those patients at increased risk of NSAID gastropathy who require NSAID use. The recent introduction of a combination product of diclofenac and misoprostol may make its use convenient and cost-effective enough to allow more common usage.

More recent literature proposes that the H^+/K^+ ATPase inhibitors that reduce acid secretion (e.g., omeprazole) may also be effective in preventing NSAID gastropathy.[96] Data suggest that a combination of such inhibitors plus an NSAID reduces the risk of gastric toxicity to the same degree as use of a COX-2-selective inhibitor alone.[97]

Other concepts in GI protection while using NSAIDs have been explored. Because of their weak peripheral anti-inflammatory effect (while still preserving a central analgesic benefit), some have proposed that the R enantiomers of NSAIDs may be effective analgesics with fewer side effects. However, studies of the R enantiomers of flurbiprofen, etodolac, ketoprofen, and ibuprofen reveal that all have some GI effects. Furthermore, after systemic administration, conversion of the R form to the S form can occur, so the selective benefits might be limited.[7] Another concept involves the role of nitric oxide, which is a critical mediator of GI mucosal defense. Promising results showed fewer gastric lesions with NSAIDs that had NO-releasing moieties associated while maintaining or enhancing analgesic effect.[7]

Renal Toxicity: Renal impairment has been reported to occur in as many as 18% of patients using ibuprofen, whereas acute renal failure has been shown to occur in about 6% of patients using NSAIDs in another study.[98,99] Forms of renal impairment with NSAIDs include a reduction in renal perfusion due to inhibition of prostaglandin formation, acute interstitial nephritis, and nephrotic syndrome.

Prostaglandin regulation of renal blood flow is clinically significant in patients with heart failure, renal insufficiency, or liver disease, but not in normal patients.[100] Hence, reduced renal blood flow with subsequent medullary ischemia may result from NSAID use in susceptible individuals.[101] PGE_2 and PGI_2 can act as direct vasodilators or can attenuate the vasoconstrictive effects of angiotensin II, renal sympathetic nerve activity, or catecholamines, thus providing increased renal blood flow in the presence of those countering stimuli.[102] Prostaglandins are synthesized in various parts of the nephron in both the cortical and medullary regions.[103] PGI_2 is found in large amounts in the cortex while PGE_2 is found in significant amounts in the tubules and medullary interstitial cells. Since prostaglandins are synthesized as needed and have no distant effects outside the kidney, they appear to function as autocoids.[104] Not all prostanoids are vasodilators: PGH_2 and TXA_2 are both potent renal vasoconstrictors.[105] Hence, the renal response to an NSAID may be contingent on the relative amounts of PGE_2, PGI_2, PGH_2, and TXA_2 present.

The subcategory of patients who may have renal impairment in response to NSAID use are considered to be in a renal prostaglandin-dependent state (RPDS). These patients have elevated renal sympathetic nerve and/or angiotensin II activity. Animal studies demonstrating RPDS include those with volume depletion, low cardiac output, hepatic cirrhosis, renal ischemia, aminoglycoside toxicity, unilateral or subtotal nephrectomy, hypertension, and diabetes.[102] Animal data must be interpreted carefully, though. Based on human data, the renal response to NSAIDs is no different in people following nephrectomy compared to those with two intact kidneys.[106]

The resulting decline in glomerular filtration rate from NSAID use in susceptible individuals can lead to increased water and electrolyte reabsorption in the proximal tubule.[107] This in turn can antagonize antihypertensive therapies and even exacerbate congestive heart failure.[101,108] NSAIDs vary markedly in their effect on blood pressure, although one review cited naproxen and indomethacin as producing significant rises in blood pressure while another study demonstrated that naproxen in fact has a minimal effect on antihypertensive drug therapy.[109,110] It should be noted that most studies do not show a significant effect of NSAIDs on blood pressure in normal individuals, and even the effect in hypertensive patients is only mild. Such mild effects can, however, raise patients' blood pressures into the clinically high range.[111]

Salsalate and other nonacetylated salicylates have been touted as being less nephrotoxic, but this may purely be the result of their relatively weak inhibition of COX compared to other NSAIDs; when given in amounts sufficient to inhibit PG formation significantly, reductions in GFR are not much different from other NSAIDs.[102] Sulindac has theoretical advantages in the patient at risk for NSAID renal toxicity: it does not block PGE_2 or prostacyclin in the kidney due to local inactivation of the active metabolite in the kidney and liver, and thus should not impair renal blood flow.[112,113] On the other hand, some question the renal safety profile of sulindac, noting that accumulation of the active metabolite could occur over time in the patient with impaired renal function, thereby negating the renal sparing effect.[102] It should be noted that even the most efficient NSAIDs can only inhibit 60% to 80% of renal PG synthesis, so a large amount of prostaglandins can remain functional during NSAID use and a decline in renal function may not always be the result of PG formation inhibition.[102]

Acute renal injury from NSAID use has been reported. For example, it is possible in acute overdose of ibuprofen to induce acute renal failure with tubular necrosis.[114] Allergic nephritis to NSAIDs can occur within 2 to 13 days of use and is accompanied by fever, skin eruptions, and serum IgE elevations. Tubulointerstitial nephritis with proteinuria can then occur, and treatment consists of steroids and dialysis. However, not all cases will recover, and since all NSAIDs are protein bound, they are not easily dialyzed.[115] However, considering the enormous number of users of NSAIDs, the incidence of NSAID-induced acute interstitial nephritis is extremely low.[116]

Minimal change nephrotic syndrome has also been reported in about 10% to 12% of patients on NSAIDs. Many NSAIDs may be involved with this syndrome, and discontinuing the drug typically results in complete remission in a few weeks. The drug may be taken for months before the proteinuria is detected. Progression to renal failure has been reported but is extremely rare.[116]

At present there is no evidence that the COX-2-selective inhibitors confer any additional safety benefit in terms of renal toxicity. The same caution when using nonselective agents should be applied when using the COX-2-selective drugs. It is known that COX-2 is constitutively expressed in the kidneys and probably plays a role in both renal blood flow as well as in sodium and water balance.[117]

Hematologic Toxicity: As noted above, arachidonic acid is converted into prostaglandin endoperoxides PGG_2 and PGH_2 by the action of COX. These are in turn converted to thromboxane A_2 (TXA_2) in platelets from the action of thromboxane synthase, but in vascular endothelium they are converted to prostacyclin (PGI_2) by the action of prostacyclin synthase. Thromboxane A_2 functions as a platelet activator and vasoconstrictor, whereas prostacyclin is a platelet inhibitor and vasodilator. Furthermore, activated platelets divert some of their endoperoxides to vascular cells ("endoperoxide steal") to further provide substrate for PGI_2 formation.[118] Platelet activity is therefore the result of a constant balance between the effects of PGI_2 in the endothelium and TXA_2 in the platelets. By inhibiting the formation of TXA_2, NSAIDs inhibit platelet activation. Aspirin covalently acetylates COX causing irreversible inhibition, which is significant in the case of platelets since without a nucleus they are unable to form additional COX. It therefore takes 7 to 10 days for platelets to recover from the effect of aspirin by the formation of new platelets.[118] However, vascular endothelium is capable of creating more COX, so the effect of aspirin on platelet function can be profound.[119] Clinically, however, bleeding times tend to normalize sooner than expected after aspirin use because of the release of large numbers of uninhibited platelets from bone marrow in response to the induced coagulopathy.[118]

It should be noted that while in vitro studies of platelet function changes to NSAIDs have provided much information, it is ultimately the clinical effect in patients that is of greatest interest. The clinical test primarily used to assess clinical platelet function is the bleeding time, but this test is highly operator dependent and is subject to much technical artifact.[118] In addition, its usefulness in preoperative screening of platelet function to predict intraoperative bleeding has been put in serious doubt, and there is question as to whether bleeding assessed on the forearm relates to bleeding in other areas of the body.[120–122]

Nonaspirin NSAIDs, unlike aspirin, induce a reversible platelet inhibition that resolves when the drug is mostly eliminated.[123] A single dose of 300 to 900 mg of ibuprofen can block platelet aggregation 2 hours after administration, but the effect is largely gone by 24 hours.[124] Sulindac also can produce changes in platelet aggregation that are gone by 24 hours, and similar findings have been seen with diclofenac.[118] Platelet effects of long-acting NSAIDs such as piroxicam, though, can last for several days after the drug is discontinued.[125] Overall, nonaspirin NSAIDs cause "transient, dose-dependent, and modest bleeding time abnormalities," which often do not exceed normal limits.[118]

Studies have shown variable clinical effects of the NSAIDs on bleeding. In one study of patients undergoing total hip replacement surgery 140 patients had more intraoperative and postoperative blood loss when using NSAIDs than those who did not.[126] Other studies have confirmed that finding and noted more complications in patients using NSAIDs with half-lives longer than 6 hours.[127] On the other hand, no difference was found in clinical blood loss during total hip replacement or transurethral resection of the prostate in patients on diclofenac compared to those on placebo preoperatively in other studies.[128,129]

Most NSAIDs potentiate the anticoagulant activity of warfarin either by displacing the protein-bound drug or by inhibiting metabolism by hepatic microsomal enzymes.[118] For this reason they should be used with caution in patients on oral anticoagulants, especially in the elderly who been shown to have a significant increase in bleeding and hospitalizations when the two are used in combination.[130]

Almost by definition, COX-2-selective inhibitors have no effect on platelet function even in supratherapeutic doses. This is due to the lack of COX-2 in the platelets. Numerous studies examining bleeding time as well as more sensitive assays fail to demonstrate any changes in platelet aggregation or bleeding time even with several days of usage at high doses with these medications.[131–133] This gives these selective agents a particular advantage in their usage perioperatively, since increased bleeding from their use is not an issue (see below).

Hepatic Toxicity: Hepatic-related side effects of NSAIDs have been reported to occur in 3% of patients receiving the drugs.[134,135] The prevalence of minor increases in hepatic enzymes during NSAID use has been cited as 1% to 15%, and is considered by many to be a "class effect" of NSAIDs.[136] The mechanism by which almost all NSAIDs produce hepatoxicity seems to be immunologic or metabolic, with dose related toxicity being seen in aspirin and acetaminophen (paracetamol). Most NSAIDs produce hepatocellular injury with only a few causing cholestatic or mixed injury.[136]

Regarding specific NSAIDs, sulindac has been implicated as having a higher risk compared to most other NSAIDs of producing hepatic damage, although the injury was usually found to be mild and reversible.[136] Reports associating the use of diclofenac with fulminant hepatitis have appeared in both US and European literature, although it is not clear whether the incidence of diclofenac induced hepatitis is higher than for other NSAIDs.[137,138] More recently (1998), bromfenac was removed from the US market following the appearance of several cases of lethal or near-lethal hepatic damage. In almost all cases patients took the medication for longer than the recommended 10-day maximum, but it was believed that further efforts to limit its use would not be effective. The mechanisms of such hepatotoxicity are not clear, but it seems advisable to follow liver function tests in patients on long-term NSAID therapy.[139]

Effects on Bone Healing: Both COX-1 and COX-2 have been shown to play a role in bone healing following fracture.[140] It would therefore seem that NSAIDs inhibit bone healing. In fact, this feature had been previously utilized to limit heterotopic bone formation following orthopedic procedures.[141] On the other hand, numerous case series over the years failed to show any impact of NSAID use on fracture healing.[142–145] One study from the UK did show an association between nonunion of femur fractures and NSAIDs, but it was not possible to determine whether the NSAIDs contributed to the nonunions or whether the nonunions merely required the use of NSAIDs to control pain.[146]

Retrospective reviews of failed lumbar fusions in patients show a strong association with perioperative ketorolac usage, and animal studies following this confirmed that NSAIDs could reduce the rate of successful fusion.[147] This effect on bone healing appears to depend at least in part on duration of dosing, as fewer doses seemed to cause less effect on fusion rates.[148] This observation has triggered significant concern regarding the impact of NSAIDs perioperatively in any procedure involving bone healing.

Much of the current data comes from animal models of fracture healing. Results from these studies sometimes conflict, but some tend to indicate that nonselective NSAIDs have a greater effect on inhibiting bone healing than do the COX-2-selective inhibitors, although even the COX-2-selective inhibitors have an effect.[149] Overall, it would appear that for lumbar fusion it might be best to minimize NSAID and perhaps even COX-2-selective inhibitor usage, but whether the effect has clinical significance for other orthopedic procedures or fracture healing is unclear. The use of these drugs for decades in treating the pain following fracture without negative effect tends to support their continued but careful use in that area, although some suggest this apparent lack of effect is because the delay in healing is only transient and hence has not been observed (and therefore probably not meaningful anyway).[150] Also of interest is that there is repeated evidence in the orthodontic literature that NSAIDs have no impact on bone healing, although this could be due to a relative lack of mechanical loading and stress in this model.[151–153]

Asthma: Although not a toxicity per se, there is a subpopulation of patients who demonstrate severe bronchospasm in response to taking nonselective NSAIDs. This condition, termed aspirin-induced asthma (AIA), is present in about 10% of asthmatics. Typically these patients suffer from more severe asthma and all already steroid dependent. The reaction is not a true allergy: skin testing is negative and the only way to document its presence is by exposure to a nonselective NSAID.[154]

The mechanism appears to be from the diversion of arachidonic acid breakdown from the COX pathway to the lipooxygenase pathway. Patients with AIA may have increased levels of leukotriene C4 synthase in the bronchial walls. When a nonselective NSAID is given, more arachidonic acid is available to be broken down by lipooxygenase, and therefore more substrate is available to the overproduced C4 synthase. In turn this produces leukotriene C4 and other leukotrienes that then trigger bronchospasm.[155]

The COX-2-selective inhibitors in theory should not trigger this reaction since the arachidonic acid can still be broken down through the remaining COX-1 pathway thereby avoiding the complete diversion to the lipooxygenase system. Studies on limited numbers of patients have confirmed that in patients with known AIA who develop bronchospasm to aspirin there is no bronchospasm in response to either rofecoxib or celecoxib.[156,157]

SPECIFIC DRUGS

It should be noted that while traditionally the NSAIDs have been classified by chemical structure, such classification does not reflect the clinical effect or side-effect profile of these agents. For that reason, classification schemes by elimination half-life or by COX inhibition selectivity (COX-1 vs. COX-2) have been proposed. However, since even these methods have not been widely recognized as clinically useful, the traditional scheme has been used here (Table 16-4).

Salicylates

ASPIRIN: The best-studied and most commonly used NSAID, aspirin has an elimination half-life that changes from 2.5 hours at low doses to 19 hours at high doses. It is well absorbed by the stomach and small intestine with peak blood levels 1 hour after an oral dose. There is then rapid conversion of aspirin to salicylates from a high first-pass effect that occurs in both the wall of the small intestine and the liver. Of all the NSAIDs, aspirin has been associated with the unique but dangerous condition, Reye's syndrome. This combination of seizures, coma, and sometimes death has been associated with the use of aspirin during a viral illness in children.[158]

DIFLUNISAL: Possibly better tolerated in the GI system due to the fact that it is not metabolized to salicylic acid in plasma. It has a short half-life relative to aspirin.

CHOLINE MAGNESIUM TRISALICYLATE (CMT) AND SALSALATE: Both are nonacetylated salicylates that have minimal effect on platelet function and less effect on GI mucosa than their acetylated counterparts. They produce similar analgesia and blood levels of salicylate to those of the acetylated class. However, both are recognized as weak analgesics for acute pain as evidenced by the lack of published studies for their use in that area.

Acetaminophen: This is a *para*-aminophenol derivative with analgesic and antipyretic properties similar to those of aspirin. Antipyresis is likely from direct action on the hypothalamic heat-regulating centers via inhibiting action of endogenous pyrogen. Although equipotent to aspirin in inhibiting central prostaglandin synthesis, acetaminophen has no significant peripheral prostaglandin synthetase inhibition. Doses of 650 mg have been shown to be more effective than doses of 300 mg, but little additional benefit is seen at doses above 650 mg indicating a possible ceiling effect. It has few side effects in the usual dosage range: there is neither significant GI toxicity nor platelet functional changes that occur with acetaminophen use. It is almost entirely metabolized in the liver, and the minor metabolites are responsible for the hepatotoxicity seen in overdose. Inducers of the P-450 enzyme system in the liver (such as alcohol) increase the formation of metabolites and hence increase hepatotoxicity.

Acetic Acid Derivatives: This group of NSAIDs contains two subclasses: pyrroleacetic acids and phenylacetic acids (of which only diclofenac is approved for use in the USA so far).

INDOMETHACIN: This has good oral and rectal absorption, although the extent of absorption varies widely between patients. There is also a large interpatient variability in elimination half-life, due to extensive enterohepatic recirculation of the drug. Its clinical use is somewhat limited by a relatively high incidence of side effects.

SULINDAC: This was approved for use in the USA in 1978 after several years of use in Europe; it was the result of a search for a drug similar to indomethacin but with less toxicity. The lower GI toxicity with sulindac may be the result of the fact that sulindac is an inactive pro-drug which is converted after absorption by liver microsomal enzymes to sulindac

TABLE 16-4. **CLASSIFICATION OF NSAIDs BY CHEMICAL STRUCTURE**

Class	Generic Name	Example Brand Name (USA)
Propionic acids	Naproxen Flurbiprofen Oxaprozin Ibuprofen Ketoprofen Ketorolac	Naprosyn, Anaprox, Alleve Ansaid Daypro Motrin Orudis, Oruvail Toradol
Indoleacetic acids	Sulindac Indomethacin Etodolac	Clinoril Indocin Lodine
Phenylacetic acids	Diclofenac Bromfenac	Cataflam, Voltaren Duract
Salicylic acids	Salsalate Diflunisal Choline magnesium trisalicylate (CMT)	Disalcid, Monogesic, Salflex Dolobid Trilisate
Napthylalkanone	Nabumetone	Relafen
Oxicam	Piroxicam Meloxicam	Feldene Mobic
Anthranilic acid	Mefenamic acid Meclofenamate	Ponstel
Pyrroleacetic acid	Tolmetin	Tolectin
Pyrazolone	Phenylbutazone	
COX-2 selective	Celecoxib Rofecoxib Valdecoxib Etoricoxib Parecoxib Lumericoxib	Celebrex Vioxx Bextra Arcoxia (ex-USA) Dynastat (ex-USA) Prexige (in development)

disulfide, which appears to be the active metabolite. However, one study demonstrated a relatively high rate of GI hemorrhage with sulindac.[159] As mentioned previously, sulindac was considered in previous studies to be the least nephrotoxic of the NSAIDs, but more recent studies have failed to support that contention.[160,161]

TOLMETIN AND ETODOLAC: Both claim fewer side effects than other NSAIDs. Etodolac was approved for use in the USA in 1993. It demonstrates notable COX-2 selectivity.

KETOROLAC: This is currently the only parenteral NSAID for clinical analgesic use in the USA. Although indomethacin has been available as an injectable form for years, it was pursued only in low dose as a treatment for patent ductus arteriosus.

Ketorolac demonstrates analgesia well beyond its anti-inflammatory properties (its anti-inflammatory properties are between that of indomethacin and naproxen; the analgesia is 50 times that of naproxen). It has antipyretic effects 20 times that of aspirin, and thus can mask temperatures when given routinely to patients postoperatively. Several studies have demonstrated efficacy comparable or exceeding that of morphine for moderate postoperative pain treatment but with fewer side effects.[162,163] It has also been shown to be a potential alternative to fentanyl for intraoperative use.[164] Although ketorolac prolongs bleeding time, it does not do so excessively, although case reports of postoperative bleeding associated with intraoperative ketorolac use have been reported.[165,166] Oral ketorolac was approved for use in the USA approximately three years after the parenteral form and has an efficacy similar to that of naproxen and ibuprofen.[167] However, while the parenteral form is given in a loading dose of 60 mg followed by 30 mg IM every 6 hours, the oral dose is limited to 10 to 20 mg due to GI toxicity, and it is recommended that the duration of therapy also be very limited.

DICLOFENAC: This differs from the other NSAIDs by having a high first-pass effect, and hence a lower oral bioavailability. As mentioned previously, it may also have a significantly higher incidence of hepatotoxicity than the other NSAIDs. A parenteral form has been used in Europe, with one study showing it effective in reducing opioid requirements and reducing pain after thoracotomies.[168]

Propionic Acid Derivatives: This class contains ibuprofen, fenoprofen, ketoprofen, flurbiprofen, and naproxen. A newer drug in this class is oxaprozin, which stands out for its once-daily dosing but has no other distinct advantage over other NSAIDs.[169]

Oxicam Derivatives: The only two NSAIDs in this class in clinical use are piroxicam and meloxicam. Unlike other NSAIDs, piroxicam has a slow time to peak serum concentrations following oral dosing: 5.5 hours. It is also notable for its long elimination half life of 48.5 hours, so it may take up to a week to achieve steady-state blood concentrations, although it does also allow once-daily dosing. As noted above, some consider the long half-life to be a major factor in piroxicam's significant GI toxicity profile.

It should be noted that some publications incorrectly identify meloxicam as a COX-2-selective inhibitor. When tested in clinical trials, its selectivity to inhibit COX-2 vs. COX-1 was only around 10-fold. Further, there was inhibition of platelet thromboxane production after oral treatment at both 7.5 mg/day and 15 mg/day. Further, although some data suggest less GI toxicity with meloxicam at 7.5 mg/day, doses at 15 mg/day have been shown in endoscopic studies to be similar in GI effect to piroxicam. These data suggest that there is a dose dependency to meloxicam's tendency to inhibit COX-2, and that doses used in acute pain appear to render the drug nonselective.[170]

Pyrazolone Derivatives: The only one in clinical use in this class is phenylbutazone. Although a very effective anti-inflammatory and analgesic, it has been associated with aplastic anemias and agranulocytosis and hence its long-term use is not recommended. It is thus not often clinically used.

Anthranilic Acid Derivatives: These NSAIDs are unique in that they not only block prostaglandin synthesis but also the tissue response to prostaglandins. Mefenamic acid has been associated with severe pancytopenia and many other side effects. Hence, therapy is not to be for more than one week.[171] Meclofenamate has a high incidence of GI toxicity and hence is also not a first-line drug.

Naphthylalkanones: This class of NSAID is most noted for relative COX-2 selectivity and for being of a "nonacidic" chemical structure unlike other clinically used NSAIDs, although some describe its structure as similar to that of naproxen. This nonacidic form supposedly minimizes topical injury to the gastric mucosa.[83] The only clinically available

NSAID in this class is nabumetone. Nabumetone is a pro-drug, with only 35% of the drug converted to its active form (6-methoxy-2-naphthyl acetic acid, 6-MNA) after oral administration and none of the parent drug being measurable in plasma after oral administration because of the rapid biotransformation.[172]

The relative COX-2 selectivity of nabumetone has been assumed to mean that the side effects related to COX-1 inhibition will be much less with this agent. Some studies have shown its use to result in fewer gastric lesions than aspirin, naproxen, or ibuprofen, but direct comparisons to other NSAIDs cannot be assumed from this limited information. One study in female volunteers using nabumetone for 7 days in a crossover study found three subjects during its use to have developed a bleeding time of over 15 minutes; an absolute lack of significant effect on COX-1-related systems cannot therefore be assumed.[173]

HIGHLY SELECTIVE COX-2 INHIBITORS

The introduction of the highly selective COX-2 inhibitors such as celecoxib, rofecoxib, valdecoxib, etoricoxib, and lumericoxib reflects a new direction in NSAID technology. By definition, these products do not inhibit COX-1 in supratherapeutic concentrations, and their primary advantages are in reduced GI morbidity and complete lack of effect on platelet function. Effects on bone healing may be less, but renal effects should be assumed to be the same as nonselective NSAIDs, with the possible exception of rofecoxib (see below).

All products are analgesic, anti-inflammatory, and antipyretic. Rofecoxib has a bioavailability of about 0.93, but because of low water solubility bioavailability studies of celecoxib are not available. The effective half-lives of rofecoxib and celecoxib are about 11 and 17 hours, respectively. It should be noted that there is no evidence that either drug is less prone to renal toxicity than other NSAIDs. The most recently approved of this class in the USA was valdecoxib, with a bioavailability of 0.83 and an elimination half-life of 8.11 hours.[13] However, because of valdecoxib's higher affinity to the COX-2 enzyme, only once-daily dosing is possible. As with the NSAIDs, there is a dose response to these agents, with lower doses used for chronic pain and higher doses for acute pain. It should also be noted that both celecoxib and valdecoxib are contraindicated in patients with known sulfa allergy.

Currently, only one selective COX-2 inhibitor is available for parenteral use, parecoxib. Approved in Europe and Central/South America, it is a pro-drug that once given parenterally is converted in the liver to valdecoxib. Current data suggest an efficacy similar to ketorolac but without the platelet effect and with greatly reduced GI toxicity.

Evidence suggests that rofecoxib possesses a unique cardiovascular and renal toxicity profile compared to the other selective agents. An increased incidence of nonfatal myocardial infarction was noted in a large multicenter trial (VIGOR) relative to naprosyn, along with an increased incidence of hypertension and peripheral edema at high doses (50 mg/day). While no single study demonstrated statistical significance, at least two more studies (unpublished, but cited on the FDA website www.fda.gov) showed that even lower doses (12.5 to 25 mg/day) might be associated with higher rates of MI relative to nabumetone and naprosyn.[174] Epidemiologic data are conflicting: while a large Medicaid database review revealed that only the higher dose was associated with cardiac events,[175] another epidemiologic review indicated all doses were associated with increased risks of acute MI.[176] The significance and mechanism of this finding are unclear, as similar findings have not yet been found with other COX-2-selective drugs in clinically used dosages. One proposed mechanism was an increase in coagulability: since only COX-2 is inhibited, this means that prostacyclin in endothelium may be inhibited (allowing enhanced platelet adherence) while platelets' ability to aggregate is unaffected. The net effect would be slight tendency toward a hypercoagulable state. However, no evidence of this phenomenon has been shown (e.g., through increased deep venous thrombosis or through measured tests of coagulation) and the lack of MI issues in other COX-2-selective inhibitors raises doubts about this explanation.[177]

COMBINATION DRUGS

In an effort to enhance the efficacy and safety of NSAID analgesia, other drugs have been formulated in combination with NSAIDs. Formulations of ibuprofen containing hydrocodone are available, and more recently diclofenac has also been formulated in a combination with misoprostol. Caffeine, long sold in combination with acetaminophen and aspirin in over-the-counter analgesia preparations, has also been studied in combination with ibuprofen.[178,179] The effect of the added analgesia from the caffeine is measurable but not substantial. The enhanced NSAID analgesia seen in combination with caffeine is likely not the result of alterations in absorption or distribution of the NSAID.[180]

ROLE IN ACUTE PAIN MANAGEMENT

The value of NSAIDs in acute pain management is unquestioned, and has been reviewed extensively in the literature for a wide range of acute injuries as well as for the pain following a variety of surgical procedures.[181] NSAIDs play a key role in multimodal analgesia, often providing critical synergy to opioid analgesia. Opioids, notorious in producing side effects (e.g., sedation) despite insufficient analgesia,[182] can be reduced in their postoperative requirements by about 20% to 40% if NSAIDs are used.[183] While the reduction in opioid usage sometimes is enough to reduce the severity of side effects,[184] this is not consistently demonstrated. However, the quality of analgesia is often improved with the addition of NSAIDs regardless of the lack of impact on opioid side effects.[185–187]

Three areas are important to consider when utilizing NSAIDs for perioperative pain: dosing, timing, and toxicity. As mentioned earlier, while the NSAIDs demonstrate a ceiling effect in terms of analgesic efficacy, there remains a dose–response relationship up to that ceiling.[188] For chronic use it is generally recommended to use the lowest effective dose of an NSAID to achieve analgesia, but when attempting to decrease postoperative opioid use and prevent severe pain it is probably best (at least initially) to utilize the maximum dose that is clinically safe for a given patient. Even intravenous NSAIDs, such as ketorolac or parecoxib, require at least 10 to 20 minutes for onset of analgesia,[189] and if the dose used were insufficient another 10 to 20 minutes would be required for the "top-up" dose to become effective. Since sedation, nausea, and respiratory depression are not a concern with NSAIDs, it seems best to make the initial dose maximal when possible.

Timing is another important aspect of NSAID dosing. While the topic of preemptive analgesia remains controversial, most data seem to support that in the clinical setting it does not matter whether analgesia is given before or after surgical insult.[190] However, there is little question that analgesia given before the patient experiences pain will produce greater satisfaction than allowing the patient to experience pain before administering analgesics. Patients' recall of pain depends in large part on the most severe pain experienced rather than the average pain.[191] NSAIDs are optimally suited for this situation, since the lack of sedation and respiratory depression allows their administration in a maximal dose before or during an anesthetic, allowing the patient to emerge with less pain. High-dose opioids can delay emergence and so are often limited near the end of surgery. NSAIDs could also be administered to maximum benefit any time before a regional anesthetic or local anesthetic wears off, again keeping the pain controlled before it becomes severe.[192]

Unfortunately, toxicity issues particularly relevant to the postsurgical patient often limit their use. NSAIDs given prior to or during surgery or even immediately postoperatively are often not desired by the surgeon due to the effect on platelets and bleeding. This problem can be circumvented, however, by use of the COX-2-selective inhibitors since they are totally devoid of platelet inhibitory effects. Studies confirm efficacy at least as good as that offered by nonselective NSAIDs, whether given orally preoperatively, postoperatively, or any time intravenously.[189,193,194] The analgesic effects of the COX-2 inhibitors have been demonstrated following bunionectomy,[195] oral surgery,[196] total joint operations,[197,198] spinal,[199] gynecologic,[200] and abdominal surgery.[201]

Another area of concern is renal toxicity, which may pose a greater risk in patients undergoing surgery; the reduced renal blood flow from anesthesia and blood loss combined with exposure to other renal toxic agents (aminoglycoside antibiotics, intravenous radiographic dyes, etc.) all can increase the risk of NSAID renal toxicity. Patients with compromised renal function or with one kidney might not be considered candidates for NSAIDs, even if COX-2 selective. Ketorolac was banned in many European countries as a result of several cases of postoperative renal failure associated with its use.

Other issues, such as bone healing effects of the NSAIDs, must also be considered. However, one should be aware that there are data suggesting that COX-2-selective inhibitors might even help tendon healing, so not all aspects of these drugs in orthopedic surgery are detrimental.[202]

FUTURE TRENDS

NSAIDs continue to offer analgesia that can either supplement or sometimes surpass that offered by opioids. However, the existence of serious side effects involving hematologic, GI, renal, and hepatic systems should be mentioned to patients placed on these medications. Concerns with bone healing may also be an issue in orthopedic patients receiving these medications for prolonged periods postoperatively. Such risks must also be weighed carefully against the benefits of these agents particularly when long-term use is anticipated.

It is hoped that with improved understanding of the role of prostaglandins in nociception and normal human physiology that drugs manipulating them can be developed which are safer and more effective than those currently available.

NSAIDs may be able to be developed that have effects isolated to the CNS, producing analgesic benefits with complete lack of the peripheral toxic effects. Development of nitric oxide NSAIDs may also significantly reduce some peripheral toxicity of the NSAIDs.[203] With the discovery of COX-3, there may be reason to identify even more isoenzymes that may provide even greater selectivity of NSAIDs in focusing only on those systems involved in pain and analgesia.

KEY POINTS

- NSAIDs are antihyperalgesic compounds related by their ability to decrease prostaglandin formation through inhibition of COX following tissue injury. Their mechanism of action for analgesia is largely based on actions in the CNS, although peripheral mechanisms likely are synergistic. The analgesic (antihyperalgesic) benefits are not necessarily related to their anti-inflammatory capabilities.
- There are two major isoforms of COX. COX-1 is largely constitutive and is responsible for the production of prostaglandins involved in protecting the GI tract and facilitating platelet aggregation. COX-2 is an inducible form created in the presence of inflammation, and is largely responsible for the production of prostaglandins involved in pain and inflammation. The COX-2-selective inhibitors, by virtue of leaving COX-1 alone, are capable of producing the same antihyperalgesic effect of the nonselective NSAIDs but without affecting platelet function and with a decreased morbidity on the GI tract.
- Nonselective NSAID toxicity is seen in reduced platelet aggregation (bleeding) and NSAID gastropathy with gastroduodenal ulcers. However, additional toxicity that is seen with both selective COX-2 inhibitors as well as NSAIDs occurs with reduced bone healing, reduced renal function (in low perfusion states), and rare hepatic toxicity. Aspirin-induced asthma, however, does not seem to be triggered by COX-2-selective inhibitors.
- The NSAIDs are extremely effective in enhancing opioid analgesia postoperatively, consistently reducing opioid requirements while providing better pain control. COX-2-selective inhibitors provide the additional advantage in the surgical setting of not affecting platelet function, and so will not affect bleeding if given pre- or intraoperatively.

REFERENCES

1. Clive D, Stoff J: Renal syndromes associated with nonsteroidal anti-inflammatory drugs. N Engl J Med 310:563–572, 1984.
2. Anti-arthritic medication usage: United States, 1991. Stat Bull Metropol Insur Co 73:25–34, 1992.
3. Garner A: Adaptation in the pharmaceutical industry, with particular reference to gastrointestinal drugs and diseases. Scand J Gastroenterol 27(Suppl 193):83–89, 1992.
4. Larkai E, Smith J, Lidsky M et al: Gastroduodenal mucosa and dyspeptic symptoms in arthritic patients during chronic nonsteroidal anti-inflammatory drug use. Am J Gastroenterol 82:1153–1158, 1987.
5. Singh G: Gastrointestinal complications of prescription and over-the-counter nonsteroidal anti-inflammatory drugs: A view from the ARAMIS database. Arthritis, Rheumatism, and Aging Medical Information System. Am J Therapeutics 7:115–21, 2000.
6. Plotz P: Aspirin and salicylate. In Kelly W, Harris E, Ruddy S, Sledge C (eds): Textbook of Rheumatology. W.B. Saunders, Philadelphia, 1981, pp 740–767.
7. Wallace J: Nonsteroidal anti-inflammatory drugs and gastroenteropathy: The second hundred years. Gastroenterology 112:1000–1016, 1997.
8. Vane J: Inhibition of prostaglandin synthesis as a mechanism of action for aspirin-like drugs. Nature New Biol 231:232–235, 1971.
9. Flower R, Moncada S, Vane J: Analgesic-antipyretics and anti-inflammatory agents; drugs employed in the treatment of gout. In Gilman A, Goodman L, Rall T, et al (eds): The Pharmacological Basis of Therapeutics, ed 7. Macmillan, New York, 1985.
10. Björkman R: Central antinociceptive effects of nonsteroidal and antiinflammatory drugs and paracetamol. Experimental studies in the rat. Acta Anaesthes Scand 39(Suppl):9–44, 1995.
11. Parr G, Darekar B, Fletcher A, et al: Joint pain and quality of life: Results of a randomized trial. Br J Clin Pharmacol 27:235–242, 1989.
12. Eisenberg E, Berkey C, Carr D, et al: Efficacy and safety of nonsteroidal antiinflammatory drugs for cancer pain: A meta-analysis. J Clin Oncology 12:2756–2765, 1994.
13. Physicians' Desk Reference, ed 58. Thompson PDR, Montvale, NJ, 2004.
14. McCormack K, Brune K: Dissociation between the antinociceptive and anti-inflammatory effects of the nonsteroidal anti-inflammatory drugs. A survey of their analgesic efficacy. Drugs 41:533–547, 1991.
15. Svensson C, Yaksh T: The spinal phospholipase–cyclooxygenase–prostanoid cascade in nociceptive processing. Annu Rev Pharmacol Toxicol 42:553–583, 2002.
16. Ferreira S: Prostaglandins, aspirin-like drugs and analgesia. Nature 240:200–203, 1972.
17. Levine JD, Lau W, Kwiat G, Goetzl EJ. Leukotriene B4 produces hyperalgesia that is dependent upon polymorphonuclear leukocytes. Science 225:743, 1984.
18. McCormack K: The spinal actions of nonsteroidal anti-inflammatory drugs and the dissociation between their anti-inflammatory and analgesic effects. Drugs 47(Suppl): 28–45, 1994.
19. Byers MR, Bonica JJ. Peripheral pain mechanisms and nociceptor plasticity. In Loeser JD, Butler SH, Chapman CR, Turk DC (eds): Bonica's Management of Pain, ed 3. Lippincott Williams & Wilkins, Philadelphia, PA, 2001, pp 27–72.
20. Vasko M: Prostaglandin-induced neuropeptide release from spinal cord. Prog Brain Res (Neth) 104:367–380, 1995.
21. England S, Bevan S, Docherty R: PGE2 modulates the tetrodotoxin-resistant sodium current in neonatal rat dorsal root ganglion neurones via the cyclic AMP-protein kinase A cascade. J Physiol 495:429–440, 1996.
22. Ahmadi S, Lippross S, Neuhuber W, Zeilhofer H: PGE(2) selectively blocks inhibitory glycinergic neurotransmission onto rat superficial dorsal horn neurons. Nature Neurosci 5:34–40, 2002.
23. Vasko M: Prostaglandin-induced neuropeptide release from spinal cord. Prog Brain Res 104:367–380, 1995.
24. Samad TA, Moore KA, Sapirstein A, et al: Interleukin-1beta-mediated induction of Cox-2 in the CNS contributes to inflammatory pain hypersensitivity. Nature 410:471–475, 2001.
25. Brune K: Spinal cord effects of antipyretic analgesics. Drugs 47(Suppl 5):21–27, 1994.
26. DeWitt D, Meade E, Smith W: PGH synthase isoenzyme selectivity: The potential for safer nonsteroidal antiinflammatory drugs. Am J Med 95(Suppl 2A):40–43, 1993.
27. Simmons D, Xie W, Chipman J, et al: Multiple cyclooxygenases: Cloning a mitogen-inducible form. In Bailey JM (ed): Prostaglandins, Leukotrienes, Lipoxins, and PAF. Plenum Press, New York, 1991, pp 67–78.
28. Kujubu D, Reddy S, Fletcher B, Herschman H: Expression of the protein product of the prostaglandin synthase-2/TIS10 gene

in mitogen-stimulated Swiss 3T3 cells. J Biol Chem 268: 5425–30, 1993.

29. Crofford L: COX-1 and COX-2 tissue expression: Implications and predictions. J Rheumatol 24(S9):15–19, 1997.

30. Zhu X, Conklin D, Eisenach JC: Cyclooxygenase-1 in the spinal cord plays an important role in postoperative pain. Pain 104:15–23, 2003.

31. Botting R: Mechanism of action of acetaminophen: Is there a cyclooxygenase 3? Clin Infect Diseases 31:S202–210, 2000.

32. Simmons D: Variants of cyclooxygenase-1 and their roles in medicine. Thrombosis Res 110:265–268, 2003.

33. Bela K, Snipes J, Isse T, et al: Putative cyclooxygenase-3 expression in rat brain cells. J Cerebral Blood Flow Metab 23:1287–1292, 2003.

34. Ziel R, Krupp P: The significance of inhibition of prostaglandin synthesis in the selection of non-steroidal anti-inflammatory agents. Int J Clin Pharmacol Biopharm 12:186–191, 1975.

35. Abramson S: Therapy with and mechanisms of nonsteroidal anti-inflammatory drugs. Curr Opin Rheumatol 3:336–340, 1991.

36. Ferreira S: Prostaglandins: Peripheral and central analgesia. In Bonica JJ, Lindblom U, Iggo A (eds): Advances in Pain Research and Therapy, vol 5. Raven Press, New York, 1983.

37. Willer J, De Broucker T, Bussel B: Central analgesic effects of ketoprofen in humans: Electrophysiological evidence for a supraspinal mechanism in a double-blind and cross-over study. Pain 38:1–7, 1989.

38. Carlsson K, Monzel W, Jurna I: Depression by morphine and the non-opioid analgesic agents metamizol, lysine acetylate and paracetamol, of activity in rat thalamus neurons evoked by electrical stimulation of nociceptive afferents. Pain 32:313–326, 1988.

39. Taiwo Y, Levine J: Prostaglandins inhibit endogenous pain control mechanisms by blocking transmission at spinal noradrenergic synapses. J Neurosci 8:1346–1349, 1988.

40. Fabbri A, Cruccu G, Sperti P, et al: Piroxicam-induced analgesia: Evidence for a central component which is not opioid mediated. Experientia 48:1139–1142, 1992.

41. McCormack K, Brune K: Dissociation between the anti-nociceptive and anti-inflammatory effects of the nonsteroidal anti-inflammatory drugs: A survey of their analgesic efficacy. Drugs 41:533–547, 1991.

42. Malmberg A, Yaksh T: Hyperalgesia mediated by spinal gluta-mate or substance P receptor blocked by spinal cyclo-oxygenase inhibition. Science 257:1276–79, 1992.

43. Catania A, Arnold J, Macaluso A, et al: Inhibition of acute inflammation in the periphery by central action of salicylates. Proc Natl Acad Sci USA 88:8544–8547, 1991.

44. Taiwo Y, Levine J: Prostaglandins inhibit endogenous pain control mechanisms by blocking transmission at spinal noradrenergic synapses. J Neurosci 8:1346–1349, 1988.

45. Carlsson K, Jurna I: Central analgesic effect of paracetamol manifested by depression of nociceptive activity in thalamic neurons of the rat. Neurosci Lett 77:339–343, 1987.

46. Shyu K, Lin M: Hypothalamic monoaminergic mechanisms of aspirin-induced analgesia in monkeys. J Neural Transm 62: 285–293, 1985.

47. Carlsson K, Helmreich J, Jurna I: Activation of inhibition from the periaqueductal grey matter mediates central analgesic effect of metamizol (Dipyrone). Pain 27:373–390, 1986.

48. Vescovi P, Passeri M, Gerra G, Grossi E: Naloxone inhibits the early phase of diclofenac analgesia in man. Pain Clinic 19:151–155, 1987.

49. Bannwarth B, Netter P, Pourel J, et al: Clinical pharmacokinetics of nonsteroidal anti-inflammatory drugs in the cerebrospinal fluid. Biomed Pharmacother 43:121–126, 1989.

50. Netter P, Lapicque F, Banwarth B, et al: Diffusion in intra-muscular administered ketoprofen into the cerebrospinal fluid. Eur J Pharmacol 29:319–321, 1985.

51. Tegeder I, Niederberger E, Vetter G, et al: Effects of selective COX-1 and -2 inhibition on formalin-evoked nociceptive behaviour and prostaglandin E2 release in the spinal cord. J Neurochem 79:777–786, 2001.

52. Aronoff D, Neilson E: Antipyretics: Mechanisms of action and clinical use in fever suppression. Am J Med 111:304–315, 2001.

53. Day R, Graham G, Williams K, Brooks P: Variability in response to NSAIDs – Fact or fiction? Drugs 36:643–651, 1988.

54. Day R, Graham G, Williams K, et al: Clinical pharmacology of non-steroidal anti-inflammatory drugs. Pharmacol Ther 33:384–433, 1987.

55. Dukes M, Lunde I: The regulatory control of non-steroidal anti-inflammatory drug preparations within individual rheumatology private practices. J Rheumatol 16:1253–1258, 1989.

56. Kurumbail R, Stevens A, Gierse J, et al: Structural basis for selec-tive inhibition of cyclooxygenase-2 by anti-inflammatory agents. Nature V 384:644–648, 1996.

57. Fosslien E: Biochemistry of cyclooxygenase (COX)-2 inhibitors and molecular pathology of COX-2 in neoplasia. Crit Rev Clin Lab Sci 37:431–502, 2000.

58. Carabaza A, Cabré F, Rotllan E, et al: Stereoselective inhibition of inducible cyclooxygenase by chiral nonsteroidal antiinflamma-tory drugs. J Clin Pharmacol 36:505–512, 1996.

59. Geisslinger G, Schaible H: New insights into the site and mode of antinociception action of flurbiprofen enantiomers. J Clin Pharmacol 36:513–520, 1996.

60. Mauleon D, Artigas R, Garcia M, Carganico G: Preclinical and clinical development of dexketoprofen. Drugs 52(Suppl 5): 24–45, 1996.

61. Verbeeck R, Blackburn J, Lowewen G: Clinical pharmacokinetics of nonsteroidal anti-inflammatory drugs. Clin Pharmacokinet 8:297–331, 1983.

62. Denson D, Katz J: Nonsteroidal antiinflammatory agents. In Raj P (ed): Practical Management of Pain, ed 2. Mosby Year Book, St Louis, 1992, pp 606–619.

63. Adams S: Non-steroidal, anti-inflammatory drugs, plasma half-lives, and adverse reactions. Lancet 2:1204–1205, 1987.

64. Murray M, Brater D: Non-steroidal anti-inflammatory drugs. Clinics Geriat Med 6:365–397, 1990.

65. Levy G, Tsuchiya T: Salicylate accumulation kinetics in man. N Engl J Med 287:430–432, 1972.

66. Hayes A: Therapeutic implications of drug interactions with acetaminophen and aspirin. Arch Intern Med 141:301–304, 1981.

67. Brune K: Clinical relevance of nonsteroidal anti-inflammatory drug pharmacokinetics. Eur J Rheumatol Inflamm 8:18–23, 1987.

68. Bloom B: Direct medical costs of disease and gastrointestinal side effects during treatment for arthritis. Am J Med Suppl 2A:20–24, 1988.

69. Gabriel S, Fehring R: Trends in the utilization of non-steroidal anti-inflammatory drugs in the United States, 1986–1990. J Clin Epidemiol 45:1041–1044, 1992.

70. Katz J, Daltroy L, Brennan T, et al: Informed consent and the prescription of nonsteroidal antiinflammatory drugs. Arthritis Rheum 35:1257–1263, 1992.

71. Griffin M, Ray W, Schaffner W: Non-steroidal anti-inflamma-tory drug use and death from peptic ulcer in elderly persons. Ann Intern Med 109:359–363, 1988.

72. Nuki G: Pain control and the use of non-steroidal analgesic anti-inflammatory drugs. Br Med Bull 46:262–278, 1990.

73. Weinblatt M: Nonsteroidal anti-inflammatory drug toxicity: increased risk in the elderly. Scand J Rheumatol Suppl 91: 9–17, 1991.

74. Clark D, Ghose K: Neuropsychiatric reactions to nonsteroidal anti-inflammatory drugs. The New Zealand experience. Drug Safety 7:460–465, 1992.

75. Fries J, Williams C, Bloch D: The relative toxicity of nonsteroidal antiinflammatory drugs. Arthritis Rheum 34:1353–1360, 1991.

76. Smalley W, Griffin M: The risks and costs of upper gastrointestinal disease attributable to NSAIDs. Gastroenterol Clin North Am 25:373–396, 1996.

77. Morgan G, Poland M, DeLapp R: Efficacy and safety of nabumetone vs. diclofenac, naproxen, ibuprofen, and piroxicam in the elderly. Am J Med 95:19S–27S, 1993.

78. Fries J: NSAID gastropathy: The second most deadly rheumatic disease? Epidemiology and risk appraisal. J Rheumatol 18(Suppl 28):6–10, 1991.

79. Smalley W, Griffin M, Ray W: Costs for treatment of upper gastrointestinal disease attributable to nonsteroidal anti-inflammatory drug (NSAID) use in the elderly Medicaid recipients. Gastroenterology 104:A194, 1993.

80. Singh G: Recent considerations in nonsteroidal anti-inflammatory drug gastropathy. Am J Med 105:31S–38S, 1998.

81. Roth S: Non-steroidal anti-inflammatory drugs: Gastropathy, deaths and medical practice. Ann Intern Med 109:353–354, 1988.

82. Caruso I, Bianchi Porro G: Gastroscopic evaluation of anti-inflammatory agents. BMJ 1:75–78, 1980.

83. Scheiman J: NSAIDs, gastrointestinal injury, and cytoprotection. Gastroenterol Clin North Am 25:279–296, 1996.

84. Gabriel S, Jaakkimainen L, Bombardier C: Risk for serious gastrointestinal complications related to use of nonsteroidal anti-inflammatory drugs. A meta-analysis. Ann Intern Med 115:787–796, 1991.

85. Laine L: *Helicobacter pylori*, gastric ulcer, and agents noxious to the gastric mucosa. Gastroenterol Clin North Am 22:117–125, 1993.

86. Smale S, Tibble J, Sigthorsson G, Bjarnason I: Epidemiology and differential diagnosis of NSAID-induced injury to the mucosa of the small intestine. Best Practice Res Clin Gastroenterol 15:723–738, 2001.

87. Bjarnason I: Experimental evidence of the benefit of misoprostol beyond the stomach in humans. J Rheumatol Suppl 20:38–41, 1990.

88. Tibble JA, Sigthorsson G, Foster R, Bjarnason I: Comparison of the intestinal toxicity of celecoxib, a selective COX-2 inhibitor, and indomethacin in the experimental rat. Scand J Gastroenterol 35:802–807, 2000.

89. Sievert W, Stern A, Lambert J, Peacock T: Low dose antacids and nonsteroidal anti-inflammatory drug-induced gastropathy in humans. J Clin Gastroenterol 13(Suppl 1):S145–148, 1991.

90. Roth S, Bennett R, Mitchell C, et al: Cimetidine therapy in non-steroidal anti-inflammatory drug gastropathy. Arch Int Med 147:1799–1801, 1987.

91. Ehsanullah R, Page M, Tildesley G, et al: Prevention of gastroduodenal damage induced by non-steroidal anti-inflammatory drugs: Controlled trial of ranitidine. BMJ 297:1017–1021, 1988.

92. Rachmilewitz D: The role of H2-receptor antagonists in the prevention of NSAID-induced gastrointestinal damage. Aliment Pharmacol Ther 2:65–73, 1988.

93. Robinson M, Mills R, Euler A: Ranitidine prevents duodenal ulcers associated with non-steroidal anti-inflammatory drug therapy. Aliment Pharmacol Ther 5:143–150, 1991.

94. Agrawal N, Roth S, et al: Misoprostol compared with sucralfate in the prevention of nonsteroidal anti-inflammatory drug induced gastric ulcer. Ann Intern Med 115:195–200, 1991.

95. Miglioli M, Porro G, Vaira D, et al: Prevention with sucralfate gel of NSAID-induced gastroduodenal damage in arthritic patients. Am J Gastroenterol 91:2367–2371, 1996.

96. Agrawal N, Dajani E: Prevention and treatment of ulcers induced by nonsteroidal anti-inflammatory drugs. J Assoc Acad Minor Phys 3:142–148, 1992.

97. Chan F, Hung L, Bing S, et al: Celecoxib vs diclofenac and omeprazole in reducing the risk of recurrent ulcer bleeding in patients with arthritis. N Engl J Med 347(26):2104–2110.

98. Murray M, Brater D: Adverse effects of nonsteroidal drugs on renal function. Ann Intern Med 112:559–560, 1990.

99. Corwin H, Bonventre J: Renal insufficiency associated with nonsteroidal anti-inflammatory agents. Am J Kidney Dis 4:147–152, 1984.

100. Dunn M, Simonson M, Davidson E, et al: Non-steroidal anti-inflammatory drugs and renal function, J Clin Pharmacol 28:524–529, 1988.

101. Carmichael J, Shankel S: Renal effects of nonsteroidal anti-inflammatory drugs. Am J Med 78:992–1000, 1985.

102. Zambraski E: The effects of nonsteroidal anti-inflammatory drugs on renal function: Experimental studies in animals. Sem Nephrol 15:205–213, 1995.

103. Sraer J, Siess W, Moulonguet-Doleris L, et al: In vitro prostaglandin synthesis by various rat renal preparations. Biochim Biophys Acta 15:45–52, 1982.

104. Palmer B, Henrich W: Clinical acute renal failure with nonsteroidal anti-inflammatory drugs. Sem Nephrol 15:214–227, 1995.

105. Kato, Iwana Y, Okumura K, et al: Prostaglandin H_2 may be the endothelium-derived contracting factor released by acetylcholine in the aorta of the rat. Hypertension 15:475–481, 1990.

106. Mizuiri S, Takano M, Hayashi I, et al: Effects of prostaglandins on renal function in uninephrectomized humans. Nephron 63:429–433, 1993.

107. Donker A, Arisz L, Brentjens J, et al: Effect of indomethacin on kidney function and plasma renin activity in man. Nephron 16:288–296, 1976.

108. Davis A, Day R, Begg B: Interactions between non-steroidal anti-inflammatory drugs and anti-hypertensive diuretics. Aust NZ J Med 16:537–546, 1986.

109. Weiss Y, et al: Maintenance of blood pressure control in elderly hypertensives on ketoprofen. Scand J Rheumatol Suppl 91:37–44, 1991.

110. Pope J, Anderson J, Felson D: A meta-analysis of the effects of nonsteroidal anti-inflammatory drugs on blood pressure. Arch Intern Med 153:477–484, 1993.

111. Mene P, Pugliese F, Patrono C: The effects of nonsteroidal anti-inflammatory drugs on human hypertensive vascular disease. Sem Nephrol 15:244–252, 1995.

112. Clabattoni G, Pugliese F, Cinotti G, Patrono C: Renal effects of antiinflammatory drugs. Eur J Rheumatol 3:210–221, 1980.

113. Eriksson L, Bostrom H: Deactivation of sulindac-sulphide by human renal microsomes. Pharm Toxicol 62:177–183, 1988.

114. Perazella M, Buller G: Can ibuprofen cause acute renal failure in a normal individual? Am J Kidney Dis 18:600–602, 1991.

115. Shibasaki T, et al: Clinical characterization of drug-induced allergic nephritis. Am J Nephrol 11:174–180, 1991.

116. Kleinknecht D: Interstitial nephritis, the nephrotic syndrome, and chronic renal failure secondary to nonsteroidal atni-inflammatory drugs. Sem Nephrol 15:228–235, 1995.

117. Brater D: Effects of nonsteroidal anti-inflammatory drugs on renal function: Focus on cyclooxygenase-2 selective inhibition. Am J Med 107:65S–71S, 1999.

118. Schafer A: Effects of nonsteroidal antiinflammatory drugs on platelet function and systemic hemostasis. J Clin Pharmacol 35:209–219, 1995.

119. Jaffe E, Weksler B: Recovery of endothelial cell prostacyclin production after inhibition of low doses of aspirin. J Clin Invest 63:532–535, 1979.

120. Burns E, Lawrence C: Bleeding time: a guide to its diagnostic and clinical utility. Arch Pathol Lab Med 113:1219–1224, 1989.

121. Lind S: The bleeding time does not predict surgical bleeding. Blood 77:2547–2552, 1991.

122. McGurk M, Dinsdale R: A comparison of template bleeding time with mucosal petechiometry as a measure of the platelet

function defect induced by aspirin. Br J Oral Maxillofac Surg 29:173–175, 1991.

123. Kantor T: Peripherally-acting analgesics. *In* Kuhar M, Pasternak G (eds): Analgesics: Neurochemical, Behavioral, and Clinical Perspectives. Raven Press, New York, 1984, pp 289–312.

124. McIntyre B, Philp R, Inwood J: Effect of ibuprofen on platelet function in normal subjects and hemophilic patients. Clin Pharmacol Ther 24:616–621, 1978.

125. Weintraub M, Case K, Kroening B: Effects of piroxicam on platelet aggregation. Clin Pharmacol Ther 23:134–135, 1978.

126. An H, Mikhail W, et al: Effects of hypotensive anesthesia, non-steroidal antiinflammatory drugs, and polymethylmethacrylate on bleeding in total hip arthroplasty patients. J Arthroplasty 6:245–250, 1991.

127. Connelly C, Panush R: Should nonsteroidal antiinflammatory drugs be stopped before elective surgery? Arch Intern Med 151:1963–1966, 1991.

128. Lindgren U, Djupsjo H: Diclofenac for pain after hip surgery. Acta Anaesthesiol Scand 56:28–31, 1985.

129. Bricker S, Savage M, Hanning C: Perioperative blood loss and nonsteroidal antiinflammatory drugs: An investigation using diclofenac in patients undergoing transurethral resection of the prostate. Eur J Anaesthesiol 4:429–434, 1987.

130. Shorr R, Ra W, Daugherty J, Griffin M: Concurrent use of nonsteroidal antiinflammatory drugs and oral anticoagulants places elderly persons at high risk for hemorrhagic peptic ulcer disease. Arch Intern Med 153:1665–1670, 1993.

131. Greenberg H, Gottesdiener K, Huntington M, et al: A new cyclooxygenase-2 inhibitor, rofecoxib (VIOXX), did not alter the antiplatelet effects of low-dose aspirin in healthy volunteers. J Clin Pharmacol 40:1509–1515, 2000.

132. Leese P, Hubbard R, Karim A, et al: Effects of celecoxib, a novel cyclooxygenase-2 inhibitor, on platelet function in healthy adults: A randomized, controlled trial. J Clin Pharmacol. 40:124–132, 2000.

133. Leese P, Talwalker S, Kent J, Recker D: Valdecoxib does not impair platelet function. Am J Emerg Med 20:275–281, 2002.

134. Kromaann-Anderson H, Pedersen A: Reported adverse reactions to and consumption of nonsteroidal anti-inflammatory drugs in Denmark over a 17-year period. Danish Med Bull 35:187–192, 1988.

135. Rabinovitz M, Van Thiel D: Hepatotoxicity of nonsteroidal anti-inflammatory drugs. Am J Gastroenterol 87:1696–1704, 1992.

136. Fry S, Seeff L: Hepatotoxicity of analgesics and antiinflammatory agents. Gastroenterol Clin North Am 24:875–905, 1995.

137. Helfgott S, Sandberg-Cook J, Zakim D, Nestler J: Diclofenac associated hepatotoxicity. JAMA 264:2660–2662, 1990.

138. Babany G, Bernau J, Danaw G, et al: Fulminating hepatitis in a woman taking glafenine and diclofenac. Gastroenterol Clin Biol 9:185, 1991.

139. Gay G: Another side effect of NSAIDs. JAMA 264:2677–2678, 1990.

140. Gerstenfeld L, Thiede M, Seibert K, et al: Differential inhibition of fracture healing by non-selective and cyclooxygenase-2 selective nonsteroidal anti-inflammatory drugs. J Orthop Res 21:670–675, 2003.

141. Neal B: Non-steroidal anti-inflammatory drugs for preventing heterotopic bone formation after hip arthroplasty (Cochrane Review). *In* The Cochrane Library, Issue 4, Update Software, Oxford, 2001.

142. Perlman M, Thordarson D: Ankle fusion in a high risk population: An assessment of nonunion risk factors. Foot Ankle Int 20:491–496, 1999.

143. Alho A: Internally fixed femoral neck fractures. Early prediction of failures in 203 elderly patients with displaced fractures. Acta Orthop Scand 70:141–144, 1999.

144. Bhandari M: Reamed versus nonreamed intramedullary nailing of lower extremity long bone fractures: A systematic overview and meta-analysis. J Orthop Trauma 14:2–9, 2000.

145. Karladani A: The influence of fracture etiology and type of fracture healing: A review of 104 consecutive tibial shaft fractures. Arch Orthop Trauma Surg 121:325–328, 2001.

146. Giannoudis PV, et al: Nonunion of the femoral diaphysis. The influence of reaming and non-steroidal anti-inflammatory drugs. J Bone Joint Surg Br 82:655–658, 2000.

147. Maxy R, Glassman S: The effect of nonsteroidal anti-inflammatory drugs on osteogenesis and spinal fusion. Regional Anesthesia Pain Med 26:156–158, 2001.

148. Glassman S, Rose S, Dimar J, et al: The effect of postoperative nonsteroidal anti-inflammatory drug administraton on spinal fusion. Spine 23,834–838, 1998.

149. Gerstenfeld L, Thiede M, Seibert K, et al: Differential inhibition of fracture healing by non-selective and cyclooxygenase-2 selective nonsteroidal anti-inflammatory drugs. J Orthop Res 21:670–675, 2003.

150. Einhorn T: Do inhibitors of cyclooxygenase-2 impair bone healing? J Bone Mineral Res 17:977–979, 2002.

151. Jeffcoat M: The effect of systemic flurbiprofen on bone supporting dental implants. JADA 126:305–311, 1995.

152. Brägger U: Effect of the NSAID flurbiprofen on remodelling after periodontal surgery. J Periodontal Res 32:375–382, 1997.

153. Bichara J: The effect of postsurgical naproxen and a bioabsorbable membrane on osseous healing in intrabony defects. J Periodontol 70:869–877, 1999.

154. Szczeklik A, Nizankowska E, Mastalerz L, Szabo Z: Analgesics and asthma. Am J Therap 9:233–243, 2002.

155. Salvi S, Krishna T, Sampson A, Holgate S: The anti-inflammatory effects of leukotriene-modifying drugs and their use in asthma. Chest 118:1470–1476, 2000.

156. Dahlen B, Szczeklik A, Murray J: Celecoxib in patients with asthma and aspirin intolerance. N Engl J Med 344:142, 2001.

157. Szczeklik A, Nizankowska E, Bochenek G, et al: Safety of a specific COX-2 inhibitor in aspirin-induced asthma. Clin Experim Allergy 31:219–225, 2001.

158. Farrell G: Liver disease produced by non-steroidal anti-inflammatory drugs. *In* Farrell G (ed): Drug-induced Liver Disease. Churchill-Livingstone, Edinburgh, 1994, p 371.

159. Carson J, Strom B, Morse M, et al: The relative gastrointestinal toxicity of the non-steroidal anti-inflammatory drugs. Arch Int Med 147:1054–1059, 1987.

160. Roberts D, Gerber J, Barnes J, et al: Sulindac is not renal sparing in man. Clin Pharmacol Ther 38:258–265, 1985.

161. Quintero E, Gines P, Arroyo V, et al: Sulindac reduces the urinary excretion of prostaglandins and impairs renal function in cirrhosis with ascites. Nephron 42:298–303, 1986.

162. Stouten E, Armbruster S, Houmes R, et al: Comparison of ketorolac and morphine for postoperative pain after major surgery. Acta Anaesthesiol Scand 36:716–721, 1992.

163. Brown C, Mazzulla J, Mok M, et al: Comparison of repeat doses of intramuscular ketorolac tromethamine and morphine sulfate for analgesia after major surgery. Pharmacotherapy 10:45S–50S, 1990.

164. Bosek V, Smith D, Cox C: Ketorolac or fentanyl to supplement local anesthesia? J Clin Anesth 4:480–483, 1992.

165. Greer I: Effects of ketorolac tomethamine on hemostasis. Pharmacotherapy 10:71S–76S, 1990.

166. Garcha I, Bostwick J: Postoperative hematomas associated with Toradol [letter]. Plast Reconstr Surg 88:919–920, 1991.

167. Forbes J, et al: Evaluation of ketorolac, ibuprofen, acetaminophen, and an acetaminophen–codeine combination in post-operative oral surgery pain. Pharmacotherapy 10:94S–105S, 1990.

168. Rhodes M: Nonsteroidal antiinflammatory drugs for postthoracotomy pain. J Thorac Cardiovasc Surg 103:17–20, 1992.

169. Miller L: Oxaprozin: A once-daily nonsteroidal anti-inflammatory drug. Clin Pharm 11:591–603, 1992.

170. Roberts L, Morrow J: Analgesic–antipyretic and antiinflammatory agents and drugs employed in the treatment of gout. *In* Hardman J, Limbird L (eds): Goodman & Gilman's The Pharmacological Basis of Therapeutics, ed 10. McGraw-Hill, New York, 2001, p 714.

171. Med Lett 14:31, 1972.

172. Dahl S: Nabumetone: A "nonacidic" nonsteroidal antiinflammatory drug. Ann Pharmacother 27:456–463, 1993.

173. Freed M, Audet P, Zariffa N, et al: Comparative effects of nabumetone, sulindac, and indomethacin on urinary prostaglandin excretion and platelet function in volunteers. J Clin Pharmacol 34:1098–1108, 1994.

174. FDA Advisory Committee Briefing Document, NDA 21-042, s007 VIOXX Gastrointestinal Safety. Source www.fda.gov, 8 February 2001.

175. Ray W, Stein C, Daugherty J, et al: COX-2 selective nonsteroidal anti-inflammatory drugs and risk of serious coronary heart disease. Lancet 360:1071–1073, 2002.

176. Solomon D, Schneeweiss S, Glynn R, et al: The relationship between selective COX-2 inhibitors and acute myocardial infarction. Abstract 1823 presented at the Am Coll of Rheumatology, September 2003.

177. Baigent C, Patrono C: Selective cyclooxygenase 2 inhibitors, aspirin, and cardiovascular disease. Arthritis Rheumatism 48:12–20, 2003.

178. Forbes J, Beaver W, Jones K, et al: Evaluation of caffeine on ibuprofen analgesia in postoperative oral surgery pain. Clin Pharmacol Ther 49:674–684, 1991.

179. McQuay H, Angell K, Carroll D, et al: Ibuprofen compared with ibuprofen plus caffeine after third molar surgery. Pain 66:247–251, 1996.

180. Castaneda-Hernandez G, Castillo-Mendez M, Lopez-Munoz F, et al: Potentiation by caffeine of the analgesic effect of aspirin in the pain-induced function impairment model in the rat. Can J Physiol Pharmacol 72:1127–1131, 1994.

181. Jin F, Chung F: Multimodal analgesia for postoperative pain control. J Clin Anesthesia 13:524–539, 2001.

182. Paqueron X, Lumbroso A, Mergoni P, et al: Is morphine-induced sedation synonymous with analgesia during intravenous morphine titration? Br J Anaesthesia 89:697–701, 2002.

183. Camu F, Vanlersberghe C: Pharmacology of systemic analgesics. Best Practice Res Clin Anaesthesiol 16:475–488, 2002.

184. Alexander R, El-Moalem H, Gan T: Comparison of the morphine-sparing effects of diclofenac sodium and ketorolac tromethamine after major orthopedic surgery. J Clin Anesthesia 14:187–192, 2002.

185. Mather L: Do the pharmacodynamics of the nonsteroidal anti-inflammatory drugs suggest a role in the management of postoperative pain? Drugs 44(Suppl 5):1–12, 1992.

186. Camu F, Beecher T, Recker D, Verburg K: Valdecoxib, a COX-2-specific inhibitor, is an efficacious, opioid-sparing analgesic in patients undergoing hip arthroplasty. Am J Therap 9:43–51, 2002.

187. Munro H, Walton S, Malviya S, et al: Low-dose ketorolac improves analgesia and reduces morphine requirements following posterior spinal fusion in adolescents. Can J Anaesthesia 49:461–466, 2002.

188. Eisenberg E, Berkey C, Carr D, Mosteller F: Efficacy and safety of nonsteroidal antiinflammatory drugs for cancer pain: A meta-analysis. J Clin Oncol 12:2756–2765, 1994.

189. Barton S, Langeland F, Snabes M, et al: Efficacy and safety of intravenous parecoxib sodium in relieving acute postoperative pain following gynecologic laparotomy surgery. Anesthesiology 97:306–314, 2002.

190. Steen M, Kehlet H, Jørgen Berg D: A qualitative and quantitative systematic review of preemptive analgesia for postoperative pain relief: The role of timing of analgesia. Anesthesiology 96:725–741, 2002.

191. Stone A, Broderick J, Kaell A, et al: Does the peak-end phenomenon observed in laboratory pain studies apply to real-world pain in rheumatoid arthritics? J Pain 1:212–217, 2000.

192. Reuben S, Bhopatkar S, Maciolek H, et al: The preemptive analgesic effect of rofecoxib after ambulatory arthroscopic knee surgery. Anesthesia Analgesia 94:55–59, 2002.

193. Matheson A, Figgitt D: Rofecoxib: A review of its use in the management of osteoarthritis, acute pain and rheumatoid arthritis. Drugs 61:833–865, 2001.

194. Clemett D, Goa K: Celecoxib: S review of its use in osteoarthritis, rheumatoid arthritis and acute pain. Drugs 59:957–980, 2000.

195. Desjardins PJ, Shu VS, Recker DP, et al: A single preoperative dose of valdecoxib, a new cyclooxygenase-2 specific inhibitor, relieves post-oral surgery or bunionectomy pain. Anesthesiology 97:565–573, 2002.

196. Daniels SE, Desjardins PJ, Talewaker S, et al: The analgesic efficacy of valdecoxib vs. oxycodone/acetaminophen after oral surgery. JADA 133:611–621, 2002.

197. Malan TP, Marsh G, Hakki SI, et al: Parecoxib sodium, a parenteral cyclooxygenasae 2 selective inhibitor, improves morphine analgesia and is opioid-sparing following total hip arthroplasty. Anesthesiology 98:950–956, 2003.

198. Buvanendran A, Kroin JS, Tuman KJ, et al: Effects of perioperative administration of a selective cyclooxygenase 2 inhibitor on pain management and recovery of function after knee replacement: A randomized controlled trial. JAMA 290:2411–2418, 2003.

199. Reuben SS, Connelly NR: Postoperative analgesic effects of celecoxib or rofecoxib after spinal fusion surgery. Anesth Analg 91:1221–1225, 2000.

200. Barton SF, Langeland FF, Snabes MC, et al: Efficacy and safety of intravenous parecoxib sodium in relieving acute postoperative pain following gynecologic laparotomy surgery. Anesthesiology 97:306–314, 2002.

201. Sinatra RS, Shen QJ, Halaszynski T, et al: Preoperative rofecoxib oral suspension as an analgesic adjunct after lower abdominal surgery: The effects of an effort-dependent pain and pulmonary function. Anesth Analg 98:135–140, 2003.

202. Forslund C, Bylander B, Aspenberg P: Indomethacin and celecoxib improve tendon healing in rats. Acta Orthop Scand 74:465–469, 2003.

203. Monck N: NO-naproxen (AstraZeneca). Idrugs 6:593–599, 2003.

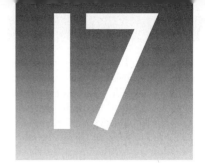

Muscle Relaxants

Onur Melen, M.D.

Muscle relaxants are a pharmacologically diverse group of agents that are used for various medical purposes. They may be classified into the following three broad categories:

1. Neuromuscular blocking agents, which are used as an adjunct to general anesthesia to facilitate endotracheal intubation and muscle relaxation during surgery and mechanical ventilation.
2. Antispasticity drugs, which are indicated for treatment of spasticity and associated, sometimes painful, flexor and extensor spasms due to disorders of the central nervous system (CNS).
3. Drugs that are useful in short-term relief of pain and muscle spasm associated with acute musculoskeletal conditions.

This chapter discusses the drugs in the second and third categories.

ANTISPASTICITY DRUGS

Spasticity is an involuntary increase in muscle tone that occurs during muscle stretch. It is defined as a motor disorder characterized by an increase in tonic stretch reflexes, exaggerated tendon jerks, cutaneous nociceptive and flexor withdrawal reflexes, Babinski's response, and contractures. Its pathophysiology is not entirely clear. Spasticity is mediated peripherally by muscle spindle primary Ia fibers, which mediate monosynaptic reflex arc, and centrally through reticulospinal and vestibulospinal pathways. Accumulating evidence suggests that spasticity is primarily caused by long-term reduction in inhibition rather than in increase in excitation of alpha motor neurons. Current hypotheses suggest that decreased presynaptic inhibition of primary Ia afferent terminals, decreased reciprocal inhibition of antagonistic motor neurons, decreased nonreciprocal inhibition, and dysfunction of Ia inhibitory interneurons are the principal mechanisms of spasticity. Presynaptic inhibition is mediated by gamma-aminobutyric acid (GABA), a major inhibitory neurotransmitter in the CNS. GABA reduces the amount of neurotransmitter release by Ia fiber terminals and

inhibits sensory signals from muscle spindles. There are two types of GABA receptors. The more prominent is GABA-A, which forms an integral part of multiple units of ligand-gated chloride ion channels. Most of the rapid inhibitory transmission in the CNS is believed to be mediated by these chloride channels.[1,2] The second type of receptor is GABA-B, which is less represented than GABA-A receptors. GABA-B is believed to regulate ion channels. Glycine is another neurotransmitter released by inhibitory interneurons and is found to be reduced in spastic experimental animals.

Drugs that reduce spasticity act either centrally to enhance inhibitory neurotransmission (benzodiazepines and anticonvulsants, baclofen and tizanidine) or peripherally on contractile elements of the skeletal muscle (dantrolene, botulinum toxin).

CENTRALLY ACTING MUSCLE RELAXANTS

Benzodiazepines: Benzodiazepines have unique pharmacodynamic and pharmacokinetic properties that allow their use for various therapeutic purposes. They are administered as sedatives, anxiolytics, hypnotics, anticonvulsants, and muscle relaxants. Only diazepam (Valium) and to a much lesser extent, clonazepam (Klonopin) are used as muscle relaxants.

MECHANISM OF ACTION: The effects of benzodiazepines virtually all result from their action on the CNS. They exert their antispastic function by enhancing presynaptic inhibition in the spinal cord. Their targets are inhibitory neurotransmitter receptors that are directly activated by GABA. The majority of GABA neurons are interneurons. Experiments have demonstrated that benzodiazepines act presynaptically on the interneurons to facilitate the release of GABA and its binding to GABA-A receptor. Benzodiazepines are considered to be indirect GABA-ergic agents. They increase the gain of inhibitory transmission mediated by GABA-A receptors.[3,4] As a result, the chloride channels open within the receptor chloride channel complex, magnifying chloride ion currents. This leads to hyperpolarization of Ia afferent terminals at their synapses with GABA-ergic interneurons in the spinal cord.

The net result is decreased transmitter release from Ia afferents to motor neurons, and reduced motor neuron output.

DIAZEPAM: Diazepam is the most widely used benzodiazepine as a muscle relaxant. It can be administered alone or in combination with other muscle relaxants. It is most effective in patients with spinal cord disease and injury but less so in those with cerebral palsy and spastic hemiplegia due to stroke. Painful, persistent, and disabling muscle spasms seem to respond to diazepam better than periodic flexor spasms. In addition, diazepam is valuable in the treatment of tetanus, stiff-person syndrome, and occasionally in alleviating local muscle spasms and pain due to inflammatory joint disease and radiculopathy. Diazepam induces hypotonia without interfering with locomotion, but it often produces decreased muscle strength. This side effect along with its potential to cause somnolence, dizziness, and sedation makes nonambulatory patients better candidates for treatment with diazepam.

PHARMACOKINETICS, DOSE, AND TOXICITY: Diazepam is absorbed from the gastrointestinal system reaching the effective blood level in 30 minutes and the peak level within 3 hours. The half-life of a single dose is about 8 hours. It is detoxified by the liver and excreted in urine and feces. It crosses the placenta and is found in breast milk.

The usual starting dose of oral diazepam is 2 mg twice daily. Depending on the patient's sensitivity and tolerance, the dose can be raised in increments of 2 to 4 mg per week to a maximum total daily dose of 20 to 30 mg. Smaller doses are often not very effective in reducing the muscle tone but most patients do not show good tolerance of doses higher than 15 to 20 mg, no matter how slowly the dose is escalated. Limiting side effects are dizziness, somnolence, lassitude, confusion, increased reaction time, memory loss, ataxia, and digestive disturbance. Sometimes adverse psychological effects are encountered such as anxiety, irritability, euphoria, hypomania, depression, paranoia, and suicidal ideation. Concomitant use of CNS-acting drugs such as baclofen, barbiturates, and narcotics potentiate the side effects. Long-term use of diazepam carries the risk of dependence. Incidents of allergic and hematologic reactions and hepatotoxicity are low. Abrupt termination of diazepam therapy may lead to serious withdrawal symptoms, such as delirium, and seizures.[5,6] Parenterally administered diazepam has little role in the long-term treatment of spasticity, but it is valuable in tetanus as an adjunct to antitoxin and antibiotics. Up to 120 mg per day of diazepam can be administered when ventilatory support is available.

CLONAZEPAM: Clonazepam is primarily used to suppress myoclonus, akinetic, and petit mal seizures, and more recently panic disorders. Its use in spasticity is less common. It may be useful in alleviating nocturnal spasms and in reducing spasticity in children with cerebral palsy.[7] In an open trial clonazepam's antispastic effects were compared to baclofen. They were found to be equally efficacious and the side-effect profile was worse in clonazepam leading to more discontinuation.[8]

Anticonvulsants: Recent research suggested that anticonvulsants Gabapentin (Neurontin) and Tiagabine (Gabitril) may have antispastic properties.[9–13] Several studies have shown that Gabapentin in doses of 1,200 mg per day or more may be efficacious in reducing muscle tone in patients with multiple sclerosis and spinal cord injury.[9–11] Gabapentin has a favorable side-effect profile but can cause somnolence and dizziness.

Tiagabine, a novel presynaptic GABA uptake inhibitor, was shown in a study to relieve spasticity in children with uncontrollable seizures and spasticity.[12]

Baclofen (Lioresal)

MECHANISM OF ACTION: Baclofen is structurally similar to GABA. It is a GABA-B receptor agonist. Baclofen is an overall powerful neuronal depressant that exerts its action by binding to presynaptic GABA-B receptors in the dorsal horn of the spinal cord, the brain stem, and other CNS sites. The site of its antispastic action is the spinal cord. By binding to GABA-B receptors, it suppresses the release of excitatory neurotransmitters and inhibits excitatory afferent terminals that are involved in monosynaptic and polysynaptic reflex activity at the spinal cord level.[13–15] In high concentrations baclofen may block the postsynaptic action of excitatory neurotransmitters.[16] In addition, baclofen appears to have an inhibitory effect on the release of excitatory neurotransmitters from nociceptive afferent neural endings that originate in the skin.[17]

Baclofen is indicated and is particularly useful in the treatment of spasticity of the spinal cord origin. Patients with cord injury and multiple sclerosis are prime candidates. The efficacy of baclofen in the treatment of spastic hemiplegia due to various cerebral lesions is far less certain. Some patients with generalized or cervical dystonia, upper motor neuron disease, and stiff-person syndrome may particularly benefit from baclofen. It provides a long-term reduction in spasticity and decreases the frequency of flexor spasms in addition to alleviating the pain associated with them. Reduction of flexor spasms at night allows patients to enjoy uninterrupted sleep. Release of adductor and flexor contractions facilitates nursing care. Modest muscle weakness appears in some patients but baclofen has little overall effect on locomotion.

Antispastic effects of baclofen and diazepam are similar. Baclofen is usually preferred over diazepam because it causes less sedation, which allows its use at maximum effective doses.

PHARMACOKINETICS, DOSE, AND TOXICITY: Baclofen is available in 10 mg tablets. Usual starting dose is 5 mg, three times a day. The dose can be doubled every 3 to 4 days to a maximum daily dose of 80 to 100 mg, if needed and tolerated.

In a single dose baclofen is rapidly absorbed. The serum half-life is about 4 hours. About 30% is bound to serum proteins and deaminated in the liver. The remainder is excreted unchanged in the urine and feces. Only a small fraction crosses the blood–brain barrier.

Baclofen is a safe drug and is tolerated well even in large doses. Somnolence and dizziness are the most frequent side effects and in larger doses, confusion, ataxia, and even hallucinations may appear, especially in patients with cerebral lesions. Rarely does baclofen trigger seizure activity in epileptic patients. Abrupt withdrawal should be avoided because of risks of increased flexor spasms, hallucinations, and seizures.

Because of low lipid solubility, baclofen does not cross the blood–brain barrier in sufficient amount to reach high concentrations in cerebrospinal fluid (CSF), even when given in large doses. Devices have been developed to deliver baclofen directly into the target sites in the spinal cord. Administrating baclofen intrathecally offers the advantage of achieving rapid and sustainable effective CSF levels and reaching the receptor sites in the spinal cord without risking systemic side effects.

Intrathecal baclofen is delivered using an infusion system that consists of an implantable pump, an intrathecal catheter, and an external programmer with a programmer head. The pump is implanted into the abdominal wall and the catheter is inserted into the lumbar intrathecal space. Communication with the pump is accomplished via a radiotelemetric link between the external programmer and the pump. Dosage titration can be selected with the programmer. Before placement of the pump, a trial dose is given and the patient is observed for several hours. If decreased spasticity is observed, the patient is selected for pump placement.

Intrathecal baclofen is effective in reducing spasticity in patients with spinal cord injury and multiple sclerosis.[18,19] Its usefulness in cerebral palsy, spastic hemiplegia due to stroke or cerebral injury, upper motor neuron disease, and dystonia has not yet been fully established.

Although intrathecal baclofen often eliminates the need for other antispasticity medications, it can still be used in conjunction with others in selective patients. Rare complications of intrathecal baclofen therapy include drowsiness, orthostatic hypotension, and pump-related complications such as malfunction, kinking, dislodgement, disconnection, breakage, and wound infection.

Tizanidine (Zanaflex)
MECHANISM OF ACTION: Tizanidine is a newly introduced muscle relaxant. Structurally, it is an imidazoline derivative. Pharmacologically, it is a centrally acting alpha$_2$ adrenergic agonist. Because of the pharmacologic and clinical evidence of its concomitant antinociceptive properties, it has gained acceptance in the treatment of both spasticity and rheumatologic conditions associated with painful muscle spasms.[20]

Animal experiments have revealed that tizanidine suppresses polysynaptic excitation of dorsal horn neurons in the spinal cord and depresses polysynaptic reflexes in spontaneous neuronal activity, probably by reducing the release of excitatory neural transmitters (glutamate, aspartate) from presynaptic sites.[21]

Tizanidine exhibits a high affinity for alpha$_2$ adrenergic receptors. This property, along with the structural similarity of tizanidine to alpha$_2$-agonist clonidine (which has a mild antispastic action of its own), raises the possibility that the muscle relaxant function is at least partly mediated by the adrenergic system. The action of tizanidine may include inhibition on locus ceruleus firing and subsequent inhibition of the cerulospinal pathway, which normally exert a facilitatory effect on synaptic activity in the spinal cord. Finally, evidence suggests a possible postsynaptic action at the excitatory amino acid receptors.[21] Because of its unique and various actions at different level, tizanidine induces hypotonia without undue muscle weakness.

Animal studies have demonstrated antinociceptive activity of tizanidine, mediated by inhibition of A and C fiber activity, as well as selective inhibition of dorsal horn neurons to nociceptive stimulation.[22,23]

Well-controlled studies have revealed the effectiveness of tizanidine as an antispastic agent in about a third to half of patients with multiple sclerosis, spinal cord injury, motor neuron disease, and stroke.[24,25] It is most beneficial in reducing the frequency of muscle spasms and clonus, but is less consistent in reducing the muscle tone. Assessment of neurologic

functions and functional disability scores has failed to reveal consistent and significant treatment effects. Tizanidine provided little impact on scores of activities of daily living. When compared to baclofen, the results with tizanidine were about equal in most parameters assessed, except tizanidine caused less muscle weakness. Comparison with diazepam favors tizanidine in all parameters including side effects (particularly sedation). Tizanidine was better tolerated than diazepam and baclofen.[26]

PHARMACOKINETICS, DOSE, TOXICITY: Tizanidine is supplied in 4 mg tablets. It is completely absorbed through the gastrointestinal tract and has a half-life of approximately 2.5 hours. Peak plasma levels are reached in 1.5 hours after a single dose. It is 30% bound to plasma proteins, metabolized by the liver, and excreted in the urine and feces.

Reported side effects include asthenia, headache, digestive disturbance, somnolence, dry mouth, and hallucinations. About 80% of patients complain of at least one of the side effects and about 25% discontinue taking it. Although blood pressure and pulse rates are not adversely affected by tizanidine, it is recommended to administer the drug very carefully with other antihypertensive agents and not with other alpha$_2$-agonists. No consistent hematologic crises have been encountered in clinical trials but mild elevation of liver enzymes have been observed.

The recommended starting dose is 4 mg once daily. The dose may be raised in increments of 4 to 6 mg/week to a total daily regimen of 36 mg. Tizanidine can be used as a single agent or given in combination with diazepam or baclofen, although the efficacy of combination does not differ significantly from that of the single agent. In some patients combination therapy may offer long-term benefit if it allows reduction of each medication's daily dose and, therefore, its side effects.

PERIPHERALLY ACTING ANTISPASTICITY DRUGS

Dantrolene (Dantrium)
MECHANISM OF ACTION: Dantrolene is structurally an imidazoline derivative and is classified as a direct acting muscle relaxant. Its primary action is on the contractile elements of the muscle. Although some of its side effects such as mental depression, confusion, and dizziness suggest a CNS effect, a central antispasticity property of dantrolene has not been identified.

In resting muscle calcium is stored in sarcoplasmic reticulum. For muscle contraction to take place, calcium has to be released from sarcoplasmic reticulum to activate myosin adenosine triphosphatase (ATPase) and excitation–contraction coupling. Dantrolene blocks the release of calcium and disassociates excitation–contraction coupling leading to hypotonia and muscle weakness.[27] Heightened reflex activity and clonus are also reduced. Unless it is given in very large doses, the effect of dantrolene on myocardium and smooth muscle is negligible.

Dantrolene is primarily used to treat spasticity. It is indicated in patients with spinal cord injury, multiple sclerosis, cerebral palsy, and stroke. It is of particular benefit to patients who are nonambulatory and have prolonged muscle contractions due to chronic spasticity. Relief of spasticity and fixed contractions aids nursing care, enhances physical rehabilitation, and restores residual function. Ambulatory patients benefit less from dantrolene, because the induced muscle weakness interferes with the patient's ability to ambulate. Dantrolene is not indicated in the treatment of skeletal muscle spasm and pain resulting from rheumatologic disorders.

Intravenous dantrolene is indicated in the treatment of malignant hyperthermia, a potentially life-threatening condition triggered by succinylcholine and inhalation anesthetics.[28] Oral or intravenous dantrolene is a useful adjunct to dopamine agonists in the treatment of neuroleptic malignant syndrome, brought about by dopamine depleting agents, such as psychotropic drugs. This syndrome is characterized by encephalopathy, muscle rigidity, fever, autonomic disturbance, leukocytosis, and elevated creatinine phosphokinase concentration. By its direct action on the muscle, dantrolene reduces the muscle rigidity and limits muscle fiber breakdown and elevation of creatinine phosphokinase levels.[29,30]

PHARMACOKINETICS, DOSE, AND TOXICITY: Oral dantrolene is absorbed slowly and incompletely. It is metabolized by the liver to hydroxyl and amino derivatives and excreted in the urine. Risk of physical dependence and tolerance is low.

Standard oral starting dose for treatment of chronic spasticity is 25 mg twice daily. If needed, the dose can be raised to a maximum daily dose of 400 mg over a period of 3 to 4 weeks. If no response is demonstrated after a month, the drug should be discontinued.

The most frequent side effects of dantrolene are drowsiness, dizziness, muscle weakness, and occasional fatal or nonfatal hepatotoxicity. It is advisable to conduct liver function tests before initiating therapy and monitor liver functions through the course of the treatment.

Botulinum Toxin: Botulinum toxin (BTX) has recently been added to the list of agents for treatment of spasticity and painful muscle spasms. It was first introduced in the late 1970s to treat strabismus. Later its usefulness was recognized in the treatment of a variety of disorders, characterized by involuntary, inappropriate, and excessive muscle activity.

Botulinum neurotoxin is produced by a Gram negative anaerobic bacterium, *Clostridium botulinum*. There are seven serologically distinct serotypes of the toxin, designated A, B, C, D, E, F, and G. *Clostridium botulinum* is widespread in the environment. Its spores germinate under anaerobic conditions and cause occasional outbreaks of botulism. Human disease is brought about by either ingestion of contaminated food or by wound infection. Only types A, B, E, and F strains cause human disease.

A purified and attenuated form of the toxin is available for clinical use and marketed in three different preparations: BTX-A (Botox), Dysport (in Europe) and BTX-B (Myobloc). Preparation is achieved by establishing and growing cultures of *Clostridium botulinum* in a fermenter. The cultures are then harvested and diluted with human serum albumin and subsequently either vacuum dried (Botox) or freeze dried (Dysport) and packaged in vials. The toxin is kept in a refrigerator until its use. The potency of the product is determined by in vivo mouse assays. One unit of BTX is defined by the amount of toxin that can kill 50% (LD_{50}) of a group of test mice. The units are not equivalent in different products.

MECHANISM OF ACTION: BTXs primary action is on the neuromuscular junction. It acts on peripheral cholinergic nerve endings and inhibits the release of acetylcholine from presynaptic terminals leading to muscle relaxation. When injected into the muscle it causes reversible denervation atrophy followed by reinnervation and full return of function in about three months.[31,32] BTX does not cross the blood–brain barrier and therefore has no effect on central cholinergic pathways.

In addition to neuromuscular blocking effect, BTX has other properties. It is capable of inhibiting transmitter release from pre- and postganglionic cholinergic nerve endings of the autonomic nervous system. Experiments have suggested two additional effects of BTX, one on the afferent limb of the motor system and the other analgesic effect on the sensory system. It has been proposed that BTX-A can modify the sensory feedback loop to the CNS either by reducing muscle activity or by blocking intrafusal fibers and thereby reducing muscle spindle activity. The end result would be diminished Ia afferent input to the central nervous system.[33–36]

The analgesic effect of BTX may not solely be the result of muscle relaxation. In addition to altering afferent nerve transmission, BTX may have an effect on the nociceptor system and may reduce inflammatory pain by inhibiting release of neuropeptides such as substance P and perhaps other neuromodulators.[37,38]

Currently BTX is used for various conditions. These are:

- Focal dystonias (cervical dystonia, blepharospasm, laryngeal dystonia, oral mandibular dystonia, limb dystonia).
- Nondystonic excessive muscle contractions (hemifacial spasm, spasticity, bruxism, tics, tremors, stuttering, stiff-person syndrome).
- Headaches (migraine, tension headache).
- Myofascial pain.
- Hyperhidrosis.
- Genitourinary disorders (detrusor-sphincter dyssynergia).
- Gastrointestinal disorders (achalasia, constipation, esophageal sphincter spasm).

There are many advantages of BTX treatment over medical and surgical procedures for chronic conditions. BTX is easily administered in office and well tolerated by patients. Adverse reactions are usually local, such as pain, mild and of short duration. The toxin may diffuse in small amounts to neighboring muscles with unintended consequences, such as dysphagia during treatment of cervical dystonia. Occasionally, the toxin may spread to more distant muscles. Although it causes electromyographic changes, it rarely produces disabling weakness.[39] There have been no reports of sustained generalized weakness in patients who have been treated with BTX over many years. Systemic side effects such as flu-like symptoms and idiosyncratic reactions rarely occur. BTX does not lead to permanent tissue injury as do some surgical procedures utilized in the treatment of dystonias and spasticity. Doses can be easily adjusted for optimum response and minimal side effects.

Patients experience improvement within the first week of treatment. The average duration of benefit is approximately three months. About 10% of the treated patients do not respond at all (primary nonresponders). Another 10% to 15% develop resistance to treatment because of antibody formation.

Patients with myasthenia gravis, Lambert–Eaton syndrome, and motor neuron disease should not be treated with BTX. It is also not recommended during pregnancy and in lactating women.

BTX is most commonly used to treat focal dystonias predominantly cervical dystonia (spasmodic torticollis) and blepharospasm. Efficacy and safety of BTX for treatment of cervical dystonia has been established by controlled and open label studies.[40,41] About 70% to 80% of patients respond favorably to BTX demonstrating reduction in dystonic spasms and pain as well as improvement in function of the head and neck.[42–45] Most important factors in administration of BTX is knowledge of the anatomy of the cervical muscles and identification of muscles responsible for the abnormal movement and posture. Some complex cases may require EMG guidance for localization of target muscles. The dose of BTX depends on the number of muscles involved in cervical dystonia, their size, and severity of the spasms. Usual doses delivered range from 200 to 400 units for BTX-A (Botox) and 7,500 to 20,000 units BTX-B (Myobloc).

BTX is very effective in the treatment of blepharospasm, an idiopathic focal dystonia, characterized by tonic and clonic spasms of the orbicularis oculi muscles. This results in forceful eye closure rendering some patients functionally blind. Short- and long-term results of BTX trials indicate 70% to 80% favorable response rates.[46,47] The dose range is 15 to 30 units of BTX-A per eye injected subcutaneously around the orbicularis oculi muscles at four or five different sites.

Hemifacial spasm is another condition which is very responsive to BTX.[48,49] It is a disorder of the facial nerve manifested by involuntary clonic and tonic contractions of the facial muscles. The most common cause is compression of the facial nerve at the brain base by an aberrant blood vessel. Orbicularis oculi, zygomaticus, orbicularis oris, and platysma are the usual muscles targeted for injection. The usual dose distributed to those muscles ranges between 25 and 40 units of BTX-A.

Another condition that is disabling and refractory to medical treatment but responsive to BTX is limb dystonia. Inappropriate and involuntary muscle contractions and posturing impair the control of the desired action of the hands and feet. A variant of limb dystonia is task-specific dystonia. The best-known forms of task specific dystonia are writer's cramp and musician's cramps. Although trials have found that BTX is generally useful, it remains an individual therapy benefiting selective patients.[50] BTX injection to the limbs are often problematic, because the relief of excessive muscle spasm may only be possible when the muscles are made very weak, thus impairing the patient's ability to use the limbs for other tasks.

The therapeutic application of BTX has been extended to spasticity. It has been found useful in multiple sclerosis, traumatic brain injury, cerebral palsy, spinal cord injury, and stroke.[51–59] Reduction of muscle tone in the muscles not only provides comfort to the patient but also improves function and makes nursing care easier.

Injection of spastic adductor muscles of the thigh with up to 400 units of BTX-A reduces the tone, improves passive abduction, and maximum distance between the knees. It helps sitting, positioning, hygiene, bladder catheterization, and enhances overall nursing care in nonambulatory patients. Painful muscle spasm may also be alleviated.

Injecting the lower extremity muscles such as soleus, medial and lateral gastrocnemius, tibialis posterior, and extensor hallucis longus improves spastic foot drop, ankle position at rest, and range of active and passive motion. Equinovarus and equinovalgus deformities can be partially corrected thus improving positioning and sometimes gait.

BTX can be administered to a spastic upper extremity in hemiplegia. Injection of elbow and wrist flexors in a dose range of 75 to 200 units of BTX-A may increase range of motion and function. In all of these conditions BTX can be used along with other conventional antispasticity drugs without adverse interaction and can therefore serve as a useful supplemental therapeutic agent.

DRUGS USED IN SHORT-TERM RELIEF OF PAIN AND MUSCLE SPASM

Cyclobenzaprine Hydrochloride (Flexeril): Cyclobenzaprine is a tricyclic amine salt. It relieves skeletal muscle spasm of local origin without interfering with muscle strength. It is indicated for relief of muscle spasm and pain associated with acute, painful musculoskeletal conditions. It is ineffective in spasticity due to CNS disease. Cyclobenzaprine does not act directly on muscle or neuromuscular junction. Studies indicate that the primary action of cyclobenzaprine is on the brain stem. Pharmacologic studies in animals show a similarity between the effects of cyclobenzaprine and those of the tricyclic antidepressants, such as norepinephrine potentiation, sedation, and peripheral and central anticholinergic effects. Cyclobenzaprine improves signs and symptoms of skeletal muscle spasm, reduces local pain and tenderness, and helps increase range of motion. It is recommended for short-term therapy, as information is not available on its long-term effectiveness. Cyclobenzaprine is available in 10 mg tablets. The standard daily dose is 30 to 40 mg, taken for 2 or 3 weeks. The most common side effects are drowsiness, dizziness, and dry mouth. It may interact with monoamine oxidase inhibitors.

Chlorzoxazone (Paraflex): Chlorzoxazone is a centrally acting agent, although its exact mode of action has not been clearly identified. Experimental data suggest that the primary site of action is the spinal cord, where it inhibits polysynaptic reflex pathways that are involved in the production of increased tone.

Chlorzoxazone is indicated for short-term treatment of muscle spasm associated with acute, painful musculoskeletal conditions. Spasticity due to CNS disease is not relieved by this agent.

Chlorzoxazone is available in 250 mg caplets. The usual effective dose is 1,000 to 2,000 mg/day. It is generally well tolerated. Various side effects include digestive disturbance, dizziness, drowsiness, and hepatotoxicity.

Carisoprodol (Soma): Carisoprodol produces muscle relaxation, probably by inhibiting interneuronal activity in the descending reticular activating system and the spinal cord. Some of its effect may be related to its sedative action. No direct action on skeletal muscle or neuromuscular junction has been identified.

Carisoprodol is recommended for use of relief of discomfort and pain in acute musculoskeletal conditions. It is not indicated to treat spasticity.

Carisoprodol is marketed in 350 mg tablets. A combination of 200 mg of carisoprodol and 325 mg of aspirin is also available. The usual recommended daily dose is 350 mg 3 to 4 times a day. The most frequent side effects are drowsiness, ataxia, tremor, irritability, insomnia, confusion, and disorientation. An occasional patient may experience tachycardia and postural hypotension.

Methocarbamol (Robaxin, Robaxisal): The mechanism of action of methocarbamol is not clear. Although it is primarily used for relief of discomfort associated with acute painful musculoskeletal conditions, methocarbamol has no proven muscle relaxant effect. It is believed that methocarbamol acts as a primary CNS depressant.

Methocarbamol is available in 500 and 750 mg tablets. The usual recommended daily dose is 3 to 4 g. Side effects include drowsiness, light-headedness, dizziness, and nausea.

REFERENCES

1. Ragan CL, McKernan RM, Wafford K, et al: Gamma-aminobutyric acid – A (GABA-A) receptor/ion channel complex. Biochem Soc Trans 21:622–626, 1993.
2. Twyman RE, Rogers CJ, MacDonald RL: Differential regulation of gamma-aminobutyric acid receptor channels by diazepam and phenobarbital. Ann Neurol 25:213–220, 1989.
3. Biggio G, Costa E (eds): Symposium: GABA and benzodiazepine receptor subtypes: molecular biology, pharmacology, and clinical aspects. Adv Biochem Psychopharmacol 46:1–239, 1990.
4. Pole P: Electrophysiology of benzodiazepine receptor ligands: Multiple mechanisms and sites of action. Prog Neurobiol 31:349–423, 1988.
5. Roth T, Roches TA: Issues in the use of benzodiazepine therapy. J Clin Psychiatry 53(Suppl 6):14–18, 1992.
6. Woods JH, Katz JL, Winger G: Benzodiazepines: Use, abuse, and consequences. Pharmacol Review 4:15–347, 1992.
7. Dahlin M, Knuttson E, Nergardh A: Treatment of spasticity in children with low dose benzodiazepine. J Neurol Sci 117:54–60, 1993.
8. Cendrowski W, Sobczyk W: Clonazepam, baclofen, and placebo in the treatment of spasticity. Eur Neurol 16:257–262, 1997.
9. Priebe MM, Sherwood AM, Graves DE, et al: Effectiveness of gabapentin in controlling spasticity: A quantitative study. Spinal Cord 35:171–175, 1997.
10. Gruenthal M, Mueller M, Olson WI, et al: Gabapentin for the treatment of spasticity in patients with spinal cord injury. Spinal Cord 35:686–689, 1997.
11. Cutter NC, Scott DD, Johnson JC, Whiteneck G: Gabapentin effect on spasticity in multiple sclerosis: A placebo controlled randomized trial. Arch Phys Med Rehabil 81:164–169, 2000.
12. Holden KR, Titus MO: The effect of trigabine on spasticity in children with intractable epilepsy: A pilot study. Pediat Neurol 21:728–730, 1999.
13. Bowery NG, Hill DR, Hudson AL, et al: Baclofen decreases neurotransmitter release in the mammalian CNS by action at a novel GABA receptor. Nature 283:92–94, 1980.
14. Krain JS, Penn RD, Bissinger RL, et al: Reduced spinal reflexes following intrathecal baclofen in the rabbit. Exp Brain Res 54:191–194, 1984.
15. Mueller H, Zierski J, Drake D, et al: The effect of intrathecal baclofen in electrical muscle activity in spasticity. J Neurol 234:234–352, 1987.
16. Baxter TJ, Carlen PL: Pre and postsynaptic effects of baclofen in the rat hippocampal slices. Brain Res 341:195–199, 1985.
17. Hwang AS, Wilcox GL: Baclofen, gamma-aminobutyric acid B receptors and substance P in the mouse spinal cord. J Pharmacol Exp Ther 248:1026–1033, 1989.
18. Penn RD: Intrathecal baclofen for spasticity of spinal origin: Seven years of experience. J Neurosurg 77:236–240, 1992.
19. Coffey RJ, Cahill D, Steers W, et al: Intrathecal baclofen for intractable spasticity of spinal origin: Results of a long-term multicenter study. J Neurosurg 78:26–232, 1993.
20. Coward DM: Trizanidine: Neuropharmacology and mechanism of action. Neurology 44(Suppl 9):6–11, 1994.
21. Davies J: Selective depression of synaptic transmission of spinal neurons in the cat by a new, centrally acting muscle relaxant, 5-chloro-4-(2 imidazolin-2-yl-amino)-2, 1, 3-benzothiadiazole (DS 103-282). Br J Pharmacol 76:473–481, 1982.
22. Davies J, Johnson SE: Selective antinociceptive effects of tizanidine (DS 103-282), a centrally acting muscle relaxant on dorsal horn neurons in the feline spinal cord. Brit J Pharmacol 82:409–421, 1984.
23. Villanueva L, Chitour D, LeBars D: Effects of tizanidine (DS 103-282) on the dorsal horn convergent neurons in the rat. Pain 35:187–197, 1988.
24. Smith C, Birnbaum G, Carter JL, et al and US Tizanidine Study Group: Tizanidine treatment of spasticity caused by multiple sclerosis. Results of a double blind, placebo controlled trial. Neurology 44(Suppl 9):34–43, 1994.
25. Nance PW, Baugaresti J, Shellenberger K, et al and the North American Tizanidine Study Group: Efficiency and safety of tizanidine in the treatment of spasticity in patients with spinal cord injury. Neurology 44(Suppl 9):44–52, 1994.
26. Lataste X, Emre M, Davis C, et al: Comparative profile of tizanidine in the management of spasticity. Neurology 44:(Suppl 9):53–59, 1994.
27. VanWinkle WB: Calcium release from skeletal muscle sarcoplasmic reticulum, site of action of dantrolene sodium? Science 193:1130–1131, 1976.
28. Rosenberg H, Fletcher JE: Malignant hyperthermia. In Azar I (ed): Muscle Relaxants: Side Effects and Rational Approach to Selection (Clinical Pharmacology Series), vol 7. Marcel Dekker, New York, 1987, pp 115–148.
29. Addonizio G, Susman VL, Roth SD: Neuroleptic malignant syndrome: Review of analysis of 115 cases. Biol Psychiatry 22:1004–1020, 1987.
30. Pearlman CA: Neuroleptic malignant syndrome: A review of the literature. J Clin Psychopharmocol G:257–273, 1986.
31. Alderson K, Holds JB, Anderson RL: Botulinum induced alteration of nerve–muscular interactions in the human orbicularis oculi following treatment for blepharospasm. Neurology 61:1800–1805, 1991.
32. DePavia A, Meunier FA, Molg Aoki KA, Dolly JO: Functional repair of motor end-plates after botulinum neurotoxin type A poisoning. Biphasic switch of synaptic activity between nerve sprouts and their parent terminals. Proc Natl Acad Sci USA 96:3200–3205, 1999.
33. Ludlow CI, Hallett M, Sedory SE, et al: The pathophysiology of spasmodic dysphonia and its modification by botulinum toxin. In Barrardelli A, Benecke R, Manfredi M, Marsden CM (eds): Motor Disturbances II. Academic Press, New York, 1990, pp 273–288.
34. Zwirner P, Murry T, Swenson M, et al: Effects of botulinum toxin therapy in patients with adductor spasmodic dysphonia: acoustic, aerodynamic, and video endoscopic findings. Laryngoscope 102:400–406, 1992.
35. Brin MF, Blitzer A, Stewart C, Fahn S: Treatment of spasmodic dysphonia (laryngeal dystonia) with local injections of botulinum toxin: review and technical aspects. In Blitzer A, Brin MF, Sasaki CT, et al (eds): Neurologic Disorders of the Larynx. Thieme, New York, 1992, pp 214–228.
36. Rosales RI, Arimura K, Takenaga S, et al: Extrafusal and intrafusal muscle effects in experimental botulinum toxin-a injection. Muscle-Nerve 19:488–496, 1996.
37. Aoki KR: Pharmacology and immunology of botulinum toxin serotypes. J Neurol 248(Suppl 1):3–10, 2001.

38. Cui M, Aoki KR: Botulinum toxin type A (BTX-A) reduces inflammatory pain in the rat formalin model. Cephalalgia 20:414 (abstr), 2000.

39. Lange DJ, Rubin M, Greene PE, et al: Distant effect of locally injected botulinum toxin: A double blind study of single fiber EMG changes. Muscle Nerve 14:672–675, 1991.

40. Greene P: Controlled trials of botulinum toxin for cervical dystonia: A critical review. *In* Jankovic J, Hallett M (eds): Therapy with Botulinum Toxin. Marcel Dekker, New York, 1994, pp 279–287.

41. Poewe W, Wissel J: Experience with botulinum toxin in cervical dystonia. *In* Jankovic J, Hallett M (eds): Therapy with Botulinum Toxin. Marcel Dekker, New York, 1994, pp 267–278.

42. Tsui JKC: Botulin toxin as a therapeutic agent. Pharmacol Ther 72:13–24, 1996.

43. Muchau A, Bhatia KP: Uses of botulin toxin injections in medicine today. BMJ 320:161–165, 2000.

44. Jankovic J, Schwartz K: Botulinum toxin injection for cervical dystonia. Neurology 40:227–280, 1990.

45. Poewe W, Schelosky L, Kleedorfer B, et al: Treatment of spasmodic torticollis with local injection of botulinum toxin. One year follow-up in 37 patients. J Neurol 239:21–25, 1992.

46. Dutton JJ, Buckley EG: Long-term results and complications of botulinum A toxin in the treatment of blepharospasm. Ophthalmology 95:1529–1534, 1988.

47. Jankovic J, Brin MF: Drug therapy, therapeutic uses of botulinum toxin. N Engl J Med 324:1186–1194, 1991.

48. Savino PJ, Sergott RC, Bosley TM, et al: Hemifacial spasm treated with botulinum A toxin injection. Arch Ophthalmol 103:1305–1306, 1985.

49. Biglan AW, May M, Bowes RA: Management of facial spasm with clostridium botulinum toxin, type A (Oculinum). Arch Otolaryngol 114:1407–1412, 1988.

50. Tsui JK, Bhatt M, Calnes, et al: Botulinum toxin in the treatment of writer's cramp: A double blind study. Neurology 43:183–185, 1993.

51. Borg-Stein J, Pine ZM, Miller JR, et al: Botulinum toxin for the treatment of spasticity in multiple sclerosis: New observations. Am J Phys Med Rehabil 72:364–368, 1993.

52. Hyman N, Barnes M, Bhakata B, et al: Botulinum toxin (Dysport) treatment of hip adductor spasticity in multiple sclerosis: A prospective, randomized, double blind, placebo controlled, dose ranging study. J Neurol Neruosurg Psychiatry 68:707–712, 2000.

53. Dengler R, Neyer U, Wohlfahrt K, et al: Local botulinum toxin in the treatment of spastic foot drop. J Neurol 239:375–378, 1992.

54. Fehlings D, Rang M, Glazier J, et al: An evaluation of botulinum-A toxin injections to improve upper extremity function in children with hemiplegic cerebral palsy. J Pediatr 137:331–337, 2000.

55. Koman LA, Mooney JF, III, Smith BP, et al: Botulinum toxin type A neuromuscular blockade in the treatment of lower extremity spasticity in cerebral palsy: A randomized, double blind, placebo controlled trial. BOTOX study group. J Pediatr Orthop 20:108–115, 2000.

56. Bakheit AM, Thilmann AF, Ward AB, et al: A randomized, double-blind, placebo-controlled, dose-ranging study to compare the efficacy and safety of three doses of botulinum toxin type A (Dysport) with placebo in upper limb spasticity after stroke. Stroke 31:2402–2406, 2000.

57. Bhakta BB, Cozens JA, Chembelain MA, et al: Impact of botulinum toxin type A in disability and career burden due to arm spasticity after stroke: A randomized double blind placebo controlled trial. J Neurol Neurosurg Psychiatry 69:217–221, 2000.

58. Burbaud P, Wiart L, Dubos JL, et al: A randomized, double blind, placebo controlled trial of botulinum toxin in the treatment of spastic foot in hemiparetic patients. J Neurol Neurosurg Psychiatry 61:265–269, 1996.

59. Simpson DM, Alexander DN, O'Brien CF, et al: Botulinum toxin type A in the treatment of upper extremity spasticity: A randomized, double-blind, placebo-controlled trial. Neurology 46:1306–1310, 1996.

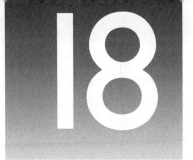

Pharmacology for the Interventional Pain Physician

B. Todd Sitzman, M.D., M.P.H.,
Yuan Chen, M.D.,
R. Rallo Clemans, M.D.,
Scott M. Fishman, M.D., and
Honorio Benzon, M.D.

It is imperative that the interventional pain physician has a thorough understanding of all drugs used in his or her practice. This chapter reviews the clinical pharmacology, pharmacokinetics, possible side effects, and cautions of drugs most commonly used in interventional pain medicine. These drug categories reviewed include radiocontrast agents, local anesthetics, corticosteroids, and botulinum toxin. Radiocontrast agents and local anesthetics are extensively reviewed elsewhere in this text; therefore, their coverage is limited in this chapter.

Regardless of one's familiarity with the pharmacology of a specific classification of medication, a review of each drug's most current product information is well advised. This information is located within published manufacturer information on the medication's package insert, and can often be found within a current Physicians' Desk Reference®.[1] It should also be stressed that there are inherent risks associated with any drug. As such, drugs should be administered only when there is a clinical indication and when the prospects of patient benefit outweigh the risks involved. Additionally, drugs should be administered in the smallest dose that will reliably produce the desired effect. An increased total dose or volume should not be used to compensate for inadequate injection technique.

RADIOCONTRAST AGENTS

Radiographic contrast agents serve a diagnostic role by aiding in the localization of anatomic structures and needle placement under X-ray guidance, such as fluoroscopy. As X-ray beams pass through the body they are attenuated by the different anatomic structures through which they pass. Each structure has an attenuation coefficient dependent on its thickness and the energy level of the X-ray radiation source.[2] Iodinated compounds provide greater X-ray attenuation relative to tissue and bone, and thus decrease the amount of radiation reaching the detector (e.g., fluoroscopic image intensifier). Conventional "iodinated" contrast agents provide radiopacity by way of a triiodinated benzoate anion. Because these iodine atoms are loosely bound, there is a significant amount of unbound iodine in solution leading to a high osmolality. Clinically, the use of first-generation contrast agents is limited by their extremely high osmolar concentration—up to eight times the physiologic level. The higher the osmolality of a conventional contrast agent the greater the physiologic toxicity (e.g., hemodynamic instability and patient discomfort). This led to the development of "second-generation" radiocontrast agents, also known as "nonionic" contrast agents. Although referred to as nonionic, these drugs contain iodine atoms that are tightly bound to a benzene ring with a minimal amount of free iodine. Their higher iodine to particle ratio leads to comparable radiation attenuation with a lower osmolality. The osmolality of these agents is near physiologic (300 mOsmol/kg water) and are more commonly used in spinal injections.

Examples of two commonly used radiocontrast agents include iopamidol (Isovue-M®) and iohexol (Omnipaque®). Each agent is commercially available in preparations of varying ionic concentration and osmolality (Table 18-1, Fig. 18-1).[3,4]

Both iopamidol and iohexol are absorbed rapidly into the bloodstream from intrathecal, epidural, and paraspinal tissues. Plasma levels can be measured within one hour of injection with nearly the entire remaining drug reaching systemic circulation

TABLE 18-1. **RADIOCONTRAST AGENTS USED FOR SPINAL INJECTIONS**

Agent	Concentration (W/V %)	Ionic Concentration (mg iodine/mL)	Osmolality (mOsmol/kg H_2O)
Isovue-M®			
Isovue-M 200	iopamidol 41%	200	300
Isovue-M 300	iopamidol 61%	300	616
Omnipaque®			
Omnipaque 180	iohexol 39%	180	360
Omnipaque 240	iohexol 52%	240	510
Omnipaque 300	iohexol 65%	300	672

within 24 hours.[3,4] Both agents undergo minimal, if any, metabolism, deiodination, or biotransformation. Excretion is greater than 90% renal.

Adverse reactions associated with radiocontrast agents may be from one of three possible etiologies: chemotoxic, osmolar, and allergic. Note that these reactions are relatively rare with the use of "nonionic" rather than the conventional ionic radiocontrast agents (Table 18-2[5]).

The vast majority of severe adverse reactions occur within 15 minutes of exposure to the contrast agent.[6] Therefore, it is imperative to observe all patients receiving contrast agents for a minimum of 30 to 60 minutes following injection. When an allergic reaction is suspected, treatment should be prompt and aggressive using current basic and advanced life support therapies.[7] These measures include oxygen, intravenous fluids, antihistamines (H_1- and H_2-blockers), adrenergic drugs (epinephrine), and corticosteroids.

In patients with a known previous allergic reaction to radiocontrast agents, pretreatment options to minimize a subsequent reaction should be exercised. A recommended regimen, beginning 12 hours prior to contrast exposure is outlined in Table 18-3.[8,9]

LOCAL ANESTHETICS

Local anesthetics (LAs) reversibly interrupt neural conduction by blocking sodium channels located on internal neuronal membranes. This results in inhibition of sodium permeability

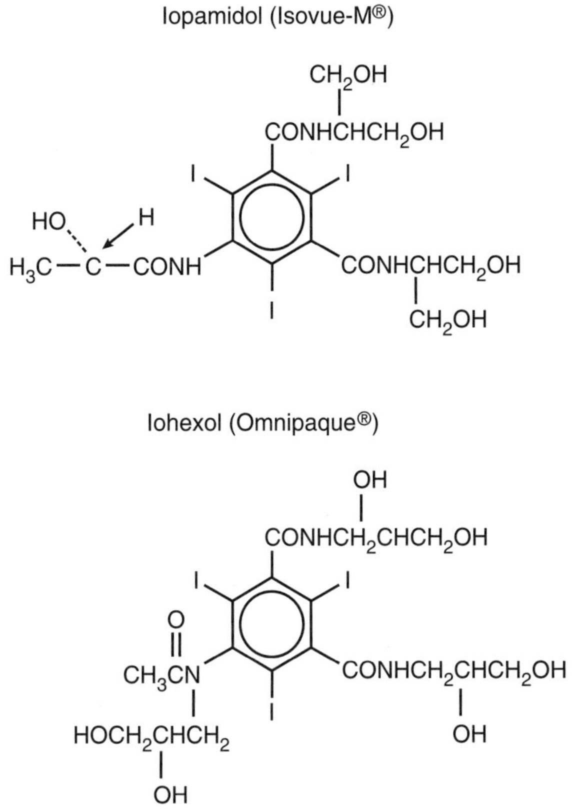

Iopamidol (Isovue-M®)

Iohexol (Omnipaque®)

FIGURE 18–1. Chemical structures of iopamidol and iohexol.

TABLE 18-2. **POTENTIAL ADVERSE REACTIONS ASSOCIATED WITH CONTRAST AGENTS**[5]

A. Chemotoxic
  1. Thyrotoxicosis
  2. Nephrotoxicity

B. Hyperosmolality: rare when used at concentrations that approximate physiologic osmolality
  1. Erythrocyte damage
  2. Endothelial damage and thrombosis
  3. Vasodilation of arteriolar and capillary vasculature (feeling of warmth, discomfort)
  4. Hypervolemia
  5. Cardiac depression

C. Allergic
  1. Vasomotor (warmth, flush)
  2. Cutaneous (scattered hives, severe urticaria)
  3. Bronchospasm (wheezing)
  4. Cardiovascular (hypotension)
  5. Vagal (bradycardia, hypotension, nausea)
  6. Anaphylactoid reaction (angioedema, urticaria, bronchospasm, hypotension)

TABLE 18-3. PRETREATMENT REGIMEN FOR PREVIOUS RADIOCONTRAST ALLERGIC REACTIONS

A. 12 hours pre-contrast exposure
  1. Prednisone 20 to 50 mg p.o.
  2. Ranitidine 50 mg p.o.
  3. Diphenhydramine 25 to 50 mg p.o.

B. 2 hours pre-contrast exposure
  1. Prednisone 20 to 50 mg p.o.
  2. Ranitidine 50 mg p.o.
  3. Diphenhydramine 25 to 50 mg p.o.

C. Immediate pre-injection
  1. Diphenhydramine 25 mg i.v.

necessary for action potential propagation.[10] LAs are weak bases classified on their ester- or amide-type chemical structures. Amide-type LAs have more widespread use in spinal diagnostic and therapeutic injections. Therefore this chapter focuses on the amide-type LAs lidocaine and bupivacaine.[11,12] Readers are directed elsewhere in this text (Chapter 67) for a more extensive review of LA pharmacology.

The clinical action of a LA is often described by its potency, speed of onset, and duration of action. In simplistic terms, a LA's potency is related to lipid solubility, its speed of onset related to pK_a, and duration of action related to protein binding. However, a thorough understanding of LA physiochemical properties is necessary when LAs are used for diagnostic and or prognostic purposes (Table 18-4).

The **potency** of a LA is related to its lipid solubility, which is often described by its in vitro octanol:water partition coefficient.[13] The more lipophilic a LA, the more readily it permeates neuronal membranes, resulting in greater sodium channel binding affinity. Bupivacaine is more potent than lidocaine with a 9-fold greater octanol:water partition coefficient (27.5 versus 2.9).

The **speed of onset** of most LAs is dependent on the dissociation constant (pK_a) and the local tissue's pH. The pK_a is the pH at which a specific drug is half ionized and half in its neutral, unionized form. It is the unionized form that more readily diffuses across the nerve membrane. Therefore, a LA whose pK_a approximates physiologic tissue pH will have a faster onset of action. Another factor affecting speed of onset is the pH of the LA preparation itself. Commercially available

LA preparations containing vasoconstrictors (e.g., epinephrine) are often adjusted to an acidic pH with the addition of hydrochloric salts to enhance the stability of the LA–vasoconstrictor solution. For this reason, clinicians are advised to note the pH of the LA preparation that they are using. If the pH is acidic, and a more rapid onset of action is desired, small amounts of sodium bicarbonate ($NaHCO_3$ to LA volume ratio of 1:20) may be added.[14,15]

The **duration of action** is multifactorial and dependent on the site of injection, the presence of vasoconstrictors, the lipid solubility of the LA itself, and the dose administered. The duration of LA action in clinical practice is not primarily a function of its protein binding. Protein binding is strictly the mode by which LAs are transported in the blood, but the time to vascular absorption has a greater impact on LA duration of action in clinical practice. Longer-acting LAs are often more lipid soluble and hence are more slowly "washed out" from neural membranes, both in vitro and in vivo. The duration of LA action also depends on the absorption from the site of injection. The more vascular the site of injection (subcutaneous > intercostal > caudal > epidural > peripheral nerve > intrathecal), the more rapidly the LA is absorbed into the bloodstream, distributed, metabolized, and excreted.

LA chemical structure, ester or amide, determines its metabolism. Ester-type LAs (e.g., procaine, benzocaine) undergo rapid metabolism via plasma pseudocholinesterase yielding *para*-aminobenzoic acid (PABA) as a metabolic byproduct. PABA has been implicated as an allergenic source with ester-type LAs. Amide-type LAs undergo oxidative dealkylation via the hepatic cytochrome P450 enzyme system as well as conjugation. As such, the clearance of lidocaine and bupivacaine is highly dependent on hepatic blood flow, extraction, and enzyme function. Caution with the use of large volumes of amide-type LAs is advised in patients with liver dysfunction.

Adverse reactions associated with LAs may arise from direct toxicity, reaction to an added vasoconstrictor or preservative, or allergic reaction (Table 18-5). Toxicities result from high blood levels of LA usually as a consequence of accidental intravascular injection, increased uptake from perivascular areas, or overdosage.

Prevention of LA-related adverse reactions is contingent on both appropriate dosage administration (dependent on concentration and volume) and clinical vigilance for early detection of toxic reactions. Additionally, preventive measures such as aspiration for blood prior to injection and administration of contrast agent prior to LA injection (i.e., to assess for vascular uptake) are often utilized to minimize the risk of inadvertent intravascular injection.

TABLE 18-4. PHYSIOCHEMICAL PROPERTIES OF LOCAL ANESTHETIC AGENTS USED IN SPINAL INJECTIONS[16]

Agent	Available Concentration (%)	Onset	Duration (hours)	pK_a (25°C)	pH of Plain Solutions	Recommended Maximal Single Dose (mg) w/o Epi
Lidocaine	0.5, 1, 1.5, 2, 5	Fast	1–2	7.7	6.5	300
Bupivacaine	0.25, 0.5, 0.75	Slow	2–4	8.1	4.5–6	175

TABLE 18-5. ADVERSE REACTIONS ASSOCIATED WITH LOCAL ANESTHETICS[16]

A. Central nervous system (CNS) toxicity. Initial symptoms are usually excitatory as a result of blockade of central inhibitory pathways. In order of appearance, CNS symptoms include:
  1. Numbness of the tongue or foreign taste
  2. Light-headedness
  3. Auditory disturbances
  4. Muscular twitching
  5. Unconsciousness
  6. Convulsions
  7. Coma
  8. Respiratory arrest
  9. Cardiovascular depression

B. Cardiovascular toxicity. Most LAs will not produce cardiovascular toxicity until blood levels are twice that needed to produce seizures.[17] LAs bind to and inhibit cardiac sodium channels, with bupivacaine binding more avidly and for a longer duration than lidocaine[18]

C. Neuronal toxicity[19,20]
  1. Preservative related (e.g., sodium metabisulfite)
  2. Concentration related (e.g., 5% lidocaine)

D. Vasoconstrictor reaction: due to inadvertent vascular injection or uptake of epinephrine. These are commonly misdiagnosed as allergic reactions
  1. Tachycardia
  2. Elevated blood pressure
  3. Headache
  4. Apprehension

E. Allergic reaction: more common with ester-type LAs[21]
  1. Vasomotor (warmth, flush)
  2. Cutaneous (scattered hives, severe urticaria)
  3. Bronchospasm (wheezing)
  4. Cardiovascular (hypotension)
  5. Vagal (bradycardia, hypotension, nausea)
  6. Anaphylactoid reaction (angioedema, urticaria, bronchospasm, hypotension)

Treatment of an adverse reaction should be prompt and aggressive, based on the severity of symptoms. Central nervous system (CNS) toxicities necessitate supportive therapies (i.e., airway, breathing, circulation, supplemental oxygen), but may also require pharmacological intervention. Seizures may be terminated with an intravenous benzodiazepine (midazolam 0.05 to 0.1 mg/kg) or with an intravenous short-acting barbiturate (thiopental 1 to 2 mg/kg). Signs and symptoms of cardiovascular toxicity should be treated as aggressively as possible using Advanced Cardiac Life Support guidelines.[7] Note that in the setting of LA-induced ventricular dysrhythmias, amiodarone rather than lidocaine should be used. Lastly, allergic reactions to amide-type LAs are rare. If one is suspected, treatment should include administration of intravenous fluids, antihistamines (H_1- and H_2-blockers), adrenergic drugs (epinephrine), and corticosteroids.

CORTICOSTEROIDS

Corticosteroids exert effects on many important physiologic functions. Some of these include regulation of carbohydrate, protein, and lipid metabolism; fluid and electrolyte balance; cardiovascular, immune, endocrine, and nervous system effects; and effects on kidney and muscle. Corticosteroids have widespread pharmacologic actions, which provide therapeutic benefits but may have serious side effects. Naturally occurring corticosteroids are classified into three functional groups: mineralocorticoids, glucocorticoids, and adrenal androgens, all produced by the adrenal cortex.

Mineralocorticoids are 21-carbon-atom structures produced in the outer zona glomerulosa of the adrenal cortex. Aldosterone, the primary mineralocorticoid, is responsible for fluid and electrolyte balance and can lead to striking effects on the cardiovascular system.

Glucocorticoids (GCS), the most important naturally occurring one being cortisol, are 21-carbon-atom structures produced by the inner adrenal cortex (zona reticularis). GCS derive their name from their function: increasing blood glucose levels by stimulating hepatic gluconeogenesis while increasing protein synthesis in muscle. The focus of this chapter is on the anti-inflammatory effects of GCS. As pain medicine practitioners we must become familiar with GCS side effects, which, despite the use of relatively small doses, may be troublesome.

The hormones produced by the adrenal cortex are all part of a family of compounds derived from the cyclopentanoperhydrophenanthrene ring structure (Fig. 18-2). This structure includes three cyclohexane rings and one cyclopentane ring.[22] Steroids exert a variety of physiologic effects, and small modifications of the basic steroid structure can lead to significant differences in function and side effects. It is important to understand common characteristics as well as unique properties of individual compounds.

All human steroids are derived from cholesterol. Most of the cholesterol for adrenal use (i.e., corticosteroid production) is provided by the circulating plasma lipoproteins. Cholesterol is primarily in the form of low-density lipoprotein (LDL) with some contribution from high-density lipoprotein HDL.[22] Cortisol (hydrocortisone) is the active, natural GCS produced by the body (Fig. 18-3).[23] Modifications at sites on the molecule produce synthetic analogues with different properties such as

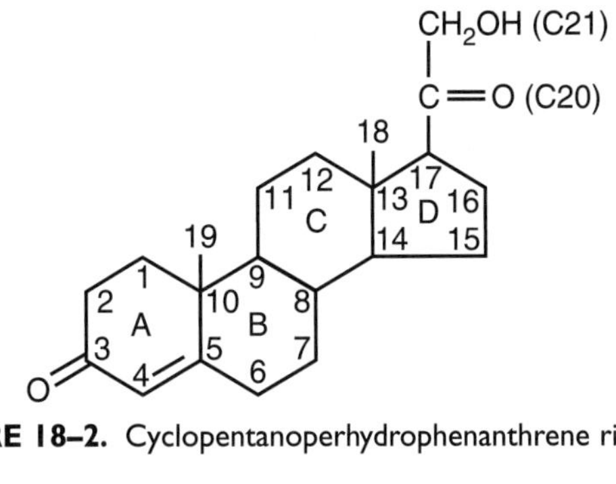

FIGURE 18–2. Cyclopentanoperhydrophenanthrene ring.

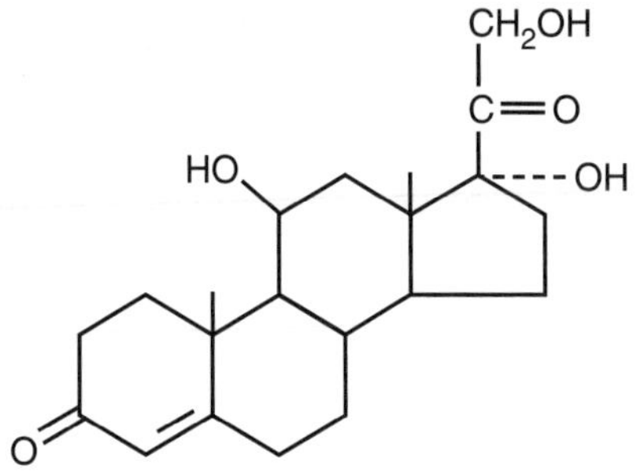

FIGURE 18–3. Cortisol.

varying mineralocorticoid activity and anti-inflammatory potency. Relative biological potency of synthetic analogues is compared with cortisol in Table 18-6.

Cortisol has a half-life of 70 to 90 minutes. Changes in structure alter metabolism, causing steroid analogues to have different half-lives.[23] The biological half-life represents the time for one half the given drug's serum concentration to "disappear" from circulation. Half-life, however, is a poor indicator of duration of action, which is best reflected by period of ACTH suppression after a single dose. Short-acting GCS have duration of action of 8 to 12 hours, intermediate of up to 36 hours, and long-acting of over 48 hours.[24]

Depending on the physiologic effects desired, the use of a steroid with differing physiochemical properties may be advantageous. For example, betamethasone and dexamethasone exhibit prolonged anti-inflammatory and hypothalamic–pituitary–adrenal suppression and are therefore suited for the treatment of disorders requiring inhibition of ACTH secretion. However, their use would not be advised in a clinical situation requiring a rapid physiologic effect, such as an allergic emergency.[25] One must also keep in mind relative mineralocorticoid potencies, which could have profound effects in patients with impaired cardiovascular function.[24]

GCS secretion is regulated by interactions between the hypothalamus, pituitary, and adrenal glands. During "nonstress" periods, cortisol synthesis depends on interactions that stimulate afferent signals to the CNS. These include baroreceptors, chemoreceptors, nociceptors, as well as emotional stimuli. The thalamus, hypothalamus, medulla, and pons receive input from these receptors and convey signals to the hypothalamic paraventricular nucleus, which increases corticotropin-releasing hormone (CRH) synthesis.[26] CRH is the most important regulator of corticotropin (ACTH) secretion. ACTH is synthesized as a part of a large precursor molecule, proopiomelanocortin (POMC) that is processed into several peptides.[27] The principal peptide produced in the anterior pituitary is ACTH. ACTH stimulates the zona fasciculata cells of the adrenal cortex to increase steroid synthesis and release of cortisol occurs within 5 minutes.[26]

ACTH is secreted in episodic bursts resulting in varying plasma ACTH levels at different times of the day. Plasma ACTH and, consequently, cortisol levels are highest in the early morning.[22] Recent estimates of GCS secretion are about 5 to 10 mg/m^2 of cortisol per day.[28] The effect of acute physical or psychological stress activates the hypothalamic–pituitary–adrenal axis. Surgery is one of the most potent activators of the axis. In periods of severe stress cortisol synthesis can increase 5- to 10-fold.[28]

Negative feedback occurs by circulating plasma cortisol, which inhibits both ACTH secretion and POMC gene transcription. Plasma cortisol also inhibits CRH release from the hypothalamus by binding to steroid receptors in the CNS. Other inhibitory mechanisms on CRH release include atrial natriuretic factor and substance P. Hypoperfusion of the adrenal gland, and some medications, can also inhibit cortisol synthesis.[26]

The hypothalamus is first to be suppressed by steroid dosing but the first to recover after therapy. ACTH levels return to normal after several months. The adrenals are last to be suppressed and the slowest to recover. Therefore, they may not normalize for 6 to 12 months. Patients may be vulnerable to stress caused by surgery or infection during one or more years after long-term therapy. Therefore, patients receiving long-term steroid therapy should be given a parenteral dosing of hydrocortisone prior to stressful situations.

TABLE 18-6. PROPERTIES OF SYNTHETIC CORTISOL ANALOGUES

Drug	GCS Potency (mg)	Mineralocorticoid Activity	Duration of Action (hours)	Plasma Half-life (minutes)
Short acting				
Cortisone	25	1	8–12	60
Hydrocortisone	20	0.8	8–12	90
Intermediate acting				
Prednisone	5	0.25	24–36	60
Prednisolone	5	0.25	24–36	200
Methylprednisolone	4	0	24–36	180
Triamcinolone	4	0	24–36	300
Long acting				
Dexamethasone	0.75	0	36–54	200
Betamethasone	0.6	0	36–54	200

Circulating GCS is 90% bound to cortisol binding globulin (transcortin), which is present in a small amount but has high affinity for GCS.[26] Cortisol binding globulin is, therefore, saturated first. Albumin, which has low binding affinity but is abundant in serum, also binds GCS. The free fraction is the amount of steroid that is active. Any decrease in albumin causes higher free steroid level, and therefore increased risk of toxicity.[24] From the serum, steroids passively diffuse through target cell membranes and form complexes with cytoplasmic GCS receptors.

Mechanisms of Gene Regulation: GCS affect gene regulation in three distinct ways: induction of transcription, inhibition of transcription, as well as nontranscriptional effects.

INDUCTION OF TRANSCRIPTION:

GCS receptors and other steroid hormone receptors are part of a supergene family of DNA binding proteins that regulate gene transcription. They have a hormone-binding site and a DNA-binding site and are expressed in most cells.[29] The inactive receptor is bound to a large protein complex which keeps the GCS receptor in a conformation that facilitates GCS binding and prevents the inactive receptor from localizing to the nucleus.[29] Once GCS binds to the receptor, the large protein complex dissociates and the hormone–receptor complex acquires the ability to bind to DNA. This activated complex migrates to the nucleus where it binds DNA and affects gene expression. It has been suggested that the number of steroid responsive genes per cell is between 10 and 100. In the nucleus GCS receptors bind to DNA at certain promoter regions of steroid-responsive genes. This binding changes the rate of transcription of the gene by changing the configuration of DNA, exposing previously masked areas, causing increased binding of transcription factors.[29]

INHIBITION OF TRANSCRIPTION:

GCS receptor–DNA complex also causes gene repression by other, less well understood mechanisms.[29]

NONTRANSCRIPTIONAL EFFECTS:

Corticobinding protein (CBP) that is not bound to GCS can bind to target tissues. GCS can than bind to CBP–receptor complex and activate adenylyl cyclase and the cAMP-dependent transduction pathway.

Metabolism: In the liver most steroid hormones are inactivated by the *reduction* of the delta double bond (which is usually in conjunction with a 3-ketone) by 5-alpha reductase. This is the rate-limiting step in cortisol metabolism. *Oxidation* occurs by removal of side chains, conversion of the 11-beta hydroxyl group to a ketone, and conversion of C21-hydroxyl to a carboxylic acid. *Hydroxylation* occurs to a minor extent to produce a highly water-soluble product, whereas *conjugation* renders metabolites of cortisol more water-soluble. Cirrhosis and certain medications may limit hepatic metabolism of GCS. Most cortisol is eliminated by renal excretion of hepatic metabolites.[22] The kidney is the major site of extrahepatic metabolism. Cortisol is converted to cortisone here. Nevertheless, less than 1% of cortisol is renally eliminated.

Physiologic Effects: Replacement therapy and treatment of pain, allergic states, or undesirable inflammatory processes are the most important uses of GCS. Replacement corticosteroids may be given by oral, inhaled, or parenteral routes. GCS absorption through the gastrointestinal tract occurs in the jejunum and peak plasma levels are seen in 30 to 90 minutes.[24] GCS replacement in periods of stress may be necessary for patients who have received GCS in the last 6 months.[26]

It is generally assumed that corticosteroids relieve pain by reducing inflammation; however, there are additional explanations of how they affect pain transmission and perception. Persistent noxious stimulation leads to enhanced responsiveness of dorsal horn neurons. This central sensitization is likely due to the increased production of prostaglandins. When administered neuraxially, corticosteroids may block the development of this hyperalgesic state. Corticosteroids have also been shown to block nociceptive C fiber transmission. By directly stabilizing neural membranes, GCS prevent the development of ectopic discharges from neuromas.[30,31]

Inflammation is the body's way of mobilizing appropriate cell populations to the site of injury. Excessive inflammation, however, can be detrimental. Varying levels of GCS exist in the circulation at all times. We can make use of this "natural remedy" to treat certain inflammatory states. The inflammatory cascade is initiated with tissue injury. Neurohumoral signals that initiate an inflammatory response also activate transcription factors, which stimulate the production of enzymes and cytokines associated with inflammation.[32] These inflammatory mediators are released and activate the endothelium, resulting in an influx of inflammatory cells into the site of injury.[32] Prostanoids are formed by hydrolysis of arachidonic acid (AA) from membrane glycerophospholipids by phospholipase A2.[33] Free AA is then converted to prostaglandin G2 and then to PGH_2 by PGH synthase. This enzyme, which occurs in two isoforms, is referred to as cyclooxygenase (COX)-1 and COX-2. PGH_2 is then converted to different prostanoids.[33]

Some of the cytokines resulting from the cascade are: IL-1, IL-4, IL-13, TNF-alpha (activate the endothelium), IgE (activates mast cells and release of TNG-alpha); IL-3, IL-5, GM-CSF, interferon-gamma (prolong eosinophil survival, increase adhesion molecule expression, potentiate eosinophil degranulation); and chemokines (induce cell migration and activate certain cell types).[32]

During the inflammatory response cells release a number of mediators, which stimulate the brain to activate the hypothalamic–pituitary–adrenal axis. This results in an increased level of cortisol in circulation, to help balance the inflammatory response.[32] GCS are the most potent agents in controlling inflammation, primarily as a result of altering gene transcription.[29]

GCS suppress inflammation by the following methods:

1. Maintain microcirculation integrity by causing a reduction in endothelial permeability. This occurs by the inhibition of TNF-alpha and IL-1, IL-4, and IL-13 release from infiltrating cells and by the inhibition of nitric oxide synthase.[32]
2. Maintain cell membrane integrity by preventing sequestration of intracellular water.[25]
3. Decrease the influx of inflammatory cells by inhibiting chemokines.[32]
4. Reduce the life of certain inflammatory cells (e.g., eosinophils) by inhibiting the production of GM-CSF, IL-3, and IL-5.[29,32]

5. Up-regulate the transcription of anti-inflammatory genes (lipocortin, neutral endopeptidase, and inhibitors of plasminogen activator).[32]

6. Suppress the transcription of genes involved in inflammation: cytokine genes (collagenase, elastase, plasminogen activator, nitric oxide synthase, cyclooxygenase type II, and most cytokine and chemokine genes) and the genes for their receptors.[29,32,33]

7. Secondary effects by induction of enzymes that metabolize inflammatory mediators.[29]

Side Effects: GCS are widely used by physicians of nearly all medical specialties. Short courses of GCS therapy (<3 weeks) are considered safe. Side effects from short-term therapy are rare and usually short-lived[24] (Table 18-7).

The use of GCS injections, either with or without LA, in management of back pain and joint arthropathies is widely accepted. Despite small doses, systemic absorption of the steroid from the epidural space may result in depression of plasma cortisol levels.[41] Knight and Burnell reported several cases of Cushing's syndrome induced by multiple epidural steroid injections when the cumulative dose exceeded 200 mg of methylprednisolone. There have also been case reports of decreased insulin sensitivity (in normal as well as diabetic individuals) and Cushing's syndrome after a single epidural steroid injection.[42] These reports describe patients with typical cushingoid appearance, proximal muscle weakness (steroid myopathy), and decreased serum cortisol levels indicating adrenal suppression.[41,43] Early recognition of these effects should allow for discontinuation of the GCS in a timely manner.

Long-term therapy, with GCS doses near physiologic levels, is relatively safe. However, when supraphysiologic replacement is needed, there is a dose-related increase in the incidence of adverse effects. Especially at risk are people with difficulty metabolizing GCS, such as alcoholics, patients with liver disease, or patients with hypoalbuminemia. These conditions may result in larger amounts of circulating drug. Risk is also increased when the dose is not adjusted for patients with lower BMI.[24]

Major adverse effects of long-term GCS therapy include Cushing's syndrome, a reversible metabolic syndrome with physical findings including obesity, impaired glucose tolerance or diabetes, hypertension, and gonadal dysfunction.

The effects on carbohydrate and protein metabolism, which promote hyperglycemia, have a teleologic role to protect glucose-dependent cerebral function. Induction of hepatic enzymes stimulates the formation of glucose, peripheral utilization of glucose is decreased, and there is an antagonism of insulin effects. This promotes glucose storage as glycogen. Normally this may cause worsening of preexisting diabetes, which resolves when GCS are discontinued; however, new-onset diabetes may also occur.[23,25] Increased plasma triglycerides secondary to insulin insufficiency may also occur. Weight gain may be related to increased appetite and fluid retention, occurring preferentially in the face, posterior neck and trunk.[24]

Electrolyte abnormalities such as hypokalemia may also occur, usually when using GCS with strong mineralocorticoid effects.[24] Edema and hypertension may take place as a result of sodium retention and vasoconstriction. Vasoconstriction results from GCS potentiation of norepinephrine and opposition of natural vasodilators such as histamine. At greatest risk are those with preexisting hypertension and those treated with GCS for longer than 2 weeks.[24]

Osteoporosis occurs by steroid inhibition of intestinal absorption of calcium and an increase in renal excretion of calcium, which may result in hyperparathyroidism. This stimulates osteoclast activity resulting in bone resorption and osteoblast inhibition, which inhibits synthesis of bone. At highest risk are female patients who are postmenopausal, alcoholic, or hypoalbuminemic. Calcium supplements, calcitonin, bisphosphonates, and exercise are treatments for this side effect.[24]

Steroid-induced myopathy is uncommon, but seen mostly with fluorinated agents such as triamcinolone, betamethasone, and dexamethasone.[24,26] The etiology is unclear; however, it may result from decreased glucose and amino acid uptake by affected muscles. It is characterized by predominant involvement of the proximal (pelvic girdle) muscles. Treatment is physical therapy and decreasing or discontinuing the dose.

Cataracts and glaucoma may occur with chronic treatment. Children are the group most at risk. Glaucoma is caused by swelling of collagen strands at the angle of the anterior chamber of the eye causing resistance to outflow of aqueous humor. The treatment is to discontinue the steroid treatment and monitor intraocular pressure closely.[24]

Nausea, vomiting, and PUD may result from decreased enteral mucosal cell production. Antacid use or taking medication with food may decrease these symptoms. Esophagitis may occur and may be related to reflux or overgrowth of

TABLE 18-7. POTENTIAL ADVERSE REACTIONS ASSOCIATED WITH CORTICOSTEROIDS[34–40]

Fluid retention
Elevated blood pressure
Mood changes
Hyperglycemia
Generalized erythema/facial flushing
Menstrual irregularities
Gastritis/peptic ulcer disease
Hypothalamic–pituitary–adrenal axis suppression
Cushing's syndrome (obesity, impaired glucose tolerance or diabetes, hypertension, and gonadal dysfunction)
Bone demineralization
Steroid myopathy/weakness
Allergic reaction

candida albicans. Pancreatitis is uncommon and may be related to increased viscosity of pancreatic secretions and obstruction.[24]

The hematologic effects of GCS result from an influx of granulocytes from bone marrow thereby increasing the number of circulating leukocytes, but not total number of leukocytes.[24] Immunosuppression results in the inhibition of natural killer cells and the migration of macrophages and neutrophils. Wound healing may also be delayed secondary to inhibition of fibroblasts and collagen production.

CNS effects are variable and may include insomnia, mood changes (from mild anxiety to psychosis), and may theoretically aggravate preexisting epilepsy.[22,44] Several other purported adverse reactions have been reported following corticosteroid injection. Sterile meningitis and arachnoiditis has been reported following intrathecal injection of methylprednisolone—although possibly related to the polyethylene additive of the preparation.[45] Although rare, anaphylactoid reactions have been reported following intravenous, intramuscular, and soft-tissue corticosteroid injections.[46–48] The "succinate" salts of hydrocortisone and methylprednisolone have been most implicated, with absence of any allergic-type reaction following administration of acetate or phosphate salts of the same corticosteroid. Any type of anaphylactic reaction should be treated promptly and aggressively with supportive therapies (i.e., airway, breathing, circulation, supplemental oxygen), including advanced cardiac life support measures when indicated.[7]

Lastly, coadministration of corticosteroids with preservative-containing LAs (e.g., methylparabin-, propylparaben-, and phenol-containing LAs) may result in flocculation of the steroid. Injection of a steroid precipitate poses a theoretical risk of mechanical damage to soft-tissue (cartilage, tendon, joint), neural, and vascular structures. An inadvertent injection of a steroid precipitate into the artery of Adamkiewicz during a thoracic or upper-lumbar level transforaminal epidural steroid injection could result in spinal cord ischemia leading to profound lower extremity motor deficits, even paraplegia. For this reason, the injectionist should always visually inspect the injectate for compatibility if a corticosteroid is mixed with a preservative-containing LA.

BOTULINUM TOXIN THERAPY

History and Early Clinical Development: Botulinum toxins are potent neurotoxins produced by the Gram-negative anaerobic bacterium *Clostridium botulinum*. They produce flaccid paralysis by blocking acetylcholine release at the neuromuscular junction. There are eight botulinum neurotoxin subtypes. The A, B, C1, D, E, F, and G subtypes are neurotoxins. The C2 subtype is not.

Early development of botulinum toxin began during World War II. Although much of this initial work was carried out on botulinum toxin A (BTA), other types of botulinum toxin (BT) were also studied. The purpose was to develop a polyvalent toxoid for immunization purposes. After the war, a crystallized form of BTA became available and stimulated considerable scientific interest. Scott initiated efforts to study BT in a monkey model of strabismus in the late 1960s and reported clinical use in correcting strabismus in humans in the early 1980s.[49]

In 1989 the FDA approved BTA for use in treating strabismus, blepharospasm, and hemifacial spasm. In December 2000

botulinum toxin B (BTB) was FDA-approved for use in treating cervical dystonia. BTs have been used in a vast array of clinical problems: achalasia, anismus, benign prostatic hypertrophy, dysphonia, dystonias, essential tremor, hyperhidrosis, kyphoscoliosis, low back pain, migraine and tension-type headache, myofascial pain, pancreatitis, pelvic floor disorders, rectal fissures, sialorrhea, spasticity, temporomandibular joint syndrome, urinary sphincter dysfunction, wrinkles, and various other movement disorders.

Among the seven botulinum neurotoxins, type A and type B have been introduced into clinical practice. Type A is available in the USA as Botox (Allergan, Inc., Irvine, CA) and in several other countries as Dysport (Ipsen Ltd, Berkshire, UK). Type B is available in the USA as Myobloc (Elan Pharmaceuticals, San Diego, CA) and in European countries as NeuroBloc (Elan Pharmaceuticals, San Diego, CA).

Structure and Mechanism of Action of BTs: BTs are synthesized as single-chain polypeptides and are activated by proteolytic enzymes in a cleaving process (Fig. 18-4). The cleaved heavy chain is responsible for high-affinity docking of the neurotoxin to the presynaptic nerve terminal receptor, enabling the internalization of the bound toxin into the cell.[50] The light chain is a zinc-dependent endopeptidase that cleaves membrane proteins responsible for docking acetylcholine vesicles on the inner side of the nerve terminal membrane. The cleavage of these proteins irreversibly precludes fusion of the vesicles with the nerve membrane, thereby preventing release of neurotransmitters into the neuromuscular junction.[51]

Type A BT appears to be the most potent of the subtypes, and, when injected clinically, has the longest duration of action. While type B and F have limited clinical use, and others are the subject of further study, the multiple differences thus far observed suggest that the subtypes are not interchangeable.

Pharmacological effect of BTs occurs in three stages: binding, internalization, and proteolysis.[52]

BINDING: The binding of BTs to the motor endplate presynaptic membrane is a two-stage process.[53,54] The C-terminal region of the heavy chain binds in a serotype-specific manner to receptors on the axon terminals of cholinergic neurons. Binding is irreversible and is independent of nerve activity.[55] Specific gangliosides have been proposed as the receptors, as well as specific proteins.[56,57]

INTERNALIZATION: Binding of the neurotoxin induces the formation of an endosome that carries the toxin into the axon terminal. Internalization of the bound toxin occurs by receptor-mediated endocytosis. Once formed, the contents of the endosome become increasingly acidic, most likely by normal cellular mechanisms. The decrease in pH within the endosome prompts a configurational change in the toxin, which then forms a channel through the membrane. The channel allows all or part of the toxin to enter the cytosol.[58] This process is pH dependent.

PROTEOLYSIS (FIG. 18-5): The exceptional potency of the botulinum neurotoxins has long suggested that a catalytic effect is involved. In the cytosol the proteolytic effects occur. BT types A, E, and C cleave synaptosome-associated protein-25 (SNAP-25). Types B, D, F, and G cleave the synaptic protein synaptobrevin, also known as vesicle-associated membrane

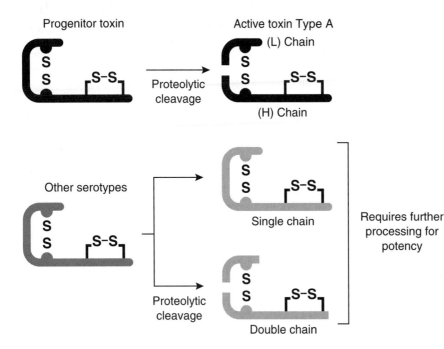

FIGURE 18–4. Structures of botulinum toxins.

protein (VAMP). Type C also cleaves syntaxin.[59] Each of these protein substrates participates in the formation of the exocytotic SNARE (soluble N-ethylmaleimide-sensitive factor attachment protein receptor) complex, which is essential for fusion of acetylcholine-containing vesicles with the presynaptic membrane, a prerequisite for acetylcholine release. SNAREs form coiled bundles that bridge the membrane of the synaptic vesicle with the plasma membrane by an interaction between VAMP, which is anchored in the vesicle membrane, and syntaxin, which is anchored in the plasma membrane, perhaps preceded by an interaction between VAMP and SNAP-25.[60]

The effects of the botulinum neurotoxins are due to irreversible inhibition of the release of acetylcholine from cholinergic nerve terminals, including those of motor neurons, preganglionic sympathetic and parasympathetic neurons, and postganglionic parasympathetic nerves.

Recovery: Functional denervation is observable for 6 weeks up to 6 months following injection, but typically lasts for 3 to 4 months. During peak effect, muscle histology shows evidence of atrophy and increased variation of fiber size following BT administration. Recovery of functional innervation is associated with histological evidence of neuronal sprouting, reinnervation and enlargement of some endplates, along with the formation of new smaller endplates. There is also an increase in the number of muscle fibers innervated per axon, with some fibers coming to be innervated by more than one axon. Recovery is complete after allowing sufficient time for regrowth.[61] Fiber size, and presumably neuromuscular function, returns to essentially normal, even after multiple cycles of injection and recovery.[62]

Because of the incidental findings of the effectiveness of BTs in nonmuscle-related disorders, researchers have proposed other potential mechanisms of these toxins. One of the most exciting hypotheses regarding the mechanism of analgesia after the use of BT suggests that there may be a direct effect of BT on noncholinergic neurons, resulting in reduced release of glutamate,

substance P, CGRP, and other substances.[63] The injection of subcutaneous nonparalytic doses of BTA into the paws of rats exposed to the formalin experimental pain model was associated with a lack of observable decline in motor behavior compared with controls. However, there was clear evidence of reduced pain behavior compared to controls, as well as a reduction in the release of glutamate release and the expression of C-fos in the dorsal spinal cord.[64]

Antibody Formation: The incidence of antibody formation was reported in 32 patients with spasmodic torticollis who received repeated injections of BTA.[65] Four patients (12.5%) produced antibodies after 2 to 9 months of treatment. Since the dose range used in blepharospasm is much less than that used in cervical dystonial spasmodic torticollis, the incidence of antibody formation is far less. Based upon the data from a number of studies, the incidence of antibody formation with BTA for the treatment of cervical dystonia is probably less than 5%.[66]

Since BTA and BTB display quite different chemical compositions, it has long been felt that the antibody cross reactivity between the two is extremely small.[67] Nonetheless concern has been expressed over the potential problem of neutralizing antibody formation with lower potency and shorter-acting BT serotypes. Higher toxin doses and frequent injections appear to be associated with neutralizing antibody formation.[68]

Preparation and Dosages: BTs are measured in units. One unit is defined as the LD_{50} in female Swiss Webster mice. Botox is supplied in freeze-dried powder of 100 ± 10 U w/ 0.5 mg human albumin and 0.9 mg NaCl per vial. It needs to be reconstituted with preservative-free saline into volume of dilution 1 to 8 ml/100 U. The manufacturer recommends consuming the product within 4 hours of reconstitution. Myobloc is available in ready to use solution of 2,500, 5,000, and 10,000 U per vial with a shelf life of up to 36 months refrigerated and 9 months at room temperature. The estimated human lethal dose of Botox is about 2,800 to 3,500 U for a

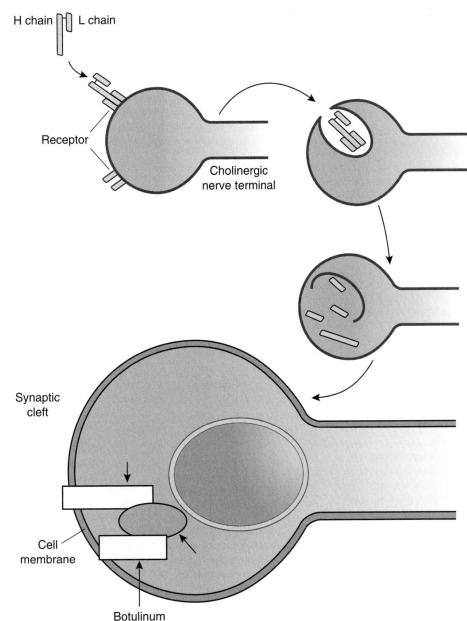

FIGURE 18–5. Mechanisms of action of botulinum toxins.

70 kg adult. The recommended adult dose is 50 to 100 U. The LD_{50} of Myobloc in humans is 144,000 U. The ideal dose and number of injection sites has not been elucidated. Myobloc has been used safely at as much as 15,000 to 20,000 U per visit.

BOTULINUM TOXIN CLINICAL APPLICATIONS

Cervical Dystonia: This is the most common focal dystonia, characterized by intermittent or continuous spasms of the sternocleidomastoid, trapezius, and other cervical muscles. About 70% of patients with cervical dystonia report pain as a principal complaint. Controlled clinical trials in cervical dystonia suggest a dramatic effect of BT injections in controlling the pain component of this syndrome. Not surprisingly, improvements in movement and range of motion (ROM) were also demonstrated. Supporting these findings is a survey of

19 studies in which BT was used for the treatment of cervical dystonia.[69] The mean weighted percentage of patients reporting an improvement in pain was 76% (range 50 to 100% for the 16 studies reporting pain results; $N = 938$ patients). Per-muscle doses of BT ranged from 40 to 120 U of Botox, while per-treatment doses ranged between 100 and 374 U.

Tempomandibular Disorder: Although the pathologies of tempomandibular disorder (TMD) may be arthrogenic or myogenic, the symptoms of these disorders are similar and most commonly manifest as pain in the orofacial region. In preliminary studies BTs have been successfully used to treat these disorders. The treatments involved injection of Botox 5 to 25 U into medial pterygoid and temporalis, 5 to 10 U into masseter, or Myobloc of 1,000 to 3,000 U into these muscles.[70–72]

Headaches: The primary headache disorders consist of migraine, tension-type headache, and cluster headache. Although cluster headache is rare, migraine and tension-type headache are extremely common. The current therapeutic approach to migraine and tension-type headache consists of acute and/or prophylactic treatments that offer substantial relief for many patients but are less than satisfactory for many others.

MIGRAINE: The possible efficacy of BT in relieving migraine was noted serendipitously in certain patients who were receiving type A injections for cosmetic treatment of facial wrinkles. Several of these patients reported coincident improvement in their headaches, which prompted an open-label trial of BT in patients with migraine.[73] The investigators enrolled 106 subjects who had been identified retrospectively as having gained relief from migraine after cosmetic treatment with BT, along with other patients who had primary headache disorders. All were treated prospectively with BTA. Treatment was judged effective on the basis of headache symptom reduction. Fifty-one percent of patients reported complete elimination of headaches (mean duration of benefit 4.1 months) after the BT injections, and 27 (38%) had partial responses (mean duration of benefit 2.7 months). Silberstein et al.[74] and Brin et al.[75] conducted double-blind, placebo-controlled trials to assess the efficacy of this treatment. Compared with vehicle treatment, subjects in the 25 U BTA treatment group showed significantly fewer migraine attacks per month, a reduced maximum severity of migraines, a reduced number of days using acute migraine medications, and reduced incidence of migraine-associated vomiting.

Opida[76] conducted an open-label evaluation of the efficacy of BTB in treating transformed migraine headaches. Forty-seven patients who qualified for the study had at least four headaches and several days of disabling headaches within a 4-week baseline period. Treatment entailed doses of 5,000 U of BTB injected into three or more muscles. Injection sites were chosen on the basis of pain distribution, trigger points, and frown lines. Sixty-four percent of 47 patients reported improvement in headache intensity and severity. For all 47 patients, the mean headache frequency decreased significantly from baseline to week 4.

TENSION HEADACHE: Freund and Schwartz[77] conducted a retrospective study of 21 patients with chronic tension-type headache (based on IHS criteria) who also had palpable muscle tenderness of the scalp or upper neck. Patients received botulinum BTA 100 U over five sites representing muscle points most tender to palpation in the scalp and upper neck. Eighteen patients experienced a greater than or equal to 50% reduction in headache frequency.

Smuts et al[78] conducted a randomized, double-blind, placebo-controlled trial of BTA on 37 patients with tension-type headache. Patients received type A 100 U or placebo, divided among six injection sites: two in the temporal muscles and four in the cervical muscles. Patients kept a diary of headache intensity and frequency and medication use, starting 1 month before treatment and continuing for 3 months after injections were administered. The actively treated group showed a trend toward decreased headache severity over the 3 months after injection. This improvement reached statistical significance at month 3 relative to the pretreatment month.

Similarly, the number of headache-free days was greater at month 3 than at baseline. The Chronic Pain Index, a subjective indicator of pain intensity, also reflected improvement in the actively treated patients but not in the placebo group.

Alternative explanations for the efficacy of BT in headache invoke its possible neurogenic effects (both peripheral and central). BT affects the release of several neurotransmitters and also affects the parasympathetic nervous system. It is therefore possible that the toxin has an antinociceptive effect that is separate from its effect on muscle activation. Several lines of evidence support this view. Jankovic and Schwartz[79] noted that pain improved long before any reduction in muscle spasm could be detected in a large series of patients with cervical dystonia. Aoki and Cui[80] have found that BTA reduced inflammatory pain in the rat formalin model (formalin injected subcutaneously into the paw). Finally, BT appears to decrease the release of inflammatory peptides such as substance P.[63] If this explanation is correct, BT may prove useful in a wide variety of painful conditions, including those in which muscle tension is not a contributing factor.

Whiplash Injury: Whiplash-associated disorders (WADs) occur as a result of trauma and are often due to motor vehicle accidents and sports injuries. Cervical injury is attributed to rapid extension followed by neck flexion. The exact pathophysiology of WAD is uncertain but probably involves some degree of aberrant muscle spasms and may produce a wide range of symptoms. BTA has been studied in small trials of patients with WAD and has generally been found to relieve pain and improve range of motion. In addition, recent preliminary data from a small trial showed that BTB produced almost immediate pain relief for most patients with postwhiplash headache. Freund and Schwartz conducted a pilot study exploring the potential benefits of relaxing selected neck muscles with BTA.[81,82] In this randomized, placebo-controlled trial, 28 subjects with chronic grade 2 WAD received injections of BTA 100 U or saline placebo. Each subject received five injections of 0.2 mL each into one or more of the following sites: splenius capitis, rectus capitis, semispinalis capitis, and trapezius, bilaterally. The five injection sites were chosen by palpation and corresponded to the five most tender cervical muscular points. At 2 weeks after injection the treatment group showed a trend toward improvement in ROM and a reduction in pain. At 4 weeks after injection this group was significantly improved from preinjection levels ($p < 0.01$). The placebo group did not demonstrate any significant changes at any time after treatment. The functional index revealed a trend toward improvement in the treatment group but the results were not significant. Additional data were gathered for a 3-month follow-up period but have not yet been published. The treatment group continued to demonstrate significant pain reduction and improved ROM at 2 months ($p < 0.05$) and 3 months ($p < 0.05$).

BTB is also being evaluated for several painful conditions, including postwhiplash headaches. An open-label study evaluating BTB for the treatment of 31 patients with disabling headaches after injury was recently conducted.[83] Patients had pain radiating from the occipital region to the orbit region that had lasted longer than 5 months. They also had restricted head flexion, rotation, and side bending. Before treatment, all patients rated their pain as severe (mean score 9.4 on a 0 to 10 numeric rating scale (NRS)). They received injections of BTB

5,000 U divided equally among the suboccipital muscles (rectus capitis posterior major and minor, obliquus capitis inferior and superior). Seventy-one responded favorably to treatment, reporting a decrease in headache pain and frequency.

Hemifacial Pain: Caused by vascular irritation or compression of the facial nerve leading to the brainstem, hemifacial spasm is characterized by intermittent clonic or tonic contractions of the muscles supplied by the facial nerve. It is usually a chronic, progressive disease, and generally presents unilaterally. Only 8% of study participants reported meaningful benefit from any of these agents. Surgical microvascular decompression of the facial nerve can effectively cure the condition in most cases, but serious potential complications, such as permanent facial weakness or hearing loss, deter many patients from undergoing this procedure.[84]

BT has become the treatment of choice for hemifacial spasm.[84,85] Almost all patients show substantial improvement, and the effects appear to last for up to 5 months. The most common adverse effects are transient ptosis and facial weakness. The initial dose of Botox is 1.25 to 2.5 U (0.05 to 0.1 mL) injected into abnormally contracting muscles, rarely exceeding 5 U in a single location. For BTB the initial dose is 125 to 250 U per muscle site (total dose 750 to 5,000 U).[86]

Low Back Pain: Chronic low back pain is the second most common illness reported by patients in the USA and accounts for substantial morbidity and health-care resource utilization. Many back and spine stressors can contribute to tissue injury, resulting in acute or chronic pain. Foster et al.[87] have published results in the medical literature for a randomized, placebo-controlled study of BTA for treatment of back pain. Other data have been presented showing variable results for the use of BTA for treatment of back pain, some failing to show statistical significance of efficacy.[88,89] In a recent prospective open-label study, BTB was evaluated for safety and efficacy as a treatment for chronic low back pain.[83] Study participants had been experiencing back spasms and back pain without radiating leg pain for at least 6 months. They also had reduced back flexion, rotation, or side bending of the lumbar area. However, small patient populations, different study designs, and differing pathologies contributing to back pain make it difficult to extrapolate results across studies. As yet, there have been no randomized, placebo-controlled studies of BTB for use in back pain. Current information about the use of BTs for treatment of back pain are encouraging but larger, rigorously designed studies using similar outcome measures are needed to better characterize its efficacy.

Myofascial Pain: Myofascial pain syndrome (MFPS) is characterized by painful muscles with increased tone and stiffness containing trigger points (TPs), which are tender firm nodules, or taut bands, usually 3 to 6 mm in diameter. Palpation produces aching pain in localized reference zones. Mechanical stimulation of the taut band by needling or brisk transverse pressure will produce a localized muscle twitch.[90] Trigger point palpation will often elicit a "jump sign," an involuntary reflex-like recoil or flinching by the patient that is disproportionate to the pressure applied.[91] In a small but carefully designed double-blind, crossover study of six patients with MFPS, injections of BT or placebo showed a clear benefit of BT. Patients were selected on the basis of focal pain involving the cervical paraspinal or shoulder girdle muscles, and had discrete trigger points, which when palpated reproduced a typical pattern of radiating pain for that patient. Patients with diffuse pain or neurological deficits were excluded. Patients were randomly injected with either BT (50 U in 4 mL normal saline) or normal saline alone on two occasions separated by at least 8 weeks. Trigger points were identically injected in the 2 or 3 sites affected on both occasions. Subjects were not told when to expect any relief, and were followed up at weekly intervals for 4 weeks and at 8 weeks after treatment. During the study, other medications for pain relief were not permitted. In addition to investigator palpation and grading of trigger points, pain was assessed both subjectively (visual analogue scale) and by the application of a pressure algometer to determine pain threshold in kilograms. A positive response was defined as a reduction from baseline of more than 30% on at least two occasions. Four of six patients responded in this manner. Onset of response occurred within the first week following BT injection, but not at the 30-minute observation time. Mean duration of response was 5 to 6 weeks. One subject responded to both BT and saline, and one subject's pain threshold following BT had not returned to baseline by the time of the placebo injection. Results between the two treatment regimens were statistically significant in favor of BT and suggest that additional clinical testing for this indication is warranted.

Piriformis Syndrome: This is thought to involve the piriformis muscle because of its close proximity to the sciatic nerve. It is associated with buttock, hip, and lower limb pain and occurs predominantly in women. On clinical examination, palpation of the buttocks at a point midway between the sacrum and greater trochanter of the hip reproduces the patient's usual pain. Maneuvers that activate the piriformis muscle are also painful. Freiberg's maneuver of forceful internal rotation of the extended thigh elicits buttock pain by stretching the piriformis muscle. Active hip flexion, adduction (or abduction), and internal rotation exacerbate symptoms. Medical treatment of piriformis muscle syndrome includes therapeutic stretch, ultrasound, massage, manipulation, and oral analgesic agents.[92–98] Caudal epidural steroid injections, local perineural and intramuscular steroid injections, and surgical resection of the muscle have also been reported as effective treatment.[99–102] In the randomized double-blinded study of Fishman et al.[102] 65%, 32%, and 6% of patients had 50% pain reduction in 200 U of Botox, in LA with steroid, and placebo groups, respectively. Childers et al.[103] conducted a randomized, crossover, double-blind pilot study that showed significant pain reduction up to 10 weeks in the Botox (5 U/kg) treatment group.

Summary: The goal of treatment in MPS should be the restoration of function by diligent use of massage and physical therapy, preferably without using narcotic or nonnarcotic analgesics. If these measures fail, LAs with steroids should be injected up to a maximum of three times in six weeks. If the pain is relieved but returns quickly, a trial of BT injection therapy may provide longer lasting benefit. Besides providing a longer period of pain relief, this strategy may facilitate physical therapy and promote long-term improvement in quality of life.

BTs appear to be a useful treatment in refractory MFPS and headache. Presumably BTs work by breaking the spasm/pain cycle giving the patient a window period for traditional conservative measures to facilitate healing of the injured tissue.

Moreover, several studies suggest that a direct antinociceptive effect distinct from any reduction in muscle spasm may be at play. The major benefit of BTs compared with standard therapies is duration of response.

BTs should not be used as a first line treatment for MFPS or headache. However, in refractory cases where nothing else has worked, it may offer a chance for improvement or cure not otherwise available.

During the last decade, BTs have been widely used as a safe and effective treatment for many different disorders. This treatment has also demonstrated benefit in many other neurologic and nonneurologic disorders. The benefit of BT for its approved indications is clearly related to its ability to cause muscle paralysis in overactive spastic muscles. Dosage should be selected on an individualized basis, depending on the disorder being treated, the size of the muscle, and various other factors.

REFERENCES

1. Physicians Desk Reference, ed 58. Medical Economics Company, Montvale, NJ, 2004.
2. Morris TW, Katzberg RW: Intravenous contrast media: Properties and general effects. *In* Katzberg (ed): The Contrast Media Manual. Williams & Wilkins, Baltimore, 1992, pp 1–18.
3. Product Information: Isovue®, iopamidol. Bracco Diagnostics, Princeton, NJ, revised August 1999.
4. Product Information: Omnipaque®, iohexol. Nycomed Inc., Princeton, NJ, revised July 1996.
5. Grainger RG: Intravascular contrast media. *In* Grainger RG, Allison DJ (eds): Diagnostic Radiology, ed 2. Churchill Livingstone, New York, 1992, pp 11–22.
6. Grainger RG: Annotation: Radiological contrast media. Clin Radiol 38:3–5, 1987.
7. American Heart Association in collaboration with International Liaison Committee on Resuscitation: Guidelines 2000 for Cardiopulmonary Resuscitation and Emergency Cardiovascular Care: International Consensus on Science. Anaphylaxis. Circulation 102(Suppl I):I241–243, 2000.
8. Lasser EC, Berry CC, Talner LB, et al: Pre-treatment with corticosteroids to alleviate reactions to intravenous contrast media. N Engl J Med 317:845–849, 1987.
9. Bush WH: Treatment of acute reactions to contrast media. *In* Katzberg (ed): The Contrast Media Manual. Williams & Wilkins, Baltimore, 1992, pp 19–27.
10. Butterworth JF, Strichartz GR: Molecular mechanisms of local anesthesia: A review. Anesthesiology 72:711–734, 1990.
11. Product Information: Lidocaine hydrochloride injection. Abbott Laboratories, North Chicago, IL, revised January 2001.
12. Product Information: Bupivacaine hydrochloride injection. Abbott Laboratories, North Chicago, IL, revised September 1999.
13. Strichartz GR, Sanchez V, Arthur GR, et al: Fundamental properties of local anesthetics: II. Measured octanol:buffer partition coefficients and pKa values of clinically used drugs. Anesth Analg 71:158–170, 1990.
14. Ririe DG, Walker FO, James RL, et al: Effect of alkalinization of lidocaine on median nerve block. Br J Anaesth 84:163–168, 2000.
15. DiFazio CA, Carron H, Grosslight KR, et al: Comparison of pH-adjusted lidocaine solutions for epidural anesthesia. Anesth Analg 65:760–764, 1986.
16. Covino BG, Wildsmith JAW: Clinical pharmacology of local anesthetic agents. *In* Cousins MJ, Bridenbaugh PO (eds): Neural Blockade in Clinical Anesthesia and Management of Pain, ed 3. Lippincott-Raven, Philadelphia, PA, 1998, pp 97–128.
17. Reiz S, Nathan S: Cardiotoxicity of local anaesthetic agents. Br J Anaesth 58:736–746, 1986.
18. Chernoff DM: Kinetic analysis of phasic inhibition of neuronal sodium currents by lidocaine and bupivacaine. Biophys J 58:53–68, 1990.
19. Gissen AJ, Datta S, Lambert D: The chloroprocaine controversy. Is chloroprocaine neurotoxic? Reg Anesth 9:135, 1984.
20. Lambert LA, Lambert DH, Strichartz GR: Irreversible conduction block in isolated nerve by high concentrations of local anesthetics. Anesthesiology 80:1082–1093, 1994.
21. deShazo RD, Nelson HS: An approach to the patient with a history of local anesthetic hypersensitivity: Experience with 90 patients. J Allergy Clin Immunol 63:387–394, 1979.
22. Orth D, Kovacs W: The adrenal cortex. *In* William's Textbook of Endocrinology, ed 9. WB Saunders, Philadelphia, 1998, pp 517–664.
23. Dluhy R, Lauler D, Thorn G: Pharmacology and chemistry of adrenal glucocorticoids. Med Clinics North Am 57:1155–1165, 1973.
24. Nesbitt LT: Minimizing complications from systemic glucocorticosteroid use. Dermatol Clinics 13:925–939, 1995.
25. Melby J: Clinical pharmacology of systemic corticosteroids. Ann Rev Pharmacol Toxicol 17:511–527, 1977.
26. Burchard K: A review of the adrenal cortex and severe inflammation: Quest of the eucorticoid state. J Trauma 51: 800–814, 2001.
27. Orth D: Medical progress: Cushing's syndrome. N Engl J Med 332:791–803, 1995.
28. Coursin D, Wood K: Corticosteroid supplementation for adrenal insufficiency. JAMA 287:236–240, 2002.
29. Barnes P, Adcock I: Anti-inflammatory actions of steroids: molecular mechanisms. Trends Pharmacol Sci 14:436–441, 1993.
30. Abram S: Treatment of lumbosacral radiculopathy with epidural steroids. Anesthesiology 91:1937, 1999.
31. Devor M, Govrin-Lippmann R, Raber P: Corticosteroids suppress ectopic neural discharge originating in experimental neuromas. Pain 22:127–137, 1985.
32. Schwiebert L, Beck L, et al: Glucocorticosteroid inhibition of cytokine production: Relevance to antiallergic actions. J Allergy Clin Immunol 97:143–152, 1996.
33. Santini G, Patrignani P, Sciulli M, et al: The human pharmacology of monocyte cyclooxygenase 2 inhibition by cortisol and synthetic glucocorticoids. Clin Pharmacol Therap 70:475–483, 2001.
34. Product Information: Hydrocortone® acetate, hydrocortisone acetate. Merck & Co., Inc., West Point, PA, February 1997.
35. Product Information: Hydrocortone® phosphate, hydrocortisone phosphate. Merck & Co., Inc., West Point, PA, February 1997.
36. Product Information: Kenalog®-40 injection, triamcinolone acetonide. Bistal-Myers Squibb Co., Princeton, NJ, revised April 2001.
37. Product Information: Aristocort® Forte, trimacinolone diacetate. Lederle Parenterals, Inc., Carolina, Puerto Rico, April 1999.
38. Product Information: Depo-Medrol®, methylprednisolone acetate. Pharmacia & Upjohn Co., Kalamazoo, MI, revised March 1999.
39. Product Information: Decadron® phosphate injection, dexamethasone sodium phosphate. Merck & Co., Inc., West Point, PA, October 1996.
40. Product Information: Celestone® Soluspan®, betamethasone sodium phosphate and betamethasone acetate. Schering Corporation, Kenilworth, NJ, revised October 1999.
41. Boonen S, Van Distel G, Westhovens R, Dequeker J: Steroid myopathy induced by epidural triamcinolone injection. Br J Rheumatol 34:385–386, 1995.
42. Ward A, Watson J, Wood P, et al: Glucocorticoid epidural for sciatica: Metabolic and endocrine sequelae. Rheumatology 41:68–71, 2002.
43. Tuel S, Meythaler J, Cross L: Cushing's syndrome from epidural methylprednisolone. Pain 40:81–84, 1990.

44. Orth D: Medical progress: Cushing's syndrome. N Engl J Med 332:791–803, 1995.

45. Nelson DA: Dangers from methylprednisolone acetate therapy by intraspinal injection. Arch Neurol 45:804–806, 1988.

46. Goldstein DA, Zimmerman B, Spielberg S: Anaphylactic response to hydrocortisone in childhood: A case report. Ann Allergy 55:599–600, 1985.

47. Freedman MD, Schocket AL, Chapel N, et al: Anaphylaxis after intravenous methylprednisolone administration. JAMA 245:607–608, 1981.

48. Peller JS, Bardana EJ: Anaphylactoid reaction to corticosteroid: Case report and review of the literature. Ann Allerg 54:302–305, 1985.

49. Scott AB: Botulinum toxin injection of eye muscles to correct strabismus. Trans Am Ophthalmol Soc 79:734–770, 1981.

50. Sakaguchi G: Clostridium botulinum toxins. Pharmacol Ther 19:165–194, 1983.

51. Putnam FW, Lamanna C, Sharp DG: Physicochemical properties of crystalline botulinum type A toxin. J Biol Chem 176:401–412, 1948.

52. DasGupta BR: Structure and biological activity of botulinum neurotoxin. J Physiol (Paris) 84:220–228, 1990.

53. Montceucco C: How do tetanus and botulinum toxins bind to neuronal membranes? Trends Biochem Sci 11:314–317, 1986.

54. Evans DM, Williams RS, Shone CC, et al: Botulinum neurotoxin type B: Its purification, radioiodination and interaction with rat-brain synaptosomal membranes. Eur J Biochem 154:409–416, 1986.

55. Evans DM, Williams RS, Shone CC, et al: Botulinum neurotoxin type B: Its purification, radioiodination, and interaction with rat-brain synaptosomal membranes. Eur J Biochem 154:409–416, 1986.

56. Schengrund C-L, DasGupta BR, Ringler NJ: Binding of botulinum and tetanus neurotoxins to ganglioside GT1b and derivatives thereof. J Neurochem 57:1024–1032, 1991.

57. Kozaki S, Ogasawara J, Shimote Y, et al: Antigenic structure of Clostridium botulinum type B neurotoxin and its interaction with gangliosides, cerebrosides, and free fatty acids. Infect Immunol 55:3051–3056, 1987.

58. Poulain B, Tauc L, Maisery EA, et al: Neurotransmitter release is blocked intracellularly by botulinum neurotoxin, and this requires uptake of both toxin polypeptides by a process mediated by the larger chain. Proc Natl Acad Sci USA 85:4090–4094, 1988.

59. Blasi J, Chapman ER, Link E, et al: Botulinum neurotoxin A selectively cleaves the synaptic protein SNAP25. Nature 365:160–163, 1993.

60. Hay JC: SNARE complex structure and function. Exp Cell Res 271:10–21, 2001.

61. Borodic GE, Ferrante R: Histologic effects of repeated botulinum toxin over many years in human orbicularis oculi muscle. J Clin Neuro-Ophthalmol 12:121–127, 1992.

62. Borodic GE, Ferrante RI, Pearce LB, Alderson K: Pharmacology and histology of the therapeutic application of botulinum toxin. In Jankovic J, Hallett M (eds): Therapy with Botulinum Toxin. Marcel Dekker, New York, 1994, pp 119–157.

63. McMahon HT, Foran P, Dolly JO, et al: Tetanus toxin and botulinum toxins type A and B inhibit glutamate, gamma-aminobutyric acid, aspartate, and met-enkephalin release from synaptosomes. J Biol Chem 267:21338–21343, 1992.

64. Cui ML, Khanijou S, Rubino J, et al: Botulinum toxin A inhibits the inflammatory pain in the rat formalin model [abstract]. Soc Neurosci 26:656, 2000.

65. Racz GB: Botulinum toxin as a new approach for refractory pain syndromes. Pain Digest 8:353–356, 1998.

66. Porta M, Perretti A, Gamba M, et al: The rationale and results of treating muscle spasm and myofascial syndromes with botulinum toxin type A. Pain Digest 8:346–352, 1998.

67. Abrams BM: Tutorial 36: Myofascial pain syndrome and fibromyalgia. Pain Digest 8:264–272, 1998.

68. Lang AM: Botulinum toxin for myofascial pain. In Advancements in the Treatment of Neuromuscular Pain. Johns Hopkins University Office of Continuing Medical Education Syllabus, 1999, Chapter 5, pp 23–28.

69. Poewe W, Wissel J: Experience with botulinum toxin in cervical dystonia. In Jankovic J, Hallett M (eds): Therapy with Botulinum Toxin. Marcel Dekker, New York, 1994, pp 267–278.

70. To EW, Ahuja AT, Ho WS, et al: A prospective study of the effect of botulinum toxin A on masseteric muscle hypertrophy with ultrasonographic and electromyographic measurement. Br J Plast Surg 54:197–200, 2001.

71. Jensen R: Pathophysiological mechanisms of tension-type headache: A review of epidemiological and experimental studies. Cephalalgia 19:602–621, 1999.

72. Freund BJ, Schwartz M: A focal dystonia model for subsets of chronic tension headache. Cephalalgia 20:433, 2000.

73. Binder WJ, Brin MF, Blitzer A, et al: Botulinum toxin type A (BOTOX) for treatment of migraine headaches: An open-label study. Otolaryngol Head Neck Surg 123:669–676, 2000.

74. Silberstein S, Mathew N, Saper J, et al: Botulinum toxin type A as a migraine preventive treatment. Headache 40:445–450, 2000.

75. Brin MF, Swope DM, O'Brien C, et al: Botox for migraine: Double-blind, placebo-controlled, region-specific evaluation [abstract]. Cephalalgia 20:421, 2000.

76. Opida C: Open-label study of Myobloc (botulinum toxin type B) in the treatment of patients with transformed migraine headaches. J Pain 3(Suppl 1):10, 2002.

77. Freund BJ, Schwartz M: A focal dystonia model for subsets of chronic tension headache. Cephalalgia 20:433, 2000.

78. Smuts JA, Baker MK, Smuts HM, et al: Prophylactic treatment of chronic tension-type headache using botulinum toxin type A. Eur J Neurol 6:S99–102, 1999.

79. Jankovic J, Schwartz K: Botulinum toxin injections for cervical dystonia. Neurology 40:277–280, 1990.

80. Aoki KR, Cui M: Botulinum toxin type A: Potential mechanisms of action in pain relief. Presented at the 37th Annual Meeting of the Interagency Botulinum Research Coordinating Committee, Asilomar, CA, 17–20 October 2000.

81. Freund B, Schwartz M: Treatment of whiplash associated neck pain with botulinum toxin A: A pilot study. J Rheumatol 27:481–484, 2000.

82. Freund B, Schwartz M: Use of botulinum toxin in chronic whiplash-associated disorder. Clin J Pain 18:S163–S168, 2002.

83. Opida CL: Open-label study of Myobloc™ (botulinum toxin type B) in the treatment of patients with post-whiplash headaches. Poster 204 presented at the International Conference on Basic and Therapeutic Aspect of Botulinum and Tetanus Toxins, Hannover, Germany, June 2002.

84. O'Day J: Use of botulinum toxin in neuro-ophthalmology. Curr Opin Ophthalmol 12:419–422, 2001.

85. Tsui JKC: Botulinum toxin as a therapeutic agent. Pharmacol Ther 72:13–24, 1996.

86. WE MOVE. Practical considerations for the clinical use of botulinum toxin type B: A self-study continuing medical education activity [online course]: Available at www.mdvu.org.

87. Foster L, Clapp L, Erickson M, Jabbari B: Botulinum toxin A and chronic low back pain. Neurology 561:1290–1293, 2001.

88. Knusel B, DeGryse R, Grant M, et al: Intramuscular injection of botulinum toxin type A (BOTOX) in chronic low back pain associated with muscle spasm. Presented at 17th Annual Scientific Meeting, American Pain Society, San Diego, CA, 5–8 November 1998.

89. Porta M, Perretti A, Gambia M, et al: The rationale and results of treating muscle spasm and myofascial syndromes with botulinum toxin type A. Pain Digest 8:346–352, 1998.

90. Travell JG, Simons DG: Myofascial Pain and Dysfunction: The Trigger Point Manual. Williams and Wilkins, Baltimore, 1983.

91. Cheshire WP, Abashian SW, Mann ID: Botulinum toxin in the treatment of myofascial pain syndrome. Pain 59:65–69, 1994.

92. Fishman LM, Zybert PA: Electrophysiologic evidence of piriformis syndrome. Arch Phys Med Rehabil 73:359–364, 1992.

93. Simons DG, Travell JG: Myofascial origins of low back pain: 3. Pelvic and lower extremity muscles. Postgrad Med 73:99–108, 1983.

94. Retzlaff EW, Berry AH, Haight AS, et al: The piriformis muscle syndrome. J Am Osteopath Assoc 73:799–807, 1974.

95. TePoorten BA: The piriformis muscle. J Am Osteopath Assoc 69:50–160, 1969.

96. Hallin RP: Sciatic pain and the piriformis muscle. Postgrad Med 74:69–72, 1983.

97. Mullin V, de Rosayro M: Caudal steroid injection for treatment of piriformis syndrome. Anesth Analg 71:705–707, 1990.

98. Barton PM: Piriformis syndrome: A rational approach to management. Pain 47:345–352, 1991.

99. Benzon HT, Katz JA, Benzon HA, Iqbal MS: Piriformis syndrome anatomic considerations, a new injection technique and a review of literature. Anesthesiology 98:1442–1448, 2003.

100. Park HW, Jahng JS, Lee WH: Piriformis syndrome: A case report. Yonsei Med J 32:64–68, 1991.

101. Fishman LM, Dombi GW, Michaelsen C, et al: Piriformis syndrome: Diagnosis, treatment and outcome. A ten year study. Arch Phys Med Rehabil 83:295–301, 2002.

102. Fishman LM, Anderson C, Rosner B: Botox and physical therapy in the treatment of piriformis syndrome. Am J Phys Med Rehabil 81:936–942, 2002.

103. Childers M, Wilson D, Gnatz S, et al: Botulinum toxin type A use in piriformis muscle syndrome: A pilot study. Am J Phys Med Rehabl 81:751–759, 2002.

19

Diagnostic Nerve Blocks
(Including Local Anesthetic Infusions)

Robert E. Molloy, M.D., and
Kenneth D. Candido, M.D.

Diagnostic nerve blocks provide important clinical information when interpreted in the light of the problem-oriented pain history and comprehensive neurological physical examination. Many causes of the etiology of a painful syndrome are not readily apparent, even when competent and experienced clinicians have evaluated the patient, diagnostic radiological information, and the results of laboratory and psychological testing. It therefore behoves the prudent practitioner to have a fundamental appreciation of the applicability of diagnostic nerve blocks particularly when considering whether a given patient is a candidate for therapeutic nerve blocks, radiofrequency lesioning, or neurolytic blocks. Since pain is a totally subjective phenomenon, what is needed to identify the neural pathway subserving it is some sort of objective diagnostic test. A description of the classic approach to differential nerve blocks follows.

CLASSIC DIFFERENTIAL NERVE BLOCKS

Differential neural blockade may provide the essential information necessary for verifying a particular diagnosis or delineating a treatment plan of management. This technique relies upon the selective blockade of one neurologic modality without blocking the others, and is divided into two clinical approaches. The basis for the *anatomic approach* is the actual anatomical separation of somatic and sympathetic nervous system fibers, so that an injection of local anesthetic solution blocks one modality without affecting the others. The basis for the *pharmacologic approach* is the presumed difference in the sensitivities of the various types of nerve fibers to local anesthetics, so that an injection of local anesthetic solutions in different concentrations may selectively block different types of fibers. While the techniques of differential neural blockade are appealing based upon their simplicity, the techniques are controversial largely because of the changing state of knowledge regarding factors determining nerve conduction and nerve blockade by local anesthetics as well as our new-found appreciation of the complexities of chronic pain.[1–3]

The foundation for differential neural blockade is nerve fiber length and fiber diameter. Nerve fiber length determines relative susceptibilities of a given fiber to local anesthetic concentrations, and nerve fiber diameter determines the modalities subserved by the fiber (Table 19-1).

There are four subclasses of A fibers: A-alpha, A-beta, A-gamma, and A-delta. A-alpha fibers subserve motor function and proprioception. A-beta fibers subserve touch and pressure. A-gamma fibers subserve muscle spindle tone. A-delta fibers subserve pain and temperature sensations. B fibers are thin myelinated, preganglionic autonomic nerves; and the unmyelinated C fibers subserve pain and temperature. C fibers are thinner than the myelinated A and B fibers and have a lower conduction velocity than the others (Table 19-1). The simplest example of the pharmacologic approach with the most discrete end points is the *differential spinal block*. Differential spinal block attempts to block separately sympathetic, sensory, and motor systems for the subsequent determination of the etiology of an individual's lower abdominal or lower extremity pain mechanism. After obtaining informed and written consent, an intravenous catheter is secured and a crystalloid infusion is begun as for any subarachnoid block. A full complement of noninvasive hemodynamic monitors is applied and baseline vital signs are recorded. In the conventional differential spinal block four solutions are prepared and labeled A, B, C, and D. Solution A contains no local anesthetic (placebo); solution B contains 0.25% procaine; solution C contains 0.5% procaine; and solution D contains 5.0% procaine. These solutions are injected sequentially (obviously this is labor and time intensive as the effects of each solution must completely dissipate prior to injecting the subsequent solution in sequence) through a 25- to 27-gauge spinal needle, which has been introduced in standard fashion at the L2–3 or L3–4 interspace. There are four basic interpretations of the differential spinal block (Table 19-2) as follows:

Psychogenic pain. If the injection of the placebo solution (solution A) relieves the patient's pain, the pain is tentatively classified as psychogenic, depending upon the duration of relief. For prolonged or permanent relief, the pain is probably truly psychogenic, whereas if the pain relief is temporary, the response is likely a placebo reaction.

Sympathetic pain. If the patient does not obtain relief following the placebo injection, but does obtain relief from

TABLE 19-1. CLASSIFICATION OF NERVES BY FIBER SIZE AND RELATION OF FIBER SIZE TO FUNCTION AND SENSITIVITY TO LOCAL ANESTHETICS*

Group/Subgroup	Diameter (μm)	Conduction Velocity (m/s)	Modalities Subserved	Sensitivity to Local Anesthetics (%)†
A (myelinated)				
A-alpha	15–20	8–120	Large motor, proprioception	1.0
A-beta	8–15	30–70	Small motor, touch, pressure	↓
A-gamma	4–8	30–70	Muscle spindle, reflex	↓
A-delta	3–4	10–30	Pain, temperature	0.5
B (myelinated)	3–4	10–15	Preganglionic autonomic	0.25
C (unmyelinated)	1–2	1–2	Pain, temperature	0.5

* Subarachnoid procaine.
† Vertical arrows indicate intermediate values, in descending order.

0.25% procaine (solution B), the mechanism subserving the patient's pain is likely mediated by the sympathetic nervous system. This presumes that there are clinical signs of complete sympathetic block and no detectable sensory changes.

Somatic pain. If the patient does not obtain relief following the injection of placebo or 0.25% procaine, but 0.5% procaine does provide significant relief, this typically indicates that the pain is subserved by A-delta fibers and/or C fibers, and is therefore classified as somatic. The caveat, of course, is that the patient did exhibit signs of sympathetic nervous system blockade following the injection of 0.25% procaine, and that the pain relief is accompanied by analgesia or anesthesia in the areas of concern. This is important because of the variability in C_m for B fibers that is known to exist. If the patient has an elevated C_m for B fibers, pain relief from 0.5% procaine might be due to a sympathetic block rather than a sensory block.

Central pain. If the injections of solutions A, B, and C fail to resolve the patient's pain, 5% procaine (solution D) is then injected to block all modalities. If solution D does relieve the pain, the mechanism is still considered to be somatic, and it is presumed that the patient has an elevated C_m for A-delta

and C fibers. However, if there is no relief following the injection of the 5% solution, the pain is classified as central in origin, with the four possible subclassifications as noted in Table 19-2.

The *modified differential spinal block* was developed to overcome the disadvantages inherent in the conventional differential block and is, in essence, an observational process that is the reverse of the classic approach. In the modified block, only solutions A and D are injected through the spinal needle. If the patient obtains no or only partial relief following the injection of solution A (placebo), then 2 mL of 5% procaine (solution D) are injected through the spinal needle. The needle is then removed, and the patient is placed supine. The modified differential block is less labor intensive than the classic approach and has proven to be as efficacious as the former in the clinical setting. The proposed interpretation of the modified differential spinal is as follows:

- If the patient's pain is relieved after injection of solution A, the interpretation is the same as in the conventional differential spinal technique.

TABLE 19-2. INTERPRETATION OF CLASSIC DIFFERENTIAL SPINAL BLOCK

Solution Injected	Intended Blockade	Pain Relief	Interpretation
Saline	None	If yes	Placebo responder or psychogenic mechanism
0.25% Procaine	Sympathetic	If yes	Sympathetic mechanism
0.5% Procaine	Sensory	If yes	Somatic mechanism
5% Procaine	Motor	If none	Central mechanism*

* A central mechanism may be due to a CNS lesion above the level of block; true psychogenic pain; malingering; or encephalization (original peripheral pain mechanism becomes self-sustaining at central level).
Data from Winnie and Candido.[1–3]

- If the patient does not obtain relief following the injection of solution D (5% procaine), the diagnosis is considered to be the same as in the conventional approach whereby the patient fails to get relief following injection of all solutions (A through D).
- If the patient obtains complete pain relief after injection of solution D, the pain is considered to be somatic and/or sympathetic in nature. At this point the regression of blockade becomes important, as 5% procaine blocks motor, sensory, and sympathetic fibers. Therefore, the patient is queried as to the return of his or her pain concomitant with the regression of, first, motor block, followed by sensory block regression, and, ultimately, by sympathetic block regression.
- If the pain returns when the patient again appreciates pinprick as sharp (recovery from analgesia), the mechanism is considered to be somatic (subserved by A-delta fibers and/or C fibers).
- If the pain relief persists for a prolonged period after recovery from analgesia, the mechanism is considered to be mediated by the sympathetic nervous system (mediated by B fibers).

The *differential epidural block* was developed by Raj[4] in an effort to circumvent the possibility of producing post lumbar puncture cephalgia following the differential spinal block and to allow for better assessment of incident pain if a catheter is placed. The basis for the procedure is identical to that of the differential spinal block, with the technique relying upon placement of a standard 18- or 20-gauge Tuohy-type epidural needle into the epidural space at L2–3 or L3–4 as described above for the differential spinal block. Four solutions are sequentially injected, with solution A still indicating a placebo (typically normal saline solution), and solution B containing 0.5% lidocaine, presumed to be the mean sympathetic blocking concentration of lidocaine in the epidural space. Solution C is 1% lidocaine, presumed to be the mean sensory blocking concentration of lidocaine, and solution D is 2% lidocaine, a concentration intended to block all modalities. The sequence of injections is identical to that proposed for the conventional differential spinal block, with the same patient observations being made following the injection of each of the solutions in sequence.

There are two shortcomings of the technique, as proposed by Raj, however. First, because of the delay in onset of blockade of each modality using the epidural approach (as compared with subarachnoid administration of local anesthetic), a significantly longer period would be required between injections, thus increasing the time-intensive nature of the procedure. Second, if local anesthetics fail to give discrete endpoints when administered in the subarachnoid space, they do so even more frequently when administered epidurally, therefore tending to further "muddy the waters" in assessing the response of patients to each injection. Again, however, the technique may be modified as for differential spinal block so that only two solutions, A and D, may be administered sequentially as above for differential spinal block.

The *anatomic approach to differential block* is the other modality described. The utility of the technique is that, unlike differential spinal block (and to a lesser extent differential epidural block), painful conditions affecting *any* body region may be addressed (including but not limited to the lower abdomen and lower extremities). The anatomic approach relies upon three injections: a placebo, a sympathetic nerve block, and a somatic sensory and motor block. The sympathetic block is carried out at a site where the sympathetic fibers are anatomically separate from sensory and motor fibers, and can thus be blocked independently of one another. The various sympathetic and somatic block procedures vary depending upon the painful area to be evaluated (Table 19-3). Whereas the anatomic approach certainly has applicability for head and neck and upper extremity pain, the differential epidural approach may be preferred for thoracic pain to minimize the likelihood of pneumothorax resulting from thoracic paravertebral blocks used in the anatomic approach.

TABLE 19-3. ANATOMIC DIFFERENTIAL BLOCK: PROCEDURAL SEQUENCE

Site of Pain	Block Performed First After Placebo	Sympathetic Block	Somatic Block
Head	Sympathetic	Stellate ganglion	Trigeminal I, II, III; C2; occipital nerve
Neck	Sympathetic	Stellate ganglion	Cervical plexus or specific nerve
Arm	Sympathetic	Stellate ganglion	Brachial plexus or specific nerve
Chest	Somatic	Thoracic sympathetic	Intercostal nerve or paravertebral somatic
Abdomen	Somatic	Celiac plexus	Intercostal nerve or paravertebral somatic
Pelvis	Somatic	Hypogastric plexus	Paravertebral somatic or intercostal nerve
Leg	Sympathetic	Lumbar sympathetic	Lumbosacral plexus or specific nerve

Data from Winnie and Candido.[1–3]

As an example of a modified anatomic approach to differential block for the patient with upper extremity pain, a *differential brachial plexus block* approach might be chosen. Two sequential injections are made into the perivascular compartment at the interscalene (for shoulder pain), subclavian (for pain between the shoulder and the wrist), or axillary level (for pain in the lower forearm to the fingers). One injection consists of normal saline solution; the other consists of 2% chloroprocaine. The same observations are made as for differential spinal block. If the patient obtains pain relief following the injection of saline, the pain is considered to be of "psychogenic" origin, with the same considerations applying as previously mentioned. If pain disappears following the chloroprocaine injection, the pain is considered to be either sympathetic or somatic. The pain is considered to be somatic if it returns once the sensory block dissipates; but if pain relief persists after the sensory block dissipates, it is considered to have a sympathetic nervous system origin. If the patient continues to experience pain, even in the face of complete sensory and motor block, the pain is considered to be central, with the same considerations as previously mentioned above for differential spinal block.

Limitations of Differential Blocks: Despite the seemingly objective nature of differential neural blockade as a means of confirming a diagnosis when a patient's pain is obvious, as well as its role in establishing a diagnosis when there appears to be no demonstrable cause, some difference of professional opinion exists regarding its ultimate utility.[5,6] Some authors argue that the use of a nerve block to identify a nerve pathway that is the source of an individual's ongoing pain assumes three potentially false premises: (1) pathology causing pain is located in an exact peripheral location and impulses from this site travel via a unique and consistent neural route, (2) injection of a local anesthetic totally and selectively abolishes sensory function of intended nerves, and (3) relief of pain following local anesthetic block is due solely to block of the target neural pathway. These assumptions are limited by certain complexities of the anatomy, physiology, and psychology of pain perception, and the effect of local anesthetics on impulse conduction (Table 19-4). The resultant potential limitations of diagnostic blocks have been reviewed by Hogan and Abram,[6] and examples are provided below and in Table 19-4.

A peripheral nerve block performed proximal to the site of an injury may not interrupt pain due to spontaneous discharge from dorsal root ganglion (DRG) cells. However, a nerve block distal to the site of nerve injury may interrupt propagated antidromic C fiber activity that maintains peripheral receptor sensitization. Selective sympathetic block may produce multiple indirect effects, interrupting receptor sensitization, peripheral inflammation, or neuroma firing. Spinal block may interrupt superficial fibers of the descending inhibitory system. Stress-induced analgesia may occur during a diagnostic block procedure due to activation of descending inhibitory spinal tracts. Blocking one limb of converging inputs may relieve pain but fail to identify a major underlying pain source. The response to diagnostic block may be unpredictable in the presence of central sensitization; and block of an adjacent uninjured nerve may relieve allodynia in its distribution. Relief after sympathetic block may be due to subtle somatic block that is not clinically obvious. A typically less than complete local anesthetic neural block may produce an apparently negative diagnostic somatic block. Differential pharmacologic

block by local anesthetic is unpredictable and may not be reliably produced. Neuropathic pain may be relieved by systemic effects of absorbed local anesthetics. The reader is referred to the review by Hogan and Abram[6] for additional details.

ROLE OF DIAGNOSTIC BLOCKS

Boas and Cousins have listed seven aspects of a patient's pain that may be profitably investigated using nerve blocks.[7] These are the foundation for the following discussion (Table 19-5).

TABLE 19-4. DIAGNOSTIC BLOCKS: LIMITATIONS

Potential limitations due to altered primary afferent nerve activity
- Receptor sensitization by tissue factors
- Spontaneous discharge from DRG* proximal to injury
- Propagation of antidromic activity distal to site of nerve injury
- Sympathetic influences on receptor sensitization, inflammation, or neuroma firing

Potential limitations due to altered spinal processing
- Peripheral nerve block alters balance of large fiber and C fiber input to dorsal horn
- Spinal block of superficial fibers of descending inhibitory system
- Acute activation of descending inhibitory tracts by stress of nerve block procedure
- Presence of conditioned descending stimulatory modulation, which may persist
- Pain dependent on converging inputs from two sources, not both apparent

Potential limitations due to central plasticity
- Unpredictable response to block of conditioning afferent input with central sensitization
- Block of afferents may normalize dorsal horn responsiveness, leading to prolonged relief
- Block of adjacent uninjured nerve may relieve pain in its area if altered central processing
- Block of injured nerve may not relieve deafferentation pain if there is DRG* receptive field expansion

Potential limitations due to local anesthetic effects
- Relief after sympathetic block may be due to subtle undetected somatic block
- Intended profound somatic blocks typically less than complete neural block
- Differential pharmacologic block by local anesthetics is unpredictable, with varying degrees of overlapping partial block of each sensory modality
- Systemic effects of absorbed local anesthetics on neuropathic pain

* DRG, dorsal root ganglion.
Data from Hogan and Abram.[6]

TABLE 19-5. DIAGNOSTIC NERVE BLOCKS

Questions to be addressed by nerve blocks
1. Anatomic location and source of pain
2. Visceral versus somatic origin of trunk pain
3. Sympathetic versus somatic origin of peripheral pain
4. Identify referred pain syndromes
5. Segmental levels of nociceptive input
6. Painful muscle spasm versus fixed contracture deformity
7. Diagnosis of central pain states

Data from Boas and Cousins.[7]

Anatomic Location of Pain Source: Direct injection of local anesthetics into tender superficial or deep tissues may clearly delineate the source of pain. Examples include nerve entrapment syndromes including radiculopathies, post-traumatic neuroma formation, myofascial trigger points, and focal muscle spasm. Prompt, complete pain relief on at least two separate occasions may confirm the diagnosis, although said pain relief does not guarantee that myofascial pain is the principle cause. Other confounding factors include the possibility of placebo effects and systemic uptake of local anesthetics, as well as spread to adjacent nerves/structures.

Facet joint diagnostic blockade is probably most accurately performed by medial branch nerve block. The greatest specificity for a positive response to a facet denervation procedure is achieved when the diagnosis is established via highly controlled anesthetic blocks.[8] The gold standard used here is the subsequent carefully recorded short- to longer-term response to a facet denervation procedure.

With sciatica the sensitivity of selective nerve root block is very high, with only a moderate level of specificity being demonstrated.[8] Additionally, diagnostic selective nerve root injections may be a useful tool in the diagnosis of radicular pain in atypical presentations, particularly when diagnostic imaging and clinical examinations do not correlate.[9,10] However, North et al. found that the specificity and sensitivity of nerve root blocks are very low (9% to 42% sensitivities) specific to the diagnosis of "sciatica".[11] Selective nerve root block was most helpful as a negative predictor for the presence of nerve root compression if the block result was negative. Pain relief with blockade of a spinal nerve cannot distinguish between pathology of the proximal nerve in the intervertebral foramen or pain transmitted from distal sites by that nerve.[6] The same group (North et al.) found the strongest association between the relief of sciatica and relief by medial branch posterior ramus (facet) blocks.

The diagnosis of third occipital nerve headache after whiplash injury in cases where there is no distinguishing feature on history or physical examination is typically made by local anesthetic C2–3 facet joint blocks.[12] The false-positive rate, however, of anesthetic blocks of the medial branches of the cervical dorsal rami in the diagnosis of cervical zygapophysial joint pain is high (27%; 95% confidence interval 15% to 38%). This seriously detracts from the specificity of the block.[13] Some evidence exists that local anesthetic peripheral nerve blocks may provide useful diagnostic information in cases of peripheral mononeuropathy.[14] However, pain relief

following paravertebral spinal nerve injection does not predict success by neuroablative surgery, either by dorsal rhizotomy or dorsal root ganglionectomy.[6]

Visceral Versus Somatic Trunk Pain: The origin of pain in the chest, abdomen, or pelvis may be evaluated by diagnostic blocks. A somatic source may be confirmed by injections into costochondral tissue, truncal muscles, or intercostal nerves. Persistent postoperative truncal wound pain may also be evaluated by muscle and neuroma infiltration. Rectus abdominis muscle entrapment of cutaneous nerves may also be isolated. If it can be established that pain is visceral in origin, treatment may be directed towards exploration of abdominal or pelvic organs, or towards denervation of visceral structures, if an untreatable malignancy is encountered. Celiac plexus block, hypogastric plexus block, intercostal nerve block, or local infiltration techniques have all been employed in the diagnosis of painful states involving the viscera and the trunk.[15] However, given the relatively large volume of local anesthetic employed for blocks such as that of the celiac plexus, systemic local anesthetic effects and local spread in the abdomen to adjacent structures cannot be dismissed with any certainty.

Sympathetic Versus Somatic Peripheral Pain: When sympathetic nerve activity is suspected to play an important role in a patient with chronic pain, sympathetic blocks may help confirm the diagnosis. Diagnostic sympathetic blocks should be performed at anatomic sites separate from somatic nerve fibers. These include the cervicothoracic and lumbar sympathetic chain. Confirmation of pain relief and complete sympathetic block on two occasions with different local anesthetics may establish the presence of a sympathetically maintained pain state. Failure to obtain relief is consistent with sympathetically independent pain (SIP). This distinction is descriptive of a pattern of response with potential therapeutic implications; however, it does not indicate a separate disease process. Somatic nerve blocks may assist in the diagnosis of specific musculoskeletal or neuropathic pain syndromes, as described previously.

Referred Pain States: Somatic–somatic pain states may be identified if injection of the original pain site simultaneously relieves pain in the referral zone. This phenomenon can be seen when medial branch blocks for facet syndrome relieve distal buttock and thigh pain, or when injection of active trigger points for myofascial pain provides relief of distant somatic referred pain.

Segmental Levels of Nociceptive Input: Determining the spinal segments associated with somatic or visceral pain, coupled with knowledge of the segmental innervation of body tissues, may indirectly aid in locating the bodily structures involved. Either paravertebral somatic or intercostal nerves may be progressively blocked until all pain is relieved. Repeated blocks with fluoroscopic guidance are essential to making an accurate diagnosis.

Central Pain States: Central pain arises from the brain or spinal cord. It may occur after a central lesion or as a result of abnormal central modulation of nociceptive and non-nociceptive input. Examples include thalamic syndrome after cerebrovascular accident and traumatic spinal cord injury.

The classic response seen with a central pain state is inadequate analgesia after multiple peripheral blocks. Inadequate pain relief is expected after epidural anesthesia to a segmental level that supplies the painful area, as well as poor analgesia with systemic or intraspinal opioids. However, temporary relief of central pain has occurred following diagnostic spinal anesthesia, such as relief of lower but not upper extremity pain in a patient with hemiplegia after a cerebral infarction.[16] Neuropathic pain associated with lesions of the peripheral nervous system may also be associated with altered central processing of nociception. This pain is often relieved with spinal or plexus anesthesia, and it may have a partial response to opioid analgesics.[17,18] Both central and peripheral neuropathic pain may be relieved by intravenous local anesthetic administration.[19,20]

Psychogenic pain has been given an important place in the interpretation of differential blocks. Failure to relieve pain with complete sensory and motor block of the segmental levels associated with the painful area suggests the presence of supraspinal mechanisms. It does not of itself allow the specific diagnosis of either central pain or a psychogenic pain syndrome. Temporary pain relief after a placebo block is a common phenomenon, which allows only for the diagnosis of placebo responder. Observations of unusual responses, such as prolonged dramatic analgesia after a placebo injection or the presence of excessive pain behaviors, may correlate with the clinical impression formed during the initial history and physical examination.

Prognostic Blocks: Local anesthetic blocks may be used to evaluate patients with cancer pain as potential candidates for neurolytic blocks, such as celiac plexus block for the visceral pain of pancreatic cancer.[21] Opioid or local anesthetic injections help predict the response to an implanted apparatus for intraspinal drug administration in similar patients with cancer pain. A single block or repeated local anesthetic blocks may be used before a contemplated neurodestructive procedure is undertaken. Failure to obtain adequate analgesia will prevent an unnecessary operation. Once initial postblock analgesia is achieved, the patient can experience the extent of pain relief and the presence of any unpleasant side effects, such as numbness and dysesthesias, prior to accepting a neurodestructive procedure. However, positive prognostic blocks do not reliably predict long-lasting analgesia, without deafferentation pain, after neurodestructive procedures in patients with chronic nonmalignant pain.[22,23]

ADDITIONAL TECHNIQUES OF DIAGNOSTIC BLOCK

Sacroiliac Joint Injections: That the sacroiliac joint may be a source of low back pain is rarely disputed: what is disputed is the value of performing diagnostic nerve blocks to verify clinical suspicion of the joint being involved as a factor in the etiology of the patient's symptoms.[24] Unfortunately, intra-articular spread of local anesthetic is necessary to achieve efficacy, and this is rarely achieved without adjacent spread of the injectate. Pain relief following injection may be related to infiltration of the sacroiliac joint ligament or sacrospinalis muscle, thus giving the incorrect impression that the joint is the source of the pain. Groin pain seems to be a distinguishing characteristic of patients who respond favorably to sacroiliac joint injection.[25] Unfortunately, no historical or physical examination findings demonstrate sufficient specificity to allow for reliable clinical diagnosis of sacroiliac joint pain; and there is no gold standard, verifying the presence of this diagnosis, to which the results of sacroiliac joint injection can be compared.[8]

Intervertebral Disc Injections: Pain may arise from the annulus of the intervertebral disc, and discography may be a useful technique of determining the internal structure of the disc. Identifying a particular disc as the source of a patient's pain is difficult due to overlap in innervations and due to similar pain arising from facet pathology. Although discography with evaluation of induced pain can discern structurally abnormal and sensitive discs, this does not establish whether the test identifies the source of the patient's pain.[6] One report implies that the diagnostic accuracy in predicting surgical outcomes following discography was 91% at cervical levels, and 82% for lumbar levels.[26] Discography is most accurate and beneficial when the diagnosis of discogenic pain is highly probable, based on sequential analysis of the history, physical examination, and imaging studies.[8]

Selective Sympathetic Blockade: Lumbar sympathectomy may be performed to relieve lower extremity ischemic pain due to advanced peripheral vascular disease. This therapeutic intervention may be preceded by a prognostic lumbar sympathetic block (LSB) using a local anesthetic agent. The presence of an acceptable increase in skin temperature following LSB further supports performance of a therapeutic lumbar sympathectomy (by radiofrequency lesion or by neurolytic blockade) designed to increase blood flow to the ischemic extremity (see Chapter 81). The role of the efferent sympathetic nervous system in persistent pain states is often unclear. Particularly in patients who have received the diagnoses of complex regional pain syndrome, reflex sympathetic dystrophy, or sympathetically maintained pain, there often is a dearth of diagnostic evidence to support the clinical findings. Because of this, historically, sympathetic blocks have been utilized to provide diagnostic insight and to guide therapy. The purpose of diagnostic sympathetic block is to selectively interrupt sympathetic nervous system control of vasculature, while leaving somatic pathways unchallenged. The intended endpoint, complete sympathetic block in an extremity, has proven to be an elusive goal. Stellate ganglion blockade may fail to produce sympathetic denervation of the upper extremity due to the multiple sites of sympathetic nerve activity that bypass the ganglion. Production of Horner's syndrome is no guarantee that sympathetic flow to the hand has been interrupted.[27,28] Also, at lumbar levels there are multiple pathways of sympathetic fibers including collateral chains and crossover connections that may allow persistent sympathetic innervation to reach the lower extremities, hence minimizing the validity of selective lumbar sympathetic nerve blocks in effecting a diagnosis. Unfortunately, the degree of sympathetic nervous system dysfunction does not correlate with the response of pain to sympathetic blockade, nor does the response correlate with serum norepinephrine levels.[29–31]. Therefore, although clinicians continue to employ sympathetic blocks for diagnosis and treatment of many diverse painful states, the evidence does not support their use diagnostically.

Intravenous Regional Sympathetic Block: Intravenous regional blocks (IVR) using bretylium and guanethidine have been administered to patients with suspected sympathetically mediated pain syndromes. Both agents inhibit release of norepinephrine from nerve terminals, and guanethidine depletes tissues of it. Regional sympathetic block follows these procedures, and the patient's response during the post block period may indicate the extent to which the pain is mediated by the sympathetic nervous system. Since there is a high correlation between relief of pain following IV phentolamine and IVR guanethidine, it is likely that each agent is producing analgesia by a sympatholytic mechanism.[32] Unfortunately, there is no indication that a given patient who responds favorably to IVR sympatholysis will have a long-term beneficial effect following either a series of blocks or from systemically administered antisympathetics.

Local Anesthetic Infusions: Intravenous lidocaine hydrochloride has been used in the diagnosis of neuropathic pain states. Patients who respond favorably to IV lidocaine infusions may be placed on oral congeners of lidocaine, notably mexiletine or tocainide for prolonged management. Studies suggest that there is selective peripheral and central analgesia produced by intravenous lidocaine in neuropathic pain states.[33] While at least four studies document the analgesic effect of oral mexiletine in individuals who responded favorably to IV lidocaine,[34–37] there is one randomized and controlled study that indicates the ability of IV lidocaine to diagnose predictably potential responders to oral mexiletine.[38]

Intravenous Phentolamine: Phentolamine, an α-adrenergic blocking agent, has been administered intravenously in an attempt to determine if a patient's pain is sympathetically mediated. Response to IV phentolamine should indicate patients who might expect positive response to systemic or transdermal sympatholytic agents. Unfortunately, phentolamine has demonstrated local anesthetic properties, possibly biasing the analgesia that results from its use.[39,40] Additionally, the role of α-receptors in sympathetically mediated pain is poorly quantified.[41] Other reports suggest that phentolamine response may not differ appreciably from placebo response.[42,43] Considered alone, the phentolamine test is not very specific or sensitive (for diagnosing sympathetically mediated pain).[6]

PREREQUISITES FOR OPTIMAL DIAGNOSTIC BLOCK

The physician must make a complete evaluation of the patient prior to undertaking any diagnostic nerve block. A comprehensive history should include a pain diary, a history of the present pain, and all previous diagnostic workup and therapy information. A complete neurological and general physical examination including a functional evaluation should be undertaken. Results of diagnostic studies and psychological evaluations are reviewed. A physician who is knowledgeable about pain syndromes and diagnostic procedures must then determine if a diagnostic block is indicated and document the specific goal to be achieved with the selected procedure. Communication with the patient is necessary to obtain informed consent, ensuring that the true goals and limitations of the block are understood. The patient must be monitored for any major regional anesthesia or conduction block.

The following modifications to regional anesthesia procedures may improve the reliability of diagnostic nerve block:

- Limit the use of pre-procedure sedatives and analgesics to ensure that the patient remains communicative at all times.
- Limit the volumes of local anesthetics to minimize the likelihood of spread to adjacent, unwanted sites.
- Make liberal use of radiography including fluoroscopy, computed tomography (CT) scans, contrast material, ultrasonography, and plain film X-rays to improve accuracy.
- Employ a peripheral nerve stimulator with a variable output to locate target nerves precisely for plexus and peripheral nerve block.
- Repeat positive blocks with a local anesthetic of different duration, if the first block is successful, in an attempt to correlate the duration of pain relief to that of the expected duration of the local anesthetic.
- Maintain detailed observations and records of the effects of the diagnostic block.
- Record the patient's pain scores at rest and with function, as well as vital signs, sensory and motor examination findings, signs of sympathetic nervous system function, and the presence of pain behaviors both before and after the diagnostic block.
- Ask the patient to maintain records of neurologic symptoms, degree of pain relief, pain scores, activity levels, and analgesic intake following discharge.

Interpretation of Block Results: It is important to understand the limits of diagnostic blocks. They are not intended to be therapeutic, and they have little diagnostic value unless considered within the framework of all other information obtained about the patient. Careful observation of the patient's response to blockade must be made and recorded. The extent of motor, sensory, and sympathetic block must be assessed by neurologic testing and correlated with the degree of pain relief and functional improvement over time. Conclusions about various aspects of the patient's pain may then be made, considering all of the information mentioned previously.

Pitfalls in Evaluating Results: Pain relief due to an unintended action of a block can be classified as a false-positive response. False-positive results may occur due to a placebo response, systemic effects of local anesthetics, spread of agent to adjacent tissues or nerves, unreliable patient report of block effects, and temporary alterations in central processing due to lack of normal afferent input.[7] Placebo response occurs in about 30% of patients and should always be considered after a positive diagnostic block. A report of differential spinal block for chronic pain has noted this response in just less than 20% of patients.[44] The presence of a placebo response has no reliable diagnostic significance. Confirmatory facet blocks with different local anesthetics have documented a false-positive rate for uncontrolled blocks in 27% to 38% of patients.[13,45] Systemic effects of local anesthetics may be expected to influence neuropathic pain states, particularly after use of large doses.[46] Distal block of afferent sensory input to the spinal cord may temporarily relieve pain due to a proximal or central lesion.[16–18,47] This implies that normal sensory input is activating a sensitized central neuronal pathway, and it is temporarily interrupted by the diagnostic block.

False-negative responses may occur when a block fails to relieve pain. This may result from an incomplete block, the presence of alternative pain pathways, unappreciated referred pain syndromes, unreliable patient report of block effects, and diagnostic testing performed at inappropriate times.[7] Blocks may be incomplete due to deficiencies in technique, particularly when reduced volumes of local anesthetics are used to achieve selective block. Failure to select all the pertinent neural pathways may result in apparent failure, particularly for painful joints that have multiple, overlapping innervations. Failure to document complete block of desired target nerve fibers in the expected location will also lead to apparent failure. It is not unusual for sympathetic or somatic blocks to be less than complete. Referred somatic pain phenomena may lead to failure to block the correct source of somatic pain initially. For example, back and leg pain may be due to lumbar disc herniation or degeneration, or to piriformis muscle syndrome, facet joint disease, sacroiliac joint dysfunction, ligamentous strain or tear, or myofascial pain, requiring radically different diagnostic somatic blocks to be performed. Diagnostic blocks should not be performed unless the patient is experiencing significant pain; the extent of pain relief should be evaluated when the maximum local anesthetic effect has been achieved.

Diagnostic nerve blocks can be useful aids in the workup and management of chronic pain states, particularly when the specific diagnosis remains in doubt following an exhaustive clinical evaluation. However, as stated by Hogan and Abram, these blocks are informative only in proportion to the care with which they are performed and the thoroughness with which the response is evaluated; and the findings should be interpreted cautiously.[6]

KEY POINTS

- Pain relief after local anesthetic blockade does not reliably predict successful neurodestructive surgery, i.e., long-lasting analgesia without deafferentation pain.
- Prognostic local anesthetic blocks may be used to evaluate patients for neurolytic block. A negative response to blockade may be extremely valuable in preventing an unnecessary neurodestructive procedure.
- Relief of neuropathic pain with intravenous lidocaine appears to predict potential responders to oral mexilitine therapy.
- Placebo response occurs frequently and should be considered after a positive diagnostic block.
- After an initial positive block, confirmatory medial branch blocks with a different local anesthetic demonstrate a 27% to 38% false-positive rate.
- It is not unusual for sympathetic or somatic nerve blocks to be less than complete. This should be considered after a negative diagnostic block.

REFERENCES

1. Winnie AP, Candido KD: Diagnostic tools available for pain management. *In* Raj PP (ed): Pain Medicine. A Comprehensive Review, ed 2. Mosby, St Louis, 2003, p 195.
2. Winnie AP, Candido KD: Differential neural blockade for the diagnosis of pain. *In* Waldman SD (ed): Interventional Pain Management, ed 2. WB Saunders, Philadelphia, 2001, p 162.
3. Winnie AP, Candido KD: Differential neural blockade in the diagnosis of pain mechanisms. *In* Raj PP (ed): Practical Management of Pain, ed 3. Mosby, St Louis, 2000, p 427.
4. Raj PP: Sympathetic pain mechanisms and management. Second Annual Meeting of the American Society of Regional Anesthesia, Hollywood, FA, 10–11 March 1977.
5. Hogan QH, Abram SE: Neural blockade for diagnosis and prognosis. A review. Anesthesiology 86:216–241, 1997.
6. Hogan QH, Abram SE: Diagnostic and prognostic neural blockade. *In* Cousins MJ, Bridenbaugh PO (eds): Neural Blockade in Clinical Anesthesia and Management of Pain, ed 3. Lippincott-Raven, Philadelphia, 1998, pp 837–877.
7. Boas RA, Cousins MJ: Diagnostic neural blockade. *In* Cousins MJ, Bridenbaugh PA (eds): Neural Blockade in Clinical Anesthesia and Management of Pain, ed 2. JB Lippincott, Philadelphia, 1988, p 885.
8. Saal JS: General principles of diagnostic testing as related to painful lumbar spine disorders: A critical appraisal of current diagnostic techniques. Spine 27:2538–2545, 2002.
9. Huston CW, Slipman CW: Diagnostic selective nerve root blocks: Indications and usefulness. Phy Med Rehab Clin N Am 13:545–565, 2002.
10. Pang WW, Ho ST, Huang MH: Selective lumbar spinal nerve block. A review. Acta Anaesthesiol Sin 37:21–26, 1999.
11. North RB, Kidd DH, Zahurak M, et al: Specificity of diagnostic nerve blocks: A prospective, randomized study of sciatica due to lumbosacral spine disease. Pain 65:77–85, 1996.
12. Lord SM, Barnsley L, Wallis BJ, et al: Third occipital nerve headache: A prevalence study. J Neurol Neurosurg Psychiatry 57:1187–1190, 1994.
13. Barnsley L, Lord S, Wallis B, et al: False-positive rates of cervical zygapophysial joint blocks. Clin J Pain 9:124–130, 1993.
14. Abram SE: Neural blockade for neuropathic pain. Clin J Pain 16(Suppl 2):S56–S61, 2000.
15. Gallegos NC, Hobsley M: Recognition and treatment of abdominal wall pain. J R Soc Med 82:343, 1989.
16. Crisolgo PA, Neal B, Brown R, et al: Lidocaine-induced spinal block can relieve central poststroke pain: Role of the block in chronic pain diagnosis. Anesthesiology 74:184, 1991.
17. Kibler RF, Nathan PW: Relief of pain and paresthesia by nerve blocks distal to a lesion. J Neurol Neurosurg Psychiatry 23:91, 1960.
18. Loh L, Nathan PW, Schott G: Pain due to lesions of the central nervous system removed by sympathetic block. BMJ 282:1026, 1981.
19. Boas RA, Covino BG, Shahnarian A: Analgesic response to iv lidocaine. Br J Anaesth 54:501, 1982.
20. Woolf C, Weisenfeld-Hollin Z: The systemic administration of local anesthetics produces a selective depression of C-afferent fiber evoked activity in the spinal cord. Pain 23:361, 1985.
21. Bonica JJ, Buckley FP: Regional anesthesia with local anesthetics. *In* Bonica JJ (ed): The Management of Pain, ed 2. Lea & Febiger, Philadelphia, 1990, p 1883.
22. Loeser JD: Dorsal rhizotomy for the relief of chronic pain. J Neurosurg 36:745, 1972.
23. Tasker R: Deafferentation and causalgia. *In* Bonica JJ (ed): Advances in Pain Research and Treatment. Raven Press, New York, 1980, p 305.
24. Fortin JD, Dwyer AP, West S, et al: Sacroiliac joint: Pain referral maps upon applying a new injection/arthrography technique: I. Asymptomatic volunteers. Spine 19:1475, 1994.
25. Schwarzer C, April CN, Bogduk N: The sacroiliac joint in chronic low back pain. Spine 20:31, 1995.
26. Simmons EH, Segil C: An evaluation of discography in the localization of symptomatic levels in discogenic disease of the spine. Clin Orthop 108:57, 1975.
27. Malmqvist EL, Bengtsson M, Sorensen J: Efficacy of stellate ganglion block: A clinical study with bupivacaine. Reg Anesth 17:340, 1992.

28. Ready LB, Kozody R, Barsa JE, et al: Side-port needles for stellate ganglion block. Reg Anesth 7:160, 1982.

29. Loh L, Nathan PW: Painful peripheral states and sympathetic block. J Neurol Neurosurg Psy 41:664, 1978.

30. Tahmoush AJ, Malley J, Jennings JR: Skin conductance, temperature and blood flow in causalgia. Neurology 33:1483, 1983.

31. Drummond PD, Finch PM, Smythe GA: Reflex sympathetic dystrophy: The significance of differing plasma catecholamine concentrations in affected and unaffected limbs. Brain 114:2025, 1991.

32. Arner S: Intravenous phentolamine test: Diagnostic and prognostic use in reflex sympathetic dystrophy. Pain 46:17, 1991.

33. Rowlingson JC, DiFazio CA, Foster J, Carron H: Lidocaine as an analgesic for experimental pain. Anesthesiology 52:20, 1980.

34. Peterson P, Kastrup J: Dercum's disease (adiposa dolorosa): Treatment of the severe pain with intravenous lidocaine. Pain 28:77, 1987.

35. Vickers ER, Cousins MJ: Neuropathic orofacial pain: 2. Diagnostic procedures, treatment guidelines and case reports. Aust Endod J 26:53–63, 2000.

36. Scott RM: Mexiletine and vascular headaches. Aust N Z J Med 93:92, 1981.

37. Dirks J, Fabricius S, Petersen KL, et al: The effect of systemic lidocaine on pain and secondary hyperalgesia associated with the heat/capsaicin sensitization model in healthy volunteers. Anesth Analg 91:967–972, 2000.

38. Galer BS, Harle J, Rowbotham MC: Response to intravenous lidocaine infusion predicts subsequent response to oral mexiletine: a prospective study. J Pain Symptom Manage 12:161–167, 1996.

39. Northover BJ: A comparison of the electrophysiological actions of phentolamine with those of some other antiarrhythmic drugs on tissues isolated from the rat heart. Br J Pharmacol 80:85, 1983.

40. Ramirez JM, French AS: Phentolamine selectively affects the fast sodium component of sensory adaptation in an insect mechanoreceptor. J Neurobiol 21:893, 1990.

41. Ochoa J, Verdugo R: Reflex sympathetic dystrophy: Definitions and history of the ideas; a critical review of human studies. In Low PA (ed): The Evaluation and Management of Clinical Autonomic Disorders. Little, Brown, Boston, 1993, pp 473–492.

42. Verdugo R, Rosenblum S, Ochoa J: Phentolamine sympathetic blocks mislead diagnosis. Soc Neurosci 17(abstr):107, 1991.

43. Fine PG, Roberts WJ, Gillette RG, et al: Slowly developing placebo responses confound tests of intravenous phentolamine to determine mechanisms underlying idiopathic chronic low back pain. Pain 56:235, 1994.

44. Jacobson L, Chabal C, Mariano AJ, et al: Persistent low-back pain is real: However, diagnostic spinal injections are not helpful in its evaluation. Clin J Pain 8:237, 1992.

45. Schwarzer AC, April CN, Derby R, et al: The false-positive rate of uncontrolled blocks of the lumbar zygapophyseal joints. Pain 58:195, 1994.

46. Ekblom A, Hansson P, Lindblom U, et al: Does a regional nerve block change cutaneous perception thresholds outside the anesthetic area? Implications for the interpretation of diagnostic blocks. Pain 50:163, 1992.

47. Xavier AV, McDaniel J, Kissin I: Relief of sciatic radicular pain by sciatic nerve block. Anesth Analg 67:1177, 1988.

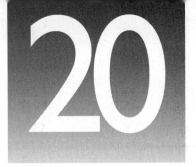

Neurosurgical Procedures for Treatment of Intractable Pain

Robert M. Levy, M.D., Ph.D.

Modern neurosurgical procedures for pain were first attempted in the latter part of the 19th century. Letievant first described sectioning of the cranial and peripheral nerves to alleviate pain in his book "Traite de Sections Nerveuses" in 1873. In 1891 Horsley performed a gasserian neurectomy for trigeminal neuralgia; Frazier perfected this technique in 1928. The first spinal dorsal rhizotomy was reported by Abbe in 1889 and the first successful chordotomy was performed by Spiller and Martin in 1912. Leriche, in his 1939 book "La Chirurgie de la Douleur," is credited with the development of sympathectomy. Moniz first performed frontal lobotomy for pain control in 1936. From these sentinel reports has grown a significant experience in the ablation of neural structures to control medically intractable pain. This chapter attempts to present a concise review of the current status of neroblative procedures used in the management of chronic pain; neuromodularity procedures are discussed elsewhere in this volume.

PERIPHERAL NERVE PROCEDURES

Spinal Dorsal Rhizotomy: Attempts at pain control through invasive procedures were initially directed at the peripheral nervous system. After Abbe performed the first spinal posterior rhizotomy in 1889, enthusiasm for the procedure spread quickly. At the height of its popularity, spinal dorsal rhizotomy was used for a wide variety of pain syndromes. Cervicothoracic dorsal rhizotomy was performed for angina pectoris, intractable headaches, and facial pain, and it became widely used for failed back surgery syndrome, paraplegic pain, pelvic cancer, postherpetic neuralgia, and post-thoracotomy pain. More recently percutaneous radiofrequency methods of spinal rhizotomy have been devised to minimize the risks of extensive laminectomies. Dorsal rhizotomy was thought to have great analgesic potential based on the early neuroanatomic principles that suggested that the dorsal roots carry only sensory

fibers, whereas ventral roots carry only motor fibers. The more recent demonstration of unmyelinated sensory fibers in the ventral root may explain the often unsatisfactory results of these procedures; sensory pain fibers entering via the ventral route escape interruption by dorsal rhizotomy. Histologic sprouting, both in the intact cutaneous nerves and the spinal cord dorsal horn adjacent to denervated regions, may also allow transmission of nociceptive information despite dorsal rhizotomy. The possibility that nociceptive afferents bypass the dorsal spinal roots and that dorsal horn neurons have modifiable receptive fields may further account for the poor success rate of dorsal rhizotomy for pain control.

Despite decades of experience, it is difficult to define clearly the indications for rhizotomy. Nonetheless, there is consistent failure of dorsal rhizotomy for post-thoracotomy pain, post-herpetic neuralgia, failed back surgery syndrome, and post-paraplegia pain. Current indications for open dorsal rhizotomy include neuropathic pain of the chest wall associated with allodynia, treated by thoracic rhizotomy; cancer pain of the pelvis, rectum; and pain in a functionally useless limb, treated by a multi-level rhizotomy.[1] Patients medically unfit for open laminectomy can benefit from percutaneous rhizotomy. Benign intractable monoradicular pain in the cervical thoracic pain of malignant origin may be effectively treated with percutaneous rhizolysis.

Prior to dorsal rhizotomy, a trial block of the selected roots with local anesthesia should be performed; nonetheless, transient pain relief with a local block does not guarantee long-term pain relief. If local blocks are successful, open dorsal rhizotomy is performed using a routine laminectomy technique. Due to overlapping dermatomal innervation, one or two roots above and below the targeted dermatome should be sectioned. The percutaneous approach for dorsal rhizotomy was introduced in 1974 by Uematsu and colleagues and the techniques in localization of invertebral foramen are well described.[2–]

The technique combines the use of a thermistor-monitored electrode, a fluoroscopic image intensifier, a nerve stimulator, and a radiofrequency lesion generator. Uematsu and co-workers recommend graded increments of heating using the thermocoagulator at 50 to 90°C for 90 to 120 seconds. Potential but rare complications of rhizotomy include wound infection, meningitis, hemorrhage, spinal cord infarction, trauma to the spinal cord, and cerebral spinal fluid leak. Postrhizotomy dysesthesias and anesthesia dolorosa are also potential complications of this denervation procedure.

There is considerable variability in the reported effectiveness of open dorsal rhizotomy; few outcome studies of percutaneous dorsal rhizotomy are available. Ten studies published between 1969 and 1986 reported on a total of 1,173 patients; the mean success rate was 59%, with a range from 28% to 100%. Four significant reports have been published on the results of percutaneous dorsal rhizotomy, but the number of subjects has been small and outcome definitions are not consistent. Nonetheless, these authors reported success rates ranging from 52% to 93%.

Dorsal Root Ganglionectomy: Scoville first reported an extradural approach to dorsal roots and dorsal root ganglions in 1966. Smith began performing dorsal root ganglionectomies using the rationale that simple dorsal rhizotomies failed because some of the pain impulses traveled via the dorsal root ganglia to the sympathetic chain and entered the spinal cord at a higher level.[5] With the exception of a small number of cell bodies of nociceptive fibers in the ventral root, dorsal root ganglionectomy should overcome the anatomic limitations of spinal rhizotomy by removing nearly all nociceptive cell bodies.

Possible indications for dorsal root ganglionectomy include perineal or chest wall pain secondary to cancer; peripheral pain of thoracic and abdominal origin; and thoracic postherpetic pain.[1] Although mixed results have been reported in the setting of failed back surgery syndrome,[6–9] North reported long-term follow-up of at least 5 years with only 15% success.

Preoperative screening with local anesthetic blockade of the spinal ganglia along with control placebo injection should be performed. Failure of the block should preclude ganglionectomy. However, complete pain relief from preoperative blockade does not guarantee surgical success. As with other segmental neuroblative procedures, ganglionectomy is performed at the involved level as well as at levels above and below, to cover the desired dermatomes. As with the dorsal rhizotomy, the risks of ganglionectomy may include disruption of the vascular supply, hemorrhage, infection, cerebrospinal fluid leak, wound dehiscence, and other possible complications of spinal surgery. Postganglionectomy dysesthesias and anesthesia dolorosa have been reported.[6–9] Eleven series have been reported from 1966 to 1991, representing 237 patients treated with dorsal root ganglionectomy. Reported success rates varied from 0% to 100%; the mean reported success rate was 61%.

Facet Denervation: Goldthwait first described pain from disorders of the facet joint in 1911. The innervation of the facet comes from radicular spinal nerves. The posterior primary ramus of the spinal nerve divides into a medial and lateral branch; the medial branch innervates the facet joint. With this anatomic understanding, Rees advanced the concept of percutaneous facet denervation and later communicated a 99.8% success rate without mortality or major morbidity in 1,000 procedures.[10]

Others have since reported lesser success with this procedure. Multiple modifications of the procedure, including the use of radiofrequency thermocoagulation, have since been described. Although no unanimity of opinion exists, patients with chronic mechanical back pain with no other treatable cause in whom conservative management has failed may be candidates for percutaneous facet denervation. Critical for patient selection is the response to a local, selective facet block with local anesthetic. Pain relief should be complete or nearly complete and should be achieved consistently with repeated trials. The technique for percutaneous facet denervation is well described.[11,12] Repeating this procedure at least one level above and below the desired target is required for lasting pain relief. Complications from reported series are rare.[13–16] Beside the risks involved in all percutaneous operative procedures, superficial burns from failure of insulation and acute radiculitis have been reported. From 1971 until 1990, 10 reports were published of 1,990 patients treated with facet denervation procedures. Success rates ranged from 21% to 99%; the mean success rate was 62%.

Peripheral Neurectomy: In 1828 Wood first used the term "neuroma" to describe the pathologic condition characterized by a bulbous terminal of injured nerves, and Mitchell coined the term "causalgia" in 1872 to describe the chronic pain after nerve injury experienced by veterans of the Civil War. Although resection of the involved peripheral nerve is, at first glance, an appealing approach, overwhelming clinical and physiologic evidence has accrued against the use of neurectomy for the management of chronic pain.[4] Thus, most peripheral nerves consist of mixed motor and sensory fibers, and sectioning the nerve may result in both motor deficits and total anesthesia. With the resulting significant sensory loss, denervation hypersensitivity or anesthesia dolorosa may develop. Neuromas may form at the transsected nerve stump. Furthermore, pain relief following neurectomy is often short lived due to adjacent sprouting of sensory nerves.

Today, peripheral neurectomy has a limited role in the management of chronic pain. Cranial neurectomy has proved to be of little value in the treatment of trigeminal neuralgia, headaches, or atypical facial pain. Neurectomy has failed to relieve consistently phantom limb, chest wall, or abdominal pain. However, there are a few selected situations in which peripheral neurectomy may be of value, including pain due to a neuroma in a weight-bearing area, pain due to a neuroma in continuity from an entrapment or a traumatized nerve, and pain due to severe intractable meralgia paresthetica.[4] Proper patient selection is the most important predictor of successful neurectomy or neuroma excision. Thorough history and physical examination; sympathetic, thermal, and mechanical testing; electromyelography/nerve conduction velocity studies; and diagnostic nerve blocks should be performed. At surgery, the neuroma can be best located with the help of the Tinel's sign. The neuroma is excised and the proximal nerve stump is implanted into muscle or bone marrow. External or internal neurolysis is reserved for treatment of neuroma-in-continuity, when preservation of function is desired. The addition of nerve transposition may be performed to avoid repeated trauma to the nerve stump or proximal nerve.

Postoperative dysesthesias following neurectomy are possible; anesthesia dolorosa is rare. For neuroma-in-continuity, the nerve function may be disrupted and a new neurologic deficit may occur. Between 1976 and 1995, seven large series have reported the results of peripheral neurectomy and/or neuroma resection in 443 patients. The mean reported success rate was 71%.

Sympathectomy: Leriche first performed a sympathectomy for lower extremity trophic ulcers and was the first to implicate the sympathetic nervous system in chronic pain states.[17] Pathogenic studies of causalgia and sympathetic dystrophy soon postulated the formation of "artificial synapses" following nerve injury and suggested that tonic efferent sympathetic impulses jumped to the adjoining injured and poorly myelinated fibers. More recently abnormal increases in the firing rate of regenerating transsected fibers, especially in response to norepinephrine, have been observed as has the successful use of regional guanethidine blocks in patients with causalgia and sympathetic dystrophy. The development of endoscopic approaches and both percutaneous radiofrequency and chemical techniques for the production of lesions have made sympathectomy a safer treatment option.

Sympathectomy for relief of chronic pain is currently indicated only in a handful of conditions involving the limbs and abdominal viscera. These include pain due to causalgia, reflex sympathetic dystrophy, peripheral vascular disease, and Raynaud's disease. Sympathectomy may also be considered for abdominal visceral pain due to chronic pancreatitis or pancreatic carcinoma. Failure of conservative therapy, a thorough preoperative assessment, and both therapeutic and diagnostic sympathetic blocks should be performed prior to surgical sympathectomy. The techniques for sympathectomy are well described and include upper thoracic ganglionectomy, lower thoracic sympathectomy or splanchnicectomy, and lumbar sympathectomy. Transthoracic endoscopic and stereotactic percutaneous approaches are also currently employed.[18,19] Complications of upper thoracic ganglionectomy include wound infection, pneumonia, pneumothorax, cerebrospinal fluid leak, Horner's syndrome, spinal cord injury, and empyema. Pleural tears, wound infections, empyema, and paraplegia due to vascular disruption have been reported in splanchnicectomy. For lumbar sympathectomy, the major neurologic complication is sexual dysfunction in men who have undergone bilateral procedures. Postsympathectomy neuralgia consisting of severe, deep aching and burning pain in the proximal limb is not an infrequent complication of sympathectomy. Although it may occur in up to 20% of cases of sympathectomy, this phenomenon usually subsides spontaneously within 6 months. The reported success rate of sympathectomy varies from 59% to 89% for causalgia and sympathetic dystrophy and from 67% to 100% for pancreatic pain. For other chronic pain syndromes, the results of sympathectomy are less vigorous. Despite reports of 60% success for treatment of pain for Raynaud's disease, other series report quite poor rates of success. Discouraging results have also been reported for postamputation pain. The effectiveness of lumbar sympathectomy for ischemic rest pain or claudication remains unclear.

Lesions of the Dorsal Root Entry Zone: With the knowledge that spontaneous discharges from neurons occurred within the spinal cord dorsal horn on deafferentation, Nashold and co-workers in 1976 attempted to produce a lesion in the substantia gelatinosa to alleviate phantom pain.[20] Sindou and colleagues[21] reported a similar operation using open microsurgical techniques.

Current theory suggests that the pathologic responses associated with deafferentation, allodynia, hyperalgesia, and hyperesthesia result from the facilitation of incoming signals, which occurs in the dorsal horn. Thus, the goal of producing a lesion in the dorsal root entry zone (DREZ) is to destroy the site of pathologic processing at which such facilitation occurs.

DREZ lesioning is currently considered primarily for pain due to brachial or lumbosacral plexus avulsions. It may also be effective in treating the segmental pain secondary to spinal cord injury, postherpetic neuralgia amputation or phantom limb pain, and pain due to malignancy and in certain facial pain syndromes.

A number of different methods have been devised to produce lesions in the DREZ, including the microsurgical ablation first described by Sindou and others,[21] laser destruction, and radiofrequency heating. Currently, radiofrequency lesioning is the most popular method; lesions are made by heating the electrode to 75°C for 15 seconds. Bernard and co-workers[22] have expanded the use of DREZ lesions to the nucleus caudalis for severe postherpetic neuralgia and severe intractable facial pain, in which the lesions are made from the upper rootlets of C2 to an area just rostral to the level of the obex.

Complications of DREZ lesioning include weakness of the ipsilateral leg, reduction of proprioception, loss of pain and temperature sensation beyond the painful limb, and impotence. In addition, the inherent risks of intradural spinal surgery such as cerebrospinal fluid leak, infection, hemorrhage, infarction, and wound dehiscence, may also be encountered.

DREZ lesions for pain control following brachial plexus avulsion injuries have been reported in 341 patients from 1984 until 1993. Success rates range from 29% to 100%; the mean reported success rate of these studies was 66%. Of the 130 reported cases of patients treated with DREZ lesions for spinal cord injury pain, 65 patients (50%) had good results. Pain relief was excellent for segmental pain and poor for distal pain. The results of DREZ lesions for postherpetic neuralgia are generally disappointing, ranging from 20% to 50%. Patients usually gain early relief only to experience recurrence of the pain. For phantom limb pain, the average success rate of DREZ lesioning is 37%. The experience of DREZ lesions in the nucleus caudalis for treatment of facial pain is very limited; good results may be obtained in patients with facial pain due to postherpetic neuralgia, brain stem infarction, or multiple sclerosis, but not for anesthesia dolorosa or peripheral trigeminal neuralgia.

SPINAL CORD ABLATIVE PROCEDURES FOR CHRONIC PAIN

Commissural Myelotomy: Based on the anatomic concept that fibers carrying nociceptive information cross at the anterior commissure of the spinal cord, Armour in 1926 performed the first commissural myelotomy for pain. Commissural myelotomy involves interruption of decussating spinothalamic fibers in the anterior commissure with the expectation that this will produce bilaterally symmetrical analgesia at the level of myelotomy. Additional extensive areas of pain relief caudal to the lesion, without associated sensory changes, are often observed. The primary indication for commissural myelotomy is intractable bilateral pain in the lower half of the body, particularly due to malignancy. Myelotomy is especially valuable for patients with midline pain that is unresponsive to spinal opioids.

Complications occur in 5% to 10% of patients and include dysesthesias, motor weakness, gait ataxia, and bladder dysfunction. The risks inherent to intradural spinal surgery must also be considered. Approximately 350 cases of open commissural myelotomy have been reported; the range of reported success rates varies from 20% to 100%, with a mean of approximately 65%. Although the total cases performed via percutaneous technique is smaller, the success rate is very similar.

The use of neuroaugmentative devices has reduced the use of the commissural myelotomy, and the indications for its use currently are quite limited. As has been suggested by the results just mentioned, this procedure has the potential to produce a favorable outcome in a selected group of patients who do not have malignant disease and do not respond to other less invasive therapies.

Anterolateral Cordotomy: Spiller performed the first open thoracic cordotomy in 1912; since that time the procedure has been carefully described and refined.[23] Mullan and associates introduced the percutaneous method of performing an anterolateral cordotomy in 1963,[24] and Rosomoff and co-workers developed a percutaneous radiofrequency technique in 1965.[25] Anterolateral cordotomy leads to loss of contralateral pain and temperature sensation without loss of position or light touch sensation. In general, pain sensitivity is diminished within two to three levels below the level of cordotomy.

In the past, anterolateral cordotomy was used for a variety of painful conditions that were medically intractable. With greater knowledge of its long-term complications and newer neuroaugmentative techniques, anterolateral cordotomy is rarely used and is reserved for medically intractable pain due to cancer in patients whose life span is less than 3 years.

Numerous publications have described the techniques of open anterolateral cordotomy.[26] Following C2 hemilaminectomy or appropriate high thoracic bilateral laminectomy, the dura is opened and the dentate ligament identified. The lateral attachment of the dentate ligament is cut to allow for mobilization of the cord. A cordotomy knife is inserted just ventral to the dentate ligament, and this quadrant of the spinal cord is sectioned. In the percutaneous approach[27] patients are placed in supine position and, under local anesthesia, an 18-gauge needle is introduced into the subarachnoid space under fluoroscopic guidance, aimed just anterior to the dentate ligament between C1 and C2. Following myelographic confirmation of the needle position, an electrode is introduced through the needle into the parenchyma of the cord, and the target location is confirmed with the use of electrical stimulation. When the appropriate target is identified, a radiofrequency lesion is made.

The mortality rate for open anterolateral cordotomy has been reported in a different series to range from 3% to 20%. Cervical cordotomies and bilateral cordotomies have a higher mortality rate than that of thoracic and unilateral cordotomies. Respiratory complications occur in about 10% of the cases. Motor impairment is reported in 10% to 15% of patients for unilateral lesions and up to 39% when bilateral procedures are performed Dysfunctions of micturition and defecation as a complication vary widely. Postcordotomy dysesthesias occur in up to 11% of patients. The complication rate for the percutaneous approach is much lower; motor deficit (3%), ataxia (3%), bladder or sexual dysfunction (3%), respiratory problems (1%), and postcordotomy dysesthesia (1%) are all uncommon following percutaneous cordotomy.

From 1966 to 1977 three large series reported the results of open cordotomy in 712 patients; the mean reported success rate was 75%. From 1966 to 1988 seven large series reported the results of percutaneous cordotomy in 6,665 patients; the mean reported success rate was 73%. For bilateral procedures, the success rates were marginally lower. As with many other ablative procedures for pain, this rate of success decreases as the time of follow-up is lengthened. Thus, although 3-month pain control was reached in 84% of patients in one study, the long-term success rate at 5 to 10 years was 37%.[27]

INTRACRANIAL ABLATIVE PROCEDURES

The introduction of stereotactic techniques together with advances in neuroimaging and computer technology have revolutionized intracranial ablative procedures. Today, intracranial ablative procedures can be done accurately and safely under local anesthesia. Modern intracranial ablative techniques include producing lesions in the brainstem pain pathways (trigeminal tractotomy, spinothalamic tractotomy, mesencephalotomy), the diencephalon (thalamotomy, pulvinarotomy, hypothalamotomy), the telencephalon (cingulotomy or cingulumotomy), and the pituitary gland (hypophysectomy).

Most patients considered for intracranial ablative procedures have medically intractable chronic severe pain secondary to cancer, although the procedures are rarely used for pain of nonmalignant origins. In these patients, in whom pain is unresponsive to medical therapy and less invasive surgical therapies have failed, intracranial ablative procedures are contemplated. Patients with diffuse, nociceptive pain and short life expectancy tend to have the best results; it is important that they have a sufficiently clear sensorium to provide meaningful informed consent.

Traditionally, ventriculography was the method of choice for localization of the target for the placement of the lesion. Today, computer tomography (CT) or magnetic resonance imaging (MRI) guided stereotactic methods are usually used. Modern stereotactic treatment planning software can allow for careful preoperative planning of target location and trajectory. Although radiofrequency thermal lesions are the standard for intracranial ablative procedures, noninvasive radiosurgical techniques are currently under active investigation.[28]

Trigeminal Tractotomy: Sjoqvist first developed the medullary trigeminal tractotomy in 1938, which was refined by both Grant in 1941 and Sweet in 1955. In the 1960s Hitchcock and Crue developed percutaneous approaches to trigeminal tractotomy. The trigeminal nerve pain fibers traverse the medulla to the nucleus caudalis. These fibers are joined by pain fibers from cranial nerves VII, IX, and X. Medullary trigeminal tractotomy targets these fibers for pain control. This procedure has been particularly helpful in the relief of intractable pain caused by malignancy of the head and neck. For postherpetic neuralgia and anesthesia dolorosa, trigeminal tractotomy has been less effective.

Technically, this can be performed as an open or percutaneous procedure, with or without the aid of stereotaxy.[29,30] The open procedure consists of a C1 and C2 laminectomy and durotomy followed by identification of obex and dorsolateral sulcus. After identification of the trigeminal tract by evoked potentials, a careful incision is made on the dorsolateral sulcus that is 3 mm in depth, extending from 2 mm below the obex to the accessory nerve filaments. Stereotactically, the procedure can be done under local anesthesia with radiofrequency lesioning.

Complications from trigeminal tractotomy include weakness and ataxia, usually of the ipsilateral upper extremity, analgesia in the contralateral leg, Horner's syndrome, dysarthria, and hiccups. Most of these are temporary. Including patients with advanced neoplastic disease, the overall mortality rate from this procedure may be as high as 5% to 10%. The overall success rate for a combined total of 669 cases for open medullary trigeminal tractotomy is 75%, whereas that for the cases with the percutaneous approach is 82.5%; the overall complication rate is 22% to 25%.[31]

Pontine and Bulbar Spinothalamic Tractotomy: The first medullary spinothalamic tractotomy was described by Schwartz in 1941. Similar to the open anterolateral cordotomy, spinothalamic tractotomy at this level can relieve more rostral pain in the upper shoulder and neck. At the medullary level, the spinothalamic tract is located ventral to the descending trigeminal tract and dorsolateral to the inferior olivary nucleus. With the introduction of high percutaneous cervical cordotomy and DREZ lesions for the upper arm, this procedure is much less commonly used.

Current indications for medullary spinothalamic tractotomy include intractable unilateral cancer pain, especially in the upper arm, shoulder, and neck. Severe pulmonary compromise is a relative contraindication for this procedure. Technically, a suboccipital craniectomy is performed, the arch of C1 is removed, and the dura is opened on the side of the intended lesion. At a depth of 6 mm, a 4 mm incision is made transversely using the rootlets of the spinal accessory nerve as the dorsal limit. Risks may include ataxia, lateropulsion, weakness, loss of proprioception, bleeding, infection, and infarction. Some 131 cases have been reported in 14 series; the main initial success rate was 87%, which dropped to 45% on long-term follow-up. Reported morbidity and mortality were 23% and 13%, respectively.

Mesencephalotomy: Walker, in 1942, was the first to perform an operation aimed at interrupting the spinothalamic pathway in the midbrain. With their introduction of newer stereotactic methods, Wycis and Spiegel performed the first stereotactic mesencephalotomy in 1947 and reported their long-term results in 1962.[32] The anatomic regions involved in a mesencephalotomy include the spinothalamic tract and the structures medial to it, the *quintothalamic tract*. As proposed by Wycis and Spiegel, the involvement of the reticulospinal fibers in the periaqueductal gray matter just medial to the quintothalamic tract in a mesencephalotomy improves the result of the procedure.

With similar indications as for medullary spinothalamic tractotomy, trigeminal tractotomy, or high cervical cordotomy, mesencephalotomy, by interrupting both the spinothalamic and quintothalamic tracts, affects both head and body or limb pain. In addition, there is no significant contraindication to its use in patients with pulmonary dysfunction. The patients most greatly benefiting from mesencephalotomy have unilateral head and neck pain secondary to cancer. Some authors advocate its use in central pain, facial dysesthesia, or anesthesia dolorosa after unsuccessful trigeminal surgery and in postherpetic facial pain.

Mesencephalotomy is performed using stereotactic methods. A twist drill or burr hole is performed and an electrode is passed into the midbrain. Once the target site is reached, stimulation should always be done for confirmation of the location before the lesion is made.[30] Potential complications include gaze palsy, hemiparesis, and postoperative dysesthesia or anesthesia dolorosa. The overall complication rate is 22% and mortality rate is about 1.5%. In the 12 series reporting 501 cases, the mean success rate was 76%.[31]

Thalamotomy/Pulvinotomy: Wycis and Spiegel[32] first reported the use of dorsomedian thalamotomy for the treatment of pain in 1953. Several targets for thalamotomy have since been proposed including the area below the ventral posterior nuclei rostral to midbrain, the medial thalamus, the posteromedial thalamus and pulvinar, and the dorsomedial and anterior nuclei of the thalamus. Combination operations have been proposed in which lesions are placed at two different sites in the hope of controlling both the transmission of noxious stimuli and the affective component of pain.

Thalamotomy for intractable pain is controversial; some feel that this is best used for central noncancer pain, whereas others believe the only indication for thalamotomy is cancer pain. Thalamotomy is a stereotactic procedure and can be performed under local anesthesia with a low complication rate. Initial success rates for medial and basal thalamotomies have been reported to be as high as 80%, only to drop to 30% after 1 year.

Hypothalamotomy: Hypothalamotomy was first performed in 1962 by Sano for the treatment of violent aggressive behavior; in 1971 he performed posteromedial hypothalamotomy for intractable pain. The mechanism for pain relief following hypothalamotomy as well as the indications for hypothalamotomy remain unclear. In the past this procedure has been used for cancer pain involving the face, especially when the pain is accompanied by affective features such as depression, anxiety, and suffering. The ventriculographic guided technique as described by Sano consists of placing the lesion 2 mm below the anterior commissure–posterior commissure midpoint and 2 mm lateral to the wall of the third ventricle. The reported success rate in a limited number of series is 65% to 80%. No operative mortality and a 10% transient complication rate were reported.

Hypophysectomy: In 1953 Luft and Olivecrona published their pioneering work on hypophysectomy for treatment of various conditions.[33] Based on their understanding of hormonal influence on cancer, they included a number of patients with advanced cancer of the breast and prostate. To their surprise, many of these cancer patients had relief of their pain hours after the procedure. Since that time, numerous methods of pituitary destruction using the open transcranial or transsphenoidal approaches have been devised, including sectioning of pituitary stalk and the use of alcohol, radiofrequency, cryotherapy, and interstitial radiation. Currently, hypophysectomy is considered for patients with severe diffuse pain from cancer, especially of the prostate and breast.

Endocrinopathies, especially diabetes insipidus, are the most common side effects of hypophysectomy. Other potential complications include cerebrospinal fluid leak, ocular nerve palsy, visual field deficits, and, rarely, meningitis, carotid artery damage, headache, and hypothalamic dysfunction. Approximately 50% to 80% of hypophysectomy patients report excellent to good pain relief, regardless of technique;[34] this pain relief, however, appears to be relatively short-lived. For treatment of severe cancer pain, the relatively safe and technically straightforward chemical hypophysectomy should be considered.

Cingulotomy: During follow-up of psychosurgical procedures performed in the 1940s, several investigators noted that some patients who complained bitterly about pain preoperatively no longer did so afterward. One consistent target for which pain relief was noted was the cingulate gyrus, which was chosen because this area represented the frontal lobe component in Papez's limbic lobe, and it was thought at the time that the best target for affective disorders and related intractable pain would be areas involved with emotional expression. In 1962 Foltz and White[35] and Ballantine and others[36] each developed stereotactic methods for cingulotomy. The patients for which cingulotomy may be of most benefit have diffuse nociceptive pain secondary to cancer. This is especially true when the patient has a significant affective component to the pain, with prominent features of emotional suffering and depression.

Cingulotomy may be performed under general or local anesthesia using image-guided stereotactic techniques. Two frontal burr holes are made, 1.3 cm from midline and 9.5 cm posterior to the nasion. The target site for the cingulum should be about 3 cm posterior from the tip of the lateral ventricles, 1.5 cm superior to the ventricles, and 1.5 cm from the midline. Radiofrequency lesions are then made at 75°C for 60 to 90 seconds or longer for larger lesions. Some authors recommend overlapping two lesions to produce a more discrete conical lesion consistent with the shape of the cingulate gyrus at this level.

Reported complications of cingulotomy include seizures, hemorrhage, transient mania, headaches, decreased memory, and hemiplegia. Extensive neuropsychiatric testing reveals very few and minor changes after cingulotomy.[37] Major morbidity is rare for this procedure, and mortality is extremely unusual (0.1%). The overall rate of successful pain relief from cancer pain for six modern series reporting a total of 87 patients was 31%, but a 92% success rate was demonstrated when the cingulotomy was combined with another central procedure that interrupted a pain pathway. For cingulotomies performed for chronic pain of nonmalignant origin, a long-term success rate of 38% was demonstrated.[38]

SUMMARY

Although the role of intracranial ablative procedures remains poorly defined, they are clearly of value for the treatment of some difficult intractable pain syndromes. In patients who have undergone multidisciplinary pain assessment and therapy, including pharmacotherapy, physical therapy, and psychological therapy, and in whom neuroaugmentative procedures for pain control have failed, neuroablative procedures offer what is often the last hope for the relief of pain and suffering. Taking advantage of advances in our understanding of neuroanatomy, surgical technique, neuroimaging, and computer technology, most of these procedures have a low complication rate, and many can be carried out under local anesthesia. In general, with appropriate patient selection, these procedures have success rates of 50% to 80%, which is similar to those reported for most neuroaugmentative procedures. Thus, with judicious use, neuroablative procedures remain an important part of the neurosurgical armamentarium in the treatment of intractable pain.

Note to the reader: The chapter was not revised due to lack of advances in the area.

REFERENCES

1. Burchiel KJ: Neurosurgical procedures of the peripheral nerves. *In* North RB, Levy RM (eds): The Neurosurgical Management of Pain. Springer-Verlag, New York, 1997, p 133.
2. Uematsu S, Udvarhelyi G, Benson DW, et al: Percutaneous radiofrequency rhizotomy. Surg Neurol 2:319, 1974.
3. Sluijter ME, Mehta M: Treatment of chronic neck and back pain by cutaneous thermal lesions. In Lipton S, Miles J (eds): Persistent Pain: Modern Methods of Treatment. Academic Press, New York, 1981, pp 141–179.
4. Uematsu S: Percutaneous electrothermocoagulation of spinal nerve trunk, ganglion, and rootlets. In Schmidek HH, Sweet WH (eds): Operative Neurosurgical Techniques: Indications, Methods, and Results. Grune and Stratton, New York, 1988, pp 1207–1221.
5. Smith FP: Trans-spinal ganglionectomy for relief of intercostal pain. J Neurosurg 32:574–577, 1970.
6. Osgood CP, Dujovny M, Faille R, et al: Microsurgical lumbosacral ganglionectomy, anatomic rationale, and surgical results. Acta Neurochir 35:197–204, 1976.
7. Pawl RP: Microsurgical ganglionectomy for treatment of arachnoiditis related unilateral sciatica. Presented at the American Pain Society Meeting, Miami, 1982.
8. Taub A: Relief of chronic intractable sciatica by dorsal root ganglionectomy. Trans Am Neurol Assoc 105:340–343, 1980.
9. Taub A: Ganglionectomy lectures presented to the Massachusetts General Hospital (cited in Gybels JM, Sweet WH: Neurosurgical Treatment of Persistent Pain: Physiological and Pathological Mechanisms of Human Pain. S. Karger, Basel, 1989, pp 122–123).
10. Rees WES: Multiple bilateral subcutaneous rhizolysis of segmental nerves in the treatment of intervertebral disc syndrome. Ann Gen Pract 26:126–127, 1971.
11. Bogduk N, Long DM: The anatomy of the so-called "articular nerves" and their relationship to facet denervation in the treatment of low back pain. J Neurosurg 51:172–177, 1979.
12. Ingnelzi RJ: Radiofrequency lesions in the treatment of lumbar spinal pain. Contemp Neurosurg 12:1–6, 1980.
13. Lazorthes Y, Verdie JC, Lagarrugue J: Thermocoagulation percutanee des nerfs rachidiens a visee analgesique. Neurochirurgie 22:445, 1976.
14. Burton CV: Percutaneous radiofrequency facet denervation. Appl Neurophysiol 38:80–86, 1976.
15. Lora J, Long DM: So-called facet denervation in the management of intractable back pain. Spine 1:121–126, 1976.
16. Shealy CN: Percutaneous radiofrequency denervation of spinal facets: Treatment for chronic back pain and sciatica. J Neurosurg 43:448–451, 1975.
17. Leriche R: The Surgery of Pain. Baillière Tindall, London, 1939.
18. Kux M: Thoracic endoscopic sympathectomy by transthoracic electrocoagulation. Br J Surg 67:71, 1980.
19. Wilkinson HA: Percutaneous radiofrequency upper thoracic sympathectomy: A new technique. Neurosurgery 15:811–814, 1984.
20. Nashold BS, Urban B, Zorub DS: Phantom pain relief by focal destruction of the substantia gelatinosa of Rolando. Adv Pain Res Ther 1:959–963, 1976.
21. Sindou M, Fischer G, Mansuy L: Posterior spinal rhizotomy and selective posterior rhizotomy. *In* Krayenbuhl H, Maspes PE,

Sweet WH (eds): Progress in Neurological Surgery. S. Karger, Basel, 1976, pp 201–250.

22. Bernard EJ, Nashold BS, Caputi F: Clinical review of nucleus caudalis dorsal root entry lesions for facial pain. Appl Neurophysiol 51:218, 1988.

23. Schwartz HG: High cervical cordotomy: Technique and results. Clin Neurosurg 8:282–293, 1960.

24. Mullan S, Harper PV, Hekmatpanah J, et al: Percutaneous interruption of spinal-pain tracts by means of a strontium needle. J Neurosurg 20:931–939, 1963.

25. Rosomoff HL, Carroll F, Brown J, et al: Percutaneous radiofrequency cervical cordotomy technique. J Neurosurg 23:639–644, 1969.

26. Poletti CE: Open cordotomy medullary tractectomy. In Schmidek HH, Sweet WH (eds): Operative Neurosurgical Techniques: Indications, Methods, and Results. Grune and Stratton, New York, 1988, pp 1155–1168.

27. Rosomoff HL: Percutaneous spinothalamic cordotomy. In Wilkins RH, Rengachary SS (eds): Neurosurgery. McGraw-Hill, New York, 1985, pp 2446–2451.

28. Young RF, Jacques D, Rand RW, et al: Medial thalamotomy for chronic pain: A comparison of gamma knife and radiofrequency stereotactic techniques [abstract]. Neurosurgery 35:571, 1994.

29. King RB: Medullary tractotomy for pain relief. In Wilkins RH, Rengachary SS (eds): Neurosurgery. McGraw-Hill, New York, 1985, pp 2452–2454.

30. Nashold BS, Crue BL: Stereotaxic mesencephalotomy and trigeminal tractotomy. In Youmans JR (ed): Neurological Surgery, ed. 2. WB Saunders, Philadelphia, 1982, pp 3702–3716.

31. Loeser JD, Gildenberg PL: Medullary and mesencephalic tractotomy. In Bonica JJ (ed): The Management of Pain. Lea & Febiger, Philadelphia, 1990, pp 2086–2093.

32. Wycis HT, Spiegel EA: Long range results in the treatment of intractable pain by stereotaxic midbrain surgery. J Neurosurg 19:101–107, 1962.

33. Luft R, Olivecrona H: Experiences with hypophysectomy in man. J Neurosurg 10:301–316, 1953.

34. Ramirez LF, Levin AB: Pain relief after hypophysectomy. Neurosurgery 14:499–504, 1984.

35. Foltz EL, White LE: Pain relief by frontal cingulotomy. Neurosurgery 19:89–100, 1962.

36. Ballantine HT, Bouckoms AJ, Thomas EK: Treatment of psychiatric illness by stereotactic cingulotomy. Biol Psychiatr 22:807–819, 1987.

37. Corkin S, Twitchell TE, Sullivan EV: Safety and efficacy of cingulotomy for pain and psychiatric disorder. In Hitchcock ER, Ballantine HT, Meyerson BA (eds): Modern Concepts in Psychiatric Surgery. Elsevier, Amsterdam, 1979, pp 253–272.

38. Ojemann G: Frontal lobe operations for pain. In Bonica JJ (ed): The Management of Pain. Lea & Febiger, Philadelphia, 1990, pp 2096–2100.

Physical Medicine and Rehabilitation Approaches to Pain Management

Steven P. Stanos, D.O.,

Heidi Prather, D.O.,

Joel M. Press, M.D., and

Jeffrey L. Young, M.D., M.A.

Physical medicine and rehabilitation practitioners use a comprehensive approach to pain management. The treatment they provide is guided by a specific diagnosis made in an acute, subacute, or chronic setting. Pain management programs may include using medications, flexibility and strengthening exercise, aerobic exercise, modalities, orthotics, injections, and adaptive equipment. A comprehensive rehabilitation program promotes improvement in function beyond simply resolving pain symptoms. Strong emphasis is placed on the patient being an active participant in the rehabilitation process. The purpose of this chapter is to briefly review modalities and the application of therapeutic exercise and to introduce the concept of comprehensive interdisciplinary pain management.

OVERVIEW OF MODALITIES

Modalities are physical agents utilized to produce a therapeutic tissue response.[1,2] Types of modalities include heat, cold, water, sound, electricity, and electromagnetic waves. Physical medicine and rehabilitation practitioners must have a good understanding of the physiological effects of modalities to use them safely and appropriately. Modalities are most effective when applied in response to a specific diagnosis with close monitoring of the patient's response. Most importantly, modalities are an adjunctive treatment included as part of a comprehensive rehabilitation program, not an isolated treatment option.

HEAT

General Considerations: Tissue structures are warmed via three mechanisms: conduction, convection, and conversion.

Conduction is the transfer of heat directly from one surface to another. Examples include hydrocollar packs and paraffin baths. Convection is the transfer of heat due to the movement of air or water across a body surface. Examples include hydrotherapy and fluidotherapy. Conversion involves the transfer of heat via a change in energy. Examples are infrared lamps, ultrasound, and electromagnetic microwaves.

Heating a structure creates both local and distant effects. Vasodilation and increased metabolic demands promote increased blood flow with the delivery of leukocytes and oxygen and increased capillary permeability. The use of heat modalities is beneficial in assisting with pain control, muscle relaxation, and collagen extensibility. Table 21-1 summarizes the indications for heat modalities used for musculoskeletal pain management. The mechanism chosen is based on the specific diagnosis. Table 21-2 lists general contraindications and precautions for the use of therapeutic heat.

Superficial Heat: Direct heat penetration is greatest at a depth of 0.5 to 2 cm from the skin surface and depends on the amount of adipose tissue. The more commonly used modes for musculoskeletal rehabilitation include hydrocollars, whirlpools, and contrast baths. Hydrocollar packs are made in three standard sizes and are heated in stainless steel containers in water with temperatures between 65 and 90°C. The highest temperatures found during use of the packs are at the skin's surface. Towels are applied with the packs to minimize skin trauma and to maintain heat insulation. The treatment sessions usually last 20 to 30 minutes.

Hydrotherapy is heating via submersion of small or large body surface areas. The risk of elevating core body temperature

TABLE 21-1. INDICATIONS FOR THERAPEUTIC HEAT

Muscle spasm
Pain
Contracture
Hematoma resolution
Hyperemia
Increase collagen extensibility
Accelerate metabolic processes

exists when large body surface areas are heated. Water temperature should not exceed 40°C when large body surfaces are heated in a Hubbard tank as compared to up to 43°C when a patient submerges just a limb in a whirlpool. Hydrotherapy provides a gravity-eliminated environment which facilitates joint motion. Agitation created by the water flow provides sensory input.

Paraffin baths are a mixture of paraffin and mineral oil used as a treatment to deliver heat to small joints. Mineral oil creates a lower melting point for the paraffin providing increased thermal release when compared to water. The bath is kept at a temperature of 52 to 58°C for upper limb therapeutic sessions and 45 to 52°C for lower limb sessions. Paraffin bath contraindications include open wounds and severe peripheral vascular disease.

Fluidotherapy involves the placement of the extremity to be treated into a container through which hot air is blown within

TABLE 21-2. CONTRAINDICATIONS FOR THERAPEUTIC HEAT

Acute inflammation
Hemorrhage or bleeding disorders
Decreased sensation
Poor thermal regulation
Malignancy
Edema
Ischemia
Atrophic skin or scarred skin
Inability to respond to pain

a medium of a dry powder of glass beads. Benefits include the heat plus mechanical stimulation that may further help in pain control.

Deep Heat: Conversion is used to heat deep-tissue structures. Deep-heating agents include ultrasound, phonophoresis, and shortwave and microwave diathermy. Ultrasound is most commonly used, however. Ultrasound is sound waves classified within the acoustic spectrum above 20,000 Hz. It is unique in that the production of heat is due to high-frequency alternating current (0.8 to 1.0 MHz) which is converted via a crystal transducer to acoustic vibration. Energy transfer occurs due to the piezoelectric effect whereby the crystal undergoes changes in shape when voltage is applied. Selective heating is greatest when acoustic impedance is high, such as at the bone–muscle interface. Conversely, ultrasonic energy is readily conducted through homogenous structures such as subcutaneous fat or metal implants with minimal thermal effects due to the rapid removal of heat energy. Ultrasound can be safely used near metal implants. However, in the presence of methyl methacrylate and high-density polyethylene, which is often used in total joint replacements, a higher amount of ultrasound energy is absorbed so there is potential for overheating. Ultrasound can heat to depths of 5 cm below the skin surface thereby providing therapeutic benefit to bone, joint capsule, tendon, ligament, and scar tissue. Ultrasound also has some nonthermal effects. Gaseous cavitation involves gas bubbles created by high-frequency sound or turbulence. These bubbles may increase in size causing pressure changes within the tissues. Cavitation may cause movement of material, mechanical distortion, and change in cellular function. Acoustic streaming causes movement of material secondary to pressure asymmetries produced by sound as it passes through a medium. Streaming has the potential to cause plasma membrane damage and acceleration of metabolic processes. Standing waves are produced by superimposition of sound waves and can cause heating at tissue interfaces at different densities.

Ultrasound dosage is measured in watts per square centimeter (W/cm^2). Intensities of 1.0 to 4.0 W/cm^2 are most commonly used. Application is usually started at 0.5 W/cm^2 and gradually increased while the practitioner monitors the patient response. Duration of treatment is 5 to 10 minutes and is based on the size of the treatment area. Table 21-3 lists some common uses and Table 21-4 lists precautions for ultrasound.

Cryotherapy: The physiological effects of cold include vasoconstriction with reflexive vasodilation, decreased local

TABLE 21-3. COMMON USES FOR THERAPEUTIC ULTRASOUND

Contractures
Tendonitis
Degenerative arthritis
Subacute trauma

TABLE 21-4. **PRECAUTIONS FOR ULTRASOUND**

Malignancy
Open epiphysis
Pacemaker
Laminectomy site
Radiculopathy
Near brain, eyes, or reproductive organs
Pregnant or menstruating uterus
Heat precautions in general
Caution around arthroplasties, methyacrylate, or high-density polyethylene

TABLE 21-6. **PRECAUTIONS AND CONTRAINDICATIONS FOR CRYOTHERAPY**

Ischemia
Raynaud's disease or phenomenon
Cold intolerance
Insensitivity
Inability to report pain

Contrast Baths: The alternating therapeutic use of heat and cold has been described as a form of vascular exercise because of the alternating vasodilation and vasoconstriction that occurs. This creates a hyperemic response that improves circulation and fosters the healing response. Indications for contrast baths include improving range of motion, control of swelling, and assistance in pain control.

THERAPEUTIC EXERCISE

Therapeutic exercise is described in two broad categories. Exercises exist that focus on muscle flexibility and strength and aerobic exercise. A rehabilitation program to manage musculoskeletal pain and dysfunction will include all of these in addition to patient education about proper biomechanics and ergonomics. The treatment program focuses on managing a particular diagnosis when possible. Each program is customized to include specific work or sport activities.

When implementing an exercise program the specific adaptation to imposed demand (SAID) principle should be applied. The principle states that the body responds to given demands with specific and predictable adaptations. Stronger muscles develop with strength training. Oxidative capacities of skeletal muscles increase with aerobic training. Pliability of connective tissue increases with flexibility exercises. With these outcomes in mind, exercise training parameters are implemented.

Some reviews of exercise therapy for low back pain have failed to find any benefit of specific back exercises for low back pain.[3] They have shown that exercise may be useful in the treatment of chronic low back pain if they aim at improving return to normal daily activity and work. Still other reviews have shown therapeutic exercise to be beneficial for chronic, subacute, and postsurgery low back pain. Continuation of normal activities was the only interaction with beneficial effects for acute low back pain.[4] Newer studies that address exercise programs based on mechanical assessment may add more specificity to the exercise treatment program. Exercises that are adapted based on preferential direction of movement with assessment of the patient have shown much more predictable results.[5–7] All forms of exercise should address functional movement patterns that patients will need to move through during their daily, work, and sports activities.

metabolism, decreased enzymatic activity, and decreased oxygen demand. Cold decreases muscle spindle activity and slows nerve conduction velocity and therefore is often used to decrease muscle spasticity and guarding. Connective tissue stiffness and muscle viscosity is increased with cold. With these physiological effects in mind, cryotherapy is often used during the first 48 hours after an acute musculoskeletal injury. However, care must be taken when applying cold over nerves due to the potential development of neuropraxia. To minimize this, cold application should not exceed 30 minutes and efforts should be made to protect peripheral nerves in the region being treated. Cryostretch and cryokinetics refer to the use of cryotherapy to facilitate joint motion. By decreasing pain and muscle guarding, improved flexibility and function can be achieved. Tables 21-5 and 21-6 summarize general indications and contraindications for cryotherapy.

TABLE 21-5. **INDICATIONS FOR CRYOTHERAPY**

Acute trauma
Edema
Hemorrhage
Analgesia
Pain
Muscle spasm
Spasticity
Reduction of metabolic activity

Flexibility Exercises: Maintaining or regaining muscle flexibility and range of motion is an important part of a rehabilitation program. Connective tissue stretches with a small amount of force and returns to its original length when the force is removed. When the muscle fibers are straightened, more force is required to apply a stretch. Furthermore, if connective tissues are stretched to a certain length and maintained, the tension within the tissue decreases. For best results, stretching should be maintained for 30 seconds with the patient perceiving a pulling sensation rather than pain. Warming an area before stretching improves the elongation of the collagen fibers. Rapid or bouncing stretches promote tissue recoil and a sustained stretch is not achieved. The risk of excessive loading and injury also occurs with bouncing. If too much force is applied with stretching, the patient will experience muscle soreness for more than 24 hours. Other potential problems with stretching include joint subluxation or overstretching during the healing phase of tissues such as tendons and ligaments. Improper timing of stretching in such instances may result in excessive laxity. With adherence to an appropriately applied stretching program, patient flexibility should improve within 1 to 2 months.

Types of Muscle Contractions: An isometric contraction is a muscle contraction without motion. Isometric contractions are used to stabilize a joint, such as when a weight is held at waist level neither raising nor lowering it. Dynamic contractions are muscle contractions with a fixed amount of weight. They are divided into concentric and eccentric contractions. A concentric contraction occurs when the muscle length is shortened during a contraction, e.g., a biceps curl. An eccentric contraction occurs when the muscle length is increased during the contraction, i.e., the "negative" contraction. Eccentric contractions are used for decelerating or controlling motions. Isokinetic contractions are activated at a constant velocity and are artificially created by types of exercise equipment. Measurements of these contractions are often used in research settings but little relevance has been proven under real conditions. Plyometrics refers to a contraction sequence when a rapid eccentric contraction precedes a concentric contraction such as during a jump. An example is a jumper lowering the body and eccentrically loading the gluteal muscles prior to the jump which then requires concentric gluteal muscle contraction. Plyometric training can be especially useful in sport-specific rehabilitation. Strength is the maximal force generated during a single contraction while power is the amount of force generated per unit time. Power may be more important to emphasize for a person to return to maximal function. The amount of force generated by muscle contraction type from highest to lowest is: eccentric > isometric > concentric.

Strength Training: Muscle strengthening is a well-accepted part of any rehabilitation program. However, the practitioner must have a complete understanding of the functional anatomy so that the appropriate balance between agonist and antagonist muscle groups can be achieved. The amount of resistance to be applied is determined by the muscle's capability and should be assessed for each individual. Increases in cross-sectional area and hypertrophy of muscle are associated with increases in strength. Training is most effective when exercises focus on different muscle groups in rotating sessions. Improvements in strength observed during the first two weeks of training are related to neuromuscular reeducation and more efficient recruitment of muscles. Initially, 1 to 3 sets of lifting weights 8 to 12 times per week is recommended. Resistance should not be increased by more than 10% per week. If progress is not

made, the practitioner should evaluate whether the proper technique is being used, whether there is too little or too much training intensity, or there is neurogenic strength loss.

Aerobic Fitness: The patient must maintain cardiovascular fitness during rehabilitation. If the injury or dysfunction prohibits weight bearing, a nonweight-bearing aerobic activity needs to be implemented. To improve aerobic capacity, the oxidative metabolism of the muscle must be stressed. Oxygen consumption (VO_2) increases in proportion to the intensity of the exercise. VO_{2max}, the highest level of oxygen consumption achieved during exercise, is the best indicator of aerobic fitness. Intensity of exercise is the difficulty level of the exercise and is usually used in reference to maximal effort. This is typically at 40% to 85% of VO_2 max for aerobic training and 25% to 95% of one repetition maximum for strength training. The duration for aerobic training is usually greater than 15 minutes of continuous exercise. Frequency for aerobic training is usually 3 to 6 times per week while strength training is typically 3 to 5 times per week. When prescribing an aerobic program the practitioner must remember that if activity level is reduced beyond one week, aerobic conditioning decreases. Maximum oxygen consumption decreases by 25% when a patient takes three weeks of bedrest. Intensity, duration, and frequency parameters must be adjusted in the deconditioned patient. Benefits of aerobic conditioning measured by 10% to 20% increases in VO_{2max} can be noted within 8 to 12 weeks of training implementation. If improvements are not observed, their lack may be attributed to infrequent exercise sessions, too low an intensity, or too short a duration of exercise sessions.

DEVELOPING A COMPREHENSIVE REHABILITATION PROGRAM

An individualized therapeutic program aims to correct soft tissue inflexibilites and improve muscle strength deficits and imbalances, endurance, and power to the appropriate muscle groups. Consideration is given to the joint above and below the injured area which are linked together and referred to as the kinetic chain. The program should also include patient education about posture, body mechanics, and proprioception. A patient's return to activity should be monitored in a supervised setting so that any residual problems can be addressed.

A comprehensive rehabilitation program consists of an acute phase, a recovery phase, and a maintenance phase. During the acute phase, education about how to protect the injured tissue is important. A review of proper body mechanics and activities of daily living should be completed. Relative rest is important because excessive immobilization results in decreased muscle strength, endurance, and flexibility. Modalities can be used as described previously to help with pain management but should not be relied upon as the only treatment application. Also, medications should be used to facilitate the rehabilitation program by decreasing pain and inflammation. Manual therapy techniques may help modify pain by assisting in early controlled motion of the injured tissue. Mechanoreceptor activation can assist in modifying muscle tone and pain. Although orthotics can help control range of motion, warm underlying tissue, and provide proprioceptive feedback, the patient should not be encouraged to become reliant on them. Therapeutic exercise should begin during the acute phase. The direction of the initial movement pattern is based on the presumed pathology, pain pattern, and functional anatomy.

Once acute inflammation and pain have been addressed, the program focuses on the subacute or recovery phase. Goals of this phase include achievement of full range of motion that is pain-free to the affected tissue and surrounding tissues and regaining appropriate strength, balance, and proprioception. Manual techniques should focus on improving soft tissue extensibility that helps promote proper alignment of collagen fibers during healing and remodeling. These techniques may include massage, fascial stretching, traction, and joint mobilization. Myofascial release improves elasticity and motion by applying pressure in shear forces directed by fascial planes, and assists with pain control. Mobilization is also used to facilitate motion at specific joints or joint segments. These techniques may facilitate a patient's progress but again should not be relied upon solely because protracted passive treatment places the patient in a dependent role. Concern should also be given for the potential hypermobility that may result with extensively repeated treatment. A flexibility program is devised to achieve proper balance and allow the patient to achieve a neutral position, the least painful and best posture. While maintaining the posture, exercises progress from static to dynamic. Challenges to the neutral posture are afterward incorporated by gravity and then by a therapist or assistive device. Activity-specific retraining is initiated first by breaking the motion into components. Training for each component is completed before reassembling the entire motion. Cardiovascular training should be maintained adapting the method to the specific injury. Aquatic training should be considered if a nonweight-bearing activity is necessary.

The final or maintenance phase is devised as the patient returns to the work or sport-specific activity to promote continued cardiovascular fitness as well as to prevent reinjury. Education about ergonomics and equipment or adaptive devices should be in place. The patient should be able to use a home exercise program independently and know how to solve problems that may occur during this last stage of recovery.

INTERDISCIPLINARY COMPREHENSIVE PAIN MANAGEMENT TREATMENT

Patients failing to progress in the acute, subacute, and maintenance program may need referral to a more comprehensive interdisciplinary rehabilitation-based program. Patients may continue to report ongoing pain and reduced physical and psychological functioning. Progress may also be impeded by related affective distress and depressive symptoms including disturbed sleep, loss of appetite, and weight loss. In these cases treatment of chronic low back pain may not only be focused on removing an underlying organic disease, but on the reduction of disability through modification of environmental contingencies and cognitive processes. Behavioral interventions, including cognitive behavioral therapy, are a key component in interdisciplinary programs. In addition, early interventions should include trials of antidepressant medications for depressed mood and disturbed sleep. Lower-dose tricyclic and tricyclic-like antidepressants may help augment serotonin levels in the brain and improve the quality of sleep. Targeted analgesia may also involve a number of medications from a number of pharmacologic classes including anti-inflammatories, antiepileptics, muscle relaxants, and/or opioid medications.

TABLE 21-7. STAFF COMPOSITION OF AN INTERDISCIPLINARY PAIN MANAGEMENT TEAM

Physiatrist/pain medicine specialist
Nurse educator
Pain psychologist
Physical therapist
Occupational therapist
Vocational counselor
Biofeedback therapist
Therapeutic recreational therapist

The role of effective chronic opioid medication management in multidisciplinary, behaviorally based programs remains controversial.[8,9]

Comprehensive interdisciplinary rehabilitation pain treatment programs typically involve a number of health care providers including rehabilitation specialists, physical, occupational, and therapeutic recreational therapists, pain psychologists, biofeedback specialists, and nursing and vocational counselors. This interdisciplinary approach relies heavily on a coordination of services fostered by ongoing communication between team health care provider members with a goal of improving patient function at home and/or in the workplace, fostering independence, and improving psychosocial functioning (Table 21-7). Typical programs may last 7 to 8 hours per day for 3 to 4 weeks. At the completion of the program, patients are encouraged to continue utilizing pain management techniques as they return to previous levels of sport, work, and/or community function. An extensive review of the behavioral treatment for chronic low back pain has shown that it can be an effective treatment for chronic low back pain.[3,10,11]

KEY POINTS

- Pain management approaches to the patient with low back pain will need to include the use of different treatment options. Rarely is one treatment modality sufficient.
- Pain management should be the first step in restoration of function. Functional improvement is not always synonymous with alleviation of pain.
- Physical modalities (ultrasound, hot packs, etc.) may be of benefit in acute pain situations. Chronic use of these passive modalities should be discouraged.
- Exercise treatment, although not a panacea, is a helpful adjunct in treating patients with all types of pain disorders.
- Referral for comprehensive multidisciplinary treatment may be necessary for those patients failing to progress in the acute, subacute, and maintenance-based programs.
- The treatment of chronic low back pain may not only be focused on removing an underlying organic disease but on

the reduction of disability through modification of environmental contingencies and cognitive processes via the use of additional behavioral interventions.

REFERENCES

1. Basford JR: Physical agents. *In* DeLisa JA (ed): Rehabilitation Medicine: Principles and Practice, ed 2. Lippincott, Philadelphia, 1993, pp 404–423.
2. Young JL, Press JM, Cole AJ: Physical therapy options for lumbar spine pain. *In* Cole AJ, Herring SA (eds): The Low Back Pain Handbook. Hanley and Belfus, 1997, pp 125–141.
3. van Tulder MW, Ostelo R, Vlaeyen JW, et al: Behavioral treatment for chronic low back pain: A systematic review within the framework of the Cochrane Back Review Group. Spine 26:270–281, 2001.
4. Philadelphia Panel: Philadelphia Panel evidence-based clinical practice guidelines on selected rehabilitation interventions for low back pain. Phys Ther 81:1641–1674, 2001.
5. Donelson RC, Aprill, et al: A prospective study of centralization of lumbar and referred pain. A predictor of symptomatic discs and anular competence. Spine 22:1115–1122, 1997.
6. Delitto A, Snyder-Mackler L: The diagnostic process: Examples in orthopedic physical therapy. Phys Ther 75:203–211, 1995.
7. Fritz JM, Erhard RE: A nonsurgical treatment approach for patients with lumbar spinal stenosis. Phys Ther 77:962–973, 1997.
8. Harden RN: Opioid therapy: The controversy continues. Rehabil Manage 2:22–24, 1999.
9. Jamison RN, Raymond SA, Slawsby EL, et al: Opioid therapy for chronic non-cancer back pain. Spine 23:2591–2600, 1998.
10. Becker N, Sjogren P, Bech P, et al: Treatment outcome of chronic non-malignant pain patients managed in a Danish multidisciplinary pain centre compared to general practice: A randomised controlled trial. Pain 84:203–211, 2000.
11. Flor H, Fydrich T, Turk D: Efficacy of multidisciplinary pain treatment centers: A meta-analytic review. Pain 49:221–230, 1992.

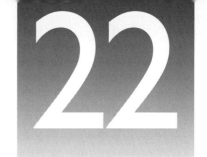

Acupuncture

Christopher M. Criscuolo, M.D., and Henry M. Liu, M.D.

Acupuncture involves the placement and manipulation of needles at various points in the body for the treatment of many medical conditions. It is a valuable tool in the management of the symptoms of disease. In this chapter we focus on the use of this ancient art in the management of pain. Although the roots of acupuncture are deeply planted in China, acupuncture has increasingly been practiced in the West. Acupuncture is an important option in today's multidisciplinary approach to the treatment of pain. There is an increasing body of scientific evidence that demonstrates efficacy similar to Western methods of disease and symptom management. While acupuncture will not replace the modern miracles of Western medicine, it has become a valuable adjunctive therapy in the multidisciplinary management of pain.

HISTORY

Origin: Acupuncture originated in China more than 2,000 years ago. Probably the first record of acupuncture therapy is in the Huang-di-nei-jing (The Yellow Emperor's Classic in Internal Medicine), written by Chi Po around 200 BC. Its popularity spread throughout ancient Egypt, the Middle East, the Roman Empire, and later into Western Europe. With the improved relations between the USA and China that occurred in the 1970s, interest in acupuncture and traditional Chinese medicine increased significantly.

Acupuncture was born out of Taoist philosophy. Tao as described by Lao-tse in the Tao-te-ching around 500 BC assumes that nature is constantly changing. The Tao, or the way, is the source of all creation and is the force behind this ever-recurring change. It acts through two opposing but balancing forces, the yin and the yang. Because people exist in a dynamic interaction with nature, they exist within the tensions created by these opposing forces. According to the philosophy, sickness occurs when these opposing forces fall out of balance, and interventions are needed to restore the harmony.

Fundamental to the practice of classic acupuncture is the concept of qi, pronounced "chee." Qi is energy. This energy flows through different channels or meridians that connect the internal body with the external environment. There are different types of qi that serve different functions. These functions are protective, nourishing, and also represent a type of energy that is hereditary in nature. The network of meridians runs longitudinally in and around the body. Each meridian is categorized as being either yin or yang and is associated with one of the body's internal organs. There are 14 principal meridians, of which 12 are paired and 2 are unpaired. Thus, when the flow of qi is unobstructed, the body is in a healthy state of balance. Obstruction of qi results in a disequilibrium of yin and yang, which is manifested as disease or pain.

The meridians emerge at the surface of the body at certain places, known as acupuncture points. These points are areas where the qi may be affected and modulated by an external agent. There are a total of 361 classic acupuncture points and they are located along the meridians. Acupuncture points are stimulated to balance the circulation of energy. Acupuncture involves choosing which points to stimulate as well as choosing how to stimulate these points, the needle being one method.

Schools of Acupuncture: Several different schools of acupuncture have developed. Although the meridians and points are universally accepted, each school differs in the choice of points as well as in the method of stimulation. These schools include classic acupuncture, formula acupuncture, acupuncture as a form of trigger-point therapy, and acupuncture as a procedure for electrical stimulation.

Classic acupuncture is the traditional practice according to the principles of Taoism. The goal is to reestablish the balanced energy state by restoring the flow of qi. Emphasis is on maintaining the wholeness of the patient. Treatment is individualized according to the patient's energy state at the time. Thus, points selected may differ from one patient to another, as well as from one treatment session to another. This individuality makes evaluations of efficacy difficult owing to the lack of comparable controls.

There are many variations of classic acupuncture. Among them is ear acupuncture, or auriculotherapy. The pinna of the ear contains a map of acupuncture points that represent the entire body. Although somatotropic mapping of musculoskeletal pain at the ear has been done,[1] controlled trials of auriculotherapy have failed to yield evidence supporting efficacy.[2]

Today, many practitioners in Asia and parts of Europe still practice classic acupuncture. However, most in the West practice formula acupuncture. Formula acupuncture emphasizes standardized treatments. Routine sets of acupuncture points are used to treat specific pain problems. Practitioners have embraced this school partly because this approach is most often employed in acupuncture research.

Another application of acupuncture is essentially trigger-point therapy. Needles are inserted around symptomatic areas. Classic principles, meridians, and acupuncture points are not adhered to. The basis of this approach is that stress or injury causes local skeletal muscle contraction, which can result in neural changes. Needling provides relief by the release of these contractures. Trigger-point therapy and its mechanism were initially described by Bonica,[3] Travell and Simons,[4] Sola,[5] and others and is discussed elsewhere in this book.

With the increasing use of acupuncture during prolonged operations in the early 1970s, Chinese practitioners began using electricity as a source of needle stimulation. At the same time, the growing popularity of the gate-control theory of pain by Melzack and Wall[6] led to electrical stimulation therapies for pain control, which in turn led to the development of the transcutaneous electrical nerve stimulation unit. Electrical stimulation is now commonly employed for needle stimulation.

Despite its initial popularity, acupuncture as a whole has remained in the realm of alternative medicine. Thanks to the efforts of Joseph M. Helms, M.D., founding president of the American Academy of Medical Acupuncture and director of the University of California at Los Angeles program in Medical Acupuncture, there are currently several thousand physicians trained to perform acupuncture. With the long-time acceptance of acupuncture in Europe and the increasing public demand in the USA, this ancient form of therapy is becoming more mainstream. We have found it to be a valuable modality to offer our patients in pain. Physiologic and clinical data to support diverse therapeutic claims have been scarce. The clinical database, although large, contains mostly anecdotal and biased information. After more than two decades of research, evidence to support the effectiveness of acupuncture in relieving pain is only beginning to surface.

MECHANISM

Research on the mechanism behind acupuncture has been problematic. During the 1970s, when interest in acupuncture began, enkephalins and endorphins were being discovered, and the roles played by the raphe-spinal structures were being elucidated. However, it has been difficult to prove an association between acupuncture and endorphin release. Bonta[7] hypothesizes that since all types of pain are not relieved by acupuncture, and that conditions other than pain are treated with this modality, that perhaps an interaction occurs between neuropeptides and cytokines to account for some beneficial effects in other disorders. Animal studies of acupuncture analgesia cannot easily be extrapolated to human models. This is in part due to the difficulty in differentiating the effects of acupuncture analgesia with stress-induced analgesia.[8] Unlike in humans, acupuncture in animals is a stressful event, resulting in the release of hormones, including endorphins and cortisol.

Furthermore, when animals are frightened they often fall into a state of insensibility and unconsciousness.[9,10] Lee et al.[11] showed that cholecystokinin-A receptors are more expressed in nonresponder rats than responder rats, while CCK-B receptor expression is similar in both groups.

Human laboratory studies have been more helpful. In an extensive review, Pomeranz[12] concluded that acupuncture appears to cause the release of various endorphins and monoamine neurotransmitters, and involves both the peripheral and central nervous systems. According to Pomeranz, acupuncture activates sensory nerve fibers in muscles that, in turn, send signals to the spinal cord. This activates other centers in the midbrain and hypothalamic–pituitary axis, causing the release of neuropeptides. Enkephalin and dynorphin, released at the level of the spinal cord, block afferent pathways. Enkephalin, produced at the midbrain, stimulates the inhibitory raphe descending system, releasing the monoamines serotonin and norepinephrine. These neurotransmitters further block spinal cord pain transmission. Finally, beta-endorphin, released from the hypothalamic–pituitary axis, produces analgesia through the systemic circulation and cerebrospinal fluid. Ulett et al.[13] conclude after an extensive review of the literature that healing in acupuncture comes about not by manipulating qi but by neuroelectric stimulation for the expression of genes responsible for the production of neuropeptides.

Peripheral nerve involvement in acupuncture had previously been established. Nathan[14] and later Han and Terenius[15] showed that infiltration of acupuncture points with local anesthetic abolished analgesia from subsequent needling. Furthermore, clinical observation showed that stimulation of denervated areas in patients with spinal cord injuries failed to produce analgesia in rostral regions. Both small and large fibers appear to be involved. It is interesting to note that acupuncture points are sites of low skin resistance and represent areas on the body where the peripheral nervous system is most accessible.[12,16]

Acupuncture appears to increase the endorphin levels in various parts of the central nervous system.[17] During acupuncture analgesia, endorphin levels rise in the blood and cerebrospinal fluid. This correlates with an elevation of messenger RNA (mRNA) levels involved in the production of endorphins.[18] It also has been demonstrated that the opioid antagonist naloxone blocks acupuncture analgesia in animals and humans.[19] Also, antibodies to endorphins block acupuncture only if placed at known analgesic sites in the central nervous system.[18] Furthermore, lesions at the arcuate nucleus (a site of 3-endorphin release) and at the periaqueductal gray matter (where high concentrations of opioid receptors reside) abolish acupuncture analgesia.[20]

It appears that different levels of stimulation produce different endorphins. Han et al.[21] demonstrated that electrical stimulation at 4 Hz produces enkephalins, whereas stimulation at 100 Hz produces dynorphin A. Furthermore, acupuncture affects many other neuropeptides and neurotransmitters.[22,23] These include dopamine, 5-hydroxytryptamine, acetylcholine, and norepinephrine. The importance of these neurotransmitters has yet to be defined. Moreover, the role of these neurotransmitters and neuropeptides in chronic pain still needs to be elucidated.

Needling tender areas as a form of trigger-point therapy is a poorly understood process. Trigger-point therapy has been reviewed by Travel and Simons[4] and Sola.[5] The goal of therapy is to release painful contractures. Studies have been performed comparing dry needling of a tender area to the injection of a local anesthetic with or without steroids, and injection of placebo. Dry needling may be just as efficacious as injection of local anesthetics.[24] Interestingly, the relief of pain in a tender area does not always relieve pain caused by a pathologic lesion at a remote site.[25] This suggests that the peripheral and central nervous systems are involved.

INDICATIONS

The best-documented effects of acupuncture are its beneficial effects on headache[26,27] and backache.[28] However, acupuncture appears to provide some benefit in various other pain syndromes. These include fibromyalgia, arthritic pain,[29,30] pain from muscle spasms, trigeminal neuralgia,[31] chronic abdominal pain,[32] pelvic pain,[33] and dental pain.[34] Further evaluation is required for reflex sympathetic dystrophy,[35] cervical neck pain,[36] cancer pain,[37] postherpetic neuralgia,[38] and migraine headache.[27] A review by Ezzo et al. showed benefit in treating osteoarthritis of the knee.[39] Acupuncture can also be used successfully in the treatment of pediatric patients with chronic pain.[40]

CONTRAINDICATIONS

Acupuncture has few absolute contraindications. However, reports of various adverse effects have generated a list of relative contraindications. Pregnancy is a relative contraindication because acupuncture may induce premature labor.[41] Specific acupuncture points can induce labor and these should be avoided. A thorough knowledge of the functions of acupuncture points is imperative if one is going to treat pregnant patients. Bleeding diathesis and anticoagulant therapy may result in prolonged bleeding and hematoma formation. Bacterial endocarditis has also been reported in patients with rheumatic heart disease.[42,43] Steroids may attenuate the effects of acupuncture, and they should be discontinued prior to therapy if possible. Eating heavy meals or drinking alcohol before a treatment is inadvisable because of the risk of vasovagal symptoms, including nausea, vomiting, and fainting. Caution should be exercised when performing acupuncture in the thoracic region in patients in whom a pneumothorax would be catastrophic, such as persons with severe lung disease. Care should be taken with electrical stimulation in patients with a cardiac pacemaker because of the risk of electromagnetic interference.[44] Finally, acupuncture can mask symptoms that are of medical importance. Therefore, treatment of certain pain syndromes, such as abdominal pain, should be performed only after a complete medical evaluation.

TECHNIQUE

No consensus exists about which of the many techniques of needle insertion is optimal. Some practitioners purport that different ways of placing the needle can produce different results. However, no evidence supports the efficacy of one technique over another.

Patients are positioned to allow adequate access for the therapist and optimal comfort for the patient. Positions include sitting as well as lying prone or supine. A lateral decubitus position may also be used. The skin must be clean. This can be accomplished with an antiseptic such as alcohol.

Some practitioners do not use antiseptic solutions prior to superficial needling except in immunocompromised patients. Prior to inserting the needle the skin at the puncture site is stretched. A sterile acupuncture needle is then inserted in a manner that minimizes discomfort. (This can be accomplished with or without rotating the needle.) Insertion can be rapid or slow. Some practitioners penetrate only the skin, whereas other techniques require penetration to muscle. There is also a technique that utilizes periosteal placement of needles. Tubular guides are available for needle insertion.

The usual angle of insertion is perpendicular or oblique. Usually the deeper the penetration, the more perpendicular the needle ought to be angled. Horizontal insertion is often used in certain areas, such as the face and chest. Many classic acupuncturists slant the needle either in the same direction or in the opposite direction of the qi along the treated meridian.

There are a total of 361 classic acupuncture points. These are well described in the literature and various manuals. Most points are located linearly along the major meridians. Each point is identified by a Chinese name, its meridian, and a number. Two methods are used in locating a specific acupuncture site. One method uses anatomic landmarks, such as bony structures, muscles, and external features. The other method uses a defined unit of measurement to locate acupuncture points from identifiable landmarks. This unit of measurement is named cun, and is defined as the distance between the joint creases of the interphalangeal joints of the patient's flexed middle finger. This distance is also equivalent to the width of the patient's thumb.

The selection of acupuncture points follows certain basic rules. Tender spots, or pressure points, are used as local acupuncture points. These are also referred to as trigger points. Distal points are selected according to the involved meridian. Certain points are also selected according to specific symptoms present. Furthermore, certain points are chosen according to the acuteness or chronicity of the problem.

The insertion of the needle may be accompanied by de qi, a painless sensation of heaviness and numbness at the site. Concomitantly, the therapist feels as if the muscle is grabbing and holding the needle. Classic therapists believe that de qi defines correct placement. Furthermore, the acupuncturist should not remove the needles until the de qi has dissipated. This is indicated by the ease with which the needle can be lifted from the underlying tissue. Others, however, report that patients who do not experience de qi often respond to acupuncture nevertheless.

After insertion, needles may be left in place or stimulated. According to traditional thinking, needle stimulation depends on the excess or deficiency of the qi. Stimulation can be continuous for a short course, such as 10 to 20 seconds, followed by the removal of the needle. The needle may also be stimulated intermittently for several seconds. A third method involves continuous stimulation of several minutes to hours or until the pain is resolved. Stimulation of needles can be accomplished manually, or with electroacupuncture stimulators. These are battery-operated units that deliver low to high frequencies of varying intensities. Some acupuncturists warm the needles after placement with a heat lamp. Moxa, a Chinese herb that is rolled into a cigar, may also be used to warm the needles. Needle removal is accomplished by applying pressure on the skin with one hand while withdrawing the needle with the other hand. Slowly twirling the needle during removal is often helpful.

Many types of needles are available. The most commonly used are stainless steel needles, but gold, silver, and copper needles are also available. The needle consists of a body or shaft with a handle. The needle shaft is used to base gauge and length measurements. Needles come in numerous sizes and lengths. Common sizes are 30 to 32 gauge, with lengths ranging from 20 to 125 mm. Shorter needles are useful with children or for shallow penetration, such as around the face. Longer needles are used for penetration of deeper structures, especially the limbs. Disposable stainless steel needles are now widely available.

Wide variation exists in the duration and course of therapy. Acute problems may involve frequent treatment. Chronic conditions may require several courses of treatment. Again, there is wide variation in treatment intervals. For chronic problems, maintenance therapy may be required.

Generalized body fatigue is a common side effect, and the patient may experience unusual sleepiness. Thus, patients should be advised to avoid strenuous activities after an acupuncture treatment. The fatigue may occur either immediately after a treatment or several hours later. The sleepiness has not been reported to interact with the somnolence that may be caused by some medications. Worsening of pain may occur 1 or 2 days after a treatment before relief is felt.

COMPLICATIONS

Although acupuncture has a long history of use and a paucity of complications has been documented, it is not free of risk. In a review, Ernst and White[45] found a total of five documented fatalities related to acupuncture. Although these appear to be rare events, the actual incidence of adverse events is unknown. Probably the most common complications with needle placement result from a vasovagal response. Nausea, pallor, dizziness, and syncope may all occur. Conservative measures for the treatment of a vasovagal response are usually adequate, but occasionally oxygen, fluids, and medications are required.

Other concerns with needle insertion include tissue trauma, dermatitis, hematoma, and infection. Pneumothorax can occur when needles are placed in the thoracic region. This is the second most often reported serious complication.[45,46] There have also been several reports of cardiac tamponade.[47] Injury to the spinal cord by an acupuncture needle has also been reported.[48] Contact and nickel dermatitis has been documented.[49,50] Kao and Chang[51] reported a case of popliteal artery pseudoaneurysm that required surgical repair.

Another rare complication is the formation of a hematoma at the site of needle insertion. To prevent a hematoma, direct pressure can be applied over the acupuncture site on removal of the needle. Placing needles deeply or near vascular structures may increase the risk of hematoma formation; caution should be exercised with patients at risk for bleeding complications.

Infections can result from the improper sterilization of needles. Hepatitis B, hepatitis C, and human immunodeficiency virus (HIV) infections have all been reported. Rampes and James[46] reported 126 cases of hepatitis associated with acupuncture; making hepatitis transmission the most often reported serious complication of acupuncture. Transmission of HIV has also been linked to acupuncture, but is not well documented.[52,53]

Bacterial infections reported include *Propionibacterium acnes*,[43] *Pseudomonas aeruginosa*,[44] and *Staphylococcus aureus*.[54]

These infections are especially significant in patients at risk for bacterial endocarditis. Infections may be minimized with the use of disposable needles.

CLINICAL DATA

Problems Associated with Acupuncture Research:
Acupuncture has been difficult to evaluate as a form therapy. This difficulty has several possible explanations.[55] First, studies determining the efficacy of acupuncture analgesia lack proper controls. In classic acupuncture the therapist may select different points for patients with the same disease. Furthermore, the therapist may change points in the same patient with each visit, depending on the patient's prior responses. This approach is not amenable to rigorous analysis. Therefore, formula acupuncture, in which treatment consists of sets of points determined by the diagnosis, has gained widespread use in clinical trials. Even so, a comparable control in the form of sham acupuncture is less than ideal because of its possible therapeutic effects.

A second reason that evaluation is problematic is the difficulty in conducting a double-blind trial. A properly conducted double-blind study is optimal for the removal of bias. However, with acupuncture, "blinding" the therapist is not possible, because any qualified therapist can easily distinguish correct from sham points. Thus, a single-blind trial may be the best alternative.

Furthermore, no standards exist for correct acupuncture therapy. The frequency and number of treatments may affect patient response. Yet, there is no accepted minimum number of treatments that defines a treatment failure. Recent studies have used one to two acupuncture treatments a week for a duration of 2 to 4 months, each session lasting 20 to 30 minutes.[31,56,57] Follow-up evaluations should be long enough, preferably greater than 6 months, to establish long-term benefits.

Finally, chronic pain is complex, and often includes psychological components. Patients often have a history of failed therapies, such as surgery, and extensive medication use. Drug abuse and drug dependency are often present.

Results of Available Data:
Since the first edition of this book, many studies have been accomplished in quality peer-reviewed journals. The evidence supporting the efficacy of acupuncture appears to be mixed. Mendelson[58] reviewed follow-up studies on acupuncture published before 1976. The studies were mostly uncontrolled and did not differentiate different pain syndromes. A review by Lewith and Machin[59] concluded that acupuncture benefited 70% of chronic pain patients, whereas sham controls resulted in 50% positive response. Placebos gave a 30% positive response rate. In a later review, Lewith[60] concluded that acupuncture works to some extent in 60% of patients with chronic pain and that these effects were greater than those of random needling or placebo treatment. Furthermore, acupuncture was as effective as physiotherapy or pharmacologic therapy for musculoskeletal pain, but caused fewer adverse reactions. Kotani et al. showed that preoperative insertion of acupuncture needles reduced postoperative analgesic requirements as well as nausea and vomiting. They also showed a reduction in the activation of the sympathoadrenal system.[61] In a randomized, investigator- and patient-blinded study by Fink et al. acupuncture was used to treat epicondylitis. They found benefit in utilizing real acupoints when compared to sham points.[62]

Richardson and Vincent[63] looked at acupuncture analgesic trials performed between 1973 and 1985. Headache and back-ache were the most commonly studied syndromes. Other studies included phantom limb pain, arthritic pain, and cervical neck pain. The extent of the therapeutic effect was mixed among the different studies. In the controlled studies about 50% to 80% of the patients showed a therapeutic response, suggesting at least short-term effectiveness of acupuncture. Follow-up periods ranged from 2 weeks to 4 months. The few studies in which patients were followed up for more than 6 months were uncontrolled and showed a relapse rate of about 50%. A more recent study of chronic low back pain that was randomized and double-blinded utilized a 9-month follow-up.[64] This study by Leibing et al. showed an improvement in both traditional acupuncture and sham acupuncture when compared to physical therapy alone. However, this also suggested a placebo effect of traditional acupuncture in low back pain. This was also concluded in a meta-analysis by Ernst et al. in 2002.[65]

Carlsson and Sjolund[56] studied the long-term effects of acupuncture on several subtypes of pain. They demonstrated that patients with nociceptive low back pain improved the most, with nearly 50% of the patients experiencing long-term pain relief. Only 32% of patients with neurogenic pain and 15% of patients with psychogenic pain benefited from acupuncture. In a review of 27 trials treating headache 23 reported positive outcomes on migraine, muscle tension headache, and mixed forms.[66] A meta-analysis by Melchart et al.[67] concluded that acupuncture has a role in the treatment of recurrent headaches but better study designs are needed.

FUTURE DIRECTION; THE NATIONAL INSTITUTES OF HEALTH CONSENSUS STATEMENT

In November of 1997 the National Institutes of Health (NIH) organized a conference of experts from various disciplines and medical specialties to evaluate and review the available literature on the use of acupuncture in treating a variety of medical conditions. During this conference a number of venues were used to examine the current status of acupuncture in American medicine. Presentations were made in both open and closed format. The culmination of this conference was a consensus statement that addressed issues such as the efficacy, a comparison with current Western treatments, and the biological effects of acupuncture. Guidance was also given as how to incorporate this ancient form of therapy into a modern health care system. Future research needs were also addressed.[68] The conclusions of this consensus statement are as follows. Acupuncture is widely practiced in the USA. While designing studies to evaluate efficacy remain a challenge, there are several entities that seem to respond to acupuncture. These include treatment for nausea and vomiting both postoperative and chemotherapy related, and dental pain. Other promising results have been seen in the treatment of headache, low back pain, asthma, menstrual cramps, fibromyalgia, and myofascial pain, among others. Acupuncture appears to be useful as an adjunct or as an alternative to current treatment strategies.[68]

SUMMARY

Acupuncture has been used as a treatment for pain for thousands of years. Although scientific data have not been able to support many of its diverse claims, there is evidence that acupuncture may be effective in relieving certain types of pain. Musculoskeletal problems, such as low back pain, and certain types of headaches seem to respond well to acupuncture. Furthermore, acupuncture appears to be effective with acute pain and spasm caused by injury. However, further clinical studies are needed to support this mode of treatment. Although the actual incidence of adverse effects is still unknown, acupuncture appears to have a low complication rate. Thus, acupuncture appears to be a safe alternative treatment for certain types of pain and has become an integral part of today's comprehensive pain therapy.

REFERENCES

1. Oleson TD, Kroenig RJ, Bresler DE: An experimental evaluation of auricular diagnosis: The somatotrophic mapping of musculo-skeletal pain at acupuncture points. Pain 8:217, 1980.
2. Melzack R, Katz K: Auriculotherapy fails to relieve chronic pain: A controlled crossover study. JAMA 251:1041, 1984.
3. Bonica JJ: Management of myofascial pain syndromes in general practice. JAMA 165:732, 1957.
4. Travel J, Simons D (eds): Myofascial Pain and Dysfunction: The Trigger Point Manual. Williams & Wilkins, Baltimore, 1983.
5. Sola AE: Treatment of myofascial pain syndromes. *In* Benedetti C, Chapman CR, Moricca G (eds): Advances in Pain Research and Therapy, vol 7. Raven Press, New York, 1984, p 467.
6. Melzack R, Wall PD: Pain mechanisms: A new theory. Science 150:971, 1965.
7. Bonta IL: Acupuncture beyond the endorphin concept? Med Hypotheses 58:221, 2002.
8. Maier SF: The opioid/nonopioid nature of stress-induced analgesia and learned helplessness. J Exp Psychol 9:80, 1983.
9. Gellup GG: Animal hypnosis: Factual status of a fictional concept. Psychol Bull 81:836, 1974.
10. Carli G, Farabollini F, Fontani G: Effects of pain, morphine, and nalaxone on the duration of animal hypnosis. Behav Brain Res 2:373, 1981.
11. Lee G, Shin M, Hong M, et al: The association of cholecystokinin-A receptor expression with the responsiveness of electroacupuncture analgesic effects in rat. Neurosci Lett 31:325, 2002.
12. Pomeranz B: Scientific basis of acupuncture. *In* Stux G, Pomeranz B (eds): Acupuncture Textbook and Atlas. Springer-Verlag, Berlin, 1987, p 1.
13. Ulett GA, Han J, Han S: Traditional and evidence-based acupuncture: History, mechanisms, and present status. South Med J 91:1115, 1998.
14. Nathan PW: Acupuncture analgesia. Trends Neurosci 7:21, 1978.
15. Han JJ, Terenius L: Neurochemical basis of acupuncture analgesia. Annu Rev Pharmacol Toxicol 22:193, 1982.
16. Baldry PE: The deactivation of trigger points. *In* Baldly FE (ed): Acupuncture, Trigger Points, and Musculoskeletal Pain. Churchill Livingstone, London, 1993, p 91.
17. Han JJ: Central neurotransmitters and acupuncture analgesia. *In* Pomeranz B, Stun G (eds): Scientific Basis of Acupuncture. Springer-Verlag, Berlin, 1988, p 10.
18. Pomeranz B: Scientific basis of acupuncture. In Stun G, Pomeranz B (eds): Basics of Acupuncture, ed 2. Springer-Verlag, Berm, 1991, p 4.
19. Mayer DJ, Price DD, Raffi A: Antagonism of acupuncture analgesia in man by the narcotic antagonist nalaxone. Brain Res 121:368, 1977.
20. Wang Q, Mao L, Han JJ: The arcuate nucleus of the hypothalamus mediates low but not high frequency electroacupuncture in rats. Brain Res 513:60, 1990.
21. Han JJ, Xie GX, Ding XZ, et al: High and low frequency electroacupuncture analgesia are mediated by different opioids. Pain 20(Suppl):S369, 1984.

22. Han JJ, Terenius L: Neurochemical basis of acupuncture analgesia. Annu Rev Pharmacol Toxicol 22:193, 1982.

23. Ungar G, Ungar A, Maim DH, et al: Brain peptides with opiate antagonistic action: Their possible role in tolerance and dependence. Psychoneuroendocrinology 2:1, 1977.

24. Frost FA, Jessen B, Siggaard-Andersen J: A control, double-blind comparison of mepivacaine injection versus saline injection for myofascial pain. Lancet 4:499, 1980.

25. Kellgren JH: Some painful joint conditions and their relation to osteoarthritis. Chin Sd 4:193, 1939.

26. Johansson V, Kosic S, Lindahl O: Effect of acupuncture in tension headache and brainstem reflexes. Adv Pain Res Ther 1:839, 1976.

27. Dowson DI, Lewith GI, Macbin D: The effects of acupuncture versus placebo in the treatment of headache. Pain 21:35, 1985.

28. Thomas M, Lundberg T: Importance of modes of acupuncture in the treatment of chronic nociceptive low back pain. Acta Anaesthesiol Scand 38:63, 1994.

29. Man SC, Barager BD: Preliminary clinical study of acupuncture in rheumatoid arthritis. J Rheumatol 1:126, 1974.

30. Christensen BV, IuhI IU, Vilbeck HC, et al: Acupuncture treatment of severe knee arthrosis: A long term study. Acta Anaesthesiol Scand 36:578, 1992.

31. Beppu S, Sato Y, Amemiya Y: Practical application of meridian acupuncture treatment for trigeminal neuralgia. Anesth Pain Control Dent 1:103, 1992.

32. Zhao J: Acupuncture at huatuojiaji points for treatment of acute epigastric pain. Tradit Chin Med 11:258, 1991.

33. Sung YF, Kutner MH, Cerine FC, et al: Comparison of the effects of acupuncture and codeine on postoperative dental pain. Anesth Analg Curr Res 56:473, 1972.

34. Dellenbach P, Rempp C, Haeringer MT, et al: Chronic pelvic pain. Another diagnostic and therapeutic approach. Gynecol Obstet Fertil 29:234, 2001.

35. Fialka V, Resch KL, Ritter-Dietrich D, et al: Acupuncture for reflex sympathetic dystrophy [letter]. Arch Intern Med 153:661, 1993.

36. Petrie JP, Langley GB. Acupuncture in the treatment of chronic cervical pain: A pilot study. Chin Exp Rheumatol 1:333, 1983.

37. Brule-Fermand S: Treatment of chronic cancer pain: Contribution of acupuncture, auriculotherapy and mesotherapy. Soins 568:39, 1993.

38. Lewith GT, Field J, Machin D: Acupuncture compared with placebo in post herpetic pain. Pain 17:361, 1983.

39. Ezzo J, Hadhazy V, Birch S, et al: Acupuncture for osteoarthritis of the knee: A systematic review. Arthritis Rheum 44:819, 2001.

40. Kemper KJ, Sarah R, Silver-Highfield E, et al: On pins and needles? Pediatric pain patients' experience with acupuncture. Pediatrics 105:941, 2000.

41. Dunn PA, Rogers D, Halford K: Transcutaneous electrical nerve stimulation at acupuncture points in the induction of uterine contractions. Obstet Gynecol 73:286, 1989.

42. Scheel O, Sundsfjord A, Lunde P, et al: Endocarditis after acupuncture and injection treatment by a natural healer. JAMA 267:56. 1992.

43. Jeffreys DB, Smith S, Brennand-Roper DA, et al: Acupuncture needles as a cause of bacterial endocarditis. BMJ 287:326, 1983.

44. Fujiwara H, Taniguchi K, Ikezono E: The influence of low frequency acupuncture on a demand pacemaker. Chest 78:96, 1980.

45. Ernst E, White A: Life-threatening adverse reactions after acupuncture: A systematic review. Pain 71:123, 1997.

46. Rampes H, James R: Complications of acupuncture. Acupunct Med 1:26, 1995.

47. Hasegawa J, Noguchi N, Yamasaki J: Delayed cardiac tamponade and hemothorax induced by an acupuncture needle. Cardiology 78:58, 1991.

48. Ernst E: The risks of acupuncture. Int J Risk Saf Med 6:179, 1995.

49. Romaguera C, Grimalt F: Contact dermatitis from a permanent acupuncture needle. Contact Dermatitis 7:156, 1981.

50. Romaguera C, Grimalt F: Nickel dermatitis from acupuncture needles. Contact Dermatitis 5:195, 1979.

51. Kao CL, Chang JP: Pseudoaneurysm of the popliteal artery: A rare sequela of acupuncture. Tex Heart Inst J 29:126, 2002.

52. Vittiecoq D, Mettetal JF, Rouzioux C, et al: Acute HIV infection after acupuncture treatments. N Eng J Med 320:250, 1989.

53. Castro KG, Lifson AR, White CR: Investigation of AIDS patients with no previously identified risk factors. JAMA 259:1338, 1988.

54. Lee RJE, McIlwain JC: Subacute bacterial endocarditis following ear acupuncture. Int J Cardiol 7:62, 1985.

55. Hsu DT: Acupuncture: A review. Reg Anesth 21:361, 1996.

56. Carlsson GB, Sjolund BH: Acupuncture and subtypes of chronic pain: Assessment of long-term results. Clin J Pain 10:290, 1994.

57. Coan RH, Wang S, Ku SC, et al: The acupuncture treatment of low back pain: A randomized controlled study. Am J Gun Med 8:181, 1986.

58. Mendelson G: Acupuncture analgesia: 1. Review of clinical studies Aust N Z J Med 7:642, 1977.

59. Lewith GT, Machin D: On the evaluation of the clinical effects in acupuncture. Pain 16:111, 1983.

60. Lewith GT: How effective is acupuncture in the management of pain? J R Coll Gen Pract 34:275, 1984.

61. Kotani N, Hashimoto H, Sato Y, et al: Preoperative intradermal acupuncture reduces postoperative pain, nausea and vomiting, analgesic requirement, and sympathoadrenal responses. Anesthesiology 95:349, 2001.

62. Fink M, Wolkenstein E, Karst M, Gehrke A: Acupuncture in chronic epicondylitis: A randomized controlled trial. Rheumatology 41:205, 2002.

63. Richardson PH, Vincent C: Acupuncture for the treatment of pain: A review of evaluative research. Pain 24:15, 1986.

64. Leibing E, Leonhardt U, Koster G, et al: Acupuncture treatment of chronic low-back pain. Pain 96:189, 2002.

65. Ernst E, White AR, Wider B: Acupuncture for back pain: Meta-analysis of randomized controlled trials and an update with data from the most recent studies. Schmerz 16:129, 2002.

66. Manias P, Tagaris G, Karageorgiou K: Acupuncture in headache: A critical review. Clin J Pain 16:334, 2000.

67. Melchart D, Linde K, Fischer P, et al: Acupuncture for recurrent headaches: A systematic review of randomized controlled trials. Cephalalgia 19:779, 1999.

68. Acupuncture. NIH Consensus Statement 3–5 November; 15:1–34, 1997.

Psychological Interventions for Chronic Pain

Jennifer A. Haythornthwaite, Ph.D., and

Leslie J. Heinberg, Ph.D.

Psychological (such as cognitive and emotional variables) and social factors have long been recognized as influencing the experience of pain. A number of important historical events have contributed to the interest in psychosocial factors such as mood, appraisal and coping, and interpersonal interactions. First, Beecher observed that the personal meaning of pain was an important determinant of the pain complaints he observed in soldiers wounded in World War II.[1] Second, the work of Melzack, Wall, and Casey on the "gate-control" theory of pain[2] stimulated much interest in the multidimensional and subjective aspects of the pain experience. Third, the pioneering work of Fordyce[3] encouraged consideration of social and environmental factors that influence both the verbal and motoric expression of pain. Fourth, the taxonomy developed by the International Society for the Study of Pain introduced a definition that included both sensory and emotional factors in the experience of pain.[4] Fifth, the publication of Turk et al.[5] of a comprehensive review of the pain literature demonstrated the influence of psychological factors on the experience of pain. This was augmented by their superb ideas for cognitive-behavioral interventions—in almost workbook form—based on the existing empirical literature.

Psychological interventions for pain management have largely grown out of two important literatures. First, early studies of laboratory pain demonstrated the importance of psychological factors in influencing the level of reported pain and pain thresholds. Second, the psychotherapy literature demonstrated the impact that psychological interventions can have on many areas of functioning and quality of life. The benefit of psychological treatments is particularly clear for anxiety and depression, which are two emotional states shown to influence the experience of pain. This chapter briefly reviews psychological interventions utilized for chronic pain, focusing primarily on the interventions that have been empirically tested through the use of clinical trials. General psychological interventions, such as psychotherapy, marital/family therapy, and general group psychotherapy, which have not been widely tested, are not included in this overview. The overall goals for psychological treatment include: (1) reducing pain and pain-related disability; (2) treating comorbid mood disturbances, particularly depression; (3) increasing perceptions of control and self-efficacy; (4) reducing pain-related disability; and (5) addressing pain-related psychosocial factors, such as the impact of pain on family and/or marital functioning (see Fig. 23-1).

BEHAVIORAL INTERVENTIONS

Learning theory, incorporating the principles of operant conditioning (e.g., reinforcement and punishment), provides the theoretical basis for behavioral interventions. Many of the techniques are adapted from behavior therapy, which has been used extensively in managing anxiety, depression, and behavioral aspects of other medical conditions.

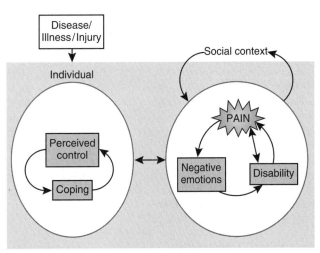

FIGURE 23-1. Key targets for psychological interventions in chronic pain.

Operant Interventions: In an operant model of pain, the primary focus of intervention is the behavior of the patient. These behaviors can include either verbal expressions of pain (e.g., complaints of pain or requests for medication), gross motor movements that are indicators of pain (e.g., grimacing or limping), or avoidance of pain-generating activities. As observable behaviors, these responses are regarded as subject to the principles of operant conditioning, which focus attention on the consequences of the behavior. Reinforcing consequences increase the likelihood that a behavior will occur in the future and punishing consequences decrease the likelihood that a behavior will occur. For example, when a patient grimaces and a loved one responds by expressing concern, grimacing may occur more frequently in the future when that loved one is present. In this case, the social attention in the form of concern reinforces the grimace. Alternatively, pain as an aversive stimulus can serve as a punishment for an activity that increases the pain. If an individual experiences pain during or following sexual intercourse and then decreases the frequency of sexual intercourse, then the pain is likely punishing sexual behavior.

The goal of operant interventions is to decrease learned pain behavior and replace these maladaptive responses with adaptive behaviors inconsistent with the sick role. Operant interventions ideally occur in an environment where there is the opportunity to control the social consequences of pain behaviors and shape new "well" behaviors. Most operant pain programs are based on inpatient units where this level of control is possible. "As needed" prescriptions are changed to fixed time intervals in order to remove the contingent relationship between complaints of pain (i.e., the pain behavior) and pain relief (i.e., the reinforcer). Pain complaints are largely ignored and well behaviors, including attending physical therapy and increasing activity level, are socially rewarded (i.e., reinforced).

Pacing and activity modulation are important components of operant behavioral pain management programs. When individuals push their activity level to a point of pain exacerbation, they are more likely to decrease their activity over time. That is, activity is punished by pain and therefore decreases over time. If an individual reports exacerbation of low back pain after 30 minutes of sitting at desk, an operant intervention would begin by having the individual get up after 20 minutes, stretch and move around for a period of time. After this duration of sitting was established with comfort, the duration of sitting would be gradually increased, possibly by only 5 minutes with each increment. Over a period of weeks, the individual may increase the comfortable duration of sitting to be 60 minutes without shifting positions or standing up. This process of gradually increasing the nature, frequency, or duration of a behavior is called "shaping." The goal of such an intervention is to increase the behavior while managing the consequences, which include removing any punishment (e.g., pain) and introducing reinforcement (e.g., social attention). The involvement of the spouse or family in treatment often occurs and these individuals are taught these principles—reinforcement/punishment and shaping—of behavior. Inclusion of the family in treatment can facilitate generalization of treatment gains from the inpatient setting to the home environment.

Relaxation Interventions: An extensive literature documents the benefits of relaxation exercises, particularly in the areas of anxiety and stress management. The goal for most relaxation techniques is nondirected relaxation accomplished through two common components: first, repetitive focus on a word, body sensation, or muscle activity; and second, a passive attitude towards thoughts unrelated to the attentional focus.[6] Common methods used for teaching relaxation include systematically tensing and relaxing specific muscle groups (e.g., progressive muscle relaxation), focusing on breathing and enhancing diaphragmatic breathing, and using guided imagery. A psychophysiological model of pain, which has received some empirical support,[7] suggests that stress or pain leads to subtle increases in muscle tension, which can exacerbate pain at the site of an injury. A primary goal of relaxation training is to break such a pain–muscle tension–pain cycle.

A panel of experts sponsored by the National Institutes of Health (NIH)[6] reviewed the empirical support for the use of relaxation techniques in the treatment of chronic pain. This panel concluded that strong evidence supports the use of these techniques for pain management and recommended the broad integration of relaxation techniques with more traditional, biomedical interventions for pain management.

Biofeedback: Biofeedback provides the individual with detailed information about a physiological process that is typically not within the individual's awareness. Through this detailed feedback, the individual can learn voluntary control over usually involuntary processes. The psychophysiological model briefly outlined above is an important underpinning for the use of biofeedback. Biofeedback for pain management usually entails providing feedback about muscle tension, typically using electromyographic (EMG) feedback from the site of the pain or a standard location such as the frontalis muscles, or feedback about skin temperature, typically using thermistors attached to the fingers.

Empirical support for the efficacy of biofeedback for pain management is limited to some specific painful conditions, including Raynaud's phenomenon, tension and migraine headaches, vulvar vestibulitis, and low back pain. Although widely used within the pain field, particularly in conjunction with relaxation training, the empirical support for its specific efficacy beyond the general effects of relaxation strategies has been demonstrated only for migraine headaches. The NIH panel mentioned above[6] found moderate evidence supporting the use of biofeedback for chronic pain management, particularly within the area of headaches. Patients often respond favorably to the sophisticated technology required to implement this intervention and the rationale often fits their own conceptualization of the pain problem, particularly since the intervention is focused on physiological responses to pain and stress.

COGNITIVE-BEHAVIORAL INTERVENTIONS

The demonstration that cognitive and emotional factors influence the experience of pain has encouraged the application of cognitive-behavioral theory and treatment to the management of chronic pain. These interventions typically include components of the behavioral model, particularly relaxation training and some components of operant conditioning. However, an emphasis is also placed on cognitive factors, such as attitudes and beliefs that underlie maladaptive emotional and behavioral responses to pain.[8] The NIH panel[6] found moderate evidence for the use of cognitive-behavioral interventions for chronic pain management, providing the strongest support in treating patients with low back pain, rheumatoid arthritis, and osteoarthritis pain, and cognitive-behavioral interventions reduce pain and increase positive coping.[9]

Coping Skills: Primary goals of these interventions include increasing perceptions of pain as a controllable experience and decreasing the use of maladaptive coping strategies, such as pain-contingent rest or use of medications. Specific pain coping skills often include some of the strategies outlined above, particularly relaxation and pacing of activity level. In this approach the emphasis is on skill development and refinement. In the case of skill development, a new skill is introduced and patients are encouraged to develop and refine the skill during low pain periods before applying the skill for actual pain management. Often the use of the skill is shaped over time, so that the skill is gradually applied to increasingly challenging (i.e., painful) episodes. Therapy focuses on problem-solving discussions of skill application. A similar approach is taken to the application of many pain coping skills, including cognitive or behavioral distraction, relaxation, pacing of activities, and the appropriate use of social support. Attention is paid to factors that increase or decrease pain and these factors guide the application of pain coping skills.

Cognitive Restructuring: Cognitive restructuring focuses on the role of cognitive factors, such as attitudes, thoughts, and beliefs, in determining emotional and behavioral responses to pain. These interventions challenge negative self-talk, such as catastrophizing (e.g., "I can't stand the pain anymore"), and replace these self-statements with more positive statements that reduce negative affect, emphasize control, and encourage adaptive coping (e.g., "This is a challenge that I have faced before and I can handle it this time"). Catastrophizing is a particularly maladaptive response to pain that has been shown to correlate with depression and disability. In the context of treatment, patients are frequently asked to monitor their thoughts about their pain, or pain-related situations, identify negative thoughts, and generate more accurate, adaptive thoughts to replace the negative thoughts. The emphasis is on balanced thinking, not necessarily positive thinking. This monitoring process is supplemented with more in-depth discussions of the underlying attitudes and beliefs contributing to the negative thoughts.

HYPNOSIS

Hypnosis typically includes an attention-focusing component similar to those identified above under relaxation strategies and a suggestion component that outlines specific goals for outcome (e.g., analgesia). Hypnosis has been most widely applied and studied with pain due to cancer, and the NIH panel concluded that strong evidence supports the use of hypnosis in reducing chronic pain due to malignancies.[6] Other data support its efficacy in treating pain due to irritable bowel syndrome, temporomandibular joint disorders, and tension headaches.

MULTIDISCIPLINARY TREATMENT
Multidisciplinary programs typically include many or most of the procedures detailed above in conjunction with other nonpsychological interventions (e.g., physical therapy). A meta-analysis of the literature[9] evaluating the efficacy of these programs demonstrated beneficial effects on pain, mood, and functioning. In addition to these important outcomes, return to work rates were higher (68% vs. 32%) and use of the health care system was lower in patients treated within these programs. Gains were found to extend well beyond treatment, lasting an average of almost 2 years. These patients were found to be functioning at a higher level than 75% of the patients treated within traditional, unimodal treatment approaches.[9]

SUMMARY

A number of psychological interventions have been empirically demonstrated to reduce pain and suffering in patients with a wide variety of chronic pain syndromes. These treatments can be broadly identified as behavioral and cognitive and have become an integral part of multidisciplinary pain treatment programs. Although most patients with chronic pain may benefit from such interventions, certain subpopulations should be targeted for referral to these programs. For example, patients reporting depression or anxiety often require these interventions. In addition, patients reporting or demonstrating excessive disability should be referred for psychological treatment. Although this impairment may be due to negative affect, family/social factors, or "secondary gain," psychological interventions often reduce disability. Problematic medication use, including dose escalation, misuse, or under-use, can also be addressed. Certain pain disorders (e.g., headaches) may be highly responsive to specific psychological interventions such as biofeedback, and such treatments should be considered a standard part of medical management. Finally, specific patient groups may not be suitable candidates for some medical or pharmacological treatment (e.g., chronic opioid therapy for the recovering substance abuser). For such individuals, psychological treatment, particularly multidisciplinary programs, may be considered an essential first-line treatment option.

REFERENCES

1. Beecher HK: Pain and some factors that modify it. Anesthesiology 12:633–641, 1951.
2. Melzack R, Wall PD: Pain mechanisms: A new theory. Science 150:971–979, 1965.
3. Fordyce WE, Fowler RS, Lehmann JF, et al: Operant conditioning in the treatment of chronic pain. Arch Phys Med Rehabil 54:399–408, 1973.
4. International Association for the Study of Pain: Pain terms: A list with definitions and notes on usage. Pain 6:249–252, 1979.
5. Turk DC, Meichenbaum D, Genest M: Pain and Behavioral Medicine: A Cognitive-Behavioral Perspective. Guilford Press, New York, 1983.
6. NIH Technology Assessment Panel: Integration of behavioral and relaxation approaches into the treatment of chronic pain and insomnia. NIH Technology Assessment Panel on Integration of Behavioral and Relaxation Approaches into the Treatment of Chronic Pain and Insomnia. JAMA 276:313–318, 1996.
7. Flor H, Birbaumer N, Schugens MM, Lutzenberger W: Symptom-specific psychophysiological responses in chronic pain patients. Psychophysiology 29:452–460, 1992.
8. Turner JA, Romano JM: Cognitive behavioral therapy. In Bonica J (ed): The Management of Pain, ed 2. Lea & Febiger, Philadelphia, 1990, pp 1711–1720.
9. Morley S, Eccleston C, Williams A: Systematic review and meta-analysis of randomized controlled trials of cognitive behaviour therapy and behaviour therapy for chronic pain in adults, excluding headache. Pain 80:1–13, 1999.

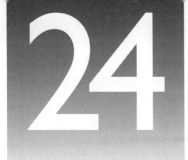

Substance Use Disorders and Detoxification

Michael R. Clark, M.D., M.P.H.

SUBSTANCE USE AND CHRONIC PAIN

The prevalence of substance use disorders in patients with chronic pain is higher than in the general population.[1,2] In a study of primary care outpatients with chronic noncancer pain who received at least 6 months of opioid prescriptions during 1 year, behaviors consistent with opioid abuse were recorded in approximately 25% of patients.[3] Almost 90% of patients attending a clinic specializing in pain management were taking medications and 70% were prescribed opioid analgesics.[4] In this population, 12% met DSM-III-R criteria for substance abuse or dependence. In another study of 414 chronic pain patients, 23% met criteria for active alcohol, analgesic, or sedative misuse or dependency; 9% met criteria for a remission diagnosis; and current dependency was most common for analgesics (13%).[5] In a review of substance dependence or addiction in patients with chronic pain the prevalence ranged from 3% to 19% in high-quality studies.[6,7]

Determining the presence of a substance use disorder usually involves the problem of how to evaluate the patient with chronic pain who is prescribed controlled substances with abuse potential.[8–11] In one study of 12,000 medical patients treated with opioids for a variety of conditions, virtually no patients without a history of substance abuse developed dependence on the medication.[12] Other studies of opioid therapy have found that patients who developed problems with their medication all had a history of substance abuse.[13,14] Inaccurate and underreporting of medication use by patients complicates assessment.[15,16] However, in patients with chronic pain who did develop new substance use disorders, the problem most commonly involved the medications prescribed by their physicians.[17,18]

The causes and onset of substance use disorders have been difficult to characterize in relationship to chronic pain. During the first five years after the onset of chronic pain, patients are at increased risk for developing new substance use disorders and additional physical injuries.[19,20] This risk is highest in patients with a history of substance abuse or dependence, childhood physical or sexual abuse, and psychiatric comorbidity.[8,21,22]

In a study of chronic low back pain patients, 34% had a substance use disorder, yet in 77% of cases the abuse was present before the onset of their chronic pain.[19,23] The mechanisms of relapse into substance abuse are not well understood and probably involve multiple factors; however, a cycle of pain followed by relief *after* taking medications is a classic example of operant reinforcement of *future* medication use that eventually becomes abuse.[24] Careful monitoring of patients is essential to prevent this complication of the treatment of chronic pain. Research in patients with substance abuse has demonstrated abnormalities in pain perception and tolerance. An increased sensitivity to pain and the reinforcing effects of relieving pain with substance use suggest a different mechanism for the development of substance abuse in patients with chronic pain.

Patients with substance use disorders have increased rates of chronic pain and are at the greatest risk for under-treatment with appropriate medications and subsequent self-medication with illicit drugs.[25,26] Almost a quarter of patients admitted to inpatient residential substance abuse treatment and over a third of patients in methadone maintenance treatment programs reported severe chronic pain, with almost half of the inpatients and two-thirds of the methadone maintenance patients suffering pain-related interference in functioning.[26] In another study of methadone maintenance therapy, patients with pain were more likely to overuse both prescribed and nonprescribed medications.[27] Patients with substance abuse and back pain were less likely to complete a substance abuse treatment program compared to those without pain.[28] Ethical principles such as beneficence, quality of life, and autonomy can provide particularly useful guidance for the use of chronic opioid therapy, recognizing that benefits should be optimized in a context of risk management.[7,29,30]

RISKS OF PHARMACOLOGICAL TREATMENT FOR CHRONIC PAIN

Opioids: Opioids are effective in the treatment of chronic nonmalignant pain, as demonstrated in randomized placebo-controlled trials, in reducing pain, pain-related disability, depression, insomnia, and physical dysfunction.[31–36] Studies of neuropathic pain show that opioids provide direct analgesic benefit, not just counteract the unpleasantness of pain.[37,38] Levorphanol reduced pain, affective distress, interference with function, and sleep difficulties in adults with neuropathic pain.[39] Continuous-release morphine decreased pain in patients with postherpetic neuralgia significantly more than tricyclic antidepressants or placebo.[40] Most experts agree that opioids with slow onset of action and longer duration of action are preferred to minimize the initial euphoria and interdose withdrawal symptoms. Extended-release oral medications and transdermal routes of administration decrease these qualities of opioids. A constant rather than intermittent "as needed" schedule should be followed, keeping the time between dosages and the individual dose amounts consistent. Opioid dependence is mediated by the actions and interactions of opioid receptors.[41] Mesolimbic dopaminergic projections to the nucleus accumbens have been implicated in the development of psychological dependence. In contrast, physical dependence on opioids is probably due to noradrenergic activity in the locus ceruleus.

However, the treatment of nonmalignant chronic pain with opioids remains a subject of considerable debate with fears of regulatory pressure, medication abuse, and the development of tolerance, creating a reluctance to prescribe opioids and, subsequently, their underutilization.[18,42–45] Fortunately, the prescribing of long-term opioids for the treatment of chronic nonmalignant pain syndromes has increased despite dramatic coverage by the public press of the various forms of abuse of these medications.[46–49] Chronic pain conditions may facilitate the development of tolerance to opioid analgesia.[50] The loss of analgesia over time can have many causes and should be carefully evaluated to determine its etiology. It is most likely due to disease progression or other changes in the patient's condition such as the development of delirium. While tolerance does occur and several mechanisms have been described, it is relatively rare in clinical practice.[51–58] The incidence of analgesic tolerance is lower with more potent opioids such as fentanyl, presumably because these agents are more receptor-specific and fewer receptors are needed to produce an analgesic effect. Tolerance to different opioid effects emerges at different rates, with constipation the most likely to persist, suggesting receptor-related differences.

Benzodiazepines: Benzodiazepines such as diazepam and clonazepam are commonly prescribed for insomnia and anxiety in patients with chronic pain but no studies have demonstrated any benefit for these target symptoms.[59,60] Only a limited number of chronic pain conditions such as trigeminal neuralgia, tension headache, and temporomandibular disorders were found to improve with benzodiazepines.[61] Clonazepam has been reported to provide long-term relief of the episodic lancinating variety of phantom limb pain.[62] A recent extensive review failed to conclude that benzodiazepines significantly improved spasticity following spinal cord injury and no evidence was found to support the analgesic efficacy of barbiturates.[63,64] Benzodiazepines have been used for the detoxification of patients with chronic pain from sedative/hypnotic medications and were superior to barbiturates for minimizing symptoms of withdrawal.[65] Higher levels of withdrawal symptoms during detoxification predicted relapse to future use of benzodiazepines.[66]

Benzodiazepines also cause cognitive impairment as demonstrated by abnormalities on neuropsychological testing and EEG.[67,68] In patients with chronic pain use of benzodiazepines and not opioids was associated with decreased activity levels, higher rates of healthcare visits, increased domestic instability, depression, and more disability days.[69] Combining benzodiazepines with opioids may cause additional problems. In methadone-related mortality, almost 75% of deaths were attributable to a combination of drug effects and benzodiazepines were present in 74% of the deceased.[70,71] Benzodiazepines have been associated with exacerbation of pain and interference with opioid analgesia, which is mediated by the serotonergic system.[72–74] Benzodiazepines also increase the rate of developing tolerance to opioids.[55]

DIAGNOSIS OF SUBSTANCE USE DISORDERS

The fourth edition of the Diagnostic and Statistical Manual of Mental Disorders of the American Psychiatric Association defines both substance abuse and dependence as maladaptive (behavioral) patterns of substance use leading to clinically significant impairment or distress.[75] Substance abuse must be accompanied by any of the following: interpersonal problems, legal problems, failure to fulfill major role obligations, and recurrent substance use in hazardous situations. Substance dependence is distinguished from abuse by more than simply a continuum of severity. In contrast to abuse, substance dependence is manifested by tolerance, withdrawal, using the substance in larger amounts or over a longer period than was intended, persistent desire or unsuccessful efforts to decrease or control substance use, spending large amounts of time in activities necessary to obtain the substance, the giving up or reduction of important activities because of substance use, and continued substance use despite knowledge of having physical or psychological problems caused or exacerbated by the substance. Making the distinct diagnosis of dependence is important because it reliably predicts more severe medical sequelae, poorer treatment outcomes, higher relapse rates, and worse overall prognosis.

Recent efforts have attempted to standardize diagnostic criteria and definitions for problematic behaviors of medication use and substance use disorders across professional disciplines (Table 24-1).[11,76–78] The core criteria for a substance use disorder in patients with chronic pain include the loss of control in the use of the medication, excessive preoccupation with the medication despite adequate analgesia, and adverse consequences associated with the use of the medication.[9] Items from the Prescription Drug Use Questionnaire that best predicted the presence of addiction in a sample of patients with problematic medication use were (1) the patients believing they were addicted, (2) increasing analgesic dose/frequency, and (3) a preferred route of administration. The diagnosis of addiction in the patient with chronic pain must demonstrate certain drug-taking behaviors that interfere with the successful fulfillment of life activities. Access to opioids may not be a specific problem because a physician has been prescribing them. If addiction is present, however, the patient may fear that opioid access will be limited and therefore try to conceal any problematic use of the medication. The presence of maladaptive behaviors is emphasized to diagnose addiction because physical dependence and tolerance should be recognized as normal physiological phenomena.

TABLE 24-1. **DEFINITIONS APPROVED BY THE AMERICAN SOCIETY OF ADDICTION MEDICINE**

Abuse	Harmful use of a specific psychoactive substance
Addiction	Continued use of a specific psychoactive substance despite physical, psychological, or social harm
Misuse	Any use of a prescription drug that varies from accepted medical practice
Physical dependence	Physiological state of adaptation to a specific psychoactive substance characterized by the emergence of a withdrawal syndrome during abstinence which may be relieved in total or in part by readministration of the substance
Psychological dependence	Subjective sense of need for a specific psychoactive substance, either for its positive effects or to avoid negative effects associated with its abstinence

Increased function and opioid analgesia without side effects, not the avoidance of high doses of opioids, are the goals of treatment.[79–84] The evaluation of a patient suspected of misusing medications should be thorough and include an assessment of the pain syndrome as well as other medical disorders, patterns of medication use, social and family factors, patient and family history of substance abuse, and a psychiatric history.[8,58] Reliance on medications that provide pain relief can result in a number of stereotyped patient behaviors that are often mistaken for addiction. Persistent pain can lead to increased focus on opioid medications. Patients may take extraordinary measures to ensure an adequate medication supply even in the absence of addiction. This may be manifested as frequent requests for higher medication doses and larger quantities of medication or seeking medication from additional sources. Patients understandably fear the reemergence of pain and withdrawal symptoms if they run out of medication. Drug-seeking behavior may be the result of an anxious patient trying to maintain a previous level of pain control. In this situation the patient's actions define pseudoaddiction that results from therapeutic dependence and current or potential undertreatment but not addiction.[2,85] These behaviors resolve once adequate opioid therapy is prescribed.

In patients with higher risk of addiction prevention begins with a treatment contract to clarify the conditions under which treatment with opioids will be provided. Elements of a contract emphasize a single physician being responsible for the prescription of the medication, and, in advance, describe for the patient all the conditions under which continued use of opioids would be inappropriate. Under optimal circumstances opioid contracts attempt to improve compliance by distributing information and utilizing a mutually designed, agreed upon

treatment plan that includes consequences for aberrant behaviors and incorporates the primary care physician to form a "trilateral" agreement with patient and pain specialist.[86–88] When there is concern that a patient will have difficulty taking medications as directed, a policy of prescribing small quantities of medications, performing random pill counts, and not refilling lost supplies should be explicitly discussed and then followed. External sources of information such as urine toxicology testing, interviews with partners and family members, data from prescription monitoring programs, and review of medical records can improve detection of substance use disorders.[89] Patients who denied using illicit substances that were detected on urine toxicology were more likely to be younger, receiving worker's compensation benefits, and have a previous diagnosis of polysubstance abuse.

The occurrence of any aberrant medication-related behaviors should prompt evaluation for addiction. Even when the diagnosis of a substance use disorder is suspected in patients taking opioids for chronic pain, behaviors such as stealing or forging prescriptions are relatively uncommon.[6,90,91] These more serious aberrant behaviors consistent with addiction also include selling medications, losing prescriptions, using oral medications intravenously, concurrent abuse of alcohol or illicit drugs, repeated noncompliance with the prescribed use of medications, and deterioration in the patient's ability to function in family, social, or occupational roles. Concerns by family or friends about the patient's pattern of medication use, an appearance suggesting intoxication, or the patient having other difficulties with functional abilities require in-depth evaluation. Any unwillingness to discuss the possibility of addiction or changes in chronic opioid therapy requires discussion about the patient's worries and possible aberrant behaviors including medication misuse.

TREATMENT OF SUBSTANCE USE DISORDERS IN PATIENTS WITH CHRONIC PAIN

In general, an active substance use disorder is a relative contraindication to chronic opioid therapy. However, it can be accomplished successfully if the clinical benefits are deemed to outweigh the risks. The treatment of this extraordinary subset of patients with chronic pain will always require considerably more effort and frustration on the part of the physician. A strict treatment structure with therapeutic goals, landmarks to document progress, and contingencies for noncompliance should be made explicit and agreed upon by the patient and all the providers of health care. The first step for the patient is acknowledging that a problem with medication use exists. The first step for the clinician is to stop the patient's behavior of misusing medications. Then, sustaining factors must be assessed and addressed. These interventions include treating other medical diseases and psychiatric disorders, managing personality vulnerabilities, meeting situational challenges and life stressors, and providing support and understanding. Finally, the habit of taking the medication inappropriately must be extinguished.

The patient should be actively participating in an addictions treatment program that will reinforce taking the medication as prescribed and examine the possible reasons for any inappropriate use. Relapse is common and patients with addiction require ongoing monitoring even if the prescription of opioids has ceased. Traditional outpatient drug treatment or 12-step programs can provide support for recovery. Relapse prevention should rely on family members or sponsors to assist the patient in getting prompt attention before further deterioration occurs. If relapse is detected, the precipitating incident should be examined and strategies to avoid another relapse should be implemented. Although the misuse of medications is unacceptable, complete abstinence is not always the most appropriate or optimal treatment of patients with chronic pain. Restoration of function should be the primary treatment goal and may improve with adequate, judicious, and appropriate use of medications.[92]

WHY IS DETOXIFICATION NECESSARY?

Detoxification does not imply that a patient has been given the diagnosis of substance use disorder such as addiction, abuse, or misuse of medications.[93] Detoxification is simply the process of withdrawing a person from a specific psychoactive substance in a safe and effective manner. While addiction may necessitate detoxification in order to begin drug rehabilitation treatment, there are many reasons that patients must undergo detoxification. Since long-term treatment will have resulted in physiological dependence, discontinuation or substantial dose reduction requires gradual tapering of the medication. In the treatment of chronic nonmalignant pain, the ongoing assessment of a therapeutic trial of medications such as opioids may result in the conclusion that the risk–benefit ratio is no longer acceptable (Table 24-2). A carefully planned and monitored detoxification will avoid a withdrawal syndrome in the patient who has become physiologically dependent on medications such as opioids or benzodiazepines.

OPIOID DETOXIFICATION

Although physiological opioid dependence can be demonstrated experimentally within 7 days, most patients will not experience withdrawal symptoms unless they have continuously taken opioids for at least several weeks. Patients with a history of physiological opioid dependence, opioid withdrawal, or any other drug withdrawal will generally be more likely to experience opioid withdrawal after shorter periods of treatment. Regardless of the total daily dose, once physiological

TABLE 24-2. INDICATIONS FOR DETOXIFICATION

Intolerable side effects
Inadequate response or benefit

Aberrant drug-related behaviors
  Non-compliance
  Loss of control of medication use
  Preoccupation with the medication
  Continued use despite adverse consequences

Refractory comorbid psychiatric illness
Lack of functional improvement or impairment   in role responsibilities

dependence is established, abrupt discontinuation of opioids will precipitate acute withdrawal. Even a reduction in dose can precipitate withdrawal to a lesser degree. Patients taking opioid analgesics on a variable schedule are at higher risk for experiencing intermittent withdrawal. Even a long overnight dosing hiatus from short-half-life opioids can cause significant withdrawal symptoms. Exacerbations of pain or intermittent withdrawal symptoms relieved by taking medications are highly reinforcing and a common factor in the failure of detoxification. Patients with these experiences will require longer tapering schedules and more support to overcome this conditioned habit.

The essential element for successful opioid detoxification is the gradual tapering of the dose of medication.[94] Opioid withdrawal is generally not dangerous except with patients at risk from increased sympathetic tone (e.g., increased intracranial pressure or unstable angina). However, opioid withdrawal is very uncomfortable and distressing to patients. Patients with pain are often particularly miserable during opioid withdrawal because of the phenomenon of rebound pain. Increases in pain can occur even if the analgesic effects of opioid therapy had not been appreciable. Although it is generally not possible to avoid discomfort completely, the goal of detoxification is to ameliorate withdrawal as much as is clinically practical. Explaining the treatment plan to patients before the detoxification begins is critical. In particular, patients should know to expect worsening of pain and should have a few concrete short-term goals to focus on, such as the improvement in withdrawal symptoms, increasing functional abilities, or an alternative analgesic trial when withdrawal has resolved. The projected length of a taper is typically a balance between the expected severity of withdrawal symptoms (increased with faster tapers) and their expected duration (shorter with faster tapers).

Setting: The inpatient setting offers more intensive monitoring, supervision, and other support that generally allows for a faster taper schedule. Indications for inpatient detoxification include the failure of outpatient detoxification attempts, medically unstable patients, comorbid psychiatric illness, unreliable or noncompliant patients, and complicated pharmacological regimens requiring taper of more than one medication or illicit drug. Usually opioid detoxification can be accomplished in the outpatient setting. Outpatient detoxification should be planned with a careful inventory of support and monitoring systems. Patients should plan not only for discomfort but also temporary emotional lability and reduction in function. Compensatory planning might include warning family and work supervisors, planning for a decrease in workload on the job, and even taking vacation or sick leave days. Extensive support with frequent monitoring substantially increases the likelihood of a successful taper.

Higher success rates have been reported for patients with better therapeutic relationships or formal treatment programs that have included a period of stabilization on long-half-life opioids and then proceed with a taper slowly over a period of months. Office visits should occur at least weekly but daily contact with the patient proves a major advantage for ensuring success. Most contact with the patient does not have to involve the physician and often can be done over the telephone. A nursing visit to check vital signs and assess the severity of withdrawal can provide enormous help to the patient. This should include allowing the patient to express discomfort and frustration but then focus on the treatment plan and the patient's progress. Formal checklists of signs and symptoms such as the Subjective Opioid Withdrawal Scale (SOWS) and the Objective Opioid Withdrawal Scale (OOWS) allow for the objective rating of withdrawal and documentation of the patient's condition over time (Table 24-3).[95] Adjustment to the treatment plan is then based on several sources of information and not just the patient's complaints.

TABLE 24-3. OPIOID WITHDRAWAL RATING SCALES

The objective opiate withdrawal scale (OOWS)
Score one point for each sign that is present during a 10-minute observation period ___ Yawning (≥1 yawn per observation period) ___ Rhinorrhea (≥3 sniffs per observation period) ___ Piloerection (gooseflesh: observe patient's arm) ___ Perspiration ___ Lacrimation ___ Mydriasis ___ Tremors (hands) ___ Hot and cold flashes (shivering or huddling for warmth) ___ Restlessness (frequent shifts of position) ___ Vomiting ___ Muscle twitches ___ Abdominal cramps (holding stomach) ___ Anxiety (from mild fidgeting to severe trembling or panic)
Total score ___ (maximum severity = 13)
The subjective opiate withdrawal scale (SOWS)
Patients should rate each symptom statement on a scale of 0−4; 0 = not at all, 1 = a little, 2 = moderately, 3 = quite a bit, 4 = extremely ___ I feel anxious ___ I feel like yawning ___ I am perspiring ___ My eyes are tearing ___ My nose is running ___ I have goose flesh ___ I am shaking ___ I have hot flashes ___ I have cold flashes ___ My bones and muscles ache ___ I feel restless ___ I feel nauseous ___ I feel like vomiting ___ My muscles twitch ___ I have cramps in my stomach ___ I feel like taking [name of opioid] now
Total score ___ (maximum severity = 64)

Agents: The primary principle for detoxification is that medication should not be prescribed by a "cookbook" approach but through ongoing patient evaluation and subsequent dosage titration.[96] The simplest strategy institutes a taper of the agent that the patient is currently using. This may be a short-half-life agent but offers the advantages of using an agent already familiar to the patient, simplifies an anxiety-filled process, and avoids the imperfect calculation of dosage equivalence and incomplete cross-tolerance. Short-half-life agents possess the disadvantage of pharmacokinetics that may not allow a smooth taper. Serum levels will fluctuate more with increasing dosing intervals. Patients will usually experience mild withdrawal within 4 to 8 hours of a dosage reduction. The severity of withdrawal will usually peak with a short-half-life agent at 8 to 36 hours; however, it can occur as late as 72 hours. When using these agents, certain procedures can minimize the risks of severe withdrawal symptoms (Table 24-4).

The preferable pharmacological strategy is to choose a long-half-life pure opioid agonist such as methadone, sustained-release morphine or oxycodone, and transdermal fentanyl patches (Table 24-5). This strategy has the primary advantage of more consistent opioid serum levels with less chance of intermittent withdrawal between doses. With a long-half-life agent, the onset of withdrawal symptoms should be expected at 12 to 24 hours although 24 to 48 hours is the usually reported time course. The severity will usually peak at 36 to 96 hours but can occur up to 1 week later. Substitution, which is often not exact, may require some initial titration to achieve dosing equivalence. An initial test dose of the agent can be given to determine the total dose needed. Switching from short- to long-half-life opioids in anticipation of detoxification may serendipitously prove an effective analgesic strategy. Side effects, intermittent withdrawal, and rebound pain may all improve such that detoxification may not be needed.

A third detoxification strategy uses the partial agonist/antagonist opioids. The agent most commonly used in this

TABLE 24-4. SHORT-HALF-LIFE OPIOID TAPER

Determine the total daily dosage being used by the patient
Adopt a fixed interval schedule with equal doses every 4–6 hours for 48 hours
Increase the prescribed dose until the patient has no opioid withdrawal symptoms for 48 hours
Taper the amount of each dose without lengthening the interval between doses
Taper the total daily dose approximately 10% every 3–7 days

Slowing the taper may be accomplished by:
    Increasing the number of days at a given total dose
    Decreasing a single dose amount while keeping the remaining doses the same
    Increasing the time between doses only if the smallest individual dose has been reached

TABLE 24-5. LONG-HALF-LIFE OPIOID TAPER

Determine the total daily dose of the prescribed agent being taken by the patient
Estimate by conversion the equivalent total daily dose of the long-half-life opioid
Adopt a fixed interval schedule with equal doses every 6–8 hours for 48 hours
Increase the prescribed dose of long-half-life opioid until the patient has no withdrawal symptoms for 3–5 days
Taper the amount of each dose unless the patient can tolerate an interval schedule of dosing every 8–12 hours
Taper the total daily dose approximately 10% every 3–7 days
Increase the number of days at a given total daily dose to slow the taper

category is buprenorphine (Table 24-6). The use of partial agonist/antagonists is designed to reduce the severity of withdrawal and cause less reinforcing drug effects. As a result, the taper should be easier and more successful. There is also less risk of respiratory depression, which is an infrequent consequence of overestimating the dosing equivalence with pure agonist substitution. When using partial agonist/antagonists such as buprenorphine, it is important to give a small test dose under supervision because of the rare precipitation of

TABLE 24-6. BUPRENORPHINE TAPER

Test for the precipitation of acute withdrawal symptoms by giving an initial dose of 0.1 mg SQ/IM or 1.0 mg SL
Determine the total daily dose of the prescribed agent being taken by the patient
Estimate the equivalent total daily dose of buprenorphine (0.2 mg SQ/IM = morphine 10 mg PO)
Adopt a fixed interval schedule with equal doses every 8–12 hours
Titrate the dosage until the patient has no withdrawal symptoms for 24–72 hours
Taper the dose and interval to 0.1 mg SQ/IM or 1.0 mg PO qd
Discontinue the medication when the patient experiences no or tolerable withdrawal symptoms

withdrawal symptoms secondary to the partial antagonist effect. If patients tolerate the test dose, then the titration of dose equivalence substitution can proceed.

Adjunctive Agents: Several nonopioid pharmacological agents are commonly used as adjunctive agents to provide patients additional relief from withdrawal symptoms (Table 24-7). Clonidine, an alpha-2-adrenergic agonist that decreases adrenergic activity, is the most commonly prescribed. Clonidine can help relieve many of the autonomic symptoms of opioid withdrawal, such as nausea, cramps, sweating, tachycardia, and hypertension, which result from the loss of opioid suppression of the locus ceruleus during the withdrawal syndrome.[97] Other adjunctive agents include nonsteroidal anti-inflammatory drugs for muscle aches, Pepto-Bismol® for diarrhea, Bentyl® for abdominal cramps, and antihistamines for insomnia and restlessness.

Schedule: Unless patients are involved with dangerous aberrant drug-taking behaviors, there is generally no urgency to shorten the duration of opioid detoxification. The longer a patient has been taking opioids, the more difficulty they are likely to have with withdrawal. The taper will then require more time to be completed. Other factors that tend to increase the difficulty and length of a taper are medical comorbidity and complexity, older age, female gender, and detoxification from multiple agents simultaneously. Detoxification is more difficult in the last stages of a taper, and it should be anticipated that decreases in the dose of opioids would need to be more gradual during this time. If a taper becomes more complicated, the schedule should be extended by decreasing dosage reductions or lengthening the intervals between reductions. As long as patients are demonstrating ongoing progress, there is generally no reason not to extend an opioid taper over several weeks or even months. Progress can be demonstrated by simple compliance with taper instructions, not using other illicit substances, improvement in side effects of opioids, and maintenance of function.

Follow-Up: The process of detoxification does not end with the completion of the opioid taper. Patients can have lingering

TABLE 24-7. ADJUNCTIVE AGENTS FOR SYMPTOMS OF OPIOID WITHDRAWAL

Symptom	Agent Type	Agent
Diarrhea	Bismuth products	Pepto-Bismol®
Rhinorrhea	Antihistamines	Diphenhydramine, Loratadine
Muscle aches	Muscle relaxants	Methocarbamol
Abdominal cramps	Anticholinergics	Dicyclomine HCl
Insomnia	Antihistamines Antidepressants	Diphenhydramine Trazodone, Doxepin

subacute withdrawal symptoms for weeks. In rare circumstances they can last for months. Insomnia and rebound pain are the most common symptoms. After the taper, patients who had difficulty with aberrant drug-taking behaviors continue to need increased levels of monitoring and supervision in their treatments because the risk of relapse is high. Patients without a history of addiction and aberrant drug-taking behaviors do not require specialized substance abuse treatment. These patients should be reassured that they do not have an addiction or the diagnosis of substance abuse/dependence. However, any detoxification precipitated by the diagnosis of addiction or medication misuse should have further evaluation and treatment. Referral to an addiction specialist is usually a helpful first step. Furthermore, active ongoing participation in the treatment prescribed for addiction should be a condition of continued pain treatment. For these patients, the prevention of relapse requires a long-term outpatient program of substance abuse rehabilitation.

BENZODIAZEPINE DETOXIFICATION

The technique of a benzodiazepine taper follows the same general principles of an opioid taper.[98,99] If patients have been using benzodiazepines only intermittently, there is generally no need for a taper. However, anyone who has been using benzodiazepines continuously for more than 2 weeks should be tapered to avoid the unpleasant experience of mild withdrawal and the risk of unexpected major withdrawal symptoms. The higher the total daily dose and the longer the duration of use, the higher the risk of significant and potentially dangerous withdrawal with abrupt cessation. The general features of benzodiazepine withdrawal are similar to those of opioid withdrawal with hyperarousal and hypersympathetic states. However, in its more specific features, the withdrawal syndrome is more like the one observed with alcohol (Table 24-8). Similarly, benzodiazepine withdrawal is much more dangerous than opioid withdrawal and includes the potential for seizures, hallucinations, hyperthermia, and delirium tremens. Like alcohol withdrawal, when untreated, severe benzodiazepine withdrawal has a high rate of morbidity and mortality.

The two main techniques for detoxification include a taper of the agent a patient has been taking and the substitution of an equivalent dose of a long-half-life agent such as diazepam or clonazepam. Another strategy for benzodiazepine detoxification utilizes phenobarbital substitution, especially in cases of complex detoxification from multiple agents such as opioids, sedative-hypnotics, and alcohol. The phenobarbital dose should be determined by a series of test doses and subsequent observation to determine the level of tolerance. It is important to note that infrequently the "second generation" benzodiazepines (clonazepam, alprazolam, oxazepam, triazolam) are not fully cross-tolerant with each other or with the more traditional agents. A patient may require higher doses than expected to avoid significant withdrawal symptoms when taking these medications. Benzodiazepine tapers will generally require more time than opioid tapers with less frequent dose reductions. A taper of 6 weeks or more, especially with long-half-life agents, is not unusual.

CONCLUSION

Patients with chronic pain are at increased risk of substance use disorders. However, it is crucial to appreciate that there are many causes for aberrant medication-related behaviors. Misuse of medication is a clinical problem that can be the result of dependence but is more likely to be the result of inadequate analgesia. This can be due to undertreatment with opioids and other analgesics, disease progression, or tolerance to medications. Eventually, instead of consulting their physician, the patient may simply take more medication. Without the proper instructions, they will often take it inappropriately. If the patient does have an addiction, they will be preoccupied with the medication, have lost control of its use, and continue taking it regardless of the negative consequences they are now suffering. This patient requires specialized evaluation and treatment in addition to the management of their chronic pain syndrome. If careful planning and common principles are applied, detoxification will facilitate the transition from ineffective or problematic treatments to other potentially more effective treatments for pain. Treatment may include drug rehabilitation but it should not be prescribed for every patient undergoing detoxification. By avoiding unpleasant or dangerous withdrawal syndromes and providing the patient with the reinforcement that all treatments should result in benefits that outweigh their risks, the therapeutic relationship will be strengthened and the chances for successful treatment optimized.

TABLE 24-8. SIGNS AND SYMPTOMS OF SEDATIVE-HYPNOTIC WITHDRAWAL

Hyperarousal	Psychiatric
Agitation	Depersonalization
Anxiety	Depression
Hyperactivity	Hyperventilation
Insomnia	Malaise
Fever	Paranoid delusions
	Visual hallucinations
Neurological	Gastrointestinal
Ataxia	Abdominal pain
Fasciculation/myoclonic jerks	Constipation
Formication	Diarrhea
Headache	Nausea
Myalgia	Vomiting
Paresthesias/dysesthesias	Anorexia
Pruritis	
Tinnitus	
Tremor	
Seizures	
Delirium	
Genitourinary	Cardiovascular
Incontinence	Chest pain
Loss of libido	Flushing
Urinary urgency, frequency	Palpitations
	Hypertension
	Orthostatic
	hypotension
	Tachycardia
	Diaphoresis

REFERENCES

1. Dersh J, Polatin PB, Gatchel RJ: Chronic pain and psychopathology: Research findings and theoretical considerations. Psychosom Med 64:773–786, 2002.

2. Weaver M, Schnoll S: Abuse liability in opioid therapy for pain treatment in patients with an addiction history. Clin J Pain 18:S61–S69, 2002.

3. Reid MC, Engles-Horton LL, Weber MB, et al: Use of opioid medications for chronic noncancer pain syndromes in primary care. J Gen Intern Med 17:238–240, 2002.

4. Kouyanou K, Pither CE, Wessely S: Medication misuse, abuse and dependence in chronic pain patients. J Psychosom Res 43:497–504, 1997.

5. Hoffman NG, Olofsson O, Salen B, Wickstrom L: Prevalence of abuse and dependency in chronic pain patients. Int J Addict 30:919–927, 1995.

6. Fishbain DA, Rosomoff HL, Rosomoff RS: Drug abuse, dependence: addiction in chronic pain patients. Clin J Pain 8:77–85, 1992.

7. Nicholson B: Responsible prescribing of opioids for the treatment of chronic pain. Drugs 63:17–32, 2003.

8. Miotto K, Compton P, Ling W, Conolly M: Diagnosing addictive disease in chronic pain patients. Psychosomatics 37:223–235, 1996.

9. Compton P, Darakjian J, Miotto K: Screening for addiction in patients with chronic pain and "problematic" substance use: Evaluation of a pilot assessment tool. J Pain Symptom Manage 16:355–363, 1998.

10. Robinson RC, Gatchel RJ, Polatin P, et al: Screening for problematic prescription opioid use. Clin J Pain 17:220–228, 2001.

11. Savage SR: Assessment for addiction in pain-treatment settings. Clin J Pain 18:S28–S38, 2002.

12. Porter J, Jick H: Addiction rate in patients treated with narcotics. N Engl J Med 302:123, 1980.

13. Portenoy RK, Foley KM: Chronic use of opioid analgesics in non-malignant pain: Report of 38 cases. Pain 25:171–186, 1986.

14. Taub A: Opioid analgesics in the treatment of chronic intractable pain on non-neoplastic origin. In Kitahata LM (ed): Narcotic Analgesics in Anesthesiology. Williams and Wilkins, Baltimore, 1982, pp 199–208.

15. Ready LB, Sarkis E, Turner JA: Self-reported vs. actual use of medications in chronic pain patients. Pain 12:285–294, 1982.

16. Fishbain DA, Cutler RB, Rosomoff HL, Rosomoff RS: Validity of self-report drug use in chronic pain patients. Clin J Pain 15:184–191, 1999.

17. Long DM, Filtzer DL, BenDebba M, et al: Clinical features of the failed-back syndrome. J Neurosurg 69:61–71, 1988.

18. Maruta T, Swanson DW, Finlayson RE: Drug abuse and dependency in patients with chronic pain. Mayo Clin Proc 54:241–244, 1979.

19. Brown RL, Patterson JJ, Rounds LA, Papasouliotis O: Substance use among patients with chronic pain. J Fam Pract 43:152–160, 1996.

20. Savage SR: Addiction in the treatment of pain: Significance, recognition and management. J Pain Symptom Manage 8:265–278, 1993.

21. Fishbain D, Cutler R, Rosomoff H: Comorbid psychiatric disorders in chronic pain patients. Pain Clin 11:79–87, 1998.

22. Aronoff GM: Opioids in chronic pain management: Is there a significant risk of addiction? Curr Rev Pain 4:112–121, 2000.

23. Polatin PB, Kinney RK, Gatchel RJ, et al: Psychiatric illness and chronic low back pain. Spine 18:66–71, 1993.

24. Fordyce W, Fowler R, Lehmann J, et al: Operant conditioning in the treatment of chronic pain. Arch Phys Med Rehab 54:399–408, 1973.

25. Gilson AM, Joranson DE: US policies relevant to the prescribing of opioid analgesics for the treatment of pain in patients with addictive disease. Clin J Pain 18:S91–S98, 2002.

26. Rosenblum A, Joseph H, Fong C, et al: Prevalence and characteristics of chronic pain among chemically dependent patients in methadone maintenance and residential treatment facilities. JAMA 289:2370–2378, 2003.

27. Jamison RN, Kauffman J, Katz NP: Characteristics of methadone maintenance patients with chronic pain. J Pain Symptom Manage 19:53–62, 2000.

28. Stack K, Cortina J, Samples C, et al: Race, age, and back pain as factors in completion of residential substance abuse treatment by veterans. Psychiatr Serv 51:1157–1161, 2000.

29. Cohen MJ, Jasser S, Herron PD, Margolis CG: Ethical perspectives: opioid treatment of chronic pain in the context of addiction. Clin J Pain 18:S99–S107, 2002.

30. Drug Enforcement Administration: A joint statement from 21 health organizations and the Drug Enforcement Administration. Promoting pain relief and preventing abuse of pain medications: a critical balancing act. J Pain Symptom Manage 24:147, 2002.

31. Ballantyne JC, Mao J: Opioid therapy for chronic pain. N Engl J Med 349:1943–1953, 2003.

32. Caldwell JR, Rapoport RJ, Davis JC, et al: Efficacy and safety of a once-daily morphine formulation in chronic, moderate-to-severe osteoarthritis pain: Results from a randomized, placebo-controlled, double-blind trial and an open-label extension trial. J Pain Symptom Manage 23:278–291, 2002.

33. Maier C, Hildebrandt J, Klinger R, et al and MONTAS Study Group: Morphine responsiveness, efficacy and tolerability in patients with chronic non-tumor associated pain – Results of a double-blind placebo-controlled trial (MONTAS). Pain 97:223–233, 2002.

34. Moulin DE, Iezzi A, Amireh R, et al: Randomised trial of oral morphine for chronic non-cancer pain. Lancet 347:143–147, 1996.

35. Roth SH, Fleischmann RM, Burch FX, et al: Around-the-clock, controlled-release oxycodone therapy for osteoarthritis-related pain: Placebo-controlled trial and long-term evaluation. Arch Intern Med 160:853–860, 2000.

36. Sittl R, Griessinger N, Likar R: Analgesic efficacy and tolerability of transdermal buprenorphine in patients with inadequately controlled chronic pain related to cancer and other disorders: A multicenter, randomized, double-blind, placebo-controlled trial. Clin Ther 25:150–168, 2003.

37. Dellemijn PL, Vanneste JA: Randomised double-blind active-placebo-controlled crossover trial of intravenous fentanyl in neuropathic pain. Lancet 349:753–758, 1997.

38. Watt JW, Wiles JR, Bowsher DR: Epidural morphine for postherpetic neuralgia. Anaesthesia 51:647–651, 1996.

39. Rowbotham MC, Twilling L, Davies PS, et al: Oral opioid therapy for chronic peripheral and central neuropathic pain. N Engl J Med 348:1223–1232, 2003.

40. Raja SN, Haythornthwaite JA, Pappagallo M, et al: Opioids versus antidepressants in postherpetic neuralgia: A randomized, placebo-controlled trial. Neurology 59:1015–1021, 2002.

41. Narita M, Funada M, Suzuki T: Regulations of opioid dependence by opioid receptor types. Pharmacol Ther 89:1–15, 2001.

42. Chabal C, Jacobson L, Chaney EF, et al: Narcotics for chronic pain: Yes or no? A useless dichotomy. Am Pain Soc J 1:276–281, 1992.

43. Morgan JP: American opiophobia: Customary underutilization of opioid analgesics. Adv Alc Sub Abuse 5:163–173, 1985.

44. Potter M, Schafer S, Gonzalez-Mendez E, et al: Opioids for chronic nonmalignant pain. Attitudes and practices of primary care physicians in the UCSF/Stanford Collaborative Research Network. University of California, San Francisco. J Fam Pract 50:145–151, 2001.

45. Schug SA, Merry AF, Acland RH: Treatment principles for the use of opioids in pain of nonmalignant origin. Drugs 42:228–239, 1991.

46. Clark JD: Chronic pain prevalence and analgesic prescribing in a general medical population. J Pain Symptom Manage 23:131–137, 2002.

47. Fanciullo GJ, Ball PA, Girault G, et al: An observational study on the prevalence and pattern of opioid use in 25,479 patients with spine and radicular pain. Spine 27:201–205, 2002.

48. Moulin DE, Clark AJ, Speechley M, Morley-Forster PK: Chronic pain in Canada – Prevalence, treatment, impact and the role of opioid analgesia. Pain Res Manag 7:179–184, 2002.

49. Turk DC, Brody MC, Okifuji EA: Physicians' attitudes and practices regarding the long-term prescribing of opioids for non-cancer pain. Pain 59:201–208, 1994.

50. Christensen D, Kayser V: The development of pain-related behaviour and opioid tolerance after neuropathy-inducing surgery and sham surgery. Pain 88:231–238, 2000.

51. Borgland SL: Acute opioid receptor desensitization and tolerance: is there a link? Clin Exp Pharmacol Physiol 28:147–154, 2001.

52. Cahill CM, Morinville A, Lee MC, et al: Prolonged morphine treatment targets delta opioid receptors to neuronal plasma membranes and enhances delta-mediated antinociception. J Neurosci 21:7598–7607, 2001.

53. Dogrul A, Zagli U, Tulunay FC: The role of T-type calcium channels in morphine analgesia, development of antinociceptive tolerance and dependence to morphine, and morphine abstinence syndrome. Life Sci 71:725–734, 2002.

54. France RD, Ruban BJ, Keefe FJ: Long-term use of narcotic analgesics in chronic pain. Soc Sci Med 19:1379–1382, 1984.

55. Freye E, Latasch L: Development of opioid tolerance – Molecular mechanisms and clinical consequences. Anasthesiol Intensivmed Notfallmed Schmerzther 38:14–26, 2003.

56. Katz NP: MorphiDex (MS:DM) double-blind, multiple-dose studies in chronic pain patients. J Pain Symptom Manage 19:S37–S41, 2000.

57. Mao J, Sung B, Ji RR, Lim G: Chronic morphine induces down-regulation of spinal glutamate transporters: Implications in morphine tolerance and abnormal pain sensitivity. J Neurosci 22:8312–8323, 2002.

58. Portenoy RK: Chronic opioid therapy in nonmalignant pain. J Pain Symptom Manage 5(Suppl 1):S46–S62, 1990.

59. Holister LE, Conley FK, Britt R, et al: Long-term use of diazepam. JAMA 246:1568–1570, 1981.

60. King SA, Strain JJ: Benzodiazepine use by chronic pain patients. Clin J Pain 6:143–147, 1990.

61. Dellemijn PL, Fields HL: Do benzodiazepines have a role in chronic pain management? Pain 57:137–152, 1994.

62. Bartusch SL, Sanders BJ, D'Alessio JG, et al: Clonazepam for the treatment of lancinating phantom limb pain. Clin J Pain 12:59–62, 1996.

63. McLean W, Boucher EA, Brennan M, et al: Is there an indication for the use of barbiturate-containing analgesic agents in the treatment of pain? Guidelines for their safe use and withdrawal management. Canadian Pharmacists Association. Can J Clin Pharmacol 7:191–197, 2000.

64. Taricco M, Adone R, Pagliacci C, Telaro E: Pharmacological interventions for spasticity following spinal cord injury. Cochrane Database Syst Rev 2:CD001131, 2000.

65. Sullivan M, Toshima M, Lynn P, et al: Phenobarbital versus clonazepam for sedative-hypnotic taper in chronic pain patients. A pilot study. Ann Clin Psychiatry 5:123–128, 1993.

66. Couvee JE, Zitman FG: The Benzodiazepine Withdrawal Symptom Questionnaire: Psychometric evaluation during a discontinuation program in depressed chronic benzodiazepine users in general practice. Addiction 97:337–345, 2002.

67. Buffett-Jerrott SE, Stewart SH: Cognitive and sedative effects of benzodiazepine use. Curr Pharm Des 8:45–58, 2002.

68. Hendler N, Cimini C, Ma T, et al: A comparison of cognitive impairment due to benzodiazepines and to narcotics. Am J Psychiatry 137:828–830, 1980.

69. Cicccone DS, Just N, Bandilla EB, et al: Psychological correlates of opioid use in patients with chronic nonmalignant pain: A preliminary test of the downhill spiral hypothesis. J Pain Symptom Manage 20:180–192, 2000.

70. Caplehorn JR, Drummer OH: Fatal methadone toxicity: signs and circumstances, and the role of benzodiazepines. Aust N Z J Public Health 26:358–362, 2002.

71. Ernst E, Bartu A, Popescu A, et al: Methadone-related deaths in Western Australia 1993–99. Aust N Z J Public Health 26:364–370, 2002.

72. France RD, Kirshman KR: Psychotropic drugs in chronic pain. In France RD, Kirshman KR (eds): Chronic Pain. American Psychiatric Association, Washington, DC, 1988.

73. Nemmani KV, Mogil JS: Serotonin–GABA interactions in the modulation of mu- and kappa-opioid analgesia. Neuropharmacology 44:304–310, 2003.

74. Sawynok J: GABAergic mechanisms of analgesia: An update. Pharmacol Biochem Behav 26:463–474, 1985.

75. American Psychiatric Association: Diagnostic and Statistical Manual of Mental Disorders, ed 4. American Psychiatric Press, Washington, DC, 1994, pp 458–462.

76. American Academy of Pain Medicine, the American Pain Society, the American Society of Addiction Medicine: Definitions related to the use of opioids for the treatment of pain. WMJ 100:28–29, 2001.

77. Chabal C, Erjavec MK, Jacobson L, et al: Prescription opiate abuse in chronic pain patients: Clinical criteria, incidence, and predictors. Clin J Pain 13:150–155, 1997.

78. Greenwald BD, Narcessian EJ, Pomeranz BA: Assessment of physiatrists' knowledge and perspectives on the use of opioids: Review of basic concepts for managing chronic pain. Am J Phys Med Rehabil 78:408–415, 1999.

79. Carey KB, Purnine DM, Maisto SA, et al: Treating substance abuse in the context of severe and persistent mental illness: Clinicians' perspectives. J Subst Abuse Treat 19:189–198, 2000.

80. Marlatt GA: Harm reduction: Come as you are. Addict Behav 21:779–788, 1996.

81. Hamilton M: Researching harm reduction – Care and contradictions. Subst Use Misuse 34:119–141, 1999.

82. Hathaway AD: Shortcomings of harm reduction: Toward a morally invested drug reform strategy. Int J Drug Policy 12:125–137, 2001.

83. Pappagallo M, Heinberg LJ: Ethical issues in the management of chronic nonmalignant pain. Semin Neurol 17:203–211, 1997.

84. Savage SR: Opioid therapy of chronic pain: Assessment of consequences. Acta Anaesthesiol Scand 43:909–917, 1999.

85. Kirsh KL, Whitcomb LA, Donaghy K, Passik SD: Abuse and addiction issues in medically ill patients with pain: Attempts at clarification of terms and empirical study. Clin J Pain 18:S52–S60, 2002.

86. Fishman SM, Bandman TB, Edwards A, Borsook D: The opioid contract in the management of chronic pain. J Pain Symptom Manage 18:27–37, 1999.

87. Fishman SM, Mahajan G, Jung S, Wilsey BL: The trilateral opioid contract: Bridging the pain clinic and the primary care physician through the opioid contract. J Pain Symptom Manage 24:335–344, 2002.

88. Fishman SM, Wilsey B, Yang J, et al: Adherence monitoring and drug surveillance in chronic opioid therapy. J Pain Symptom Manage 20:293–307, 2000.

89. Katz N, Fanciullo GJ: Role of urine toxicology testing in the management of chronic opioid therapy. Clin J Pain 18:S76–S82, 2002.

90. Sees KL, Clark HW: Opioid use in the treatment of chronic pain: Assessment of addiction. J Pain Symptom Manage 8:257–264, 1993.

91. Longo LP, Parran T, Jr., Johnson B, Kinsey W: Addiction: II. Identification and management of the drug-seeking patient. Am Fam Physician 61:2401–2408, 2000.

92. Currie SR, Hodgins DC, Crabtree A, et al: Outcome from integrated pain management treatment for recovering substance abusers. J Pain 4:91–100, 2003.

93. O'Brien C: Drug addiction and drug abuse. *In* Hardman JG, Gilman AG, Limbird LE (eds): Goodman and Gilman's the Pharmacologic Basis of Therapeutics, ed 9. McGraw Hill, 1996, pp 557–578.

94. O'Conner PG, Koster TR: Management of opioid intoxication and withdrawal. *In* Miller NS (ed): Principles of Addiction Medicine. American Society of Addiction Medicine, Chevy Chase, MD, 1994, Section XI, Chapter 5, pp 1–6.

95. Handelsman L, Cochrane KJ, Aronson MJ, et al: Two new rating scales for opiate withdrawal. Am J Drug Alcohol Abuse 13:293–308, 1987.

96. Jaffe JH: Pharmacological treatment of opioid dependence: Current techniques and new findings. Psychiatric Annals 25:369–375, 1995.

97. Fishbain DA, Rosomoff HL, Rosomoff RS: Detoxification of nonopiate drugs in the chronic pain setting and clonidine opiate detoxification. Clin J Pain 8:191–203, 1992.

98. Benzer DG: Management of sedative-hypnotic intoxication and withdrawal. *In* Miller NS (ed): Principles of Addiction Medicine. American Society of Addiction Medicine, Chevy Chase, MD, 1994, Section XI, Chapter 4, pp 1–5.

99. Benzer DG, Smith DE, Miller NS: Detoxification from benzodiazepine use: Strategies and schedules for clinical practice. Psychiatric Annals 25:180–185, 1995.

25

Pain Management in the Emergency Department

James J. Mathews, M.D.

The complaint of pain is the most common symptom presenting to the emergency department (ED).[1,2] The causes of pain encompass the entire range of human diseases, including psychological illness. The assessment of the severity of pain is subjective, and what appears to be the same problem or injury can affect each individual very differently. Several systems have been developed to quantify the degree of pain, but all rely on the patient's perception of their pain.[3,4] Practitioners must bring all their clinical acumen into play to make an appropriate decision regarding the need for and class of analgesic to use in a given circumstance.

Pain can be divided into two major categories, acute and chronic. Acute pain serves a physiologic function in that it is a warning to the patient that something is wrong, and sends the patient for help or prevents the patient from doing further harm by limiting activity. Acute pain is defined as being less than six months in duration. The bulk of this chapter is devoted to the discussion of the management of acute pain in the ED.

CHRONIC PAIN

Chronic pain serves no useful function to the patient. Patients with chronic pain can be divided into four general groups. These groups are patients with chronic pain secondary to underlying diseases such as cancer and AIDS, patients with known pain syndromes such as tic douloureux and migraine headache, chronic pain patients without an identifiable cause, and finally the group of patients that uses the complaint of chronic pain to obtain drugs or for other personal gains.

Each of these groups of patients requires a different management approach. Cancer patients with new pain or with acute worsening of their previous pain should be evaluated for a new complication and their pain aggressively managed with opiates.[5] Patients with known pain syndromes and without objective cause for their pain require an aggressive team approach, and if they are patients within one's institution, prearranged therapeutic plans should be in place for when they appear in the ED. This is particularly helpful for those patients

with sickle cell disease and frequent pain crises. The final group is a subset of pain patients that tests the patience and professionalism of emergency physicians and nurses. The majority of these patients are seeking narcotics. The diagnosis of malingering must be a diagnosis of exclusion, and cannot be made on the first visit by a patient to the ED. An appropriate workup for the patient's complaint should be done, and often needs to be repeated two or three times before the diagnosis of malingering is made. If malingering is suspected, the patient should be referred to the outpatient pain and psychiatric services for further evaluation and treatment. Each time these patients appear in the ED, the emergency physician should perform at least a basic history and physical examination, but can refuse to give further narcotics. Another approach is to use such agents as butorphanol (Stadol), which has good analgesic activity but gives little euphoria. Nonsteroidal anti-inflammatory drugs (NSAIDs) may be offered, but these patients will often refuse them or state that they cannot take them. There are no hard and fast rules as to how to handle this type of patient. All one can do is to maintain professional ethics and practice, and do the best one can by referring the patient to the appropriate outpatient services.

ACUTE PAIN

Pain is a combination of physical, chemical, and psychological factors. There is no current method to measure directly the degree of pain that a given patient is experiencing from a given injury. However, if a patient presents to the ED with a complaint of pain, an attempt should be made to quantify the patient's perception of the degree of pain. A patient's verbal report is the only way to obtain reliably a patient's evaluation of their pain. Several tools have been developed to grade a given patient's pain and the response to treatment (see Table 25-1). Pain scales should be incorporated as part of the triage process, and should be located on the record where the vitals are recorded. The severity of pain index should be recorded during the initial assessment process, and early and effective management of pain should be ensured.[6] After treatment, the assessment

TABLE 25-1. **PAIN ASSESSMENT TOOLS**

Clinical Tool	Grading Pain	When Used
Verbal quantitative scale	0 to 10 (none to worst possible)	Routine evaluation
Visual analogue device	[_____] None to worst. Patient places a mark on the line	Routine evaluation
Global satisfaction question	Are you satisfied with your pain relief? Yes/No	Useful for confused patients
Pediatric pain scales		
Observer generated	Facial expressions, crying	Neonate to age 3 and some 3–6
Draw a picture of your pain	Estimate location, intensity, and character	Over age 6 and some 3–6
Faces		Over age 6 and some 3–6
Pain thermometer	Like visual scale for adults	Over age 6 and some 3–6

should be repeated as needed. All too often this does not occur.[7]

Numerous studies have documented inadequate use of analgesic agents in the ED.[8,9] This is particularly true in the pediatric population.[10] Many patients do not receive any pain medications while in the ED, even though their primary presenting complaint was pain.[8,9,11] In addition to no analgesia, there are a number of therapeutic errors that may result in the inadequate use of analgesics in the ED. These include prescribing the wrong agent, inappropriate dosage and dosing intervals, route of administration, improper use of adjunct agents, and concern for medically induced addiction to narcotics.

Failure to give analgesics is an issue that must be addressed by education of nursing staff and physicians.[12] The goal should be adequate pain relief for all patients. Emphasis of the importance of pain control to the patient is key in this process of changing practice habits. Patient satisfaction may be directly related to adequate pain control.[13,14] In addition, the early control of acute pain appears to reduce the incidence of chronic pain syndromes, and may improve the patient's outcome.[15,16] Finally, health care providers have sworn to reduce or prevent pain and suffering.

Correction of the inappropriate usage of analgesics also requires a great deal of physician reeducation and frequently major changes in practice habits must be instituted. Severe pain generally requires the use of parenteral opioids. In the acute situation, an IV line should be established, and the dosage titrated for the individual patient. The amount required of a given opiate for adequate pain relief can vary widely from patient to patient. For example, the effective level for morphine has been reported to be as much as eight times greater from one patient to another. The IM route should be avoided, as it is painful and the onset of action is variable. If an IV route cannot be obtained, the subcutaneous route offers an excellent alternative. In addition there are newer agents that can be given by the sublingual or nasal route. Fentanyl is available in sucker form, which has great applicability in the pediatric population.

Sufentanil and butorphanol, both potent opioids, are effective when given via the nasal mucosa. Once the route and dosage is determined, it should be given at frequent enough intervals to prevent the return of pain.

There is little role for adjunct agents in the management of acute pain in the ED. The exception is the clinical circumstance of persistent nausea and vomiting following the use of opioids, or in patients with pain who also have nausea and vomiting. The practice of using an adjunct to reduce the opioid dose simply is not valid and exposes the patient to another set of side effects. This practice should be abandoned.

The risk of addiction to the opioids with medical use must be a concern for physicians, especially when treating patients with chronic pain. However, in the acute patient there seems to be little evidence for undue concern. Of 11,892 inpatients that received opioids while in the hospital, only 4 became addicted without a prior history of substance abuse.[17]

SPECIFIC PROBLEMS

Abdominal Pain: For years the conventional teaching was to avoid the use of opioids for abdominal pain until a definitive decision had been made regarding surgery. This practice arose prior to the development of modern diagnostic tools, such as computed tomography (CT) scanning, and is outdated.[18,19] The goal in patients with abdominal pain is not to achieve pain-free status, but rather to reduce the severity of the pain. Opioids given by the IV route allow for careful titration of these agents. The patient should be responsive enough to allow for subsequent examinations. Close observation of the patient's course is mandatory, especially in patients with ulcerative colitis because of the added risk of toxic megacolon. NSAIDs are effective adjunct therapy when treating biliary or renal colic.

Headache: The complaint of headache is commonly seen in the ED.[20] Many of these patients have a known history of a specific type of headache such as migraine or vascular headaches.

There are many causes of headache, and a minority of these patients may require extensive workups, including CT scanning, magnetic resonance imaging (MRI), and lumbar puncture, to rule out a life-threatening cause of headache. By far the majority of patients presenting to the ED with the complaint of headache will need only pain relief and follow-up.[21] A useful guideline to assist the emergency physician to sort through this complaint is the *Classification and Diagnostic Criteria for Headache Disorders, Cranial Neuralgias and Facial Pain* published by the International Headache Society in 1988.[22] This handbook divides headaches into 13 categories, and provides an organized approach to the diagnosis and management of the various types of headache and facial pain.

MIGRAINE: In the USA each year over 1 million patients present to emergency departments with the complaint of migraine.[23] If the patient does not have a clear and reproducible history of migraines, this diagnosis should be made with caution, and a headache workup needs to be done. If the prodromal symptoms, pattern of pain, and associated symptoms are similar to past attacks, the workup may be limited to a history and physical examination unless there is coexisting illness. Most of these patients have had failure by their usual medications to control pain prior to arrival to the ED. Therapy to relieve the pain is indicated. In mild to moderate migraine, acetaminophen or nonsteroidal agents are often effective. In more severe and persistent migraine such agents as subcutaneous sumatriptan, prochlorperazine, and chlorpromazine by the IV route may be required to relieve the pain and to counteract nausea and vomiting. Sumatriptan is contraindicated in patients with known coronary artery disease, hypertension, pregnancy, and peripheral vascular disease. The other two agents may be associated with hypotension, sedation, and dystonic reactions. Patients receiving chlorpromazine or similar agents should receive a 500 cm^3 bolus of saline prior to the drug being given to help avoid hypotension. Opioids should only be given for patients who do not get relief by other means, or in those who are unable to receive other agents. Dihydroergotamine is contraindicated in vascular disease and if sumatriptan has already been used. This agent is especially useful for those patients with a refractory attack of migraine, and, if used, the patient should first receive an antiemetic.

CLUSTER HEADACHE: Cluster headaches are seen much less commonly in the ED, and emergency physicians are often less comfortable with management of this clinical problem. If the patient is having a typical pattern of headache, there is little indication for extensive workup and treatment should be initiated to control the pain. In many cases sumatriptan will abort the attack. Frequently the patient with this problem has already used this medication, and is in need of pain control. High-flow oxygen will often end the attack. If these attempts fail, dihydroergotamine given by the IV route is effective. Numerous other agents have been used, but if the above fails neurological consultation should be considered to assist in managing this problem.

SUBARACHNOID HEMORRHAGE: Without a high index of suspicion, the emergency physician may not recognize this entity. Subarachnoid hemorrhage (SAH) has a high morbidity and mortality rate, exceeding 50%. Many of these patients will expire before they can get to medical care. Patients with SAH often deteriorate rapidly, and early diagnosis is mandatory to maximize the chances for a good outcome. The current approach is to obtain rapidly a CT to look for blood, and if this is negative, to do a lumbar puncture. CT cannot be relied on alone, as approximately 10% of acute SAH will not show blood. This percentage of false negatives may exceed 50% by one week after the acute headache.[24]

In many cases the patient describes the headache as if their head is exploding, or that the top of their head felt as if it was going to come off. These patients will frequently state that this is or was the worst headache of their life. Even if the patient has none of the other features of a SAH, these complaints should not be ignored. A patient giving this type of history should have the workup for SAH. After the emergency physician has decided the course, pain relief can be given. Nonsteroidals are contraindicated in the treatment of patients with suspected SAH because of their anticoagulation properties. Opioids are safe and effective, but should be titrated to prevent excessive sedation.

TENSION HEADACHE: This is the most common cause of headache in the ED, and is frequently associated with other medical and psychological problems. Tension headaches are also the most general and difficult to categorize. To a great extent, this is a diagnosis of exclusion, and should only be given if the practitioner is satisfied that a more serious problem is not causing the headache. This may require imaging studies. Tension headaches often have a general pattern, in that the patient complains of a band-like pressure around the head and associated neck stiffness. Other symptoms are usually absent, and if present are mild. Pain relief can usually be achieved with acetaminophen or nonsteroidals. If there is associated anxiety, mild tranquilizers may help to prevent recurrence.

OTHER CAUSES OF HEADACHE: There are numerous other disease processes that are either the direct cause of or are associated with the complaint of headache. An in-depth discussion of these is beyond the scope of this chapter. In many of these conditions associated neurological symptoms will make the complaint of headache secondary. If the headache is related to a space-occupying lesion in the brain, opioids in careful doses are very useful to relieve the patient's suffering. The patient requires rapid consultation with the appropriate specialty. For headaches associated with underlying medical diseases, such as hypertension, the treatment of the underlying problem will often relieve the headache with minimum need for analgesia. Suffice it to say, the emergency physician must use judgment when prescribing pain medications for the headache patient. Underlying causes for the headache should not be masked by the aggressive use of analgesics. However, the patient should not be denied some relief of their discomfort. Careful selection of the agent used, appropriate titration of the dosage of the agent, and proper delivery route of the drug can go a long way towards achieving these therapeutic goals without overly confusing the clinical picture.

Chest Pain: Chest pain is a frequent complaint in the ED. The causes of chest pain are myriad, and the emergency physician must make rapid clinical decisions if the pain is secondary to a life-threatening disease.[25] The three most common serious diseases presenting with chest pain are myocardial ischemia and infarction, pulmonary embolism, and dissection of the thoracic aorta. Clinical pathways, particularly for myocardial ischemia, are well established.[26] Part of these pathways is the use of morphine for the reduction of pain and anxiety. A major role of this agent is in those patients whose pain is not fully relieved by nitrates and beta-blockers. Doses should be given IV, and titrated to achieve pain relief without respiratory depression. The clinician must carefully monitor the patient to avoid hypotension. Aortic dissection commonly requires an opioid to relieve the severe pain experienced by patients with this condition. Pulmonary embolism seldom requires heavy analgesia, and good pain relief can usually be obtained with NSAIDs. If required, opioids are safe and effective.

Most of the remaining causes of chest pain are either inflammatory, such as pericarditis, or due to musculoskeletal problems. The majority of these patients will respond well to NSAIDs or to acetaminophen. Adjunct therapy of heat or cold, massage therapy, and physical therapy may be indicated in follow-up. A commonly occurring condition where NSAIDs should be avoided is in those patients with gastroesophageal reflux disorder (GERD). Acetaminophen may be used, but primary treatment with antacids and histamine blockers should be initiated.

Musculoskeletal Pain: All people experience a variety of aches and pains secondary to contusions, minor arthritis, and soft tissue sprains and strains. By far the majority of these individuals treat themselves at home with a host of over-the-counter medications of varying degrees of efficacy, and other adjunctive measures. The two over-the-counter drugs most frequently used today are ibuprophen and acetaminophen. If these patients do present to the ED, a history of what agents and the amount taken needs to be obtained by the emergency physician in order to give appropriate treatment and to avoid overdosing the patient. Icing sprains and contusions and appropriate splinting and rest of the injured extremity is mandated in the acute period, but these adjunct therapies are often overlooked during long waits in the waiting room. This group of patients comprises the largest single source of complaints regarding failure of staff to control pain.

Although there has been little research to support the use of muscle relaxants, they do appear to have a role in acute musculoskeletal injury when there is associated severe muscle spasm. Commonly used agents are orphenadrine citrate, methocarbamol, and the benzodiazepines. These agents cannot be a substitute for adequate analgesia. Oral opioids may be required in the management of severe musculoskeletal pain, especially when these patients are discharged. Acetaminophen with codeine has been used for years, but in reality codeine is a poor analgesic and has not been demonstrated to be more effective than NSAIDs or acetaminophen alone. Other oral opioids are effective in the management of severe pain, but physicians are often reluctant to prescribe them on an outpatient basis because of the fear of causing addiction. Included in this group are hydrocodone, oxycodone, and oral meperidine. These agents should be used if the pain is severe, and are generally safe to prescribe for short-term use. All of these agents do have a relatively high potential for abuse, and they should be prescribed with discretion and in limited amounts.

Patients with obvious fractures should be seen as soon as possible, and early immobilization should be obtained. This prevents further soft tissue injury and will reduce the pain. Opioids often are required to control the pain, and the safest and most effective method is titration of these agents by the IV route. Patients given IV opioids need to be monitored for respiratory depression, hypotension, and excessive euphoria. If patients require extended "road trips" to radiology for multiple X-rays or CT scanning, they should be accompanied by medical personnel to monitor their vitals and to give additional analgesia if required.

PAIN MANAGEMENT IN PEDIATRICS

It has been well demonstrated that the pediatric population is often overlooked for adequate analgesia.[10] Children over the age of five can usually tell one where it hurts, and how much. Pediatric scales have been developed and are a useful adjunct for pain assessment (see Table 25-1). Pediatric patients are often overlooked in a busy department because the bulk of their complaints are not life- or limb-threatening, and they do not openly complain. Their parents may attribute their child's fussiness to being tired and hungry, or to being frightened from being in the ED. The same attention and assessment for pain is mandated in the pediatric population, and appropriate doses of analgesics should be given. The same agents that are effective in adults are effective in children when used in proper dosage and if administered by the appropriate route.

ANALGESIA DURING PROCEDURES

The use of "OK, OK" anesthesia has little role in the practice of emergency medicine. This is a time-honored but brutal practice that has been used for everything from reduction of small joints to using force to restrain children for repair of small lacerations. Although it is impossible to do any procedure without some pain and discomfort, every attempt should be made to keep these to a minimum.[27] Adequate sedation prior to performing the procedure helps to reduce the anxiety and fear associated with procedures and reduces the memory of the event. Also it produces muscle relaxation, an important effect for major joint reduction. Numerous regimens have been developed to provide sedation, amnesia, muscle relaxation, and analgesia. The emergency physician needs to have an excellent knowledge of one or two of these regimes, and to know what side effects to expect. Patients must be monitored carefully, and specific procedures to ensure that this occurs need to be in place. The American College of Emergency Physicians has published guidelines to assist in developing the approach to safe use of procedural sedation and analgesia (PSAA), also known as conscious sedation[28] (see Table 25-2). The American Society of Anesthesiologists also recommends a period of fasting of 6 hours for solids and 2 hours for liquids prior to PSAA.[29] To date, there has been no evidence that PSAA as performed in the ED requires prolonged fasting, and prior ingestion of food is not a contraindication. If ingestion of food or liquids has occurred recently, the degree of sedation should be minimized by carefully titration of the agent(s) used to obtain PSAA.

Specific Agents
FENTANYL AND MIDAZOLAM: This combination is widely used for PSAA in both adults and children. Fentanyl is a short-acting opioid with high potency and minimal cardiovascular effects.[30] This agent has a rapid onset of action, usually within 2 minutes, and the duration of action is 30 to 40 minutes.

TABLE 25-2. RECOMMENDATIONS OF THE CLINICAL POLICIES COMMITTEE OF THE AMERICAN COLLEGE OF EMERGENCY PHYSICIANS

1. Personnel involved in the administration of agents to and monitoring of PSAA patients must understand the drugs given, have the ability to monitor properly the patient, and the necessary skills to intervene to manage the potential complications. An excellent approach is to have one support person present in addition to the provider.
2. The patient should receive a history of past or present illnesses and allergies, and limited physical examination aimed at vital signs, airway, and cardiovascular status. Recent ingestion of food is not a contraindication.
3. Initial consent to treatment is adequate, but separate consent may be obtained.
4. Advanced life support equipment and oxygen should be available. In addition, antagonists (naloxone for opiates, flumazenil for benzodiazepines) need to be present. An IV line should be obtained.
5. Patient monitoring must include frequent vital signs. Constantly monitoring pulse oximetry and cardiac monitoring are excellent options, but may not be mandatory in every circumstance. The patient's appearance and response to verbal stimuli should be watched during and after the procedure.
6. Drugs should be administered slowly and titrated to desired effect.
7. The patient should be monitored carefully during the postprocedure period. Discharge occurs when the patient responds appropriately, the vitals are stable and back to normal for the patient, respiratory function is normal, pain has been addressed, minimal nausea, and new symptoms are handled. Patients should be back to baseline before discharge or discharged to a responsible third party.

Serum half-life is approximately 90 minutes. This combination of rapid onset, high potency, and short half-life makes fentanyl an excellent agent for most ED procedures. The usual required dose is between 2 and 3 μg/kg IV for both adults and children, although more or less of the agent may be required depending on the individual's response. Because of its high potency and short half-life, fentanyl is very easy to titrate by using multiple small doses to achieve the desired effect. Fentanyl can induce severe respiratory depression, especially when used with other agents such as midazolam. This side effect is dose related, and usually appears within 5 minutes of administration of the agent. The doses used for PSAA in the ED have not been reported to cause muscular and glottic rigidity or "board chest", which has been well documented when the agent is used in general anesthetic doses of over 50 μg/kg. This reaction can be reversed by either naloxone or succinylcholine. Seizures have not been documented when using fentanyl for ED PSAA. General pruritis is not frequent with the use of fentanyl as occurs with many opioids because of histamine release, and nausea is usually minimal when compared to other opioid analgesics. Fentanyl can also be administered orally in the form of a lollipop, making it useful in children if the IV route is not possible or required. The dose is usually 10 to 15 μg/kg, and onset of action is between 12 and 30 minutes. It is not feasible to titrate fully the dosage administered when fentanyl is given by the oral route. Nausea and vomiting are more common, but major side effects of seizures and chest rigidity have not been reported.

Midazolam is so frequently used in combination with fentanyl that these two agents should be considered together. The usual dose is 0.02 to 1.0 mg/kg for adults and 0.05 to 0.15 mg/kg for children. Midazolam also has a rapid onset of action of 1 to 3 minutes and a relatively short half-life of less than 2 hours. When given IV, the drug is easily titrated to achieve the desired response. Midazolam provides excellent sedation, a beneficial hypnotic effect, muscle relaxation, amnesia, and antiseizure activity. The major side effect is respiratory depression, which is dose related and is more pronounced in the presence of other central nervous system depressants such as alcohol. The elderly and patients with chronic lung disease are more sensitive to this agent. In general, cardiovascular side effects are not seen at sedative dosages. If other agents, such as fentanyl, are used in combination with midazolam, hypotension may occur. This will usually respond to a bolus of saline solution. Occasionally children will have paradoxical agitation when midazolam is used. If the IV route is not available, midazolam may be administered by rectal suppository, orally, and by nasal insufflation. This alternative can be useful to sedate children before simple therapeutic or diagnostic procedures.

KETAMINE: Ketamine has had extensive use in PSAA and is especially useful and safe in the pediatric population.[31] It is a derivative of phencyclidine, a notorious street drug. When ketamine is used, dissociation of the limbic and thalamoneocortical systems occurs, and essentially the patient is unable to perceive pain. It does not produce muscle relaxation, and if this is required for the procedure another agent such as midazolam must be added. Hypertension may occur with the use of ketamine, especially in adults. The presence of cardiovascular disease is a relative contraindication for this agent. Emergence phenomena such as hallucinations and nightmares are common (over 50%) in the adult population, but are usually mild.

The drug should be avoided in patients with a history of personality disorders. Both of these complications are much less common in the pediatric population. Laryngospasm is a serious complication in children, especially in those less than 3 months old, and it should not be used in this age group. Laryngospasm rarely occurs in children older than 3 months. Ketamine can be given by all routes of administration, including IM. The IV route is the easiest to titrate, and the dose required is 1 to 2 mg/kg by the IV route. Onset of action is within 1 minute of IV infusion, and the duration of action is only 15 minutes. In adults, prolonged procedures require a constant infusion of ketamine at the rate of 1 to 2 mg/kg/hour, while in children repeated small doses of 0.05 to 0.1 mg/kg are given as required. This agent is an excellent first-line agent in the pediatric population, and is a good alternative to opioids in adults, especially those who are allergic to opioids.

OTHER AGENTS: Numerous agents have been used to provide PSAA. These include the short acting barbiturate propofol, the imidazole etomidate, and nitrous oxide. These agents appear to be safe and effective, but all have side effects and appear to offer no advantage over the agents previously discussed. Chloral hydrate was used extensively in children, but has little indication today because of its delayed onset of action and prolonged duration. The use of the combination of meperdine, promethazine, and chlorpromazine, known as DPT, should be dropped because of the numerous side effects that are seen with this mixture.

LOCAL ANESTHETICS

These remain a mainstay of anesthesia in the ED. The so-called "caine" drugs are divided into two classes, the esters and the amides, and the various agents have different times of onset and duration (see Table 25-3). The most commonly used in the ED are lidocaine, bipuvicaine, and mepivicaine, all of which are amides. If a patient has a history of allergy to these agents, almost invariably it will be to the ester class. Allergic reactions to the amides are exceedingly rare, and they can usually be safely used. Pain during administration is the norm. Efforts should be made to reduce this discomfort. These include using as small a needle as possible, warming the solution to be injected, slow injection of the agent, injecting through the wound edges rather than through skin, and use of topical anesthetics prior to administration. Buffering the injected solution with sodium bicarbonate has been advocated.[32] The amount of bicarbonate solution suggested for lidocaine is 1 cm^3 of bicarbonate per 10 cm^3 of lidocaine solution. All of these agents may produce central nervous system and cardiovascular toxicity if blood concentrations are too high. The potential toxic effects of the "caine" drugs include seizures and ventricular fibrillation. These tragedies can be avoided by calculating total doses before use and by careful administration of the agent.

Topical anesthesia has been used for years especially in ear, nose, and throat and dental practice. Cocaine is an excellent topical agent for such things as nosebleed because of its additional vasoconstrictor effect. A 50:50 mixture of topical tetracaine and adrenaline solutions will produce similar results. The major application for topical anesthetics is in treating lacerations in small children. The two agents used most frequently are the combination of lidocaine, epinephrine, and tetracaine (LET) in solution, and EMLA, a eutetic mixture of local anesthetic agents. This compound comes in cream form and the active ingredients are lidocaine and prilocaine. The cream is applied directly to the laceration under an occlusive dressing without pain to the child. Within 30 to 60 minutes complete anesthesia can be obtained which will last up to 5 hours. Depth of penetration is limited, and for deep wounds additional injection may be required. There are theoretical concerns about the effect of this combination on wound healing, but these concerns have largely been refuted. This agent has been a real boon to the management of lacerations in the pediatric population, and has virtually eliminated the need to tie down these patients as was done in the past.

KEY POINTS

- Pain is the most common complaint seen in the ED. The emergency physician must ensure that patients in pain are treated with appropriate analgesics as soon as is feasible.
- With modern diagnostic modalities, such as CT scanning, there is no reason to withhold pain medications for patients with abdominal pain. The goal is to reduce the pain for the patient while they are undergoing diagnostic evaluation.

TABLE 25-3. COMMON LOCAL ANESTHETICS

Agent (Trade Names)	Type of Agent	Use, Onset, and Duration
Lidocaine (Xylocaine, Dilocaine, Ultracaine)	Amide	Blocks, infiltration. Onset is rapid. Duration 90–200 minutes
Tetracaine (Pontocaine)	Ester	Spinal, topical, eye. Onset slow. Duration 180–600 minutes
Mepivacaine (Carbocaine)	Amide	Epidurals, blocks, infiltration. Onset very rapid. Duration 120–240 minutes
Bupivacaine (Marcaine)	Amide	Blocks. Onset intermediate. Duration 180–600 minutes
Procaine (Novocaine, Neocaine)	Ester	Blocks, infiltrations. Onset slow. Duration 60–90 minutes

Oversedation should be avoided to enable reliable physical examinations by consultants.

- Procedural sedation and analgesia, i.e., conscious sedation, is an integral part of the practice of emergency medicine. The emergency physician must know several of the various regimens well, and to anticipate these regimens' potential side effects and complications. Protocols for the appropriate monitoring of these patients need to be in place.

- Drug-seeking behavior is a problem in every ED. However, a patient's complaint should not be attributed to this without adequate diagnostic evaluation. Drug-seeking behavior is a diagnosis of exclusion.

REFERENCES

1. Ducharme J: Emergency pain management: A Canadian Association of Emergency Physicians (CAEP) consensus document. J Emerg Med 12:855, 1994.

2. Holleran RS: The problem of pain in emergency care: Nurs Clin North Am 37:67–78, 2002.

3. Ready LB, Edwards WT: Management of Acute Pain: A Practical Guide, International Association for the Study of Pain. IASP Publications, Seattle, 1992.

4. Guru V, Dubinski I: The patient vs. caregiver perception of acute pain in the emergency department. J Emerg Med 18:7–12, 2000.

5. Fortner BV, et al: The zero acceptance of pain (ZAP) quality improvement project: Evaluation of pain severity, pain interference, global quality of life, and pain-related costs. J Pain Symptom Manage 25:334–343, 2003.

6. Ducharme J: Acute pain in pain control: State of the art. Ann Emerg Med 35:592–603, 2000.

7. Eder SC, Sloan EP, Todd K: Documentation of ED patient pain by nurses and physicians. Am J Emerg Med 21:253–257, 2003.

8. Brown JC, et al: Emergency department analgesia for fracture pain. Ann Emerg Med 42:197–205, 2003.

9. Singer AJ, Thode HC Jr: National analgesia prescribing patterns in emergency department with burns. J Burn Care Rehabil 23:361–365, 2002.

10. Petrack EM, Christopher NC, Kriwinsky J: Pain management in the emergency department: Patterns of analgesic utilization. Pediatrics 99:711–714, 1997.

11. Vassiliadis J, Hitos K, Hill CT: Factors influencing prehospital and emergency department analgesia administration to patients with femoral neck fractures. Emerg Med 14:261–266, 2002.

12. Jones JB: Assessment of pain management skills in emergency medicine residents: The role of a pain education program. J Emerg Med 17:349–354, 1999.

13. Tanabe P, Ferket K, Thomas R, et al: The effect of standard care, ibuprophen, and distraction on pain relief and patient satisfaction in children with musculoskeletal trauma. J Emerg Nurs 28:118–125, 2002.

14. Kelly AM: Patient satisfaction with pain management does not correlate with initial or discharge VAS pain score, verbal pain rating at discharge, or change in VAS score in the emergency department. J Emerg Med 19:113–116, 2000.

15. Acute Pain Management Guideline Panel: Acute pain management: Operative and medical procedures: Clinical practice guideline, No. 92-0032. Agency for Health Care Policy and Research, Rockville, MD, US Department of Health and Human Services, February 1992.

16. Barsan WG, Tomassoni AJ, Seger D, et al: Safety assessment of high-dose narcotic analgesia for emergency department procedures. Ann Emerg Med 22:1444, 1993.

17. Porter J, Jick H: Addiction rare in patients treated with narcotics. N Engl J Med 302:123, 1980.

18. Mackaway-Jones K, Harrison M: Towards evidence based emergency medicine: Best BETS from the Manchester Royal Infirmary. Analgesia and assessment of abdominal pain. J Accid Emerg Med 17:126–129, 2000.

19. Silen W: Cope's Early Diagnosis of the Acute Abdomen, Oxford University Press, New York, 2000.

20. Centers for Disease Control and Prevention: Vital and Health Statistics of the Centers for Disease Control and Prevention/National Center of Health Statistics. National Hospital Ambulatory Medical Survey. Emergency Department Survey, 1995.

21. Diamond ML: Emergency department management of the acute headache. Clin Cornerstone 1:45–54, 1999.

22. Daroff RB: Classification and diagnostic criteria for headache disorders, cranial neuralgias and facial pain. Headache Classification of the International Headache Society. Cephalgia 8:1, 1988.

23. Diamond S, Diamond ML: Emergency treatment of migraine: Insights into current opinion. Postgrad Med 101:169, 1997.

24. Edlow JA, Caplan LR: Avoiding pitfalls in the diagnosis of subarachnoid hemorrhage. N Engl J Med 342:29, 2000.

25. Newby LK, Mark DB: Navigating the Scylla and Charybdis of chest pain management. Is a computer the answer? Am J Med 112:95, 2002.

26. Richards CR, Richell-Herren K, Mackaway-Jones K: Emergency management of chest pain: Patient satisfaction with and emergency department based six hour rule out myocardial infarction protocol. Emerg Med J 19:122–125, 2002.

27. Flood RG, Krauss B: Procedural sedation and analgesia for children in the emergency department. Emerg Med Clin North Am 21:121–139, 2003.

28. Jagoda AS: Clinical policy for procedural sedation and analgesia in the emergency department. Ann Emerg Med 31:663, 1998.

29. Gross JB, Bailey PL, Caplan RA, et al: Guidelines for sedation and analgesia by nonanesthesiologists. Anesthesiology 84:459, 1996.

30. Chudnofsky CR, Wright SW, Dronen SC, et al: The safety of fentanyl use in the emergency department. Ann Emerg Med 18:6, 1989.

31. Green SM, Johnson NE: Ketamine sedation for pediatric procedures: 2. Review and implications. Ann Emerg Med 19:1033, 1990.

32. Bartfield JM, Ford DT, Homer PJ: Buffered versus plain lidocaine for digital nerve block. Ann Emerg Med 22:216, 1993.

26

Preemptive Analgesia: Physiology and Clinical Studies

Ursula Heck, M.S., M.D., and
Veronica D. Mitchell, M.D.

During the past decade many advances have been made toward understanding the pathophysiology of nociceptive pathways. Researchers have learned more about the presence and function of nociceptors and mediators that act in the periphery, as well as those that act centrally at the level of the spinal cord. One such finding is the observation that tissue injury resulting from a noxious stimulus causes changes to occur in the periphery and in the spinal cord that lead to prolonged excitability, which is known as "hypersensitivity." This hypersensitive state can persist for days and contributes to the postoperative pain state. This process is called peripheral and central sensitization (see Chapter 1 for details).

PATHOPHYSIOLOGY OF PREEMPTIVE ANALGESIA

Transmission of nociceptive information from the periphery to the cortex depends on signal processing, sensory transduction, and integration at three levels of the central nervous system (CNS): the spinal cord, the brain stem, and the forebrain. The sensory receptors that are responsible for detecting stimuli that damage tissue, nociceptors, are activated by noxious stimuli, which include strong mechanical, thermal, and chemical stimuli, or by electrical stimulation of their axons. This leads to pain. This activation process is called sensory transduction.

POSTINJURY PERIPHERAL SENSITIZATION

Postsurgical pain is an inflammatory pain state caused by peripheral tissue damage. Surgery, a noxious stimulus, results in tissue injury, which then leads to the activation of high-threshold nociceptors, a process known as sensory transduction. The release of several chemicals and mediators from this

tissue damage, in combination with inflammatory mediators and activation of sympathetic terminals, causes an increase in the sensitivity of the transduction mechanism. In addition, the threshold of nociceptors is lowered and low-intensity stimuli can induce pain. Peripheral sensitization occurs as a summation of these processes (Fig. 26-1; see also Chapter 2).

There are a number of steps that occur on the cellular level that are responsible for this hypersensitization. (1) Vanilloid receptors (VRs) on small C fibers can be sensitized by repeated heat stimulation, capsaicin, or exposure to protons. VRs are nonselective cation channels that participate in the sensation of thermal and inflammatory pain.[1] (2) Inflammatory mediators,

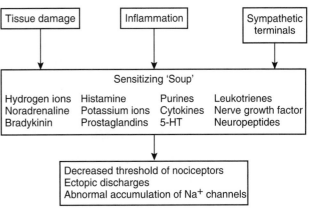

FIGURE 26-1. Mechanisms of tissue injury-induced peripheral sensitization of nociceptors.

such as PGE_2, serotonin, bradykinin, epinephrine, adenosine, and nerve growth factor (NGF), increase the magnitude of Na^+ current in sensory neuron-specific channels. In addition, NGF upregulates the expression of sensory neuron-specific channels. (3) Activation of intracellular kinases occurs (protein kinase C (PKC) or tyrosine kinase). Some of these kinases phosphorylate sensory neuron-specific sodium channels and VRs and potentiate the pro-inflammatory action of bradykinin. These changes result in an increase in the magnitude of the sodium current and a decrease in the activation threshold and in the rate of inactivation. (4) Neurogenic inflammation (vasodilation and edema) also occurs, a process mediated by calcitonin gene-related peptide (CGRP), substance P (SP) and neurokinin A. These vasoactive peptides are released from perivascular afferents.

POSTINJURY CENTRAL SENSITIZATION

CNS hypersensitivity also occurs as a result of tissue injury and may outlast the duration of the initiating nociceptive stimulus. Following a tissue injury, C fiber nociceptors are activated and action potentials are transmitted toward the spinal cord. This C fiber input causes strengthening of synapses at spinal terminals. As a result, the response of dorsal horn neurons to a particular stimulus is increased in intensity as well as duration, and many dorsal horn neurons begin to respond to stimuli outside of their original border (known as receptive-field expansion). In addition, there is a reduction in the threshold necessary to elicit a response. Clinically, we may observe primary hyperalgesia (an area of pain and increased sensitivity to external stimuli where the noxious stimulus was applied) and an area of secondary hyperalgesia (increased sensitivity in the intact surrounding area). There is evidence that demonstrates C fiber input from an injury also causes formation of anatomic connections at the spinal cord level between neurons that respond to A-beta fiber transmission and neurons that respond to A-delta and C fiber transmission. A touch stimulus could then elicit pain (known as allodynia) (see Chapter 1).

Stimulation of C nociceptors in the periphery normally activates dorsal horn neurons via the release of SP and glutamate, an excitatory amino acid, from their terminals in laminae I, II, and V. Glutamate is also released after A-beta nociceptors are stimulated following a touch stimulus. However, the dorsal horn neurons are minimally activated by an A-beta source because the glutamate receptor, the N-methyl-D-aspartate (NMDA) receptor, is normally blocked by Mg^{2+}. Intense or sustained noxious stimulation (high-frequency discharge) results in the removal of this magnesium blockade. The NMDA receptor can now respond to glutamate released from A-beta stimulation and activate dorsal horn neurons. Ca^{2+} can then enter the cell through this mechanism, but also enters through voltage-gated calcium channels and stimulation of other glutamate receptors. PKC is then activated and phosphorylates NMDA receptors, which leads to a prolongation of this touch-evoked pain state (Fig. 26-2; see also Chapter 2).

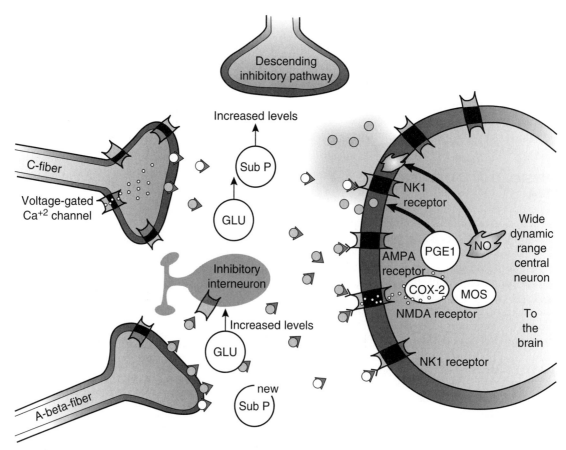

FIGURE 26-2. Mechanisms of central sensitization.

GENOTYPIC AND PHENOTYPIC CHANGES

C fiber stimulation elicits genetic changes (e.g., c-fos gene) at the spinal cord level, thereby leading to changes in the phenotype of primary afferent nociceptors. An increase in expression of VRs and sensory neuron-specific Na+ channels has been found in response to injury. These Na+ channels are found in peripheral axons and in the central terminals of primary afferent nociceptor neurons. Traumatic injury causes a redistribution and increase in the number of sensory neuron-specific Na+ channels proximal to the site of injury. These changes can persist for months.[2] Tissue injury also causes a down-regulation of SP and CGRP by C fibers and A-delta fibers, expression of SP and CGRP by A-beta fibers, and "sprouting" of A-beta fibers from the deeper laminae in the dorsal horn (III and IV) to lamina II. Hence, a non-noxious stimulus like brushing of the skin may now cause c-fos expression and may elicit pain. Additional neuronal changes elicited by tissue injury include the expression of alpha adrenoreceptors and sprouting of sympathetic axons into the dorsal root ganglion (DRG). Primary afferents can then discharge in response to circulating catecholamines.

It is well known that the phenomena of peripheral and central sensitization that occur following stimulation of nociceptors and the release of mediators as a result of tissue damage contribute to the postoperative pain state. Research, in the past, has focused on comparing the analgesic effects of certain techniques that were applied in the postoperative period. More recently, because of our developed understanding of central sensitization, an interest in observing the analgesic effects of techniques applied pre- and intraoperatively was born. The concept of preemptive analgesia was introduced in 1983 by Woolf who demonstrated through experimental studies that postinjury pain hypersensitivity results via a central mechanism.

Further widespread clinical interest in this subject occurred following publication of an editorial by Wall in 1988 based on clinical studies that suggested that preoperative analgesic techniques may decrease postoperative pain. The hypothesis was that interrupting the pathway between the nociceptive stimulus and the spinal cord resulted in prevention of spinal cord changes (i.e., neuroplasticity). This in turn led to the concept of "preemptive analgesia," that is, the idea that therapies can be applied prior to a noxious event (e.g., surgical incision), in order to prevent or reduce the magnitude and duration of postoperative pain, pathologic pain (allodynia, hyperalgesia, and hyperpathia), and/or the development of chronic pain.

Despite convincing experimental studies and encouraging animal studies, human studies have continued to demonstrate controversial and inconsistent results. A review of older studies reveals that they did not truly test the hypothesis of preemptive analgesia. They were not designed to compare the effects of an identical analgesic technique applied preoperatively or postoperatively to comparable patient groups. More recent trials, although well designed, demonstrate varying times at which the antinociceptive technique was initiated and varying durations of application. All of these factors most likely contribute to the reason why we have seen a lack of evidence supporting this concept of preemptive analgesia.

CLINICAL STUDIES

A close review of the research in the area of preemptive analgesia reveals essentially three types of general approaches. The first category involves comparison between a specific preoperative therapy in one group of patients (experimental group) with an untreated second group (control group). The second type of study compares the efficacy of a specific therapy when given preoperatively vs. postoperatively. The third type of trial has involved observation of the effects of continuous analgesic therapy administered through the perioperative period. Attention is focused on the last two types of studies, as the first type does not adequately address the true concept of preemptive analgesia.

A review of 80 randomized controlled clinical trials[3] (1983–2000) of preemptive analgesia for acute or chronic postoperative pain including only trials with identical or nearly identical analgesic regimens initiated before vs. after surgical incision showed some statistical improvement in postoperative pain relief in or at certain time points in 24 of the 80 trials. A total of 3,761 patients were studied. The trials were stratified according to the type of drug: nonsteroidal anti-inflammatory drugs (NSAIDs), intravenous opioids, parenteral NMDA receptor antagonists, epidural analgesia (single dose or continuous), caudal analgesia, and peripheral local anesthetics (Tables 26-1 to 26-3). The postoperative effectiveness was evaluated through quantitative analysis for pain relief using pain scores, time to first analgesic request, and consumption of supplementary analgesics between the preemptive and post surgical group. For the quantitative analysis the average pain scores within the first 24 hours postoperatively were chosen. A lack of evidence for benefit was found in the preemptive trials for treatment with NSAIDs, intravenous opioids, intravenous ketamine, peripheral local anesthetics, and caudal analgesia for postoperative pain relief. The only two existing dextromethorphan trials were positive for a preemptive effect. Single-dose epidural studies showed some benefit, although in most of the trials these were small improvements. The results for continuous epidural infusion revealed statistically improved pain scores but did not support preemptive analgesia being of greater benefit than applying the analgesic technique after the onset of surgery.

One oral adjuvant medication that seems to have potential for inducing preemptive analgesia is gabapentin. Dirks et al.[4] performed a randomized, double-blind, placebo-controlled study in 70 patients who received a single 1,200 mg dose of gabapentin vs. placebo 1 hour prior to undergoing unilateral radical mastectomy with axillary dissection. Total morphine consumption was substantially reduced and pain during movement at 2 hours postoperatively and 4 hours postoperatively was significantly reduced in the gabapentin group.[1]

A review of clinical randomized controlled trials from 1950 to 1994 done earlier with some overlap to the previous study[5] based on the same inclusion criteria (preemptive treatment vs. treatment given after incision) showed similar results. Most of the trials involving NSAIDs were performed with oral surgery patients.[6–9] The results were consistent and showed no measurable difference between the same dose given preoperatively vs. postoperatively. The studies using local anesthetics are divided into trials of epidural (spinal) analgesia, nerve blocks, and wound infiltration. Dahl et al.[10,11] compared epidural bolus and infusion of a local anesthetic and opioid combination pre- and postoperatively. Pryle et al.[12] compared local anesthetics with adrenaline given pre- and postoperatively. Rice et al.[13] compared caudal blocks pre- and postsurgery, and Dierking et al.[14] compared inguinal field blocks involving

TABLE 26-1. **PRESURGERY vs. POSTSURGERY NONOPIOID ADJUVANTS**[3]

Study (Year)	Treatment Tested	Surgical Procedure	No. of Patients	Preemptive Analgesia?
Fletcher et al. (1995)[20]	Ketorolac (IV)	Total hip replacement	40	Yes
Rogers et al. (1995)[20]	Ketorolac (IV)	Abdominal hysterectomy	58	No
Romsing et al. (1998)[20]	Ketorolac	Tonsillectomy	40	No
Adam et al. (1999)[20]	Ketamine	Total mastectomy	128	No
Mathisen et al. (1999)[20]	Ketamine	Lap cholecystectomy	40	No
Cabell (2000)[20]	Ketorolac	Gyn laparoscopy	49	No
Meningaux et al. (2000)[20]	Ketamine	Arthroscopic acl repair	30	No
Flath et al. (1987)[5]	Flurbiprofen (PO)	Endodontic treatment	60	No

These studies were selected based on receiving a 5 out of 5 score on the quality scale determined by the authors of the review article. The quality scale evaluated three areas: randomization, blinding, and reasons for subject withdrawals.

TABLE 26-2. **PRESURGERY vs. POSTSURGERY INTRAVENOUS OPIOIDS**[3]

Study (Year)	Treatment Tested	Surgical Procedure	No. of Patients	Preemptive Analgesia?
Mansfield et al. (1996)[20]	Morphine	Abdominal hysterectomy	40	No
Sarantopoulos and Fassoulaki (1996)[20]	Sufentanil	Abdominal hysterectomy	39	No
Millar et al. (1998)[20]	Morphine	Abdominal hysterectomy	60	No

These studies were selected based on receiving a 5 out of 5 score on the quality scale determined by the authors of the review article. The quality scale evaluated three areas: randomization, blinding, and reasons for subject withdrawals.

TABLE 26–3. **PRESURGERY vs. POSTSURGERY LOCAL ANESTHESIA**[3]

Study (Year)	Treatment Tested	Surgical Procedure	No. of Patients	Preemptive Analgesia?
Katz et al. (1994)[20]	Bupivacaine (single-dose epidural)	Lower abdominal surgery	42	Yes
Ke et al. (1998)[20]	Bupivacaine	Gyn laparoscopy	49	Yes
Ejlersen et al. (1992)[14]	Lidocaine (incisional)	Inguinal hernia repair	37	Yes
Orntoft et al. (1994)[20]	Bupivacaine	Tonsillectomy	24	No
Likar et al. (1999)[20]	Ropivacaine	Tonsillectomy	39	No

These studies were selected based on receiving a 5 out of 5 score on the quality scale determined by the authors of the review article. The quality scale evaluated three areas: randomization, blinding, and reasons for subject withdrawals.

epidural anesthetics. No evidence of a preemptive effect was found. Several researchers have explored the effects of local anesthetic wound infiltration administered preoperatively and postoperatively. The only study that showed a benefit for the preemptive group was conducted by Ejlersen et al.[15] They observed that patients who had received preincisional infiltration (5 minutes prior to incision) had a significantly longer time until remedication. Turner and Chalkiadis[16] compared infiltration after induction with infiltration after surgery and found no significant differences between the groups. Some studies involving presurgical vs. post surgical administration of opioids have demonstrated a preemptive analgesic effect, whereas others have not. Richmond et al.[17] found significantly reduced patient-controlled analgesia (PCA) intravenous morphine consumption for the first 24 hours in the group who had received intravenous morphine at induction compared to the same dose via the same route at closure. This effect however was reversed in the following 24 hours. Katz et al.[18] compared epidural fentanyl infusion administered preoperatively or postoperatively and found significantly lower PCA morphine consumption from 12 to 24 hours following surgery in the preemptive group but no difference in the VAS scores. Wilson et al.[19] found no difference in analgesic outcome measures (VAS scores and PCA intravenous morphine consumption) in patients who received intravenous alfentanyl at induction or after skin incision.

Why then, despite convincing evidence for preemptive analgesia in experimental studies, have we not been able to demonstrate consistently this phenomenon in humans? One such reason may lie in the fact that some of the clinical studies, by nature of their design, may be somewhat faulty. The surgical incision is not a single one-time noxious stimulus, but a constant barrage of C fiber and A-delta fiber input into the spinal cord. If the analgesic technique applied prior to the incision initially blocked this input, as the effects of the technique begin to wear off, nociceptive information would then reach the spinal cord, thereby causing hypersensitization. In addition, central sensitization is not only induced during surgery but also postoperatively by inflammatory processes, therefore possibly negating any beneficial effect that could have initially occurred. Also, many studies included the use of premedications or intraoperative analgesic adjuvants, as well as nitrous oxide, which all have a well-known preemptive analgesic effect. This could have made it difficult to detect significant differences between the control and experimental groups.

A second reason for the lack of strong evidence supporting preemptive analgesia in clinical studies may be that no objective standard exists to measure pain. Pain severity and opioid consumption are often used in clinical trials as measures of outcome. However, opioid consumption is not a reliable index, as no proportionality exists between postoperative pain intensity and analgesic requirement. Opioid consumption is not only a reflection of pain intensity, but is also profoundly influenced by various psychological factors including anxiety level, mood, and expectation of recovery. In addition, opioid plasma concentration and analgesic response curves vary tremendously amongst individuals.

A third reason that preemptive analgesia is not an obvious phenomenon in clinical trials may be that it is extremely difficult to block completely noxious input from reaching the spinal cord despite the analgesic technique used. Researchers have used plasma cortisol levels as a determinant of the stress response to determine if complete neural blockade occurs during surgery. One researcher showed that only a block extending from T4 to S5 prevented a rise in cortisol levels following lower abdominal surgery.[20]

SUMMARY

Postoperative pain management has improved tremendously with the development of PCA and continuous epidural analgesia. It remains, however, suboptimal for a certain number of patients. The potential of preemptive analgesia seems to be great but the optimal technique has not yet been identified. Neuroplasticity is a well-recognized phenomenon but is not yet fully understood. As we develop a better understanding of this process through more research, additional studies looking at the effects of preemptive analgesia will be performed. It also seems likely, based on current knowledge, that a complete block of afferent input combined with a multimodal approach may prove to be most effective. It is because of the potential that preemptive analgesia has to revolutionize the field of pain medicine that, despite unconvincing clinical trials, it continues to be an area of great interest and exploration.

KEY POINTS

- Postoperative pain results from peripheral and central sensitization.
- The NMDA receptor responds to glutamate, an excitatory amino acid.
- The NMDA receptor is normally blocked by Mg^{2+}. Removal of this blockade leads to an influx of Ca^{2+} into the cell.
- The concept of preemptive analgesia is the idea that therapies can be applied prior to a noxious event in order to prevent or reduce the magnitude and duration of postinjury pain and/or the development of chronic pain.
- Although there are several experimental studies that support the idea of preemptive analgesia, human clinical studies have demonstrated inconsistent and controversial results.
- Older clinical trials did not adequately address the concept of preemptive analgesia because instead of comparing a therapy pre- and postoperatively, these studies compared a specific preoperative therapy in the experimental group with an untreated control group.
- Therapies that have been tested in preemptive trials include NSAIDs, intravenous opioids, intravenous ketamine, peripheral local anesthetics, caudal and epidural analgesia, dextromethorphan, and gabapentin.
- One reason that human studies have not been able to demonstrate beneficial results favoring the idea of preemptive analgesia is that there is not an objective standard for measuring pain.
- Another reason that human studies have not been able to show results in support of preemptive analgesia is that, despite the analgesic therapy used, it is nearly impossible to block completely noxious input from reaching the spinal cord.
- A third reason that preemptive analgesia is not an obvious phenomenon in clinical trials is that central sensitization is induced by inflammatory processes, and therefore a preemptive effect could be negated in the immediate postoperative period secondary to inflammation.

REFERENCES

1. Hayrunnisia B, Moskowitz MA: Mechanisms of pain modulation in chronic syndromes. Neurology 10:59, 2002.

2. Gould H, England JD, Liu ZP, Levinson SR: Rapid sodium channel augmentation in response to inflammation induced by complete adjuvant. Brain Res 802:69–74, 1998.

3. Moiniche S, Kehlet H, Dahl JB: A qualitative and quantitative systemic review of preemptive analgesia for postoperative pain relief. Anesthesiology 96(3):725–741, 2002.

4. Dirks J, Fredensborg BB, Christensen D, et al: A randomized study of the effects of single-dose gabapentin versus placebo on postoperative pain and morphine consumption after mastectomy. Anesthesiology 97(3):560–564, 2002.

5. McQuay H, Moore A: An Evidence-Based Resource for Pain Relief. Oxford Medical, 1999.

6. Flath RK, Hicks ML, Dionne RA, Pelleu GB: Pain suppression after pulpectomy with preoperative flurbiprofen. J Endodontics 13:339–347, 1987.

7. Sisk AL, Mosley RO, Martin RP: Comparison of preoperative and postoperative diflunisal for suppression of postoperative pain. J Oral Maxillofacial Surg 47:464–468, 1989.

8. Sisk AL, Grover BJ: A comparison of preoperative and postoperative naproxen sodium for suppression of postoperative pain. J Oral Maxillofacial Surg 48:674–678, 1990.

9. Gustafsson I, Nystrom E, Quiding H: Effects of preoperative paracetamol on pain after oral surgery. Eur J Clin Pharmacol 24:63–65, 1983.

10. Dahl JB, Hansen BL, Hjortso NC, et al: Influence of timing on the effect of continuous extradural analgesia with bupivacaine and morphine after major abdominal surgery. Br J Anaesth 69:4–8, 1992.

11. Dahl JB, Daugaard JJ, Rasmussen B, et al: Immediate and prolonged effects of pre- versus postoperative epidural analgesia with bupivacaine and morphine on pain at rest and during mobilization after total knee arthroplasty. Acta Anaesth Scand 38:557–561, 1994.

12. Pryle BJ, Vanner RG, Enriquez N, Reynolds F: Can pre-emptive lumbar epidural blockade reduce postoperative pain following lower abdominal surgery? Anaesthesia 48:120–123, 1993.

13. Rice LJ, Pudimat MA, Hannallah RS: Timing of caudal block placement in relation to surgery does not affect duration of postoperative analgesia in paediatric ambulatory patients. Can J Anaesth 37:429–431, 1990.

14. Dierking G, Dahl JB, Kanstrup J, et al: The effect of pre- versus postoperative inguinal field block on postoperative pain after herniotomy. Br J Anaesth 68:344–348, 1992.

15. Ejlersen E, Andersen HB, Eliasen K, Morgensen T: A comparison between pre- and postincisional lidocaine infiltration on postoperative pain. Anesth Analg 74:495–498, 1992.

16. Turner GA, Chalkiadis G: Comparison of preoperative with postoperative lignocaine infiltration on postoperative analgesia requirements. Br J Anaesth 72:541–543, 1994.

17. Richmond CE, Bromley LM, Woolf CJ: Preoperative morphine pre-empts postoperative pain. Lancet 342:73–75, 1993.

18. Katz J, Kavanagh BP, Sandler AN, et al: Preemptive analgesia – Clinical evidence of neuroplasticity contributing to postoperative pain. Anesth 77:439–446, 1992.

19. Wilson RJT, Leith S, Jackson IJB, Hunter D: Preemptive analgesia from intravenous administration of opioids. Anesthesia 49:591–593, 1994.

20. Kehlet H: Surgical stress: The role of pain and analgesia. Br J Anaesth 63:189–195, 1989.

Patient-Controlled Analgesia

Edward R. Sherwood, M.D., Ph.D., and
Honorio T. Benzon, M.D.

Patient-controlled analgesia (PCA) is a method by which patients self-administer small doses of opioid analgesics when pain is experienced. This technique can be employed in a variety of settings and is based on the use of a microprocessor-controlled infusion pump that delivers a preprogrammed dose of medication when the patient pushes a demand button. A timer within the pump is programmed to prevent administration of additional drug until a specified amount of time, known as the lockout interval, has elapsed. Modern PCA devices allow for the programming of demand dose, lockout interval, basal continuous infusions, and limitation of dose over a 1- to 4-hour period. These devices also record patient usage information such as total number of demands and drug delivery during the previous 1-hour and 24-hour periods. This information can be useful in optimizing drug delivery based on the needs of individual patients. Most commonly, drugs are delivered via indwelling intravenous catheters. However, techniques have been developed to deliver analgesics via the intramuscular, subcutaneous, and epidural routes using PCA technology.

PCA allows patients to titrate analgesics to their needs and bypasses the unavoidable delays that occur when analgesics are provided upon request. These delays include the response time of a potentially busy nurse, screening of the appropriateness of the request, signout and preparation of the analgesic, and, finally, administration of the medication. PCA, when used properly, theoretically allows patients to maintain a narrower range of plasma drug concentration compared to intramuscular or intravenous bolus dosing. Subtherapeutic troughs and excessive peak plasma concentrations, which can be associated with significant side effects such as sedation and respiratory depression, could be avoided. However, two meta-analyses did not show a difference in adverse effects when comparing PCA use to conventional opioid dosing.[1,2] Nevertheless, PCA gives patients more control over their analgesic needs as their relative level of pain changes. Patients generally self-administer opioids appropriately, and several studies have shown that the total opioid requirements of patients using PCA are less than those of patients using conventional intramuscular dosing.[1,2] Because of the sense of control over their pain managements, patients generally report greater satisfaction with PCA than with on-demand dosing of opioids.[1,2]

A critical principle in the use of PCA is that the patient controls the amount of analgesic delivered. This is very important for the safe delivery use of PCA technology. Sedation usually precedes the respiratory depression as plasma concentrations of opioid increase within a given patient. The sedated patient has difficulty pushing the demand button and is generally unable to deliver further doses of opioids that could lead to significant respiratory depression. It is important for nursing personnel and the patient's family members to be aware of this principle so that the demand button is not pushed by anyone other than the patient. For optimal results, patients, nurses, and family members should be instructed on the basic principles of PCA use. Selected patients must be cooperative and have the ability to push the demand button. This requirement limits the use of PCA in children younger than 3 to 5 years of age and persons with some mental or physical handicaps. It is the responsibility of physicians and nursing staff to examine patients, determine whether adequate analgesia is being provided, and that undesirable side effects are minimized. Because of pharmacokinetic and pharmacodynamic variability among patients, conventional PCA settings may need to be adjusted. In addition, PCA pumps are mechanical devices that can, on occasion, malfunction. Although the safety record of PCA pumps is excellent, incidences of excessive medication delivery have been reported.[3,4] However, experience has shown that over-sedation and respiratory depression are less common with PCA than with conventional intramuscular or intravenous dosing.

The use of basal infusion with PCA is controversial. Theoretically, continuous opioid infusion in association with PCA might provide more constant plasma opioid levels and improve analgesia. However, some studies have shown that addition of a basal infusion rate does not improve patients' ability to sleep or rest comfortably and does not alter scores for pain, fatigue, and anxiety.[5] The number of patient demands, number of supplemental bolus doses, and total opioid use were also not changed in patients receiving basal infusions of opioids. One study demonstrated improved patient comfort with a continuous basal infusion.[6] The disadvantage of a basal infusion is that most programming errors that have resulted in adverse side effects occurred during the use of basal infusions.[5] In addition, use of basal infusions bypasses the basic safety mechanism of patient control. Specifically, in a sedated patient, delivery of opioid continues at a basal rate and may put the patient at higher risk of respiratory depression. However, the use of basal infusions in patients with high opioid requirements may be appropriate, but careful patient selection is essential.

Several opioids have been used effectively with PCA pumps. The ideal analgesic for use with PCA would have a rapid onset of action, high efficacy, and intermediate duration of action without significant accumulation of drug or metabolites over time. Morphine, hydromorphone and meperidine most closely fit these criteria and are the most widely used agents in PCA pumps. However, a variety of agonist and agonist–antagonist opioids have been used in PCA pumps and the agent used should be tailored to the clinical setting. The typical dosing, lockout, and infusion parameters for PCA opioids are indicated in Table 27-1.

APPLICATIONS OF PATIENT-CONTROLLED ANALGESIA

PCA is most commonly used for the management of postoperative pain. However, PCA also can be used for the management of labor pain, post-traumatic pain, cancer pain, and pain associated with myocardial infarction.

LABOR PAIN

Parenteral opioid administration is a viable option for providing labor analgesia when epidural analgesia is not available or is contraindicated. However, most studies show that opioids delivered by PCA are inferior to epidural analgesia in the management of labor pain.[7,8] Nevertheless, some parturients do not want epidural analgesia or have clinical conditions that contraindicate its use. In this situation PCA should be considered. Many parturients wish to limit the use of medications and avoid excessive sedation before delivery. Compared with bolus intramuscular or intravenous dosing, PCA provides the ability to titrate analgesic needs as labor progresses and is better titrated against the large variability in analgesic requirements among parturients. Other advantages of PCA in the parturient include superior pain relief, less maternal sedation and respiratory depression, lower placental drug transfer, less need for antiemetics, and higher patient satisfaction compared to bolus intramuscular dosing.[9] However, one major concern with the use of parenteral opioids during labor and delivery is the potential depression of fetal ventilation and neurological activity during the postdelivery period. The use of epidural anesthesia decreases or eliminates fetal exposure to depressant drugs and may also improve placental perfusion and fetal oxygenation during labor.[10] However, in patients that are not

TABLE 27-1. GUIDELINES REGARDING BOLUS DOSES, LOCKOUT INTERVALS, AND CONTINUOUS INFUSIONS FOR PARENTERAL ANALGESICS WHEN USED WITH A PCA SYSTEM

Drug	Bolus (mg)	Lockout Interval (minutes)	Continuous Infusion (mg/hour)
Agonists			
Fentanyl	0.015–0.05	3–10	0.02–0.1
Hydromorphone	0.1–0.5	5–15	0.2–0.5
Meperidine	5–15	5–15	5–40
Methadone	0.5–3	10–20	–
Morphine	0.5–3	5–20	1–10
Oxymorphone	0.2–0.8	5–15	0.1–1
Sufentanil	0.003–0.015	3–10	0.004–0.03
Agonists–antagonists			
Buprenorphine	0.03–0.2	10–20	–
Nalbuphine	1–5	5–15	1–8
Pentazocine	5–30	5–15	6–40

The addition of a basal infusion is controversial (see text).

candidates for epidural analgesia, PCA has been shown to decrease cord opioid levels compared with conventional bolus dosing and most studies have not demonstrated significant fetal depression after its use for labor analgesia. Recently some investigators have advocated the use of shorter-acting opioids such as fentanyl, alfentanil, and remifentanil in PCA pumps for laboring parturients, partly as a mechanism to decrease neonatal depression in the postdelivery period.[11,12] In order to minimize fetal depression many practitioners discontinue PCA once the mother's cervix is completely dilated.

PAIN CONTROL IN PEDIATRIC PATIENTS

PCA is a safe and effective means of controlling pain in adolescents and young children. The most important factor in determining the success of PCA in pediatric patients is the ability of the patient to understand the basic principles of PCA use. Most children older than 7 years of age can use PCA independently. Children aged 4 to 6 years can use PCA pumps with the encouragement of parents and nursing staff. However, the failure rate in this age group is high. Children younger than 4 years of age are not good candidates for PCA use. Some investigators have advocated parental assistance for PCA use by young children. However, this practice bypasses the basic safety mechanism of patient control and has been discouraged in the postoperative setting. If parent-controlled analgesia is to be considered in the postoperative setting, then a formal parent education program should be implemented along with close observation by nursing staff.

Basal opioid infusions have also been used successfully by some practitioners in the pediatric population for control of postoperative pain. However, some studies have shown an increased incidence of hypoxemia in children receiving continuous opioid infusions with PCA.[13] Therefore, continuous infusions should be used with caution in the pediatric population and pulse-oximetry, as a mechanism of detecting opioid-induced respiratory depression, should be considered. Concurrent administration of drugs with respiratory depressant effects should also be viewed with caution. Typical PCA dosing for children is shown in Table 27-2.

CANCER PAIN

PCA is useful for cancer pain management in the inpatient setting for both children and adults. In contrast to postoperative pain management the use of continuous opioid infusions for the management of cancer pain is very effective and is encouraged.

TABLE 27-2. PCA DOSING IN CHILDREN

Drug	Bolus (μg/kg)	Lockout (minutes)	Infusion (μg/kg/hour)
Morphine	10–20	7–15	10–20
Meperidine	100–200	7–15	100–200
Fentanyl	0.1–0.2	7–15	0.1–0.2

The addition of a basal infusion to PCA is controversial (see text).

In the pediatric cancer patient population parental assistance with PCA use is also encouraged.[13] The dosages of opioid used in the management of cancer pain often far exceed those used in the postoperative setting. Parenteral opioids provide an important option for patients with moderate to severe cancer pain and are a good alternative to spinal opioids. A recent study showed changing the route of opioid administration, including the use of PCA-administered parenteral opioids is an important strategy for patients that exhibit refractory cancer pain.[14] The use of methadone in PCA pumps, a practice not commonly advocated during the postoperative period, is also an important consideration in treating patients with intractable cancer pain.[15]

KETAMINE ADDED TO MORPHINE FOR PATIENT-CONTROLLED ANALGESIA

The side effects of opioids, including nausea, sedation, and respiratory depression, and the development of tolerance even during the very early stage of treatment led investigators to add an adjunctive medication including ketamine.[16] Ketamine is an N-methyl-D-aspartate (NMDA) antagonist, and NMDA receptors are involved in the hyperexcitability of spinal cord nociceptive neurons induced by C fiber stimulation.[17,18] In addition, ketamine inhibits voltage-gated sodium and potassium channels and the reuptake of serotonin and dopamine.[18] The addition of a small dose of ketamine (250 μg/kg) in addition to intravenous morphine provided rapid and sustained analgesia in postoperative patients whose pain was not relieved by >0.1 mg/kg morphine.[19] The preoperative administration of intravenous ketamine followed by the intravenous infusion of ketamine lowered the visual analogue pain scores and decreased the epidural analgesic consumption of patients who underwent renal surgery.[20] In this study the incidence of nausea and pruritus were more frequent in the control group (patient-controlled epidural analgesia, PCEA, morphine plus saline infusion). In an elegant study on postoperative intravenous PCA after spine and hip surgery investigators found the ideal ratio of morphine and ketamine to be 1:1 and a lockout interval of 8 minutes.[16] It remains to be seen whether ketamine will be used more frequently in conjunction with intravenous PCA or PCEA.

KEY POINTS

- PCA allows patients to titrate analgesics to their needs and bypasses the delays that occur when analgesics are provided upon request.
- The patient should control the use of the PCA device. This is important for patient safety; a sedated patient has difficulty pushing the demand button. The ability to push the demand button limits the use of PCA for patients younger than 3 to 5 years of age and patients with mental and physical handicaps.
- The use of a basal infusion is controversial in the postoperative setting. Studies showed the addition of a basal infusion did not improve the patient's ability to sleep and not alter the scores for pain, fatigue, and anxiety. For cancer pain, the use of a continuous infusion is encouraged. The superiority of an additional basal infusion is probably related to the higher analgesic requirements in patients with cancer pain.

- The ideal analgesic for PCA use is one with a rapid onset of action, high efficacy, and intermediate duration of action. Morphine and hydromorphone best fit these criteria.
- The major disadvantage of using opioid PCA during labor is the potential depression of fetal ventilation and neurologic activity.
- The efficacy of PCA in the pediatric population is related to the ability of the patient to understand the basic principles of PCA use. Children older than 7 years can safely use PCA.
- The addition of ketamine appears to improve the efficacy of morphine intravenous PCA. Ketamine is an NMDA antagonist and NMDA receptors are involved in spinal cord hyperexcitability from C fiber stimulation.

REFERENCES

1. Ballantine J, Carr D, Chalmers T, et al: Postoperative patient-controlled analgesia: Meta-analysis of initial randomized control trials. J Clin Anesth 5:182–193, 1993.
2. Walder B, Schafer M, Henzil I, et al: Efficacy and safety of patient-controlled opioid analgesia for acute postoperative pain. A quantitative systematic review. Acta Anaesthesiol Scand 45:795–804, 2001.
3. Tamsen A, Hartvig P, Fagerlund C: Patient-controlled analgesic therapy: Clinical experience. Acta Anesthesiol Scand; Suppl 26:157–161, 1982.
4. Ashburn M, Love G, Pace N: Respiratory-related critical events with intravenous patient-controlled analgesia. Clin J Pain 10:52–56, 1994.
5. Parker R, Holtmann B, White P: Effects of continuous opioid infusion with PCA therapy on patient comfort and analgesic requirements after abdominal hysterectomy. Anesthesiology 76:362–367, 1992.
6. Smith G: Management of post-operative pain. Can J Anaesth 362–366, 1989.
7. Sharma S, Alexander J, Messick G, et al: Cesarean delivery: A randomized trial of epidural analgesia versus intravenous meperidine analgesia during labor in nulliparous women. Anesthesiology 96:546–551, 2002.
8. Head B, Owen J, Vincent R: A randomized trial of intrapartum analgesia in women with severe preeclampsia. Obstet Gynecol 99:452–457, 2002.
9. Isenor L, Penny-MacGillivray T: Intravenous meperidine infusion for obstetric analgesia. J Obstet Gynecol Neonatal Nurs 22:349–356, 1993.
10. Mattingly J, D'Alessio J, Ramanathan J: Effects of obstetric analgesics and anesthetics on the neonate: A review. Paediatr Drugs 5:615–627, 2003.
11. Thurlow J, Laxton C, Dick A, et al: Remifentanil by patient-controlled analgesia compared with intramuscular meperidine for pain relief in labor. Br J Anesth 88:374–378, 2002.
12. Morley-Forster P, Reid W, Vandeberghe H: A comparison of patient-controlled analgesia fentanyl and alfentanil for labor analgesia. Can J Anesth 47:113–119, 2000.
13. Berde C, Sethna N: Drug therapy: Analgesics for the treatment of pain in children. N Engl J Med 347:1094–1103, 2002.
14. Enting R, Oldenmenger W, van der Rijt, et al: A prospective study evaluating the response of patients with unrelieved cancer pain to parenteral opioids. Cancer 94:3049–3056, 2002.
15. Fitzgibbon D, Ready L: Intravenous high-dose methadone administered by patient controlled analgesia and continuous infusion for the treatment of cancer pain refractory to high-dose morphine. Pain 73:259–261, 1997.
16. Sveticic G, Gentilini A, Eichenberger U, et al: Combinations of morphine with ketamine for patient-controlled analgesia. Anesthesiology 98:1195–1205, 2003.
17. Petrenko AB, Yamakura T, Baba H, Shimoji K: The role of N-methyl-D-aspartate (NMDA) receptors in pain: A review. Anesth Analg 97:1108–1016, 2003.
18. Hocking G, Cousins MJ: Ketamine in chronic pain management: An evidence-based review. Anesth Analg 97:1730–1739, 2003.
19. Weinbroum AA: A single small dose of postoperative ketamine provides rapid and sustained improvement in morphine analgesia in the presence of morphine-resistant pain. Anesth Analg 96:789–795, 2003.
20. Kararmaz A, Kaya S, Karaman H, et al: Intraopeartive intravenous ketamine in combination with epidural analgesia: Postoperative analgesia after renal surgery. Anesth Analg 97:1092–1096, 2003.

Intrathecal Opioid Injections for Postoperative Pain

Jeffrey M. Richman, M.D., and
Christopher L. Wu, M.D.

Over the past two decades the use of single-dose intrathecal (IT) opioids has become commonplace in anesthetic practice. Since the first described use of IT morphine in 1979, hundreds of case reports and clinical investigations have been published on the IT administration of opioids. Human and animal studies have elucidated the mechanism of action of IT opioids, side-effect profiles, dose–response pharmacology, adjuvant agents, and clinical uses for a wide range of surgical cases. Common uses of IT opioids for postoperative analgesia include obstetric and gynecologic surgery, orthopedic joint and spine procedures, thoracic and vascular procedures, cardiac bypass, pediatric surgery, urologic procedures, and abdominal procedures. Use of IT opioids has also been reported in the treatment of chronic pain.

MECHANISMS OF ACTION OF INTRATHECAL OPIOIDS

Nociceptive information is transmitted by multiple afferent neurons with small-diameter unmyelinated fibers playing a major role in the transmission of pain. Central terminals of small unmyelinated fibers are located in Rexed's laminae I, II, and III.[1] Opioid receptors exist in Rexed's laminae I, II, and V in the dorsal horn of the spinal cord. This provides the anatomic basis for selective analgesia by opioids injected into the cerebrospinal fluid (CSF). Spinal cord analgesia is likely mediated by μ and κ receptors. Experimental studies have shown that substance P is released into the CSF by electrical stimulation.[1] This release is inhibited by the administration of morphine into the CSF. Inhibition may be mediated by gamma-aminobutyric acid (GABA) presynaptically and glycine postsynaptically in vivo.

The pharmacologic properties of the different opioids determine their onset, duration of action, and side effects (Table 28-1). Lipophilicity (versus hydrophilicity) is the key property affecting the speed of onset and duration of action. The highly lipid-soluble drugs such as fentanyl and sufentanil have a faster onset but shorter duration of action when used intrathecally.[2,3] Shortly after injection, CSF levels are barely detectible as the drug is quickly distributed to the spinal cord.[3]

TABLE 28-1. CHARACTERISTICS OF INTRATHECAL OPIOIDS

Opioid	Oil–Water Partition Coefficient*	Typical Adult Intrathecal Dose	Onset of Analgesia (minutes)	Duration of Analgesia (minutes)
Morphine	1.4	0.05–0.6 mg	30–60	480–1440
Meperidine	39	10–100 mg	2–12	60–400
Fentanyl	816	10–50 μg	5–10	30–120
Sufentanil	1727	2.5–12.5 μg	3–6	60–180

*A higher number reflects increased lipophilicity.

This may result in a more segmental spread of analgesia and a lower concentration reaching the brain, decreasing the risk of delayed respiratory depression. Morphine, which is hydrophilic, has a slower onset and longer duration of action, and remains detectable in the CSF long after injection. Delayed respiratory depression may be more likely with morphine than other lipophilic drugs as morphine remains in the CSF long enough to circulate rostrally to the brainstem and respiratory centers.

Only meperidine has strong enough local anesthetic properties to be used as a sole agent for surgery. IT injection of meperidine produces spinal anesthesia that is qualitatively similar to that achieved with conventional local anesthetics.[4] It is likely the combined action of its local anesthetic properties and its opioid receptor binding that allows meperidine to be used as the sole agent in spinal anesthesia. The onset of action for meperidine is similar to that of fentanyl despite being significantly less lipid soluble; however, its duration is longer than fentanyl. Meperidine has a shorter duration of action than morphine as meperidine dissipates from the CSF four times faster than morphine.[4]

ADVANTAGES OF INTRATHECAL OPIOIDS

There are several advantages inherent to the use of IT opioids compared to intravenous and epidural opioids or IT and epidural local anesthetics (Table 28-2). Equianalgesic doses of IT opioids are typically a small fraction of those used for intravenous or epidural use.[5] The resultant serum levels, especially with morphine, are barely detectable, thus limiting the systemic effects while maximizing the analgesic properties.[5,6] In contrast, the dose of epidural opioids is approximately 10 times that of a comparable IT dose, which may result in systemic analgesic levels of drug and increased levels of sedation.[1,5] The duration of analgesia for a hydrophilic opioid such as morphine is greater compared to intravenous epidural administration.[1,7] A single IT injection of morphine 0.04 to 0.5 mg will provide up to 15 to 24 hours of analgesia.[8–11] With the relative ease and reliability of cannulating the IT space compared to the epidural space, IT morphine may be more of an ideal analgesic in certain situations. IT opioids may also provide an advantage over epidural catheters in operations where anticoagulation will be started immediately postoperatively, necessitating the removal of the epidural catheter.

Opioids per se do not cause adverse hemodynamic changes when applied intrathecally and may not attenuate the neuroendocrine stress response even when administered in extremely large doses (4.0 mg).[12] Local anesthetics applied neuraxially will produce a sympathectomy with resultant vasodilation, and hypotension. In addition, opioids do not cause motor blockade or sensory loss, allowing early and safe ambulation.[13] IT opioids do provide a sparing effect on local anesthetics, allowing lower doses to be used intrathecally or epidurally while still maintaining adequate analgesia.[14] Meperidine, an opioid with local anesthetic properties, has been used effectively as the sole agent for spinal anesthesia.[4]

SIDE EFFECTS OF INTRATHECAL OPIOIDS

Unfortunately, IT opioids are not without a significant number of adverse effects (Table 28-3). Most of these are dose dependent and may be more common for intrathecally administered agents than by other routes. They are less common in patients who are chronically exposed to opioids. Most, but not all, side effects are mediated via interaction with opioid receptors.

The most feared complication is respiratory depression and arrest. Shortly following the first description of the use of IT morphine in humans, cases of delayed respiratory depression were reported. Large doses of up to 20 mg had been used in the early 1980s with an alarmingly high rate of respiratory depression.[1] It has been demonstrated that the risk of respiratory depression is dose related,[15] with few instances of clinically significant depression reported at doses less than 0.4 mg of IT morphine.[16] Respiratory depression, however, has been noted at even smaller doses on rare occasions.[17]

The incidence of respiratory arrest is difficult to quantify, although from the available literature it appears to be <1% for IT opioids.[18,19] In fact, the incidence of respiratory depression is <1% for opioids regardless of the route of administration.[19] Respiratory depression typically occurs within minutes to hours for the lipophilic opioids (fentanyl, sufentanil) with early respiratory depression (minutes) not being reported with

TABLE 28-2. **ADVANTAGES OF INTRATHECAL OPIOIDS**

Long duration of action
Small doses required for equianalgesic effect
Almost undetectable vascular absorption
Ease of cannulating the intrathecal space
Minimal hemodynamic changes
No motor blockade
No sensory loss

TABLE 28-3. **SIDE EFFECTS OF INTRATHECAL OPIOIDS**

Common	Uncommon
Mild respiratory depression	Respiratory arrest
Pruritus	Generalized muscle rigidity
Sedation	Nystagmus
Nausea	Epileptic seizure
Vomiting	Myoclonus
Urinary retention	Hyperalgesia Neurotoxicity Water retention

a hydrophilic opioid such as morphine. For morphine, delayed respiratory depression characteristically occurs 6 to 12 hours after administration but has been reported up to 19 hours after IT injection.[20] Clinically significant respiratory depression has never been reported beyond 19 hours after IT morphine administration. Considerable hypoventilation may occur following IT morphine even in the presence of a "normal" pulse oximetry and respiratory rate. Sedation may be another indicator of impending respiratory depression, although only arterial blood gas analysis will routinely identify hypercarbia. Supplemental oxygenation may prevent hypoxemia but may not correct the underlying etiology, especially when obstruction of the airway (e.g., obstructive sleep apnea) is implicated.

The risk of respiratory depression increases with the addition of systemic opioids or sedatives, increasing age, lack of opioid tolerance (i.e., opioid-naive state), obesity, and sleep apnea.[1,8,21] With hydrophilic opioids, respiratory depression occurs after the migration of opioid in the CSF with subsequent interaction with opioid receptors in the ventral medulla.[20] Naloxone has been used effectively to treat respiratory depression from IT opioids, although there is a case report of naloxone-resistant respiratory depression.[17] Naloxone will most likely need to be readministered or used as a continuous infusion due to its relatively short half-life. Long-acting opioid antagonists have also been used for treatment and prevention of respiratory depression.

The risk of postoperative respiratory depression after the use of IT opioids has stirred debate about whether intensive care unit-like monitoring is required after patients leave the postanesthesia care unit. With lipid-soluble opioids, this is not as much of an issue, as delayed respiratory depression would be highly unlikely. The risk of delayed respiratory depression from IT morphine, however, has prompted some institutions to require admission to a monitored unit for all patients receiving IT morphine. Observational data indicate that respiratory depression from opioids (from any route of administration) is <1%,[19] is not higher with IT or neuraxial administration, and rarely occurs with IT morphine doses of <0.4 mg. A higher dose may be acceptable for opioid-tolerant patients. In addition, the requirement of monitored beds may prevent a significant number of patients who would benefit from IT opioids from receiving them. Patients with comorbitities such as sleep apnea, sedation, pulmonary disease and mental status changes should be monitored closely after receiving IT opioids. IT morphine should not be used for ambulatory surgery.

The most common side effect of IT opioids is pruritus.[20] Pruritus is usually noted in the facial areas innervated by the trigeminal nerve; however, itching may be generalized. Although IT opioid-induced pruritus is likely due to cephalad migration of the drug and interaction with opioid receptors in the trigeminal nucleus located superficially in the medulla,[20] the exact etiology is not clear. The incidence has been reported anywhere from 20% to 100% in various studies and may be dose dependent.[13,20,22,23] It is difficult to determine differences in incidence of pruritus among the different opioids due to methodologic issues; however, it appears that patients who receive morphine have a higher incidence of pruritus than those who receive fentanyl.[20,24] The obstetric patient population has one of the highest incidences of pruritus.[20,22,23,25,26] Despite the relatively high incidence of pruritus, very few patients actually request treatment as pruritus is typically noted as a side effect often only if the clinician inquires about it.

Itching is not histamine mediated nor is it related to systemic absorption of the drug. Antihistamines are minimally effective as a treatment; however, their sedating properties may relieve symptoms in some patients. Opioid receptor antagonists, such as naloxone, and opioid agonists–antagonists are effective in the treatment for pruritus.[20,27,28] Low-dose intravenous naloxone may be effective in attenuating pruritus but does not generally decrease the analgesic efficacy of IT opioids.[21,29] Long-acting opioid receptor antagonists, such as nalbuphine, naltrexone, and nalmefene, do reduce itching when given prior to IT morphine, but appear to shorten the duration and possibly quality of pain relief. Propofol in a 20 mg dose may relieve pruritus without affecting analgesia, but is less effective than μ receptor antagonists.[28] Ondansetron may be an effective agent for treating spinal or epidural morphine-induced pruritus.[30] Prophylactic ondansetron 0.1 mg/kg intravenous (IV) has also been shown to reduce the incidence of pruritus after IT morphine.[31]

Nausea and vomiting are also common and troublesome side effects after IT opioid injection. Although the incidence is lower than that seen with pruritus, patients may require treatment more frequently. Nausea occurs in approximately 20% to 40% of patients receiving IT opioids.[20] Although the underlying mechanism is not related to systemic absorption, the incidence is comparable to IV and epidural administration. Nausea usually occurs within 4 hours of injection and may be more likely when IT morphine is utilized.[20] Numerous studies have shown a slight correlation between dose and nausea and vomiting, while others have failed to show a connection, with the mechanism likely due to the cephalad migration of drug and subsequent interaction with opioid receptors in the area postrema.[1,20] Naloxone is generally effective in the treatment of nausea and vomiting induced by IT opioids. Long-acting opioid antagonists may not be as effective in treating nausea, but there may be a benefit if given prophylactically.[24,27,32,33]

Urinary retention following IT opioids is much more common than after equivalent doses given intravenously. The incidence of urinary retention varies considerably but occurs most frequently in males.[20] Urinary retention induced by IT opioids is not dose related, may be more frequent when IT morphine is administered, and is likely related to opioid receptor-induced inhibition of sacral parasympathetic nervous system outflow, resulting in detrusor relaxation and an increase in bladder capacity.[20] Naloxone may be effective in treatment, although bladder catheterization is frequently required.[20,34]

Sedation is a dose-dependent side effect of IT opioids that occurs with all opioids.[8] The incidence may be higher with sufentanil than other opioids.[20,35,36] Respiratory depression should always be suspected when sedation occurs following IT opioids.[8,20] The difference in levels of sedation from IT, IV, and epidural routes is not well documented, but appears to be common regardless of route of delivery. Opioid receptor antagonists are effective in decreasing the level of sedation.[27] Chronic opioid use may decrease the incidence of sedation.

Herpes simplex labialis virus reactivation has been reported following IT morphine, although a causal relationship is not well established at this time.[37,38] Neuraxial (epidural) morphine has also been postulated to cause reactivation of herpes, although no mechanism has been clearly identified. Opioids reach the sensory ganglia where the herpes virus lies dormant and may reactivate the virus through an unknown interaction.[37]

There are numerous other rare side effects linked with IT opioids in the literature. Generalized muscle rigidity in a neonate was reported following IT fentanyl during cesarean delivery.[39] Muscle rigidity and myoclonic movements, not mediated by opioid receptors, are also reported in adults.[20] Nystagmus, double vision, and convulsive movements of the eyelids have been described.[17] Epileptic seizure has also been reported following an IT morphine bolus.[40] Large doses of IT morphine may cause hyperalgesia in laboratory animals.[20]

CLINICAL USES OF INTRATHECAL OPIOIDS FOR POSTOPERATIVE ANALGESIA

Numerous case reports, randomized clinical trials, and dose–response studies have been completed over the last two decades related to the use of IT opioids for postoperative pain management for a variety of procedures including obstetric, orthopedic, abdominal, pediatric, and cardiac surgeries. The great majority of trials have evaluated the use of IT morphine due to its long-lasting analgesic effects. The lipophilic opioids do play a role in postoperative analgesia; however, their relatively short duration may limit their use for single-dose IT administration in the management of postoperative pain.

There are more studies on the use of IT opioids in postoperative obstetric patients (excluding labor analgesia) than in any other patient population. In general, there has been a trend toward using lower doses of hydrophilic opioids, which provide reasonable levels of postoperative analgesia with a lower incidence of side effects (Table 28-4). Milner et al. demonstrated that 0.1 mg of IT morphine produces analgesia comparable to a dose of 0.2 mg but with significantly less nausea and vomiting.[41] A dose–response study comparing the use of

TABLE 28-4. DOSE–RESPONSE STUDIES OF INTRATHECAL MORPHINE

Study (Author, Year)	Study Population (n)	Trial Design	Doses Examined (mg)	Optimal Dose (mg)
Jacobson et al., 1988	ORTHO (33)	DB, RCT	0, 0.3, 1, 2.5	0.3–1
Boezaart et al., 1999	ORTHO (60)	DB, RCT	0.2, 0.3, 0.4	0.3
Kirson et al., 1989	GU (10)	DB, RCT	0, 0.1, 0.2	0.1
Sarma and Bostrom, 1993	GYN (80)	DB, RCT	0, 0.1, 0.3, 0.5	0.3
Yamaguchi et al., 1990	GI (139)	RCT	0, 0.04, 0.06, 0.08, 0.10, 0.12, 0.15, 0.20	0.06–0.12
Jiang et al., 1991	OB (63)	RCT	0, 0.025, 0.05, 0.075, 0.1, 0.125	0.075–0.125
Milner et al., 1996	OB (50)	RCT	0.1, 0.2	0.1
Kelly et al., 1998*	OB (80)	RCT	0, 0.125, 0.25, 0.375	–
Palmer et al., 1999	OB (108)	DB, RCT	0, 0.025, 0.05, 0.075, 0.1, 0.2, 0.3, 0.4, or 0.5	0.1
Sarvela et al., 2002	OB (150)	DB, RCT	0.1, 0.2	0.1

*Diamorphine.
DB, double blind; GI, abdominal; GU, urologic; GYN, gynecologic; OB, obstetric (cesarean section); ORTHO, orthopedics; RCT, randomized controlled trial.
Boezaart AP, Eksteen JA, Spuy GV, et al: Intrathecal morphine. Double-blind evaluation of optimal dosage for analgesia after major lumbar spinal surgery. Spine 24:1131–1137, 1999. Jacobson L, Chabal C, Brody MC: A dose–response study of intrathecal morphine: Efficacy, duration, optimal dose, and side effects. Anesth Analg 67:1082–1088, 1988. Jiang CJ, Liu CC, Wu TJ, et al: Mini-dose intrathecal morphine for post-cesarean section analgesia. Ma Zui Xue Za Zhi 29:683–689, 1991. Kelly MC, Carabine UA, Mirakhur RK: Intrathecal diamorphine for analgesia after caesarean section. A dose finding study and assessment of side-effects. Anaesthesia 53:231–237, 1998. Kirson LE, Goldman JM, Slover RB: Low-dose intrathecal morphine for postoperative pain control in patients undergoing transurethral resection of the prostate. Anesthesiology 71:192–195, 1989. Milner AR, Bogod DG, Harwood RJ: Intrathecal administration of morphine for elective Caesarean section. A comparison between 0.1 mg and 0.2 mg. Anaesthesia 51:871–873, 1996. Palmer CM, Emerson S, Volgoropolous D, et al: Dose–response relationship of intrathecal morphine for postcesarean analgesia. Anesthesiology 90:437–444, 1999. Sarma VJ, Bostrom UV: Intrathecal morphine for the relief of post-hysterectomy pain – A double-blind, dose–response study. Acta Anaesthesiol Scand 37:223–227, 1993. Sarvela J, Halonen P, Soikkeli A, et al: A double-blinded, randomized comparison of intrathecal and epidural morphine for elective cesarean delivery. Anesth Analg 95:436–440, 2002. Yamaguchi H, Watanabe S, Motokawa K, et al: Intrathecal morphine dose–response data for pain relief after cholecystectomy. Anesth Analg 70:168–171, 1990.

0.125, 0.25, or 0.375 mg of diamorphine for cesarean section demonstrated improved postoperative analgesia with the two higher doses at the cost of increasing pruritus and vomiting.[22] When comparing 0.1 mg and 0.2 mg doses of IT morphine to 3 mg of epidural morphine, Sarvela and colleagues concluded that the dose of 0.1 mg of IT morphine provided optimal postoperative analgesia for cesarean section patients.[23] A comparative study on patients undergoing cesarean section found that 0.25 mg of IT diamorphine was equivalent to 5 mg of epidural diamorphine. Sufentanil (10 μg) improves intraoperative analgesia in patients undergoing cesarean section and prolongs the duration of analgesia but at the cost of increased hypotension and pruritus.[42]

Lower extremity orthopedic cases are frequently ideal candidates for regional anesthesia and possibly IT opioids due to the presence of significant postoperative pain, which can be difficult to control. Morphine 0.3 mg IT significantly reduces pain and IV morphine patient-controlled analgesia (PCA) requirements compared to placebo following knee arthroplasty in patients undergoing bupivicaine spinal anesthesia with no significant difference in hypoxemia or apnea between the groups.[43] A dose–response study in patients undergoing major lumbar spinal surgery demonstrated that 0.3 to 0.4 mg of IT morphine provided superior analgesia compared to a dose of 0.2 mg and although the arterial carbon dioxide tension was higher in the group who received 0.4 mg of IT morphine, no clinical signs of respiratory depression were noted.[16] The use of high-dose IT morphine (10 to 20 μg/kg) has been reported to provide excellent analgesia without significant respiratory depression in patients undergoing spinal fusion with instrumentation.[44] Patients who received doses of 20 μg/kg of IT morphine remained pain free longer, required less additional narcotic, and had fewer respiratory complications.[44] Blackman et al. used a dose of 7 to 19 μg/kg in teenage patients undergoing spinal arthrodesis and found that pain relief lasted from 8 to over 40 hours, but there was a relatively high incidence (>10%) of respiratory depression as defined by an arterial carbon dioxide tension of >60 mmHg.[45] IT morphine is clearly beneficial in reducing the opioid requirements in patients undergoing orthopedic surgery, but the optimal dose is not clear. For patients who are opioid-tolerant, higher doses are probably acceptable while doses of <0.3 mg may be ideal for opioid-naive individuals.

IT opioids have also been used in cardiac surgery. While IT morphine has been demonstrated to provide pain relief following coronary artery bypass grafting (CABG), the fear of bleeding complications in a patient who is fully heparinized may have limited the use of this technique. IT opioids have been used in many studies of patients undergoing heart surgery with CABG without the development of epidural hematoma. An IT dose of 5 μg/kg morphine produces superior analgesia compared to IV PCA morphine over 24 hours in patients having off-pump CABG, although extubation times were significantly longer in the IT morphine group.[46] Alhashemi et al. also found that larger doses (0.5 mg) of IT morphine prolonged extubation time but improved analgesia.[47] They concluded that 250 μg is the optimal dose of IT morphine to provide significant postoperative analgesia without delaying tracheal extubation.[47] When compared to patients who received IV sufentanil, cardiac surgery patients who received 8 μg/kg of IT morphine had superior postoperative analgesia.[48] The differences in opioid-related side effects were similar in the two

groups and the time to extubation was nearly identical. Thus, the use of IT morphine appears to be effective in providing improved analgesia in patients undergoing cardiac surgery; however, time to extubation may be prolonged.

An ample amount of literature now exists describing the use of IT opioids in pediatric patients. It is important to note that the standard doses often used in adults may be excessive in children. In a dose–response study using 0, 2, or 5 μg/kg of IT morphine in children 9 to 19 years of age undergoing a spinal fusion the two IT opioid groups had superior postoperative analgesia, with the 2 and 5 μg/kg doses having a similar effectiveness and side-effect profile.[49] A retrospective study of 52 pediatric patients receiving either IT morphine or IV PCA nalbuphine for upper abdominal or thoracic surgery concluded that IT morphine provided superior pain relief without an increase in serious complications.[50] Although more dose–response studies are needed in pediatric patients, IT morphine in doses less than 10 μg/kg has been demonstrated to be effective in children at least 6 months of age.

IT opioid combinations will provide superior analgesia versus systemic opioids in patients undergoing vascular and thoracic procedures. Compared to those who received IV PCA morphine, patients who received a mixture of either 20 μg of sufentanil with 0.2 mg of morphine or 50 μg of sufentanil with 0.5 mg of morphine have improved pain control with minimal side effects other than an increased frequency of urinary retention.[7,10] Although epidural analgesia with local anesthetics and opioids is likely superior to IT opioids in decreasing pulmonary complications after thoracotomy,[51] IT opioids may be a good alternative to epidural analgesia in situations where an epidural catheter cannot be maintained.

IT opioids have been demonstrated to provide excellent analgesia in abdominal procedures. A dose–response trial evaluating doses of IT morphine ranging from 0 to 0.2 mg in patients undergoing cholecystectomy concluded that 0.06 to 0.12 mg was the optimal dose range for maximal analgesia with minimal side effects such as respiratory depression, vomiting, or pruritus.[9] The use of low-dose IT morphine (0.075 to 0.1 mg) in providing adequate postoperative pain control was confirmed in a subsequent study.[52] Low-dose (0.1 mg) IT morphine was also found to be adequate for the relief of pain in postpartum women undergoing tubal ligation.[53] For abdominal hysterectomy, a dose of 0.1 mg of IT morphine was found to be ineffective and a dose of 0.3 mg was recommended as providing superior analgesia with the fewest side effects.

ADJUVANTS TO INTRATHECAL OPIOIDS

Numerous studies have been published that have used other IT agents in combination with IT opioids to improve analgesia while minimizing side effects. Most of these adjuncts are analgesics that do not interact with opioid receptors. Other adjunct agents are used to alleviate or prevent side effects of IT opioids, but may have varying degrees of analgesic properties.

Clonidine, an alpha-2 receptor agonist, has been used to improve analgesia in combination with IT opioids as well as IT local anesthetics. Clonidine increases the duration of sensory and motor blockade from bupivicaine spinal anesthesia through several mechanisms.[54] Alpha-2 adrenergic agonists administered intrathecally may increase the antinociceptive threshold by activating descending noradrenergic pathways in the spinal cord.[55] This inhibits nociceptive neuron firing in the substantia gelatinosa and inhibits spinal substance P release.[55] Alpha-2 receptors mediating spinal analgesia are postsynaptic. The clinical data on the analgesic interaction between clonidine and opioids are equivocal. Grace and colleagues did not demonstrate any additional pain relief when 75 μg of IT clonidine was coadministered with 0.5 mg of IT morphine.[55] Another study also failed to demonstrate a benefit from the addition of oral clonidine to IT morphine.[56] In contrast, using a lower dose of IT morphine, Goyagi and Nishikawa demonstrated a decreased requirement for supplemental analgesia in patients receiving 5 μg/kg of oral clonidine.[57] Gautier et al. found that 30 μg of clonidine combined with 2.5 to 5 μg of sufentanil produced significantly longer analgesia than sufentanil alone.[36] A review of the current data suggests that clonidine is more likely to improve analgesia when combined with lower doses of IT morphine rather than large doses. Most of the evidence indicates that lower doses of 15 to 30 μg may be equally efficacious as larger doses while decreasing side effects including sedation, hypotension, and bradycardia. Although the mechanism of potentiation appears to be mediated in the spinal cord, oral and IV administration of clonidine may also be effective in conjunction with IT opioids.[57]

SUMMARY

IT opioids have been shown to be a safe and effective method of postoperative pain control. The benefit of long-lasting, noncyclic pain relief obtained with IT hydrophilic opioids, along with the lack of hemodynamic effects and motor blockade, makes this an excellent option for some patients. Adverse reactions, including nausea, vomiting, pruritus, respiratory depression, urinary retention, and sedation, should be monitored in patients receiving IT opioids and may be easily treated with currently available pharmacologic agents. The wide variety of surgical procedures that can benefit from IT opioids offers many opportunities for their use. It is certainly not the ideal technique in many cases, but when used appropriately it can have great benefit to patients.

KEY POINTS

- The pharmacologic properties of IT opioids reflect the extent of the hydro- versus lipophilicity of the specific opioid: lipophilic opioids (fentanyl and sufentanil) have a shorter onset and duration of action whereas hydrophilic opioids (morphine) have a delayed onset and prolonged duration of action (and certain side effects such as delayed respiratory depression).
- Like opioids administered by other routes, IT opioids may result in widely recognized opioid-related side effects such as nausea, vomiting, pruritus, sedation, and respiratory depression. The incidence of respiratory depression from clinically relevant doses of IT opioids is not greater than that given by other routes. Frequent monitoring of patients who have received IT opioids is recommended; however, the need for an intensive care-like unit setting for postoperative monitoring of these patient is controversial.
- Delayed respiratory depression is more likely with use of hydrophilic opioids; however, it is much less likely with the currently clinically used doses which are lower than those used one to two decades previously. The following factors may contribute to the development of respiratory depression

after IT opioid administration: opioid-naive state, concurrent use of systemic opioids or sedatives, increasing age, and sleep or obstructive sleep apnea.

REFERENCES

1. Cousins MJ, Mather LE: Intrathecal and epidural administration of opioids. Anesthesiology 61:276–310, 1984.
2. Grass JA: Sufentanil: Clinical use as postoperative analgesic – Epidural/intrathecal route. J Pain Symptom Manage 7:271–286, 1992.
3. Hansdottir V, Hedner T, Woestenborghs R, et al: The CSF and plasma pharmacokinetics of sufentanil after intrathecal administration. Anesthesiology 74:264–269, 1991.
4. Ngan Kee WD: Intrathecal pethidine: Pharmacology and clinical applications. Anaesth Intensive Care 26:137–146, 1998.
5. Dahström B: Pharmacokinetic and pharmacodynamics of epidural and intrathecal morphine. Int Anesthesiol Clin 24:29–42, 1986.
6. Sjöstrom S, Tamsen A, Persson MP, et al: Pharmacokinetics of intrathecal morphine and meperidine in humans. Anesthesiology 67:889–895, 1987.
7. Liu N, Kuhlman G, Dalibon N, et al: A randomized, doubleblinded comparison of intrathecal morphine, sufentanil and their combination versus IV morphine patient-controlled analgesia for postthoracotomy pain. Anesth Analg 92:31–36, 2001.
8. Bailey PL, Rhondeau S, Schafer PG, et al: Dose–response pharmacology of intrathecal morphine in human volunteers. Anesthesiology 79:49–59, 1993.
9. Yamaguchi H, Watanabe S, Motokawa K, et al: Intrathecal morphine dose–response data for pain relief after cholecystectomy. Anesth Analg 70:168–171, 1990.
10. Mason N, Gondret R, Junca A, et al: Intrathecal sufentanil and morphine for post-thoracotomy pain relief. Br J Anaesth 86:236–240, 2001.
11. Sarma VJ, Boström UV: Intrathecal morphine for the relief of post-hysterectomy pain – double blind, dose–response study. Acta Anaesthesiol Scand 37:223–227, 1993.
12. Chaney MA, Smith KR, Barclay JC, et al: Large-dose intrathecal morphine for coronary artery bypass grafting. Anesth Analg 83:215–222, 1996.
13. Slappendel R, Weber EW, Benraad B, et al: Itching after intrathecal morphine: Incidence and treatment. Eur J Anaesthesiol 17:616–621, 2000.
14. Mulroy MF, Larkin KL, Siddiqui A: Intrathecal fentanyl-induced pruritus is more severe in combination with procaine than with lidocaine or bupivacaine. Reg Anesth Pain Med 26:252–256, 2001.
15. Clergue F, Montembault C, Despierres O, et al: Respiratory effects of intrathecal morphine after upper abdominal surgery. Anesthesiology 61:677–685, 1984.
16. Boezaart AP, Eksteen JA, Spuy GV, et al: Double-blind evaluation of optimal dosage for analgesia after major lumbar spinal surgery. Spine 24:1131–1137, 1999.
17. Krenn H, Jellinek H, Haumer H, et al: Naloxone-resistant respiratory depression and neurologic eye symptoms after intrathecal morphine. Anesth Analg 91:432–433, 2000.
18. Ferouz F, Norris MC, Leighton BL: Risk of respiratory arrest after intrathecal sufentanil. Anesth Analg 85:1088–1090, 1997.
19. Etches RC: Respiratory depression associated with patient-controlled analgesia: A review of eight cases. Can J Anaesth 41:125–132, 1994.
20. Chaney MA: Side effects of intrathecal and epidural opioids. Can J Anaesth 42:891–903, 1995.
21. Johnson A, Bengtsson M, Soderlind K, et al: Influence of intrathecal morphine and naloxone intervention on postoperative ventilatory regulation in elderly patients. Acta Anaesthesiol Scand 36:436–444, 1992.

22. Kelly MC, Carabine UA, Mirakhur RK: Intrathecal diamorphine for analgesia after Cesarean section. Anaesthesia 53:231–237, 1998.

23. Sarvela J, Halonen P, Soikkeli A, et al: A double-blinded, randomized comparison of intrathecal and epidural morphine for elective Cesarean delivery. Anesth Analg 95:436–440, 2002.

24. Ozalp G, Guner F, Kuru N, et al: Postoperative patient-controlled epidural analgesia with opioid bupivicaine mixtures. Can J Anaesth 45:938–942, 1998.

25. Wilson DJ, Douglas MJ: Neuraxial opioids in labour. Baillière's Clin Obstet Gynaecol 12:363–376, 1998.

26. Hallworth SP, Fernando R, Bell R, et al: Comparison of intrathecal and epidural diamorphine for elective Caesarean section using a combined spinal-epidural technique. Br J Anaesth 82:228–232, 1999.

27. Abboud TK, Lee K, Zhu J, et al: Prophylactic oral naltrexone with intrathecal morphine for Cesarean section: Effects on adverse reactions and analgesia. Anesth Analg 71:367–370, 1990.

28. Charuluxananan S, Kyokong O, Somboonviboon W, et al: Nalbuphine versus propofol for treatment of intrathecal morphine-induced pruritus after Cesarean delivery. Anesth Analg 93:162–165, 2001.

29. Johnson A, Bengtsson M, Loftstrom JB, et al: Influence of postoperative naloxone infusion on respiration and pain relief after intrathecal morphine. Reg Anesth 13:146–151, 1988.

30. Borgeat A, Stirnemann HR: Ondansetron is effective to treat spinal or epidural morphine-induced pruritus. Anesthesiology 90:432–436, 1990.

31. Yeh HM, Chen LK, Lin CJ, et al: Prophylactic intravenous ondansetron reduces the incidence of intrathecal morphine-induced pruritus in patients undergoing Cesarean delivery. Anesth Analg 91:172–175, 2000.

32. Ward RC, Lawrence RL, Hawkins RJ, et al: The use of nalmefene for intrathecal opioid-associated nausea in postpartum patients. AANA J 70:57–60, 2002.

33. Pellegrini JE, Bailey SL, Graves J, et al: The impact of nalmefene on side effects due to intrathecal morphine at Cesarean section. AANA J 69:199–205, 2001.

34. Niemi L, Pitkanen MT, Tuominen MK, et al: Comparison of intrathecal fentanyl infusion with intrathecal morphine infusion or bolus for postoperative pain relief after hip arthroplasty. Anesth Analg 77:126–130, 1993.

35. Nelson KE, Rauch T, Terebuh V, et al: A comparison of intrathecal fentanyl and sufentanil for labor analgesia. Anesthesiology 96:1070–1073, 2002.

36. Gautier PE, De Kock M, Fanard L, et al: Intrathecal clonidine combined with sufentanil for labor analgesia. Anesthesiology 88:651–656, 1998.

37. Ross A: Intrathecal morphine and herpes reactivation. Anaesth Intensive Care 21:126, 1993.

38. Pennant JH: Intrathecal morphine and reactivation of oral herpes simplex. Anesthesiology 15:167, 1991.

39. Bolisetty S, Kitchanan S, Whitehall J: Generalized muscle rigidity in a neonate following intrathecal fentanyl during Caesarean delivery. Intensive Care Med 25:1337, 1999.

40. Kronenberg MF, Laimer I, Rifici C, et al: Epileptic seizure associated with intracerebroventricular and intrathecal morphine bolus. Pain 75:383–387, 1998.

41. Milner AR, Bogod DG, Harwood RJ: Intrathecal administration of morphine for elective Caesarian section: A comparison between 0.1 mg and 0.2 mg. Anaesthesia 51:871–873, 1998.

42. Lin BC, Lin PC, Lai YY, et al: The maternal and fetal effects of the addition of sufentanil to 0.5% spinal bupivacaine for Cesarean delivery. Acta Anesthesiol Sin 36:143–148, 1998.

43. Cole PJ, Craske DA, Wheatley RG: Efficacy and respiratory effects of low-dose spinal morphine for postoperative analgesia following knee arthroplasty. Br J Anaesth 85:233–237, 2000.

44. Urban MK, Jules-Elysee K, Urquhart B, et al: Reduction in postoperative pain after spinal fusion with instrumentation using intrathecal morphine. Spine 27:535–537, 2002.

45. Blackman RG, Reynolds J, Shively J: Intrathecal morphine: Dosage and efficacy in younger patients for control of postoperative pain following spinal fusion. Orthopaedics 14:555–557, 1991.

46. Jara FM, Kalush J, Kilaru V: Intrathecal morphine for off-pump coronary artery bypass patients. Heart Surgery Forum 4:57–60, 2001.

47. Alhashemi JA, Sharpe MD, Harris CL, et al: Effect of subarachnoid morphine administration on extubation time after coronary artery bypass graft surgery. J Cardiothorac Vasc Anesth 14:639–644, 2000.

48. Zarate E, Latham P, White PF, et al: Fast-track cardiac anesthesia: Use of remifentanil combined with intrathecal morphine as an alternative to sufentanil during desflurane anesthesia. Anesth Analg 91:283–287, 2000.

49. Gall O, Aubineau JV, Berniere J, et al: Analgesic effect of low-dose intrathecal morphine after spinal fusion in children. Anesthesiology 94:447–452, 2001.

50. Krechel SW, Helikson MA, Kittle D, et al: Intrathecal morphine for postoperative pain control in children: A comparison with nalbuphine patient controlled analgesia. Paediatric Anaesth 5:177–183, 1995.

51. Ballantyne JC, Carr DB, deFerranti S, et al: The comparative effects of postoperative analgesic therapies on pulmonary outcome: Cumulative meta-analyses of randomized, controlled trials. Anesth Analg 86:598–612, 1998.

52. Motamed C, Bouaziz H, Franco D, et al: Analgesic effect of low-dose intrathecal morphine and bupivacaine in laparoscopic cholecystectomy. Anesthesia 55:118–124, 2000.

53. Campbell DC, Riben CM, Rooney ME, et al: Intrathecal morphine for postpartum tubal ligation postoperative analgesia. Anesth Analg 93:1006–1011, 2001.

54. Brunschwiler M, Van Gessel E, Forster A, et al: Comparison of clonidine, morphine or placebo mixed with bupivacaine during continuous spinal anaesthesia. Can J Anaesth 45:735–740, 1998.

55 Grace D, Bunting H, Milligan KR, et al: Postoperative analgesia after co-administration of clonidine and morphine by the intrathecal route in patients undergoing hip replacement. Anesth Analg 80:86–91, 1995.

56. Mayson KV, Gofton EA, Chambers KG: Premedication with low dose oral clonidine does not enhance postoperative analgesia of intrathecal morphine. Can J Anaesth 47:752–757, 2000.

57. Goyagi T, Nishikawa Y: Oral clonidine premedication enhances the quality of postoperative analgesia by intrathecal morphine. Anesth Analg 82:1192–1196, 1996.

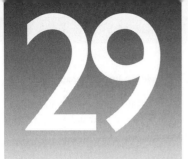

Epidural Opioids for Postoperative Pain

Zenobia Casey, M.D., and
Christopher L. Wu, M.D.

The use of epidural opioids, either as a single injection or continuous infusion, is an important analgesic option for the treatment of postoperative pain. The clinician can choose from a range of available epidural opioids, each with its own pharmacokinetic profile that allows titration to the specific clinical scenario. Despite some of the side effects associated with epidural opioid administration, there are many advantages of using epidural opioids for analgesia including some data that suggest an improvement in some clinically oriented patient outcomes.

PHARMACOLOGY OF EPIDURAL OPIOIDS

An opioid administered into the epidural space will diffuse into the surrounding tissues including epidural fat and veins. Opioids that diffuse into epidural fat are no longer available to bind to opioid receptors and thus cannot produce analgesia. Opioids administered into the epidural space can generally produce analgesia via two mechanisms (spinal and supraspinal/systemic analgesia). To produce supraspinally mediated analgesia, epidural opioids may be absorbed into plasma and redistributed to the brainstem via the bloodstream.[1] To produce spinally mediated analgesia, epidural opioids must diffuse through the spinal meninges (dura mater and, more importantly, arachnoid mater) into the cerebrospinal fluid (CSF). The interactions between the physiochemical properties of the spinal meninges and epidural opioids are complex and the permeability of an epidurally administered opioid through the spinal meninges is dependent on many factors including the lipid solubility of the opioid.[1] Once inside the CSF, epidural opioids interact with spinal opioid receptors located in lamina II of the dorsal horn of the spinal cord and achieve antinociception via presynaptic reduction of afferent neurotransmitter release and postsynaptic hyperpolarization of dorsal horn neurons.

One of the key pharmacologic properties of an epidurally administered opioid that determines its analgesic and side-effect profile is the extent of its lipophilicity. After single-dose epidural administration, lipophilic opioids, such as fentanyl and sufentanil, generally have a relatively faster onset but shorter duration of action when compared to that of more hydrophilic opioids such as morphine and hydromorphone. The extent of lipophilicity also affects the side-effect profile of the individual opioid with relatively rapid clearance from the CSF of lipophilic opioids which may limit the development of certain side effects such as delayed respiratory depression.[2,3]

Unlike opioids that are injected intrathecally and expected to produce analgesia via a spinal mechanism, epidural opioids do not consistently produce analgesia predominantly through a spinal mechanism. The degree to which lipophilic opioids produce analgesia via a spinal or supraspinal mechanism is still somewhat controversial.[1,4] Although some data suggest that epidural fentanyl for labor analgesia may produce a selective spinal analgesic effect,[1,5] it is generally thought that lipophilic opioids (especially when administered in a continuous infusion) will produce analgesia primarily by systemic uptake and redistribution of the lipophilic opioid to brainstem opioid receptors.[1] The systematic nature of epidurally administered lipophilic opioid is especially obvious when a continuous infusion is used for a prolonged period of time.[6] On the other hand, it is clear that the primary analgesic site of action for hydrophilic opioids is selectively spinal.[7,8] Once the epidurally administered hydrophilic opioid has penetrated the dural membrane into the CSF, the opioid will remain within the CSF to produce spinal analgesia and spread cephalad or rostrally in the CSF (due in part to its low lipid solubility) to act at the brainstem.[8] The rostral spread of hydrophilic opioid to the brainstem may be associated with facial pruritus, nausea, and sedation.[9]

INJECTION OF SINGLE-DOSE EPIDURAL OPIOIDS

A single-dose injection of neuraxial opioids can provide effective postoperative analgesia as a sole analgesic agent or in combination with other agents (e.g., local anesthetics or alpha-2 agonists); however, the analgesic profile (duration of analgesia and side effects) is dependent primarily on the degree of lipophilicity (versus hydrophilicity) with hydrophilic agents such as morphine and hydromorphone producing a longer duration of analgesia versus lipophilic agents such as fentanyl and sufentanil. The pharmacokinetic differences in analgesia between the hydrophilic and lipophilic opioid should be tailored to the surgical procedure to optimize analgesia and minimize side effects. For instance, a single injection of a hydrophilic opioid like morphine typically provides 12 to 18 hours of analgesia and would be useful for postoperative analgesia in surgical inpatients with appropriate monitoring of side effects. In outpatient surgery a lipophilic opioid like fentanyl may be more appropriate, as its analgesic onset is more rapid and duration of action is shorter (thus minimizing the risk of delayed respiratory depression) than hydrophilic opioids.

Both lipophilic and hydrophilic opioids may provide effective postoperative analgesia when administered in a single dose. When compared to intravenous fentanyl boluses, epidural fentanyl given via an epidural bolus for the first 20 hours after surgery has been shown to provide adequate pain relief as well as inhibiting physiologic, hormonal, and metabolic responses observed in the postoperative period as indicated by lower blood glucose levels, arterial blood pressure, and plasma cortisol levels.[10] A single epidural bolus of a lipophilic opioid like fentanyl may be administered to provide a rapid (onset within 5 to 10 minutes) but relatively transient (up to 4 hours) postoperative analgesia. Diluting the epidural dose of fentanyl (typically 50 to 100 µg) in at least 10 mL of preservative-free normal saline may hasten onset and prolong the duration of analgesia possibly as a result of an increase in the initial spread and diffusion of fentanyl.[2,11]

A single epidural dose of a hydrophilic opioid is especially efficacious for prolonged postoperative analgesia.[12] Epidural morphine when administered as a single bolus has been shown

to provide effective postoperative analgesia for a variety of procedures including cesarean sections and major abdominal vascular surgery.[12,13] Combining a hydrophilic opioid (e.g., morphine) and a lipophilic opioid (e.g., sufentanil) in a single epidural injection combines the short onset time produced by the lipophilic opioid and the long duration of analgesia produced by the hydrophilic opioid.[14]

Epidural analgesia may also provide preemptive analgesia, provided by administering an analgesic prior to nociceptive stimuli.[15] Epidural opioids given preoperatively in conjunction with ketamine result in a reduction in postoperative pain interventions, including an increase in epidural dosing.[16] Epidural administration (either as a single shot or continuous infusion) of a hydrophilic opioid is especially effective in scenarios where the epidural catheter location is not congruent with the surgical incision (e.g., lumbar epidural catheter for thoracic surgery). The doses of epidural morphine may need to be decreased for elderly patients and thoracic catheter sites.[2,17,18] Commonly used dosages for epidural administration of opioids are provided in Table 29-1.

CONTINUOUS INFUSION OF EPIDURAL OPIOIDS

Continuous infusions of epidural opioids will provide effective postoperative pain control for a variety of surgical procedures. When used alone for postoperative pain control, analgesic infusions of epidural opioids will not generally cause motor block or hypotension from sympathetic blockade which may be seen in patients receiving a local anesthetic-based epidural regimen.[19] Similar to that seen with single-dose administration, there are important clinical differences between continuous epidural infusions of lipophilic (fentanyl, sufentanil) and hydrophilic (morphine, hydromorphone) opioids.

Although the precise site of analgesic action (spinal versus supraspinal/systemic) for continuous epidural infusions of lipophilic opioids has not yet been elucidated, many randomized controlled trials suggest that the epidural infusions of lipophilic opioids produce analgesia primarily via a supraspinal/systemic mechanism.[20–22] In these trials there were no differences in plasma concentrations, side effects, or pain scores between those receiving either intravenous or epidural infusions of fentanyl.[20,21] Despite the presence of a trial suggesting a benefit of continuous epidural infusions of fentanyl,[23] the overall advantage of administering continuous epidural infusions of lipophilic opioids alone is minimal with the possible exception of obstetric analgesia.[1,19]

On the other hand, continuous epidural infusions of hydrophilic opioids produce analgesia primarily via a spinal mechanism.[24] Similar to that seen with single-dose epidural administration of a hydrophilic opioid, continuous infusions of hydrophilic opioids may be particularly effective in providing postoperative pain control where either the epidural catheter insertion is not congruent with the site of surgery or side effects (e.g., hypotension, motor block) limit the ability to use an epidural local anesthetic-based analgesic regimen. Use of a continuous epidural infusion of morphine may provide superior analgesia when compared to systemic opioids[6,25] or intermittent boluses of epidural morphine.[24,26]

Although continuous infusions of epidural opioids may be used alone and are effective in controlling postoperative pain, continuous infusions of epidural opioids are more commonly

TABLE 29-1. COMMON DOSES OF EPIDURAL OPIOIDS*

	Single Dose	Continuous Infusion
Fentanyl	50–100 µg	25–100 µg/hour
Sufentanil	10–50 µg	10–20 µg/hour
Alfentanil	0.5–1 mg	0.2 mg/hour
Morphine	1–5 mg	0.1–1 mg/hour
Diamorphine	4–6 mg	–
Hydromorphone	0.5–1 mg	0.1–0.2 mg/hour
Meperidine	20–60 mg	10–60 mg/hour
Methadone	4–8 mg	0.3–0.5 mg/hour

* Doses based on use of neuraxial opioid alone. Lower doses may be effective when administered to the elderly or when injected in the cervical or thoracic region.

administered in conjunction with a local anesthetic. This combination may confer analgesic advantages over infusions using either a local anesthetic alone or opioid alone although the incidence of side effects may or may not be diminished.[9,27–29] The choice of opioid varies among clinicians: many will choose to use a lipophilic opioid (fentanyl 2 to 5 μg/mL or sufentanil 0.5 to 1 μg/mL) as part of a patient-controlled epidural analgesic regimen to allow for rapid titration of analgesia;[2,19,24] however, use of a hydrophilic opioid (morphine 0.05 to 0.1 mg/mL or hydromorphone 0.01 to 0.05 mg/mL) as part of a local anesthetic–opioid epidural analgesic regimen may also provide effective postoperative analgesia.[2,24]

SIDE EFFECTS OF EPIDURAL OPIOIDS

Similar to that seen when administered systemically, epidural opioids exhibit side effects of respiratory depression, pruritus, nausea, and vomiting. Many of these side effects appear to be dose dependent; however, the side-effect profile is slightly different between lipophilic and hydrophilic epidural opioids. Hypotension is rarely directly attributable to epidural opioids and the difference in heart rate and mean arterial blood pressure between systemic opioid and epidural opioid administration is minimal.[30] It is important to always consider other causes for the side effects (e.g., hypovolemia and bleeding for hypotension) before automatically attributing the etiology to epidural opioids. In addition, standing orders and nursing protocols for monitoring of neurologic status (e.g., sensory and motor function) and side effects with physician notification of critical parameters should be standard for all patients receiving continuous infusions of epidural opioids.

Respiratory Depression: Respiratory depression may occasionally occur after administration of epidural opioids. Respiratory depression associated with epidural (and intrathecal) administration of opioids is dose dependent and the incidence is typically reported from 0.1% to 0.9%.[31–36] The incidence of respiratory depression with epidural opioids (when used in appropriate doses) is not higher than that seen with systemic administration of opioids. Use of continuous infusions of epidural opioids also is not associated with a higher incidence of respiratory depression than that seen after systemic opioid administration.[31,36] There is some controversy as to whether patients receiving continuous epidural infusions of hydrophilic opioids need intensive care-like monitoring to detect respiratory depression; however, several large-scale studies have demonstrated the relative safety of continuous epidural infusions of hydrophilic opioids on regular surgical wards where the incidence of respiratory depression was less than 0.9%.[32,35,37,38] Factors that may increase the risk of developing respiratory depression in patients who have received epidural opioids include thoracic surgery, presence of comorbidities, increasing age, an opioid-naive state, and concomitant use of systemic opioids and sedatives.[36]

There are differences in the respiratory depressant profile between epidural lipophilic and hydrophilic opioids. Lipophilic opioids administered in the epidural space are associated with early (typically within 2 hours of administration) rather than later (more than 2 hours after administration) respiratory depression as lipophilic opioids are rapidly absorbed systemically from the epidural venous plexus and delivered to the brain and respiratory centers; thus, the onset and resolution of respiratory depression from lipophilic opioids occurs relatively quickly.

On the other hand, the onset of respiratory depression after epidural administration of hydrophilic opioids is generally slower than that seen with epidural administration of lipophilic opioids. Hydrophilic epidural opioids are primarily delivered to the brain via relatively slower rostral migration in the CSF rather than the more rapid systemic absorption of lipophilic opioids. Cephalad spread of hydrophilic opioids typically occurs within 12 hours following injection.[36] Respiratory depression from epidural administration of hydrophilic opioids can occur later, typically within 6 to 12 hours after injection. Assessing the patient's respiratory rate alone may not be a reliable predictor of a patient's ventilatory status or impending respiratory depression.[33] Administration of naloxone (0.1 to 0.4 mg increments) is generally effective in reversing respiratory depression; however, a continuous infusion of naloxone (0.5 to 5 μg/kg/hour) may be needed since the duration of action of naloxone is shorter than that of the respiratory depressant effect of epidural opioids.[2,36]

Nausea and Vomiting: Nausea and vomiting occurs in 20% to 50% of patients after a single dose of epidural opioid[9,39,40] and the overall incidence in those receiving continuous infusions of epidural opioids is reported at 45% to 80%.[41–43] The development of opioid-induced nausea and vomiting after administration of epidural opioids appears to be dose dependent.[44–46] Nausea and vomiting from epidural opioids is the result of interaction with opioid receptors in the area postrema and chemotactic trigger zone of the medulla. With epidurally administered hydrophilic opioids, nausea and vomiting may be related to the cephalad migration of opioid within the CSF to the area postrema in the medulla.[9] Treatment of epidural opioid-induced nausea and vomiting may include the use of naloxone, droperidol, metaclopramide, dexamethasone, transdermal scopolamine, and even a small dose of propofol.[41,47–49]

Pruritus: The etiology of epidural opioid-induced pruritus is unclear and may be related to activation of an "itch center" in the medulla, interaction with opioid receptors in the trigeminal nucleus or nerve roots, or changes in the sensory modulation of the trigeminal and upper cervical spinal cord with cephalad migration of the opioid; however, opioid-induced pruritus does not appear to be associated with peripheral histamine release.[9] Pruritus from epidural opioids may occur in as many as 60% of patients compared to a 15% to 18% incidence with systemic opioid use.[50–52] Whether epidural opioid-induced pruritus is dose dependent is uncertain with some systematic data indicating no evidence of a dose-dependent relationship[50] but other studies suggesting the presence of such a relationship.[53,54] Naloxone, naltrexone, nalbuphine, and droperidol appear to be effective in the treatment of epidural opioid-induced pruritus.[51] Use of epidural morphine is associated with postpartum reactivation of herpes simplex labialis.[55]

Urinary Retention: Administration of epidural opioids may result in urinary retention which is related to a decrease in detrusor muscle strength contraction secondary to spinal opioid receptor activation.[9] When compared to that administered systemically (approximately 18%),[9,50] the incidence of urinary retention from epidurally administered opioids appears to be much higher (70% to 80%).[53,56] The development of urinary

TABLE 29-2. OUTCOMES STUDIES OF EPIDURAL MORPHINE VERSUS SYSTEMIC OPIOIDS FOR POSTOPERATIVE ANALGESIA

Study (Author, Year)	Study Population (n)	Trial Design	Morbidity (EA vs. SYST)	Mortality (EA vs. SYST)
Park et al., 2001	ABD (1021)	RCT	22% vs. 37%*	Combined data
Tsui et al., 1997	ABD–THOR (578)	RCT	EA improved pulmonary (EA: 13% vs. 25%; $P = 0.002$) and CV (EA: 21% vs. 43%; $P < 0.001$) outcomes and LOS (EA: 22 ± 20 vs. 30 ± 37; $P = 0.005$)	EA: 8% vs. 14%; $P = 0.038$
Major et al., 1996	ABD (65)	OBS	Improvement in EA for CV ($P = 0.0002$) and pulmonary ($P = 0.019$) outcomes and LOS ICU ($P = 0.024$)	None reported
Liu et al., 1995	ABD (54)	RCT	No difference in GI recovery between epidural and systemic opioids	None reported
Beattie et al., 1993	Mixed (55)	RCT	Improvement in EA for CV ischemia (EA: 17.2% vs. 50%; $P = 0.01$) and tachyarrhythmias (EA: 20.7% vs. 50%; $P < 0.05$)	None reported
Her et al., 1990	ABD (49)	OBS	Improvement in EA for need for ventilatory support ($P = 0.0002$), respiratory failure ($P = 0.018$), and LOS ICU (EA: 2.7 days vs. 3.8 days; $P = 0.003$)	None reported
Hasenbos et al., 1987	THOR (129)	RCT	Improvement in EA for pulmonary complications (EA: 12.1% vs. 38%)	
Rawal, 1984	ABD	RCT	Improvement in EA for pulmonary complications (EA: 13% vs. 40%), GI function (EA: 56.7 ± 3.1 hours vs. 75.1 ± 3.1 hours; $P < 0.05$), and LOS (EA: 7 ± 0.5 days vs. 9 ± 0.6 days; $P < 0.05$)	None reported

* Data represented are a subgroup (aortic aneurysm repair) of the study which showed no overall difference. Morbidity and mortality data combined.

ABD, abdominal surgery; CV, cardiovascular; EA, epidural morphine analgesia; GI, gastrointestinal; ICU, intensive care unit; LOS, length of stay; OBS, observational trial; RCT, randomized controlled trial; SYST, systemic opioid analgesia; THOR, thoracic surgery.

Beattie WS, Buckley DN, Forrest JB: Epidural morphine reduces the risk of postoperative myocardial ischaemia in patients with cardiac risk factors. Can J Anaesth 40:532–541, 1993. Hasenbos M, van Egmond J, Gielen M, et al: Post-operative analgesia by high thoracic epidural versus intramuscular nicomorphine after thoracotomy: III. The effects of per- and post-operative analgesia on morbidity. Acta Anaesthesiol Scand 31:608–615, 1987. Her C, Kizelshteyn G, Walker V, et al: Combined epidural and general anesthesia for abdominal aortic surgery. J Cardiothorac Anesth 4:552–557, 1990. Liu SS, Carpenter RL, Mackey DC, et al: Effects of perioperative analgesic technique on rate of recovery after colon surgery. Anesthesiology 83:757–765, 1995. Major CP Jr, Greer MS, Russell WL, et al: Postoperative pulmonary complications and morbidity after abdominal aneurysmectomy: A comparison of postoperative epidural versus parenteral opioid analgesia. Am Surg 62:45–51, 1996. Park WY, Thompson JS, Lee KK: Effect of epidural anesthesia and analgesia on perioperative outcome: A randomized, controlled Veterans Affairs cooperative study. Ann Surg 234:560–569, 2001. Rawal N, Sjostrand V, Christoffersson E, Dahlstrom B, Awill A, Rydman H. Comparison of intramuscular and epidural morphine for postoperative analgesia in the grossly obese: influence on postoperative ambulation and pulmonary function. Anesth Analg 63:583–92, 1984. Tsui SL, Law S, Fok M, et al: Postoperative analgesia reduces mortality and morbidity after esophagectomy. Am J Surg 173:472–478, 1997.

retention does not appear to be dose dependent.[56,57] Low-dose naloxone may be effective in treating epidural opioid-induced urinary retention but at the risk of reversing analgesia.[58]

PATIENT OUTCOMES AND EPIDURAL MORPHINE

The use of a local anesthetic-based epidural anesthetic–analgesic technique is associated with a decrease in perioperative morbidity and mortality.[59] The analgesic and physiologic benefits of a local anesthetic-based epidural solution may be attributed in part to the attenuation or even complete suppression of perioperative pathophysiology. Unlike local anesthetics, use of an opioid-based epidural analgesic solution typically can only confer partial attenuation of perioperative pathophysiology despite the superior analgesia provided by epidural morphine versus systemic opioids. Thus, the effect of epidural morphine on patient outcomes may not be as apparent when compared to that using a local anesthetic-based solution.

Administration of epidural morphine may modify the perioperative stress response, although to a lesser extent when compared to local anesthetics.[60] Unlike that seen with local anesthetics, use of epidural morphine will still allow transmission of nociceptive information through the central nervous system. Because of the inability to suppress completely the neuroendocrine stress response, epidural opioids do not consistently prevent the perioperative increases in cortisol, epinephrine, or glucose but may attenuate increases in levels of norepinephrine.

Despite the fact that epidural morphine can only partially attenuate perioperative pathophysiology, there are data suggesting an improvement in patient outcomes with the perioperative use of epidural morphine compared to systemic opioids (Table 29-2). Some relatively large-scale randomized trials suggest that epidural morphine for postoperative analgesia may decrease perioperative mortality.[61–63] Randomized data also suggest that postoperative epidural morphine analgesia when compared to systemic opioids may decrease both cardiovascular and pulmonary complications.[61–64] In addition, a meta-analysis examining the effects of various analgesic regimens on pulmonary outcomes revealed that use of epidural morphine (versus systemic opioids) will decrease the incidence of postoperative atelectasis.[65] However, use of epidural morphine either alone or as part of a local anesthetic–morphine infusion does not facilitate return of postoperative gastrointestinal function when compared to systemic opioids.[59]

SUMMARY

Epidurally administered opioids are a valuable analgesic option in the treatment of postoperative pain. The lipid solubility of the specific epidural opioid is a primary determinant of its clinical analgesic (and side-effect) profile. Single-dose hydrophilic opioids can provide prolonged pain relief in an inpatient surgical population whereas lipophilic opioids will provide postoperative pain relief of a shorter duration. Continuous infusions of hydrophilic opioid alone provide effective postoperative analgesia even when the catheter insertion site is not congruent to the incision site. Continuous infusions of lipophilic opioid alone will not provide a selective spinal site of action but because of the titratability, lipophilic opioid infusions

are most commonly seen as part of a local anesthetic–opioid solution in patient-controlled epidural analgesia. Hydrophilic opioids, particularly morphine, may improve patient outcomes especially in high-risk patients.

KEY POINTS

- As seen with intrathecal opioids, the pharmacologic properties of epidurally administered opioids reflect the extent of the hydro- versus lipophilicity of the specific opioid: lipophilic opioids (fentanyl and sufentanil) have a shorter onset and duration of action whereas hydrophilic opioids (morphine, hydromorphone) have a delayed onset and prolonged duration of action (and certain side effects such as delayed respiratory depression).
- Epidural opioids exhibit the same side effects (respiratory depression, pruritus, nausea, and vomiting) as opioids given systemically. Many of these side effects appear to be dose dependent; however, the side-effect profile is slightly different between lipophilic and hydrophilic epidural opioids. The incidence of respiratory depression is similar regardless of the route of administration (epidural versus systemic). Certain groups of patients may be at higher risk for developing respiratory depression after epidural administration of opioids.
- The clinician should consider the analgesic and side-effect profile of epidural lipophilic and hydrophilic opioids and tailor these for individual clinical scenarios (e.g., avoiding a long-acting hydrophilic opioid such as morphine for ambulatory surgery).
- Unlike neuraxially administered local anesthetics, use of epidural morphine can only partially attenuate perioperative pathophysiology. However, perioperative use of epidural morphine (versus systemic opioids) may result in an improvement in patient outcomes such as cardiovascular–pulmonary complications and even mortality in some studies.

REFERENCES

1. Bernards CM: Understanding the physiology and pharmacology of epidural and intrathecal opioids. Best Prac Res Clin Anaesthesiol 16:489–505, 2002.
2. Grass JA: Epidural analgesia. Problems in Anesthesia 10:45–67, 1998.
3. Hamber EA, Viscomi CM: Intrathecal lipophilic opioids as adjuncts to surgical spinal anesthesia. Reg Anesth Pain Med 24:255–263, 1999.
4. Cooper DW: Can epidural fentanyl induce elective spinal hyperalgesia? Anesthesiology 93:1153, 2000.
5. D'Angelo R, Gerancher JC, Eisenach JC, et al: Epidural fentanyl produces labor analgesia by a spinal mechanism. Anesthesiology 88:1519–1523, 1998.
6. Loper KA, Ready LB: Epidural morphine after anterior cruciate ligament repair: A comparison with patient-controlled intravenous morphine. Anesth Analg 68:350–352, 1989.
7. Bernards CM: Rostral spread of epidural morphine: The expected and the unexpected. Anesthesiology 92:299–301, 2000.
8. Angst MS, Ramaswamy B, Riley ET, et al: Lumbar epidural morphine in humans and supraspinal analgesia to experimental heat pain. Anesthesiology 92:312–324, 2000.
9. Chaney MA: Side effects of intrathecal and epidural opioids. Can J Anaesth 42:891–903, 1995.

10. Salomaki TE, Leppaluoto J, Laitinen JO: Epidural versus intravenous fentanyl for reducing hormonal, metabolic, and physiologic responses after thoracotomy. Anesthesiology 79:672–679, 1993.

11. Birnbach DJ, Johnson MD, Arcario T, et al: Effect of diluent volume on analgesia produced by epidural fentanyl. Anesth Analg 68:808–810, 1989.

12. Fuller JG, McMorland GH, Douglas MJ, et al: Epidural morphine for analgesia after cesarean section: A report of 4880 patients. Can J Anaesth 37:636–640, 1990.

13. Connelly NR, DuBose R, Brull SJ: Use of single-dose epidural morphine in a patient undergoing an abdominal aortic aneurysm resection. J Clin Anesth 2:272–275, 1990.

14. Dottrens M, Rifat K, Morel DR: Comparison of extradural administration of sufentanil, morphine and sufentanil–morphine combination after caesarean section. Br J Anaesth 69:9–12, 1992.

15. Subramaniam B, Pawar DK, Kashyap L: Pre-emptive analgesia with epidural morphine or morphine and bupivacaine. Anaesth Intensive Care 28:392–398, 2000.

16. Subramaniam K, Subramaniam B, Pawar DK, et al: Evaluation of the safety and efficacy of epidural ketamine combined with morphine for postoperative analgesia after major upper abdominal surgery. J Clin Anesth 13:339–344, 2001.

17. Ready LB, Chadwick HS, Ross B: Age predicts effective epidural morphine dose after abdominal hysterectomy. Anesth Analg 66:1215–1218, 1987.

18. Mulroy MF: Epidural opioid delivery methods: Bolus, continuous infusion, and patient-controlled epidural anesthesia. Reg Anesth 21(6S):100–104, 1996.

19. Wheatley RG, Schug SA, Watson D: Safety and efficacy of postoperative epidural analgesia. Br J Anaesth 87:47–61, 2001.

20. Loper KA, Ready LB, Downey M, et al: Epidural and intravenous fentanyl infusions are clinically equivalent after knee surgery. Anesth Analg 70:72–75, 1990.

21. Sandler AN, Stringer D, Panos L, et al: A randomized, double-blind comparison of lumbar epidural and intravenous fentanyl infusions for postthoracotomy pain relief. Analgesic, pharmacokinetic, and respiratory effects. Anesthesiology 77:626–634, 1992.

22. Guinard JP, Mavrocordatos P, Chiolero R, et al: A randomized comparison of intravenous versus lumbar and thoracic epidural fentanyl for analgesia after thoracotomy. Anesthesiology 77:1108–1115, 1992.

23. Salomaki TE, Laitinen JO, Nuutinen LS: A randomized double-blind comparison of epidural versus intravenous fentanyl infusion for analgesia after thoracotomy. Anesthesiology 75:790–795, 1991.

24. de Leon-Casasola OA, Lema MJ: Postoperative epidural opioid analgesia: What are the choices? Anesth Analg 83:867–875, 1996.

25. Malviya S, Pandit UA, Merkel S, et al: A comparison of continuous epidural infusion and intermittent intravenous bolus doses of morphine in children undergoing selective dorsal rhizotomy. Reg Anesth Pain Med 24:438–443, 1999.

26. Rauck RL, Raj PP, Knarr DC, et al: Comparison of the efficacy of epidural morphine given by intermittent injection or continuous infusion for the management of postoperative pain. Reg Anesth 19:316–324, 1994.

27. Jorgensen H, Wetterslev J, Moiniche S, et al: Epidural local anaesthetics versus opioid-based analgesic regimens on postoperative gastrointestinal paralysis, PONV and pain after abdominal surgery. Cochrane Database Syst Rev 4:CD001893, 2000.

28. Hjortso NC, Lund C, Mogensen T, et al: Epidural morphine improves pain relief and maintains sensory analgesia during continuous epidural bupivacaine after abdominal surgery. Anesth Analg 65:1033–1036, 1986.

29. Vercauteren M, Meert TF: Isobolographic analysis of the interaction between epidural sufentanil and bupivacaine in rats. Pharmacol Biochem Behav 58:237–242, 1997.

30. Correll D, Viscusi E, Grunwald Z, et al: Epidural analgesia compared with intravenous morphine patient-controlled analgesia: Postoperative outcome measures after mastectomy with immediate TRAM flap breast reconstruction. Reg Anesth Pain Med 26:444–449, 2001.

31. Etches RC: Respiratory depression associated with patient-controlled analgesia: A review of eight cases. Can J Anaesth 41:125–132, 1994.

32. de Leon-Casasola OA, Parker B, Lema MJ, et al: Postoperative epidural bupivacaine–morphine therapy. Experience with 4,227 surgical cancer patients. Anesthesiology 81:368–375, 1994.

33. Bailey PL, Rhondeau S, Schafer PG, et al: Dose–response pharmacology of intrathecal morphine in human volunteers. Anesthesiology 79:49–59, 1993.

34. de Leon-Casasola OA, Parker BM, Lema MJ, et al: Epidural analgesia versus intravenous patient-controlled analgesia. Differences in the postoperative course of cancer patients. Reg Anesth 19:307–315, 1994.

35. Ready LB, Loper KA, Nessly M, et al: Postoperative epidural morphine is safe on surgical wards. Anesthesiology 75:452–456, 1991.

36. Mulroy MF: Monitoring opioids. Reg Anesth 21(6S):89–93, 1996.

37. Stenseth R, Sellevold O, Breivik H: Epidural morphine for postoperative pain: Experience with 1085 patients. Acta Anaesthesiol Scand 29:148–156, 1985.

38. Rygnestad T, Borchgrevink PC, Eide E: Postoperative epidural infusion of morphine and bupivacaine is safe on surgical wards. Organisation of the treatment, effects and side-effects in 2000 consecutive patients. Acta Anaesthesiol Scand 41:868–876, 1997.

39. Wang JJ, Tzeng JI, Ho ST, et al: The prophylactic effect of tropisetron on epidural morphine-related nausea and vomiting: a comparison of dexamethasone with saline. Anesth Analg 94:749–753, 2002.

40. Tzeng JI, Hsing CH, Chu CC, et al: Low-dose dexamethasone reduces nausea and vomiting after epidural morphine: A comparison of metoclopramide with saline. J Clin Anesth 14:19–23, 2002.

41. Gedney JA, Liu EH: Side-effects of epidural infusions of opioid bupivacaine mixtures. Anaesthesia 53:1148–1155, 1998.

42. White MJ, Berghausen EJ, Dumont SW, et al: Side effects during continuous epidural infusion of morphine and fentanyl. Can J Anaesth 39:576–582, 1992.

43. Nakata K, Mammoto T, Kita T, et al: Continuous epidural, not intravenous, droperidol inhibits pruritus, nausea, and vomiting during epidural morphine analgesia. J Clin Anesth 14:121–125, 2002.

44. Kelly MC, Carabine UA, Mirakhur RK: Intrathecal diamorphine for analgesia after caesarean section. A dose finding study and assessment of side-effects. Anaesthesia 53:231–237, 1998.

45. Milner AR, Bogod DG, Harwood RJ: Intrathecal administration of morphine for elective Caesarean section. A comparison between 0.1 mg and 0.2 mg. Anaesthesia 51:871–873, 1996.

46. Kirson LE, Goldman JM, Slover RB: Low-dose intrathecal morphine for postoperative pain control in patients undergoing transurethral resection of the prostate. Anesthesiology 71:192–195, 1989.

47. Choi JH, Lee J, Choi JH, et al: Epidural naloxone reduces pruritus and nausea without affecting analgesia by epidural morphine in bupivacaine. Can J Anaesth 47:33–37, 2000.

48. Moscovici R, Prego G, Schwartz M, et al: Epidural scopolamine administration in preventing nausea after epidural morphine. J Clin Anesth 7:474–476, 1995.

49. Borgeat A, Wilder-Smith OH, Saiah M, et al: Subhypnotic doses of propofol relieve pruritus induced by epidural and intrathecal morphine. Anesthesiology 76:510–512, 1992.

50. Walder B, Schafer M, Henzi I, et al: Efficacy and safety of patient-controlled opioid analgesia for acute postoperative pain.

A quantitative systematic review. Acta Anaesthesiol Scand 45:795–804, 2001.

51. Kjellberg F, Tramer MR: Pharmacological control of opioid-induced pruritus: A quantitative systematic review of randomized trials. Eur J Anaesthesiol 18:346–357, 2001.

52. Bucklin BA, Chestnut DH, Hawkins JL: Intrathecal opioids versus epidural local anesthetics for labor analgesia: A meta-analysis. Reg Anesth Pain Med 27:23–30, 2002.

53. Ko MC, Naughton NN: An experimental itch model in monkeys: Characterization of intrathecal morphine-induced scratching and antinociception. Anesthesiology 92:795–805, 2000.

54. Herman NL, Choi KC, Affleck PJ, et al: Analgesia, pruritus, and ventilation exhibit a dose–response relationship in parturients receiving intrathecal fentanyl during labor. Anesth Analg 89:378–383, 1999.

55. Slappendel R, Weber EW, Dirksen R, et al: Optimization of the dose of intrathecal morphine in total hip surgery: A dose-finding study. Anesth Analg 88:822–826, 1999.

56. Boyle RK: A review of anatomical and immunological links between epidural morphine and herpes simplex labialis in obstetric patients. Anaesth Intensive Care 23:425–432, 1995.

57. O'Riordan JA, Hopkins PM, Ravenscroft A, et al: Patient-controlled analgesia and urinary retention following lower limb joint replacement: Prospective audit and logistic regression analysis. Eur J Anaesthesiol 17:431–435, 2000.

58. Wang J, Pennefather S, Russell G: Low-dose naloxone in the treatment of urinary retention during extradural fentanyl causes excessive reversal of analgesia. Br J Anaesth 80:565–566, 1998.

59. Liu S, Carpenter RL, Neal JM: Epidural anesthesia and analgesia. Their role in postoperative outcome. Anesthesiology 82:1474–1506, 1995.

60. Kehlet H: Modification of responses to surgery by neural blockade. In Cousins MJ, Bridenbaugh PO (eds): Neural Blockade in Clinical Anesthesia and Management of Pain, ed 3. Lippincott-Raven, Philadelphia, 1998, p 129.

61. Tsui SL, Law S, Fok M, et al: Postoperative analgesia reduces mortality and morbidity after esophagectomy. Am J Surg 173:472–478, 1997.

62. Park WY, Thompson JS, Lee KK: Effect of epidural anesthesia and analgesia on perioperative outcome: A randomized, controlled Veterans Affairs cooperative study. Ann Surg 234:560–569, 2001.

63. Hasenbos M, van Egmond J, Gielen M, et al: Post-operative analgesia by high thoracic epidural versus intramuscular nicomorphine after thoracotomy: III. The effects of per- and postoperative analgesia on morbidity. Acta Anaesthesiol Scand 31:608–615, 1987.

64. Beattie WS, Buckley DN, Forrest JB: Epidural morphine reduces the risk of postoperative myocardial ischaemia in patients with cardiac risk factors. Can J Anaesth 40:532–541, 1993.

65. Ballantyne JC, Carr DB, deFerranti S, et al: The comparative effects of postoperative analgesic therapies on pulmonary outcome: Cumulative meta-analyses of randomized, controlled trials. Anesth Analg 86:598–612, 1998.

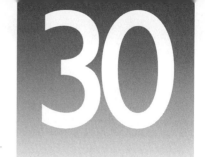
Intraarticular and Intraperitoneal Opioids for Postoperative Pain

Kenneth D. Candido, M.D.,

Antoun Nader, M.D., and

Honorio T. Benzon, M.D.

INTRAARTICULAR OPIOIDS

The use of arthroscopic techniques in orthopedic surgery has gained a preeminent role as diagnostic and therapeutic procedures for the knee, hip, ankle, shoulder, and hand. Arthroscopy is typically an outpatient procedure, and although touted as being less painful than open surgical procedures, is nevertheless associated with postoperative pain that is at times severe. Oral and systemic analgesics, including opioids and nonsteroidal anti-inflammatory drugs (NSAIDs), have been used with varying degrees of success to combat postoperative pain, but with various attendant side effects also reported. The intraarticular (IA) injection of local anesthetics and adjuvants has been considered efficacious in modulating postoperative pain, but support for their routine use is limited. IA local anesthetics have demonstrated modest, and short-acting efficacy in a systematic review of the literature.[1] Mu-agonist opioids, most notably morphine, have support for use in moderate to severe pain when administered IA, but whether the resultant analgesia is due to a local or systemic effect is debatable.[2–5] NSAIDs have consistently demonstrated a benefit in modulating postoperative pain when injected IA, yet there is a concern that they may inhibit or retard bone healing. The use of the alpha-2 agonist clonidine IA has demonstrated a modest and limited reduction in postoperative pain, although the same controversy exists as to whether these benefits are mediated systemically or are local phenomena. Other agents, such as ketamine, corticosteroids, and neostigmine, are currently undergoing IA trials but current support for their use is sparse.

Intraarticular Morphine: Morphine is the prototypical mu-receptor opioid agonist to which all other opioids are compared.

In humans morphine produces analgesia, sedation, euphoria, and a reduction in the ability to concentrate on a task. Other sensations include nausea, subjective feeling of warmth, dry mouth, and pruritis, particularly perinasally. Systemically administered morphine increases pain thresholds and modifies the perception of noxious stimulation. In contrast to nonopioid analgesics, morphine is effective against pain arising from visceral structures in addition to that arising from skeletal muscles, joints, and integument. Peak effect occurs in about 45 to 90 minutes, and duration of action is about 4 hours.

A significant number of papers have been dedicated to the injection of IA morphine sulfate, most notably into the knee joint following diagnostic arthroscopy. This subject has produced significant controversy in the published literature: some investigators demonstrated a benefit to IA morphine following knee arthroscopy[6–9] while others did not.[10–14] Niemi et al. in a randomized and double-blinded study showed that the need for postoperative ketoprofen was less after 1 mg morphine compared to IA saline.[15] Khoury et al. demonstrated that morphine alone or combined with bupivacaine IA provided postoperative analgesia of delayed onset but of remarkably long duration, and longer than that provided by IA bupivacaine alone.[16] Similar results were observed by Jaureguito et al.[17] The injection of local anesthetic (bupivacaine) and morphine after knee surgery provided superior analgesia than either agent alone.[18] In another study the combination of morphine and bupivacaine IA provided superior postoperative analgesia when compared to IA saline, IA morphine, or IA bupivacaine, as determined by pain scores (visual analogue scale, VAS) and analgesic use.[19]

IA morphine may not provide comparable analgesia to that provided by continuous peripheral nerve blocks following surgical arthroscopy of the knee. When IA morphine (1 mg) was compared to IA bupivacaine or continuous lumbar plexus (3-in-1) blocks for postoperative analgesia after knee arthroscopy, the lumbar plexus blocks were found to be superior to the IA morphine or IA local anesthetic.[20]

Other local anesthetics besides bupivacaine have also been compared to IA morphine. When compared to IA morphine alone (1 or 5 mg) or morphine plus ropivacaine (5 mg and 75 mg), IA ropivacaine alone (150 mg) was noted to provide superior analgesia after knee arthroscopy but only in the early postoperative period.[21] No difference was noted in the pain scores or the tramadol consumption between the groups by 24 and 48 hours postoperatively.[21]

Other adjuvant agents such as clonidine and ketorolac were compared to morphine, either alone or in combination with morphine. A combination of clonidine (1 μg/kg), 30 mL of bupivacaine (0.25%), and morphine (3 mg) provided superior postoperative analgesia compared to the IA bupivacaine or either adjunct used in combination with the local anesthetic.[22] In comparison, ketorolac and morphine administered together IA did not improve postoperative analgesia when compared to either agent given alone IA, although both proved efficacious in reducing postoperative pain after arthroscopic meniscus repair.[23] Another study compared IA morphine/bupivacaine with IA morphine/bupivacaine combined with systemic (intramuscular) diclofenac (75 mg). The group who received the combination therapy demonstrated the lowest VAS scores and lowest postoperative fentanyl use after knee arthroscopy.[24]

A nonpharmacologic adjunct to IA morphine was suggested by Whitford et al. They found that analgesia was superior in a group of patients in whom the thigh tourniquet was maintained for 10 minutes after the IA morphine administration.[25] The optimum analgesic dose of IA morphine appears to be 1 to 2 mg.[26] Doses up to 5 mg have been used, but do not appear to confer any specific advantage to more modest ones. As to the optimal time of administering morphine IA for knee surgery, it was found that analgesia was superior when the IA morphine (3 mg) was given before incision compared to its administration postoperatively.[27]

The type of arthroscopic knee surgery may be a factor in determining the efficacy of IA morphine. A prospective, randomized, double-blind study compared "low inflammatory surgery" (arthroscopy, menisectomy) and "high inflammatory surgery" (anterior cruciate ligament (ACL) reconstruction, lateral release, patellar shaving, plicae removal).[28] IA bupivacaine (25 mL, 0.25%), morphine (5 mg), or saline was administered at the end of surgery and postoperative pain scores and ketorolac usage were followed. Bupivacaine IA proved more effective in mediating pain in the "low inflammatory" group while morphine IA was better in the "high inflammatory" group. The results are interesting in that the selection of the IA agent may depend on the nature of the surgical procedure.[28] Earlier studies showed the efficacy of IA morphine after ACL ("high inflammatory") surgery.[29,30] Unfortunately, other studies showed no benefit from IA morphine following ACL reconstruction when compared to femoral nerve block,[31] epidural block,[32] or multimodal analgesia using NSAIDs, external cooling, and IA bupivacaine.[33]

There is some controversy in interpreting the literature on the efficacy of IA morphine after arthroscopic knee surgery. In an attempt to clarify the apparent discrepancies, Jadad et al. described a 5-point qualitative scale to assess the efficacy of this intervention.[3] In a subsequent review of the literature assessing the IA effects of morphine, Kalso and co-workers noted only four studies that scored more than 4 points on this 5-point scale.[2] These investigators did not perform a meta-analysis of the information since they believed there was a lack of an adequate number of high-quality studies. Their conclusion was that morphine probably had a mild effect on postoperative pain when injected IA in humans. In the review by Gupta et al. all human studies were included in their meta-analysis unless there was compelling reason to exclude them.[4] Their analysis led them to conclude that a definite but mild analgesic effect of morphine was evident for up to 24 hours postoperatively. Furthermore, they felt that this analgesic effect was probably not dose dependent, nor could a systemic effect of IA morphine be excluded. A recent review by Kalso et al. looked at all studies in which the postoperative pain was ≥5 on a 10-point VAS.[5] In doing so, they excluded all studies wherein the postoperative pain intensity was "mild." They concluded that IA morphine has definite analgesic properties in cases where postoperative pain intensity is moderate to severe. On the other hand, Meiser and Laubenthal argued that their review of 34 randomized, controlled studies concerning IA morphine after knee surgery would not support meta-analysis of the data since study designs differ substantially.[34]

Any study that attempts to promulgate an antinociceptive action of IA morphine (or similar mu-agonist opioids) should hypothesize its mechanism of action. Stein et al. used immunocytochemistry and autoradiography and found that synovial opioid peptides and opioid receptors are abundant in pronounced synovitis. Furthermore, they deduced that opioids expressed in inflamed tissues do not produce tolerance to peripheral morphine analgesia, and that there is no major downregulation of peripheral opioid receptors. They extrapolated this information to suggest that IA opioids might have a role in mediating chronic arthritis pain and other inflammatory conditions.[35] Keates et al. used radioligand binding to determine whether opioid binding sites could be induced during inflammatory states produced in the radiocarpal joints of canines.[36] They found that opioid binding site densities in articular and periarticular tissues in inflammatory states were approximately 100 times larger than the respective published densities in brain tissues, leading them to speculate that the use of IA opioids has a scientifically valid basis.[36] Similar findings were noted in a study using a rat model of inflammation that demonstrated the potency of IA morphine did not diminish during the onset of induced arthritis.[37] Perfusion of inflamed rat knee joints with exogenous endorphin-1 produced a significant reduction in synovial vascular permeability and a fall in protein exudation. Destruction of knee joint unmyelinated afferent nerve fibers by capsaicin treatment significantly attenuated the anti-inflammatory effects of endorphin-1, suggesting that the peptide (and, hence, perhaps exogenously administered opioid analgesics) acts via a neurogenic mechanism.[38]

The effects of IA opioids may be mediated through the G-protein-coupled receptors affecting the cAMP pathway. Elvenes et al., using immunodetection polymerase chain reaction and Western blotting, demonstrated that human osteoarthritic cartilage and cultured chondrocytes possess the mu-opioid receptor. Stimulation of chondrocytes with beta-endorphin resulted in decreased phosphorylation of the transcription factor cAMP responsive element binding protein (CREB), an effect reversible by naloxone.[39] Studies such as these have led other investigators to hypothesize that IA morphine might be beneficial in the treatment paradigm of patients suffering from chronic arthritis states. Indeed, synovial leukocyte counts are reduced following IA morphine but not following IA saline, indicating that morphine may have anti-inflammatory effects in chronic osteoarthritis of the knee.[40] Likar et al. found in a double-blind, cross-over study that IA morphine provided outstanding and long-lasting analgesia in patients suffering from chronic ostoearthritis of the knee.[41]

Morphine has been used IA following other types of surgical procedures besides knee arthroscopy, including total knee arthroplasty (TKA),[42] rotator cuff repair,[43] shoulder arthroscopy,[44] and ankle arthroscopy.[45] In a group of 37 patients undergoing TKA, IA morphine 1 mg and postoperative intravenous patient-controlled analgesia (PCA) was compared to epidural morphine and a PCA only group. There was no difference between the three groups with regard to VAS scores, morphine requirements, or stress hormone levels, indicating that IA morphine for TKA offers no benefit over epidural analgesia or PCA analgesia.[42] Following open rotator cuff repair under interscalene brachial plexus block, three groups of patients received IA boluses of 0.25% bupivacaine with 1 mg morphine, 50 μg fentanyl, or 10 μg sufentanil added. The IA morphine proved superior to the other two opioids with regard to pain scores and rescue opioid doses over the first 24 hours.[43] However, following shoulder arthroscopy for subacromial decompression in 32 patients, IA morphine 5 mg was only equivalent to a saline IA injection.[44] The difference in the results following shoulder surgery may represent a preferential effect of morphine in the "high inflammatory" surgeries (open procedures) compared to "low inflammatory" states (arthroscopy). When IA morphine was added as a component of multimodal analgesia following arthroscopic ankle surgery, there was a significant reduction in pain, joint swelling, time of immobilization, duration of sick leave, and return to physical activity. Attributing the success of this modality to the morphine (5 mg) is limited by the fact that the morphine was added to bupivacaine (15 mg) and methylprednisolone (40 mg). Which of these adjuncts was most efficacious or how the combination was more successful than either agent alone was not investigated.[45]

In summary, there is significant clinical evidence that supports the use of IA morphine following certain types of knee manipulation, including arthroscopic surgery.

Intraarticular Meperidine: Meperidine is a synthetic opioid agonist at mu and kappa opioid receptors derived from phenylepiperidine. Several analogues are derived from meperidine including fentanyl, sufentanil, alfentanil, and remifentanil. Structurally, meperidine is similar to atropine, and it possesses a mild atropine-like antispasmodic effect. It is about one-tenth as potent as morphine and its duration of pharmacologic action is about 2 to 4 hours.

Meperidine has been injected IA in doses of 10 to 200 mg, alone or in combination with local anesthetics and tenoxicam. In a study comparing IA local anesthetic (lidocaine 2%) plus meperidine (10 mg) with local anesthetic plus meperidine (10 mg) and tenoxicam (20 mg) the authors found that the latter regimen provided superior pain relief from 4 hours postoperatively onwards.[46] A study limitation includes the lack of a control local anesthetic group. Westman et al. conducted a series of studies on IA meperidine for knee and ankle arthroscopy analgesia. They compared IA meperidine to

prilocaine in ankle arthroscopy. The use of IA meperidine resulted in lower VAS pain scores at rest but not during movement.[47] When IA or intramuscular meperidine (10 mg) was compared to morphine (1 mg) or fentanyl (10 μg) for knee arthroscopy, no difference between the groups was noted although there was a tendency for improved analgesia in the IA meperidine group.[48] The same group demonstrated that IA meperidine was superior to prilocaine for analgesia following knee arthroscopy, at least in the 100 mg and 200 mg meperidine groups.[49] However, there was significant systemic absorption and side effects at these doses, negating any definitive determination as to whether or not the effects were centrally mediated or locally mediated. In another study by the same investigators IA meperidine (200 mg) was compared to meperidine plus epinephrine and a control group receiving IA local anesthetic only for knee arthroscopy.[50] Epinephrine did not extend additional benefit to the meperidine group, which had the best analgesia 1 to 4 hours postoperatively. It appears from the studies by Westman et al. that IA meperidine is effective following knee surgery in doses of about 100 to 200 mg. It is not certain whether the local anesthetic properties of meperidine influenced the results or whether a systemic effect resulted from the generous doses (200 mg) used in the studies.

Intraarticular Fentanyl: Fentanyl is a phenylpiperidine derivative synthetic opioid agonist that is structurally related to meperidine. As an analgesic, fentanyl is about 75 to 100 times more potent than morphine. A single dose of fentanyl administered intravenously has a more rapid onset than morphine and a shorter duration of clinical effect, although the elimination half-life is longer than that of morphine.

IA fentanyl has been studied in doses ranging from 10 to 100 μg. IA bupivacaine was noted to provide superior analgesia compared to IA fentanyl in the immediate postoperative period, for up to 2 hours, following knee arthroscopy. There was no difference in the analgesic efficacy between the two groups after 2 hours.[51] In direct comparison to IA morphine, IA fentanyl does not appear to confer particular advantages for postoperative analgesia after knee arthroscopy. While Varkel et al. showed that fentanyl 50 μg IA was superior to 3 mg morphine IA beginning 1 hour postoperatively and persisting up to 8 hours, the postoperative pain in both treatment groups was rated as mild, and the difference in VAS pain scores was not significant.[52] Soderlund et al. used small IA doses of fentanyl (10 μg), morphine (1 mg), or meperidine (10 mg) for knee arthroscopy and found no difference in the postoperative analgesia between the different opioids.[48] This study included 7 groups of 10 patients each, including a placebo group control, and no parameter was significantly different between any of the groups studied. When compared to 1 mg morphine IA, fentanyl 100 μg IA failed to provide equivalent analgesia for up to 48 hours postoperatively when either agent was added to 10 mL of 0.25% bupivacaine following knee arthroscopy.[53]

It might be expected that sufentanil would provide results similar to those of fentanyl when used IA since sufentanil is a thienyl analogue of fentanyl. However, sufentanil has a greater affinity for opioid receptors than fentanyl, and is about 12 times as potent.[54] Sufentanil is extensively protein bound (92.5% vs. fentanyl at 79% to 87%) and is highly lipid soluble. Its elimination half-life is intermediate between that of fentanyl and alfentanil.[55] Vranken et al.[56] compared IA sufentanil, 5 or 10 μg, and intravenous saline vs. IA saline and intravenous sufentanil 5 µg for knee arthroscopy. The IA sufentanil significantly reduced pain levels and postoperative consumption of analgesics. The larger dose of sufentanil (10 µg) did not provide additional analgesia over the smaller dose.[56]

In conclusion, IA fentanyl analgesia in doses up to 100 µg or sufentanil up to 5 µg both appear to be modestly successful in modulating nociception after knee arthroscopy. However, the studies to date do not justify their routine inclusion in periarticular injectates, particularly when compared to IA morphine.

INTRAPERITONEAL OPIOIDS

Unlike the studies on IA opioids where several clinical studies were performed, there is little clinical evidence supporting the use of opioid analgesics via the intraperitoneal (IP) route. Many studies on IP analgesia have been conducted in animals, and extrapolation to the human postsurgical arena is at best tentative. IP opioids have been studied following laparoscopic gynecologic surgery, laparoscopic cholecystectomy, and open intraabdominal procedures. Results are inconclusive in the majority of cases.

Animal Studies Supporting Intraperitoneal Opioid Administration: Niv et al. hypothesized that the simultaneous application of morphine intrathecally and intraperitoneally would produce a synergistic effect, similar to that noted when morphine is given simultaneously into the spinal cord and cerebral ventricles.[57] Using male Wistar rats, they determined that there was a supraadditive antinociceptive effect of the combined therapy.[57] Intrathecal and IP remifentanil, alfentanil, and morphine were examined in a rat model tested for hind-paw thermal withdrawal latency. All opioids demonstrated a dose-dependent analgesic response after intrathecal or IP administration. The order of IP potencies in the study was remifentanil > alfentanil > morphine, while the duration of analgesia was morphine >> alfentanil > remifentanil.[58] The side-effect profiles were best with morphine > alfentanil > remifentanil.[58] The clinical significance of these findings may be simply that the highly lipid-soluble agents are potent analgesics when administered IP, but are also associated with greater risk. Reichert et al. evaluated possible preemptive analgesic effect of IP opioids in a mouse visceral pain model. While a potent antinociceptive effect was demonstrated by IP morphine administered prior to IP acetic acid (a frequently used model of inflammation), intravenous morphine had no effect when given preemptively. This supports the concept of IP opioids acting during inflammatory states via a peripheral opioid receptor mechanism.[59] The IP administration of the N-methyl-D-aspartate (NMDA) antagonist ketamine in rats resulted in a synergistic effect to spinally administered fentanyl as assessed by the tail-flick test, but not by the electrical current threshold test.[60] In that study, IP ketamine served as a chemical cofactor to augment spinal analgesia induced by fentanyl. IP fentanyl, morphine, and oxycodone all reduced tail-flick latency in a group of male Wistar rats that was significantly more potent when the simultaneous IP administration of the neurosteroid alphadolone accompanied each agent. The steroid alone had no effect as an antinociceptive agent when given IP, implying that certain agents may augment IP antinociception produced by opioids.[61]

Human Studies on Intraperitoneal Opioids: IP opioids have been used following laparoscopic cholecystectomy,[62–64] laparoscopic gynecologic surgery,[65,66] and after open intraabdominal procedures.[67]

Schulte-Steinberg et al.[62] found that neither interpleural nor IP morphine administration reduced analgesic requirements following laparoscopic cholecystectomy surgery. In their study of 110 patients in 6 groups, only interpleural bupivacaine (0.25%, 30 mL) proved efficacious in that regard. O'Hanlon et al.,[63] however, noted a reduction in pain scores and analgesic requirements in a group of 46 patients who received IP meperidine plus bupivacaine compared to a similar group who received the meperidine intramuscularly plus IP bupivacaine. The only adverse effect noted was an increased rate of nausea in the IP meperidine group.[63] In a double-blind, randomized study IP bupivacaine (0.25%, 30 mL) and morphine (2 mg) was shown to provide early (first 6 hours postoperatively) analgesia superior to IP saline or IP bupivacaine plus intravenous morphine.[64] After the first 6 hours, however, the analgesia was superior in the group who received IP bupivacaine and intravenous morphine.[64] In summary, some studies support the use of IP morphine or meperidine after laparoscopic cholecystectomy, while another study suggests that interpleural analgesia is superior to IP opioid administration.

Morphine and meperidine have also been used following laparoscopic gynecologic surgery. In patients undergoing tubal ligation surgery, Colbert et al.[65] noted that a combination of IP meperidine (50 mg) and bupivacaine (0.125%, 80 mL) resulted in lower pain scores than IP bupivacaine and intramuscular meperidine. On the other hand, Keita et al.[66] did not observe improvement in pain scores or analgesic requirements when 3 mg morphine was added to 20 mL bupivacaine 0.5% IP in a group of patients who underwent laparoscopic gynecologic surgery.

In a randomized study wherein IP morphine 50 mg was administered to 15 patients undergoing major abdominal surgery the analgesia was inferior to that provided by the same dose of morphine given intravenously.[67] The one benefit of the IP morphine was a reduction in morphine-6-glucuronide levels when compared to intravenous morphine, implying a difference in pharmakokinetics between the two routes of administration.[67]

In summary, a few clinical studies supported the use of IP meperidine after laparoscopic procedures. The role of IP morphine after laparoscopic and major abdominal surgeries is not well defined because of the scarcity of clinical data.

KEY POINTS

- IA morphine has been shown to provide improved analgesia after knee arthroscopy when compared to local anesthetic alone or to saline placebo.
- IA morphine may be more beneficial for use in "high inflammatory" arthroscopic knee surgery (e.g., anterior cruciate ligament reconstruction, lateral release, patella shaving, and plicae removal) than for use in "low inflammatory" surgery (knee arthroscopy for meniscectomy).
- IA morphine has not shown promising results after shoulder arthroscopy or total knee arthroplasty, and its use following ankle arthroscopy remains to be defined.
- IA fentanyl, sufentanil, and meperidine have less support for use following arthroscopic surgery than does the use of IA morphine.

- There is some suggestion that IP meperidine plus bupivacaine is beneficial following laparoscopic cholecystectomy and gynecologic surgery.
- The IP administration of morphine has not been demonstrated in human studies to exert a beneficial effect following laparoscopic surgery.

REFERENCES

1. Møiniche S, Mikkelsen S, Wetterslev J, et al: A systematic review of intra-articular local anesthesia for postoperative pain relief after arthroscopic knee surgery. Reg Anesth Pain Med 24:430–437, 1999.
2. Kalso E, Tramer MR, Carroll D, et al: Pain relief from intra-articular morphine after knee surgery: A qualitative systematic review. Pain 71:127–134, 1997.
3. Jadad AR, Moore RA, Carroll D, et al: Assessing the quality of reports of randomized clinical trials: Is blinding necessary? Control Clin Trials 17:1–12, 1996.
4. Gupta A, Bodin L, Holmstrom B, et al: A systematic review of the peripheral analgesic effects of intraarticular morphine. Anesth Analg 93:761–770, 2001.
5. Kalso E, Smith L, McQuay HJ, et al: No pain, no gain: Clinical excellence and scientific rigor – Lessons learned from IA morphine. Pain 98:269–275, 2002.
6. Stein C, Comisel K, Haimerl E, et al: Analgesic effect of intra-articular morphine after arthroscopic knee surgery. N Engl J Med 325:1123–1126, 1991.
7. Joshi GP, McCarroll SM, O'Brien TM, Lenane P: Intraarticular analgesia following knee arthroscopy. Anesth Analg 76:333–336, 1993.
8. Heine MF, Tillet ED, Tsueda K, et al: Intra-articular morphine after arthroscopic knee operation. Br J Anaesth 73:413–415, 1994.
9. Kanbak M, Akpolat N, Ocal T, et al: Intraarticular morphine administration provides pain relief after knee arthroscopy. Eur J Anaesthesiol 14:153–156, 1997.
10. Heard SO, Edwards WT, Ferrari D, et al: Analgesic effect of intraarticular bupivacaine or morphine after arthroscopic knee surgery: A randomized, prospective, double-blind study. Anesth Analg 74:822–826, 1992.
11. Raja SN, Dickstein RE, Johnson CA: Comparison of postoperative analgesia effects of intraarticular bupivacaine and morphine following arthroscopic knee surgery. Anesthesiology 77:1143–1147, 1992.
12. Ruwe PA, Klein I, Shields CL: The effect of intraarticular injection of morphine and bupivacaine on postarthroscopic pain control. Am J Sports Med 23:59–64, 1995.
13. Hege-Scheuing G, Michaelsen K, Buhler A, et al: Analgesia with intra-articular morphine following knee joint arthroscopy? A double-blind, randomized study with patient-controlled analgesia. (German) Anaesthesist 44:351–358, 1995.
14. Christensen O, Christensen P, Sonnenschein C, et al: Analgesic effect of intraarticular morphine. A controlled, randomised and double-blind study. Acta Anaesthesiol Scand 40:842–846, 1996.
15. Niemi L, Pitkanen M, Tuomenen M, et al: Intraarticular morphine for pain relief after knee arthroscopy performed under regional anesthesia. Acta Anaesthesiol Scand 38:402–405, 1994.
16. Khoury GF, Chen AC, Garland DE, Stein C: Intraarticular morphine, bupivacaine, and morphine/bupivacaine for pain control after knee videoarthroscopy. Anesthesiology 77:263–266, 1992.
17. Jaureguito JW, Wilcox JF, Cohn SJ, et al: A comparison of intraarticular morphine and bupivacaine for pain control after outpatient knee arthroscopy. A prospective, randomized, double-blind study. Am J Sports Med 23:350–353, 1995.
18. Allen GC, St Amand MA, Lui AC, et al: Postarthroscopy analgesia with intraarticular bupivacaine/morphine. A randomized clinical trial. Anesthesiology 79:475–480, 1993.
19. Boden BP, Fassler S, Cooper S, et al: Analgesic effect of intra-articular morphine, bupivacaine, and morphine/bupivacaine after arthroscopic knee surgery. Arthroscopy 10:104–107, 1994.
20. De Andres J, Bellver J, Barrera L, et al: A comparative study of analgesia after knee surgery with intraarticular bupivacaine, intraarticular morphine, and lumbar plexus block. Anesth Analg 77:727–730, 1993.
21. Muller M, Burkhardt J, Borchardt E, Buttner-Janz K: Postoperative analgesic effect after intra-articular morphine or ropivacaine following knee arthroscopy – A prospective randomized, double blinded study (German). Schmerz 15:3–9, 2001.
22. Joshi W, Reuben SS, Kilaru PR, et al: Postoperative analgesia for outpatient arthroscopic knee surgery with intraarticular clonidine and/or morphine. Anesth Analg 90:1102–1106, 2000.
23. Reuben SS, Connelly NR: Postarthritic meniscus repair analgesia with intraarticular ketorolac or morphine. Anesth Analg 82:1036–1039, 1996.
24. Gurkan Y, Kilickan L, Buluc L, et al: Effects of diclofenac and intra-articular morphine/bupivacaine on postarthroscopic pain control. Minerva Anestesiol 65:741–745, 1999.
25. Whitford A, Healy M, Joshi GP, et al: The effect of tourniquet release time on the analgesic efficacy of intraarticular morphine after arthroscopic knee surgery. Anesth Analg 84:791–793, 1997.
26. Juelsgaard P, Dalsgaard J, Felsby S, Frokjaer J: Analgesic effect of 2 different doses of intra-articular morphine after ambulatory knee arthroscopy. A randomized, prospective, double-blind study. (Danish) Ugeskr Laeger 155:4169–4172, 1993.
27. Reuben SS, Sklar J, El-Mansouri M: The preemptive analgesic effect of intraarticular bupivacaine and morphine after ambulatory arthroscopic knee surgery. Anesth Analg 92:923–926, 2001.
28. Marchal JM, Delgado-Martinez AZ, Poncela M, et al: Does the type of arthroscopic surgery modify the analgesic effect of intraarticular morphine and bupivacaine? A preliminary study. Clin J Pain 19:240–246, 2003.
29. Joshi GP, McCarroll SM, McSwiney M, et al: Effects of intraarticular morphine on analgesic requirements after anterior cruciate ligament repair. Reg Anesth 18:254–257, 1993.
30. Brandsson S, Karlsson J, Morberg P, et al: Intraarticular morphine after arthroscopic ACL reconstruction: A double-blind placebo-controlled study of 40 patients. Acta Orthop Scand 71:280–285, 2000.
31. McCarty EC, Spindler KP, Tingstad E, et al: Does intraarticular morphine improve pain control with femoral nerve block after anterior cruciate ligament reconstruction? Am J Sports Med 29:327–332, 2001.
32. Dauri M, Polzoni M, Fabbi E, et al: Comparison of epidural, continuous femoral block and intraarticular analgesia after anterior cruciate ligament reconstruction. Acta Anaesthesiol Scand 47:20–25, 2003.
33. Reuben SS, Steinberg RB, Cohen MA, et al: Intraarticular morphine in the multimodal analgesic management of postoperative pain after ambulatory anterior cruciate ligament repair. Anesth Analg 86:374–378, 1998.
34. Meiser A, Laubenthal H: Clinical studies on the peripheral effect of opioids following knee surgery. A literature review (German). Anaesthesist 46:867–879, 1997.
35. Stein C, Pfluger M, Yassouridis A, et al: No tolerance to peripheral morphine analgesia in presence of opioid expression in inflamed synovia. J Clin Invest 98:793–799, 1996.
36. Keates HL, Cramond T, Smith MT: Intraarticular and periarticular opioid binding in inflamed tissue in experimental canine arthritis. Anesth Analg 89:409–415, 1999.
37. Buerkle H, Pogatzki E, Pauser M, et al: Experimental arthritis in the rat does not alter the analgesic potency of intrathecal or intraarticular morphine. Anesth Analg 89:403–408, 1999.
38. McDougall JJ, Baker CL, Hermann PM: Attenuation of knee joint inflammation by peripherally administered endorphin-1. J Mol Neurosci 22:125–138, 2004.

39. Elvenes J, Andjelkov N, Figenschau Y, et al: Expression of functional mu-opioid receptors in human osteoarthritic cartilage and chondrocytes. Biochem Biophys Res Commun 311:202–207, 2003.

40. Stein A, Yassouridis A, Szopko C, et al: Intraarticular morphine versus dexamethasone in chronic arthritis. Pain 83:525–532, 1999.

41. Likar R, Schafer M, Paulak F, et al: Intraarticular morphine analgesia in chronic pain patients with osteoarthritis. Anesth Analg 84:1313–1317, 1997.

42. Klasen JA, Opitz SA, Melzer C, et al: Intraarticular, epidural, and intravenous analgesia after total knee arthroplasty. Acta Anaesthesiol Scand 43:1021–1026, 1999.

43. Tetzlaff JE, Brems J, Dilger J: Intraarticular morphine and bupivacaine reduces postoperative pain after rotator cuff repair. Reg Anesth Pain Med 25:611–614, 2000.

44. Henn P, Steuer K, Fischer A, Fischer M: Effectiveness of morphine by periarticular injections after shoulder arthroscopy (German). Anaesthesist 49:721–724, 2000.

45. Rasmussen S, Kehlet H. Intraarticular glucocorticoid, morphine and bupivacaine reduce pain and convalescence after arthroscopic ankle surgery: A randomized study of 36 patients. Acta Orthop Scand 71:301–304, 2000.

46. Elhakim M, Nafie M, Eid A, et al: Combination of intra-articular tenoxicam, lidocaine, and pethidine for outpatient knee arthroscopy. Acta Anaesthesiol Scand 43:803–808, 1999.

47. Westman L, Valentin A, Engstrom B, et al: Local anesthesia for arthroscopic surgery of the ankle using pethidine or prilocaine. Arthroscopy 13:307–312, 1997.

48. Soderlund A, Westman L, Ersmark H, et al: Analgesia following arthroscopy: A comparison of intra-articular morphine, pethidine and fentanyl. Acta Anaesthesiol Scand 41:6–11, 1997.

49. Soderlund A, Boreus LO, Westman L, et al: A comparison of 50, 100 and 200 mg of intra-articular pethidine during knee joint surgery, a controlled study with evidence for local demethylation to norpethidine. Pain 80:229–238, 1999.

50. Ekblom A, Westman L, Soderlund A, et al: Is intra-articular pethidine an alternative to local anesthetics in arthroscopy? A double-blind study comparing prilocaine with pethidine. Knee Surg Sports Traumatol Arthrosc 1:189–194, 1993.

51. Pooni JS, Hickmott K, Mercer D, et al: Comparison of intra-articular fentanyl and intra-articular bupivacaine for post-operative pain relief after knee arthroscopy. Eur J Anaesthesiol 16:708–711, 1999.

52. Varkel V, Volpin G, Ben-David B, et al: Intraarticular fentanyl compared with morphine for pain relief following arthroscopic knee surgery. Can J Anaesth 46:867–871, 1999.

53. Uysalel A, Kecik Y, Kirdemir P, et al: Comparison of intraarticular bupivacaine with the addition of morphine or fentanyl for analgesia after arthroscopic surgery. Arthroscopy 11:660–663, 1995.

54. Scott JC, Cooke JE, Stanski DR: Electroencephalographic quantitation of opioid effect: Comparative pharmacodynamics of fentanyl and sufentanil. Anesthesiology 74:34–42, 1991.

55. Bovill JG, Sebel PS, Blackburn CL, et al: The pharmacokinetics of sufentanil in surgical patients. Anesthesiology 61:502–506, 1984.

56. Vranken JH, Vissers KC, de Jongh R, Heylen R: Intraarticular sufentanil administration facilitates recovery after day-case knee arthroscopy. Anesth Analg 92:625–628, 2001.

57. Niv D, Nemirovsky A, Rudick V, et al: Antinociception induced by simultaneous intrathecal and intraperitoneal administration of low doses of morphine. Anesth Analg 80:886–889, 1995.

58. Buerkle H, Taksh TL: Comparison of the spinal actions of the mu-opioid remifentanil with alfentanil and morphine in the rat. Anesthesiology 84:94–102, 1996.

59. Reichert JA, Daughters RS, Rivard R, Simone DA: Peripheral and preemptive opioid antinociception in a mouse visceral pain model. Pain 89:221–227, 2001.

60. Nadeson R, Tucker A, Bajunaki E, Goodchild CS: Potentiation by ketamine of fentanyl antinociception: I. An experimental study in rats showing that ketamine administered by non-spinal routes targets spinal cord antinociceptive systems. Br J Anaesth 88:685–691, 2002.

61. Winter L, Nadeson R, Tucker AP, Goodchild CS: Antinociceptive properties of neurosteroids: A comparison of alphadolone and alphaxalone in potentiation of opioid antinociception. Anesth Analg 97:798–805, 2003.

62. Schulte-Steinberg H, Weninger E, Jokisch D, et al: Intraperitoneal versus intrapleural morphine or bupivacaine for pain after laparoscopic cholecystectomy. Anesthesiology 82:634–640, 1995.

63. O'Hanlon DM, Colbert S, Ragheb J, et al: Intraperitoneal pethidine versus intramuscular pethidine for the relief of pain after laparoscopic cholecystectomy: Randomized trial. World J Surg 26:1432–1436, 2002.

64. Hernandez-Palazon J, Tortosa JA, Nuno de la Rosa V, et al: Intraperitoneal application of bupivacaine plus morphine for pain relief after laparoscopic cholecystectomy. Eur J Anaesthesiol 20:891–896, 2003.

65. Colbert ST, Moran K, O'Hanlon DM, et al: An assessment of the value of intraperitoneal meperidine for analgesia postlaparoscopic tubal ligation. Anesth Analg 91:667–670, 2000.

66. Keita H, Benifla JL, Le Bouar V, et al: Prophylactic ip injection of bupivacaine and/or morphine does not improve postoperative analgesia after laparoscopic gynecologic surgery. Can J Anaesth 50:362–367, 2003.

67. Kalman SH, Jensen AG, Nystrom PO, Eintrei C: Intravenous versus intraperitoneal morphine before surgery to provide postoperative pain relief. Acta Anaesthesiol Scand 41:1047–1053, 1997.

31

Pediatric Postoperative Pain

Patrick K. Birmingham, M.D., F.A.A.P.

Historically under-recognized and undertreated, pediatric pain management has improved dramatically over the last 10 to 15 years. Advances in pain assessment, pharmacologic studies of opioid and nonopioid analgesics in children, and the development of physician-directed hospital-based acute pain services have been important factors in this development.

ANATOMIC AND PHYSIOLOGIC DIFFERENCES

The rational use of analgesics in pediatric patients, particularly neonates and infants, requires recognition of maturational changes that take place after birth in both body composition and core organ function.

Total body water represents about 80% of body weight in full-term newborns. This drops to 60% of body weight by 2 years of age, with a large proportional decrease in extracellular fluid volume. The larger extracellular and total body water stores in infancy lead to a greater volume of distribution for water-soluble drugs. Newborns have smaller skeletal muscle mass and fat stores, decreasing the amount of drug bound to inactive sites in muscle and fat. These stores increase during infancy.

Cardiac output is higher in infants and children than adults, and is preferentially distributed to vessel-rich tissues such as the brain, allowing for rapid equilibration of drug concentrations. Immaturity of the blood–brain barrier in early infancy allows increased passage of more water-soluble medications such as morphine. This combination of increased blood flow to the brain and increased drug passage through the blood–brain barrier can lead to higher central nervous system (CNS) drug concentrations and more side effects at a lower plasma concentration.

Renal and hepatic blood flow is also increased in infants relative to adults. As glomerular filtration, renal tubular function, and hepatic enzyme systems mature, generally reaching adult values within the first year of life, increased blood flow to these organs leads to increased drug metabolism and excretion.

Both the quantity and binding ability of serum albumin and alpha-1 acid glycoprotein (AAG) are decreased in newborns relative to adults. This may result in higher levels of unbound drug, with greater drug effect and toxicity at lower overall serum levels. This has led to lower local anesthetic dosing recommendations in neonates and young infants, although neonates have shown the ability to increase acutely AAG levels while on continuous local anesthetic infusions. The difference in serum protein quantity and binding ability disappears by approximately 6 months of age.

Neurotransmitters and peripheral and central pathways necessary for pain transmission are intact and functional by late gestation, although opiate receptors may function differently in the newborn than in adults. Cardiorespiratory, hormonal, and metabolic responses to pain in adults have also been well documented to occur in neonates.

The spinal cord and dura mater in the newborn infant extend to approximately the third lumbar (L3) and third sacral (S3) vertebral level, respectively, and reach the adult levels of approximately L1 and S1–2 by about 1 year of age. The lower-lying spinal cord in young infants is thus theoretically more vulnerable to injury during needle insertion at mid- to upper lumbar levels. The intercristal line connecting the posterior superior iliac crests, used as a surface landmark during needle insertion, crosses the spinal column at the S1 level in neonates versus the L4 or L5 level in adults. There is less and more loosely connected fat in the epidural space in infants versus adults, explaining in part the relative ease with which epidural catheters inserted at the base of the sacrum can be threaded to lumbar or thoracic levels in infants and small children.

PAIN ASSESSMENT

Depending on developmental age and other factors, the pediatric patient may be unable or unwilling to verbalize or quantify pain like his or her adult counterpart. Nonetheless, a number of developmentally appropriate pain assessment scales have been designed for use in both infants and children (Table 31-1). Specialized self-reporting scales are available for children and can be used in patients as young as 3 years of age (Fig. 31-1). Behavioral or physiologic measures are available for younger ages.

TABLE 31-1. **AGE AND MEASURES OF PAIN INTENSITY**

Age	Self-Report Measures	Behavior Measures	Physiologic Measures
Birth to 3 years	Not available	Of primary importance	Of secondary importance
3 to 6 years	Specialized developmentally appropriate scales available	Primary if self-report not available	Of secondary importance
>6 years	Of primary importance	Of secondary importance	

From McGrath PJ, Beyer J, Cleeland C, et al: Report of the subcommittee on assessment and methodologic issues in the management of pain in childhood cancer. Pediatrics 86:816, 1990. Reproduced with permission from Pediatrics.

NONOPIOID ANALGESICS

Acetaminophen: Acetaminophen (paracetamol) is very commonly used in pediatric patients, alone or in combination with other analgesics. It is often administered rectally in the perioperative period in infants or children for whom oral intake is not an option. More recent studies indicate higher dosing, at least initially, is needed if given rectally (Table 31-2). Suppository insertion prior to surgical incision does not appear to significantly alter acetaminophen kinetics and may result in more timely analgesia in the early postoperative period. Higher-dose rectal acetaminophen has been shown to be equianalgesic to intravenous ketorolac following tonsillectomy and to have a significant opioid-sparing effect in children undergoing outpatient surgery. An intravenous prodrug form of acetaminophen is also available in some parts of the world.

Acetaminophen dosing in premature and term neonates is less well defined. Despite age-related differences in elimination pathways, overall elimination in small studies is similar between neonates, children, and adults. Dose-dependent hepatotoxicity is the most serious acute side effect of acetaminophen administration. Acute hepatotoxicity appears to be less common and less likely to be fatal in children than adults.

Nonsteroidal Anti-inflammatory Drugs: Nonsteroidal anti-inflammatory drugs (NSAIDs) are also widely administered to children. Studies of intravenous, intramuscular, and rectal NSAID administration in pediatric surgical patients demonstrate reduced postoperative pain scores and decreased supplemental analgesic requirements. Intravenous ketorolac is used widely in children, with a generally good safety record. The clinical significance of NSAID effects on bleeding remains controversial, leading to its avoidance by some in procedures such as tonsillectomy. Bleeding, renal damage, and gastritis are more likely to occur with prolonged administration and in the presence of coexisting disease. The clinical significance of NSAID inhibitory effects on osteogenesis following bone surgery, as documented in animal studies, remains unclear. Acetaminophen and NSAIDs are often given in combination, as they work by different mechanisms and their toxicity does not appear to be additive.

Aspirin (Acetylsalicylic Acid): Aspirin is not used for postoperative pain management in infants and children because of a highly significant association with Reye syndrome. Reye syndrome is an acute, fulminant, and potentially fatal hepatoencephalopathy that occurs in children with influenza-like illness or varicella, who ingest aspirin-containing medications.

Faces Pain Rating Scale

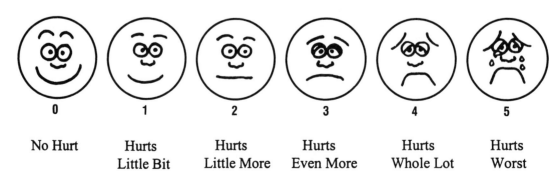

0	1	2	3	4	5
No Hurt	Hurts Little Bit	Hurts Little More	Hurts Even More	Hurts Whole Lot	Hurts Worst

FIGURE 31-1. The Wong–Baker Faces Pain Rating Scale. This rating scale is recommended for children aged 3 years and older. It is explained to the child that each face is for a person who feels happy because the person has no pain (hurt) or sad because the person has some or a lot of pain. The child is asked to choose the face that best describes how he or she is feeling. (From Wong D: Whaley and Wong's Essentials of Pediatric Nursing, ed 5. Mosby-Year Book, St Louis, MO, 1997, p 1215. Reproduced with permission.)

TABLE 31-2. ACETAMINOPHEN (PARACETAMOL) AND NSAID DOSING

Oral acetaminophen	10–15 mg/kg every 4–6 hours (max. 1 g per dose and 90 mg/kg/day up to 4 g)
Rectal acetaminophen	35–45 mg/kg loading dose,* then 20 mg/kg every 6 hours thereafter†
Intravenous acetaminophen	15–30 mg/kg every 4–6 hours‡
Oral ibuprofen	4–10 mg/kg every 6–8 hours (max. 600 mg/dose)
Oral tramadol	1–2 mg/kg every 6 hours (max. dose 100 mg)
Intravenous/intramuscular ketorolac	0.5 mg/kg (max. 15 mg if <50 kg, max. 30 mg if >60 kg) every 6 hours, for <5 days

* Dosing in neonates and young infants not well defined and may be less.
† No evidence of accumulation at 24 hours.
‡ Lower range of this dose is recommended in infants less than 10 days old.
Dose ranges are approximate and may vary depending on individual patient assessment.

OPIOID ANALGESIA

Oral, parenteral, and epidural opioids are widely employed in infants and children to optimize postoperative comfort. Codeine is given orally in a dose of 0.5 to 1 mg/kg and often in combination with acetaminophen for mild to moderate pain. Parenteral opioids are still given on an as-needed basis to some patients, but alternative means of opioid delivery have been increasingly employed over the last 15 years.

Patient-Controlled Analgesia: Patient-controlled analgesia (PCA) is used in children as young as 5 to 6 years of age, with morphine the most commonly used and studied opioid, and hydromorphone and fentanyl more commonly used alternatives (Table 31-3). Compared to prn intramuscular opioids, PCA has been shown to be safe in children and provide more effective analgesia with greater patient satisfaction. A low-dose continuous or "background" infusion is sometimes added for patients following major surgery to optimize analgesia.

Parent/Nurse-Assisted Analgesia: The concept of PCA has been expanded to allow parent- or nurse-assisted analgesia in select cases in which the patient is unwilling or unable, because of age, developmental delay, or physical disability, to operate the PCA button. This technique is used with caution as it does away with one of the safety features of PCA, in that the patient is theoretically less likely to self-overdose. While more commonly used in infants and children with cancer treatment-related pain, such as oral mucositis with bone marrow transplantation, it has also been safely used for postoperative analgesia.

Continuous Intravenous Infusions: Continuous intravenous opioid infusions are used alone (or in combination with PCA) to provide pain relief following pediatric surgery. Compared to adults given morphine, neonates and premature infants have a longer elimination half-life, lower plasma clearance, and marked interindividual variability in plasma morphine concentration. For a given dose, they will achieve a higher plasma concentration for a longer duration. By approximately 6 to 12 months of age, the kinetics of morphine and fentanyl approach adult values, and children soon thereafter demonstrate increased plasma clearance and a shorter elimination half-life. Continuous morphine infusion rates and patient age ranges are summarized in Table 31-4.

REGIONAL ANALGESIA

"Single-Shot" Caudals: One of the most widely used pediatric regional techniques for postoperative analgesia is the "single-shot" caudal (SSC). Its popularity stems in part from

TABLE 31-3. PATIENT-CONTROLLED ANALGESIA PARAMETERS

	Morphine	Hydromorphone	Fentanyl
Loading dose (over 1–10 minutes)	0.05–0.20 mg/kg	1–2 µg/kg	0.5–2.0 µg/kg
Demand dose	0.01–0.02 mg/kg	1–2 µg/kg	0.2–0.4 µg/kg
Lockout time	5–15 minutes	5–15 minutes	5–15 minutes
Four-hour limit (optional)	0.30–0.40 mg/kg	30–50 µg/kg	6–10 µg/kg
Continuous infusion (optional)	0.01–0.02 mg/kg/hour	1–2 µg/kg/hour	0.2–0.4 µg/kg/hour

Dose ranges are approximate; selection of opioid and actual parameters depends on assessment of individual patient.
Adapted from Birmingham PK: Recent advances in acute pain management. Curr Prob Pediatr 25:99–112, 1995. Reproduced with permission.

TABLE 31-4. **CONTINUOUS INTRAVENOUS MORPHINE INFUSION FOR POSTOPERATIVE ANALGESIA IN INFANTS AND CHILDREN**

Age Range of Subjects (EGA)	Infusion (μg/kg/hour)	Comments	Number of Subjects
1–18 days (32–40 weeks)	15	Some patients mechanically ventilated	20
1–49 days (35–41 weeks)	6–40	Some patients mechanically ventilated; seizures at 32 and 40 μg/kg/hour; recommend rate of 15 μg/kg/hour	12
3 months–12 years	14–21	Less total morphine than with time-contingent IM morphine	20
<1–14 years	10–40	Spontaneously ventilating	121
14 months–17 years	10–30	Postoperative cardiac; able to wean from mechanical ventilation	44
1–15 years	20	Superior to IM morphine	20
1–16 years	10–40	Superior to IM morphine	46
3–22 years	20–40	Cerebral palsy patients	55

EGA, estimated gestational age at birth; IM, intramuscular.
Adapted from Birmingham PK, Hall SC: Drug infusions in pediatric anesthesia. *In* Fragen RF (ed): Drug Infusions in Anesthesiology, ed 2. Lippincott-Raven, Philadelphia, 1996, pp 193–224. Reproduced with permission.

the readily palpable landmarks and relative ease of caudal block insertion in infants and children versus adults. SSC is used in infants and children up to approximately 10 to 12 years of age having surgery from lumbosacral to mid-thoracic dermatome levels with anticipated moderate postoperative pain. Bupivacaine in concentrations of 0.125% to 0.25% is the most commonly used and studied local anesthetic for SSC. Injection volumes of 0.5 to 1.5 mL/kg will provide analgesia for upper lumbar to mid-thoracic levels, respectively. An upper volume limit of 20 mL is generally used. The maximum recommended dose is 2.5 to 3.0 mg/kg, with an upper limit of 1.25 mg/kg recommended in infants less than 4 months of age. A test dose of 0.1 mL/kg (maximum 3 mL) of local anesthetic with 1:200,000 epinephrine (5 μg/kg) is used to ensure correct needle or catheter position. An increase in T wave amplitude, heart rate (>10 beats per minute), or systolic blood pressure (>10% increase) within 60 seconds of administration is considered a positive test dose. It is unclear whether block

TABLE 31-5. **SUGGESTED PEDIATRIC EPIDURAL DOSING GUIDELINES**

Medicine	Age Group	Bolus	Infusion
Bupivacaine	Infants <4 months	≤1.25 mg/kg initial bolus	≤0.2 mg/kg/hour
Bupivacaine	Older infants and children	≤2.5–3.0 mg/kg initial bolus	≤0.4–0.5 mg/kg/hour
Fentanyl	Infants and children	1–2 μg/kg initial bolus	0.2–2.0 μg/kg/hour
Morphine	Infants <6 months	10–25 μg/kg q 6–24 hours	≤2.5 μg/kg/hour
Morphine	Older infants and children	20–50 μg/kg q 6–24 hours	≤5.0 μg/kg/hour
Clonidine	Infants and children	0.5–2 μg/kg initial bolus	≤0.2–1 μg/kg/hour

These are approximate dose ranges. Actual dose selected depends on individual patient assessment.

placement at the beginning versus the end of the procedure prolongs postoperative analgesia.

Although usually used alone, bupivacaine can be combined epidurally with 1 to 2 µg/kg fentanyl, 20 to 50 µg/kg morphine, or 1 to 2 µg/kg of the alpha-2-adrenergic agonist clonidine. Delayed respiratory depression up to 22 hours can occur with epidural morphine. Greater risk is seen in children less than 1 year of age and when parenteral opioids have also been given.

Continuous Epidural Infusions: Epidural local anesthetic infusions with or without opioids or alpha-2 agonists have been used in infants and children for postoperative analgesia. Bolus and infusion rate recommendations for bupivacaine, fentanyl, morphine, and clonidine are listed in Table 31-5. Lower infusion rates are generally recommended in neonates and infants less than 4 to 6 months old. This is because of lower protein binding and consequently higher free fractions of drug, and because of pharmacokinetic differences potentially resulting in higher plasma levels and prolonged drug half-life. Substitution of other opioids, such as those with mixed agonist–antagonist effects, may minimize clinical side effects. As a rule, optimal analgesia is obtained with the catheter tip positioned at or near the dermatomes to be blocked. It is possible in infants and smaller children to thread caudally inserted catheters to lumbar or thoracic levels. Catheter insertion may take place following induction of general anesthesia in infants and children who are unable or unwilling to cooperate with catheter placement while awake or sedated. Patient-controlled epidural analgesia has been successively used in children as young as 5 years of age.

Peripheral nerve blocks also play an important role in pediatric postoperative pain relief. Ilioinguinal/iliohypogastric, penile, femoral, digital, and head and neck blocks are often done to provide analgesia in suitable candidates.

KEY POINTS

- Anatomic and physiologic differences in neonates and young infants necessitate lower doses of epidural local anesthetics and intravenous opioids up to 4 to 6 months of life.
- Behavioral or physiologic measures of pain intensity are available for infants and children unable to self-report their pain.
- Aspirin is not routinely used for postoperative pain control in children because of an association with Reye's syndrome, a potentially fatal hepatoencephalopathy.
- Epidural analgesia by single injection or following epidural catheter insertion is commonly employed in infants and young children following induction of general anesthesia.
- Intravenous and epidural PCA can be used in children as young as 5 to 6 years of age.
- Nurse- or parent-assisted analgesia can be used in select circumstances for children unable or unwilling to operate a PCA button.

FURTHER READING

Dalens B: Regional Anesthesia in Infants, Children, and Adolescents, ed 1. Williams & Wilkins, Baltimore, 1995.

Schechter NL, Berde CB, Yaster M: Pain in Infants, Children and Adolescents, ed 1. Williams & Wilkins, Baltimore, 2002.

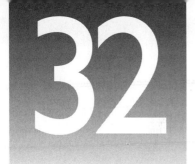

Pain Management During Pregnancy and Lactation

Cynthia A. Wong, M.D.

Complaints of pain occur in almost all pregnant and lactating women. Treatment of pain during pregnancy and lactation may affect the fetus or nursing child. Analgesics are commonly ingested during pregnancy.[1] Almost all drugs administered to the mother cross the placenta to the fetus, or are secreted in breast milk. The mechanisms of transport are similar to the transport of drugs across any membrane.[2] Diffusion is primarily passive and the concentration in the umbilical vein or breast milk depends on the concentration gradient, the lipid solubility of the drug, its degree of ionization, and protein binding, and the diffusion capacity of the membrane (this may change as pregnancy progresses).[3] The effects on the fetus or nursing child will depend on the gestational age or age, as well as the amount and duration of drug exposure, and the specific drug.

Because most drugs cross the placenta and into breast milk, and because the effect of these drugs on the fetus is difficult to ascertain, every effort should be made to minimize maternal exposure to drugs and use nonpharmacologic therapies to treat pain. When drugs are necessary, the benefit should justify the risk (e.g., the untreated illness may pose a greater risk to the fetus than the medications used to treat the illness)[4] and the minimum effective dose should be used.

DRUGS DURING PREGNANCY

Pharmacokinetic Changes During Pregnancy: The myriad physiologic changes of pregnancy influence drug absorption, distribution, and elimination.[1] Changes in gastrointestinal function can alter oral drug absorption. Renal elimination is generally increased because of an increase in glomerular filtration rate. Hepatic metabolism may be increased, unchanged, or decreased, and the increase in total body water may alter drug distribution and peak concentrations. Protein binding is usually decreased; however, the free drug concentration may be unchanged because of increased drug clearance.

Transfer of Drugs Across the Placenta: The amount of drug that crosses the placenta depends on maternal cardiac output, fetal cardiac output, placental binding, and placental metabolism, as well as factors that influence passive diffusion across the placenta.[5] Maternal plasma levels of a drug depend on the site of administration (e.g., oral, intravascular, or epidural space), the total dose, the dosing interval, and other drugs that may be coadministered (e.g., epinephrine). The amount of drug to which the fetus is exposed also depends on fetal metabolism (fetal blood carrying drugs away from the placenta passes first through the fetal liver), fetal protein binding (about half of maternal protein binding), and the distribution of fetal cardiac output (fetal distress results in redistribution of blood flow to the vital organs).[3]

In general, good studies of human drug transfer and exposure are limited. Interspecies differences in placental anatomy and function make animal model comparisons with humans risky. Ethical concerns have limited studies in pregnant women. Most studies of the placental transfer of anesthetic agents administered to the mother intrapartum report single measurements of drug concentration in the maternal and umbilical vein serum at the time of delivery (the fetal:maternal or F/M ratio). The measured fetal concentration does not reflect the effects of drug passage through the fetal liver, or the possibility of altered pharmacokinetics and pharmacodynamics in the fetus compared to the mother.

Teratogenicity: Possible adverse effects on the fetus of in utero drug exposure include structural malformations, acute neonatal intoxication or neonatal abstinence syndromes, intrauterine fetal death, altered fetal growth, and neurobehavioral teratogenicity.[6] A major determinant of the effect of a drug on the fetus is the gestational age of the fetus. Traditionally, teratogenic effects of drugs have been defined as structural malformations. However, functional and behavioral effects are also likely to occur, and are much harder to identify. In addition, effects of fetal drug exposure may be delayed and only apparent later in life.[2] The mechanisms by which drugs cause teratogenicity are poorly understood, and may be direct or indirect (direct effect on the mother indirectly effects the fetus). There is interspecies variation in the ability of a drug to cause a specific congenital defect (e.g., thalidomide is not teratogenic in nonprimates).

The period of classic teratogenesis corresponds with the critical period of organogenesis and begins approximately 31 days after the last menstrual period until about 71 days after the last period.[7] Exposure to teratogens before 31 days results in an all-or-none effect (survival without a defect or loss of pregnancy). Fetal development, particularly the central nervous system, continues into the second and third trimesters, and indeed after birth. Therefore, fetal drug exposure at this time is not risk free.

Information on the teratogenic potential of many drugs comes from large-survey studies. These studies are often flawed because of reporting bias. They often do not control for other variables, including environmental exposures, exposure to multiple drugs (including alcohol, tobacco, nonprescription and illicit drugs), and the influence of the disease itself. Case reports of an association between in utero drug exposure and fetal anomalies are more likely to be published than if no anomaly occurred.[8]

Food and Drug Administration Risk Classification: The US Food and Drug Administration (FDA) requires labeling of drugs using the Pregnancy Category System (Table 32-1). The FDA recognizes that this system is not always helpful to the prescribing physician and pregnant patient. For example, going from Category A to X does not necessarily mean increased risk of teratogenicity. While only 20 to 30 commonly used drugs are proven teratogens in humans, over 70 are listed as Category X and all new medications are classified as Category C.[9] Discussion is currently underway at the FDA on methods to improve this system.[10]

Specific Drugs: Aspirin use during pregnancy may be associated with an increased risk of gastroschisis. Pregnant women should not use aspirin (>150 mg/day) regularly.[9] Ibuprofen and naproxen during the first trimester do not appear to be teratogenic.[11,12] Prostaglandin inhibitors have been associated with narrowing of the ductus arteriosus in utero. This effect increases with gestational age, although it appears reversible when the medication is stopped.[2,9] Aspirin and other prostaglandin inhibitors may decrease amniotic fluid volume secondary to decreased fetal urine output, and they may prolong pregnancy and labor. An increased incidence of neonatal intracranial hemorrhage has been found in premature infants whose mothers ingested aspirin near birth. For these reasons full-dose aspirin and nonsteroidal anti-inflammatory drug (NSAID) therapy should be avoided in the third trimester.[2,13] If a mild analgesic is indicated during pregnancy, acetaminophen is the drug of choice.

TABLE 32-1. **US FOOD AND DRUG ADMINISTRATION PREGNANCY CATEGORY SYSTEM**

Category	Description	Drugs
A	Adequate, well-controlled studies in pregnant women have not shown an increased risk of fetal abnormalities	
B	Animal studies have revealed no harm to the fetus; however, there are no adequate and well-controlled studies in pregnant women. Or Animal studies have shown an adverse effect, but adequate and well-controlled studies in pregnant women have failed to demonstrate a risk to the fetus	Acetaminophen; butorphanol, nalbuphine; caffeine; fentanyl,* methadone,* meperidine,* morphine,* oxycodone,* oxymorphone;* ibuprofen, naproxen, indomethacin; prednisone, prednisolone
C	Animal studies have shown adverse fetal effects and there are no adequate and well-controlled studies in pregnant women. Or No animal studies have been conducted and there are no adequate and well-controlled studies in pregnant women	Amitriptyline; aspirin, ketorolac; betamethasone; codeine,* propoxyphene,* hydrocodone;* gabapentin; lidocaine; propranolol; sumatriptan
D	Studies, adequate and well controlled or observational, in pregnant women have demonstrated a risk to the fetus. However, the benefits of therapy may outweigh the potential risk	Imipramine; carbamazepine; cortisone; diazepam; phenobarbital; phenytoin, valproic acid
X	Studies, adequate and well controlled or observational, in animals and pregnant women have demonstrated positive evidence of fetal abnormalities. The use of the product is contraindicated in women who are or may become pregnant	Ergotamine

* Opioid agonists and agonist–antagonists are considered Risk Category D when used at high doses near term.

There is no evidence that maternal opioid agonist or agonist–antagonist exposure during pregnancy is teratogenic.[13,14] Chronic in utero exposure to opioids may lead to neonatal abstinence syndrome. Acetaminophen combined with hydrocodone or oxycodone may be used to treat mild or moderate pain during pregnancy.

Bupivacaine and lidocaine were not associated with risk of teratogenicity in the Collaborative Perinatal Project.[14] The incidence of fetal anomalies was increased two-fold in women who were exposed to mepivacaine; however, this group included a very small number of women, and so it is difficult to draw any conclusions from the data.

Several surveillance studies have found an association between maternal steroid use and orofacial clefts,[2] while others have not.[14] A limited trial of epidural steroid therapy is probably associated with minimal fetal risk.[13] The placenta inactivates prednisolone (the biologically active form of prednisone).[7]

Other adjuvant medications are often used in the treatment of chronic pain. The selective serotonin reuptake inhibitors (SSRIs) have not been associated with increased risk of fetal or neonatal anomalies.[15,16] There is no evidence that tricyclic antidepressant drugs are teratogenic.[17] The anticonvulsants phenytoin, carbamazepine, and valproic acid all have been associated with fetal dysmorphic syndromes and should only be used when the risk outweighs the benefit.[9]

Ergotamine is contraindicated in pregnancy, as it may be teratogenic, and it also causes uterine contractions. There is no evidence that beta-blockers are teratogenic; however, they may be associated with intrauterine growth retardation.[7,13]

DRUGS DURING LACTATION

The amount of drug to which an infant is exposed during lactation depends on a number of maternal and infant factors. Maternal factors include maternal dose and dosing interval, the elimination half-life of the drug, the infant nursing pattern (volume and timing), and the amount of drug that actually crosses into breast milk.[18] The milk to plasma (M:P) ratio is an index of the amount of drug that is excreted into breast milk. Breast milk is slightly more acidic than plasma, and therefore passive diffusion favors drugs that are weak bases, lipid soluble,

and have low protein binding.[1] The amount of drug to which the infant is actually exposed depends on infant pharmacokinetics, which may differ from maternal pharmacokinetics. The infant plasma concentration is generally 1% to 2% of the milk concentration.[13] Even when the M:P ratio approaches one, the infant plasma concentration rarely attains therapeutic levels.

Because the volume of colostrum is small, nursing neonates are exposed to minimal amounts of the drugs administered to the mother in the postpartum period.[13] Most milk is made during and immediately following nursing. Administration of drugs shortly after nursing, and avoiding long-acting drugs, may help minimize infant exposure. For mothers taking chronic medications, the in utero exposure is greater than the exposure during lactation. In general, the lowest effective dose should be used, and older drugs with a history of widespread use should be chosen.[19] It is best to use drugs that do not have an active metabolite.

American Academy of Pediatrics: The American Academy of Pediatrics encourages breast-feeding. A recent policy statement summarizes the Committee on Drugs review of this topic and categorizes drugs into risk categories for nursing infants (Table 32-2). Most drugs are compatible with nursing. The following should be considered when prescribing drugs to lactating women:[20]

- Is drug therapy really necessary?
- The safest drug should be chosen, e.g., acetaminophen rather than aspirin for mild analgesia.
- If there is a possibility of risk to the infant, then one should considering monitoring infant serum levels of the drug.
- Having the mother take the medication just after she has breast fed the infant or before the infant is due to sleep can minimize drug exposure.

Specific Drugs: Acetaminophen is considered the safest analgesic for nursing mothers. The infant of a mother taking acetaminophen 4 g/day was exposed to less than 5% the therapeutic infant dose.[19] There is controversy as to the use of aspirin in nursing mothers. Intermittent use should not pose a risk, but infants of mothers receiving chronic aspirin therapy

TABLE 32-2. SUMMARY OF RISK CATEGORIES FOR DRUGS FOR NURSING INFANTS

Category	Drugs
Drugs for which the effect on nursing infants is unknown but may be of concern	Benzodiazepines, tricyclic antidepressants, serotonin reuptake inhibitors
Drugs that have been associated with significant effects on some nursing infants and should be given to nursing mothers with caution	Aspirin, ergotamine
Maternal medication usually compatible with breast feeding	Acetaminophen, anticonvulsants, beta-blockers, local anesthetics, nonsteroidal anti-inflammatory drugs, opioid agonists, opioid agonists–antagonists, steroids, sumatriptan

Modified from the American Academy of Pediatrics 2001 Policy Statement: Transfer of drugs and other chemicals into human milk. Pediatrics 108:776–789, 2001.

should be observed for adverse side effects.[19] NSAIDs are considered compatible with nursing.[19,20]

Opioid agonist and agonist–antagonists cross freely into breast milk. The American Academy of Pediatricians considers opioids compatible with breast-feeding. These drugs undergo significant first-pass metabolism in the infant. However, infant plasma concentrations may be high enough to be associated with predictable side effects in the infant. Patient-controlled intravenous meperidine administered for postcesarean delivery analgesia had a negative impact on neonatal neurobehavioral scores compared to morphine.[21] The infants of nursing mothers ingesting opioids, particularly meperidine, should be monitored for adverse effects.

Less than 1% of the maternal dose of prednisone or prednisolone is recovered in breast milk.[2] Even at high maternal doses, this is unlikely to be enough to suppress infant adrenal function.[8]

The anticonvulsants carbamazepine, phenytoin, and valproic acid may be used safely during lactation. The American Academy of Pediatrics classifies tricyclic antidepressants as drugs whose effects on the nursing infant are of potential concern. Although very low serum concentrations of amitriptyline and imipramine are detected in the serum of nursing infants,[9] long-term studies are lacking.[18]

Maternal administration of beta-blockers results in subtherapeutic levels in nursing infants.[1] Ergotamine has been associated with neonatal convulsions and gastrointestinal disturbances and should not be used in nursing mothers.[13] The use of sumatriptan during lactation has not been well studied. Infant exposure can be avoided by pumping and discarding milk for 8 hours after injection.[13] Serum concentrations of propranolol in the nursing infant are less than 1% of the therapeutic dose.[13]

IMAGING DURING PREGNANCY

Ionizing radiation to the uterus should be avoided if at all possible until after the 15th week of pregnancy.[22] The two factors that determine the possible effects of radiation exposure on the developing fetus are the gestational age and fetal dose of absorbed radiation. During the preimplantation stage radiation exposure may be lethal to the embryo, but is unlikely to have a teratogenic effect. Magnetic resonance imaging (MRI) should be avoided if possible during the first trimester.[23] However, MRI is indicated during pregnancy when other nonionizing imaging methods, e.g., ultrasonography, are unsatisfactory, and the information obtained would otherwise require exposure to ionizing radiation.

PAIN SYNDROMES DURING PREGNANCY AND LACTATION

Musculoskeletal Pain: Back pain is very common during pregnancy and after delivery, occurring in about 50% of women.[24,25] The hormonal changes that are associated with pregnancy lead to widening of the sacroiliac synchondroses and pubic symphysis.[13] The pain is located lateral to the lumbosacral junction, and may radiate to the posterior thigh (but not leg or foot), making it difficult to differentiate from radicular pain. It often occurs when moving in bed.

Back pain during pregnancy may be accentuated lumber lordosis.[26] An MRI study showed that the prevalence of

disc herniation is not increased in pregnancy,[27] although herniation may occur. Direct pressure of the fetus on the lumbosacral plexus may be the cause of lower extremity symptoms.[25]

Few of the strategies commonly used to prevent and treat low back pain are universally effective.[13] Traditional conservative techniques should be tried first, including instruction on proper body mechanics, back exercises, relaxation training, special pillows to support the pregnant abdomen, and referral to a physical therapist. Acetaminophen is the drug of choice for minor back pain. The short-term use of NSAIDs may be appropriate during the first and second trimesters. Severe back pain may require opioid therapy. Epidural steroid injection(s) may be indicated for acute radicular pain consistent with lumbar nerve root compression.[13]

Headache: Migraine headaches are unusual during pregnancy. The initial presentation of a migraine-like headache in pregnancy should prompt a search for another serious cause.[28]

SUMMARY

Pain is frequent during pregnancy and during lactation. Often conservative therapy, or therapy with acetaminophen is adequate. The risk/benefit of using other pain treatment modalities should be assessed. Consideration should be given to the adverse fetal or neonatal effects of untreated pain.

REFERENCES

1. Loebstein R, Lalkin A, Koren G: Pharmacokinetic changes during pregnancy and their clinical relevance. Clin Pharmacokinet 33:328–343, 1997.
2. Briggs GG, Freeman RK, Yaffe SJ: Drugs in Pregnancy and Lactation, ed 6. Lippincott Williams & Wilkins, Philadelphia, 2002.
3. Santos AC, Finster M: Local anesthetics. *In* Chestnut DH (ed): Obstetric Anesthesia Principles and Practice, ed 2. Mosby, St Louis, 1999, pp 209–232.
4. Czeizel AE: Drug use during pregnancy [letter]. Lancet 357:800, 2001.
5. Herman NL: The placenta: Anatomy, physiology, and transfer of drugs. *In* Chestnut DH (ed): Obstetric Anesthesia: Principles and Practice, ed 2. Mosby, St Louis, 1999, pp 57–74.
6. American Academy of Pediatrics Committee on Drugs: Use of psychoactive medication during pregnancy and possible effects on the fetus and newborn. Pediatrics 105:880–887, 2000.
7. Niebyl JR: Nonanesthetic drugs during pregnancy and lactation. *In* Chestnut DH (ed): Obstetric Anesthesia Principles and Practice, ed 2. Mosby, St Louis, 1999, pp 235–248.
8. Rayburn WF: Connective tissue disorders and pregnancy. Recommendations for prescribing. J Reprod Med 43:341–349, 1998.
9. Hansen WF, Peacock AE, Yankowitz J: Safe prescribing practices in pregnancy and lactation. J Midwifery Womens Health 47:409–421, 2002.
10. Frederiksen MC: The drug development process and the pregnant woman. J Midwifery Womens Health 47:422–425, 2002.
11. Slone D, Siskind V, Heinonen OP, et al: Aspirin and congenital malformations. Lancet 1:1373–1375, 1976.
12. Ostensen M, Ostensen H: Safety of nonsteroidal antiinflammatory drugs in pregnant patients with rheumatic disease. J Rheumatol 23:1045–1049, 1996.

13. Rathmell JP, Viscomi CM, Bernstein IM: Managing pain during pregnancy and lactation. *In* Raj PP (ed): Textbook of Regional Anesthesia. Churchill Livingstone, New York, 2002, pp 196–211.

14. Heinonen OP, Slone D, Shapiro S: Birth Defects and Drugs in Pregnancy. Publishing Sciences Group, Littleton, MA, 1977.

15. Goldstein DJ, Corbin LA, Sundell KL: Effects of first-trimester fluoxetine exposure on the newborn. Obstet Gynecol 89:713–718, 1997.

16. Nulman I, Rovet J, Stewart DE, et al: Neurodevelopment of children exposed in utero to antidepressant drugs. N Engl J Med 336:258–262, 1997.

17. Stewart DE: Antidepressant drugs during pregnancy and lactation. Int Clin Psychopharmacol 15:S19–S24, 2000.

18. Bar-Oz B, Nulman I, Koren G, et al: Anticonvulsants and breast feeding: A critical review. Paediatr Drugs 2:113–126, 2000.

19. Spigset O, Hagg S: Analgesics and breast-feeding: Safety considerations. Paediatr Drugs 2:223–238, 2000.

20. American Academy of Pediatrics Committee on Drugs: Transfer of drugs and other chemicals into human milk. Pediatrics 108:776–789, 2001.

21. Wittels B, Glosten B, Faure EA, et al: Postcesarean analgesia with both epidural morphine and intravenous patient-controlled analgesia: Neurobehavioral outcomes among nursing neonates. Anesth Analg 85:600–606, 1997.

22. Berlin L: Radiation exposure and the pregnant patient. Am J Roentgenol 167:1377–1379, 1996.

23. Nicklas AH, Baker ME: Imaging strategies in the pregnant cancer patient. Semin Oncol 27:623–632, 2000.

24. Ostgaard HC, Andersson GB, Karlsson K: Prevalence of back pain in pregnancy. Spine 16:549–552, 1991.

25. Fast A, Shapiro D, Ducommun EJ, et al: Low-back pain in pregnancy. Spine 12:368–371, 1987.

26. MacEvilly M, Buggy D: Back pain and pregnancy: A review. Pain 64:405–414, 1996.

27. Weinreb JC, Wolbarsht LB, Cohen JM, et al: Prevalence of lumbosacral intervertebral disk abnormalities on MR images in pregnant and asymptomatic nonpregnant women. Radiology 170:125–128, 1989.

28. Chancellor AM, Wroe SJ, Cull RE: Migraine occurring for the first time in pregnancy. Headache 30:224–227, 1990.

Pain Control in the Critically Ill Patient

Michael L. Ault, M.D., and
Robert Gould, M.D.

The concepts of sedation and analgesia are inexorably intertwined in the intensive care unit (ICU). The formal definition of sedation is: "the act of calming, especially by the administration of a sedative drug; the state of being calm."[1] Perhaps a more basic viewpoint of this concept of sedation is by viewing it as a three-component goal consisting of anxiolysis, hypnosis, and amnesia. Certainly, anxiolysis and hypnosis are difficult to achieve in a patient experiencing significant pain. Thus, it is easy to understand how the concepts of sedation and analgesia have become interdependent. However, this close relationship between these two distinct goals should not confuse the clinician as to the specific aim of therapy. By understanding the tools for appropriate patient assessment and the pharmacologic agents available to accomplish these goals, one can better choose the appropriate agents for sedation and analgesia in the ICU.

GOAL ASSESSMENT

Currently two frequently used scoring systems exist to assess sedation in the ICU. These are the Ramsay Sedation Score and the Riker Sedation-Agitation Scale (Tables 33-1 and 33-2). Of the two, the Ramsay Sedation Score is the most simplistic and allows a numeric score from 1 to 6 to be generated based on motor responsiveness of the patient.[2] The Riker Sedation-Agitation Scale uses a numeric score from 1 to 7 to assess the level of patient sedation and is especially adapted to warn the clinician of "unarousable" and "dangerous agitation" levels of patient sedation, which is not provided by the Ramsay Sedation Score (Table 33-2).[3] Clinicians should be aware that a high numeric score from the Ramsay Sedation Score (representative of heavily sedated patients) is similar to a low numeric score from the Riker Sedation-Agitation Score.

BENZODIAZEPINES

Within the ICU the most commonly used benzodiazepines are midazolam, lorazepam, and midazolam. Benzodiazepines interact with the gamma-aminobutyric acid (GABA) receptor creating an increase in intracellular chloride concentration and subsequent hyperpolarization of the cellular membrane. This hyperpolarization of neuronal membranes explains the utility of the pharmacologic agents as sedatives in addition to their frequent use as anticonvulsants.

Diazepam may possess the most enduring track record for use as a sedative. Its original formulation in propylene glycol made its use difficult secondary to the frequent venous irritation and thrombophlebitis associated with its use. This has been overcome in more recent years by the use of a fat emulsion. Additionally, it is important to note that the hepatic metabolism of diazepam results in the production of an active metabolite known as desmethyldiazepam. Because patients with hepatic dysfunction may experience a significant increase in the duration of action of this already "long-acting" benzodiazepine, the

TABLE 33-1. RAMSAY SEDATION SCORE

Awake levels	1	Patient anxious, agitated, restless, or both
	2	Patient cooperative, oriented, and tranquil
	3	Patient responds to verbal commands
Asleep levels	4	Brisk response to a light glabellar tap or loud auditory stimulus
	5	Sluggish response to a light glabellar tap or loud auditory stimulus
	6	No response to a light glabellar tap or loud auditory stimulus

TABLE 33-2. RIKER SEDATION-AGITATION SCALE (SAS)

Score	Description	Examples
7	Dangerous agitation	Pulling at endotracheal tube, trying to remove catheters, climbing over bedrail, striking at staff, thrashing side-to-side
6	Very agitated	Does not calm despite frequent verbal reminding of limits, requires physical restraints, biting endotracheal tube
5	Agitated	Anxious or mildly agitated, attempting to sit up, calms down to verbal instructions
4	Calm, cooperative	Calm, easily arousable, follows commands
3	Sedated	Difficult to arouse, awakens to verbal stimuli or gentle shaking but drifts off again, follows simple commands
2	Very sedated	Arouses to physical stimuli but does not communicate or follow commands, may move spontaneously
1	Unarousable	Minimal or no response to noxious stimuli, does not communicate or follow commands

titration of diazepam to achieve appropriate levels of sedation in the critically ill patient is often challenging given the dynamic environment in which patient care occurs.

Lorazepam is used more frequently in the ICU. Metabolism of lorazepam via hepatic glucuronidation results in inactive metabolites making its elimination more predictable than diazepam. Because of the predictable pharmacokinetics of this drug and its relative low cost, its use in the ICU is quite common. It is essential for the clinician to note that this "intermediate-acting" benzodiazepine will require consistent vigilance in its use to prevent oversedation, but nonetheless it provides predictable pharmacokinetics in a cost-efficient manner.

Midazolam is frequently used in the preoperative and intraoperative areas secondary to its water-soluble characteristics that allow the drug to become highly lipid soluble at physiologic pH. Thus, it has a rapid onset. Despite these characteristics, the drug relies on the hepatic microsomal system for metabolism, and because of this it has a variable pharmacokinetic profile making reliable termination of its effects difficult to predict. Additionally, it possesses an active metabolite, alpha-hydroxymidazolam, which may prolong its duration of action in patients with renal disease.

PROPOFOL

Like benzodiazepines, propofol is also a GABA receptor agonist. Because propofol pharmacokinetics are unchanged in patients with renal or hepatic metabolism, it allows for rapid metabolism and frequent neurologic assessment of the patient while maintaining adequate sedation.[4] Propofol also acts as a vasodilator and will decrease blood pressure in addition to its dose-dependent respiratory depression. Despite these drawbacks, the drug allows for shorter durations of intubation when compared to other sedatives.[5]

Propofol is prepared with a lipid emulsion carrier that may support bacterial growth after unintentional contamination.[6]

Additionally, long-term infusion may lead to hypertriglyceridemia and pancreatitis. Thus, vigilance for these issues is essential in patients receiving this drug for sedation.

DEXMEDETOMIDINE

Dexmedetomidine is an α_2-agonist with an affinity for the α_2 receptor (1620:1 α_2/α_1 activity) that is much higher than that of clonidine (220:1 α_2/α_1 activity). The drug has been recently introduced into clinical practice and has properties that make it very useful as an ICU sedative agent. The activation of the α_{2A}-receptor results in significant analgesia that reduces the need for supplemental opioids.[7,8] The major advantage of this is that the α_2-agonists carry virtually no respiratory depressant effects, pruritus, or nausea.[9]

As with clonidine, a hypnotic effect is produced by dexmedetomidine that resembles induction of normal sleep. The hypnotic effect of dexmedetomidine is unique in that patients, when left undisturbed, will sleep; but when aroused, they will follow commands and be cooperative.[10] This effect is mediated by activation of the α_{2A}-receptor in the locus ceruleus. This characteristic requires some acclamation of ICU staff to caring for patients that are not rendered completely unconscious by the "sedation" regimen. Attention to environmental control becomes essential and should include minimization of disturbing noises, and timing of procedures and interventions to correspond with normal light–dark (i.e., sleep) cycles. The α_2-agonists have mild antegrade amnestic and anxiolytic properties;[10,11] thus, the need for other agents (e.g., benzodiazepines) may be relatively less important for these purposes.

Some adverse effects of α_2-agonists include enhancement of vagal effects by creating a pharmacologic sympathectomy (mediated by the α_{2A}-receptor).[12] This can result in a reduction in heart rate, which, depending upon the clinical situation, can be either beneficial or detrimental. If given rapidly in

TABLE 33-3. **COMPARISON OF THE SEDATIVE DRUGS USED IN THE INTENSIVE CARE UNIT**

Property	Lorazepam	Midazolam	Propofol	Dexmedetomidine
Rapid onset	−	+	+	±
Short duration	−	±	+	−
Minimal cardiovascular/respiratory depression	+	±	−	++
Inactive metabolites	+	−	+	+
Elimination minimally dependent on renal function	−	−	+	−
Few adverse side effects	+	+	±	+
No association tolerance or withdrawal	−	−	−	?
Inexpensive	+	±	−	−

−, drug is devoid of, or displays minimal activity; +, prominent drug action; ±, drug is intermediate in responsiveness.

high dose, the α_{2B}-stimulation can result in transient hypertension followed by hypotension mediated by the α_{2A}-receptor in the peripheral vascular system. However, the hemodynamic effects of α_2-agonists are relatively similar to those induced by other drugs used commonly in sedation regimens. Table 33-3 compares dexmedetomidine with other commonly used sedatives.

BUTYROPHENONES

Butyrophenones are often used as adjuncts to sedation regimens. These agents do not provide respiratory depression and are typically used to provide sedation to patients who have a significant component of psychosis or confusion contributing to their agitation. These agents possess mild α-antagonist properties as well as the ability to prolong the QT interval. Additionally, they may also have extrapyramidal effects and can trigger neuroleptic malignant syndrome. Luckily, such idiosyncratic effects are rarely seen, and these agents remain helpful in providing sedation in many ICU patients.

Appropriate attention to analgesia must be the first step in all sedation protocols because most patients (even nonsurgical critically ill patients) experience pain ranging from backaches due to prolonged supine positioning to invasive monitors that penetrate skin, muscle, and bone.[13] The lack of appropriate analgesia may lead to hypesthesia and paradoxical agitation in the face of other sedative drug administration. Once adequate analgesia has been established, the remainder of the sedation regimen should be targeted at maintaining patient comfort, behavioral control, and an appropriate degree of amnesia. The value of a standardized approach to sedation and the productive nature of interdisciplinary collaboration have been demonstrated clearly in terms of improved outcomes when such an approach is utilized.[14,15]

ANALGESIA

Patients are agitated for multiple reasons; however, inadequate pain control is the most common. Pain control can be established with any of a number of analgesic agents including opioids (morphine, fentanyl, dilaudid, etc.), nonsteroidal antiinflammatory agents, and opioid agonist–antagonist agents. Despite what is often believed to be adequate pain control and the euphoric effects of most narcotics, some patients continue to suffer agitation secondary to pain from often unrecognized sources such as prolonged immobility, chest tubes, and pressure points. To provide an adequate pain control regimen, the ICU care team must have the right tools in terms of assessment, documentation, and control of pain.[16] With these tools to assess and treat pain, better outcomes such as a quicker and more positive return to health can be expected.[17]

ANALGESIC AGENTS

Aspirin, Acetaminophen, and Nonsteroidal Antiinflammatory Drugs: These pharmacologic agents are recommended first-line therapy for the treatment of pain.[18] Despite this recommendation, their use in the ICU on a short-term basis is a frequently forgotten adjunct to pain control. Although opioids remain the mainstay of analgesia in the ICU, nonsteroidal anti-inflammatory agents such as ketorolac have been shown to have an efficacy comparable to moderate doses of commonly used opioids.[19] Nonetheless, clinical concerns often limit their usefulness, particularly in the postsurgical population.

Opioids: A careful understanding of the properties of individual opioids is essential to the appropriate use of these agents in the ICU. Most commonly, the full agonists morphine, hydromorphone, and fentanyl remain the most frequently chosen analgesics for the critically ill patient population. While popular in the past, meperidine is generally not advised as a long-term opioid to be used in the ICU due to accumulation of its neuroexcitatory metabolite, normeperidine, which can cause seizures.

Both morphine and hydromorphone have a half-life of 2 to 3 hours in healthy volunteers. However, metabolism of both these drugs may be influenced by the presence of underlying liver disease, renal disease, or alterations in protein binding. Thus, vigilance must be used when utilizing these agents in long-term infusions, as accumulation of their metabolites can lead to much difficulty in appropriate dosing.

Because critically ill patients often have altered peripheral blood flow, the use of intravenous dosing over intramuscular, subcutaneous, or transdermal delivery systems is often preferred. Demand-based patient-controlled analgesia (PCA) is often useful in allowing appropriate opioid dosing for pain control without oversedation and respiratory depression. Because of their underlying critical illness, many patients in the ICU do not possess the level of cognitive interaction required for appropriate PCA opioid dosing. Thus, the use of continuous opioid infusions has become quite popular.

Both morphine and meperidine possess histamine-releasing side effects. For critically ill patients in dire need of preload reduction (i.e., acute congestive heart failure), this vasodilating side effect can be quite beneficial. However, the vagolytic side of meperidine often prohibits its utility in an adult patient population with concomitant coronary artery disease. For some patients (i.e., those with brochospastic disease or severe hypotension), avoidance of the histamine-releasing side effects of these drugs can be quite beneficial.

Fentanyl is a high-potency opioid often used in the critically ill patient population. Its relative short duration of action often necessitates its use as an infusion. However, careful monitoring to avoid needless infusion of opioid in patients without pain is essential. Close chemical relatives of fentanyl include sufentanil and alfentanil. Their metabolism is less predictable than that of fentanyl, and their increased cost often makes these agents second-line choices. Remifentanil is, of course, an ultra-short-acting opioid with metabolism occurring by nonspecific esterases. Thus, it may have the most predictability of all of the opioid agents, but its cost for long-term ICU use is truly prohibitive. Table 33-4 provides a summary of opioid characteristics.

NEUROMUSCULAR BLOCKING AGENTS

A discussion of neuromuscular blocking agents may seem inappropriate when considering pain control in the ICU.

TABLE 33-4. PHYSICOCHEMICAL CHARACTERISTICS AND PHARMACOKINETICS OF COMMONLY USED OPIOID AGONISTS IN ADULTS

Parameter	Morphine	Meperidine	Fentanyl	Sufentanil	Alfentanil	Remifental
pK_a	7.9	8.5	8.4	8.0	6.5	7.26*
Amount nonionized (pH 7.4) (%)	23	7	8.5	20	89	58*
λ_{ow}	1.4	39	816	1757	128	17.9†
Protein binding (%)	35	70	84	93	92	66–93*
Clearance (mL/minute)	1050	1020	1530	900	238	4000
Vd_{ss} (L)	224	305	335	123	27	30
Rapid distribution half-life ($T_{1/2}\pi$, minutes)			1.2–1.9	1.4	1.0–3.5	0.4–0.5
Slow redistribution half-life ($T_{1/2}\alpha$, minutes)	1.5–4.4	4–16	9.2–19	17.7	9.5–17	2.0–3.7
Elimination half-life ($T_{1/2}\beta$, hours)	1.7–3.3	3–5	3.1–6.6	2.2–4.6	1.4–1.5	0.17–0.33

* Unpublished information from Glaxo. JG Bovill, personal communication.
† Glass PSA, Gan TJ, Howell S: A review of the pharmacokinetics and pharmacodynamics of remifentanil. Anesth Analg 89:S7–S14, 1999.
λ_{ow}, octanol:water partition coefficient; Vd_{ss}, steady-state volume of distribution.
Adapted from Bovill JG: Pharmacokinetics and pharmacodynamics of opioid agonists. Anaesth Pharmacol Rev 1:22, 1993.

TABLE 33-5. **NEUROMUSCULAR BLOCKING DRUGS FOR INTENSIVE CARE UNIT (ICU) USE**

Selected Benzylisoquinolinium Drugs (Trade Name)	Tubocurarine (Curare)	Cistacurium (Nimbex)	Atracurium (Tracrium)	Doxacurium (Nuromax)	Mivacurium (Mivacron)
Introduced (year)	1942	1995	1983	1991	1992
ED_{95} dose (mg/kg)	0.51	0.05	0.25	0.025–0.030	0.075
Initial dose (mg/kg)	0.2–0.3	0.20	0.4–0.5	Up to 0.1	0.15–0.25
Duration (minutes)	80	45–60	25–35	120–150	10–20
Infusion described	Rare	Yes	Yes	Yes	Yes
Infusion dose (μg/kg/minute)	–	2.5–3.0	4–12	0.3–0.5	9–10
Recovery (minutes)	80–180	90	40–60	120–180	10–20
Renal excretion (%)	40–45	Hofmann elimination	5–10 (uses Hofmann elimination)	70	Inactive metabolites
Renal failure	Increased effect	No change	No change	Increased effect	Increased duration
Biliary excretion (%)	10–40	Hofmann elimination	Minimal (uses Hofmann elimination)	Unclear	–
Hepatic failure	Minimum change to mild increased effect	Minimal to no change	Minimal to no change	?	Increased duration
Active metabolites	No	No	No, but can accumulate laudanosine	?	No
Histamine release hypotension	Marked	No	Minimal but dose dependent	None	Minimal but dose dependent
Vagal block tachycardia	Minimal	No	No	No	No
Ganglionic blockade hypotension	Marked	No	Minimal to none	No	No
Prolonged ICU block	?	Rare	Rare	Rare	?
Estimated US ICU use	Rare	Increasing	Minimal	Infrequent	Rare; NR
Cost (24-hour estimate)	NR	Decreasing	Decreasing	Intermediate	Very costly

Continued

TABLE 33-5. **NEUROMUSCULAR BLOCKING DRUGS FOR INTENSIVE CARE UNIT (ICU) USE—CONT'D**

Selected Aminosteroids (Trade Name)	Pancuronium (Pavulon)	Vecuronium (Arduan)	Pipecuronium (Arduan)	Rocuronium (Zemuron)	Rapacuronium (Raplon)
Introduced (year)	1972	1984	1991	1994	1999
ED$_{95}$ dose (mg/kg)	0.07	0.05	0.05	0.3	1.5
Initial dose (mg/kg)	0.1	0.1	0.085–0.1	0.6–1.0	1.5–2.0
Duration (minutes)	90–100	35–45	90–100	30	15–20
Infusion described	Yes	Yes	No	Yes	NR
Infusion dose (μg/kg/minute)	1–2	1–2	0.5–2.0	10–12	NR
Recovery (minutes)	120–180	45–60	55–160	20–30	30
Renal excretion (%)	45–70	50	50+	33	Significant
Renal failure	Increased effect	Increased effect, especially metabolites	Increased duration	Minimal	Accumulation of Org 9488 (active, potent metabolite)
Biliary excretion (%)	10–15	35–50	Minimal	>75	?
Hepatic failure	Mild increased effect	Variable, mild	Minimal	Moderate	?
Active metabolites	Yes: 3-OH and 17-OH-pancuronium	Yes: 3-desacetyl-vecuronium	Not reported	No	Yes: 3-OH-rapacuronium
Histamine release hypotension	None	None	None	None	Yes: 2–3% incidence bronchospasm
Vagal block tachycardia	Modest to marked	No	No	Some at higher doses	Mild tachycardia
Ganglionic blockade hypotension	No	No	No	No	Mild hypotension
Prolonged ICU block	Yes	Yes	No reports	No reports	NR
Estimated US ICU use	Variable	Decreasing	Uncommon	Variable	NR
Cost (24-hour estimate)	Inexpensive	Decreasing	Rarely used	More costly	NR

NR, not recommended.
Modified with permission from Prielipp RC, Coursin DB: Applied pharmacology of common neuromuscular blocking agents in critical care. New Horiz 2:34–47, 1994.

However, once again, the frequent use of neuromuscular blocking agents and confusion about their mechanism of action warrants some discussion. With the aggressive use of analgesic and sedation regimens in the ICU, neuromuscular blockade use has declined significantly over the past 10 to 15 years. The recognition of prolonged weakness and paralysis in critically ill patients secondary to use of neuromuscular blocking agents is a well-described phenomenon.[20,21] Additionally, the use of corticosteroids concomitantly has been shown to increase the risk of this complication, now termed acute quadriplegic myopathy.

In order to avoid this complication it is essential to have some understanding of the pharmacophysiology of neuromuscular blocking agents. The release of acetylcholine at the neuromuscular junction is caused by transmission of an action potential along the motor nerve. Once this action potential reaches the end of the motor nerve, acetylcholine is released into the neuromuscular junction, thereby stimulating muscle contraction. It is important to realize, however, that it is the nicotinic acetylcholine receptor subtype that is involved in conversion of the neural stimulus to muscle activity. Thus, by providing an agent that binds to the nicotinic acetylcholine receptor and prevents acetylcholine from binding, muscular response can be prevented. On rare occasions, such an effect is desired in the ICU, and neuromuscular blockade by nicotinic acetylcholine receptor antagonists is desired.

One of the most common reasons to utilize neuromuscular blocking agents in the ICU is patient–ventilator dyssynchrony. Such dyssynchrony can result in increased airway pressures which may predispose the patient to ventilator-induced lung injury. Additionally, adequate oxygenation and ventilation can become extremely difficult in many patients with dyssynchrony. In the past the most frequent form of treatment for this problem was administration of neuromuscular blockade. However, it is essential to realize that these drugs do not provide analgesia. They merely provide paralysis. Thus, not only does it become difficult to assess pain, agitation, and mental status, these agents can actually worsen patient anxiety by preventing patient movement in the presence of inadequate sedation. As one can imagine, many patients would find such a situation emotionally distressing. Thus, frequently the best approach to treatment of these patients consists of increasing opioid delivery to the patient. Since opioids provide respiratory depression, patient–ventilator dyssynchrony can be ameliorated by the use of an agent that will depress the patient's ventilatory drive without risking the side effects of prolonged paralysis from a neuromuscular blocking agent.

In addition to treating dyssynchrony, neuromuscular blocking agents are also used to decrease oxygen consumption in patients with tenuous oxygen supply versus demand. Such individuals may benefit from neuromuscular paralysis by decreasing metabolic oxygen consumption needs to a minimum. Individuals with evidence of anaerobic metabolism despite maximal maneuvers to increase tissue oxygen delivery may be able to return to a state of aerobic metabolism. Such treatment with a neuromuscular blocking agent must not be viewed as definitive, but, rather, a temporary means of controlling an oxygen supply versus demand imbalance.

The use of neuromuscular blocking agents to provide control of highly agitated patients who present a significant risk to themselves of self-harm may also benefit from short-term use of neuromuscular blocking agents. Patients who are at high risk of life-threatening self-extubation and those who remain uncooperative with potentially life-saving diagnostic studies may be appropriate candidates for the use of short-term neuromuscular blockade when attempts at maximal analgesia and sedation have failed. Additionally, in appropriate candidates, neuromuscular blockade can be used to facilitate endotracheal intubation or central venous catheterization when prior attempts at sedation have failed.

In addition to the risk of prolonged weakness due to neuromuscular blockade, the decision to use neuromuscular blocking agents in patients with a history of frequent tonic–clonic seizures or status epilepticus must occur only after careful consideration. It is important to realize that intact neuromuscular function provides the clinician with a constant monitor of potentially life-threatening seizure activity. However, in the patient who has received a neuromuscular blocking agent, this monitor is now unavailable. Thus, a risk exists that the patient may develop cerebral seizure activity without the awareness of health care providers. Such unrecognized, untreated prolonged cerebral seizure activity can then lead to irreversible neurologic injury and even brain death.

Understanding the metabolism and potential side effects of neuromuscular blocking agents such as potential hypotension, histamine release, and vagolysis is essential to the appropriate use of these agents. Table 33-5 provides a summary of the pharmacokinetic and pharmacodynamic properties of commonly used neuromuscular blocking agents.

SUMMARY

Maintaining sedation and analgesia is an extremely important goal in the care of critically ill patients. However, this aspect of their care frequently becomes lost in the myriad of physiologic derangements encountered in the critically ill patient. All sedation regimens have potentially adverse side effects that can endanger the patient's well-being and can prolong their clinical course.[22] In order to design a proper sedation regimen multiple critical endpoints and factors must be considered. These include duration of desired sedation, drug side effects, potential complications of the sedation regimen, and costs; such costs include not only the drugs alone, but also the aforementioned side effects and complications. Thus, it is essential that all members of the critical care team be aware of the sedation and analgesia plan, adhere to it, and be aware of the potential shortcomings of the plan so that appropriate adjustments can be made as the patient's condition changes or adverse effects emerge. Only with a systematized and consistent approach to sedation can one provide efficacious and cost-effective care to the tenuous patients who require this method of management.

REFERENCES

1. Stedman's Medical Dictionary, ed 23. Williams and Wilkins, Baltimore, MD, p 1267.
2. Ramsay M, Savege T, Simpson B, et al: Controlled sedation with alphaxalon–alphadolone. BMJ 2:656–659, 1974.
3. Riker RR, Picard JT, Fraser GL: Prospective evaluation of the Sedation-Agitation Scale for adult critically ill patients. Crit Care Med 27:1325–1329, 1999.
4. Shapiro BA, Warren J, Egol AB, et al: Practice parameters for intravenous analgesia and sedation for adult patients in the intensive care unit: An executive summary. Crit Care Med; 23: 1596–1600, 1995.

5. Young C, Knudsen N, Hilton A, Reves JG: Sedation in the intensive care unit. Crit Care Med 28:854–866, 2000.

6. Bennett S, McNeil M, Bland L, et al: Postoperative infections traces to contamination of an intravenous anesthetic, propofol. N Engl J Med 333:147–154, 1995.

7. Hall JE, Uhrich TD, Barney JA, et al: Sedative, amnestic, and analgesic properties of small-dose dexmedetomidine infusions. Anesth Analg 90:699–705, 2000.

8. Maze M, Fujinaga M: α_2 Adrenoceptors in pain modulation: Which subtype should be targeted to produce analgesia? Anesthesiology 92:934–936, 2000.

9. Kamibayashi T, Maze M: Clinical uses of α_2-adrenergic agonists. Anesthesiology 93:1345–1349, 2000.

10. Hall JE, Uhrich TD, Barney JA, et al: Sedative, amnestic, and analgesic properties of small-dose dexmedetomidine infusions. Anesth Analg 90:699–705, 2000.

11. Sullinen J, Haapallona A, Viltamaa A, et al: Adrenergic α_{2C}-receptors modulate the acoustic startle reflex, prepulse inhibition and aggression in mice. J Neurosci 18:3035–3042, 1998.

12. Lakhlani PP, MacMillan LB, Guo Tz, et al: Substitution of a mutant α_{2A}-adrenergic receptor via "hit and run" gene targeting reveals the role of this subtype in sedative, analgesic and anesthetic-sparing responses in vivo. Proc Natl Acad Sci USA 94:9950–9955, 1997.

13. Peruzzi WT: Sedation of the critically ill: Goals, plans, and cost-effectiveness. Crit Care Med 25:1942, 1997.

14. Brook AD, Ahrens TS, Schaiff R, et al: Effect of a nursing-implemented sedation protocol on the duration of mechanical ventilation. Crit Care Med 27:2609–2615, 1999.

15. Saura P, Blanch L, Mestre J, et al: Clinical consequences of the implementation of a weaning protocol. Intensive Care Med 22:1052–1056, 1996.

16. Stevens DS, Edwards WT: Management of pain in intensive care settings. Surg Clin North Am 79:371–386, 1999.

17. Watling SM, Dasta JF, Seidl EC: Sedatives, analgesics, and paralytics in the ICU. Ann Pharmacother 31:148–153, 1997.

18. Agency for Healthcare Policy and Research: Acute Pain Management: Operative or Medical Procedure and Trauma. US Department of Health and Human Services, Rockville, MD.

19. Gillis JC, Brogden RN: Ketorolac. A reappraisal of its pharmacodynamic and pharmacokinetic properties and therapeutic use in pain management. Drugs 53:139–188, 1997.

20. Segredo V, Caldwell JE, Mathay MA, et al: Persistent paralysis in critically ill patients after long-term administration of vecuronium. N Engl J Med 327:524–528, 1992.

21. Watling SM, Dasta JF: Prolonged paralysis in intensive care unit patients after the use of neuromuscular blocking agents: A review of the literature. Crit Care Med 5:884–893, 1994.

22. Lowson SM, Sawh S: Adjuncts to analgesia: Sedation and neuromuscular blockade. Crit Care Clin 15:119–141, 1999.

Classification of Headache

Atif B. Malik, M.D.,

Burak Alptekin, M.D., and

Zahid H. Bajwa, M.D.

Headache is amongst the most common medical complaints. The oldest known medical manuscript, the Ebers Papyrus, discovered at Thebes, Egypt, describes a cure for the headache consisting of using a ceramic crocodile with herbs stuffed into its mouth and tying it around the head of the patient. One may wonder if it was the compression around the head that was more effective than the crocodile. Headaches were also a noted problem among the immortal Greek gods. Zeus, father of all the gods, was struck down with such an excruciating headache that he begged Hepaestus, god of the blacksmiths, to split his skull open with an axe.

DIFFERENTIAL DIAGNOSIS OF HEADACHES

With persistent, recurrent headaches, the history becomes of primary importance in establishing the proper diagnosis. Important factors to consider include:

- Onset
- Duration
- Periodicity
- Timing
- Localization
- Intensity
- Character
- Precipitating factors
- Accompanying symptoms and signs
- Response to therapy

The exact description of the nature, duration, and timing of the headache often permits the correct diagnosis. Prior to the criteria of the International Headache Society (IHS), there was confusion related to terminology, and various headache classifications. For clinical purposes, headaches are divided into two broad categories: primary headaches and secondary headaches. Primary headaches are those with no organic or structural etiology, which include migraine, cluster, tension, and rebound headaches. Secondary headaches are indicative of an underlying structural lesion. Thus, it is also helpful to understand the structures that can be a source of pain when stimulated. These structures include middle meningeal artery, dural sinuses, dural folds including falx cerebri, and the proximal segments of pial arteries.

PRIMARY HEADACHES

Migraine

CLINICAL FEATURES: Migraine usually features recurring headaches in genetically prone individuals that are typically unilateral, ranging in pain from moderate to severe. Migraine is associated with various combinations of symptoms that include nausea, vomiting, autonomic symptoms, and sensitivity to light, smell, and sound. Migraine attacks can occur at any time of the day or night, but severe attacks frequently occur upon arising in the morning. Episodes last from several hours to days (4 to 72 hours) and are often disabling. Even routine activity or slight head movement can exacerbate the pain. Pain can migrate from one part of the head to another and may radiate to the neck or shoulder. Most patients also experience scalp tenderness during and/or after an attack.

Migraine is three times more common in women than men, tends to run in families, and is typically a disorder of young, primarily healthy women. The genetic association is about 70% among first-degree relatives.[1] Migraine without aura is the most common type, accounting for approximately 80% of these headaches. Migraine is an episodic headache that may be classified into three types:[2]

1. Migraine with aura (old term classic migraine).
2. Migraine without aura (old term common migraine).
3. Migraine variants (retinal migraine, ophthalmoplegic migraine, familial hemiplegic migraine).

MIGRAINE WITH AURA: Migraine with aura is commonly referred to as a classic migraine. Prior to the onset of this headache, a patient may experience several forms of visual, sensory, and motor symptoms. The visual symptoms include flashes of light (photopsia), wavy linear patterns on the visual fields (fortification spectra), scintillating scotoma, or blurred vision. Symptoms of aura can last from 5 to 60 minutes, but typically average 15 to 20 minutes. The headache is commonly described as unilateral throbbing or pulsatile. The side affected in each episode may be different.

Nausea, vomiting (less common), photophobia, phonophobia, irritability, and malaise are common symptoms. During the headache phase of migraine, patients prefer to lie quietly in a dark room. A history of certain triggers can be elicited. Common triggers include certain foods, fasting, hormonal changes, head trauma, physical exertion, fatigue, lack of sleep, drugs, stress, and barometric changes.

If the headache is always on the same side, then a structural lesion needs to be excluded by careful history, neurologic examination, and possibly imaging studies. Having a history of recurrent typical attacks and determining the provoking agent are important because a secondary headache can sometimes mimic migraine. A new headache, or change in character of the headache, even if it appears typical by history, should always evoke a broad differential diagnosis and the possibility of a structural lesion.

MIGRAINE WITHOUT AURA: Migraine without aura is a recurring headache disorder with attacks lasting 4 to 72 hours. Typically it is unilateral, pulsating, moderate to severe in intensity, aggravated by routine physical activity, and associated with nausea, photophobia, phonophobia, and less commonly vomiting.

MIGRAINE VARIANTS: *Familial hemiplegic migraine (FHM)* is a rare type of migraine that is inherited as an autosomal dominant disorder. It is a type of migraine with aura associated with hemiplegia, which typically resolves. About 50% of families with FHM are linked to a chromosome 19p13 or 1q locus in the CACNA 1A gene that encodes neuronal Ca^{2+} channels.[3] By definition, at least one relative must have identical attacks. Cerebellar ataxia may be associated with FHM and manifests at the same chromosome linkage, the 19p locus. There is also some evidence that chromosome 19p FHM locus may even be involved in patients with nonhemiplegic migraine.

Basilar migraines were previously referred to as Bickerstaff's migraine or syncopal migraine. Predominantly effecting children and adolescents, this less common form of a migraine can be seen at any age and has strong relation to menses. Basilar migraines have been described by the IHS as migraine with aura symptoms that clearly originate from the brain stem or from both occipital lobes. Symptoms associated with basilar migraines may include vertigo, confusion, dysarthria, paresthesias, weakness, double vision, and incoordination.

Migraine without headache, also called aura without the headache, tends to occur in patents that have a history of migraines with aura. As they get older the auras continue without subsequent headache attack. A vertebrobasilar migraine may present without experiencing a headache, but with vertebrobasilar symptoms such as vertigo, dizziness, confusion, dysarthria, tingling of extremities, and incoordination. Thromboembolic event should be considered if symptoms persist.

Ophthalmoplegic migraine is a type of migraine that is associated with transient extraocular muscle palsies. Most cases of well-defined ophthalmoplegic migraine occur before the age of 10 without a strong family history.

Retinal migraine is also referred to as anterior visual pathway migraine, ocular migraine, and ophthalmic migraine. This headache is associated with at least two attacks of monocular scotoma or blindness lasting less than 60 minutes with normal ophthalmologic examination outside of the attack. This is fully reversible, but if clinically indicated, embolism should be ruled out at the initial presentation. Retinal migraine as a diagnosis for transient blindness of monocular pattern should be reached as a diagnosis of exclusion.

EPIDEMIOLOGY OF MIGRAINE: A 1993 survey done in the USA revealed that migraine was the primary cause of 150 million lost workdays and 329,000 lost school days each year.[4] Migraines affect 6% of males and 17% of females in the USA. Prior to puberty, migraine prevalence is similar in both sexes but after puberty it is much higher in women. There is a decline in the incidences of migraines after the age of 40. In the USA, Caucasian women have the highest incidence of migraines, while Asian women have the lowest incidence. The female-to-male ratio increases from 2.5:1 at puberty to 3.5:1 at the age of 40. After the age of 40, the ratio declines. Currently, 1 of 6 American women experience migraine headaches. The incidence of migraine in women of reproductive age has increased over the last 20 years.

Tension-Type Headache: Tension-type headache (TTH) is the most common headache syndrome. A simple clinical rule is that TTHs are characterized as head pain devoid of typical migrainous features that does not worsen with daily activity. According to the IHS classification system, the term TTH replaces previous terms used of muscle contraction headaches, tension headaches, and chronic daily headaches. TTHs feel like pressure or tightness around the head and have a tendency to wax and wane in intensity. The IHS further subcategorized TTH into two groups, episodic and chronic, by the frequency of the attacks. Patients are diagnosed with episodic tension-type headache (ETTH) if the number of days with headaches is less than 180 per year and less than 15 per month. Headache of frequency in excess of these numbers is termed chronic tension-type headache (CTTH).

EPISODIC TENSION-TYPE HEADACHE: ETTH patients have recurrent episodes of headaches that last anything from 30 minutes to 7 days. Nausea is absent, but patients may experience photophobia or phonophobia if the pain worsens and remains untreated. The pain is described as pressing/tightening, bilateral, mild to moderate intensity, and does not worsen with activity. This type of headache is further subcategorized by the IHS if pericranial muscle tension is present or absent. This is probably not relevant in the clinic but important for research since EMG is required to measure quantitatively muscle tension.

CHRONIC TENSION-TYPE HEADACHE: In comparison, CTTH criteria include headaches present for a minimum of at least 15 days a month, for at least 6 months. Like ETTH, the pain characteristics are the same; however, CTTH may be associated with migrainous features. Like ETTH, CTTH may be subcategorized with or without pericranial muscle tension. Some patients may have overlapping features of both migraine and TTHs. Those individuals are hard to label satisfactorily with a single diagnosis. Clinical features that appear to be most predictable of migraines compared with TTHs include nausea, photophobia, phonophobia, and exacerbation by physical activity. Food triggers are also more common with migraine than TTH. There is a high correlation between analgesic abuse of over-the-counter analgesics, muscle relaxants, acetaminophen, aspirin, opioids, barbiturates, and benzodiazepines in these chronic headache sufferers. As a general rule, psychological factors play a more important role in individuals suffering from TTH compared to patients with either migraine or cluster headache.

EPIDEMIOLOGY OF TENSION-TYPE HEADACHE:
The 1-year prevalence has been variably reported from 30% to 90% for TTH. Lifetime prevalence ranges between 30% and 78%, peaking in the fourth decade with gender distribution of 63% males and 86% females. In a 1998 study women had a higher 1-year ETTH prevalence than men in all age, race, and education groups. Prevalence peaks in the 30 to 39 year age group in both men (42.3%) and women (46.9%).[5] Whites had a higher 1-year prevalence than African Americans in men (40.1% vs. 22.8%) and women (46.8% vs 30.9%). Prevalence increased with increasing educational levels in both sexes. The 1-year period prevalence of CTTH was 2.2%; prevalence was higher in women and declined with increasing education. Of subjects with ETTH, 8.3% reported lost workdays because of their headaches. Subjects with CTTH reported more lost workdays compared with subjects with ETTH.

Cluster Headache:
Cluster headaches are characterized by repetitive headaches that occur for a week to several months at a time and are followed by periods of remission. Although pathogenesis remains unclear, there is a striking circadian annual periodicity of these headaches. Some authors have raised the question of the possibility that the hypothalamic center is the site of initiation.[6] The pain begins quickly without any warning and reaches a crescendo within 10 to 15 minutes. If untreated a typical cluster headache lasts from 30 minutes to 3 hours with a mean of 60 minutes. Frequency of attacks varies between each person during the "cluster period." Pain is always unilateral, remaining on one side of the head during a single cluster. The pain can switch sides during the next cluster. The pain is usually deep, excruciating, continuous, and explosive in quality. Occasionally the pain may be pulsatile and throbbing. The pain usually begins in or around the eye or temple. Less commonly the pain may start in the face, neck, ear, or hemicranium. Some patients report superimposed paroxysms of stabbing "ice pick" like pain in the periorbital region, which lasts for a few seconds and occurs once or several times in rapid succession. Most patients feel agitated or restless, in contrast to migraine sufferers who tend to rest in a dark, quiet room.

Cluster headaches are often associated with ipsilateral lacrimation, redness of the eye, stuffy nose, rhinorrhea, sweating, and pallor. Focal neurologic symptoms are rare other than Horner's syndrome. Over 50% of sufferers report sensitivity to alcohol during a cluster period, which ceases when the cluster ends. The use of alcohol, histamine, or nitroglycerine during an attack of cluster headache may worsen the attack.

EPISODIC CLUSTER HEADACHE:
Episodic cluster headache (ECH) typically lasts several weeks and occurrences are separated by a remission period of at least 2 weeks. Of all the different types of cluster headaches from which people suffer, ECHs account for the majority of headaches.

CHRONIC CLUSTER HEADACHE:
Chronic cluster headache (CCH) attacks continue for longer than 1 year without remission, or remission is less than 2 weeks. Patients with CCH have regular attacks that are often provoked by histamine, nitroglycerine, or alcohol. Either form of cluster headache can transform into the other. Attacks tend to reoccur at the same hour each day for the duration of a single cluster; attacks occur between 9 pm and 9 am in most patients.

CHRONIC PAROXYSMAL HEMICRANIA:
Chronic paroxysmal hemicrania (CPH) syndrome is much like a cluster headache but the symptoms are shorter in duration and are more frequent. This syndrome tends to occur more frequently among women than men (ratio 6:1) and there is complete resolution with indomethacin. Pain is usually severe, unilateral, and lasts 2 to 45 minutes. CPH may also have associated conjunctival injection, rhinorrhea, ptosis, eyelid edema, and lacrimation.

EPIDEMIOLOGY OF CLUSTER HEADACHE:
Cluster headache affects about 0.4% of the general population and the male-to-female ratio is 5 to 1. It can occur at any age but usually begins in the late twenties. The peak age of onset is between 25 and 50 years but approximately 10% of patients experience their first cluster attack in their sixties.[7] Approximately 90% have episodic cluster and 10% chronic cluster (cluster period lasts for more than 1 year without remission or remission lasts less than 14 days).

Miscellaneous Headaches:
These are headaches unassociated with structural lesions and tend to be self-explanatory. These include:

- Idiopathic stabbing headache: "ice-pick" pains.
- External compression headache: "swim-goggle" headache.
- Cold stimulus headache: brought on by exposure to cold temperature.
- Benign cough headache: brought on by coughing.
- Benign exertional headache: "weight-lifter's" headache.
- Benign sex headache (coital/orgasmic cephalalgia).

SECONDARY HEADACHES

Secondary headaches are related to organic or structural etiologies. Some of the common forms in which secondary headaches manifest are discussed below.

Headache Associated With Head Trauma
ACUTE POST-TRAUMATIC HEADACHE: This type of headache can be part of the postconcussion syndrome, which presents with a wide spectrum of symptoms. These usually develop within 2 weeks after loss of consciousness or post-traumatic amnesia for more than 10 minutes.[8] There are subtle abnormalities in the neurologic examination, neuropsychological testing, or imaging studies that are done on patients. The headaches usually resolve within 2 months.

CHRONIC POST-TRAUMATIC HEADACHE: This type has the same presentation as acute post-traumatic headache, but persists for more than 2 months.[8] Patients may complain of vague headaches, fatigue, memory problems, and irritability for months or years after the traumatic event.

Headache Associated with Vascular Disorders

INTRACRANIAL HEMATOMA: Many of the patients with acute subdural hematoma have alterations of consciousness, and headaches that may have been underreported. There is wide variation of headaches from chronic subdural hematomas that range from mild to severe and paroxysmal to constant. Unilateral headaches usually occur on the same side of the subdural hematoma. Acceleration–deceleration forces associated with riding on a roller coaster without direct head trauma can tear bridging veins leading to a subdural hematoma. These may also be seen in severe whiplash injuries without direct head trauma. Classic epidural hematoma occurs after head injury to the temporoparietal region with or without initial loss of consciousness. This is usually followed by a lucid interval that deteriorates into coma within 12 hours of the injury. Chronic epidural hematoma may be associated with persistent headache, nausea, vomiting, and memory impairment consistent with a postconcussion syndrome.

SUBARACHNOID HEMORRHAGE: Headache following subarachnoid hemorrhage can be acute, severe, and continuous. They are usually associated with nausea, vomiting, meningismus, and sometimes loss of consciousness. The classic presentation of headache related to subarachnoid hemorrhage includes sudden onset, severe "blinding" head pain, stiff neck, vomiting, and altered mental status. The patient may have severe pain that is bilateral and present with neck stiffness and fever. Subarachnoid blood is usually found on lumbar puncture, if it is performed. As the majority of computed tomography scans reveal subarachnoid blood, lumbar puncture is not automatically indicated.

Characteristic focal deficits that develop are dependent on the location of the ruptured vessel or aneurysm. One example is the third nerve palsy that often follows rupture of a posterior communicating artery aneurysm.

UNRUPTURED ANEURYSMS AND ARTEROVENOUS MALFORMATIONS: Although unruptured aneurysms are usually asymptomatic these may also produce headache by compressing neighboring structures, or by rapid growth or a small leak from the aneurysm. When the headache pattern is completely stereotyped throughout life, strong suspicion should be raised as to the possibility of an arterovenous malformation rather than migraine with aura. Arterovenous malformations on occasion can be of the etiology of sudden onset of headaches and should be suspected when headache occurs with accompanying neurologic signs.[9]

TEMPORAL ARTERITIS OR GIANT CELL ARTERITIS: Temporal arteritis (TA) or giant cell arteritis (GCA) are systemic disorders characterized by an inflammatory obliterative arteritis, particularly, but not exclusively, involving branches of the external carotid and ophthalmic arteries. These disorders are well known to cause anterior ischemic optic neuropathy and ophthalmoplegia. The most common initial symptom is headache, often accompanied by diffuse aches and pains in the back and shoulders (polymyalgia rheumatica). The headache is characterized by gradual onset of head soreness or burning discomfort that progresses into a diffuse, often severe and well-localized constant pain. There may be exquisite tenderness of the scalp and blood vessels particularly in the temporal region. The headache is usually worse at night, and may be especially aggravated by exposure to cold. It must be actively sought in any recent-onset headache patient presenting after the age of 50, particularly in those with systemic symptoms. Approximately half of untreated cases progress to blindness. An elevated sedimentation rate is considered indispensable in diagnosing TA, although temporal artery biopsy is considered the gold standard diagnostic procedure.

CAROTID ARTERY PAIN: Carotid artery pain is usually associated with Horner's syndrome, transient ischemic symptoms, or neck pain. There may be tenderness, swelling, visible pulsations, and pain over the affected side. The headache may begin after an endarterectomy.

VENOUS THROMBOSIS: The classic presentation of cortical vein thrombosis occurs along with seizures and headaches. There may be neurologic deficits depending upon what venous areas are affected. The headache may be focal or diffuse.

ARTERIAL HEADACHE: Chronic moderate hypertension does not cause headache but acute hypertension can present with headache and other symptoms of hypertensive encephalopathy. New-onset headache has been associated with pheochromocytoma. Patients with this tumor have headaches that occur when the diastolic blood pressure suddenly increases more than 25% above normal. There may be associated sweating, palpitations, and anxiety. Headaches also occur with malignant hypertension, pre-eclampsia, and eclampsia. These headaches usually resolve once blood pressure normalizes.

Headache Associated with Nonvascular Intercranial Disorder

HIGH CEREBROSPINAL FLUID PRESSURE (PSEUDOTUMOR CEREBRI): High cerebrospinal fluid (CSF) pressure is associated with diffuse headache in nearly all patients when CSF pressure rises above 200 mm. Typically, these headaches are transiently relieved by lumbar puncture in this disorder. Additional symptoms may include spinal and radicular pain or facial pain. Symptoms may occasionally be the presenting complaints. Many patients complain of headache long after papilledema and raised intracranial pressure have resolved.

LOW CEREBROSPINAL FLUID PRESSURE (POSTLUMBAR PUNCTURE HEADACHE): Up to 30% of patients develop a headache following lumbar puncture. The size of the needle used, the amount of fluid withdrawn, and multiple punctures are all factors that influence the development of a headache. Lumbar puncture headaches usually begin within 48 hours and are dramatically positional. Pain is relieved when the patient lies down with their feet elevated to a higher level than the head. This headache is best described as extremely painful or "bursting" and usually worse in the occipital region and forehead, but may extend into the neck and shoulders. The headache usually lasts for 2 to 3 days, but may persist for as long as 2 weeks. It is very rare for lumbar puncture headache to last for many months.

INTRACRANIAL NEOPLASM: Headaches associated with intracranial tumors are initially paroxysmal, wake patient from their sleep at night, and are associated with projectile vomiting. With time, the headaches may become continuous and intensify with activities that increase intracranial pressure (e.g., Valsalva maneuver, coughing, sneezing). Foramen magnum tumors are present with occipital headache. Headaches worsen in the supine position and are relieved by standing up. Headaches related to chronic hydrocephalus are diffuse and can also radiate down the neck.

Headache Associated with Substance Use or Withdrawal

Patients who develop a new form of headache in close temporal relation to substance use or substance withdrawal is specified and the criteria listed below:

HEADACHE ASSOCIATED WITH FOOD: It is important to establish that a substance really induces a headache. There are a variety of substances and particular foods and alcohol that may precipitate vascular headache. Some well-known types of syndromes associated with headaches include hot dog headache, Chinese restaurant syndrome, and vitamin-A-induced headache.

HEADACHE ASSOCIATED WITH CHRONIC SUBSTANCE USAGE: These headaches occur daily after exposure to a substance for more than 3 months. This type of headache is chronic (>15 days/month) and disappears within 1 month of withdrawal of the agent. This category includes ergotamine-induced headache, and analgesics abuse headache.

HEADACHE FROM SUBSTANCE WITHDRAWAL: The acute type is most often associated with alcohol (hangover). The headache associated with substance withdrawal is described as a bilateral, symmetrical, throbbing headache. The chronic type is associated with ergotamine, caffeine, or narcotics.

Headache Associated with Infection or Fever:

Septicemia, bacteremia, and fever are also commonly associated with headache. The most intense, prolonged headaches associated with infections are those that accompany typhoid fever, typhus fever, and influenza. Headache is dull, deep, aching, and generalized, but is often worse, especially at the beginning, in the back of the head. The pain increases in intensity with physical effort and is worse in the latter part of the day.

Headache Associated with Metabolic Disorder:

These headaches are associated with derangements of metabolism.

- Hypoxia. Intense throbbing headache, sensation of fullness of the head, flushed face, photophobia, injection of the ocular mucosa, and cyanosis.
- Decompression headache. Decompression sickness appears when a sudden change in the pressure of ambient gases, to which the subject has become equilibrated, occurs. A sudden reduction in pressure of 45% is usually sufficient to cause symptoms.
- Headache associated with high altitude. Headaches occur within 24 hours after sudden assent to altitudes above 3000 meters and, according to IHS coding criteria, are associated

with at least one or other symptoms typical of high altitude, namely Cheyne Stokes respirations at night, desire to overbreathe, and dyspnea.
- Hypercapnia. Retention of CO_2 causes vasodilatation and diffuse headache. Chronic hypercapnia from pulmonary disease and situations such as the Pickwickian syndrome are often accompanied by increased intracranial pressure and severe diffuse headache, similar to that seen in pseudotumor cerebri.
- Hypoglycemia. Headaches may be precipitated by attacks of hunger and by fasting.
- Dialysis. Headaches occur with varying degrees of severity during dialysis in about 70% of dialyzed patients.

HEADACHE NOT CLASSIFIED BY IHS

Chronic Daily Headache: Chronic daily headache (CDH) has not been satisfactorily characterized by the IHS. Siberstein et al. proposed that CDH is a group of disorders that includes CTTH, transformed migraine (TM), new daily persistent headache (NDPH), and hemicrania continua (HC).[10] CDH is essentially CTTH that persists more than 4 hours per day, and occurs 15 or more days per month. CDH usually evolves over several months or years. There is usually a slow increase in tension-type headache symptoms and concomitant decrease in migraine features. CDH can also occur as the result of polypharmacy or analgesic abuse in some patients.[11]

REFERENCES

1. Kors EE, Haan J, Ferrari MD: Genetics of primary headaches. Curr Opin Neurol 12:249–254, 1999.
2. Olesen J; Headache Classification Committee of the International Headache Society: Classification and diagnostic criteria for headache disorders, cranial neuralgia, and facial pain. Cephalalgia 8(Suppl 7):1–96, 1988.
3. Ducros A, Denier C, Joutel A, et al: The clinical spectrum of familial hemiplegic migraine associated with mutations in a neuronal calcium channel. N Engl J Med 345:17–24, 2001.
4. Lipton RB, Stewart WF: Migraine in the United States: Epidemiology and health care utilization. Neurology 43(Suppl 3):6–10, 1993.
5. Schwartz BS, et al: Epidemiology of tension-type headache. JAMA 279:381–383, 1998.
6. Jarrar RG, Black DF, Dodick DW, Davis DH: Outcome of trigeminal nerve section in the treatment of chronic cluster headache. Neurology 60:1360–1362, 2003.
7. Mathew NT: Advances in cluster headache. Neurol Clin 8:867–890, 1990.
8. Haas DC: Chronic post-traumatic headaches classified and compared with natural headaches. Cephalalgia 16:486–493, 1996.
9. Troost TB: Neuro-Ophthalmology, ed 3. JB Lippincott, Philadelphia, 2000.
10. Siberstein SD, Lipton RB, Solomon S, Mathew NT: Classification of daily and near-daily headaches: Proposed revisions to the HIS criteria. Headache 34:1–7, 1994.
11. Mathew NT: Transformed migraine, analgesic rebound, and other chronic daily headaches. Neurol Clin 15:167–186, 1997.

Migraine Headache and Cluster Headache

Jack M. Rozental, M.D., Ph.D., M.B.A.

MIGRAINE HEADACHE

Epidemiology: Migraine headache represents a very common benign headache syndrome; it is sometimes referred to as a vascular headache. Approximately two-thirds of migraines occur in women. The prevalence in North America, ascertained through epidemiologic studies, is 12% to 17.6% in females and 4% to 6% in males. Prior to puberty, the prevalence of migraine in boys and girls is similar; during and after adolescence, the prevalence increases more rapidly in girls. Prevalence increases up to the age of about 40, after which it decreases; the decrease becomes steeper in women as they approach menopause. Among those with severe migraine, about 25% have four or more migraines per month. More than 80% of patients with severe migraines experience headache-related disability which ranges from decreased productivity to time off work during an attack. The cost in productivity may exceed $20 billion per year in the USA. Although the cause of migraines is unknown, the risk of suffering from migraines is about 50% higher among those who have a first-degree relative with migraines; however, genetic factors appear to account for fewer than 50% of all migraines.[1-4]

Pathophysiology: The pain-generating structures of the head include the venous sinuses, meningeal and large cerebral arteries, basal meninges, muscles, skin, and cranial nerves V, IX, and X. A plexus of largely unmyelinated fibers arises from the trigeminal ganglion and innervates the cerebral and pial arteries, the venous sinuses, and the dura mater; this plexus is referred to as the trigeminovascular system. A similar plexus arises from the dorsal roots of the upper three cervical nerves and innervates comparable structures in the posterior fossa. The neurons in the trigeminovascular system contain substance P, one of the major nociceptive neurotransmitters of primary sensory neurons; calcitonin gene-related peptide (CGRP), a peptide that causes vasodilatation and when infused intravenously into susceptible individuals triggers headache; and neurokinin A. When the trigeminal ganglion is stimulated, these peptide neurotransmitters are released near the blood vessels they innervate, a process that results in vasodilatation with consequent extravasation of plasma, or so-called sterile neurogenic inflammation. Leakage of plasma proteins from the dilated blood vessels in turn act on the trigeminal nerve endings with the end result of sterile neurogenic inflammation being the perception of pain in and around the head. Neurogenic inflammation is blocked by substances that act as agonists on a subset of serotonin (5-hydroxytryptamine, or 5-HT) receptors: the 5-HT_{1D} and 5-HT_{1B} receptors. The major drugs used to abort acute migraine attacks are agonists at the $5\text{-HT}_{1D/1B}$ receptors. Intravenous infusions of serotonin can also abort a migraine attack. Drugs that act as agonists at these sites are thought to reduce neurogenic inflammation by causing vasoconstriction and by inhibiting the trigeminal nerve endings. Agonists at the $5\text{-HT}_{1D/1B}$ receptors include ergot alkaloids (ergotamine, dihydroergotamine), triptans (sumatriptan and others), and maybe aspirin and indomethacin. Similarly, stimulation of pain-generating structures in the head activates neurons in the trigeminal nucleus caudalis and in the dorsal horn at the upper cervical levels.[5-7]

Thus, stimulation of the trigeminal ganglion, through release of neurotransmitters, results in increased cerebral and extracerebral blood flow. Stimulation of the dorsal raphe nucleus, a serotonergic nucleus in the midbrain, also increases cerebral blood flow. In contrast, stimulation of the nucleus caeruleus, the major source of central noradrenergic input, causes a decrease in cerebral blood flow.

Pain interneurons in the spinal cord and brainstem use enkephalins and γ-aminobutyric acid (GABA) as neurotransmitters. An ascending serotonergic pathway in the midbrain raphe region relays painful stimuli to the ventroposteromedial (VPM) thalamus via the quintothalamic tract. A descending endogenous pain modulating system originates in the periaqueductal gray region of the midbrain, one of whose major relay structures is the nucleus raphe magnus in the medulla. After this relay, the descending pain modulating system connects with the spinal tract of the trigeminal nerve and the dorsal horns of the first through third cervical nerves. Stimulation of the periaqueductal gray region causes headache. The major neurotransmitters of this pain modulating system are norepinephrine, serotonin, and enkephalins.[5,6]

In patients who have migraine with aura it is thought that the cortex, particularly the occipital cortex, is hyperexcitable. This hyperexcitability may relate to decreased intracellular magnesium levels, to a dysfunction of brain mitochondria, or to abnormal calcium channels. Thus, the aura phase of migraine begins as a wave of cortical neural excitation, accompanied by hyperemia, and is followed by an electrical wave of spreading neural depression and oligemia in the cortex. During the oligemic phase, blood flow remains above the ischemic threshold. This process most commonly originates in the occipital cortex; hence the visual nature of most migrainous auras. This spreading depression advances over the involved cortex at a rate of 2 to 6 mm/minute, a rate similar to that of the developing aura. Neither the spreading neural excitation and hyperemia nor the ensuing spreading depression and oligemia respect vascular territories and are thus thought to represent neural, not vascular, phenomena.[8] The trigeminovascular system might be activated through polysynaptic pathways from the activated cortex, or directly by the same mechanism that causes the aura.[5] Aura usually precedes, but sometimes accompanies, the headache phase of migraine. Spreading neural depression and oligemia in the cortex are thought not to occur in migraine without aura.

A growing body of evidence points to the importance of dopamine in the pathophysiology of migraine and its associated symptoms.[9] Dopamine receptor hypersensitivity may be responsible for the nausea, vomiting, hypotension, and dizziness that frequently accompany, and sometimes characterize, attacks of migraine. These symptoms can be elicited by low doses of dopamine or by dopamine agonists—especially in migraneurs. Antiemetics, most of which are dopamine receptor antagonists (especially at the D2 receptor), are frequently useful, and sometimes effective in and of themselves in treating migraine attacks.

Diagnosis: The diagnosis of migraine is made by a suggestive clinical history and a normal neurologic examination (see Table 35-1). The classic description of migraine is that of a

TABLE 35-1. INTERNATIONAL HEADACHE SOCIETY DIAGNOSTIC CRITERIA FOR MIGRAINE

Migraine without aura	At least five headache attacks Headache lasts 4–72 hours Has at least two of the following, but no weakness: • Unilateral • Pulsating • Moderate to severe • Aggravated by routine physical activity Has at least one of the following: • Nausea • Vomiting • Photophobia • Phonophobia
Migraine with aura (a headache with the characteristics of migraine without aura follows or accompanies the aura)	At least two headache attacks Headache lasts 4–72 hours Has at least one of the following reversible symptoms, but no weakness: • Positive or negative visual symptoms like flickering lights, spots, lines, or loss of vision (such as blurred vision, a scotoma, homonymous hemianopsia) • Positive or negative sensory symptoms like tingling or numbness • Dysphasia
Basilar migraine	At least two attacks of migraine with an aura whose reversible symptoms are brainstem or bihemispheric in origin (but without weakness) Symptoms can include: • Dysarthria • Dizziness or vertigo • Tinnitus with or without hypacusia • Diplopia • Visual symptoms in both temporal or nasal fields • Ataxia • Decreased level of consciousness • Bilateral paresthesias

Continued

TABLE 35-1. INTERNATIONAL HEADACHE SOCIETY DIAGNOSTIC CRITERIA FOR MIGRAINE—CONT'D

Aura without headache	At least two attacks of symptoms typical of auras, such as visual, sensory, or speech disturbance, without weakness, that are not followed by a headache and that resolve completely within 1 hour
Hemiplegic migraine	At least two attacks Aura of fully reversible motor weakness and one of the following: • Positive or negative visual symptoms • Positive or negative sensory symptoms • Dysphasia If at least one first- or second-degree relative has a migrainous aura that includes motor weakness it is familial hemiplegic migraine and is associated with a mutation in the neuronal calcium channel If no first- or second-degree relative has migrainous aura that includes motor weakness it is sporadic hemiplegic migraine Frequently accompanied by symptoms of basilar type migraine

From The International Classification of Headache Disorders, 2nd edition. Cephalalgia 24(Suppl 1):1–150, 2004.

recurrent headache lasting 4 to 72 hours, of moderate to severe intensity, pulsating, aggravated by routine physical activity, and associated with nausea, photophobia, and/or phonophobia. The major subtypes of migraine are migraine with aura and migraine without aura. The most frequent migrainous aura consists of visual symptoms such as bright spots, dark spots, tunnel vision, or zigzag lines (fortification spectra). Other common auras include numbness or paresthesias in one arm or side of the body. The aura is followed (or sometimes accompanied) by an intense, crescendo head pain, frequently unilateral or retro-ocular; it may be described as pounding, throbbing, pressure-like, exploding, stabbing, or vise-like.[10] Migrainous auras, particularly visual ones, occasionally occur independently of pain; these are called migraine equivalents. Typically, the headache phase lasts from 30 minutes to 1 day. Occasionally the headache becomes intractable and lasts a week or longer: this is status migrainosus. Migraines are usually accompanied by other symptoms, such as photophobia, phonophobia, osmophobia, and nausea with or without emesis. There seems to be a slightly increased risk for stroke among migraneurs.[11]

A migraine whose aura seems to originate in the brainstem or involve both hemispheres is called basilar migraine.[12] A typical aura in basilar migraine might present with hemianopsia or even blindness (which could be bitemporal or binasal). Following, or independent of the visual phenomena, patients may complain of vertigo, dysarthria, diplopia, tinnitus, ataxia, a decreased level of consciousness, or bilateral sensory (paresthesias) or subjective motor symptoms (there should be no objective weakness). Some patients present with other types of auras such as a dysphasia, and as such may resemble a transient ischemic attack (TIA), a stroke, or an evolving neurologic catastrophe. Some patients develop severe headache, sometimes described as exploding, related to exertion: these are exertional migraines. Exertional migraines can develop while engaged in heavy work or sports, lifting weights, or during sexual climax[13] (the latter are more frequent in males). On the other hand, a severe ocular headache that presents with ophthalmoplegia (usually of the oculomotor nerve and includes a dilated pupil) is no longer considered an "ophthalmoplegic migraine." The ophthalmoplegia can last hours to months and is now believed to represent an inflammatory neuritis or the Tolosa–Hunt syndrome.[10] Painful ophthalmoplegia usually has a dramatic presentation and always warrants a careful evaluation.[14]

Given a typical history and reasonable clinical judgment, a migraine can be recognized and treated as such. Occasionally the clinical circumstance requires that the physician be more circumspect and make an effort to exclude other causes for headache that, if left undiagnosed and untreated, will result in an adverse patient outcome. Some other causes for headache include a cerebral aneurysm with or without subarachnoid hemorrhage, vascular malformations with or without hemorrhage, venous thrombosis, central nervous system infections, space-occupying lesions, increased intracranial pressure, vascular dissection, and arteritis.[10,14,15]

Treatment: Migraines can be treated abortively (after they start) or prophylactically (with daily medication aimed at reducing the frequency or intensity of the headaches).

ACUTE MIGRAINE HEADACHES (ABORTIVE TREATMENT):
The following are drugs that are useful for the treatment of acute migraine headaches (abortive treatment).

A. Triptans[16] (Imitrex, Maxalt, Zomig, Frova, Relpax, Amerge) are 5-HT$_{1D/1B}$ receptor agonists. These drugs are available in a variety of forms; for example: Imitrex is available in an autoinjector, as a tablet, and as a nasal spray; Maxalt and Zomig are available as tablets and as orally disintegrating tablets; Zomig is also available as a nasal spray. In general, injectable preparations have a quicker onset of action, followed by nasal sprays, orally disintegrating tablets, and tablets that must be swallowed. These different formulations allow treatment to be tailored to the patient's needs. Patients whose headaches are accompanied by significant nausea and vomiting, or whose productivity depends on a timely return to work, might prefer an injectable preparation or a nasal spray. Orally disintegrating tablets also are useful in patients with significant nausea and vomiting. Approximately 60% to 80% of patients achieve significant relief from a triptan; however, the headache will recur in up to one-third of patients. A second dose of the same preparation, taken 2 to 24 hours after the first, may again provide significant relief. A triptan should not be used again for at least 24 hours after the second dose. Triptans should not be administered within 24 hours of another substance with vasoconstricting properties (e.g., another triptan, ergotamine, dihydroergotamine, or isometheptane). Triptans should not be administered within 2 weeks of discontinuation of a monoamine oxidase inhibitor or methysergide. Triptans should not be prescribed to patients with ischemic or other heart disease or uncontrolled hypertension; the author avoids them in patients with complicated auras such as dysphasias. The major side effects of triptans include a sensation of chest pressure, flushing, tingling, dizziness and dysphoria. These usually resolve in less than 1 hour. Vasoconstrictor drugs should be avoided during pregnancy and are relatively contraindicated in basilar-type migraine. Although each of the triptans has unique pharmacokinetic properties, in the author's experience there is little practical difference between them. That said, the different formulations allow treatment to be individualized and if a patient does not respond well to, or suffers unacceptable side effects from, one triptan they may tolerate or respond better to another.

B. Ergotamine tartrate is an older drug with 5-HT agonist activity that also is very effective for migraine.[14,17] One to two tablets are taken at the onset of the headache or aura, followed by 1 tablet every 30 minutes until the headache is gone or until a maximum of 5 tablets per headache or 10 tablets per week have been consumed. If consumed in excess, ergotamine-containing preparations can cause vasospastic complications and are emetogenic. Vasoconstrictor drugs should be avoided during pregnancy.

C. Isometheptane (Midrin) is another older but effective drug with 5-HT agonist activity.[14,17] One to two capsules are taken at the onset of the headache or aura, followed by 1 tablet every hour until the headache is gone or until a maximum of 5 capsules per headache or 10 capsules per week have been consumed. Isometheptane has fewer vasospastic complications than ergotamine.

D. Preparations containing butalbital (such as Fioricet, which also contains acetaminophen and caffeine, or Fiorinal, which contains aspirin and caffeine) are effective and can be used alone or together with one of the vasoconstricting abortive drugs (a triptan, ergotamine, or isometheptane). One to two tablets can be taken every 4 hours as needed. Barbiturate-containing preparations cause drowsiness and can be habit forming if used excessively.[14,17]

E. Narcotic-containing preparations, such as those with codeine, hydromorphone, or hydrocodone (in combination with aspirin or acetaminophen), are used frequently, perhaps too frequently. Narcotics in the emergency room or in any other setting should be used only as drugs of last resort. Narcotics bind opiate receptors and mask pain, but they do not bind serotonin receptors and therefore do not interrupt the putative pathophysiologic mechanism of migraine. The short- and long-term complications associated with the frequent use of narcotics argues that they should be used sparingly at best.[14,17]

F. Antinauseants, such as prochlorperazine, chlorpromazine, or metoclopramide, by virtue of their effect on serotonin receptors are effective against migraine pain. Their action as antagonists of the D2 dopamine receptor helps control the associated gastrointestinal symptoms and this makes them excellent adjuvant drugs.[14,17]

G. Dihydroergotamine (DHE), previously available only for parenteral use, is now also available as a 4 mg/mL nasal spray. Administered by the intravenous or intramuscular route, the dose should not exceed 2 to 3 mg in 24 hours. Administered over one or several days, intravenous DHE is still the treatment of choice for the treatment of status migrainosus. Vasoconstrictor drugs should be avoided during pregnancy and are relatively contraindicated in basilar-type migraine.[14,17]

H. Nonsteroidal anti-inflammatory drugs (NSAIDs) work for some patients with mild to moderate migraine pain. Ketorolac, which can be administered intramuscularly, and indomethacin, which also is available as a suppository, may be particularly useful. Some patients with mild headache or headaches that do not last long respond well to over-the-counter analgesic preparations.[14,17]

I. Corticosteroids are sometimes useful when used for a limited time and under strict medical supervision. They can be used alone or with other abortive medication for the relief of an intractable migraine (status migrainosus). Both short- and long-term use of steroids entails significant potential for morbidity.[14,17]

CHRONIC USE OF DRUGS: The chronic use (averaging at least 3 times per week over a prolonged period of time) of any of the triptans, NSAIDs, acetaminophen, butalbital, narcotics, ergotamine, DHE, and isometheptane can lead to development of a medication overuse, or rebound, headache syndrome.[15,18–21] Chronic use of these compounds by patients should be discouraged. Prophylactic regimens generally are not effective in the setting of rebound. The treatment of medication overuse headache is discontinuation of all analgesics (including triptans, ergots, etc.). Painkiller withdrawal frequently results in a temporary but dramatic exacerbation of the pain which can last several days. The physiologic washout period, during which patients may continue to experience frequent headaches, lasts at least 2 weeks; patients should continue to refrain from analgesic medications for a total of 3 months although the physician should use judgment with respect to treatment of an occasional breakthrough migraine during that period. It stands to reason that patients should be advised against using analgesics more than twice per week over a prolonged period of time. If patients require analgesics at least twice per week, they should be offered a prophylactic regimen.

PROPHYLACTIC TREATMENT: The following are drugs that are useful for prophylactic treatment.

A. Beta-blockers, such as propranolol, metoprolol, atenolol, timolol, and nadolol, are frequently effective first-line prophylactic drugs.[17,22] In most healthy people 60 to 80 mg once per day of a long-acting propranolol preparation can be started and the dosage can be adjusted as necessary. Side effects include dizziness from bradycardia or hypotension, fatigue, depression, worsening of symptoms in patients with asthma or chronic obstructive pulmonary disease, gastrointestinal distress, blunting of hypoglycemic symptoms in patients with diabetes, and vivid dreams.

B. Anticonvulsants such as valproic acid (Depakote and Depakote ER) and carbamazepine have been used as prophylaxis against migraine for a long time; however, efficacy is also increasingly being reported for other anticonvulsants.[17,23] Among the newer anticonvulsants finding favor in the prophylaxis of migraine are Topamax, Neurontin, and Lamictal. The usual starting dose for Depakote ER is 500 mg per day; the dose should be adjusted as necessary at 2 to 4 week intervals. Valproic acid can cause weight gain, hair loss, tremor, abdominal distress, and easy bruisability. Although a frequent side effect of Topamax is mental confusion, another is weight loss, which has made this drug increasingly popular. In addition, Topamax is an inhibitor of carbonic anhydrase and it has been reported to be useful in treating the syndrome of idiopathic increased intracranial pressure (previously called pseudotumor cerebri).

C. Antidepressants, particularly amitriptyline at a starting dose of 10 to 25 mg at bedtime, are very active prophylactic drugs.[17] Most patients who respond to tricyclic antidepressants (amitriptyline, nortriptyline, imipramine, or desipramine) usually do so at doses of 25 to 200 mg at bedtime; occasionally a patient may require more. Tricyclics help induce sleep, which may constitute one of the mechanisms by which they help migraneurs. The major side effects from tricyclics relate to their anticholinergic action and include a dry mouth, excessive daytime sleepiness, dizziness, urinary retention, glaucoma, cardiac arrhythmias, and photosensitization. The specific serotonin reuptake inhibitors (SSRIs) might be tried in patients who do not respond or who develop intolerable side effects from tricyclic drugs. The major side effects of the SSRIs include jitteriness, tremors, gastrointestinal distress, decreased libido, and occasionally headaches. In addition, these drugs are relatively contraindicated in patients who use triptans, as they may suffer from excessive serotonin stimulation (serotonin syndrome). The association between migraine and depression (depressed patients have more migraines and migraines are a risk factor for depression) make antidepressants a good first choice for prophylaxis.

D. Calcium channel blockers, such as verapamil, are occasionally useful as prophylactic agents.[17] Calcium channel blockers are worth a try when first-line agents fail; they also appear to be more useful in patients with cluster headaches.

E. Lithium carbonate may be useful in patients with frequent migraines who do not respond to more traditional prophylactic regimens.[17] The major indication for lithium is in the treatment of an ongoing cluster headache.

F. When used for short periods of time (1 or 2 weeks), aspirin (650 mg) or indomethacin (25 to 50 mg) taken at bedtime can be effective as adjuvants to other prophylactic drugs.[17]

G. Although still controversial, a botulinum toxin A injection into the frontalis, temporalis, and glabellar muscles has been reported to increase significantly the number of headache-free days in some patients with chronic migraine. The beneficial effect may last up to 90 days postinjection. This treatment approach requires additional study before it can be recommended for the general migraine population.

SELF-HELP STRATEGIES: The following are self-help strategies that can minimize the incidence of migraines.[14]

A. If the patient consumes caffeinated beverages (coffee, tea, soda, cocoa), one can limit total caffeine to less than 400 mg per day and regularize the intake to include weekends, vacations, and holidays (to avoid caffeine withdrawal).

B. One can avoid foods high in tyramine, a substance metabolized to serotonin, which is thought to play a role as a migraine trigger. Some foods high in tyramine are chocolate, aged cheeses, yogurt, sour cream, soy sauce, chicken liver, banana, avocado, nuts, and yeast extracts (including beer).

C. Foods high in nitrates can be avoided, as these might precipitate a migraine by virtue of their vasodilating properties. Some foods high in nitrates include processed meats (hot dogs, salami, bacon, ham, sausage, corned beef) and other canned, smoked, or aged meats.

D. Some patients are sensitive to certain food additives. Two examples include monosodium glutamate, frequently used in restaurants and added to cooked, packaged, and canned foods as a flavor enhancer, and aspartame (Nutrasweet). These substances contain glutamate, an excitatory neurotransmitter.

E. Many migraneurs are sensitive to alcoholic beverages.[15] Alcohol tends to dilate blood vessels.

F. Miscellaneous, but not unusual, causes of migraine include new medications,[15] stressful situations, poststress situations, lack of adequate rest or changes in sleep habit, allergies, and noncompliance with a prophylactic regimen. Patients should not allow themselves to become dehydrated, either during a headache or between headaches. If bright light is an irritant during or between headaches, patients should wear optical-quality sunglasses that block at least 85% of incident sunlight (and 100% of ultraviolet light) when outdoors.

CLUSTER HEADACHE

Cluster headaches, unlike migraine, affect predominantly males in a ratio of 3:1 or 4:1 (males:females). The prevalence is 0.1% to 0.3% of the population. A family history of cluster is not as frequent as a family history of migraine. In the majority of cases attacks begin between the ages of 20 and 40.

Pathophysiology: The pathophysiologic mechanism of cluster headaches is not known. Some investigators believe that cluster headache lies within a continuum of head pains that include cluster and severe migraine at one extreme and tension-type headache at the other. Thus, at least to some degree, the underlying mechanism of most chronic, recurring headache syndromes would be shared. Some of the clinical features of cluster, which seem to reflect local vasoactive phenomena, support the argument that neurogenic inflammation also plays a role in this headache type.[5,24,25]

Diagnosis: Cluster headache is diagnosed by a suggestive clinical history and a normal neurologic examination. Typically, severe pain, which lasts between 10 and 90 minutes, awakens the patient. The pain is unilateral and periorbital; it may include the temple, forehead, and cheek. The syndrome is accompanied by lacrimation, conjunctival injection, nasal stuffiness, ptosis (with or without eyelid edema), and miosis ipsilateral to the pain. During a cluster phase, the headaches, which can be single or multiple in a 24-hour period, occur with circadian predictability and tend to have a similar duration. Unlike patients with migraine, who seek a dark, quiet environment, patients with cluster tend to pace, scream, or appear agitated; nausea and vomiting are uncommon. A bout of cluster may last several days or several months.[10] An attack can be provoked by alcohol. Chronic paroxysmal hemicrania is considered by some to be a variant of cluster that occurs more frequently in women.[26] The duration of a cluster headache tends to be shorter than that of paroxysmal hemicrania.

Treatment: In general, the drugs that are used to treat migraine are useful in cluster except that the role for treatment aimed at aborting an acute headache is limited because the attack has usually run its course by the time the agent has exerted its effect.[14,24] Therefore, cluster is best treated early on with prophylactic drugs with the aim of interrupting the cluster. The major limitation of drugs aimed at interrupting the cluster (drugs used in migraine prophylaxis) is their slow onset of action, with most requiring 2 to 4 weeks to demonstrate activity at the initial dose, and similar intervals for subsequent dose adjustments.

INTERRUPTING THE CLUSTER: The following are drugs that are useful for interrupting the cluster.

A. Calcium channel blockers, such as verapamil, are occasionally useful and frequently prescribed.[27] Verapamil usually requires administration at relatively high doses, 240 to 480 mg/day, to be effective.

B. Anticonvulsants such as valproic acid (Depakote and Depakote ER) and carbamazepine can be useful to help abort a cluster.[24] The usual starting dose for Depakote ER is 500 mg per day; the dose should be adjusted as necessary at 2-week intervals. Valproic acid can cause weight gain, hair loss, tremor, and abdominal distress.

C. Lithium carbonate can be useful in patients with cluster; in fact, cluster remains the major indication for lithium in the treatment of headaches.[24]

D. Antidepressants, particularly amitriptyline at a starting dose of 10 to 25 mg at bedtime, are sometimes added to an anticluster regimen but there is no good evidence for their activity. Tricyclics help induce sleep, which may constitute one of the mechanisms by which they help patients with cluster. The major side effects from tricyclics relate to their anticholinergic effects and include a dry mouth, excessive daytime sleepiness, dizziness, urinary retention, glaucoma, cardiac arrhythmias, and photosensitization.[24]

E. Beta-blockers, such as propranolol, metoprolol, atenolol, timolol, and nadolol, are also used frequently for cluster.[24] In most healthy people 60 to 80 mg once per day of a long-acting propranolol preparation can be started and the dosage can be adjusted as necessary. Side effects include dizziness from bradycardia or hypotension, fatigue, depression, worsening of symptoms in patients with asthma or chronic obstructive pulmonary disease, gastrointestinal distress, blunting of hypoglycemic symptoms in patients with diabetes, and vivid dreams.

F. Corticosteroids are useful as adjuvants to other drugs in breaking a cluster.[24] They should be started simultaneously with one of the other prophylactic drugs. Corticosteroids are to be used for a limited time and under strict medical supervision. Both short- and long-term use of steroids entails significant potential for morbidity.

G. Given the regularity and sometimes circadian predictability of the headache onset during a cluster, ergotamine, isometheptane, a triptan, or a NSAID can be administered up to several hours prior to an anticipated attack, for example at bedtime. When used for a limited time, this strategy can be useful to prevent a headache until the prophylactic drugs become effective.[16,28]

H. Among the NSAIDs, indomethacin appears to be more active than others. It also can be used in anticipation of a headache to block its onset. Indomethacin can be administered in doses up to 150 mg/day but tends to irritate the gastric mucosa. Other NSAIDs might work for some patients with milder headaches. In general, the onset of action of oral formulations tends to occur at about the time the current headache has run its course.

TREATMENT OF AN ACUTE HEADACHE: The following are approaches to the treatment of an acute headache:

- As stated above, the onset of action of most analgesics tends to occur at about the time the current headache has run its course. However, inhaled oxygen remains the standard for treatment of an acute cluster headache.[29,30] Oxygen should be administered at 8 L/minute through a non-rebreather mask for 10 to 15 minutes as soon after the onset of the attack as feasible. The treatment can be repeated after a brief interval. Patients should be prescribed the oxygen for home use.
- It is not clear if parenteral or nasal formulations of a triptan might be useful in this setting, especially for headaches of longer duration.[16,28]

REFERENCES

1. Lipton RB, Silberstein SD, Stewart WF: An update on the epidemiology of migraine. Headache 34:319–328, 1994.
2. Lipton RB, Stewart WF: Migraine in the United States: Epidemiology and healthcare use. Neurology 43(Suppl 3):6–10, 1993.
3. Stewart WF, Lipton RB: Work related disability: Results from the American Migraine Study. Cephalalgia 16:231–238, 1996.
4. Stewart WF, Lipton RB, Ottman R: Familial risk of migraine: A population-based study. Neurology 41:166–172, 1997.
5. Welch KMA: Contemporary concepts of migraine pathogenesis. Neurology 61:S2–S8, 2003.
6. Moskowitz MA: Neurogenic inflammation in the pathophysiology and treatment of migraine. Neurology 43(Suppl 3):16–20, 1993.
7. Moskowitz MA: Neurovascular and molecelular mechanisms in migraine headache. Cerebrovasc Brain Metab Rev 5:150–177, 1993.
8. Lauritzen M. Pathophysiology of the migraine aura: The spreading depression theory. Brain 177:199, 1994.
9. Peroutka SH: Dopamine and migraine. Neurology 49:650–656, 1997.
10. The international classification of headache disorders, 2nd edition. Cephalalgia 24(Suppl 1):1–150, 2004.
11. Milhaud D, Bogousslavsky J, van Melle G, Liot P: Ischemic stroke and active migraine. Neurology 57:1805–1811, 2001.
12. Neuhauser H, Leopold M, von Brevern M, et al: The interrelations of migraine, vertigo and migrainous vertigo. Neurology 56:436–441, 2001.
13. Frese A, Eikermann A, Frese K, et al: Headache associated with sexual activity: Demography, clinical features, and comorbidity. Neurology 61:796–800, 2000.
14. Silberstein SD, Lipton RB, Goadsby PJ: Headache in Clinical Practice, ed 2. Isis Medical Media, London, 2002.
15. Lipton RB, Silberstein SD, Saper JR, et al: Why headache treatment fails. Neurology 60:1064–1070, 2003.
16. Ferrari MD, Roon KI, Lipton RB, Goadsby PJ: Oral triptans (serotonin 5-HT$_{1B/1D}$ agonists) in acute migraine treatment: A meta-analysis of 53 trials. Lancet 358:1668–1675, 2001.

17. Denier HC, Limmroth V: The management of migraine. Rev Contemp Pharmacother 5:271–284, 1994.

18. Katsarava Z, Limmroth V, Finke M, et al: Rates and predicators for relapse in medication overuse headache: A 1-year prospective study. Neurology 60:1682–1683, 2003.

19. Zwart JA, Hagen K, Svebak S, Holmen J: Analgesic use: A predicator of chronic pain and medication overuse headache. Neurology 61:163–164, 2003.

20. Lipton RB, Bigal ME: Chronic daily headache. Neurology 61:154–155, 2003.

21. Warner JS: Analgesic rebound as a cause of hemicrania continua. Neurology 48:1540–1541, 1997.

22. Holroyd KA, Penzien DB: Propranolol in the management of recurrent migraine: A meta-analytic review. Headache 31:33–44, 1991.

23. Hering R, Kuritzky AA: Sodium valproate in the prophylactic treatment of migraine: A double blind study versus placebo. Cephalalgia 12:81–84, 1992.

24. Bahra A, May A, Goadsby PJ: Cluster headache. Neurology 58:354–361, 2002.

25. Montagna P, Lodi R. Cortelli P, et al: Phosphorous magnetic resonance spectroscopy in cluster headache. Neurology 48:113–118, 1997.

26. Peres MFP, Silberstein SD, Nahmias S, et al: Hemicrania continua is not that rare. Neurology 57:948–951, 2001.

27. Gabe U, Spiering CLH: Prophylactic treatment of cluster headache with verapamil. Headache 29:167–168, 1989.

28. Wilkinson F, Pffafenrath V, Schenen J, et al: Migraine and cluster headache: Their management with sumatriptan: A critical review of the current experience. Cephalalgia 15:337–357, 1995.

29. Fogan L: Treatment of cluster headache: A double blind comparison of oxygen vs air inhalation. Arch Neurol 42:362–363, 1985.

30. Kudrow L: Response of cluster headache attack to oxygen inhalation. Headache 21:1–4, 1981.

Tension-Type Headache, Chronic Tension-Type Headache, and Other Chronic Headache Types

Jack M. Rozental, M.D., Ph.D., M.B.A.

EPIDEMIOLOGY

Tension-type headache (TTH) is the most common headache type and also the most difficult to classify.[1] Many different, and equally vague, terms have been applied to this headache or to what probably are variants of the same syndrome. Headaches in general are thought to affect more than 90% of the population at one time or another, with about 15% of those fitting the description of migrainous or vascular headache. This leaves about 70% of the population with some variant of TTH.[2] Moreover, almost all patients with migraine, cluster headache, trigeminal nerve neuralgias, and other recurring cephalgic syndromes have interposed TTH.[3-5]

DIAGNOSIS

The pain of a TTH tends to be duller, less intense, and less localized than that of a migraine or a cluster attack. The pain usually lasts several hours to a day, but it may continue for days or weeks. During a severe TTH patients can experience photophobia, phonophobia, nausea, and occasionally emesis. Pain referred to the neck is common; patients also frequently complain of "a knot in the neck," but the neurologic examination should be normal.[6]

The major variants of TTH are those with disorder of the pericranial muscles, those without disorder of the pericranial muscles, and chronic TTH (CTTH) (with or without disorder of the pericranial muscles). Those with disorder of the pericranial muscles are characterized by tenderness on palpation of those muscles, increased activity on electromyography (EMG), or both.

TTH without disorder of the pericranial muscles lacks those characteristics.

CTTH, previously called chronic daily headache, is diagnosed in a patient with a headache frequency of 15 days per month or 180 headaches per year averaged over a 6-month period.[6] A common variety of TTH occurs in patients with headaches of any sort in whom these temporarily exacerbate and become more frequent. Patients begin taking analgesic preparations (e.g., nonsteroidal anti-inflammatory drugs (NSAIDs), acetaminophen, aspirin, narcotics, ergot derivatives, triptans) on a regular basis (generally three times or more per week) and eventually develop medication overuse, or rebound, headaches.[7-10] It stands to reason that patients should be advised against using analgesics more than twice per week over a prolonged period of time. If they require analgesics at least twice per week, they should be offered a prophylactic regimen. Fibromyalgia and the myofascial pain syndrome also are associated with frequent or chronic daily headaches.

A particularly severe, persistent, or unusual headache should always prompt consideration of alternative explanations, and, when appropriate, these should be investigated thoroughly.[1,3,6,11] For example, temporal arteritis should be considered in an elderly patient with a persistent headache of recent onset whether or not other typical elements are present in the history and physical examination. In these patients an erythrocyte sedimentation rate (ESR) should be ordered immediately, and consideration should be given to treatment with a corticosteroid and to a temporal artery biopsy. Likewise, one would not want to miss an infectious meningitis. One must be vigilant for the sentinel bleed of an aneurysm, an undiagnosed intracranial vascular malformation, a subdural hematoma, acute hydrocephalus, venous thrombosis, or an arterial dissection. Idiopathic intracranial hypertension (previously called pseudotumor cerebri) usually presents in overweight young women with chronic headaches, a normal examination, a normal scan and papilledema—although a subset of these patients do not have papilledema.[6,12] The diagnosis is made when a lumbar puncture reveals an otherwise normal fluid under high pressure (at least 20 to 25 cmH$_2$O). Therefore, when dictated by clinical judgment, imaging, lumbar puncture, or other tests deemed necessary are indicated.

PATHOPHYSIOLOGY OF TENSION-TYPE HEADACHE

The pathophysiologic bases for TTH and CTTH are unknown. Some investigators believe that TTH lies at one end of a physiologic spectrum that includes severe migraine and cluster at one end and TTH at the other. Under this assumption, at least to some degree, the underlying mechanism of most chronic, recurring headache syndromes would be shared.[13–15] The relationship between tenderness of the pericranial muscles, EMG recordings from those muscles, and headaches is not straightforward. The muscle contraction theory of TTH relates pain to prolonged contraction, or spasm, of cervical or pericranial muscles. Again, no objective data support the theory. Most patients with a headache, migrainous or TTH, have pericranial muscle tenderness or sore spots; however, many individuals without headache also have them. There is no particular distinguishing characteristic among patients with headache, pericranial muscle tenderness, and increased EMG activity in those muscles. In fact, even pericranial muscle tenderness and the level of EMG activity in those muscles do not correlate. On the other hand, during a headache, patients with a more severe headache tend to have more tender pericranial muscles.

The relationship between cervicogenic disorders and headache is similarly unclear, although most painful disorders of the neck are associated with some sort of headache. Cervical pain can be referred to the head from intervertebral discs, interspinous ligaments, zygapophyseal joints, the periosteum, paracervical muscles, carotid and vertebral arteries, and from irritation of the C1, C2, and C3 nerve roots. The dorsal rami of the first three cervical nerve roots supply the sensory innervation to the neck and to the scalp caudal to the innervation of the trigeminal nerve, and to the meninges and arteries of the posterior fossa. Headache also can arise from pathology in the area of the foramen magnum. Some examples include a Chiari I malformation, the Dandy–Walker syndrome, atlantoaxial dislocation (e.g., from rheumatoid arthritis), Paget's disease of the bone, and basilar invagination.

TREATMENT

As with other headache types, both abortive and prophylactic treatment strategies are available for the treatment of TTH and CTTH.

Abortive Treatment Strategies: For the occasional TTH, an over-the-counter (OTC) analgesic preparation is all that is required. The number of OTC preparations continues to increase, and although they are generally safe, the lay population has little basis on which to decide how to choose among them or how to use them properly. Most people decide on a preparation either on a trial-and-error basis or are swayed by the marketing ("for tension headache," "for sinus pain," "multi-symptom relief," "PM" preparations, etc.). Several OTC analgesic preparations involve combinations of drugs (e.g., aspirin plus acetaminophen) and may contain caffeine. Caffeine combined with analgesics such as aspirin, acetaminophen, and ibuprofen enhances their analgesic effectiveness. Stronger headaches may require an analgesic (aspirin, acetaminophen, or ibuprofen) in combination with either codeine or butalbital. Some of these preparations also include caffeine. Used infrequently, the additional analgesic effectiveness obtained by adding codeine or butalbital comes with little increase in adverse effects or risk of dependence.

If aspirin or acetaminophen, with or without codeine, butalbital, or caffeine are ineffective in controlling the headache, the choice of an alternative analgesic should proceed in an orderly fashion by testing in turn members of different NSAID chemical categories at adequate doses. Indomethacin is reported to be more effective than alternative NSAIDs for pain of cephalic origin. Occasionally a patient responds well to stress management modalities or acupuncture (anyone who is going to receive acupuncture should ascertain the qualifications of the practitioner and insist on new, not sterilized, needles for every session), but it is impossible to predict accurately in whom these modalities are likely to be beneficial. The major chemical categories of NSADs include:

- Carboxylic acids—this group includes aspirin, which is an acetylated acid, as well as salsalate and choline magnesium trisalicylate, which are nonacetylated.
- Propionic acids—ibuprofen, naproxen, ketoprofen, and fenoprofen.
- Aryl and heterocyclic acids—indomethacin, diclofenac, sulindac, and tolmetin.
- Fenamic acids—mefenamic acid and meclofenamate.
- Enolic acids—piroxicam and phenylbutazone.
- Pyrrolo-pyrrole—ketorolac.
- Cyclooxygenase 2 (COX-2) inhibitors—celecoxib and rofecoxib.

Prophylactic Treatment Strategies: Fortunately, CTTH and TTH that are frequent or otherwise annoying respond to many of the agents used in migraine prophylaxis. It is possible that this reflects on the presumed common mechanism that is felt to underlie both disorders.

A. Antidepressants, particularly amitriptyline at a starting dose of 10 to 25 mg at bedtime, are active prophylactic drugs.[16] Most patients who respond to tricyclic antidepressants (amitriptyline, nortriptyline, imipramine, or desipramine) usually do so at doses of 25 to 200 mg at bedtime; an occasional patient may require more. Tricyclics help induce sleep, which may constitute one of the mechanisms by which they help. The major side effects from tricyclics relate to their anticholinergic effects and include a dry mouth, excessive daytime sleepiness, dizziness, urinary retention, glaucoma, cardiac arrhythmias, and photosensitization. The specific serotonin reuptake inhibitors (SSRIs) might be tried in patients who do not respond or who develop intolerable side effects from tricyclic drugs. The major side effects of the SSRIs include jitteriness, tremors, gastrointestinal distress, decreased libido, and occasionally headaches. In addition, these drugs are relatively contraindicated in patients who use triptans, as they may suffer from excessive serotonin stimulation (serotonin syndrome).

B. Beta-blockers, such as propranolol, metoprolol, atenolol, timolol, and nadolol, can be tried and sometimes prove effective.[17] In most healthy people 60 to 80 mg once per day of a long-acting propranolol preparation can be started and the dosage can be adjusted as necessary. Side effects include dizziness from bradycardia or hypotension, fatigue, depression, worsening of symptoms in patients with asthma or chronic obstructive pulmonary disease, gastrointestinal distress, blunting of hypoglycemic symptoms in patients with diabetes, and vivid dreams.

C. Anticonvulsants such as valproic acid (Depakote and Depakote ER) are sometimes worth a try to prophylax against frequent TTH.[18] The usual starting dose for Depakote ER is 500 mg per day; the dose should be adjusted as necessary at 2- to 4-week intervals. Valproic acid can cause weight gain, hair loss, tremor, and abdominal distress.

D. Although still controversial, a botulinum toxin A injection into the most tender pericranial muscle(s) or directly into a trigger point has been reported to increase significantly the number of headache-free days in patients with CTTH. The results are less encouraging when the injections are prescribed for TTH that does not strictly meet the criteria for CTTH. Results also are less encouraging when the injections are applied in a standardized, rather than individualized, fashion. For example, when all patients are injected into the same muscles rather than into the muscle or muscles that are specifically tender, the results are discouraging.

OTHER CHRONIC HEADACHE TYPES

Patients frequently complain of "sinus headaches."[3,4,5,19] They present after a variety of diagnostic tests have failed to corroborate the diagnosis and after one or more courses of antibiotics, antihistamines, decongestants, nasal steroids, and analgesics have failed to provide significant relief. Those patients almost invariably also self-medicate with a variety of OTC preparations the hallmark of which is that they display the words "sinus" and "relief" prominently on the label; they also combine an antihistamine, a decongestant, and an analgesic (with or without caffeine). Needless to say, these are not true sinus headaches and most of those patients have some degree of medication overuse headache at the time of presentation. Most patients complain of periorbital pain and might also experience a sensation of nasal stuffiness. Patients attribute the origin of the pain to the adjacent sinuses. However, these head pains are unaccompanied by purulent discharge, fever, or localized tenderness, and they are not seasonal. True sinus pain occurs when the ability of the sinus to drain is impaired by an acute blockage of the osteum (e.g., following an upper respiratory infection or for some anatomic reason), a bacterial infection takes hold, the mucosa becomes inflamed and pressure builds up in the sinus. One caveat is that true sinus or nasal inflammation can be a trigger for migraine. The rest of these "sinus headaches" are likely multifactorial but may represent a mild migraine in which the local sterile inflammation, perhaps mediated through the trigeminal nerve, gives the impression of sinus pressure, a TTH, or CTTH.[3,4,5,19] The care of these patients needs to be coordinated so that the various potential components of the headache are adequately addressed and treated.

Habitual snoring is increasingly being recognized as a cause of chronic daily headache.[20] Sleep-disordered breathing from, for example, sleep apnea may precipitate headaches from the resultant hypoxemia and hypercapnia. Snoring, with or without sleep apnea, can disrupt sleep architecture or interrupt sleep, either of which can result in headaches. If a history suggestive of snoring, repeated nocturnal arousals, or paroxysmal leg movements during sleep is obtained, a diagnostic polysomnogram will provide invaluable information. Treatment of the sleep disorder might not provide complete headache relief but it usually provides some. Hypnic headaches represent another syndrome of recurring head pain that awakens patients from REM sleep.[21] The headache most commonly has its onset after the age of 50, is about twice as frequent in women as in men, has its onset about 2 to 4 hours after falling asleep, and lasts about 1 hour. This headache responds best to treatment with either indomethacin or lithium.

Another uncommon headache type that may become intractable is the short-lasting, unilateral, neuralgiform headache with conjunctival injection and tearing (SUNCT).[22] This headache syndrome is characterized by frequent, short-lasting, unilateral attacks of pain around the periorbital regions and the temples. These pains are accompanied by ipsilateral signs of autonomic activation—among which conjunctival injection and tearing are a sine qua non—and which can include nasal stuffiness or rhinorrhea and eyelid edema with ptosis. SUNCT is intractable to most drugs, but recently good response has been reported after treatment with lamotrigine at doses of 125 to 200 mg/day.

REFERENCES

1. Silberstein SD, Lipton RB, Solomon S, et al: Classification of daily and near daily headaches: Proposed revisions to the IHS criteria. Headache 34:1–7, 1994.
2. Lipton RB, Scher AI, Kolodner K, et al: Migraine in the United States: Epidemiology and patterns of health care use. Neurology 58:885–894, 2002.
3. Kaniecki RG: Diagnostic challenges in headache. Migraine as the wolf disguised in sheep's clothing. Neurology 58:S1–S2, 2002.
4. Diamond ML: The role of concomitant headache types and non-headache co-morbidities in the underdiagnosis of migraine. Neurology 58:S3–S9, 2002.
5. Lipton RB, Stewart WF, Liberman J: Self-awareness of migraine. Interpreting the labels that headache sufferers apply to their headaches. Neurology 58:S21–S26, 2002.
6. The international classification of headache disorders, 2nd edition. Cephalalgia 24(Suppl 1):1–150, 2004.
7. Lipton RB, Bigal ME: Chronic daily headache. Neurology 61:154–155, 2003.
8. Katsarava Z, Limmroth V, Finke M, et al: Rates and predicators for relapse in medication overuse headache: A 1-year prospective study. Neurology 60:1682–1683, 2003.
9. Zwart JA, Hagen K, Svebak S, Holmen J: Analgesic use: A predicator of chronic pain and medication overuse headache. Neurology 61:163–164, 2003.
10. Warner JS: Analgesic rebound as a cause of hemicrania continua. Neurology 48:1540–1541, 1997.
11. Lipton RB, Silberstein SD, Saper JR, et al: Why headache treatment fails. Neurology 60:1064–1070, 2003.
12. Friedman DI, Jacobson DM: diagnostic criteria for idiopathic intracranial hypertension. Neurology 59:1492–1495, 2002.
13. Welch KMA: Contemporary concepts of migraine pathogenesis. Neurology 61:S2–S8, 2003.

14. Moskowitz MA: Neurogenic inflammation in the pathophysiology and treatment of migraine. Neurology 43(Suppl 3):16–20, 1993.

15. Moskowitz MA: Neurovascular and molecular mechanisms in migraine headache. Cerebrovasc Brain Metab Rev 5:150–177, 1993.

16. Denier HC, Limmroth V: The management of migraine. Rev Contemp Pharmacother 5:271–284, 1994.

17. Holroyd KA, Penzien DB: Propranolol in the management of recurrent migraine: A meta-analytic review. Headache 31:33–44, 1991.

18. Hering R, Kuritzky AA: Sodium valproate in the prophylactic treatment of migraine: A double blind study versus placebo. Cephalalgia 12:81–84, 1992.

19. Cady RK, Schreiber CP. Sinus headache or migraine? Neurology 58:S10–S14, 2002.

20. Scher AI, Lipton RB, Stewart, WF: Habitual snoring as a risk factor for chronic daily headache. Neurology 60:1366–1368, 2003.

21. Evers S, Goadsby PJ: Hypnic headache. Neurology 60:905–909, 2003.

22. D'Andrea G, Granella F, Ghiotto N, Nappi G: Lamotrigine in the treatment of SUNCT syndrome. Neurology 57:1723–1725, 2001.

Postdural Puncture Headache and Spontaneous Intracranial Hypotension

**John D. Moore, M.D., and
Honorio T. Benzon, M.D.**

Postdural puncture headache (PDPH) and spontaneous intracranial hypotension (SIH) are two distinct clinical entities with similar presentations, pathophysiologies, and treatments. The most obvious similarity is the pathognomonic symptom of a postural headache worse when sitting or standing and relieved when supine. The most important distinction is the initiating event often obvious in PDPH and more obscure in SIH. Although PDPH and SIH headache are separate entities, they share a common presentation and treatment.

CLINICAL PRESENTATION

PDPH was classically described by August Bier in 1898, following a spinal anesthetic, as a severe headache worse with standing or sitting and reduced in the recumbent position. Bier correctly speculated that the headache may have been caused by the loss of cerebrospinal fluid (CSF) during the spinal anesthetic placement.[1] An orthostatic headache following dural puncture is pathognomonic. The absence of an orthostatic component should lead to a search for other causes, leaving PDPH as a diagnosis of exclusion. The headache is characteristically occipital and/or frontal and always bilateral. Symptoms associated with both PDPH and SIH can include nausea, vomiting, photophobia, diplopia, visual changes, auditory changes including hypoacusis, tinnitus, and mental status changes including dementia.[2–10] Subdural hematomas and hygromas, intracerebral hemorrhage, and seizures have also been reported.[11–13] Two case reports of Bell's palsy associated with PDPH are believed to be coincidental.[4] There is one report of arm pain as the presenting symptom.[14] The headache usually presents within the first 48 hours following a dural puncture; however, later presentations are not uncommon.[7]

Similar to PDPH in its clinical presentation, SIH is more exotic to the anesthesiology community. First described by Schaltenbrand in 1938 as *spontaneous aliquorrhea*, it was an obscure diagnosis of exclusion, generally by the neurology community.[15] However, with increasing use of magnetic resonance imaging (MRI) of the brain in the workup for headaches and recognition of the characteristic presentation of meningeal thickening and enhancement the diagnosis has become more common.[16,17] It is believed that SIH is secondary to a spontaneous idiopathic dural tear in the spinal region with extravasations of the CSF. Congenital subarachnoid or Tarlov cysts have been cited as a potential site of dural weakness and rupture.[18] Similar to PDPH, this loss of CSF leads to intrathecal CSF hypovolemia and the associated postural symptoms. The term SIH can be misleading since there are reports of SIH following closed spinal manipulation, associated with intradural thoracic disc herniation and secondary to bony pathology of the spine.[19–21] There is also a proposed correlation between connective tissue disorders such as Marfan's syndrome with associated dural weakening and SIH.[18,22,23] The most common site of idiopathic dural tears is in the thoracic, cervicothoracic, and thoracolumbar junctions of the spine.[18,24] Although the symptomatology, proposed pathophysiology, and treatments are identical to PDPH, the diagnosis of SIH is more complicated since there is no associated history of a dural puncture. Identification of the dural tear is crucial both for diagnosis and localization of the level to be treated.[18] The underlying mechanism and affected population is also distinct from PDPH. SIH continues to be more commonly seen in the neurology community that has studied it most extensively.

PATHOPHYSIOLOGY

The pathophysiology of a low CSF volume headache is not completely understood. There are several proposed hypotheses. One is based on the Monro–Kellie rule and another on mechanical traction. Both hypotheses accept that CSF escapes through a known or probable dural puncture at a rate that exceeds CSF production. This is in contrast to earlier rejected hypotheses for SIH based on reduced CSF production or increased CSF absorption, both of which have not been observed.[25] The Monro–Kellie rule is that in an intact skull the sum of the volumes of brain, CSF, and intracranial blood are constant.[26] The average CSF production is 500 mL/day with an average intrathecal volume of 150 mL. The uncompensated loss of CSF in PDPH and SIH leads to a subarachnoid deficit of CSF and often a reduction in the subarachnoid pressure. The normal CSF opening pressure is 70 to 180 mmH$_2$O. Although CSF hypotension (CSF pressure less than 60 mmH$_2$O) is often noted, the significance of the reduction in subarachnoid pressure is unclear since it does not consistently correlate with the presentation of headache.[27,28] Neither is the headache related to the amount of CSF leaked.[29] It is probable that the headache is related to *sudden alterations in CSF volume*, as proposed by Raskin.[30] Raskin theorized that the sudden loss of CSF volume and the change in pressure differential between the inside and outside of the intracranial venous structures result in venous dilatation.

The direct traction hypothesis states that the reduction in CSF total volume especially in the spinal region allows the brain to shift caudally placing traction on the pain-sensitive intracranial structures and causing cerebral vasodilatation that produces the classic headache symptoms. This is supported by MRI studies of both SIH and PDPH that demonstrate a caudal shift in the brain toward the foramen magnum.[31] Pain-sensitive intracranial structures include the dura, cranial nerves, and bridging veins. The bridging veins and the dura are innervated by the ophthalmic branch of the trigeminal nerve, which refers pain to the frontal region. In addition to causing pain, traction on bridging veins can cause a tear in the vein and lead to a subdural hemorrhage.[32] The posterior fossa structures are innervated by the glossopharyngeal and vagus nerves that refer pain to the occipital region. Traction of the vagus nerve can also stimulate the chemoreceptor regions of the medulla causing nausea and vomiting. Finally traction on the upper three cervical nerves presents as occipital, cervical, and shoulder pain and stiffness. Schabel et al. reported one case of arm pain following dural puncture that resolved with an epidural blood patch (EBP).[14] In addition to generating pain, traction or pressure on the abducens nerve (CN VI) can cause nerve palsy with paralysis of the lateral rectus muscle; this can manifest as diplopia. Another proposed mechanism for the visual changes is secondary to crowding of the optic chiasm, observed on the MRI of patients with intracranial hypotension.[33] Finally oculomotor nerve (CN III) and trochlear nerve (CN IV) palsies have been attributed to intracranial hypotension due to brainstem compression and ischemia.[5]

In contrast, the Monro–Kellie hypothesis proposes that a reduction in intracranial CSF volume is compensated for by increased intracranial blood volume, since the brain volume is stable.[26,28] In accordance with the Monro–Kellie rule this increase in blood volume causes cerebral vasodilatation which activates the trigeminovascular system, similar to migraine attacks. The input reaches the thalamus through the quinto-thalamic tract and refers pain to the ophthalmic branch and the first three cervical roots. This hypothesis is supported by MRI observations of contrast enhancement of the thickened meninges in SIH and PDPH secondary to dural venous dilation.[34]

It is further supported by the fact that PDPH often responds to vasoconstrictors such as caffeine. However, the efficacy of sumatriptan has not been established. Further evidence of a shift in intracranial volumes is multiple reports of subdural hematomas, subdural hygromas, and intracranial hemorrhage associated with SIH and PDPH. Decreased intracranial pressure is probably a secondary cause since not all patients with classic PDPH have intracranial hypotension.[27]

The auditory changes noted after dural puncture may be related to changes in CSF pressure. The CSF and the perilymph of the cochlea are in direct communication through the cochlear aqueduct. A reduction in the CSF pressure translates to a reduction in the perilymph pressure that leads to an imbalance between the perilymph and endolymph pressures. This imbalance causes a reduction in the response to the auditory input that manifests as hypoacusis.[4,35]

ROLE OF THE ARACHNOID MATTER IN THE PATHOGENESIS OF CSF LEAK

The concept of dural puncture as the cause of CSF leakage and the importance of dural fiber orientation to the needle bevel is unique to the anesthesia literature and is not supported by the anatomical literature. Reina et al. demonstrated that the dura mater is composed of 78 to 82 overlapping layers in multiple orientations, therefore making a hole exclusively parallel or across the fibers is impossible.[36] Furthermore, as early as 1938 Weed postulated that the arachnoid might be the barrier between the dura and the CSF.[37] In 1967 Waggener and Beggs, based on electron microscopy observations, labeled the arachnoid membrane as a physiological barrier impermeable to CSF.[38] However, it was in Nabeshima's electron microscopy study of the meninges that he demonstrated the presence of tight junctions, similar to those found in capillary endothelium of the brain, only in the outer arachnoid layer. Because of this unique characteristic Nabeshima labeled this layer as the arachnoid barrier layer. The cells of the dura do not contain tight junctions.[37] Nabeshima and Reese further demonstrated that this barrier layer prevented high molecular weight substances from leaving the CSF.[39] Schachenmayr and Friede stated that the arachnoid barrier layer is the true boundary of the CSF compartment that prevents the exchange of CSF with the extra-arachnoid compartments.[40] Vandenabeele et al. stated that the arachnoid barrier cell layer is the only effective meningeal barrier.[41] In the light of these anatomical observations the concept of exclusive dural puncture to access the CSF and cause a CSF leak is not correct. In a study to differentiate the comparative permeability of the three meningeal layers Bernards and Hill found the arachnoid mater to be the principal diffusion barrier to CSF.[42] The findings were summarized by stating that if the dura were the primary diffusion barrier then the CSF would collect in the subdural space.[43] Although anesthesiologists probably mean to include puncture of the arachnoid when they discuss PDPH, the importance of arachnoid puncture for CSF access should be emphasized.

DIAGNOSIS

The diagnosis of a PDPH is primarily based on the history of a dural puncture or possible dural puncture. Secondly, a postural component to the headache is a pathognomonic sign in the absence of which another diagnosis should be actively investigated.[44] In contrast, the diagnosis of SIH is primarily based on physical examination and is a diagnosis of exclusion, also with a postural headache as the pathognomonic sign. The headache is always bilateral. These factors will largely establish the diagnosis of PDPH and SIH that can be accompanied by a multitude of signs and symptoms. Although imaging studies are not necessary to diagnose PDPH, in SIH they can be an important adjunct. On MRI of the brain with gadolinium, there is a characteristic meningeal thickening and enhancement, and a possible caudad shift of the brain toward the foramen magnum.[34] In SIH there are MRI reports of associated pituitary gland enlargement and decreased ventricle volume. Further investigation with a radionuclide cisternography is often indicated in SIH to document the lack of ascent of the tracer dye and, if possible, to identify the level of the dural leak.[18,45] A diagnostic dural puncture to measure CSF opening pressure may not be necessary if the clinical presentation is diagnostic. In CSF hypovolemia, CSF analysis reveals increased protein content, up to 200 mg/dL has been reported, and a lymphocytic pleocytosis up to 40 cells/mL.[46] This is believed to be secondary to meningeal inflammation.

Since the diagnoses of PDPH and SIH are largely based on a thorough history and physical examination, it is important to note that certain critical signs and symptoms may indicate concomitant intracranial pathology. The most important of these signs is a changing pattern of the headache. For example, the headache is no longer postural; it becomes constant; it becomes localized unilaterally; or there is new-onset nausea and vomiting. Another critical change is increasing neurological alterations, which include sedation, seizures, and new-onset motor and/or sensory deficits. The presence of these signs and symptoms necessitates neurology consult and additional diagnostic studies. Based on case reports, the differential diagnosis of PDPH or SIH with changing symptomatology should include intracerebral hemorrhage, eclampsia, and cerebral venous thrombosis.[13,47–50]

INCIDENCE

The incidence of PDPH ranges from 1% to 75%.[51] The determinants of this difference in incidence include the needle size, the needle tip design, and the orientation of the needle bevel during dural puncture. The smaller needle diameters correlate with a lower incidence of PDPH. This is understandable since the larger the hole in the dura the greater the leakage of CSF. The range is from 75% PDPH with a 17-gauge needle to 2.7% with a 27-gauge needle. The reduced incidence of PDPH with a smaller-gauge needle should be placed in the context of an increased failure rate and increased difficulty of use of smaller-diameter needles. It is important to realize that most unintentional dural punctures during epidural anesthesia occur with a 17-gauge Tuohy needle. In an in vitro study comparing epidural needle diameter and CSF leakage Angle et al. found reduced CSF leakage with a 20-gauge versus a 17-gauge Tuohy needle puncture.[52] The effect of needle tip design is less intuitive. There is a lower incidence of PDPH with a non-cutting blunt tip design such as the Whitacre or Sprotte needle when compared with a cutting needle design such as the Quincke needle. In fact, there is a lower incidence of PDPH with a larger-diameter blunt tip needle when compared with a smaller-diameter cutting needle. One study showed a 2.7% incidence of PDPH with a 27-gauge Quincke needle versus

1.2% incidence with a 25-gauge Whitacre needle.[51] The proposed mechanism behind this difference is that a blunt tip needle compresses the dural fibers, which then more easily close after needle removal, versus a cutting tip needle, which cuts the dural fibers. Electron microscopy studies show that a blunt tip needle produces an irregular hole in the dura versus the clean puncture observed with a cutting needle. From this observation it is proposed that an increased inflammatory reaction occurs with the blunt tip needle that promotes hole closure thus reducing the amount of CSF leakage.

The orientation of the bevel to the dura during dural puncture has been proposed as a factor affecting the amount of CSF leakage and the incidence of PDPH. In an in vitro study Cruickshank and Hopkinson showed a 21% reduction in the leakage of CSF if the bevel was parallel to the long axis of the spinal cord.[53] Norris et al. in a study of 1,558 parturients compared the risk of dural puncture and PDPH between orienting the epidural needle parallel or perpendicular to the long axis of the dura during epidural catheter placement. Although both groups had a similar incidence of dural puncture, patients in the parallel orientation group reported less PDPH and required fewer EBPs. It was proposed that the parallel orientation separated the dural fibers rather than cutting them.[54] This mechanism is contrary to the electron microscopy observation that the dura is a laminated structure whose layers are arranged concentrically around the cord.[36]

Independent risk factors of PDPH include a higher incidence in females versus males, pregnancy, a higher incidence in the age group 20 to 50 years, and a higher incidence in patients with lower body mass index.[7] PDPHs are rare in children or adolescents and in patient's older than 60 years of age.[55,56] Vercauteren et al. referred to a higher incidence of PDPH after diagnostic dural punctures performed by neurologists and neuroradiologists.[57] This is most likely due to the use of larger-gauge needles to document the opening pressure and to facilitate the injection of viscous contrast material. There is also a higher incidence in patients with a headache prior to the dural puncture and a history of prior PDPH. The most widely quoted incidence of PDPH during labor analgesia/anesthesia is between 1% and 2.6%.[51] In a retrospective review van de Velde et al. found no increased incidence of PDPH with combined spinal epidural (CSE) anesthetics versus epidural only anesthetics in parturients.[58]

Although the incidence of SIH is low, there is increasing awareness of this diagnosis. Mokri has proposed a possible correlation between connective tissue disorders, meningeal diverticula, and increased incidence of SIH. Although meningeal abnormalities are known to be associated with Marfan's syndrome, neurofibromatosis, and autosomal dominant polycystic kidney disease, no increased incidence of SIH has been observed in this population.[22]

PREVENTION

Prevention of PDPH centers around needle selection and bevel orientation during dural/arachnoid puncture. Needle selection should be guided by the fact that smaller-diameter needles have a lower incidence of PDPH. Blunt tip needles have a lower incidence of PDPH when compared with comparable diameter cutting tip needles.[59] It has been shown that bevel orientation parallel to the long axis of the spinal cord has a lower incidence of PDPH.[54] Another proposed method to reduce the incidence of PDPH during spinal placement, based on Hatfalvi's observations, is to use a paramedian approach at an angle equal to or greater than 35° with the bevel facing the dura during puncture. In in vitro studies he found that this puncture angle produces a valve that closes with increased subarachnoid pressure and theoretically prevents CSF leakage.[60] In a comparative outcome study of known wet taps with 18-gauge Tuohy needles Ayad et al. found that placing an intrathecal catheter through the dural puncture reduced the incidence of PDPH. Furthermore they found that leaving the catheter in place for 24 hours after delivery reduced the incidence to only 3%.[61] Other proposed preventive procedures include prophylactic EBPs and epidural saline injections and infusions. In a small study Charsley and Abram found that intrathecal injection of 10 mL normal saline reduced the incidence of PDPH.[62] These efforts to prevent a PDPH following dural puncture should be viewed with the perspective that only 24% of patients with dural puncture by a 22-gauge needle will develop a PDPH. Bed rest as a preventative measure is not effective and can prevent the early diagnosis and treatment of a PDPH.

TREATMENT

Treatment for a PDPH and SIH should only be initiated once the diagnosis has been clearly established based upon history, physical examination, and appropriate diagnostic tests. Treatment options should be balanced with the understanding that 85% of PDPHs last less than 5 days, and, although rare, PDPHs can be associated with significant morbidity.[11] The initial treatment regime is commonly pharmacological noninvasive therapy. Recumbent bed rest relieves the symptoms of PDPH but has no therapeutic benefit. Aggressive hydration is a common therapy despite the fact that there are no studies to support its effectiveness. Medications reported beneficial in the treatment of PDPH include the methylxanthines caffeine and theophylline, sumatriptan, adrenocorticotropic hormone, and corticosteroids. Caffeine, a potent central nervous system stimulant, causes cerebral vasoconstriction, and is the most widely used pharmacological therapy. Caffeine is administered as an oral dose of 300 mg or intravenously as 500 mg in 500 to 1000 mL normal saline over 2 hours; the intravenous dose can be repeated over the next 2 to 4 hours.[63] Although caffeine is safe and effective, there have been reports of seizures, anxiety, and arrhythmias associated with its use.[64] Caffeine is contraindicated in patients with a history of seizure disorder and in patients with pregnancy-induced hypertension. The effect of caffeine is transient and the dose must be repeated since it does not address the underlying pathology.[65] Theophylline, another cerebral vasoconstrictor effective in the treatment of PDPH, is not widely used. Sumatriptan 6 mg subcutaneously has been found effective in a very limited study; however, its use is controversial and there are no conclusive scientific trials to support its usage.[66,67] Adrenocorticotropic hormone and corticosteroids therapy has been reported on a limited basis but is not widely utilized as a first-line therapy.

Once the pharmacological options have been exhausted without relief and the patient is unable to wait for the natural resolution of the headache, more invasive options can be explored. The gold standard treatment for both PDPH and SIH is an EBP. Due to specific patient concerns numerous variations on the EBP have been developed; however, the standard and most common treatment remains the epidural autologous blood patch. The indication for an EBP is to treat a known or probable dural tear that is causing the patient's symptoms, a postural headache being the most prominent. Following a diagnostic or therapeutic procedure, the level of the dural puncture is usually obvious. In SIH the level of the dural leak is usually in the thoracic, cervicothoracic, or thoracolumbar junction region and may be confirmed by radionuclide cisternography.[18] Intracranial CSF leaks rarely cause symptoms.

The contraindications to an EBP are similar to those for any spinal or epidural procedure. The first is patient refusal in general or for a specific reason. In the case of concerns of Jehovah's Witnesses about blood transfusions there are reports of alternative patching materials.[7] Secondly, the patient's coagulation status must be assessed and considered within normal limits in order to reduce the risk of an epidural hematoma.[68] Finally it is not recommended to place an EBP in a septic patient, or through a localized infection due to the obvious concern of seeding the epidural space. It is also widely accepted to not place an epidural in a febrile patient.[69] Concerns about an EBP in HIV-positive patients are unfounded since HIV crosses the blood–brain barrier early in the course of the disease.[70]

The mechanism of EBP is controversial; however, it is generally believed to be twofold. There is an initial early effect, which occurs within minutes, secondary to compression of the dura toward the cord and reduction in the intradural volume. Szeinfeld et al. demonstrated that EBP blood spreads both longitudinally and circumferentially thus enveloping the entire dural sac.[71] The reduction in the spinal intradural volume shifts the CSF cephalad, thus resuspending the brain and reducing traction. In agreement with the Monro–Kellie rule, this intracranial shift in CSF also reduces the intracranial blood volume and cerebral vasodilatation. Due to this early effect, patients often report rapid relief following an EBP. However, using postepidural blood patch MRI, Beards et al. demonstrated that the compressive mass effect of a blood patch has resolved at 7 hours post patch.[72] A second more lasting effect is due to sealing of the dural/arachnoid tear with a gelatinous plug. This sealing of the dural/arachnoid hole prevents further loss of CSF and allows for regeneration and restoration of the CSF volume. The plug acts as a bridge until permanent repair of the dural/arachnoid hole occurs.[73] The occurrence of this second effect is more variable and accounts for the failure of EBPs despite initial relief. Another proposed mechanism of the EBP is the deactivation of adenosine receptors secondary to the acute increase in the epidural and subarachnoid pressures after the blood patch.[30]

The proposed risk factors for EBP failure include placement sooner than 24 hours after dural puncture, and performance of the procedure with residual lidocaine in the epidural space.[74–76] Due to the proposed mechanical plugging nature of the patch, it is recommended to avoid increases in intrathecal pressure until natural healing of the dural/arachnoid tear has occurred. A repeat blood patch often has more lasting benefit due to both the patch effect and performance of the blood patch later in the natural time course of healing of the dural/arachnoid tear. There are no documented long-term effects of epidural blood patch. Blanche and Ong were unable to find any conclusive impact of an EBP on the efficacy of future epidural anesthetics.[77,78] The technique of an EBP, first described by Gormley in 1960, is straightforward based on the placement of a single-shot epidural.[79] It usually requires two people, one to locate the epidural space and the other to obtain the blood. Obviously, sterility is of the greatest importance both during epidural space localization and during blood collection. The patient position during the procedure can be sitting or lateral decubitus depending on the difficulty in locating the epidural space and patient ability to tolerate the upright position. Selection of the level of placement should be guided by the observation that 15 mL of blood preferentially spreads cephalad six segments and caudad three segments, or one spinal segment per 1.6 mL of blood.[71] It is therefore common to select a site caudad to the suspected dural tear. Colonna-Romano and Linton report of a lumbar EBP successfully used to treat a PDPH due to a C6–C7 cervical dural puncture.[80] This may be related to the increase in the subarachnoid pressure and the resultant cerebral vasoconstriction as well as deactivation of the brain adenosine receptors. Because of anatomical considerations more caudad levels also have a reduced risk of direct cord compression. Although historically different volumes of blood have been used, the ideal target volume is 20 mL.[81] This is the most widely accepted and cited volume if the patient tolerates placement. If the patient complains of excessive back or leg pain or pressure during injection, especially in thoracic EBPs for SIH, less volume can be placed. These radicular symptoms are due to direct nerve pressure from the injected blood volume.[71] Due to the risk of blood clotting in the syringe it is widely accepted to locate the epidural space prior to venipuncture and blood collection. The most common site of blood collection is the antecubital veins due to their size and reduced risk of collapse. After the EBP, the patient should remain supine with the legs slightly elevated. An intravenous fluid can be administered during this time. In a small study Martin et al. found that 2 hours in the supine position post-EBP provided 100% relief versus 60% relief in patients who remained supine for only 30 minutes.[82] Although initial relief can be as high as 100%, the overall long-term relief of PDPH from an initial EBP is between 61% and 75%.[9,83] The effectiveness of the EBP is reduced by the larger size of the needle causing the dural tear.[84] Alternative dural patching materials include epidural fibrin glue and epidural Dextran-40.[85,86] Although both of these materials were reported as successful, they are not widely used due to cost and safety concerns, especially when compared to autologous blood. Mindful of these concerns, Dextran-40 may be an alternative in patients who are Jehovah's Witnesses.[7]

Alternatives to the epidural blood patch include epidural saline bolus and/or infusions, and surgical exposure and repair of the dural tear. Epidural saline bolus or infusions have not been shown to be an effective alternative and often require more interventions with a lower success rate. Binder et al. reported success using a continuous intrathecal saline infusion to treat the worsening neurological symptoms of SIH until the level of the dural tear could be identified and treated with an EBP.[87] Surgical exposure and repair of a dural tear is a more invasive procedure generally reserved for severe cases of SIH or PDPH that have not responded to an EBP. One limitation to surgical repair is that the exact location of the tear must be identified preoperatively, which is often difficult in SIH.

SIH is usually a chronic condition that has been exhaustively treated medically with limited success. There are reports of patients responding to corticosteroids; however, these are rare.[88] Although SIH has a similar complication profile to PDPH, the expected duration is much longer. In the light of this SIH treatment is usually more aggressive and definitive with either a percutaneous epidural patch or surgical repair of the CSF leak.[89]

Complications after an EBP are rare. The most common complication is mild low back and radicular pain following the procedure that resolves spontaneously in a few days and can be treated with nonsteroidal anti-inflammatory drugs (NSAIDs).[90,91] Other possible complications include epidural hematoma, infection, and arachnoiditis due to unintentional subdural/subarachnoid injection of the blood. There are two reported cases of facial nerve paralysis following EBP, which resolved spontaneously.[4] Mokri reports one case of symptomatic intracranial hypertension following an EBP.[92]

SUMMARY

PDPH and its management is a well-known and widely accepted entity in the anesthesia community. Less well known to anesthesiologists, SIH has an almost identical symptom, pathophysiology, and treatment profile. Unlike PDPH, there is no history of dural puncture in SIH. A postural headache is the cardinal sign that can indicate either pathology. In the light of these similarities, the diagnosis and treatment of either syndrome should be relatively straightforward. Although generally nonfatal, both entities can have significant comorbidity and should be treated seriously.

The similarities and differences between PDPH and SIH are summarized in Table 37-1.

KEY POINTS

Postdural Puncture Headache
- The crucial components of PDPH are a history of dural/arachnoid puncture and a postural bilateral headache on examination.
- The occurrence of headache after dural/arachnoid puncture is not directly related to the amount of CSF leaked or the subarachnoid pressure. The headache may be secondary to a *sudden alteration* in CSF volume and subsequent cerebral vasodilatation.
- Concomitant intracranial pathology may be present in patients with PDPH. The signs and symptoms include the presence of a significant nonpostural component of the headache, a changing pattern of the headache (postural headache becoming nonpostural in character), bilateral headache that becomes unilateral, and those with new-onset and severe nausea and vomiting.
- The prevention of headache depends mostly on size and design of the needle tip. Based on studies, the criteria guiding needle selection should be based on the smallest practical needle diameter with a non-cutting tip design.
- The initial therapy of PDPH for the first 24 hours should be conservative relying mainly on medications. Approximately 85% of PDPHs resolve spontaneously in five days.
- The initial and rapid relief from an EBP is secondary to circumferential compression of the dura and reduction of the intradural volume. This shifting of the vertebral subarachnoid CSF cephalad causes a resuspension of the cerebral structures and a reduction of the traction of the pain-sensitive intracranial structures, and decreased cerebral vasodilatation.

TABLE 37-1. SIMILARITIES AND DIFFERENCES BETWEEN POSTDURAL PUNCTURE HEADACHE (PDPH) AND SPONTANEOUS INTRACRANIAL HYPOTENSION (SIH)

	PDPH	SIH
Etiology	Dural/arachnoid tear	Dural/arachnoid tear
Neuraxial procedure	Yes	No
Site of tear	Depends on site of procedure	Thoracic, cervicothoracic, thoracolumbar
Postural	Yes	Yes
Bilateral	Yes	Yes
Subarachnoid pressure	Low or normal	Low
Meningeal enhancement on MRI	Yes	Yes
Associated findings on MRI	None, except in presence of concomitant intracranial pathology	Subdural hematoma, subdural hygroma
Predisposing factors	Age, size and design of needle, gender, obstetric population	Marfan's syndrome, connective tissue disorders
Treatment	Caffeine, EBP	Caffeine?, EBP

The lasting relief from the EBP is related to sealing of the dural/arachnoid hole.

- Caffeine and theophylline block brain adenosine receptors causing cerebral vasoconstriction. The acute increase in the subarachnoid pressure after an EBP may deactivate adenosine receptors and relieve the headache.

Spontaneous Intracranial Hypotension

- SIH is a more exotic diagnosis, largely based on clinical suspicion, history, physical examination, and intracranial MRI results. The underlying pathology is an idiopathic dural/arachnoid tear primarily in the thoracic, cervicothoracic, or thoracolumbar region.
- The signs and symptoms of SIH include a postural bilateral headache with meningeal thickening and enhancement on MRI. Diagnostic lumbar puncture usually documents the low subarachnoid pressure.
- Although identification of the level of the dural tear is ideal, it is often difficult. Lumbar cisternography rarely shows the site of the leak but documents the lack of ascent of the tracer dye and the rapid appearance of the dye in the kidneys and bladder.
- EBP is the most efficacious treatment of SIH. The site of the blood patch is done initially at the low thoracic area or at the location of the leak identified by radionucleotide cysternography. The EBP may be repeated in the mid- or high thoracic area if the initial injection was not effective. In this site, the injection of blood should be stopped when the patient complains of back pain. This is to prevent spinal cord compression.

REFERENCES

1. Bier A: Versucheuber cocainistrung des ruckenmarkes. Dtsch Zeitschr Chir 51:361–369, 1899.
2. Lybecker H, Djernes M, Schmidt JF: Postdural puncture headache (PDPH): Onset, duration, severity, and associated symptoms: An analysis of 75 consecutive patients with PDPH. Acta Anaesthesiol Scand 39:605–612, 1995.
3. Portier F, de Minteguiaga C, Racy E, et al: Spontaneous intracranial hypotension: A rare cause of labyrinthine hydrops. Ann Otol Rhinol Laryngol 111:817–820, 2002.
4. Day CJE, Shutt LE: Auditory, ocular, and facial complications of central neural block: A review of possible mechanisms. Reg Anesth 21:197–201, 1996.
5. Brady-McCreery KM, Speidel S, Hussein MA, et al: Spontaneous intracranial hypotension with unique strabismus due to third and fourth cranial neuropathies. Binocul Vis Strabismus Q 17:43–48, 2002.
6. Hong M, Shah GV, Adams KM, et al: Spontaneous intracranial hypotension causing reversible front temporal dementia. Neurology 58:1258–1287, 2002.
7. Munnur U, Suresh MS: Backache, headache, and neurologic deficit after regional anesthesia. Anesth Clin N Am 21:71–86, 2003.
8. Pakiam ASI, Lee C, Lang AE: Intracranial hypotension with parkinsonism, ataxia, and bulbar weakness. Arch Neurol 56:869–872, 1999.
9. Duffy PJ, Crosby ET: The epidural blood patch: Resolving the controversies. Can J Anaesth 46:878–886, 1999.
10. Wong AYC, Irwin MG. Postdural puncture tinnitus. Br J Anaesth 91:762–763, 2003.
11. Gaucher DJ Jr, Perez JA Jr: Subdural hematoma following lumbar puncture. Arch Intern Med 162:1904–1905, 2002.

12. Noronha RJ, Sharrack B, Hadjivassiliou M, et al: Subdural haematoma: A potentially serious consequence of spontaneous intracranial hypotension. J Neurol Neurosurg Psychiatry 74:752–755, 2003.

13. Benzon HT: Intracerebral hemorrhage after dural puncture and epidural blood patch: nonpostural and noncontinuous headache. Anesthesiology 1984; 60(3):258–259.

14. Schabel JE, Wang ED, Glass PS: Arm pain as an unusual presentation of postdural puncture intracranial hypotension. Anesth Analg; 91:910–912, 2000.

15. Schaltenbrand VG: Neuere anschauungen zur pathophysiologie der liquorzirkulation. Zentralbl neurochir 3:290–299, 1938.

16. Mokri B, Posner JB: Spontaneous intracranial hypotension: The broadening clinical and imaging spectrum of CSF leaks. Neurology 55:1771–1772, 2000.

17. Rabin BM, Roychowdhury S, Meyer JR, et al: Spontaneous intracranial hypotension: Spinal MR findings. Am J Neuroradiol 19:1034–1039, 1998.

18. Diaz JH: Epidemiology and outcome of postural headache management in spontaneous intracranial hypotension. Reg Anesth Pain Med 26:582–587, 2001.

19. Beck J, Raabe A, Seifert V, et al: Intracranial hypotension after chiropractic manipulation of the cervical spine. J Neurol Neurosurg Psychiatry 74:821–822, 2003.

20. Rapport RL, Hillier D, Scearce T, et al: Spontaneous intracranial hypotension from intradural thoracic disc herniation. Case report. J Neurosurg 98(Suppl 3):282–284, 2003.

21. Eross EJ, Dodick DW, Nelson KD: Orthostatic headache syndrome with CSF leak secondary to bony pathology of the cervical spine. Cephalalgia 22:439–443, 2002.

22. Ferrante E, Citterio A, Savino A, et al: Postural headache in a patient with Marfan's syndrome. Cephalagia 23:552–555, 2003.

23. Mokri B, Maher CO, Sencakova D: Spontaneous CSF leaks: Underlying disorder of connective tissue. Neurology 58:814–816, 2002.

24. Mokri B: Spontaneous intracranial hypotension. Curr Pain Headache Rep 5:284–291, 2001.

25. Mokri B: Headaches caused by decreased intracranial pressure: Diagnosis and management. Curr Opin Neurol 16:319–326, 2003.

26. Mokri B: The Monro-Kellie hypothesis: Applications in CSF volume depletion. Neurology 56:1746–1748, 2001.

27. Marshall J: Lumbar-puncture headache. J Neurol Neurosurg Pschiatr 13:71–74, 1950.

28. Miyazawa K, Shiga Y, Hasegawa T, et al: CSF hypovolemia vs. intracranial hypotension in "spontaneous intracranial hypotension syndrome". Neurology 60:941–947, 2003.

29. Iqbal J, Davis LE, Orrison WW. An MRI study of lumbar puncture headaches. Headache 35:420–422, 1995.

30. Raskin NH: Lumbar puncture headache: A review. Headache 30:197–200, 1990.

31. Koss SA, Ulmer JL, Hacein-Bey L: Angiographic features of spontaneous intracranial hypotension. Am J Neuroradiol 24:704–706, 2003.

32. Haines DE, Harkey HL, Al-Mefty O: The "subdural" space: A new look at an outdated concept. Neurosurgery 32:111–120, 1993.

33. Horton JC, Fishman RA: Neurovisual findings in the syndrome of spontaneous intracranial hypotension from dural cerebrospinal fluid leak. Ophthalmology 2:244–251, 1994.

34. Brightbill TC, Goodwin RS, Ford RG: Magnetic resonance imaging of intracranial hypotension syndrome with pathophysiological correlation. Headache 40:292–299, 2000.

35. Lybecker H, Andersen T, Helbo-Hansen HS: The effect of epidural blood patch on hearing loss in patients with severe postdural puncture headache. J Clin Anesth 7:457–464, 1995.

36. Reina MA, Dittmann M, Garcia AL, et al: New perspectives in the microscopic structure of human dura mater in the dorsolumbar region. Reg Anesth 22:161–166, 1997.

37. Nabeshima S, Reese TS, Landis DMD, et al: Junctions in the meninges and marginal glia. J Comp Neurol 164:127–170, 1975.

38. Waggener JD, Beggs J: The membranous coverings of neural tissues: An electron microscopy study. J Neuropath Exp Neurol 26:412–426, 1967.

39. Nabeshima S, Reese TS: Barrier to proteins within the spinal meninges. J Neuropath Exp Neurol 31:176–177, 1972.

40. Schachenmayr W, Friede RL: The origin of subdural neomembranes: I. Fine structure of the dura–arachnoid interface in man. Am J Path 92:53–68, 1978.

41. Vandenabeele F, Creemers J, Lambrichts I: Ultrastructure of the human spinal arachnoid mater and dura mater. J Anat 189:417–430, 1996.

42. Bernards CM, Hill HF: Morphine and alfentanil permeability through the spinal dura, arachnoid, and pia mater of dogs and monkeys. Anesthesiology 73:1214–1219, 1990.

43. Bernards CM: Human dura mater permeability. Can J Anaesth 41:1125, 1994.

44. Candido KD, Stevens RA: Post-dural puncture headache: Pathophysiology, prevention and treatment. Best Pract Res Clin Anaesthesiol 17:451–469, 2003.

45. Khurana RK: Intracranial hypotension. Semin Neurol 16:5–10, 1996.

46. Chung SJ, Kim JS, Lee MC: Syndrome of cerebral spinal fluid hypovolemia. Neurology 55:1321–1327, 2000.

47. Benzon HT, Iqbal M, Tallman MS, et al: Superior sagittal sinus thrombosis in a patient with postdural puncture headache. Reg Anesth Pain Med 28:64–67, 2003.

48. Marfurt D, Lyrer P, Ruttimann U, et al: Recurrent post-partum seizures after epidural blood patch. Br J Anaesth 90:247–250, 2003.

49. Noronha RJ, Sharrack B, Hadjivassiliou, et al: Subdural haematoma: A potentially serious consequence of spontaneous intracranial hypotension. J Neurol Neurosurg Psychiatry 74:752–755, 2003.

50. Rando TA, Fishman RA: Spontaneous intracranial hypotension: Report of two cases and review of the literature. Neurology 42:481–487, 1992.

51. Lambert DH, Hurley RJ, Hertwig L, et al: Role of needle gauge and tip configuration in the production of lumbar puncture headache. Reg Anesth 22:66–72, 1997.

52. Angle PJ, Kronberg JE, Thompson DE, et al: Dural tissue trauma and cerebrospinal fluid leak after epidural needle puncture. Effect of needle design, angle, and bevel orientation. Anesthesiology 99:1376–1382, 2003.

53. Cruickshank RH, Hopkinson SM: Fluid flow through dural puncture sites: An in vitro comparison of needle point types. Anaesthesia 44:415–418, 1989.

54. Norris MC, Leighton BL, DeSimone CA: Needle bevel direction and headache after inadvertent dural puncture. Anesthesiology 70:729–731, 1989.

55. Janssens E, Aerssens P, Alliet P: Post-dural puncture headaches in children. A literature review. Eur J Pediatr 162:117–121, 2003.

56. Matsumae M, Kikinis R, Morocz IA, et al: Age-related changes in intracranial compartment volumes in normal adults assessed by magnetic resonance imaging. J Neurosurg 84:982–991, 1996.

57. Vercauteren MP, Hoffmann VH, Mertens E, et al: Seven-year review of requests for epidural blood patches for headache after dural puncture: Referral patterns and the effectiveness of blood patches. Eur J Anaesthesiol 16:298–303, 1999.

58. Van de Velde M, Teunkens A, Hanssens M, et al: Postdural puncture headache following combined spinal epidural or epidural anaesthesia in obstetric patients. Anaesth Intensive Care 29:595–599, 2001.

59. Halpern S, Preston R: Postdural puncture headache and spinal needle design: Metaanalyses. Anesthesiology 81:1376–1380, 1994.

60. Hatfalvi BI: Postulated mechanisms for postdural puncture headache and review of laboratory models clinical experience. Reg Anesth 20:329–336, 1995.

61. Ayad S, Demian Y, Narouze SN, et al: Subarachnoid catheter placement after wet tap for analgesia in labor: Influence on the risk of headache in obstetric patients. Reg Anesth Pain Med 28:512–515, 2003.

62. Charsley M, Abram SE: The injection of intrathecal normal saline reduces the severity of postdural puncture headache. Reg Anesth Pain Med 26:301–305, 2001.

63. Camann WR, Murray RS, Mushlin PS, et al: Effects of oral caffeine on postdural puncture headache. A double blind, placebo-controlled trial. Anesth Analg 70:181–184, 1990.

64. Cohen SM, Laurito CE, Curran MJ: Grand mal seizure in a postpartum patient following intravenous infusion of caffeine sodium benzoate to treat persistant headache. J Clin Anesth 4:48–51, 1992.

65. Turnbull DK, Shepard DB: Post-dural puncture headache: Pathogenesis, prevention and treatment. Br J Anaesth 91:718–729, 2003.

66. Connelly NR, Parker RK, Rahimi A, et al: Sumatriptan in patients with postdural puncture headache. Headache 40:316–319, 2000.

67. Carp H, Singh PJ, Vadhera R, et al: Effects of the serotonin-receptor agonist sumatriptan on postdural puncture headache: Report of six cases. Anesth Analg 79:180–182, 1994.

68. Horlocker TT, Wedel DJ, Benzon HT, et al: Regional anesthesia in the anticoagulated patient: Defining the risks (2nd ASRA Consensus Conference on Neuraxial Anesthesia and Anticoagulation). Reg Anesth Pain Med 28:172–197, 2003.

69. Duffy P, Crosby ET: Epidural blood patch (EBP) and septic complication [letter]. Can J Anaesth 47:289–290, 2000.

70. Tom DJ, Gulevich SJ, Shapiro HM, et al: Epidural blood patch in the HIV-positive patient: Review of clinical experience. San Diego HIV Neurobehavioral Research Center. Anesthesiology 76:943–947, 1992.

71. Szeinfeld M, Ihmeidan IH, Moser MM, et al: Epidural blood patch: Evaluation of the volume and spread of blood injected into the epidural space. Anesthesiology 64:820–822, 1986.

72. Beards SC, Jackson A, Griffiths AG, et al: Magnetic resonance imaging of extramural blood patches: appearances from 30 min to 18 h. Br J Anaesth 71:182–188, 1993.

73. Sencakova D, Mokri B, McClelland RL: The efficacy of epidural blood patch in spontaneous CSF leaks. Neurology 57:1921–1923, 2001.

74. Loeser EA, Hill GE, Bennett GM, et al: Time vs. success rate for epidural blood patch. Anesthesiology 49:147–148, 1978.

75. Tobias MD, Pilla MA, Rogers C, et al: Lidocaine inhibits blood coagulation: Implications for epidural blood patch. Anesth Analg 82:766–769, 1996.

76. Tobias MD, Henry C, Augostides YGT: Lidocaine and bupivacaine exert differential effects on whole blood coagulation. J Clin Anesth 11:52–55, 1999.

77. Ong BY, Graham CR, Ringaert KR, et al: Impaired epidural analgesia after dural puncture with and without subsequent blood patch. Anesth Analg 70:76–79, 1990.

78. Blanche R, Eisenach JC, Tuttle R, et al: Previous wet tap does not reduce success rate of labor epidural analgesia. Anesth Analg 79:291–294, 1994.

79. Gormley JB: Treatment of post-spinal headache. Anesthesiology 21:565–566, 1960.

80. Colonna-Romano P, Linton P: Cervical dural puncture and lumbar extramural blood patch. Clinical report. Can J Anaesth 42:1143–1144, 1995.

81. Crawford JS: Experiences with the epidural blood patch. Anaesthesia 35:513–515, 1980.

82. Martin R, Jourdain S, Clairoux M, et al: Duration of decubitus position after epidural blood patch. Can J Anaesth 41:23–25, 1994.

83. Taivainen T, Pitkanen M, Tuominen M, et al: Efficacy of epidural blood patch for postdural puncture headache. Acta Anaesthesiol Scand 37:702–705, 1993.

84. Safa-Tisseront V, Thormann F, Malassine P, et al: Effectiveness of epidural blood patch in the management of post-dural puncture headache. Anesthesiology 95:334–339, 2001.

85. Kamada M, Fujita Y, Ishii R, et al: Spontaneous intracranial hypotension successfully treated by epidural patching with fibrin glue. Headache 40:844–847, 2000.

86. Souron V, Hamza J: Treatment of postdural puncture headaches with colloid solutions: An alternative to epidural blood patch. Anesth Analg 89:1333–1334, 1999.

87. Binder DK, Dillon WP, Fishman RA, et al: Intrathecal saline infusion in the treatment of obtundation associated with spontaneous intracranial hypotension: Technical case report. Neurosurgery 51:830–836, 2002.

88. Pascual LF, Santos S, Escalza I, et al: Spontaneous intracranial hypotension: Quick clinical and magnetic resonance imaging response to corticosteroids. A case report. Headache 42:359–361, 2002.

89. Benzon HT, Nemickas R, Molloy RE, et al: Lumbar and thoracic epidural blood injections to treat spontaneous intracranial hypotension. Anesthesiology 85:920–922, 1996.

90. Palmer JH, Wilson DW, Brown CM: Lumbovertebral syndrome after repeat extradural blood patch. Br J Anaesth 78:334–336, 1997.

91. Cornwall RD, Dolan WM: Radicular back pain following lumbar epidural blood patch. Anesthesiology 43:692–693, 1975.

92. Mokri B: Intracranial hypertension after treatment of spontaneous cerebrospinal fluid leaks. Mayo Clin Proc 77:1241–1246, 2002.

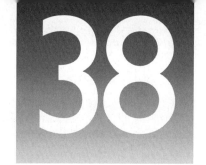

Cervicogenic Headache and Orofacial Pain

James C. Phero, D.M.D., and
Honorio T. Benzon, M.D.

CERVICOGENIC HEADACHE

Cervicogenic headache (CGH) is headache that arises from painful disorders of structures from the upper neck leading to irritation of the upper three cervical roots or their nerves and branches.[1] Sjaastad et al. introduced the term "cervicogenic headache" in 1983.[2] They published specific diagnostic criteria in 1990 and revised their criteria in 1998.[3,4] The International Headache Society (IHS) as well as the International Association for the Study of Pain (IASP) also included CGH in their diagnostic classification systems.[5,6] The diagnostic criteria set by Sjaastad et al., the IHS, and the IASP are given in Table 38-1. The characteristics of CGH, common to the diagnostic criteria of Sjaastad et al., the IHS, or the IASP, are pain that starts in the neck, mostly unilateral, aggravated by neck movement or awkward head positioning, and relieved by local anesthetic blockade of the occipital nerve. As stated, the pain starts in the neck or occipital area and may involve the hemicranium and forehead. There may be a prior history of whiplash injury or trauma. It should be noted that Sjaastad et al. considered CGH to be strictly unilateral while the IHS and IASP accepted these headaches as unilateral or bilateral.[7] Sjaastad et al. included accompanying symptoms such as nausea and vomiting, dizziness, blurred vision, photo-/phonophobia, and dysphagia as part of their criteria while the two societies did not. The IASP included relief of pain from blockade of the occipital nerves or nerve roots as part of their criteria while the IHS considered radiological abnormalities as part of their criteria.

CGH is usually confused with migraine and tension-type headache. According to Anthony[1] some patients with migraine may have a change in the character of their pain. The pain becomes more severe and develops a constant, dull aching and nonpulsatile quality. The pain spreads into the occipital area and an attack involves pain in the occipital, frontotemporal, and ocular regions of the head. The only migrainous feature is

the unilateral character of the headache. Anthony considered the following as criteria for CGH:

1. Unilateral nuchal-occipital headache, continuous or paroxysmal (neuralgic), with or without anterior radiation.
2. Headache occurring persistently on one side of the head (side-locked).
3. Circumscribed tenderness of the greater occipital nerve (GON) on the affected side as it crosses the superior nuchal line.
4. Sensory changes in the distribution of the GON (pinprick appreciation); i.e., hypo- or hyperalgesia or dysesthesia.
5. Precipitation of headache by neck movement or pressure.
6. Relief of acute attacks by blocking the GON with local anesthetic.

Anthony considered the following as criteria for migraine with CGH:

1. A history of established migraine in the past.
2. Recent increase in frequency/severity of headache with occipital radiation/origin of pain.
3. Headache always or predominantly on the same side of the head.
4. Circumscribed tenderness of the GON on the affected side as it crosses the superior nuchal line.
5. Absence of sensory changes in the area of distribution of the GON on that side.

CGH has a prevalence of 0.4% to 2.5% among the general population and 15% to 20% among patients with chronic headache.[7] There is a 4:1 female to male predominance and the mean age of patients with it is 42.9 years. The structures where the pain of CGH may originate include the posterior cranial fossa, vertebral arteries, occipital condyles, upper cervical facet joints, intervertebral discs, nerve roots, and cervical

TABLE 38-1. **CRITERIA FOR THE DIAGNOSIS OF CERVICOGENIC HEADACHE**

Criteria	Cervicogenic Headache International Study Group[4]	IHS[5]	IASP[6]
Location	Starts in the neck. Ipsilateral, vague, nonradicular neck, shoulder, arm pain or radiculopathy	Neck, occipital	Starts in neck or occiput. Forehead, temporal, hemicranium
Pain	Unilateral with no side shift. Moderate to severe. Not lancinating. Not throbbing	–	Unilateral with no side shift. Moderately severe. Varying duration
Aggravating factors	Neck movement. Awkward head position. Pressure over cervical/occipital area	Neck movement. Posture	Neck movement
Associated symptoms	Nausea/vomiting, dizziness, photo-/phonophobia, blurred vision, dysphagia	–	–
Neck trauma	Yes	–	–
Cervical spine	–	Decreased range of motion	
PE	–	Tender neck muscles	–
X-ray	–	Flexion/extension abnormalities. Fracture; tumor; rheumatoid arthritis; congenital abnormality	
Response nerves to block	Block of occipital nerves, nerve roots, or facets relieve pain	–	Blockade of occipital or nerve roots relieve pain

muscles and their bone attachments.[1,7,8] The pain may also originate from structures in the middle cervical region.

The mechanism of CGH has been ascribed to the involvement of the "cervicotrigeminal relay" (CTR) and the trigeminovascular system (TVS).[1,7] The structures implicated in CGH have their sensory innervations from the upper cervical nerve roots which enter the spinal cord and converge within the spinal tract of the trigeminal nucleus (Fig. 38-1).[7] This arrangement allows nociceptive impulses from the neck to be perceived as head pain, including pain in the temporal, frontal, and orbital regions.[7] This interconnecting system also allows pain in the frontotemporal region to be felt in the neck.[1] Neural connections between the cerebral vessels, the endogenous pain control system in the brainstem, the trigeminal nerve and its central and peripheral connections, and the upper cervical cord appear to modulate impulses from the head and neck.[9] CGH appears to involve an inflammatory component, as Marteletti reported elevated levels of interleukin-1β and tumor necrosis factor in patients with CGH.[10] Marteletti also found activation of nitric oxide synthase in CGH.

Anthony investigated the diagnostic specificity of local anesthetic blockade of the greater and lesser occipital nerves in 180 patients with headache.[1] He found that blockade of these nerves provided transient relief (1.6 to 3 hours) in 91% of the patients. The nerve block relieved not only the headache of CGH but also that of migraine headache and chronic cluster headache.[1] If blockade of the occipital nerve is a criterion for CGH, then the prevalence of CGH in patients with idiopathic headache is high. The mechanism for the effect of the occipital nerve blockade is the elimination of the sensory input to the CTR irrespective of whether the pain is in the anterior or posterior portion of the head.

The physical examination findings in patients with CGH include myofascial trigger points and decreased strength and endurance of the cervical muscles. The significance of X-ray findings in CGH is difficult to establish while electromyography does not show much abnormality.[7] In summary, there does not appear to be a specific test or clinical finding in patients with CGH.

Treatments for CGH include the use of nonsteroidal anti-inflammatory medications, occipital nerve blocks,

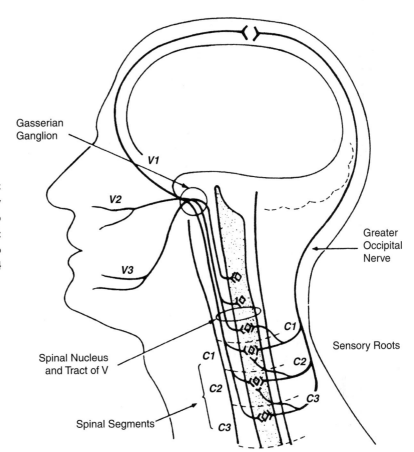

FIGURE 38-1. The pathway in cervicogenic headache. There is convergence of the sensory input from the upper cervical nerve roots into the trigeminal nucleus. (Modified from Anthony M: Cervicogenic headache: Prevalence and response to local steroid therapy. Clin Exp Rheumatol 18:S59–S64 (2 Suppl 19), 2000.

radiofrequency neurotomy of the cervical disc, epidural steroid injections, cervical manipulation, and surgery.[1,7,11–16] The studies that evaluated the efficacy of these treatments had small sample sizes, criteria for CGH were not documented, outcome measures were not standardized, and in the case of surgery the structures that were operated on were different and there was variation in the surgical procedures.

OROFACIAL PAIN

The section on orofacial pain reviews the classic orofacial pain conditions and syndromes encountered by the clinician. The practitioner addressing the complexities of orofacial pain must be cautious to avoid the pitfall of symptom management in the absence of diagnosis. The orofacial pain categories in this chapter follow the system initiated by the IASP, with some additional material supported by the IHS and the American Academy of Orofacial Pain (AAOP) (Table 38-2).

OROFACIAL PAIN OF NEUROPATHIC ORIGIN

Neuropathic pain syndromes are painful conditions caused by a lesion or dysfunction of the nervous system. The term *deafferentation pain* is used when the lesion is in the central nervous system. Orofacial pain of neuropathic origin usually results from involvement of cranial nerves (trigeminal, facial, glossopharyngeal, vagus, hypoglossal), but it is possible for these syndromes to be caused by neoplastic, post-traumatic, or inflammatory lesions.[17,18] Atypical facial pain is a global

diagnosis that contains several distinct pain syndromes, typically including neuropathic and musculoskeletal components that do not fit the category of *tic douloureux.*

Central Pain: A primary lesion of the central nervous system is an infrequent cause of orofacial pain. Central poststroke pain (thalamic pain) is the most common cause and usually presents with typical features of neuropathic pain. It has been estimated to occur in 1% to 2% of all stroke patients. The thalamus appears to be the site of this lesion in more than half of these cases. Approximately 20% of these patients develop facial pain. Facial pain may also be a feature of neoplastic conditions affecting the brain, but it is seldom seen as the presenting symptom.

Trigeminal Neuralgia
TIC DOULOUREUX: Tic douloureux is defined as a sudden, usually unilateral, severe, brief, stabbing, recurrent pain felt in the distribution of one or more branches of the fifth cranial nerve. Trigeminal root compression has been believed to be the primary cause of trigeminal neuralgia. Vascular loops compressing or contacting the trigeminal nerve at the root entry zone are observed in more than 80% of cases. The superior cerebellar artery and, in some patients, the inferior cerebellar artery are involved in this condition. Vascular anomaly, aneurysm, and bone architecture can also result in nerve compression.[19] Multiple sclerosis may also contribute to trigeminal neuralgia through segmental demyelination and microneuroma formation.

TABLE 38-2. OROFACIAL PAIN CATEGORIES

Orofacial pain of neuropathic origin
  Central pain
  Trigeminal neuralgia
    Tic douloureux
    Trigeminal neuralgia secondary to trauma
    Acute herpes zoster
    Postherpetic neuralgia
    Raeder's syndrome
  Geniculate neuralgia/Ramsay Hunt syndrome
  Nervus intermedius neuralgia/geniculate neuralgia
  Glossopharyngeal neuralgia
  Superior laryngeal neuralgia
  Hypoglossal/vagus neuralgia
  Tolosa–Hunt syndrome
  SUNCT syndrome
Non-neuropathic orofacial pain
  Extraoral pain
    Temporomandibular disorders
      Temporomandibular joint disorders
      Masticatory muscle disorders
    Carotidynia
    Sinusitis
  Intraoral pain
    Glossodynia
    Atypical odontalgia
    Burning mouth syndrome
    Cracked tooth syndrome

The paroxysmal pain attacks occur in one or more divisions of the trigeminal nerve, usually unilaterally. Trigeminal neuralgia is seldom bilateral. The pain is typically precipitated by light touch. The incidence in females is almost twice that in males. The age distribution is characterized by first occurrence in the forties, reaching a peak in the fifties. Right branches are affected more frequently than left. Pain commonly occurs according to the distribution of the second and the third branches of the trigeminal nerve, with the first branch rarely involved. Pain is always transient, lasting from seconds to as long as a few minutes. The characteristic pain is expressed as lancinating, shooting, electric shock-like, and stabbing. Between episodes, sensations are essentially normal or a slight desensitization is present. No pain or numbness is observed in the affected area between periods of paroxysmal pain. A short refractory period follows each of the pain attacks. An episode of such attacks, however, can last for months. A break in these episodes usually occurs but these attacks can return months or years later.

Trigeminal neuralgia may respond to anticonvulsant medications such as carbamazepine (Tegretol), gabapentin (Neurontin), or oxcarbazepine (Trileptal).[20] Additionally, clonazepam (Klonopin) and baclofen (Lioresal) are of benefit. Barbiturates are contraindicated in management of these cases. If an adequate dose of carbamazepine is administered without side effects, the neuralgic pain can often be completely relieved. If pain attacks are relieved by this medication and no neurologic abnormalities are present, the condition is normally diagnosed as trigeminal neuralgia. Local anesthetic injected into the trigger zone often relieves the paroxysmal episodes. However, in advanced cases, patients gradually fail to respond to this treatment. This may be due to the change of the site or intensity of nerve root compression.

TRIGEMINAL NEURALGIA SECONDARY TO TRAUMA:
Paroxysmal pain in the affected trigeminal divisions may follow trauma, surgery, and peripheral lesions.[21] Persistent burning, throbbing, or dull pain may also be observed. Peripheral neuropathy, classified as secondary trigeminal neuralgia, occurs relatively frequently after orthognathic surgery and fractures in the trigeminal distribution. Deafferentation and partial injury of peripheral nerves result in degeneration and regeneration. In cases in which this injury presents as neuritis, the pain is commonly characterized as burning. Hypoesthesia and dysesthesia are commonly observed in the affected nerve division. Allodynia and hyperalgesia are frequently observed.

ACUTE HERPES ZOSTER: TRIGEMINAL DISTRIBUTION:
If the latent varicella zoster virus remains in the trigeminal and the geniculate ganglion and the immune activity of the host declines, the infection can involve the trigeminal nerve branches and facial nerve branches, respectively. Although most patients only recognize the dermal condition because the skin symptoms are most prominent, the virus also affects nerves, vessels, bones, and other structures. Practitioners must be aware that this is essentially a recurrent viral infection of the nerve. In postmortem studies a marked loss of myelin in the peripheral nerve and sensory root is found in all patients with herpes zoster.

Trigeminal herpes zoster pain usually precedes dermal symptoms for a few days to a week, and sensory abnormality is observed in moderate and severe cases. Eruptions heal spontaneously within 3 weeks and may be associated with residual pigmentary changes in the moderate to severe cases. Induration of lymph nodes and high fever are often observed. The trigeminal nerve is involved in about 30% of all cases of herpes zoster. The first division of trigeminal nerve is affected most frequently in all dermatomal divisions. In 60% of cases of trigeminal herpes zoster vesicular eruptions occur in the first division; the second division follows in frequency, with the third being the least frequent. Ramsay Hunt syndrome is observed in 2% or 3% of cases of herpes zoster of the head. One of the most common complications in herpes zoster ophthalmicus is distorted vision (20.5%), mostly owing to corneal opacity. In some severe cases corneal ulcer results in loss of vision in the affected eye. Ophthalmoplegia, meningoencephalitis, and hemiplegia are also rarely observed. Alveolar bone can be destroyed and, in severe cases, teeth can be lost in the second and the third divisions. Some cases show symptoms of trigeminal herpes zoster and Ramsay Hunt syndrome without eruptions, or *zoster sine herpete*. These cases are very commonly misdiagnosed.

Diagnosis can be revealed by laboratory examinations. Elevated antibody level of varicella zoster virus should be observed for the diagnosis of trigeminal herpes zoster and Ramsay Hunt syndrome.[22] Clinicians should remember that some patients with symptoms similar to those of trigeminal herpes zoster and Ramsay Hunt syndrome without vesicles can be infected by varicella zoster virus, and that a proper diagnosis can be revealed only by laboratory examination findings.

POSTHERPETIC NEURALGIA: TRIGEMINAL DISTRIBUTION: Postherpetic neuralgia is characterized by chronic pain with somatosensory abnormalities that persist in the affected trigeminal divisions after eruptions of acute trigeminal herpes zoster have healed. Postherpetic neuralgia is defined as pain that persists more than 3 months after the onset of rash. The essence of the pathology of postherpetic neuralgia is denervation of the affected nerve. Skin in the severely denervated area shows anesthesia. Atrophy of dorsal horn and pathologic changes in the sensory ganglion are found on the affected side but not on the unaffected side. Central sensitization and neuroplasticity are believed to be important contributory mechanisms to postherpetic neuralgia.

Postherpetic neuralgia is characterized by burning pain with hyperalgesia, allodynia, and dysesthesia in an area affected by a previous episode of herpes zoster. The pain lasts far longer than the clinical appearance of the vesicles associated with herpes zoster. Hyperalgesia and allodynia may be observed. The diagnosis of postherpetic neuralgia is assisted by a history of eruptions in the affected area and the presence of somatosensory abnormalities. Serum varicella zoster virus antibody level is not helpful for diagnosis in chronic cases.

RAEDER'S SYNDROME: Raeder's syndrome is characterized by severe stabbing paroxysms in the first division of the trigeminal nerve with sympathetic nervous system paralysis (Horner's syndrome).[23,24] Sympatholysis is usually not accompanied by sudomotor dysfunction. The most common clinical presentation is severe, throbbing, supraorbital headache accompanied by ptosis and miosis in a middle-aged man. The headache is intermittent for several weeks or months.

Raeder's syndrome consists of two types.[24] One type is related to a lesion in the middle cranial fossa, such as a neoplasm. The other type is related to benign conditions, such as unilateral vascular headache syndromes. Raeder's syndrome may be caused by any lesion affecting the postganglionic oculosympathetic fibers distal to the bifurcation of the common carotid artery. Parasellar neoplasms often involve multiple cranial nerves, and unilateral vascular headache syndromes may be elicited by lesions of the internal carotid artery. Raeder's syndrome can be distinguished from Horner's syndrome by observing facial sweating. The combination of magnetic resonance imaging (MRI) and MR angiography is a reliable noninvasive tool to investigate the differential diagnosis of pericarotid syndrome and paratrigeminal lesions.

Geniculate Neuralgia or Ramsay Hunt Syndrome: Geniculate neuralgia is due to an acute herpetic involvement of the afferent fibers that accompany the facial nerve, usually at the geniculate ganglion level. Lancinating pains are usually felt deep in the auditory meatus and are followed a few days later with typical vesicles around the concha and the mastoid area. Facial palsy is usually associated with this condition. Typical cases of Ramsay Hunt syndrome show the triad of auricular vesicles, ipsilateral peripheral facial palsy, and vestibular/cochlear symptoms. Redness, swelling, and vesicles usually follow the pain at the auricle, external auditory canal, postauricular region, occiput, or pharynx. Treatment is as for acute herpes zoster.

Nervus Intermedius Neuralgia/Geniculate Neuralgia: This condition is noted for episodic, severe lancinating pain in the ear canal or posterior pharynx as the main presenting symptom. The etiology of nervus intermedius neuralgia is unknown. There are no lesions in the skin or mucous membrane and there are no sensory or motor deficits. It is uncommon before the fifth decade. Impingement of the nervus intermedius at the root entry zone has been demonstrated in those cases needing surgical treatment. Surgical decompression in these cases has resulted in long-term pain relief. The less intractable cases do respond to neuralgic medications such as carbamazepine.

Glossopharyngeal Neuralgia: Episodic, severe, stabbing, recurrent pains in the distribution of the glossopharyngeal nerve are the hallmark of this condition. The site of pain is confined to the tonsillar fossa. The trigger point is usually located in the faucial pillars. The pain may radiate to the external auditory meatus or to the neck. The symptoms may be associated with syncopal attacks. Vascular impingement of the nerve roots has been proposed as a central cause.

Treatment has been directed at peripheral as well as central nervous system causes. Microvascular compression is thought to be one of the primary causes of glossopharyngeal neuralgia.[25] The posterior inferior cerebellar artery is the vessel that is most commonly responsible. However, vascular decompression does not yield the same relief as with trigeminal neuralgia, indicating the possibility of other sources. Invasion or compression by parapharyngeal and posterior fossa tumors, arteriovenous malformation, and choroid plexus are reported as other causes of glossopharyngeal neuralgia.

Superior Laryngeal Neuralgia: Neuralgia of the superior laryngeal nerve is felt as sudden, brief, recurrent, lancinating pain in the throat and laryngeal area. This pain can also be felt in the deep ear and angle of the jaw and is provoked by yawning, coughing, swallowing, and gargling. In some instances symptoms of stimulation of the vagus nerve, such as salivation or hiccups, may be observed. Superior laryngeal neuralgia is more likely attributable to local lesions than to intracranial lesions. Differential diagnosis from glossopharyngeal neuralgia is often difficult because of the similarity in clinical presentation. The trigger zone is often located in the larynx. A local anesthetic block of the superior laryngeal nerve is useful for the differential diagnosis. Tumors and infections should be investigated.

Hypoglossal/Vagus Neuralgia: Neuralgia of the vagus nerve and hypoglossal nerve are rare conditions that present with paroxysmal unilateral pain affecting the angle of the jaw, thyroid cartilage, piriform sinus, and posterior aspect of the tongue. Vagal neuralgia is often brought on by acts such as yawning, coughing, or swallowing. It can be difficult to differentiate this from glossopharyngeal neuralgia or carotidynia.

Tolosa–Hunt Syndrome: This condition refers to episodic unilateral pain in the ocular area associated with ipsilateral paresis of oculomotor nerves and the first branch of the trigeminal nerve.[26] It is a condition that affects adults, usually in the fourth decade. Onset is gradual, with pain preceding the ophthalmoplegia. Trigger points are not present and there seems to be no predisposing or precipitating condition. Orbital phlebography can show the lesion in the majority of cases. The typical lesion is a narrowing or occlusion of ophthalmic venous channels around the area of the cavernous sinus. The exact pathology is unknown. The condition responds slowly but favorably to corticosteroids. The average duration of this condition is 8 to 12 weeks.

SUNCT Syndrome: SUNCT (short-lasting, unilateral, neuralgiform pain with conjunctival injection and tearing) syndrome is an idiopathic condition that is seen in adult males after the fifth decade and is associated with unilateral pain episodes lasting less than 2 minutes and affecting the orbit or periorbital area. Associated rhinorrhea, lacrimation, and conjunctival irritation are characteristic. The pain can be triggered by a variety of non-noxious stimuli and typically shows periodicity. No neurologic deficits are seen, and remissions may last for several months. The condition is resistant to classic forms of treatment.

NON-NEUROPATHIC OROFACIAL PAIN

Extraoral Pain

TEMPOROMANDIBULAR DISORDER: *Temporomandibular disorder* is a collective term that includes a number of clinical complaints involving the muscles of mastication, the temporomandibular joint (TMJ), and/or associated orofacial structures. Other commonly used terms are *Costen's syndrome, TMJ dysfunction,* and *craniomandibular disorders.* Temporomandibular disorders are a major cause of nondental pain in the orofacial region and are considered to be a subclassification of musculoskeletal disorders. In many temporomandibular disorder patients the most common source of complaint is not the TMJ but the muscles of mastication. Therefore, the terms *TMJ dysfunction* or *TMJ disorder* are actually inappropriate for many of these complaints. It is for this reason that the American Dental Association (ADA) adopted the term *temporomandibular disorder.*

Signs and symptoms associated with temporomandibular disorders are a common source of pain complaints in the head and orofacial structures. These complaints can be associated with general joint problems and somatization.[27] The primary signs and symptoms associated with temporomandibular disorders originate from the masticatory structures and are associated with jaw function. Pain during opening of the mouth or chewing is common. Some individuals report difficulty speaking or singing. Patients often report pain in the preauricular areas, face, and/or temples.[28] TMJ sounds are frequently described as clicking, popping, grating, or crepitus. This condition can produce locking of the jaw during opening or closing. Patients frequently report painful jaw muscles. They may even report a sudden change in bite coincident with the onset of the painful condition. It is important to appreciate that pain associated with most TMJ disorders is increased with jaw function. Because this is a condition of the musculoskeletal structures, functioning of these structures generally increases the pain.[29] When a patient's pain complaint is not influenced by jaw function, other sources of orofacial pain should be suspected.[30]

Temporomandibular disorders can be subdivided into two broad categories related to their primary source of pain and dysfunction. These classic subdivisions are TMJ intracapsular disorders and masticatory muscle disorders.

TEMPOROMANDIBULAR INTRACAPSULAR JOINT DISORDERS: The signs associated with functional disorders of the temporomandibular joints are probably the most common findings in a patient being examined for masticatory dysfunction. Many of these signs do not produce painful symptoms, and therefore the patient may not seek treatment. These disorders are classified in three categories: derangements of the condyle–disc complex, structural incompatibility of the articular surfaces, and inflammatory joint disorders. The first two categories have been collectively referred to as *disc-interference disorders.* The term disc-interference disorder was introduced to describe a category of functional disorders that arises from problems with the condyle–disc complex. Some of these problems are due to a derangement or alteration of the attachment of the disc to the condyle. Some problems are due to an incompatibility between the articular surfaces of the condyle, disc, and fossa. Other problems are due to the fact that relatively normal structures have been extended beyond their normal range of movement. With time, inflammatory disorders can arise from a localized protective response of the tissues that make up the TMJ. These disorders are often the result of chronic or progressive disc derangement disorders.

The two major symptoms of functional TMJ problems are joint pain and dysfunction. Joint pain can arise from healthy joint structures that are mechanically abused during function or from structures that have become inflamed. Pain originating from healthy structures is felt as sharp, sudden, and intense pain that is closely associated with joint movement. When the joint is rested, the pain resolves quickly. The patient often reports the pain as being localized to the preauricular area. If the joint structures have become inflamed, the pain is reported as constant, even at rest, yet accentuated by joint movement.

Dysfunction is common with functional disorders of the TMJ. Usually it presents as a disruption of the normal condyle–disc movement, with the production of joint sounds. The joint sounds may be a single event of short duration, known as a click. If this is loud, it may be referred to as a pop. Crepitation consists of multiple, rough, gravelly sounds, often described as grating and complicated. Dysfunction of the TMJ may also present as catching sensations during mouth opening. Sometimes the jaw can actually lock. Dysfunction of the TMJ is always directly related to jaw movement. A single click during opening of the mouth is often associated with an anteriorly displaced disc that is returned to a more normal position during the opening movement. This condition is referred to as disc displacement with reduction. When the patient closes the mouth, a second click is often felt, which represents the return of the disc to the anteriorly displaced position. For some patients the displacement of the disc progresses anteriorly, and the disc may not return to its normal relationship with the condyle during opening. This condition is referred to as disc displacement without reduction. When this occurs, the mouth often cannot be opened fully because the disc is blocking the translation of the condyle. For this reason the condition is often referred to as a closed lock.

MASTICATORY MUSCLE DISORDERS: Functional disorders of masticatory muscles are probably the most common temporomandibular disorder complaint of patients seeking treatment in the dental office. With regard to pain, these disorders are second only to odontalgia (tooth or periodontal pain) in terms of frequency. They are generally grouped into the large category *masticatory muscle disorders*.

The two major symptoms of functional TMJ problems are pain and dysfunction. The most common complaint of patients with masticatory muscle disorders is muscle pain, which may range from slight tenderness to extreme discomfort. Muscle pain, or myalgia, can arise from increased levels of muscular use. The symptoms are often associated with a feeling of muscle fatigue and tightness. Patients will commonly identify the location of the pain as broad, diffuse, and often bilateral. This complaint is quite different than the specific location of pain that is reported in intracapsular disorders. Although the exact origin of this type of muscle pain is debated, some authors suggest it is related to vasoconstriction of the relevant arteries and the accumulation of metabolic waste products in the muscle tissues. Within the ischemic area of the muscle, certain algogenic substances (e.g., bradykinins, prostaglandins) are released, causing muscle pain. However, the origins of muscle pain are far more complex than simple overuse and fatigue. Muscle pain associated with temporomandibular disorders does not seem to be strongly correlated with increased activity, such as spasm. It is now appreciated that muscle pain can be greatly influenced by central mechanisms.

The severity of muscle pain is directly related to the functional activity of the muscle involved. Therefore, patients often report that the pain affects functional activity. If the patient does not report an increase in pain associated with jaw function, the disorder is not likely related to a masticatory muscle problem, and other diagnoses should be considered. Dysfunction is a common clinical symptom associated with masticatory muscle disorders. Usually it is seen as a decrease in the range of mandibular movement. When muscle tissue has been compromised by overuse, any contraction or stretching increases the pain. To maintain comfort, the patient restricts movement within a range that does not increase pain levels. Clinically this is seen as an inability to open the mouth widely. The restriction may occur at any degree of opening, depending on where discomfort is felt. In some myalgic disorders the patient can slowly open wider, but the pain is still present and may even become worse.

Acute malocclusion is another type of dysfunction. Acute malocclusion refers to any sudden change in the occlusal position that has been created by a disorder. An acute malocclusion may result from a sudden change in the resting length of a muscle that controls jaw position. When this occurs, the patient describes a change in the occlusal contact of the teeth. The mandibular position and resultant alteration in occlusal relationships depend on the muscles involved. With functional shortening of the elevator muscles (clinically a less detectable acute malocclusion), the patient will generally complain of an inability to bite normally. It is important to remember that an acute malocclusion is the result of the muscle disorder and not the cause. Treatment should never be directed toward correcting the malocclusion. It should be aimed at eliminating the muscle disorder. When this condition is reduced, the occlusal condition returns to normal.

CAROTIDYNIA: Carotidynia is characterized by unilateral continuous aching or throbbing pain, usually starting in the ipsilateral anterior neck.[31] The pathology of carotidynia is unknown. Some cases have been reported to be associated with migraine,

aneurysm, and long intraluminal clots with incomplete vessel obstruction of the internal carotid artery. Tenderness of the carotid artery, especially around the bifurcation, is the most common feature. Palpation may aggravate head and neck pain. In cases of headache the pain complaint may resemble that of migraine. Autonomic symptoms are not observed, although some associated symptoms with migraine, such as photophobia and nausea, may be present. Episodes are superimposed on the continuous pain. Pain is precipitated by swallowing, coughing, and rotating or extending the neck. A careful review of the history and physical examination findings can lead to the diagnosis. Laboratory studies enable exclusion of other causes. Migraine, giant cell arteritis, and glossopharyngeal neuralgia should be differentiated.

SINUSITIS: Sinus pain is characterized as continuous aching or throbbing pain in the infraorbital, temporal, frontal, ear, upper molar, and/or premolar region due to inflammation of the sinuses. Pain is located unilaterally in the early stage; however, it extends to the opposite side of the face according to the involvement of the sinuses on the other side. Pain is essentially the result of inflammation, and it is exacerbated when the mucosa is swollen and the ostia of the sinuses are occluded. Acute inflammation of sinuses causes throbbing or wrenching headache; however, chronic sinusitis usually leads to dull or tender pain. Oppressive pain may be observed in the infraorbital region. Purulent discharge to the pharynx is a common finding. Rapid changes of atmospheric pressure, such as that induced by diving or traveling on airplanes, aggravate the pain. Diagnosis is not difficult if purulent discharge from the sinus ostia and radiographic opacity in ipsilateral and/or bilateral sinuses are observed. Laboratory examination shows an inflammatory pattern.

Intraoral Pain: Pain of the oral cavity has multiple causes: for example, inflammation of the dental pulp or periodontal tissue or trauma of hard and soft tissues. The headache syndromes may present as toothache.[32]

GLOSSODYNIA, ATYPICAL ODONTALGIA, AND BURNING MOUTH SYNDROME: These disorders are the oral analogues of atypical facial pain. The practitioner is uncertain as to the cause of pain in the tongue, teeth, periodontal tissues, or the whole mouth. It is important to remember that these are not conditions but syndromes, which should be diagnosed only after all other possible causes have been ruled out. These syndromes classically occur with more frequency after the fourth decade. Patients complain of continuous sore, throbbing, or burning pain in the tongue, teeth, periodontal tissues, or whole mouth. The intensity of pain is moderate. Variation of the pain is observed, and specific precipitating factors are rarely noted. No pathology or distinct somatosensory anomaly can be observed at the site of pain. Findings from thermal and mechanical (percussion) tests to the teeth in the affected area are equivocal. These syndromes often have a psychosomatic aspect.

CRACKED TOOTH SYNDROME: This pain results from an incomplete (cracked tooth) or a complete tooth fracture (split tooth).[33] A cracked tooth induces dental pulp sensitization and pulpitis, and deep periodontal pockets can give rise to severe pain. Cracked tooth syndrome is primarily seen in the molar and the premolar teeth. Vertical root fractures most frequently occur in endodontically treated posterior teeth in patients between 45 and 60 years of age.[34] When an incomplete fracture involves the dentinal layer of a vital posterior tooth, it may cause pain. Caries, inappropriate dental restoration design, overloading of the tooth, atypical root canal anatomy, and external root resorption of the tooth may predispose to this syndrome.

Location of the dentinal crack is difficult and must be guided by a precise history, thermal pulp testing, and inspection of the dentinal walls within the suspect tooth. The number, extent, and direction of the fracture lines may be ascertained readily by using transillumination and magnification. This allows the clinician to distinguish between oblique and vertical cracks. Intra-alveolar root fractures can be detected only by radiogram. The detection of a tooth fracture can be increased by taking x-rays from more than one angle. Radiolucent areas occur in the region of the root fracture more readily than in the periapical region, in a ratio of 7:1.

TREATMENT CONSIDERATIONS WITH EMPHASIS ON TRIGEMINAL NEURALGIA

Conservative Management: Pharmacotherapeutic Options: Conservative management in a multidisciplinary pain clinic seems to provide the most promising results in the majority of cases of trigeminal neuralgia. Surgical management should be considered for patients in whom conservative management has failed. Conservative management relies mainly on pharmacotherapy with the agents discussed in the following.

CARBAMAZEPINE: Carbamazepine, a tricyclic imipramine, is the drug of choice in the management of trigeminal neuralgia. The drug, however, is not without troublesome side effects and therefore must be introduced at a low dose. In the elderly it is customary to start with a 100 mg dose, which is increased gradually by 100 mg increments every 3 days until pain relief occurs or side effects supervene. Doses in the range of 800 to 1200 mg/day are usually therapeutic. Approximately 20% of patients treated with carbamazepine experience some side effects. The most common side effects, dizziness and diplopia, are neurologic, although nausea is also a frequent complaint. The most sinister side effects, however, are hematologic: anemia, thrombocytopenia, and agranulocytosis. The elderly are more susceptible to these side effects. Serious side effects are rare (2 to 6 cases per million population per year). Megaloblastic anemia is the most frequently observed hematologic side effect. Transient or persistent decreases in platelet or leukocyte counts are also frequently observed in patients receiving this drug. Allergic reactions in the form of a delayed-onset nonspecific rash are not uncommon. Routine periodic hematologic monitoring is recommended for patients taking carbamazepine. Monitoring of blood levels for therapeutic efficacy, however, is more controversial. Carbamazepine is a potent hepatic enzyme inducer and induces its own metabolism. This property of autoinduction along with its unique pharmacokinetics leads to inconsistent blood levels (i.e., correlation between the dose and serum level is poor). However, drug monitoring has been used to individualize therapy and to check for patient compliance at intervals of 6 months. A target level of 4 to 12 µg/mL has been suggested. The response of trigeminal neuralgia to carbamazepine is good in approxi-

mately 70% of patients. The majority of patients report relief within the first 2 days. Unfortunately, tolerance to therapy seems to develop over time. In such cases the patient's response can be optimized by the addition of another medication or changing to a second-line drug.

Carbamazepine is the treatment of choice for trigeminal neuralgia.[35–37] Carbamazepine was noted to be more effective than tizanidine, as effective as tocanaide, and less effective than pimozide.[38] The number-needed-to-treat for carbamazepine is 2.6,[39] supporting the efficacy of this drug in trigeminal neuralgia.

OXCARBAZEPINE: Oxcarbazepine is a keto-analogue of carbamazepine that is indicated for the treatment of partial seizures with or without secondary generalization. Similar to carbamazepine, oxcarbazepine has been successfully used in the treatment of neuropathic pain such as trigeminal neuralgia. The exact mechanism of action of oxcarbazepine is not known. It blocks the sodium channels resulting in the stabilization of neural membranes, inhibition of repetitive neuronal firing, and diminution of synaptic impulse activity. Modulation of potassium and calcium channels may also be involved. The primary pharmacologic activity of oxcarbazepine is attributed its 10-monohydroxy metabolite (MHD). An advantage of oxcarbazepine over carbamazepine is that monitoring of drug plasma levels and hematological profiles is not necessary. It is less likely than carbamazepine to cause central nervous system side effects such as dizziness or hematological abnormalities such as leukopenia.

The initial dose of oxcarbazepine for the treatment of seizures is 300 mg BID but the authors employ starting doses of 150 mg BID for chronic pain patients. The maximum dose of oxcarbazepine for seizures is 1200 mg BID. Clinically significant hyponatremia (sodium <125 mmol/L) may develop in 3% of patients treated with oxcarbazepine. A mechanism other than SIADH may be partially responsible since cases of hyponatremia without abnormal ADH levels have been observed in some of the patients. The hyponatremia typically occurs during the first 3 months of therapy. Monitoring of sodium levels should be considered if oxcarbazepine is used with other medications known to decrease sodium levels or in those with baseline hyponatremia. Normalization of sodium levels usually occurs within a few days of discontinuing the drug.

Approximately 25% to 30% of patients with carbamazepine hypersensitivity will react to oxcarbazepine, probably due to the structural similarity of the two drugs. Central nervous system adverse reactions include somnolence, dizziness, ataxia, nystagmus, and tremors. The most common gastrointestinal complaints among adults and children are nausea and vomiting. Allergic skin reactions include rash, erythema multiforme, Stevens–Johnson syndrome, and toxic epidermal necrolysis.

GABAPENTIN: Gabapentin is an anticonvulsant agent that is structurally related to the inhibitory central nervous system neurotransmitter γ-aminobutyric acid (GABA).[40,41] This drug has no direct GABA-mimetic action, and the exact mechanism of action is as yet unknown. The drug has shown immense promise in the treatment of neuropathic pain, although its use has not been based on prospective double-blind trials. There have been several case reports of its success in management of a variety of neuropathic pain syndromes, including trigeminal neuralgia. The major advantage of this new drug over carbamazepine seems to be the lack of dangerous side effects. It is not metabolized in the body nor does it cause induction of hepatic enzymes. Monitoring of blood levels is not necessary. Dosing can start at 300 mg/day (in divided doses) and can be increased gradually to a dose of 1,800 to 3,600 mg/day, until pain relief occurs or side effects are seen. The drug is well tolerated, with a less than 10% incidence of troublesome side effects. Severe side effects are not seen. The most frequent adverse effects of gabapentin therapy are sleepiness, dizziness, and ataxia. Other anticonvulsants, including phenytoin sodium, valproic acid, oxcarbazepine, and lamotrigine, have also been shown to be effective in trigeminal neuralgia. They are used as adjuvants or second-line drugs in the management of trigeminal neuralgia.

Most of the randomized clinical studies on the use of gabapentin were in patients with postherpetic neuralgia or painful diabetic neuropathy. The superiority of gabapentin over placebo was shown in these studies.[42,43]

BACLOFEN: Baclofen is a skeletal muscle relaxant that is also structurally related to GABA. In animal experiments baclofen has been shown to resemble anticonvulsants in its ability to depress excitatory synaptic transmission in the spinal trigeminal nucleus. In double-blind studies in humans it has been shown to be an effective adjuvant for management of trigeminal neuralgia.[44] Gradual dosing is recommended to avoid side effects such as ataxia, lethargy, and nausea. It is customary to start at 10 mg/day, increasing to a target dose of 40 mg/day over 2 weeks. It has been shown that L-baclofen is better tolerated than the commonly available racemic mixture.

CLONAZEPAM: Clonazepam is a benzodiazepine that is known to be effective in myoclonic epileptic states. It has been shown to be effective in patients with trigeminal neuralgia who have shown resistance to carbamazepine therapy. The level of pain control achieved, however, is not good enough for clonazepam to be considered a first-line drug. Side effects include somnolence, ataxia, and fatigue. Therapeutic effects are seen in the dose range of 1 to 4 mg/day.

OTHER AGENTS: Other agents that have been tried with some success include tocainide, mexiletine, and topical capsaicin.

Role of Psychology: As a general rule, psychological factors are more observable in atypical facial pain than in trigeminal pain. Nevertheless, all patients with trigeminal neuralgia could benefit from the assistance of a clinical psychologist who, by instructing them in the use of coping strategies, may help patients to feel control over the pain. Medical and surgical management are directed at controlling pain, whereas psychological treatment helps patients alter attitudes toward anxiety and fear.

Role of Acupuncture: Patients with trigeminal neuralgia frequently seek alternative forms of therapy. Often, these patients have experienced troublesome side effects from medical treatment or serious complications from surgery. Acupuncture is one of the alternative treatments frequently sought by patients with this condition.[45] The natural remission of trigeminal neuralgia makes it difficult to evaluate and compare the efficacy of acupuncture with that of well-established medical and surgical treatments. Ge and co-workers have published a report of the use of acupuncture in patients with trigeminal neuralgia.[46] They have claimed a high success rate, especially in patients who did not have long-standing disease. The lack of dangerous side effects seems to be its main advantage. We feel that acupuncture has a place for short-term management of pain in such patients. It should be used in patients who are intolerant to medical treatment. It may also be used as an adjuvant to optimize medical treatment.

Surgical Management: Surgical treatment should be sought only after a thorough trial of medical treatment has failed. Because surgery has no role in atypical facial pain states, diagnosis is absolutely vital. Several surgical strategies are available for management of trigeminal neuralgia, but only two methods have been shown to be consistently effective: gangliolysis and microvascular decompression.

Gangliolysis has replaced previously used neurodestructive procedures such as peripheral nerve avulsion, alcohol injections, subtemporal rhizotomy, posterior rhizotomy, and descending trigeminal tractotomy. This percutaneous procedure involves localization of the trigeminal nerve at the foramen ovale, under fluoroscopic guidance, and creation of a lesion with radiofrequency. In skilled hands the procedure has a high success rate and a low complication rate. The most feared complication is anesthesia dolorosa (painful paresthesia).

Microvascular decompression has become a popular operation among neurosurgeons for the treatment of trigeminal neuralgia. This is posterior fossa surgery and requires a general anesthetic. An operating microscope is used to delineate the vascular impingement of the nerve root as it courses through Meckel's cave to the pons.[47] The success rate of this procedure at 1 and 5 years is 85% and 80%, respectively, and the estimated half-life of the procedure is about 15 years.[48] The mortality rate is 0.5%, and other troublesome complications occur in 10% to 15% of cases. Recent advances in stereotactic surgery with the Leksell gamma knife have been extended to the management of trigeminal neuralgia, and initial results look promising.[49]

KEY POINTS

- Cervicogenic headache is a syndrome where the pain is felt at the neck and may involve the whole hemicranium. It may be misdiagnosed as migraine headache. Cervicogenic headache usually responds to blockade of the greater and lesser occipital nerves.
- The mechanism of cervicogenic headache involves the trigeminovascular system. Sensory input from the upper cervical nerve roots enters the spinal cord and converges within the spinal tract of the trigeminal nucleus. This arrangement allows pain impulses from the neck to be perceived as headache.
- Trigeminal neuralgia is characterized by a sudden, unilateral, severe, brief, stabbing pain felt in the distribution of one or more branches of the fifth cranial nerve. It has a female predominance. It may respond to the anticonvulsants, specifically carbamazepine, blockade of the involved branch of the trigeminal nerve, or to injection of trigger points. The surgical management includes gangliolysis and microvascular decompression.
- Temporomandibular disorder is a collective term that includes complaints involving the TMJ, muscles of mastication, and/or associated orofacial structures. Temporomandibular disorders are divided into TMJ intracapsular disorders and masticatory muscle disorders.

REFERENCES

1. Anthony M: Cervicogenic headache: Prevalence and response to local steroid therapy. Clin Exp Rheumatol 18:S59–S64, 2000.

2. Sjaastad O, Saunte C, Hovdahl H, et al: "Cervicogenic headache": A hypothesis. Cephalalgia 3:249–256, 1983.

3. Sjaastad O, Fredricksen TA, Pfaffenrath V. Cervicogenic headache: Diagnostic criteria. Headache 30:725–726, 1990.

4. Sjaastad O, Fredricksen TA, Pfaffenrath V. Cervicogenic headache: Diagnostic criteria. The Cervicogenic Headache International Study Group. Headache 38:442–445, 1998.

5. IHS, Headache Classification Committee of the International Headache Society: Classification and diagnostic criteria for headache disorders, cranial neuralgias, and facial pain. Cephalalgia 8:S1–S96, 1988.

6. Merskey H, Bogduk N: Classification of chronic pain. Descriptions of chronic pain syndromes and definitions of pain terms. Cervicogenic Headache, ed 2. IASP, Seattle, 1994.

7. Haldeman S, Dagenais S: Cervicogenic headaches: A critical review. Spine J 1:31–46, 2001.

8. Delfini R, Salvati M, Passacantilli E, Pacciani E: Symptomatic cervicogenic headache. Clin Exp Rheumatol S29–S32, 2000.

9. Lance JW, Lambert GA, Goadsby FJ, Duckworth JW: Brainstem influences on the cephalic circulation: Experimental data from cat and monkey of relevance to the mechanism of migraine. Headache 23:258–265, 1983.

10. Marteletti P: Proinflammatory pathways in cervicogenic headache. Clin Exp Rheumatol 18:S33–S38, 2000.

11. Nilsson N: A randomized controlled trial of the effect of spinal manipulation in the treatment of cervicogenic headache. J Manipul Physiol Ther 18:435–440, 1995.

12. Nilsson N, Christensen HW, Hartvigsen J: The effect of spinal manipulation in the treatment of cervicogenic headache. J Manipul Physiol Ther 20:326–330, 1997.

13. Hurwitz EL, Aker PD, Adams AH, et al: Manipulation and mobilization of the cervical spine. A systematic review of the literature. Spine 21:1746–1760, 1996.

14. Blume HG: Cervicogenic headaches: Radiofrequency neurotomy and the cervical disc and fusion. Clin Exp Rheumatol 18:S53–S58, 2000.

15. Reale C, Turkiewicz AM, Reale CA, et al: Epidural steroids as a pharmacological approach. Clin Exp Rheumatol 18:S65–S66, 2000.

16. Jansen J: Surgical treatment of non-responsive cervicogenic headache. Clin Exp Rheumatol 18:S67–S70, 2000.

17. Okeson JP: Orofacial Pain: Guidelines to Assessment, Diagnosis and Management, ed 3. Quintessence, Chicago, 1996.

18. Okeson JP: Management of Temporomandibular Disorders and Occlusion, ed 4. Mosby-Year Book, St Louis, 1997.

19. Yang J, Simonson TM, Ruprecht A: Magnetic resonance imaging used to assess patients with trigeminal neuralgia. Oral Surg Oral Med Oral Pathol Oral Radiol Endod 81:343, 1996.

20. Sist T, Filadora V, Miner M, et al: Gabapentin for idiopathic trigeminal neuralgia: Report of two cases. Neurology 48:1467, 1997.

21. Rappaport ZH, Devor M: Trigeminal neuralgia: The role of self-sustaining discharge in the trigeminal ganglion. Pain 56:127, 1994.

22. Tomita H, Tanaka M, Kukimoto N, et al: An ELISA study on varicella-zoster virus infection in acute peripheral facial palsy. Acta Otolaryngol 446(Suppl):10, 1988.

23. Desai BT, McHenry L Jr, Stanley JA: Raeder's syndrome. Ann Ophthalmol 7:1082, 1975.

24. Grimson BS, Thompson HS: Raeder's syndrome: A clinical review. Surv Ophthalmol 24:199, 1980.

25. Resnick DK, Jannetta PJ, Bissonnette D, et al: Microvascular decompression for glossopharyngeal neuralgia. Neurosurgery 36:64–68,1995.

26. Dornan TL, Espir ML, Gale EA, et al: Remittent painful ophthalmoplegia: The Tolosa-Hunt syndrome? A report of seven cases and review of the literature. J Neurol Neurosurg Psychiatry 42:270, 1979.

27. McCreary CP, Clark GT, Merril RL, et al: Psychological distress and diagnostic subgroups of temporomandibular disorder patients. Pain 44:29, 1991.

28. Costen JB: Syndrome of ear and sinus symptoms dependent upon functions of the temporomandibular joint. Ann Otol Rhinol Laryngol 3:1, 1934.

29. Lund JP, Widmer CG: Evaluation of the use of surface electromyography in the diagnosis, documentation, and treatment of dental patients. J Craniomandib Disord 3:125, 1989.

30. Lund JP, Widmer CG, Feine JS: Validity of diagnostic and monitoring tests used for temporomandibular disorders. J Dent Res 74:1133,1995.

31. Cannon CR: Carotidynia: An unusual pain in the neck. Otolaryngol Head Neck Surg 110:387, 1994.

32. Graff-Radford SB: Headache problems that can present as toothache. Dent Clin North Am 35:155, 1991.

33. Bender IB, Freedland JB: Clinical considerations in the diagnosis and treatment of intra-alveolar root fractures. J Am Dent Assoc 107:595, 1983.

34. Testori T, Badino M, Castagnola M: Vertical root fractures in endodontically treated teeth: A clinical survey of 36 cases. J Endod 19:87,1993.

35. Campbell FG, Graham JG, Zikha KJ: Clinical trial of carbamazepine (Tegretol) in trigeminal neuralgia. J Neurol Neurosurg Psychiatry 29:265–267, 1966.

36. Killian JM, Fromm GH: Carbamazepine in the treatment of neuralgia. Use and side effects. Arch Neurol 19:129–136, 1968.

37. Nicol CF: A four year study of Tegretol in facial pain. Headache 9:54–57, 1969.

38. Backonja MM: Anticonvulsants (antineuropathics) for neuropathic pain syndromes. Clin J Pain 16:S67–S72, 2000.

39. Jensen TS: Anticonvulsants in neuropathic pain: Rationale and clinical evidence. Eur J Pain 65:61–68, 2002.

40. Mao J, Chen LC: Gabapentin in pain management. Anesth Analg 91:680–687, 2000.

41. Nicholson B: Gabapentin in neuropathic pain syndromes. Acta Neurol Scand 101:359–371, 2000.

42. Rowbotham M, Harden N, Stacey B, et al: Gabapentin for the treatment of post-herpetic neuralgia: A multicenter double-blind, placebo-controlled study. JAMA 280:1837–1842, 1998.

43. Backonja M, Beydoun A, Edwards KR, et al: Gabapentin monotherapy for the treatment of painful neuropathy: A multicenter, double-blind, placebo-controlled trial in patients with diabetes mellitus. JAMA 280:1831–1836, 1998.

44. Fromm GH, Shibuya T, Nakata M, et al: Effects of D-baclofen and L-baclofen on the trigeminal nucleus. Neuropharmacology 29:249, 1990.

45. Xu BR, Ge SH: Observation on the effect of acupuncture treatment in 300 cases of primary trigeminal neuralgia. J Tradit Chin Med 1:51, 1981.

46. Ge S, Xu B, Zhang Y: Treatment of primary trigeminal neuralgia with acupuncture in 1500 cases. J Tradit Chin Med 11:3–6, 1991.

47. Panagopoulos K, Chakraborty M, Deopujari CE, et al: Neurovascular decompression for cranial rhizopathies. Br J Neurosurg 1:235, 1987.

48. van Loveren H, Tew J Jr, Keller JT, et al: A 10-year experience in the treatment of trigeminal neuralgia: Comparison of percutaneous stereotaxic rhizotomy and posterior fossa exploration. J Neurosurg 57:757, 1982.

49. Young RF, Vermeulen SS, Grimm P, et al: Gamma knife radiosurgery for treatment of trigeminal neuralgia: Idiopathic and tumor related [comments]. Neurology 48:608, 1997.

Overview of Low Back Pain Disorders

Rasha Snan Jabri, M.D.,
Matthew Hepler, M.D., and
Honorio T. Benzon, M.D.

EPIDEMIOLOGY

Low back pain (LBP) is one of the most common complaints in our society today. At least 60% to 90% of US adults will have LBP at some time during their lifetime and up to 50% have back pain within a given year.[1–7] Acute LBP is the fifth most common reason for all physician visits.[8,9] Although symptoms are usually acute and self-limited, LBP often recurs. Of those who develop acute LBP, 30% develop chronic LBP.[10]

LBP has great financial and socioeconomic impact in industrial countries as a growing social economic problem. The cost for direct health care is more than $20 billion annually and as much as $50 billion per year when indirect costs are included.[11,12] LBP is one of the most commonly cited problems for lost work time in industry. Back pain is the most frequently filed Workers' Compensation claim and is the most common reason for early Social Security disability in the USA for persons under the age of 45.[13] In 1990 direct medical costs for LBP exceeded $24 billion. Total annual costs for back pain increase from $35 to $56 billion when disability costs are included.[14,15]

RISK FACTORS

Epidemiological studies have reported three general classifications of risk factors to be associated with LBP: biomechanical, psychosocial, and personal. The biomechanical factors include weight lifting, lift rate, load position, reach distances, and task asymmetry. The amount of weight lifted, reach distances, task asymmetry, and lift rate have all been found to significantly increase the three-dimensional spinal loads.[16,17] The psychosocial risk factors consist of mental concentration or demands, job responsibility, lack of variety, job satisfaction, and mental stress.[18–22] Studies have investigated the impact of psychosocial factors on spine loading.[23] Personal factors have also been

identified as potential risk factors for LBP, such as physical strength, genetics, anthropometry, gender, and personality.[18,24–26] Furthermore, both psychosocial and biomechanical factors may contribute to spine loading as well as influence the loading response to the work factors.[27,28]

Epidemiological studies have shown the following factors to be associated with the development of back pain:

- Jobs requiring heavy lifting[29–31]
- Use of jackhammers and machine tools
- Operation of motor vehicles
- Cigarette smoking[29,30]
- Anxiety
- Depression
- Stressful occupations
- Women with multiple pregnancies
- Scoliosis[31]
- Obesity[32,33]
- Genetics
- Personality[34,35]

DEFINITIONS

LBP is defined as pain in the lumbosacral region localized between the costal margin and the inferior gluteal folds with or without sciatica. The Quebec Task Force on Spinal Disorders categorized patients based on the duration of symptoms:[36]

- Acute back pain: duration less than 2 to 4 weeks.
- Subacute back pain: up to 12 weeks.
- Chronic: more than 12 weeks.

Chronic pain can be classified as persistent or as multiple acute recurrences, although few studies employ this distinction.

TERMINOLOGY IN LBP

The North American Spine Society (NASS) recommended detailed definitions of lumbar disc pathology to standardize terminology among experts in the field.[37]

- Annular tear: loss of integrity of the annulus such as radial, transverse, and concentric separations.
- Bulging disc: a disc in which the contour of the outer annulus extends, or appears to extend, in the horizontal (axial) plane beyond the edges of the disc space, usually greater than 50% (180°) of the circumference of the disc and usually less than 3 mm beyond the edges of the vertebral body apophysis. Another (nonstandard) definition of bulging disc is a disc in which the outer margin extends over a broad base beyond the edges of the disc space.
- Concentric tear: tear or fissure of the annulus characterized by separation, or break, of annular fibers, in a plane roughly parallel to the curve of the periphery of the disc, creating fluid-filled spaces between adjacent annular lamellae. (See radial tear, transverse tear.)
- Contained herniation: displaced disc tissue that is wholly within an outer perimeter of uninterrupted outer annulus or capsule. Nonstandard definition: a disc with its contents mostly, but not wholly, within annulus or capsule.
- Degenerated disc: changes in a disc characterized by desiccation, fibrosis, and cleft formation in the nucleus, fissuring and mucinous degeneration of the annulus, defects and sclerosis of the endplates, and/or osteophytes at the vertebral apophysis.
- Desiccated disc: disc with reduced water content, usually primarily of nuclear tissues.
- Displaced disc: a disc in which disc material is beyond the outer edges of the vertebral body ring apophysis (exclusive of osteophytes) of the craniad and caudad vertebrae, or as in the case of intravertebral herniation, penetrated through the vertebral body endplate. The term includes, but is not limited to, disc herniation and disc migration.
- Extruded disc: a herniated disc in which, in at least one plane, any one distance between the edges of the disc material beyond the disc space is greater than the distance between the edges of the base in the same plane; or when no continuity exists between the disc material beyond the disc space and that within the disc space.
- Fissure of annulus: separations between annular fibers, avulsion of fibers from their vertebral body insertions, or breaks through fibers that extend radially, transversely, or concentrically, involving one or more layers of the annular lamellae. The terms fissure and tear are commonly used synonymously. Tear or fissure are both used to represent separations of annular fibers from causes other than sudden violent injury to a previously normal annulus, which can be appropriately termed "rupture of the annulus," which, in turn, contrasts to the colloquial, nonstandard, use of the term "ruptured disc," referring to herniation.
- Focal protrusion: protrusion of disc material so that the base of the displaced material is less than 25% (90°) of the circumference of the disc. Focal protrusion refers only to herniated discs that are not extruded and do not have a base greater than 25% of the disc circumference. Protruded discs with a base greater than 25% are "broad-based protrusions."

- Free fragment: a fragment of disc that has separated from the disc of origin and has no continuous bridge of disc tissue with disc tissue within the disc of origin. A synonymous term is sequestrated disc. Nonstandard definition: a fragment that is not contained within the outer perimeter of the annulus. Another nonstandard definition: a fragment that is not contained within annulus, posterior longitudinal ligament, or peridural membrane. Sequestrated disc and free fragment are virtually synonymous.
- Herniated disc: localized displacement of disc material beyond the normal margins of the intervertebral disc space. Nonstandard definition: any displacement of disc tissue beyond the disc space. Note: localized disc herniation means less than 50% (180°) of the circumference of the disc. Disc material may include nucleus, cartilage, fragmented apophyseal bone, or fragmented annular tissue. Herniated disc generally refers to displacement of disc tissues through a disruption in the annulus, the exception being intravertebral herniations (Schmorl's nodes) in which the displacement is through vertebral endplate.
- High intensity zone (HIZ): area of high signal intensity on T2-weighted magnetic resonance images (MRI) of the disc, usually referring to the outer annulus. Note: high intensity zones within the posterior annular substance may reflect fissure or tear of the annulus, but do not imply knowledge of etiology, concordance with symptoms, or need for treatment.
- Internal disc disruption: disorganization of structures within the disc space.
- Intra-annular displacement: displacement of central, predominantly nuclear, tissue to a more peripheral site within the disc space, usually into a fissure in the annulus. Nonstandard definition: intra-annular herniation, intradiscal herniation. Intra-annular displacement is distinguished from disc herniation, in that herniation of disc refers to displacement of disc tissues beyond the disc space. Intra-annular displacement is a form of internal disruption.
- Intravertebral herniation: a disc in which a portion of the disc is displaced through the endplate into the centrum of the vertebral body. A synonymous term is Schmorl's node.
- Normal disc: a fully and normally developed disc with no changes attributable to trauma, disease, degeneration, or aging. The bilocular appearance of the adult nucleus is considered a sign of normal maturation. Nonstandard definition: a disc that may contain one or more morphologic variants which would be considered normal given the clinical circumstances of the patient.
- Protruded disc: a herniated disc in which the greatest plane, in any direction, between the edges of the disc material beyond the disc space is less than the distance between the edges of the base, when measured in the same plane. Nonstandard definition: a disc in which disc tissue beyond the disc space is contained within intact annulus. Nonstandard: any, or unspecified type of, disc herniation. The test of protrusion is that there must be a localized (less than 50% or 180° of the circumference of the disc) displacement of disc tissue so that the distance between the corresponding edges of the displaced portion must not be greater than the distance between the edges of the base. A disc that has broken through the outer annulus at the apex, but maintains a broad continuity at the base, is protruded and uncontained.

- Radial fissure or tear: disruption of annular fibers extending from the nucleus outward toward the periphery of the annulus, usually in the craniad–caudad (vertical) plane, although, at times, with occasional horizontal (transverse) components. Occasionally a radial fissure extends in the transverse plane to include avulsion of the outer layers of annulus from the apophyseal ring.
- Ruptured annulus: disruption of the fibers of the annulus by sudden violent injury. Separation of fibers of the annulus from degeneration, repeated minor trauma, other non-violent etiology, or when injury is simply a defining event in a degenerative process should be termed fissure or tear of the annulus. Rupture is appropriate when there is other evidence of sudden violent injury to a previously normal annulus. Ruptured annulus is not synonymous with ruptured disc, which is a colloquial equivalent of disc herniation.
- Ruptured disc: Nonstandard: a herniated disc, a disc in which the annulus has lost its integrity. (See herniated disc, ruptured annulus.) Ruptured disc is used colloquially to encompass the same nonspecific meaning as the preferred term herniated disc.
- Sequestrated disc: an extruded disc in which a portion of the disc tissue is displaced beyond the outer annulus and maintains no connection by disc tissue with the disc of origin. An extruded disc may be subcategorized as "sequestrated" if no disc tissue bridges the displaced portion and the tissues of the disc of origin. If there is a fragment of disc tissue that is not continuous with parent nucleus, but still contained, even in part, by annular tissues the disc may be characterized as protruded or extruded, but not as sequestrated.
- Spondylitis: inflammatory disease of the spine, other than degenerative disease. Spondylitis usually refers to noninfectious inflammatory spondyloarthropathies.
- Spondylosis: spondylosis deformans, for which spondylosis is a shortened form. Nonstandard definition: any degenerative changes of the spine that include osteophytic enlargement of apophyseal bone. Spondylosis deformans has specific characteristics that distinguish it from intervertebral osteochondrosis. Both processes include vertebral body osteophytes.
- Spondylosis deformans: degenerative process of the spine involving essentially the anulus fibrosus and characterized by anterior and lateral marginal osteophytes arising from the vertebral body apophyses, while the intervertebral disc height is normal or only slightly decreased.
- Transverse tear: tear or fissure of the annulus, running in the axial plane (horizontally), usually limited to rupture of the outer annular attachments to the ring apophysis. Transverse tears are usually small and are located at the junction of the annulus and ring apophysis. They may fill with gas and thereby become detectable on radiographs or computed tomography (CT). They may be early manifestations of spondylosis deformans.
- Vertebral body marrow changes (Modic's classification): reactive vertebral body modifications associated with disc inflammation and degenerative disc disease, as seen on MRI. Type 1 refers to decreased signal intensity on T1-weighted spin-echo images and increased signal intensity on T2-weighted images, indicating bone marrow edema associated with acute or subacute inflammatory changes. Types 2 and 3 indicate chronic changes. Type 2 refers to increased signal intensity on T1-weighted images and isointense or increased signal intensity on T2-weighted images, indicating replacement of normal bone marrow by fat. Type 3 refers to decreased signal intensity on both T1- and T2-weighted images, indicating reactive osteosclerosis.

ANATOMY AND INNERVATION OF THE LUMBAR SPINE

The lumbar spine normally consists of five lumbar vertebrae and the sacrum. Two vertebrae and the intervertebral disc compose a motion segment. A motion segment with all its parts can be a pain generator. The intervertebral disc in adults is composed of the annulus fibrosus and the nucleus pulposus and the vertebral endplate. The annulus fibrosus consists of numerous concentric rings of fibrocartilaginous tissue. The rings are thicker anteriorly than posteriorly. The nucleus pulposus is a gelatinous loose material in the center of the disc. This material usually is under considerable pressure and is contained by the annulus. Because of the structural imbalance of the annulus, the nucleus is slightly posterior in the disc. The lumbar intervebral discs are supplied by a variety of nerves. The sinuvertebral nerves are responsible for the posterior innervations of the ventral compartment. The ramus communicans nerve innervates the ventral and lateral aspects of the disc. The pain receptors are located in:

- Ligaments of the spine
- Paraspinal musculature
- Periosteum of vertebral bodies
- Outer third of the annulus fibrosus
- Facet joints

The two main branches of the spinal nerves that provide sensory innervation to the various structures of the spine are:

- Sinuvertebral or recurrent meningeal nerve
- Medial branch of the posterior primary ramus

The first nerve to emerge is the sinuvertebral nerve which emerges from the spinal nerve just outside the intervertebral foramen and then re-enters the vertebral canal to supply the ventral half of the vertebral column, including:

- Dura mater
- Posterior longitudinal ligament
- Intervertebral discs
- Anterior longitudinal ligament

The spinal nerve then branches into its anterior and posterior primary rami; the posterior ramus branches into the medial and lateral branches. The medial branch supplies the dorsal parts of the vertebral column including the following:

- Facet joint
- Vertebral arch
- Spinous process

Note that the posterior aspect of the dura mater is not innervated. The annulus fibrosus of the intervertebral disc has diverse innervations. The dorsal aspect of the annulus fibrosus and the posterior longitudinal ligament are innervated by the sinuvertebral nerve, the dorsal and lateral side is innervated by other branches of the anterior spinal nerve; the ventral

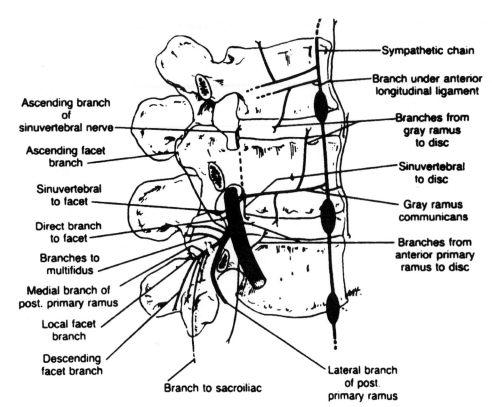

FIGURE 39-1. Segmental innervation of the lumbar spine (see text). (From Paris SV: Anatomy as related to function and pain. Symposium on Evaluation and Care of Lumbar Spine Problems. Orthop Clin North Am 14:475–489, 1983.)

and lateral side is innervated by branches of the ramus communicans nerve that connect the spinal nerve and the sympathetic trunk. The ramus communicans nerve branches from the spinal nerve just after it enters the intervertebral foramina. It runs anteriorly at the inferior third portion of the vertebral body, and connects to the sympathetic trunk before branching to the lateral and anterolateral aspects of the discs above and below. Therefore, each disc is innervated by four separate ramus communicans nerves: right and left, superior and inferior. Because of this pattern of innervation, the two ramus communicans nerves—superior and inferior—on either side should be denervated in the case of unilateral discogenic pain. The ramus communicans nerve also innervates the vertebral body.

The mechanism for transmission of a noxious stimulus from a vertebral disc is not yet completely understood. However, one hypothesis suggests that the impulse is transmitted to the sympathetic trunk via the sinuvertebral nerve and the ramus communicans nerve. The gray ramus communicans nerve provides the greatest source of disc innervation.

ETIOLOGY OF BACK PAIN

The differential diagnosis of LBP is broad and variable and includes specific and nonspecific causes. Specific LBP is defined as back pain caused by specific pathophysiological mechanism such as HNP, infection, tumor, fracture, or inflammation. Nonspecific back pain is defined as symptoms without a precise cause. Approximately 90% of all patients with LBP have a nonspecific cause and a precise pathologic anatomical cause cannot be reliably identified.[43]

In nonspecific, mechanical LBP the symptoms are thought to arise from local processes involving the spine and surrounding structures including the muscles, ligaments, facet joints, nerves, periosteum, blood vessels, and intervertebral discs. A wide range of terms are used for back pain due to mechanical causes including low back or lumbar pain/strain/sprain, lumbago, spondylosis, segmental or somatic dysfunction, ligamentous strain, subluxation, and facet joint, sacroiliac, or myofascial syndromes.

LBP arising from structures of the back can be distinguished from back pain referred from visceral diseases. In referred pain there are no signs of stiffness, and movement of the back does not increase the pain.

Mechanical Structural Back Pain Etiologies
- Spondylosis (degenerative disc disease).
- Spondylolisthesis: anterior displacement of one vertebra, typically L5, over the one beneath it.
- Spondylolysis: defect in the pars interarticularis without vertebral slippage.
- True disc herniation: presents with LBP with radiculopathy symptoms.
- Foraminal stenosis: bony material causing nerve root compression and cannot be distinguished from disc herniation symptoms.
- Facet arthropathy.
- Spinal stenosis: nonspecific LBP with typical neurogenic claudication.
- Fracture: traumatic or osteoporotic.
- Musculoligamentous: lumbar strains or sprains can be considered due to a nonspecific idiopathic musculoligamentous etiology.
- Discogenic pain: internal disc disruption and annular tear.
- Congenital disease: severe kyphosis, severe scoliosis or flat spine syndrome.

Nonmechanical Spinal Etiologies
- Neoplastic and metastatic disease.
- Infection: osteomyelitis, septic discitis, paraspinal or epidural abscess.
- Inflammatory arthritis: ankylosing spondylitis, Reiter's syndrome, psoriatic spondylitis, or inflammatory bowel disease.
- Paget's disease.
- Scheuermann's disease (osteochondrosis).

Referred Pain from Visceral Disorders
- Pelvic organs: prostatitis, endometriosis, or pelvic inflammatory disease.
- Renal disease: nephrolithiasis, pyelonephritis, or perinephric abscess.
- Vascular disease: abdominal aortic aneurysm.
- Gastrointestinal disease: pancreatitis, cholecystitis, or perforated bowel.

GUIDELINES FOR MANAGING ACUTE BACK PAIN

Most acute LBP with or without sciatica or acute disc herniation is a self-limited process and will disappear within 1 to 3 months. A comprehensive history and physical examination are important determinants in the diagnosis of LBP syndrome. Because of the high prevalence of the problem, the variation in its management, and its generally good prognosis, efforts to summarize evidence supporting common treatments for LBP and to develop recommendations have been undertaken.[45–47] In the USA the Agency for Health Care Policy and Research (AHCPR) published a guideline on acute LBP in 1994.[48] A panel of experts reviewed the available literature using strict criteria to assess the quality of the evidence. The panel focused on recommendations for the initial and subsequent evaluation and treatment of individuals with low back and/or back-related leg symptoms of less than 3 months' duration. A major finding of the guideline was that there was a paucity of reliable data on which to base treatment recommendations.

History: The history should include the patient's age, past medical and surgical history, and any history of trauma. The presence of constitutional symptoms, night pain, bone pain or morning stiffness, claudication, numbness, tingling, weakness, radiculopathy, and bowel or bladder dysfunction should be noted. The onset of pain, its location, radiation, characteristics, and severity should be assessed. Aggravating and relieving factors should be noted. Previous therapy and its efficacy, and the functional impact of the pain on the patient's work and activities of daily living should be queried. The signs and symptoms of radiculopathy, facet syndrome, and sacroiliac joint syndrome (see Chapters 42 and 43) should be noted. Finally, an assessment of social and psychologic factors that may affect the patient's pain should be made.

Physical Examination: A comprehensive general physical examination is recommended in patients with back pain. A detailed neurologic evaluation should be performed. The tests for the different syndromes causing LBP, including nerve root irritation, facet syndrome, and sacroiliac joint syndrome, are discussed in Chapters 41–43.

Red Flags: Patients with LBP should be screened for the possibility of potentially serious conditions including possible fracture, tumor, infection, or cauda equina syndrome (Table 39-1). Frequently, there are well-described "red flags" which distinguish these serious conditions from the much more frequent "benign" causes (degenerative disc disease, disc herniation, spondylolisthesis) of LBP. It is not uncommon, however, for a serious condition such as an infection or tumor to go undetected or mistaken for benign LBP without a characteristic red flag. In general, patients with "benign low back pain" should have mechanical dysfunction with pain on sitting, bending, lifting, or twisting and should improve with a short course of nonoperative treatment. Those patients with atypical symptoms or who fail to improve should be evaluated with MRI or other appropriate studies to confirm the benign diagnosis and rule out more serious conditions in the differential diagnosis. The trap of making a diagnosis that cannot be confirmed (muscle sprain or myofascial pain) should be avoided, as this is the most common reason appropriate workup is delayed and serious conditions identified late in their course.

Imaging Studies: An acute episode of LBP does not warrant immediate imaging studies unless one or more of the following is present:

- Neurologic deficit
- History of trauma
- Pain does not subside spontaneously
- Pain is severe or unusual in character
- Systemic or other injury is suspected
- History of cancer
- Corticosteroid use
- Drug or alcohol abuse
- Temperature greater than 38°C (100.4°F)
- Unexplained weight loss

In the evaluation of patients with LBP it is essential to correlate all imaging findings with the patient's symptoms and signs on physical examination. Because most imaging studies reveal abnormal findings in asymptomatic patients, a diagnosis should not be based solely on diagnostic imaging without firm correlation to the patient's symptoms.

PLAIN-FILM RADIOGRAPHY: The simple X-ray film allows the evaluation of the bony anatomy, arthritic changes of the lumbar spine, and degenerative disc disease but does not show soft tissue anatomy which requires further testing for definite diagnosis. Plain X-ray films are rarely useful in the initial evaluation of patients with acute LBP.[49,50] Studies have shown that plain X-ray films were normal or demonstrated changes of equivocal clinical significance in the majority (>75%) of patients with LBP.

Traditionally, the plain radiograph has been the first imaging test performed in the evaluation of LBP because it is relatively inexpensive, widely available, reliable, and easy to perform. The two major drawbacks of plain radiography are the difficulty in its interpretation and an unacceptably high rate of false-positive findings.[51] Plain radiographs are not required in the first month of symptoms unless the physical examination reveals specific signs of trauma or there is suspicion of tumor or infection.[52] It is important to obtain images

TABLE 39-1. POSSIBLE RED FLAGS FOR POTENTIALLY SERIOUS CONDITIONS[48]

Possible Fracture	Possible Tumor	Possible Cauda Equina Syndrome
From medical history		
Major trauma such as vehicle accident or fall from height	Age over 50 or under 20	Saddle anesthesia
Minor trauma or even strenuous lifting (in older or potentially osteoporotic patient)	Constitutional symptoms, such as recent fever or chills or unexplained weight loss	Recent onset of bladder dysfunction, such as urinary retention, increased frequency, or overflow incontinence
Substantial increase in pain or functional disability	Risk factors for spinal infection: recent bacterial infection (e.g., urinary tract infection); IV drug abuse; or immune suppression (from steroids, transplant, or HIV) Pain that worsens when supine; severe nighttime pain Substantial increase in pain or functional disability	Substantial increase in pain or functional disability
From physical examination		
Tenderness to palpation		Unexpected laxity of the anal sphincter Perianal/perineal sensory loss Major motor weakness; quadriceps (knee extension weakness); ankle plantar flexors, evertors, and dorsiflexors (foot drop)

that are free of motion or grid artifacts that display soft tissue and osseous structures of the entire lumbar spine.

Having a standard approach to evaluating radiographs can help prevent a missed diagnosis and it is crucial to develop and maintain a specific sequence of observation. The traditional sequence includes anteroposterior (AP) and lateral views of the lumbar spine, primarily to detect tumors or spinal misalignments such as scoliosis. In the AP view the indicators of a normal spine include vertical alignment of the spinous processes, smooth undulating borders created by lateral masses, and uniformity among the disc spaces. Misalignment of the spinous processes suggests a rotational injury such as unilateral facet dislocation. The AP view of the lumbar spine should include the whole pelvis allowing for evaluation of the acetabulum and heads of the femur and for the detection of possible degenerative changes in the pelvis. The lateral view provides a good image of the vertebral bodies, facet joints, lordotic curves, disc space height, and intervertebral foramen. Decreased disc space height can be indicative of disc degeneration, infection, and postsurgical condition. Unfortunately, there is a poor correlation between decreased disc height and the etiology of LBP. Anterior slippage (spondylolisthesis) of the fifth lumbar vertebra on the sacral base can be identified in lateral views.

Oblique views with the radiograph tube angled at 45° improve visualization of the neural foramina and pars interarticularis and are used to confirm suspicions generated from the initial imaging assessment. Oblique views are used to show tumors, facet hypertrophy, and spondylosis or spondylolisthesis. Flexion–extension views are helpful in assessing ligamentous and bony injury in the axial plane. The use of these views should be limited to patients who do not have other radiographic abnormalities and patients who are neurologically intact, cooperative, and capable of describing pain or early onset of neurologic symptoms. Flexion–extension views can be used in trauma patients, especially those with muscle spasm, which may be the only sign of spinal instability. When examining the lumbar spine for possible fracture it is important to include the lower portion of the thoracic spine because of the high occurrence of injury between levels T12 and L2. This region is more prone to injury because of the change in orientation of the facet joints between the thoracic spine and the lumbar spine and because it lies directly beneath the more rigid thoracic spine, which is stabilized by the rib cage.

Degenerative changes are often evident on plain radiographs caution must be used in making a diagnosis based on degenerative radiographic changes because of the high rate of asymptomatic degenerative changes. Radiographic evidence of degenerative change is most common in patients older than 40 years and is present in more than 70% of patients older than 70 years.[51] Degenerative changes have been reported to be equally present in asymptomatic and symptomatic persons.[51] The incidence of intervertebral narrowing and irregular ossification of the vertebral end plates has also been shown to be associated with increased age.[53] Even though plain radiographs usually provide little definitive information, they should be included in the screening examination for patients with certain red flags.

BONE SCINTIGRAPHY: Bone scintigraphy is useful when clinical findings are suspicious of osteomyelitis, bony neoplasm, or occult fracture. Plain radiographs, CT scans, and MRI reveal morphologic changes in bone. Bone scintigraphy detects biochemical changes through images that are produced by scanning and mapping the presence of radiographic compounds (usually technetium-99m phosphate or gallium-67 citrate). The image produced indicates bone turnover, a common occurrence in bone metastases, primary spine tumors, fracture, infarction, infection, and other metabolic bone diseases. Bone metastases normally appear as multiple foci of increased tracer uptake asymmetrically distributed. In extreme cases of bone metastases diffusely increased uptake of tracer results in every bone being uniformly illustrated and can be falsely interpreted as negative. Aggressive tumors that do not invoke an osteoblastic response, such as myeloma, can also yield a negative examination. Primary spine tumors are usually benign. Osteoid osteoma, osteoblastoma, aneurysmal bone cyst, and osteochondroma produce an active bone scan. These tumors generally affect the posterior elements of the spine. CT must be used to differentiate them and isolate their anatomic position.

Recent studies[54,55] evaluated the ability of bone scans, with the addition of single-photon emission computed tomography (SPECT), to distinguish benign lesions from malignant lesions. SPECT scan differs from bone scan because it provides a three-dimensional image that enables physicians to locate the lesion more precisely. Lesions that affect the pedicles are a strong indicator of malignancy, while lesions of the facets are likely to be benign. Lesions of the vertebral body or spinous process are just as likely to be benign as malignant and, therefore, offer little diagnostic evidence.

COMPUTED TOMOGRAPHY: CT is used to complement information obtained from other diagnostic imaging studies such as radiography, myelography, and MRI. The principal value of CT is its ability to demonstrate the osseous structures of the lumbar spine and their relationship to the neural canal in an axial plane. A CT scan is helpful in diagnosing tumors, fractures, and partial or complete dislocations. In showing the relative position of one bony structure to another, CT scans are also helpful in diagnosing spondylolisthesis. They are not as useful as MRI in visualizing conditions of soft tissue structure, such as disc infection. The data used to generate the axial images are obtained in contiguous, overlapping slices of the target area. The axial image data can be reformatted to construct views of the scanned area in any desired plane. Three-dimensional CT and CT with myelogram are reserved for more complicated problems like failed back surgery syndrome.

The limitations of CT include less detailed images and the possibility of obscuring nondisplaced fractures or simulating false ones. In addition, radiation exposure limits the amount of lumbar spine that can be scanned, and results are adversely affected by patient motion; spiral CT addresses these weaknesses because it is more accurate and faster, which decreases a patient's exposure to radiation.

MAGNETIC RESONANCE IMAGING: MRI today has become the modality of choice in the evaluation of spinal degenerative disease. MRI is superior even to CT with contrast in the distinction of bone, disc, ligaments, nerves, thecal sac, and spinal cord. On the T1-weighted image (T1WI) the disc is a fairly homogenous structure and isointense compared to muscle. On long TR images (TR is the time between consecutive 90° radiofrequency pulses) the disc becomes brighter due to its water content. The cerebrospinal fluid appears dark in the T1WI and appears white on the T2WI. The nucleus pulposus which is more hydrated than the annulus fibrosis becomes brighter than the annulus on the T2WI. Therefore the disc appears black on T1WI and white on T2WI.

MRI is the test of choice for the diagnostic imaging of neurologic structures related to LBP. MRI can evaluate soft tissue and nonbony structure pathology and disc herniation with greater accuracy than CT. For this reason, MRI remains the gold standard test in detecting early soft tissue pathologies like osteomyelitis, discitis, and epidural-type infections or hematomas. MRI is safe with no known biohazard effects. It can be problematic for patients with claustrophobia. The only contraindication to MRI is the presence of ferromagnetic implants, cardiac pacemakers, or intracranial clips. Metal stabilization devices such as plates, rods, screws, and loops used in spinal operations impose local artifacts and usually render imaging of the spinal canal almost impossible with MRI.

As with other imaging techniques, MRI can identify abnormalities in asymptomatic persons. In one study[56] MRI of 67 asymptomatic persons 20 to 80 years of age was carried out. At least one herniated disc was identified in 20% of people younger than 60 years and in 36% of those older than 60 years. Another study[57] discovered that 63% of asymptomatic persons had disc protrusion, and 13% had disc extrusion.

ELECTRODIAGNOSTIC STUDIES: Electrodiagnostic studies have only a limited role in the evaluation of acute LBP since it takes 2 to 4 weeks after the onset of symptoms before any findings are present on electromyography (EMG) or nerve conduction studies. Electrodiagnostic studies may help if the clinical findings are suggestive of radiculopathy or peripheral neuropathy. These studies help in confirming the working diagnosis and identifying the presence or absence of previous injury. They are also useful in localizing a lesion, determining the extent of injury, predicting the course of recovery, and determining whether structural abnormalities on radiographic studies are of functional significance.[58]

Psychosocial Evaluation: Screening for nonphysical factors is critical in the management of back pain. Psychological, occupational, and socioeconomic factors can complicate both assessment and treatment. Studies have revealed that patients with lower job satisfaction are more likely to report back pain and to have a protracted recovery.[59] Patients with an affective disorder (e.g., depression) or a history of substance abuse are more likely to have difficulties with pain resolution. The physician should inquire if litigation is pending since this can often adversely affect the outcome of therapy.

NONINVASIVE TREATMENTS

In acute LBP there is little or no evidence that most of the popular treatment and therapies alter the natural course of the disease. The conservative approach would be a short period of rest, analgesics, and returning to function and normal activity as soon as possible and then an exercise program to minimize reoccurrence. In chronic LBP the multidisciplinary biopsychosocial rehabilitation treatments with functional restoration have been shown to improve pain and function.[60,61]

Rest: Evidence suggests that return to normal daily activity as soon as possible is a good approach to manage acute LBP. A randomized clinical trial found that patients with two days of bed rest had clinical outcomes similar to those in patients with seven days of bed rest.[62] Studies showed that a faster return of function and ordinary activity produced faster recovery. There was no evidence that early activity had any harmful effects or led to more recurrences. Bed rest for more than a week in patients with acute LBP is not advisable. The current recommendation is two to three days of bed rest in patients with acute radiculopathy.[63]

Pharmacologic Therapy: Recent evidence in the Cochrane Collaboration Back Review,[64] which included data from 51 trials, suggests that nonsteroidal anti-inflammatory drugs (NSAIDs) are moderately effective for the short-term symptomatic relief of patients with acute LBP. There does not seem to be a specific type of NSAID that is clearly more effective than others.[65] Evidence on the use of NSAIDs in chronic LBP is still lacking.

If no medical contraindications are present, a 2- to 4-week course of an anti-inflammatory agent is suggested. Gastrointestinal prophylaxis might be necessary with the older types of NSAIDs for patients who are at risk for peptic ulcer disease. The newer NSAIDs with selective cyclooxygenase-2 inhibition have fewer gastrointestinal side effects, but they still should be used with caution in patients who are at risk for peptic ulcer or kidney disease.

The short-term use of a narcotic may be considered for the relief of acute pain. The need for prolonged narcotic therapy should prompt a reevaluation of the etiology of a patient's back pain.

The use of muscle relaxants has been shown to have a significant effect in reducing back pain, muscle tension, and increased mobility after 1 and 2 weeks.[66] All these medications can have significant adverse effects even after a short course and should be used cautiously.

Intraspinal Injections: These modalities are discussed in several chapters of this book. These interventions are innovative and backed mostly by anecdotal reports; prospective randomized studies on the efficacy of some of these procedures are still lacking.

Physical Therapy: Although there have been randomized controlled trials and systematic reviews of the effectiveness of physical intervention therapies for the management of LBP, the role of these treatments remains unclear. There are data to suggest that general exercise programs may have beneficial effects on LBP. Passive physical therapies such as heat, massage, electrical stimulation or ultrasound provide temporary comfort but no evidence of long-term improvement.[67] In general, strengthening exercise programs that facilitate weight loss appear to be helpful in alleviating LBP. Exercises that promote strengthening of the axial muscles that support the spine should be included in the physical therapy regimen. Aggressive exercise programs have been shown to reduce the need for surgical intervention.

There is limited evidence to show that specific back exercises produce clinical improvement in acute LBP. More recently, a Cochrane review[67] identified 39 studies and concluded that the data did not support the efficacy of specific exercises in the treatment of acute LBP. Waddell et al.[68] cited evidence that general exercise programs can improve pain and functional levels in those with chronic LBP. The general exercise program may be helpful for chronic LBP patients to increase return to normal daily activities and work.

Continuation of normal activities is recommended for acute LBP. National guidelines in the USA[48] and the UK[68,69] recommend a return to normal activity as soon as possible for patients with acute back pain and encourage the early access to physical therapy. Therapeutic exercises were found to be beneficial for chronic, subacute, and postsurgical LBP.

In the review by Waddell et al.[70] it was concluded that continuation of normal activities leads to less chronic disability and time off work than the traditional advice to rest and "let pain be your guide." Subsequent Cochrane reviews of the treatments for acute LBP and sciatica concluded that the "advice to stay active" has little beneficial effect for patients[71] and that, compared to bed rest, advice to stay active alone will have limited beneficial effects.[72] The treatment goals are to relieve pain, reduce muscle spasm, improve range of motion (ROM) and strength, correct postural problems, and ultimately improve functional status.

A number of rehabilitation interventions are used in the management of LBP. Among the current musculoskeletal interventions specific for LBP are body mechanics and ergonomics training, posture awareness training, strengthening exercises, stretching exercises, activities of daily living (ADL) training, organized functional training programs, therapeutic massage, joint mobilizations and manipulations, mechanical traction, biofeedback, electrical muscle stimulation, transcutaneous electrical nerve stimulation (TENS), thermal modalities, cryotherapy, deep thermal modalities, superficial thermal modalities, and work hardening.[73]

The Philadelphia Panel efforts[74] to form evidence-based clinical practice guidelines (EBCPGs) for the management of LBP were developed based on a systematic grading of the evidence determined by an expert panel, and the evidence was derived from systematic reviews and meta-analyses using the Cochrane Collaboration methodology. The finalized guidelines were circulated for feedback from practitioners to verify their applicability and ease of use for practicing clinicians.

The Philadelphia Panel recommendations[74] are in agreement with those of the AHCPR guidelines that continuation of normal activities (such as walking) is more effective than bed rest for the management of acute LBP.[75] It showed that extension, flexion, or strengthening exercises are effective for subacute and chronic LBP and for postsurgical LBP. The results for acute LBP are in full agreement with the guidelines and other reviews[76] concerning moderate effectiveness of stretching or strengthening exercises, and highly effective for the patient "to stay active."[77] Certain authors recommend return to functional and work activities as soon as possible after lumbar injury to avoid the negative effects of immobilization and bed rest prescription.[78] Task-oriented activities are recognized in rehabilitation. Patients with LBP benefit from these activities as they improve ADL for chronic LBP.[79]

There is evidence to support and recommend the use of continued normal activities for acute nonspecific LBP and therapeutic exercises for chronic, subacute, and postsurgical LBP. At the present time there is insufficient evidence regarding the definite role of thermotherapy, therapeutic massage, EMG biofeedback, mechanical traction, therapeutic ultrasound, TENS, electrical stimulation, and combined rehabilitation interventions.

Acupuncture:[80,81] Two analyses of randomized controlled trials on the role of acupuncture (one in the framework of the Cochrane Collaboration Back Review) found that there was little or no evidence that acupuncture is effective in the management of back pain. The systematic review of Van Tulder et al.[80] of 11 randomized controlled trials ($n = 542$) assessed the effects of acupuncture for the treatment of nonspecific LBP. Some of the study populations contained people with acute or unspecified LBP. Three randomized controlled trials compared acupuncture to no treatment and provided conflicting evidence. Two randomized controlled trials found that acupuncture was not more effective than trigger point injection or TENS. Eight randomized controlled trials compared acupuncture to placebo or sham acupuncture. Of the two randomized controlled trials of higher methodological quality, one did not find any difference while the other study was positive for acupuncture, although in this study the control group seemed to have more severe complaints at baseline. Five of the six remaining (lower-quality) randomized controlled trials indicated that acupuncture was not more effective than placebo or sham acupuncture. In the last study the overall conclusion was "unclear." Van Tulder et al. could not clearly conclude that acupuncture is effective in the management of back pain and could not recommend acupuncture as a regular treatment for patients with LBP. There is clearly a need for more high-quality randomized controlled trials.

Alternative Therapies (Spinal Manipulation): The exact role of spinal manipulation is not clear. Spinal manipulation proved superior to other nonconventional therapies but was not found to be more effective than traditional back pain management.[82] For patients with acute LBP, spinal manipulation conferred statistically significant benefits in comparison with sham therapy. Similar results were noted among patients with chronic LBP who received spinal manipulation when compared with sham manipulation. Assendelft et al.,[82] on the other hand, concluded that there was no evidence for increased effectiveness of spinal manipulative therapy compared with other advocated therapies for acute and chronic LBP. Massage and spinal manipulation have relatively small clinical benefits for both acute and chronic back pain. However, they are cheaper than many conventional medical techniques and adverse side effects are rare.

Cherkin et al.[83] analyzed original articles and systematic reviews of randomized controlled trials that evaluated acupuncture, massage therapy, and spinal manipulation for nonspecific back pain published since 1995. The authors concluded that "the effectiveness of acupuncture for back pain remains unclear, massage is effective for persistent back pain, spinal manipulation has small clinical benefits, similar to those of other commonly used therapies, for acute and chronic back pain." Assendelft and colleagues[82] conducted a meta-analysis of 53 published articles, representing 39 studies, which compared spinal manipulation or mobilization with another treatment or control. A total of 5,486 patients were included, with individual study sample sizes varying from 19 to 666 (median, 92). Comparison therapies included sham therapies, conventional general practitioner care (which in most cases involved the prescription of analgesics), physical therapy and exercise, and treatments (e.g., traction, bed rest, topical gel) for which there is a lack of evidence of benefits or evidence of harm. Assendelft et al.[82] concluded that spinal manipulative therapy has no statistically or clinically significant advantage over general practice care, analgesics, physical therapy, exercise, or back school for acute or chronic back pain.

Koes et al.[84] reviewed 38 trials and concluded that, although some results were encouraging, further trials were needed to establish the effectiveness of manipulation. In contrast, Shekelle et al.[85] did a meta-analysis combining data from 9 trials and concluded that manipulation could increase the rate of recovery from acute uncomplicated LBP, but that there were insufficient data to provide evidence for the effectiveness of manipulation in patients with chronic pain. The US AHCPR[48] reviewed 4 meta-analyses and 12 additional randomized trials and also concluded that manipulation could speed the recovery of patients with acute back pain and that the evidence to support the use of manipulation for radiculopathies or longer standing back pain was inconclusive. The systematic review by Assendelft et al.[86] was highly critical of the general standard of the other reviews. Nevertheless, some of the reviews reported some positive effects of manipulation.

Biofeedback Treatments: These treatments involve external feedback to translate physiological activity of muscle response (often using EMG) into visual or auditory signals that help the patient reduce muscle tension and pain. No studies have used these techniques in patients with acute symptoms, and there is limited evidence that biofeedback is ineffective for chronic LBP.[45,87]

Patient Education: It is critical that patients understand the nature of their spine disorder and their role in avoiding reinjury. The appropriate postures for sitting, driving, and lifting should be reviewed. Weight loss and healthy lifestyle should be emphasized.

SURGICAL TREATMENT

The surgical treatment of lumbar spinal disorders has made substantial advances in the last two decades. Rigid instrumentation systems, minimally invasive techniques, recombinant DNA, and joint replacement are just a few technologies that are rapidly changing what and how one treats spinal pathology. With these advances has come a corresponding increase in the rates of spine surgery; as high as 8.6/1000 Medicare enrollees in some regions of the USA.[88] Although many of these patients benefit immensely, there is a definitive complication rate which

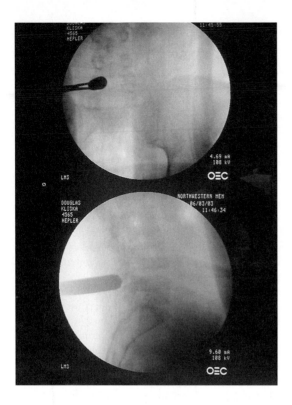

A

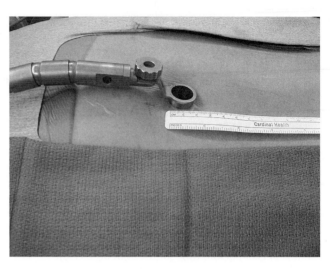

B

FIGURE 39-2. Patient undergoing endoscopic discectomy. A, AP and lateral fluoroscopic images demonstrating placement of the endoscope at the left L4–5 intralaminar level. B, METRx endoscope locked in position with flexible arm assembly. C, Postoperative picture demonstrating 18 mm incision following endoscopic discectomy.

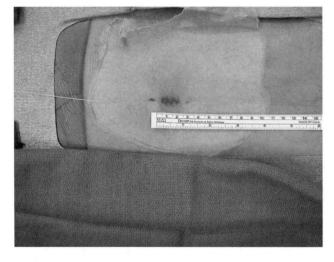

C

must be carefully weighed against potential benefits when considering surgical intervention. Validated outcome measures and randomized trials must be applied to these new techniques to assess accurately both their effectiveness and inherent risks.

LBP most commonly results from degenerative changes which produce neural compression or mechanical dysfunction. Surgical treatment, therefore, typically requires some degree of neurologic decompression and/or fusion. More recently disc replacement has demonstrated increasingly encouraging results and may, as it has in the peripheral skeleton, become a meaningful alternative to arthrodesis. This section reviews some of the various surgical treatments for spinal disorders and is organized by the underlying treatment principle rather than specific diagnosis: decompression, fusion, arthroplasty, and reconstruction. It is important to emphasize that each patient has a unique combination of pathology and expectations for treatment. Successful surgical management requires a detailed clinical evaluation with confirmatory imaging studies to identify accurately the symptomatic pathology, a careful assessment of the risks and benefits associated with any procedure, and a strict adherence to orthopedic principles while implementing treatment.

Decompression: Back pain is the fifth most common complaint leading to physician visits and the majority of these relate to disc degeneration and herniation. The disc itself may produce significant back pain and even referred pain into the groin, hip, or leg. When degenerative changes encroach upon neurologic structures they frequently produce back and leg pain from acute nerve compression in the younger patient or more insidious compression (neurogenic claudication) in the older patient population. The vast majority of these patients will improve with nonoperative management including NSAIDs, physical therapy, and injections.[89,90] For those who fail to improve with nonoperative treatment surgical decompression remains an excellent option to decompress definitively neurologic structures and relieve pain. Patients with acute and dense motor deficits should be considered for early decompression as it remains the most effective means of relieving compression and optimizing recovery, although some patients do improve with nonoperative treatment.[91]

Since Mixter and Barr's classic report in 1934[92] discectomy has become the most commonly performed spinal surgery and remains the gold standard to which all other treatments must be compared. Less invasive microdiscectomy techniques were popularized in the late 1970s permitting faster recovery and return to work with improved patient outcomes.[93,94] More recently endoscopic discectomy has been advocated as a safe and effective ambulatory procedure with superior results to other outpatient therapies (chemonucleolysis, percutaneous discectomy, and thermal coagulation). Indications include patients with primary leg pain, a positive straight leg raise, and imaging studies confirming compression at the symptomatic level. The principles of surgical treatment are decompression, mobilization of the affected nerve root, and removal of the herniated fragment. This typically includes release of the ligamentum flavum, partial laminotomy, medial facetectomy, and discectomy. Discectomy techniques differ but include at minimum removal of noncontained herniations and vertical annulotomy for removal of contained herniations. The endoscopic technique allows a limited exposure through an 18 mm tubular retractor with results comparable to microdiscectomy (Fig. 39-2). One study demonstrated complete relief of pain in 72% of patients and minimal discomfort requiring no further treatment in another 20% with a length of stay averaging 3.5 hours.[95] A separate lateral approach as described by Wiltse et al.[96] may be required to decompress the less common foraminal disc herniation.

Older patients with cumulative degenerative changes may ultimately develop symptomatic spinal stenosis (neurogenic claudication). Multiple lesions contribute to the stenosis including disc herniations/bulges, facet arthopathy, osteochondral spurs, ligament hypertrophy, and spondylolisthesis. Symptoms typically include low back and leg pain aggravated by standing and walking which must be differentiated from vascular claudication. Nonoperative treatment includes physical therapy, NSAIDs, and steroid injections. Selective nerve root blocks are helpful diagnostically as well as therapeutically as they identify symptomatic levels and may help predict response to surgical decompression (Fig. 39-3). Patients who fail to improve with nonoperative treatment are candidates for surgical decompression. Treatment often requires decompression of the central canal, lateral recess, and/or neural foramen. Determining which areas to decompress requires a careful correlation between patient symptoms and

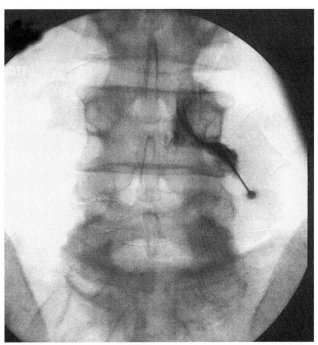

FIGURE 39-3. Fluoroscopic image of right-sided L4–5 transforaminal steroid injection. Dye injection prior to steroid demonstrating proper position and backflow along L4 nerve root sheath.

corresponding lesions on imaging studies. Studies demonstrate pain relief in 55% to 78% of patients compared to 28% of patients treated nonoperatively.[97,98] A fusion procedure may be needed in addition to decompression when there is coexisting instability (spondylolisthesis is present or more than 50% of the facet joints are resected) or the patient has primarily back pain implicating degenerative joint pain as opposed to neurogenic pain.

Lumbar Fusions: Fusion procedures have been used successfully for over 100 years but have been much more frequently performed over the last 10 to 15 years. The most common indication is disabling mechanical LBP secondary to an underlying disorder (spondylolysis, spondylolisthesis, degenerative arthritis, and scoliosis). Spine fusion is a salvage procedure in which painful degenerative joints are resected and dysfunctional motion segments stabilized. Results vary with specific pathology but many reports demonstrate good to excellent outcomes in as many as 94% of patients[99,100] (Fig. 39-4). Treating degenerative disc disease with spine fusion is far more controversial with modest success rates. Most studies demonstrate clinical improvement in 65% to 75% of patients and return to work rates in 36%.[101] The actual fusion rates also vary and range from 80% in posterolateral fusions to 97% with circumferential (360°) fusions.[102] Although achieving fusion does not always correlate with clinical improvement, patients with nonunions are more likely to have a worse outcome. In addition, patients with degenerative disc disease tend to have greater clinical improvement when the pain-generating disc is removed which can be can be accomplished with an anterior posterior spinal fusion and instrumentation (APSFI; Fig. 39-5). More recently posterior approaches such as the

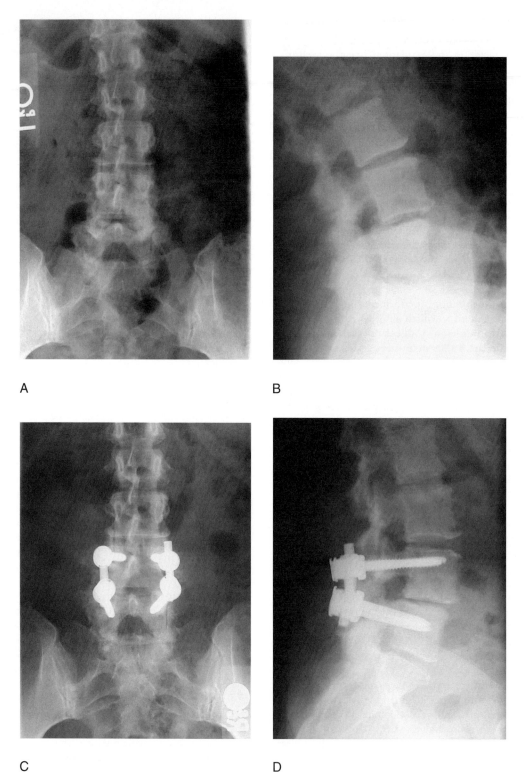

A

B

C

D

FIGURE 39-4. *A,* AP and *B,* lateral lumbar spine radiographs demonstrating grade 1 spondylolisthesis in a 47-year-old woman with disabling back and leg pain refractory to nonoperative treatment. *C, D,* Postoperative radiographs demonstrating stable fusion 1 year following posterior decompression and fusion with supplemental instrumentation. Note the robust fusion mass bridging transverse processes laterally. The patient is pain free and has returned to full level of activity including triathlons and skiing.

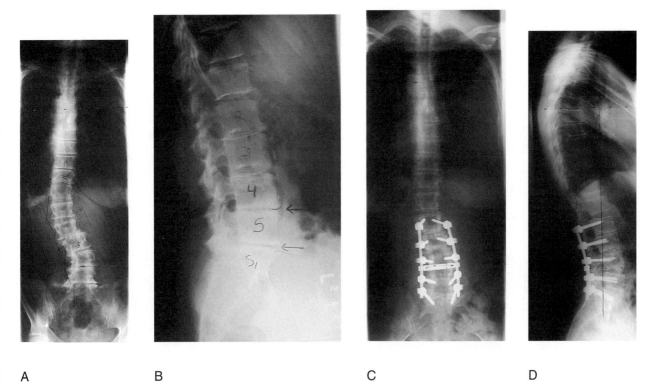

A   B   C   D

FIGURE 39-5. 64-year-old woman with degenerative scoliosis and disabling low back and radicular leg pain. *A,* AP radiograph demonstrates severe lateral listhesis at L2–3 and L3–4 resulting in symptomatic compressive neuropathy. *B,* Lateral radiograph demonstrating severe disc degeneration and consequent loss of lumbar lordosis. She was treated with anterior–posterior fusion, instrumentation, and decompression. *C,* AP radiograph demonstrates correction of lateral listhesis and tilt. *D,* Lateral film shows excellent restoration of lumbar lordosis with structural interbody allograft.

transforaminal lumbar interbody fusion (TLIF) provide the advantages of a circumferential fusion through a lower-risk posterior approach (Fig. 39-6). Clinical studies demonstrate equal or superior results with lower complication rates.[103] Various devices can be placed in the interbody space including cylindrical cages, carbon fiber devices, and bone. The highest fusion rates and clinical outcomes occur when following basic biomechanical principles (obtaining rigid fixation, loading bone under compression, and maintaining lumbar lordosis) and biologic principles with appropriate grafting material (autologous bone remains the gold standard) in a bed of vascularized tissue. Most recently recombinant human bone morphogenic protein has been shown to have similar clinical outcomes and equal or superior fusion rates in various studies.[104] This may be a useful alternative to autologous bone grafting but future studies are needed to assess the effectiveness in larger populations including multilevel cases and patients with various other risk factors.

Disc replacement arthroplasty: Although spinal fusion has been beneficial in many patients, it remains a salvage procedure that reduces motion and increases stress and consequently degeneration at adjacent levels. Disc replacement has been advocated since the 1950s, as it removes the painful and dysfunctional disc and restores physiologic motion. However, it was not until the early 1980s that a viable design began demonstrating encouraging results. Since then various implants

have emerged including ProDisc (semiconstrained device manufactured by Spine Solutions), Maverick (nonconstrained device Medtronic Sofamor Danek), and Flexcore. The Link SB Charite III is the most commonly used prosthesis with as many as 5,000 implanted worldwide. It is a nonconstrained design consisting of two cobalt–chrome endplates with a sliding polyethylene core (Fig. 39-7). The implant is anchored to the vertebral bodies by teeth and a bony ingrowth on the endplate surface. Biomechanical studies demonstrate increased motion in flexion and extension, mobility in torsion, and relative immobility in lateral bending. Primary indication is disabling LBP secondary to discogenic disc disease that has failed to improve with at least 6 months of adequate nonoperative treatment. The accurate diagnosis of discogenic back pain and identification of the symptomatic level is best confirmed by MRI and concordant pain on discography. Exclusion criteria include nerve root compression and facet arthropathy. Clinical results are good in properly selected patients with as many as 79% of patients reporting substantial improvement and 87% returning to work.[105] The postoperative rehabilitation encourages early controlled, progressive spinal motion and rapid functional recovery compared to prolonged rehabilitation in fusion patients. It is hoped that long-term studies will demonstrate continued clinical improvement and implant survivability with motion preservation and decreased adjacent degeneration. There are, however, no published prospective, randomized studies

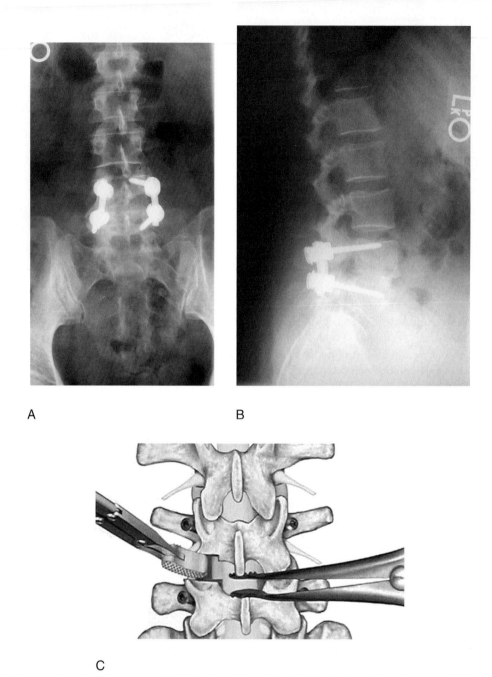

A   B

C

FIGURE 39-6. 51-year-old male with recurrent L4–5 disc herniation with disabling back and leg pain treated with revision discectomy and transforaminal lumbar interbody fusion (TLIF) L4–5. *A,* Circumferential fusion avoids exposure and fusion of transverse processes and resulting denervation of paraspinal muscles. *B,* The lateral radiograph demonstrates excellent interbody support and trabeculating bone. *C,* Technique of inserting structural allograft through transforaminal approach.

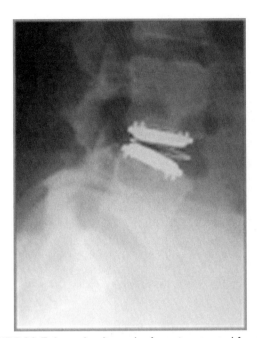

FIGURE 39-7. Lateral radiograph of a patient treated for degenerative disc disease with the Link SB Charite III at L4–5.

comparing disc replacement to fusion, although several studies are ongoing in the USA.

Spinal Reconstruction: Spinal reconstruction is necessary when a disease process destroys the structural integrity of the spine or produces a deformity, which alters normal spinal balance and biomechanics. The most common conditions requiring spinal reconstruction include trauma, infection, tumor, scoliosis, kyphosis, and increasingly iatrogenic causes from failed spinal surgery. The principles of reconstruction include resection and soft tissue release to allow realignment, anterior column support with structural grafting, rigid fixation, and biologic fusion. There are various surgical techniques employed to effect reconstruction some of which are described below.

Reconstruction frequently requires resection of diseased tissue and release of soft tissues in malaligned segments of the spine. Anteriorly, this is accomplished with vertebral body resection (corpectomy) and discectomy (Fig. 39-8). Once a corpectomy is performed the anterior column must be reconstructed with structural support. This can be accomplished with implants such as mesh cages or structural allograft or autograft. It is essential the spine is properly realigned after release to restore physiologic lumbar lordosis and thoracic kyphosis and the appropriate graft or implant length selected to maintain this sagittal balance. Most structural grafts will require some form of internal fixation to maintain stability until fusion is successfully achieved. In severe cases of spinal deformity, such as scoliosis exceeding 90°, the rib cage itself may become ankylosed and also require release in the form of

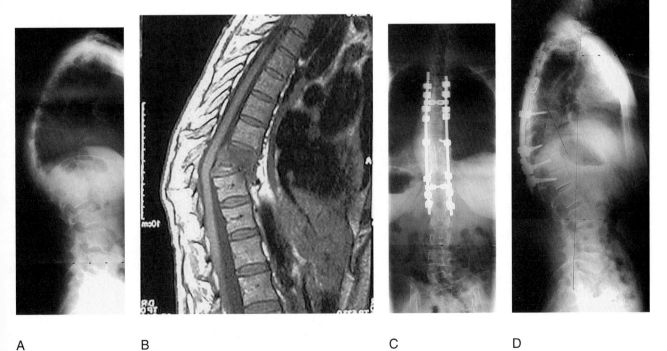

A   B   C   D

FIGURE 39-8. *A*, 43-year-old woman with blastomycosis involving T9 and T10 with progressive collapse and *B*, lower extremity weakness secondary to neurologic compromise. *C, D*, Reconstruction involved T9 and T10 vertebrectomies and anterior column support with fibular allograft and vascularized rib autograft followed by posterior fusion and instrumentation. The patient had resolution with full functional and motor recovery.

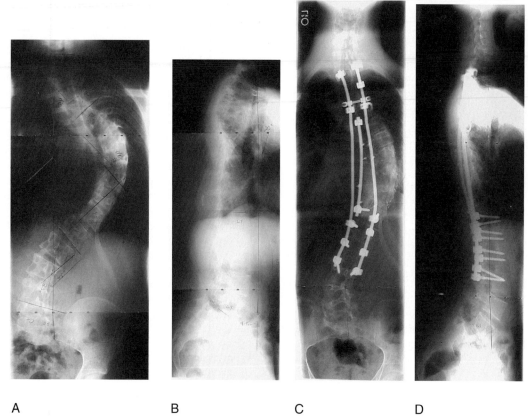

A	B	C	D

FIGURE 39-9. *A,* 22-year-old male with progressive idiopathic scoliosis, stiff right thoracic curve measuring 97°, decompensation, and FVC 37%. *B,* Lateral radiograph demonstrates thoracic lordosis and positive sagittal balance measuring 5 cm. The patient was treated with T9 vertebrectomy, internal thoracoplasties, and posterior osteotomies to release safely the stiff deformity and stabilization with fusion and instrumentation from T2 to L3. *C,* Two-year follow-up demonstrates excellent correction of scoliosis and restoration of balance in both coronal and sagittal planes. *D,* Spondylolisthesis remains asymptomatic without progression.

rib head resections to effect realignment (Fig. 39-9).[106] Such reconstruction will similarly require posterior releases. These may include chevron osteotomies which can correct sagittal and coronal malalignment,[107] rib resection or osteotomy, and pedicle subtraction osteotomy[108] (Fig. 39-10).

Once a spinal segment is properly realigned it must be rigidly fixed to maintain alignment and effect successful fusion. Modern instrumentation systems include hooks, sublaminar cables, and most frequently pedicle screws connected by rods. These "segmental" instrumentation systems allow much greater correction than earlier systems and have substantially improved the treatment of spinal deformity over the last 20 years. Nonetheless, they are subject to fatigue failure and will fracture if the spine does not go on to a solid union.

Spinal fusion remains a primary goal of most reconstruction procedures for long-term stability and function. Typically, this requires resection of articulations (disc space and facet joints), decortication of the fusion area, rigid stabilization, and an adequate volume of bone graft. The biology of lumbar fusion and bone grafts has been well characterized over the last decade and requires three key elements: precursor cells capable of transformation into bone-forming osteoblasts, osteoconductive materials (which serve as scaffolds for formation of new bone), and osteoinductive growth factors which promote differentiation of progenitor cells into osteoblasts.[109] Autologous bone graft

contains all three materials and remains the gold standard against which all other products must be compared. Limitations in the amount of graft available and morbidity associated with harvesting have led to the use of various other products including bone graft extenders (demineralized bone matrix, calcium carbonate, hydroxyapatite-tricalcium phosphate), bone graft substitutes, and more recently osteoinductive substitutes such as BMP. Although preliminary clinical studies have demonstrated promising results, these products must be validated by prospective, randomized trials and they do not replace the need for following well-established biomechanical and biological principles.

There have been tremendous advances in both the understanding and treatment of lumbar spinal disorders over the last two decades.[110] These advances have dramatically increased our ability to manage various spinal disorders with a corresponding increase in rates of surgery and devices used. Although many patients obtain substantial benefit, there are inherent and quantifiable risks that must be carefully assessed before considering surgical treatment. The injudicious use of surgery and spinal devices exposes patients to unnecessary risks and society to excessive costs. As a result, there has already been a call for restraint in the performance of such procedures.[111]

Disorders of the lumbar spine are extremely common and increasing with the age and activity of the population.

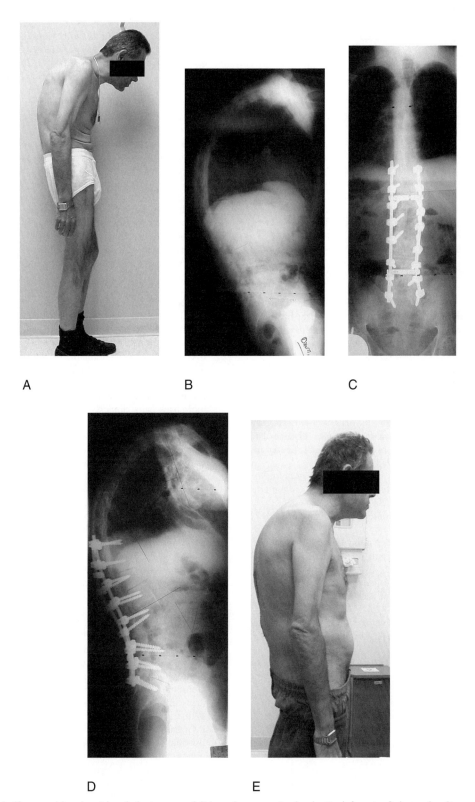

FIGURE 39-10. *A*, 42-year-old male with ankylosing spondylitis and progressive kyphotic deformity. *B*, Lateral radiographs demonstrated kyphosis involving primarily the lumbar spine. *C, D*, AP and lateral radiographs following a pedicle subtraction osteotomy of L3. *E*, Note the substantial improvement in forward gaze and neutralization of C-7 plumbline.

Fortunately, the vast majority of these patients improve with appropriately guided low-risk nonoperative care. For the small group of patients who fail to improve there is now a wide array of surgical options available. By thoroughly evaluating each patient's unique condition, carefully balancing the risks and benefits of various interventions, and employing well-established treatment principles one ensures the best chance for a satisfactory outcome.

REFERENCES

1. National Institute for Occupational Safety and Health: Musculoskeletal disorders and workplace factors: A critical review of epidemiological evidence for work-related musculoskeletal disorders of the neck, upper extremity, and low back. NIOSH technical report 97-141. National Institute for Occupational Safety and Health, US Department of Health and Human Services, Rockville, MD, 1997.
2. Frymoyer JW. Back pain and sciatica. N Engl J Med 318: 291–300, 1988.
3. Anderson GB: Epidemiological features of chronic low back pain. Lancet 354:581–585, 1999.
4. Bressler HB, Keyes WJ, Rochon PA, Badley E: The prevalence of low back pain in the elderly: A systematic review of the literature. Spine 24:1813–1819, 1999.
5. Nachemson NL: Newest knowledge of low back pain: A critical look. Clin Orthop 2798–20, 1992.
6. Andersson GBJ, Frymoyer JW (eds): The Epidemiology of Spinal Disorders, ed 2. Raven Press, New York, 1997, pp 93–141.
7. Skovron ML: Epidemiology of low back pain. Baillière's Clin Rheumatol 6:559–573, 1992.
8. McCaig LF: National Hospital Ambulatory Medical Care Survey: 1992 emergency department summary. Advance data from vital and health statistics; no 245. National Center for Health Statistics, Hyattsville, MD, 1994.
9. Hart LG, Deyo RA, Cherkin DC: Physician office visits for low back pain. Frequency, clinical evaluation, and treatment patterns from a US national survey. Spine 20:11–19, 1995.
10. Bowman JM: The meaning of chronic low back pain. AAOHN J 39:381–438, 1991.
11. Deyo RA, Cherkin D, Conrad D, Volinn E: Cost, controversy, crisis: Low back pain and the health of the public. Annu Rev Public Health 12:141–156, 1991.
12. Venning PJ, Walter SD, Stitt LW: Personal and job-related factors as determinants of incidence of back injuries among nursing personnel. J Occup Med 29:820–825, 1987.
13. Cunningham LS, Kelsey JL: Epidemiology of musculoskeletal impairments and associated disability. Am J Public Health 74: 574–579, 1984.
14. Van Tulder MW, Koes BW, Assendelft WJ, et al: The Effectiveness of Conservative Treatment of Acute and Chronic Low Back Pain. EMGO Institute, Amsterdam, 1999.
15. Deyo RA, Tsui-Wu YJ: Functional disability due to low-back pain: A population-based study indicating the importance of socioeconomic factors. Arthritis Rheum 30:1247–1253, 1987.
16. Dolan P, Kingma I, van Dieen J, et al: Dynamic forces acting on the lumbar spine during manual handling – Can they be estimated using electromyographic techniques alone? Spine 24:698–703, 1999.
17. Fathallah FA, Marras WS, Paranianpour M: An assessment of complex spinal loads during dynamic lifting tasks. Spine 23:706–716, 1998.
18. Adams MA, Mannion AF, Dolan P: Personal risk factors for first-time low back pain. Spine 24:2497–2505, 1999.
19. Bongers PM, Dewinter CR, Kompier MAJ, Hildebrandt VH: Psychosocial factors at work and musculoskeletal disease. Scand J Work Environ Health 19:297–312, 1993.
20. Burdorf A, Sorock G: Positive and negative evidence of risk factors for back disorders. Scand J Work Environ Health 23:243–256, 1997.
21. Davis KG, Heaney CA: The relationship between psychosocial work characteristics and low back pain: Underlying methodological issues. Clin Biomech 15:389–406, 2000.
22. Hoogendoorn WE, van Poppel MNM, Bongers PM, Koes BW, Bouter LM: Systematic review of psychosocial factors at work and private life as risk factors for back pain. Spine 25:2114–2125, 2000.
23. Marras WS, Davis KG, Heaney CA, et al: The influence of psychosocial stress, gender, and personality on mechanical loading of the lumbar spine. Spine 25:3045–3054, 2000.
24. Cassidy JD, Carroll LJ, Cote P: The Saskatchewan health and back pain survey—The prevalence of low back pain and related disability in Saskatchewan adults. Spine 23:1860–1866, 1998.
25. Battie MC, Videman T, Gibbons LE, et al: Determinants of lumbar disc degeneration—A study relating lifetime exposures and magnetic resonance imaging findings in identical twins. Spine 20:2601–2612, 1995.
26. Bigos SJ, Spengler DM, Martin NA, et al: Back injuries in industry: A retrospective study: III. Employee-related factors. Spine 11:252–256, 1986.
27. Marras WS, Davis KG, Heaney CA, et al: The influence of psychosocial stress, gender, and personality on mechanical loading of the lumbar spine. Spine 25:3045–3054, 2000.
28. Marras WS, Davis KG, Jorgensen M: Spine loading as a function of gender. Spine 27:2514–2520, 2002.
29. McGill SM: The biomechanics of low back injury: Implications on current practice in industry and the clinic. J Biomech 30:465–475, 1997.
30. Boshuizen HC, Verbeek JH, Broersen JP, et al: Do smokers get more back pain? Spine 18:35–40, 1993.
31. Jackson RP, Simmons EH, Stripinis D: Incidence and severity of back pain in adult idiopathic scoliosis. Spine 8:749, 1983.
32. Deyo RA, Bass JE: Lifestyle and low-back pain: The influence of smoking and obesity. Spine 14:501–506, 1989.
33. Leino PI: Does leisure time physical activity prevent low back disorders? A prospective study of metal industry employees. Spine 18:863–871, 1993.
34. Deyo RA, Loeser JD, Bigos SJ: Herniated lumbar intervertebral disk. Ann Intern Med 112:598–603, 1990.
35. Frymoyer JW: Can low back pain disability be prevented? Baillière's Clin Rheumatol 6:595–606, 1992.
36. Spitzer WO: Scientific approach to the assessment and management of activity-related spinal disorders: A monograph for clinicians. Report of the Quebec Task Force on Spinal Disorders. Spine 12(Suppl 7):1–59, 1987.
37. Fardon DF, Milette PC: Nomenclature and classification of lumbar disc pathology: Recommendations of the Combined Task Forces of the North American Spine Society, American Society of Spine Radiology, and American Society of Neuroradiology. Spine. 26:E93–E113, 2001.
38. Gordon SJ, Yang KH, Mayer PJ, et al: Mechanism of disc rupture. A preliminary report. Spine 16:450–456, 1991.
39. Williams PL, Warwick R: Gray's Anatomy. Churchill Livingstone, Edinburgh, 1980.
40. Bogduk N, Long DM: The anatomy of the so-called "articular nerves" and their relationship to facet denervation in the treatment of low-back pain. J. Neurosurg 51:172, 1979.
41. Grieve GP: Common Vertebral Joint Problems. Churchill Livingstone, Edinburgh/New York, 1981, p 10.
42. Van Tudler: Low back pain, best practice and research. Clin Rheumatol 16:761–775, 2002.
43. White AA, Gordon SL: Synopsis: Workshop on idiopathic low-back pain. Spine 7:141–149, 1982.
44. Atlas SJ, Nardin RA: Evaluation and treatment of low back pain: An evidence-based approach to clinical care. Muscle Nerve 27:265–284, 2003.

45. Scavone JG, Latshaw RF, Rohrer GV: Use of lumbar spine films. Statistical evaluation at a university teaching hospital. JAMA 246:1105–1108, 1981.

46. Burton AK, Waddell G: Clinical guidelines in the management of low back pain. Baillière's Clin Rheumatol 12:17–35, 1998.

47. Koes BW, van Tulder MW, Ostelo R, et al: Clinical guidelines for the management of low back pain in primary care. Spine 26:1504–1514, 2001.

48. US Department of Health and Human Services, Public Health Service, Agency for Health Care and Policy Research (AHCPR): Acute low back problems in adults: Assessment and treatment. AHCPR publication no. 95-0643, December 1994.

49. Scavone JG, Latshaw RF, Rohrer GV: Use of lumbar spine films. Statistical evaluation at a university teaching hospital. JAMA 246:1105–1108, 1981.

50. Scavone JG, Latshaw RF, Weidner WA: Anteroposterior and lateral radiographs: An adequate lumbar spine examination. AJR Am J Roentgenol 136:715–717, 1981.

51. Bell GR, Ross JS: Diagnosis of nerve root compression. Myelography, computed tomography, and MRI. Orthop Clin North Am 23:405–419, 1992.

52. Bigos SJ: Acute low back problems in adults. AHCPR publication no. 95–0642. US Department of Health and Human Services, Public Health Service, Agency for Health Care Policy and Research, Rockville, MD, 1994.

53. Inaoka M, Yamazaki Y, Hosono N, et al: Radiographic analysis of lumbar spine for low-back pain in the general population. Arch Orthop Trauma Surg 120:380–385, 2000.

54. Reinartz P, Schaffeldt J, Sabri O, et al: Benign versus malignant osseous lesions in the lumbar vertebrae: Differentiation by means of bone SPET. Eur J Nucl Med 27:721–726, 2000.

55. Savelli G, Chiti A, Grasselli G, et al: The role of bone SPET study in diagnosis of single vertebral metastases. Anticancer Res 20:1115–1120, 2000.

56. Boden SD, Davis DO, Dina TS, et al: Abnormal magnetic resonance scans of the lumbar spine in asymptomatic subjects. A prospective investigation. J Bone Joint Surg Am 72:403–408, 1990.

57. Boos N, Reider R, Schade V, et al: The diagnostic accuracy of magnetic resonance imaging, work perception, and psychosocial factors in identifying symptomatic disc herniations. Spine 20:2613–2625, 1995.

58. Wilbourn AJ, Aminoff MJ: AAEM minimonograph 32: The electrodiagnostic examination in patients with radiculopathies. American Association of Electrodiagnostic Medicine. Muscle Nerve 21:1612–1631, 1998.

59. Bigos SJ, Battie MC, Spengler DM, et al: A prospective study of work perceptions and psychosocial factors affecting the report of back injury. Spine 16:688, 1991.

60. Flor H, Fydrich T, Turk DC: Efficacy of multidisciplinary pain treatment centers: A meta-analytic review. Pain 49:221–230, 1992.

61. Guzman J, Esmail R, Karjalainen K, et al: Multidisciplinary rehabilitation for chronic low back pain: Systematic review. BMJ 322:1511–1516, 2001.

62. Hilde G, Hagen K, Jamtvedt G, et al: Stay active for acute, sub-acute and chronic low back pain (protocol for a Cochrane Review). The Cochrane Library, Oxford, update 2000.

63. Deyo RA, Diehl AK, Rosenthal M: How many days of bed rest for acute low back pain? A randomized clinical trial. N Engl J Med 315:1064–1070, 1986.

64. Van Tulder MW, Scholten RJ, Koes BW, Deyo RA: Nonsteroidal anti-inflammatory drugs for low back pain: A systematic review within the framework of the Cochrane Collaboration Back Review Group. Spine 25:2501–2513, 2000.

65. Moskowitz RW: The appropriate use of NSAIDs in arthritic conditions. Am J Orthop 25(Suppl 9):4–6, 1996.

66. Porter RW, Ralston SH: Pharmacological management of back pain syndromes. Drugs 48:189–198, 1994.

67. Van Tulder M, Koes B, Assendelft W, et al: Chronic low back pain: Exercise therapy, multidisciplinary programs, NSAID's back schools and behavioural therapy effective; traction not effective; results of systematic reviews. Ned Tijdschr Geneeskd 144:1489–1494, 2000.

68. Waddell G, Feder G, McIntosh G, et al: Low Back Pain Evidence Review. Royal College of General Practitioners, London, 1996.

69. Waddell G, Feder G, McIntosh G, et al: Low Back Pain Evidence Review. Royal College of General Practitioners, London, 1999.

70. Waddell G, Feder G, Lewis M: Systematic reviews of bed rest and advice to stay active for acute low back pain. Br J Gen Pract 47:647–652, 1997.

71. Hagen KB, Hilde G, Jamtvedt G, Winnem MF: The Cochrane review of advice to stay active as a single treatment for low back pain and sciatica. Spine 27:1736–1741, 2002.

72. Hagen KB, Hilde G, Jamtvedt G, Winnem MF: The Cochrane review of bed rest for acute low back pain and sciatica. Spine 25:2932–2934, 2000.

73. Nelson BW, Carpenter DM, Dreisinger TE, et al: Can spinal surgery be prevented by aggressive strengthening exercises? A prospective study of cervical and lumbar patients. Arch Phys Med Rehabil 80:20–25, 1999.

74. Philadelphia Panel: Evidence-based clinical practice guidelines on selected rehabilitation interventions for low back pain. Phys Ther 81:1641–1674, 2001.

75. Malmivaara A, Hakkinen U, Aro T, et al: The treatment of acute low back pain: Bed rest, exercises, or ordinary activity? N Engl J Med 332:351–355, 1995.

76. Guide to Physical Therapist Practice: Second Edition. Alexandria, Virginia: American Physical Therapy Association, 2001.

77. Riihimäki H: Hands up or back to work: Future challenges in epidemiologic research on musculoskeletal diseases. Scand J Work Environ Health 21:401–403, 1995.

78. Nordin M, Campello M: Physical therapy exercises and the modalities: When, what and why? Neurol Clin 17:75–89, 1999.

79. Van Tulder MW, Koes BW, Assendelft WJ, et al: The Effectiveness of Conservative Treatment of Acute and Chronic Low Back Pain. EMGO Institute, Amsterdam, 1999.

80. Van Tulder M, Cherkin D, Berman B, et al: Acupuncture for low back pain (Cochrane Review). The Cochrane Library, Oxford, 2002.

81. Van Tulder MW, Cherkin DC, Berman B, et al: The effectiveness of acupuncture in the management of acute and chronic low back pain. A systematic review within the framework of the Cochrane Collaboration Back Review Group. Spine 24:1113–1123, 1999.

82. Assendelft WJJ, Morton SC, Yu EI, et al: Spinal manipulative therapy for low back pain: A meta-analysis of effectiveness relative to other therapies. Ann Intern Med 138:871–881, 2003.

83. Cherkin DC, Sherman KJ, Deyo RA, Shekelle PG: A review of the evidence for the effectiveness, safety, and cost of acupuncture, massage therapy, and spinal manipulation for back pain. Ann Intern Med 138:898–906, 2003.

84. Koes BW, Assendelft WJ, van der Heijden GJ, et al: Spinal manipulation and mobilisation for back and neck pain: A blinded review. BMJ 303:1298–1303, 1991.

85. Shekelle PG, Adams AH, Chassin MR, et al: Spinal manipulation for low-back pain. Ann Intern Med 117:590–598, 1992.

86. Assendelft WJ, Koes BW, Knipschild PG, Bouter LM: The relationship between methodological quality and conclusions in reviews of spinal manipulation. JAMA 274:1942–1948, 1995.

87. Van Tulder MW, Koes BW, Bouter LM: Conservative treatment of acute and chronic nonspecific low back pain. A systematic review of randomized controlled trials of the most common interventions. Spine 22:2128–2156, 1997.

88. Lurie JD, Birkmeyer NJ, Weinstein JN: Rates of advanced spinal imaging and spine surgery. Spine 28:616–620, 2003.

89. Riew KD, Yin Y, Gilula L, et al: The effect of nerve-root injections on the need for operative treatment of lumbar radicular pain: A prospective, randomized, controlled, double-blinded study. JBJS 82-A:1589–1593, 2000.

90. Simotas AC, Dorey FJ, Hansraj KK, et al: Nonoperative treatment for lumbar spinal stenosis. Spine 25:197–209, 2000.

91. Dubourg G, Rozenberg S, Fautrel B, et al: A pilot study on the recovery from paresis after lumbar disc herniation. Spine 27:1426–1432, 2000.

92. Mixter WJ, Barr JS: Rupture of the intervertebral disc with involvement of the spinal canal. N Engl J Med 211:210–215, 1934.

93. Caspar W: A new surgical procedure for lumbar disc herniation causing less tissue damage through microsurgical approach. Adv Neurosurg 4:74–79, 1977.

94. Williams RW: Microlumbar discectomy: A conservative surgical approach to the virgin herniated lumbar disc. Spine 3:175–182, 1978.

95. Hilton DL: Microdiscectomy with minimally invasive tubular retractor. In Perez-Cruet MJ, Fessler RG, eds. Outpatient Spinal Surgery. St. Louis, Missouri: Quality Medical Publishing, 2002:159–170.

96. Wiltse LL, Bateman JG, Hutchinson RH, et al: The paraspinal sacro-spinalis approach to the lumbar spine. Clin Orthop 35:80, 1964.

97. Atlas SJ, Deyo RA, Keller RB, et al: The Maine lumbar spine study: III. Spine 21:1787–1794, 1996.

98. Verbiest H: Results of surgical treatment of idiopathic developmental stenosis of the lumbar vertebral canal. A review of twenty- seven years of experience. JBJS [Br] 59-B:181–188, 1977.

99. L'Heureux EA, Perra JH, Pinto MR, et al: Functional outcome analysis including preoperative and postoperative SF-36 for surgically treated adult isthmic spondylolisthesis. Spine 28:1269–1274, 2003.

100. Shapiro GS, Gaku T, Ohenaba B-A: Results of surgical treatment of adult idiopathic scoliosis with low back pain and spinal stenosis: A study of long term clinical radiographic outcomes. Spine 28:358–363, 2003.

101. Fritzell P, Hagg O, Wessberg P, et al: Lumbar fusion versus nonsurgical treatment for chronic low back pain. Spine 26:2521–2534, 2001.

102. Gertzbein SD, Betz R, Clements D, et al: Semirigid instrumentation in the management of lumbar spinal conditions combined with circumferential fusion. Spine 21:1918–1925, 1996.

103. Hee HT, Castro FP, Majd ME, et al: Anterior/posterior fusion versus transforaminal lumbar interbody fusion: Analysis of complications and predictive factors. J Spinal Disord 14:533–540, 2001.

104. Boden SD, Kang J, Sandhu H, et al: Use of recombinant human bone morphogenetic protein-2 to achieve posterolateral lumbar spine fusion in humans: A prospective, randomized clinical pilot trial: 2002 Volvo award in clinical studies. Spine 27:2662–2673, 2002.

105. Lemaire JP, Skalli W, Lavaste F, et al: Intervertebral disc prosthesis: Results and prospects for the year 2000. Clin Orthop Rel Res 337:64–76, 1997.

106. Bradford DS, Tribus CB: Vertebral column resection for the treatment of rigid coronal decompensation. Spine 22:1590–1599, 1997.

107. Voos K, Boachie-Adjei O, Rawlins BA: Multiple vertebral osteotomies in the treatment of rigid adult spinal deformities. Spine 26:526–533, 2001.

108. Thiranont N, Netrawichien P: Transpedicular decancellation closed wedge vertebral osteotomy for treatment of fixed flexion deformity of spine in ankylosing spondylitis. Spine 18:2517–2522, 1993.

109. Boden SD: Overview of the biology of lumbar spine fusion and principles for selecting a bone graft substitute. Spine 27:S26–S31, 2002.

110. Lipson SJ: Spinal-fusion surgery – Advances and concerns. N Engl J Med 350:643–645, 2004.

111. Deyo RA, Nachemson A, Mirza SK: Spinal-fusion surgery – The case for restraint. N Engl J Med 350:722–726, 2004.

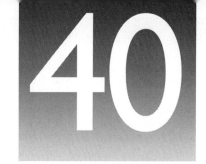

Interlaminar Epidural Steroid Injections for Lumbosacral Radiculopathy

Robert E. Molloy, M.D., and
Honorio T. Benzon, M.D.

Injections of epidural steroids have been used for more than 40 years, and their history has been reviewed in detail elsewhere.[1–6] Use of caudal steroid injection to treat sciatica in the USA was first reported by Goebert and colleagues. They reported improvement in 66% of 113 patients with sciatica given caudal epidural hydrocortisone in a prospective study.[7] Numerous other publications subsequently appeared describing the results of epidural steroid injections (ESI). The practice of lumbar ESI, performed near the level of nerve root involvement with smaller volumes of diluent, was advocated by Winnie et al. in 1972.[8] Hickey observed progressive increase in the number of responders to a series of three ESIs given every two weeks, with much greater improvements after the second and third ESI, supporting a common pattern of clinical practice.[9] The use of cervical ESI was initially summarized in three separate reports in 1986.[10–12] More precisely targeted ESI techniques have included insertion of fluoroscopically guided caudal catheters and transforaminal approaches to the lateral and anterior epidural space. Transforaminal ESI techniques are considered in Chapter 41. Controversies about indications for ESI, efficacy, safety, ideal route of administration, and benefit of fluoroscopic guidance continue.[13]

BACK PAIN AND RADICULAR PAIN

Back pain may arise from the facet joint or the paraspinal muscles in the dorsal compartment, which is innervated by the medial and lateral branches of the dorsal rami. Back pain may also arise from the anterior and posterior longitudinal ligaments and the annulus of the disc in the ventral compartment, which is innervated by the sympathetic chain and the sinuvertebral nerves. Mechanical back pain is primarily somatic pain. Annular tear may lead to continued leakage of nucleus pulposus material and associated chronic inflammation and altered central processing. Radicular pain tends to be neuropathic pain, resulting from chemical irritation and inflammation of the nerve root, which may be swollen and edematous. McCarron et al.[14] injected autologous nucleus pulposus material into the epidural space of dogs as a model for radiculopathy. They demonstrated intense inflammatory changes of the spinal cord and nerve roots, and fibrosis of the dura and epidural fat. Injection of nucleus pulposus material vs. fat in an animal model resulted in attraction of leukocytes, thrombus formation, and increased vascular permeability.[15] Disc herniation (HNP) results in release of large amounts of phospholipase A2 (PLA2),[16] which favors production of prostaglandins[17] and leukotrienes from cell membrane phospholipids, and resultant inflammation, sensitization of nerve endings, and pain generation. Elevated levels of leukotriene B4 and thromboxane B2, products of PLA2 activity, were measured in biopsies of patients operated on for lumbar disc herniation.[18] The levels of inflammatory mediators observed varied with the type of disc herniation, being highest with noncontained HNP. External pressure on nerve roots by bone can result in venous obstruction, neural edema,[19] and eventual fibrosis of the nerve and surrounding tissues. The primary indication for ESI is radicular pain due to nerve root inflammation, irritation, and edema.

DRUGS USED FOR EPIDURAL INJECTION

Most reports indicate that either methylprednisolone acetate or triamcinolone diacetate is used. The concentration of methylprednisolone is either 40 or 80 mg/mL; the therapeutic dose is 80 mg. The concentration of triamcinolone is 25 mg/mL, and the therapeutic dose is 50 mg. No study has compared the effectiveness of these two agents, and both have been reported to be effective, safe, and long acting. Most anesthesiologists dilute steroid drugs with local anesthetic or normal saline solution, and they apparently achieve equivalent results.

The volume of injectate varies with the site of injection. The injection of 6 to 10 mL has been recommended at the lumbar level to bath both the injured nerve root that is adjacent to the disc pathology and additional nearby roots that are also inflamed.[20] At the cervical level, large-volume injections have been employed but 4 to 6 mL should be adequate to bathe the cervical roots; 6 mL is the most commonly reported volume. When the caudal route is selected, a larger volume (approximately 20 to 25 mL) is selected to ensure adequate spread of injectate to the midlumbar level.

MECHANISM OF ACTION

The indication for ESI is nerve root irritation and inflammation. Nerve root edema has been observed surgically and demonstrated with computed tomographic scanning in patients with herniated discs.[21] Surgical disc samples from patients with disc herniation contain extremely high levels of PLA2.[16] This enzyme liberates arachidonic acid from cell membranes. Degenerative disc disease and tears of the annulus fibrosus may result in leakage of this enzyme from the nucleus pulposus, producing chemical irritation of the nerve roots. Olmarker and colleagues[22] observed abnormal nerve conduction and nerve fiber degeneration after epidural application of autologous nucleus pulposus in pigs; these changes were significantly reduced by intravenous administration of methylprednisolone. Lee et al.[23] studied the effect of loosely ligating lumbar nerve roots on the subsequent development of thermal hyperalgesia and elevated PLA2 levels in rats. Epidural injection of betamethasone, compared to saline, accelerated the reduction in PLA2 activity and the recovery from thermal hyperalgesia in this model.

Steroids induce synthesis of a PLA2 inhibitor, preventing release of substrate for prostaglandin synthesis. Therefore steroids can interfere with the inflammatory process at an earlier step than do systemic, nonsteroidal anti-inflammatory drugs (NSAIDs). This may benefit the many patients with a chemical rather than a compressive radicular pain syndrome and negative radiologic studies. Steroids may also decrease back pain due to inflammation and sensitization of nerve fibers in the posterior longitudinal ligament and annulus fibrosis.[6]

In addition to their anti-inflammatory effect, steroids also block nociceptive input. Corticosteroids suppress ongoing discharge in chronic neuromas and prevent the development of ectopic neural discharges from experimental neuromas.[24] This suppression of neuroma discharge has been attributed to a direct membrane action of the steroid. Local application of methylprednisolone acetate was found to block transmission in C fibers but not in Aβ fibers. The effect was reversible, suggesting direct membrane action of the steroid.[25] Steroids directly inhibit formation of adhesions and fibrosis; and they produce well-known euphoric effects.

INDICATIONS

Many authors have attempted to identify which patients are most likely to benefit from ESI. White and colleagues[26] observed how 304 patients responded to ESI and correlated these findings with the cause of their back pain. Response to ESI was predicted by nerve root irritation, recent onset of symptoms, and the absence of psychological overlay. ESI was therapeutic for patients with herniated disc and either nerve root irritation or compression. These latter two factors were also associated with efficacy in patients with spondylolisthesis or scoliosis. Relief was transient in patients with chronic lumbar degenerative disc disease or spinal stenosis. Many other studies have reported efficacy for patients with radicular pain syndromes or herniated nucleus pulposus. In a review Benzon[20] summarized the questionable benefit of ESI in patients with chronic low back pain, degenerative bony pathology, or previous back surgery.

Hacobian and associates[27] retrospectively evaluated 50 patients with lumbar spinal stenosis, back pain, or pseudoclaudication who were treated with one to three ESIs. Initial results included complete relief in 8%, partial relief in 52%, and failure in 40%. The duration of pain relief was longer than 6 months in 26%, 1 to 6 months in 33%, and less than 1 month in 40%. Overall, 60% of these patients improved, but only 15% had a prolonged response. Ciocon et al.[28] reported significant pain relief in 30 elderly patients with lumbar spinal stenosis and leg discomfort, treated with three caudal ESIs at weekly intervals and followed every 2 months for 10 months. There were significant decreases in Roland's 5-point pain-rating scale at each time interval, but this was the only outcome measure used. Patients with severe spondylolisthesis or herniated disc were excluded. In a randomized controlled trial (RCT), Fukusaki et al.[29] studied the effect of lumbar ESI on patients with degenerative spinal stenosis and neurogenic claudication, severe enough to limit ambulation to less than 20 meters. The clinical response was similar to that seen by Hacobian et al.,[27] and ESI had no beneficial effect on ambulation when compared to epidural local anesthetic alone.

Three studies have investigated predictors of response to lumbar ESI. Abram and Hopwood[30] prospectively investigated factors contributing to treatment success in 212 patients. Three factors were strongly associated with favorable response to injection: (1) advanced educational background, (2) a primary diagnosis of radiculopathy, and (3) pain duration of less than 6 months. Three factors that correlated with treatment failure were (1) constant pain, (2) frequent sleep disruption, and (3) being unemployed due to pain. Subsequently, Hopwood and Abram[31] analyzed factors associated with failure of ESI in 209 patients. There was a threefold increase in treatment failure with prolonged pain of more than 24 months' duration and with nonradicular diagnosis. A twofold increase in poor outcome was related to lack of employment because of pain, smoking, and symptom duration of 6 to 24 months.

Sandrock and Warfield[32] suggest that the five most important factors influencing the outcome of ESI are accuracy of the diagnosis of nerve root inflammation, shorter duration of symptoms, no history of previous surgery, younger age of the patient, and location of the needle at the level of pathology. Bosscher[6] recently summarized four selection criteria for ESI: they include an intention to produce short-term pain relief during physical therapy/rehabilitation; evidence of nerve root involvement; unfavorable response to 4 weeks of conservative therapy; and no contraindications to injection. Patients with radicular pain should fit into one of these categories: sensory signs and symptoms of radiculopathy; disc herniation; tumor infiltration of nerve root; postural back pain with radicular symptoms; or acute back pain and radicular symptoms superimposed on more chronic back pain.[6]

EFFICACY

Has the efficacy of ESI been established? The extensive literature on this question leaves much to be desired. Most studies were purely anecdotal, retrospective, and not randomized, controlled, or blinded. Patient populations were poorly defined and not homogeneous: patients who were studied had both acute and chronic pain, some had back surgery, and their back pain was secondary to various causes. Finally, treatment protocols were variable; outcome criteria were not well established; and timing of follow-up observations was not standard.

Investigators who reviewed the literature came to different conclusions. Although Kepes and Duncalf[1] concluded that the rationale of ESI was not proved, Benzon[2] noted it to be effective in acute lumbosacral radiculopathy. Review articles on the subject also were not in complete agreement. Spaccarelli[33] concluded that ESI was efficacious in lower extremity radicular pain syndromes at intermediate-term follow-up (2 weeks to 3 months) but that no difference could be expected at long-term follow-up. Koes and associates[34] found no suggestion of efficacy for ESI in patients with *chronic* low back pain *without* sciatica. However, they stated that 6 of 12 studies showed ESI to be more effective than the control treatment for patients *with* sciatica, while the other 6 showed it to be no better and no worse than the reference treatment. They concluded that the efficacy of ESI has not been established. This does not contradict the earlier findings of Benzon[2] that ESI may be effective in patients with acute lumbosacral radiculopathy.

A consistent verdict on treatment efficacy has not been supported by the available controlled studies. An additional analysis of this literature was published by Watts and Silagy.[35] Efficacy was defined as pain relief (at least 75% improvement) in the short term (60 days) and in the long term (1 year). ESI increased the odds ratio of pain relief to 2.61 in the short term and to 1.87 for the long-term relief of pain. Efficacy was independent of the route of administration (i.e., caudal or lumbar). This analysis provided quantitative evidence that the epidural corticosteroids are effective in the management of lumbosacral radicular pain when injected by either the lumbar or the caudal route.

There have been three prospective, randomized, double-blind, placebo-controlled studies of patients with documented herniated disc and pain present for less than 1 year who received *lumbar* ESI (Table 40-1). Dilke and associates[36] showed significantly better pain relief and better rates of return to work with ESI than with interspinous ligament saline injections at 3 months' follow-up. Snoek and colleagues[37] reported greater subjective and objective improvements after ESI compared with placebo injection, but this difference did not reach statistical significance. Their study used undiluted steroid in a 2 mL volume and evaluated patients after 24 to 48 hours (compared with 6 days in the study by Dilke and colleagues[36]). The minimum time interval for initial evaluation of response should approach 1 week. This can be derived from the observations of Green et al.[38] on the response to ESI: 37% experienced relief within 2 days, while 59% responded only after 4 to 6 days. Carette and co-workers[39] administered ESI up to 3 times and found that the differences in improvement between groups were not significant, except for improvements in the finger-to-floor distance ($P = 0.03$) and in sensory deficits at 3 weeks, and in leg pain at 6 weeks. These improvements were observed in the methylprednisolone group at 3 weeks and 6 weeks, but there were no significant differences after 3 months. ESI did not offer significant functional benefit, nor did it reduce the need for surgery in about 25% these patients within 12 months. Hopwood and Manning[40] criticized this study for selection of a patient population most likely to be sent for surgery, and for noncomparable placebo control, inadequate power, and nonstandard treatment. In a prospective randomized clinical trial Buchner et al.[41] administered three ESIs to patients with HNP who were under 50 years of age. They reported significant improvement in straight leg raising and nonsignificant improvement for pain relief and mobility after 2 weeks, but no significant benefits in the treatment group at 6 weeks and 6 months.

TABLE 40-1. RESULTS OF WELL-CONTROLLED STUDIES ON LUMBAR EPIDURAL STEROID INJECTIONS FOR PATIENTS WITH ACUTE HERNIATED DISC

Study	Type of Study	Symptom Duration	Treatments Studied and Route	Success Rate (%), Steroid vs. Control
Dilke et al.[36]	P, R, DB	≤1 year	MP, 80 mg in 10 mL NS vs. 1 mL NS, lumbar	60% vs. 31% initial pain relief; less pain, less analgesic use, and less failed return to work at 3 months
Snoek et al.[37]	P, R, DB	1–3 weeks	MP, 80 mg in 2 mL NS vs. 2 mL NS, lumbar	25% to 70% improvement in multiple outcome measures, not significantly different from 7% to 43% in placebo group
Carette et al.[39]	P, R, DB	<1 year	MP, 80 mg in 8 mL NS vs. 1 mL NS, lumbar	Less sensory deficit and leg pain; functional disability and incidence of surgery the same

P, prospective; R, randomized; DB, double blind; MP, methylprednisolone; NS, normal saline.

Bush and Hillier[42] employed *caudal* epidural steroid or normal saline injections in a randomized, double-blind, placebo-controlled study of clinically well-defined patients with radicular pain, paresthesias, and positive straight-leg raise. They found significantly better pain relief at both 4 weeks (visual analog scale 16.0 vs. 45.0) and 52 weeks (14.2 vs. 29.6) for ESI compared with placebo.

Prospective long-term follow-up studies after ESI are lacking. Persistent benefit after ESI was reported by Dilke and co-workers[36] after 3 months (36% complete and 55% partial relief); by Green and associates[38] (41% sustained relief for at least 1 year); and by Bush and Hillier[42] at 52 weeks (earlier benefit was maintained or improved), all in patients with discogenic, radicular pain. Abram and Hopwood[30] also monitored patients who received ESI and observed persistent improvement at 6 and 12 months in those who initially responded. They reported that the patients had significantly better pain reduction and better rates of return to work than patients who failed ESI. In a more heterogeneous group of patients White and co-workers[26] reported persistent improvement after 6 months in 34% of patients with acute pain and in 12% of patients with chronic pain.

CERVICAL INJECTION

Reports on the use of cervical ESI to treat cervical radiculopathy and various other diagnoses began to appear in 1986.[10–12] There have been no blinded, controlled, randomized studies to assess the efficacy of this procedure (Table 40-2).[43–45]

Stav and colleagues[43] reported on 50 patients with chronic, refractory neck and arm pain who were treated with physical therapy and continued NSAIDs. All patients had degenerative disc disease, osteoarthritis of the cervical spine, or both, with or without radiculopathy. In addition, all had had pain for

longer than 6 months. Cervical ESI proved to be superior to posterior neck intramuscular injections for short- and long-term pain relief, improved range of motion, decreased analgesic consumption, and recovery of the capacity to work. At 1 year follow-up, good to excellent results were found in 68% of the patients in the ESI group vs. 12% in the intramuscular injection group.

Ferrante and colleagues[46] attempted to find predictors of clinical outcome in a retrospective review of 100 patients who received cervical ESI. Radicular pain predicted a better outcome; radiologic diagnosis of a normal scan or of disc herniation predicted a poor outcome. The authors recommended selection of patients for cervical ESI by the presence of radicular pain and either physical or radiologic findings corresponding to the painful nerve root.

USE OF FLUOROSCOPIC GUIDANCE

Is efficacy improved when fluoroscopy is used during ESI? Many reports[47–49] suggest that needle misplacement without fluoroscopic guidance is a common reason for treatment failure with ESI. Mehta and Salmon[47] reported that placement of Tuohy needles, using a loss-of-resistance (LOR) technique to identify the lumbar epidural space, was too superficial in 17% of cases. Renfrew et al.[49] documented incorrect needle placement for caudal ESI by novice trainees 48% of the time, but also at a 15% rate by experienced practitioners. Epidural injection after correct needle placement and negative aspiration proved to be intravenous in 9.2% of cases. Manchikanti and colleagues[50] proposed that use of fluoroscopy would decrease technical failures with ESI up to 50% to 60%. Stitz and Sommer[51] reported 74% success on the first attempt at caudal needle placement in 54 patients; their initial success rate increased to 91% in the presence of easy landmarks and absence

TABLE 40-2. **RESULTS OF PROSPECTIVE REPORTS ON INTERLAMINAR CERVICAL EPIDURAL STEROID INJECTIONS***

Study	Study Design	No. of Patients	Population	Response
Stav et al.[43]	P, R, D	50	Chronic neck and arm pain for longer than 6 months, degenerative disc and cervical spine disease	68% good to very good after cervical ESI vs. 12% after IM neck injection at 1 year follow-up
Castagnera et al.[44]	P, R, C	24	Chronic cervical radicular pain for longer than 12 months, no nerve compression	71% had at least 75% decrease in VAS at 3 months
Bush and Hillier[45]	P, D	68	Cervical radiculopathy, with neurologic signs, for 1–12 months	76% pain free and 24% improved (average 2, range 1–4 on a 10-point scale)

* No well-controlled studies of cervical epidural steroid injections are available.
C, controlled; D, descriptive; P, prospective; R, randomized; VAS, visual analogue scale; ESI, epidural steroid injection; IM, intramuscular.
Adapted from Molloy RE, Benzon HT: The current status of epidural steroids. Curr Rev Pain 1:61–69, 1996.

of palpable subcutaneous air. They concluded that fluoroscopic guidance remains the gold standard for caudal epidural injection in adults. In a study of ESI without fluoroscopic guidance in 200 patients randomly assigned to injection site, 93% of lumbar and 64% of caudal injections were correctly placed.[52] The odds ratio for successful placement was reduced to 0.34 in the presence of obesity (BMI > 30 vs. BMI < 30).

Epidural needle size may influence success rate for lumbar ESI using a LOR technique. Liu and associates[53] achieved a success rate of 92% with 20-gauge Tuohy needles, significantly less than with standard 17- or 18-gauge needles. Reliability of the LOR technique was lower with increased patient age (>70 years) and male sex. Fredman and colleagues[54] reported successful blind entry into the epidural space after multiple attempts in 88% of previously operated patients; location at the intended level in just 50%; and spread of contrast to the site of pathology only 26% of the time. A retrospective review of 38 cervical ESIs detected a 53% rate of false LOR on the first attempt, unilateral spread in 51%, and ventral epidural spread in only 28%. The authors concluded that fluoroscopy with epidurography can improve accuracy of blindly performed cervical ESIs by ensuring correct needle placement and delivery of medication to the area of pathology.[55] The preponderance of evidence would suggest that use of fluoroscopy with contrast epidurography should increase accuracy of needle placement in the epidural space and targeted delivery of injected medication to the site of pathology, which may often be unilateral spread into the anterior epidural space. The most reasonable exception would be for initial lumbar ESI in younger, nonobese, nonoperated patients. The transforaminal approach has also been proposed to increase success of ESI at the lumbar and cervical levels. The efficacy and safety of this technique is considered in Chapter 41.

COMPLICATIONS

Complications of ESI may be classified as those related to epidural technique and those related to injected drugs. Technical side effects include back pain at the injection site and temporarily increased radicular pain and paresthesias without persistent morbidity. Acute anxiety, lightheadedness, diaphoresis, flushing, nausea, hypotension, and vasovagal syncope may occur, especially during procedures performed with the patient in the sitting position. Headache may occur after accidental dural puncture, the most common complication of epidural injection. In experienced hands this complication should occur in less than 1% of attempted epidural injections. MacDonald[56] cited an incidence of 0.33% for 5,685 lumbar epidural injections. Waldman[57] reported dural puncture in 0.25% of 790 cervical epidural injections. Nonpostural headache due to subarachnoid air injection has been reported; Katz and colleagues[58] reported immediate onset of headache attributed to injection of air into subdural space. Pneumocephalus has also been observed after cervical ESI.[59]

Retinal hemorrhage had been associated with rapid, large-volume caudal steroid injection performed under general anesthesia.[60] Transient blindness by the same mechanism has been reported in 10 cases after lumbar ESI.[61] Significant epidural hemorrhage appears to be rare in the absence of coagulopathy, although recent case reports after cervical ESI are of serious concern. Williams and associates[62] reported a case of acute paraplegia caused by epidural hematoma formation after a

seventh cervical ESI in a patient who had used indomethacin regularly for 6 years. Ghaly[63] reported bilateral upper extremity radicular pain with Tuohy needle insertion for cervical ESI, followed within 30 minutes by Brown–Sequard syndrome due to epidural hematoma. Stoll and Sanchez[64] observed delayed onset of acute cervical myelopathy due to a large epidural hematoma, presenting 8 days after cervical ESI, in a healthy young man without risk factors for bleeding. Early diagnosis of epidural hematoma, and immediate surgical decompression and evacuation is essential to reduce the risk of permanent neurological deficit. Reitman and Watters[65] reported the first case of anterior spinal subdural hematoma after cervical ESI. The patient developed neck pain and progressive quadriparesis within 8 hours. The postoperative course was complicated by partial recovery, meningitis, and eventual death. Two cases of intrinsic spinal cord damage and permanent neurologic symptoms developed within 24 hours after cervical ESI; intravenous sedation during the procedure appears to have interfered with patient report of acute neurological symptoms.[66]

Infectious complications of ESI include bacterial meningitis and epidural abscess. Meningitis is unlikely to develop unless unintentional dural puncture occurs. Dougherty and Fraser[67] reported two cases of bacterial meningitis after attempted ESI. One patient had accidental lumbar puncture before steroid injection; dural puncture was neither diagnosed nor ruled out with a local anesthetic test dose in the other case.

Epidural abscess was reported by Shealy[68] in 1966 after a series of four epidural injections of steroids in a patient who had coexistent local spinal metastatic disease. Cancer cells were identified in the purulent material, but no bacteria were cultured. Five other cases of epidural abscess were reported between 1984 and 1997; one after cervical, three after lumbar, and one after caudal ESI[69–73] (Table 40-3). Cultures grew *Staphylococcus aureus* in all five patients. Three patients had diabetes mellitus; two had multiple (i.e., three) injections; one had a surgical infection with *S. aureus* 2 weeks before ESI; and one had breast cancer with spinal metastasis located in the sacrum. All patients presented 3 days to 3 weeks after injection with fever, spinal pain, radicular pain, or progressive neurologic deficit; this scenario should elicit a high index of suspicion for epidural abscess. Rapid diagnosis and therapy, including surgical drainage, appears necessary if one hopes to achieve patient recovery with intact neurologic function. Magnetic resonance imaging appears to be the procedure of choice for the diagnosis of epidural abscess.[70] The combination of diabetes and steroid immunosuppression may predispose to epidural abscess formation. Two other patients developed a thoracic epidural abscess after repeated epidural injections of bupivacaine and steroid to treat neuropathic pain secondary to herpes zoster infection[74,75] (Table 40-3). Additional reports of epidural abscess after cervical[76] and lumbar[77] ESI have appeared recently; and lumbar discitis after caudal ESI[78] has also been observed.

Complications related to the drugs used for ESI include pharmacologic effects of steroids and possible neurotoxicity. Temporary development of Cushing's syndrome,[79] weight gain, fluid retention, hyperglycemia, hypertension, and congestive heart failure have all been reported after ESI. Kaposi's sarcoma was observed after intra-articular steroid injection, and it later recurred after ESI.[80] A single case of allergic reaction to ESI was reported by Simon and coworkers.[81] Very delayed onset of a cutaneous, respiratory, and gastrointestinal

TABLE 40-3. REPORTED CASES OF EPIDURAL ABSCESS AFTER EPIDURAL STEROID INJECTION

Study	Injection	Findings	Outcome	Medical History
Shealy[68]	L, ×4, M	Squamous cell cancer and inflammatory cells	Foot drop, late death due to cancer	Cancer
Chan and Leung[69]	L, ×1, T	*Staphylococcus aureus*	T8 paraplegia, near-complete recovery	Diabetes
Goucke and Graziotti[70]	L, ×3, M	*Staphylococcus aureus*	Death	Diabetes, recent postoperative staphylococcal sepsis
Waldman[71]	C, ×3	*Staphylococcus aureus*	C6-level quadriparesis	None
Mamourian et al.[72]	L, ×1	*Staphylococcus aureus*	Death	Cancer
Knight et al.[73]	S, ×2, T + P	*Staphylococcus aureus*	Paraplegia	Diabetes
Bromage[74]	Th, ×6, M	Not stated	Quadriplegia	Postherpetic neuralgia
Strong[75]	Th, ×1, M + B ×10 via 2 catheters	*Staphylococcus aureus*	Complete recovery	Resolving acute herpes zoster; two separate epidural catheters for 1 and 3 days; prophylactic oral antibiotics ×10 days
Huang[76]	C, ×1	*Staphylococcus aureus*	Complete recovery, delayed	None
Koka[77]	L ×2	*Staphylococcus aureus*	Complete recovery	Systemic lupus
Yue[78]	Caudal ×1	*Pseudomonas aeruginosa*	Successful treatment	

L, lumbar; C, cervical; S, sacral; Th, thoracic; M, methylprednisolone acetate; T, triamcinolone diacetate; B, bupivacaine; P, procaine.
Adapted from Molloy RE, Benzon HT: The current status of epidural steroids. Curr Rev Pain 1:61–69, 1996.

reaction was noted and was reproduced with subsequent exposure to triamcinolone. Adrenal suppression is a well-known result of ESI. Plasma cortisol levels are decreased for up to 3 weeks after epidural injection of 80 mg methylprednisolone acetate. Kay and colleagues[82] described the effects of three weekly epidural triamcinolone injections on the pituitary–adrenal axis in humans. Depressed levels of adrenocorticotropic hormone (ACTH) and cortisol, and abnormal cortisol response to synthetic ACTH, were noted for up to 1 month after ESI. Relative adrenal insufficiency should be considered when major surgical stress occurs within 1 month after ESI. Spinal epidural lipomatosis has been observed recently after multiple ESIs, and it may produce symptoms due to neural compression. The development and subsequent resolution of lipomas, after discontinuation of steroid injections, have been documented with serial MRI scans.[83,84]

Neurotoxicity has been attributed to spinal injections of depot steroids or to their preservatives. Adhesive arachnoiditis has been reported after repeated intrathecal steroid injections in patients with multiple sclerosis. There are no case reports of arachnoiditis after ESI alone. Abram and O'Connor[85] reviewed the risk of complications from ESI. They were unable to find a single report of arachnoiditis in 64 series describing these injections in about 7,000 patients. They did, however, collect many reports of spontaneous arachnoiditis without prior spinal injections. Aseptic meningitis has been reported three times after intrathecal steroid injection and once after ESI.[86] These patients had headache, fever, and other systemic symptoms; and their cerebrospinal fluid was characterized by low glucose with elevated protein and leukocytes.

Nelson has questioned both the efficiency and the safety of intraspinal methylprednisolone acetate.[87] He recommended against its intrathecal use because of potential polyethylene glycol toxicity. He also attempted to implicate epidural injection as dangerous because of hypothetical migration into the subarachnoid space as well as accidental subdural or intrathecal injection. He believes that this may occur often with attempted epidural injection, especially after previous injections or back surgery.

Relevant animal data on neurotoxicity after ESI are limited. MacKinnon and co-workers[88] investigated the effects of various steroids injected into or near rat sciatic nerves. Nerve injury occurred only after direct intrafascicular injection. Benzon and associates[89] examined the effect of polyethylene glycol exposure on the electrophysiology of sheathed and unsheathed rabbit nerves. They demonstrated no effect from the clinically relevant 3% or even a 10% concentration but reversible decrements in conduction at 20% and 30% and no conduction at 40%. Abram and colleagues[90] studied the effects of serial intrathecal steroid injections on the rat spinal cord, finding no demonstrable analgesia with formalin pain testing and no histologic changes 21 days after injection. They concluded that accidental intrathecal injection during attempted ESI has a low potential to cause harm.

Abram and O'Connor[85] made several recommendations to avoid further complications of ESI. They suggested a meticulous aseptic technique, especially in diabetic patients, to prevent infectious sequelae. They indicated that high-dose or repeated injections (more than one to three) have no support in the literature. They also recommended use of a local anesthetic test dose to prevent accidental, undetected intrathecal steroid injection and possible neurotoxic effects. The purported benefit to the patient must be weighed against the more likely risk of hemodynamic consequences when contemplating local anesthetic vs. saline epidural injection.

CURRENT ROLE

The efficacy of ESI has not been conclusively demonstrated, and it is unlikely that a definitive study will be completed.[40] Nevertheless, many studies have confirmed very good short- to intermediate-term success rates in selected patients. Reviews by Rowlingson,[91] Abram,[92] and Hammonds[93] state the case for continued use of this therapy as part of the overall management of patients with acute radicular pain, herniated disc, or new radiculopathy superimposed on chronic back pain or cervical spondylosis. The analysis by Watts and Silagy[35] and the review by Spaccarelli[35] support the efficacy of ESI in lumbosacral radicular pain syndromes. This conclusion is challenged but not disproved by Koes and associates.[34] The presence of nerve root irritation is required to justify use of ESI. However, this therapy may be less efficacious in patients with neurologic deficits and a large disc herniation than in those with acute radicular pain alone.[39] Thorough patient evaluation, consideration of benefits and risks, and informed patient consent are essential to active selection of patients for this treatment (Table 40-4). Reliable patient follow-up and comprehensive management of physical, occupational, and emotional rehabilitation are necessary to avoid a too narrowly focused, block-oriented approach to these patients. ESI should be avoided if there is concern about localized or systemic infection or clotting function. One should also consider the added risk of infection with diabetes and the reduced chance of success if there has been previous back surgery, prolonged symptoms, substance abuse, disability, or litigation issues.[94]

TABLE 40-4. EVALUATION CRITERIA: SELECTION OF PATIENTS FOR EPIDURAL STEROID INJECTION

	Positive Factors	Negative Predictive Factors	Increased Risk
History	Radicular pain Radicular numbness Short symptom duration Absence of significant psychological factors	Axial pain primarily Work-related injury Unemployed due to pain High number of past treatments, high number of drugs taken Compensation due to pain Litigation pending Previous back surgery Smoking history Very high pain ratings	Immunosuppression Diabetes Peptic ulcer disease Tuberculosis AIDS Bacterial infection
Examination	Dermatomal sensory loss Motor loss correlated to symptoms Positive straight leg raise	Myofascial pain prominent	
Laboratory results	Abnormal EMG findings related to symptoms Lumbar herniated disc Cervical spondylosis	Normal cervical spine imaging scans Cervical herniated disc	

Data from Rowlingson and Kirschenbaum;[12] White et al.;[26] Abram and Hopwood;[30] Hopwood and Abram;[31] Ferrante et al.;[46] Abram and Anderson;[96] and Jamison et al.[97]

The authors' technique for ESI has been described.[20] Methylprednisolone acetate 80 mg is employed as the steroid drug, with triamcinolone diacetate as the alternative choice. The diluent usually is normal saline, with the total being 5 to 10 mL at the lumbar level, 3 to 6 mL at the cervical level, and 20 mL when the caudal approach is selected. Lumbar ESI is performed as close to the level of radicular pathology as possible, often using a paramedian approach to target the lateral aspect of the interlaminar epidural space on the involved side. Cervical ESI is most often performed at the C7–T1 level. A guided epidural catheter is introduced with fluoroscopy to produce unilateral spread of injectate at higher cervical levels. A similar technique may be employed for targeted caudal or lumbar ESI.[95] The injection is not repeated if there is complete relief. If partial relief occurs a second injection is offered, but a third injection is only rarely used. Repeat injections are not offered when benefit is transient but may be considered after prolonged responses of 6 to 12 months or longer.

REFERENCES

1. Kepes ER, Duncalf D: Treatment of backache with spinal injections of local anesthetics, spinal and systemic steroids. Pain 22:33–47, 1985.
2. Benzon HT: Epidural steroid injections for low back pain and lumbosacral radiculopathy. Pain 24:277–295, 1986.
3. Haddox JD: Lumbar and cervical epidural steroid therapy. Anesthesiol Clin North Am 10:179–203, 1992.
4. Molloy RE, Benzon HT: The current status of epidural steroids. Curr Rev Pain 1:61–69, 1996.
5. Raj PP: Epidural steroid injections. In Raj PP (ed): Practical Management of Pain, ed 3. Mosby, St Louis, 2000, p 732–743.
6. Bosscher HA: Interventional techniques: Epidural steroid injections. In Raj PP (ed): Pain Medicine: A Comprehensive Review, ed 2. Mosby, St Louis, 2003, p 280–290.
7. Goebert HW, Jallo SJ, Gardner WJ, et al: Painful radiculopathy treated with epidural injections of procaine and hydrocortisone acetate: results in 113 patients. Anesth Analg 1961;40:130–134.
8. Winnie AP, Hartman JT, Meyers HL, et al: Pain clinic II: Intradural and extradural corticosteroids for sciatica. Anesth Analg 51:990–1003, 1972.
9. Hickey RF: Outpatient epidural steroid injections for low back pain and lumbosacral radiculopathy. N Z Med J 100:594–596, 1987.
10. Shulman M: Treatment of neck pain with cervical epidural steroid injection. Reg Anesth 11:92–94, 1986.
11. Purkis IE: Cervical epidural steroids. Pain Clinic 1:3–7, 1986.
12. Rowlingson JC, Kirschenbaum LP: Epidural analgesic techniques in the management of cervical pain. Anesth Analg 65:938–942, 1986.
13. Mulligan KA, Rowlingson JC: Epidural steroids. Curr Pain Headache Rep 5:495–502, 2001.
14. McCarron RF, Wimpee MW, Hudkins PG, et al: The inflammatory effect of nucleus pulposus: A possible element in the pathogenesis of low-back pain. Spine 12:760–764, 1987.
15. Olmarker K, Blomquist J, Stromberg J, et al: Inflammatogenic properties of nucleus pulposus. Spine 20:665–669, 1995.
16. Saal JS, Franson RC, Dobrow R, et al.: High levels of inflammatory phospholipase A2 activity in lumbar disc herniations. Spine 15:674–678, 1990.
17. O'Donnell JL, O'Donnell AL: Prostaglandin E2 content in herniated lumbar disc disease. Spine 21:1653–1654, 1996.
18. Nygaard O, Mellgren S, Osterud B: The inflammatory properties of contained and noncontained lumbar disc herniation. Spine 22:2484–2488, 1997.
19. Olmarker K, Rydevik B, Holm S: Edema formation in spinal nerve roots induced by experimental, graded compression. Spine 14:569–573, 1989.
20. Benzon HT: Epidural steroids. In Raj PP (ed): Practical Management of Pain, ed 2. Mosby, St Louis, 1992, p 818–828.
21. Takata K, Inoue S, Takashi K, et al: Swelling of the cauda equina in patients who have herniation of a lumbar disc: A possible pathogenesis of sciatica. J Bone Joint Surg Am 70:361–368, 1988.
22. Olmarker K, Rydevik B, Nordborg C: Autologous nucleus pulposus induces neurophysiologic and histologic changes in porcine cauda equina nerve roots. Spine 18:1425–1432, 1993.
23. Lee HM, Weinstein JN, Meller ST, et al: The role of steroids and their effect on phospholipase A2. An animal model of radiculopathy. Spine 23:1191–1196, 1998.
24. Devor M, Govrin-Lippman R, Raber P: Corticosteroids suppress ectopic neural discharge originating in experimental neuromas. Pain 22:127–137, 1985.
25. Johansson A, Hao J, Sjolund B: Local corticosteroid application blocks transmission in normal nociceptive C-fibers. Acta Anaesthesiol Scand 34:335–338, 1990.
26. White AH, Derby R, Wynne G: Epidural injections for the diagnosis and treatment of low back pain. Spine 5:78–86, 1980.
27. Hacobian A, Kahn C, Picard L, et al.: Treatment of spinal stenosis with epidural steroid injections: An outcome study. Reg Anesth 20(Suppl 2):128, 1995.
28. Ciocon JO, Galindo-Ciocon D, Amaranath L, et al: Caudal epidural blocks for elderly patients with lumbar canal stenosis. J Am Geriatr Soc 42:593–596, 1994.
29. Fukusaki M, Kobayashi I, Hara T, et al: Symptoms of spinal stenosis do not improve after epidural steroid injection. Clin J Pain 14:148–151, 1998.
30. Abram SE, Hopwood MB: What factors contribute to outcome with lumbar epidural steroids? In Bond MR, Charlton JE, Woolf CJ (eds): Proceedings of the Sixth World Congress on Pain. Elsevier, Amsterdam, 1991, pp 495–500.
31. Hopwood MB, Abram SE: Factors associated with failure of lumbar epidural steroids. Reg Anesth 18:238–243, 1993.
32. Sandrock NJG, Warfield CA: Epidural steroids and facet injections. In Warfield CA (ed): Principles and Practice of Pain Management. McGraw-Hill, New York, 1993, pp 401–412.
33. Spaccarelli KC: Lumbar and caudal epidural corticosteroid injections. Mayo Clin Proc 71:169–178, 1996.
34. Koes BW, Scholten RJPM, Mens JMA, et al: Efficacy of epidural steroid injections for low-back pain and sciatica: A systematic review of randomized clinical trials. Pain 63:279–288, 1995.
35. Watts RW, Silagy CA: A meta-analysis on the efficacy of epidural corticosteroids in the treatment of sciatica. Anaesth Intensive Care 23:564–569, 1995.
36. Dilke TFW, Burry HC, Grahame R: Extradural corticosteroid injection in management of lumbar nerve root compression. BMJ 2:635–637, 1973.
37. Snoek W, Weber H, Jorgensen B: Double blind evaluation of extradural methylprednisolone for herniated lumbar discs. Acta Orthop Scand 48:635–641, 1977.
38. Green PW, Burke AJ, Weiss CA, et al: The role of epidural cortisone injection in treatment of discogenic low back pain. Clin Orthop 153:121–125, 1980.
39. Carette S, Leclaire R, Marcoux S et al: Epidural corticosteroid injections for sciatica due to herniated nucleus pulposus. N Engl J Med 336:1634–1640, 1997.
40. Hopwood M, Manning D: Lumbar epidural steroid injections: Is a clinical trial necessary or appropriate? Reg Anesth Pain Med 24:5–7, 1999.
41. Buchner M, Zeifang F, Brocai D, et al: Epidural corticosteroid injection in the conservative management of sciatica. Clin Orthop 375:149–156, 2000.

42. Bush K, Hillier S: A controlled study of caudal epidural injections of triamcinolone plus procaine for the management of intractable sciatica. Spine 16:572–575, 1991.

43. Stav A, Ovadia L, Sternberg A, et al: Cervical epidural steroid injection for cervicobrachialgia. Acta Anaesthesiol Scand 37:562–566, 1993.

44. Castagnera L, Maurette P, Pointillart V, et al: Long term results of cervical epidural steroid injection with and without morphine in chronic cervical radicular pain. Pain 58:239, 1994.

45. Bush K, Hillier S: Outcome of cervical radiculopathy treated with periradicular/epidural corticosteroid injections: A prospective study with independent clinical review. Eur Spine J 5:319, 1996.

46. Ferrante FM, Wilson SP, Iacobo C, et al: Clinical classification as a predictor of therapeutic outcome after cervical epidural steroid injection. Spine 18:730–736, 1993.

47. Mehta M, Salmon N: Extradural block: Confirmation of the injection site by X-ray monitoring. Anaesthesia 40:1009–1012, 1985.

48. El-Khoury GY, Ehara S, Weinstein JN, et al: Epidural steroid injection: A procedure ideally performed under fluoroscopic control. Radiology 168:554–557, 1988.

49. Renfrew DL, Moore TE, Kathol MH, et al: Correct placement of epidural steroid injections: Fluoroscopic guidance and contrast administration. Am J Neuroradiol 12:1003–1007, 1991.

50. Manchikanti L, Bakhit CE, Pakanati RR, et al: Fluoroscopy is medically necessary for the performance of epidural steroids: Response. Anesth Analg 89:1330–1331, 1999.

51. Stitz M, Sommer H: Accuracy of blind versus fluoroscopically guided caudal epidural injection. Spine 24:1371–1376, 1999.

52. Price CM, Rogers PD, Prosser AS, et al: Comparison of the caudal and lumbar approaches to the epidural space. Ann Rheum Dis 2000;59:879–882.

53. Liu SS, Melmed AP, Klos JW, et al: Prospective experience with a 20-gauge Tuohy needle for lumbar epidural steroid injections: Is confirmation with fluoroscopy necessary? Reg Anesth Pain Med 26:143–146, 2001.

54. Fredman B, Nun MB, Zohar E, et al: Epidural steroids for treating "failed back surgery syndrome": Is fluoroscopy really necessary? Anesth Analg 88:367–372, 1999.

55. Stojanovic MP, Vu TN, Caneris O, et al: The role of fluoroscopy in cervical epidural steroid injections: An analysis of contrast dispersal patterns. Spine 27:509–514, 2002.

56. MacDonald R: Dr. Doughty's technique for location of the epidural space. Anaesthesia 38:71, 1983.

57. Waldman SD: Complications of cervical epidural nerve blocks with steroids: A prospective study of 790 consecutive blocks. Reg Anesth 14:149–151, 1989.

58. Katz JA, Lukin R, Bridenbaugh PO, et al: Subdural intracranial air: An unusual cause of headache after epidural steroid injection. Anesthesiology 74:615–618, 1991.

59. Simopoulos T, Peeters-Asdourian C: Pneumocephalus after cervical epidural steroid injection. Anesth Analg 92:1576–1577, 2001.

60. Ling C, Atkinson PL, Munton CGF: Bilateral retinal haemorrhages following epidural injection. Br J Opthalmol 77:316–317, 1993.

61. Young WF: Transient blindness after lumbar epidural steroid injection: A case report and literature review. Spine 27:E476–E477, 2002.

62. Williams KN, Jackowski A, Evans PJD: Epidural haematoma requiring surgical decompression following repeated cervical epidural steroid injections for chronic pain. Pain 42:197–199, 1990.

63. Ghaly RF: Recovery after high-dose methylprednisolone and delayed evacuation: A case of spinal epidural hematoma. J Neurosurg Anesthesiol 13:323–328, 2001.

64. Stoll A, Sanchez M: Epidural hematoma after epidural block: Implications for its use in pain management. Surg Neurol 57:235–240, 2002.

65. Reitman CA, Watters W, 3rd: Subdural hematoma after cervical epidural steroid injection. Spine 27:E174–E176, 2002.

66. Hodges SD, Castelberg RL, Miller T, et al: Cervical epidural steroid injection with intrinsic spinal cord damage: Two case reports. Spine 23:2137–2142, 1998.

67. Dougherty JH, Fraser RAR: Complications following intraspinal injections of steroids. J Neurosurg 48:1023–1025, 1978.

68. Shealy CN: Dangers of spinal injection without proper diagnosis. JAMA 197:1104–1106, 1966.

69. Chan ST, Leung S: Spinal epidural abscess following steroid injection for sciatica. Spine 14:106–108, 1989.

70. Goucke CR, Graziotti P: Extradural abscess following local anesthetic and steroid injection for chronic low back pain. Br J Anaesth 65:427–429, 1990.

71. Waldman SD: Cervical epidural abscess after cervical epidural nerve block with steroids. Anesth Analg 72:717–718, 1991.

72. Mamourian AC, Dickman CA, Drayer BP, et al: Spinal epidural abscesses: Three cases following spinal epidural injection demonstrated with magnetic resonance imaging. Anesthesiology 78:204–207, 1993.

73. Knight JW, Cordingley JJ, Palazzo MGA: Epidural abscess following epidural steroid and local anaesthetic injection. Anaesthesia 52:576–578, 1997.

74. Bromage PR: Spinal extradural abscess: Pursuit of vigilance. Br J Anaesth 70:471–473, 1993.

75. Strong WE: Epidural abscess associated with epidural catheterization: A rare event? Report of two cases with markedly delayed presentation. Anesthesiology 74:943–946, 1991.

76. Huang RC, Shapiro GS, Lim M, et al: Cervical epidural abscess after epidural steroid injection. Spine 29:E7–E9, 2004.

77. Koka VK, Potti A: Spinal epidural abscess after corticosteroid injections. South Med J 95:772–774, 2002.

78. Yue WM, Tan SB: Distant skip level discitis and vertebral osteomyelitis after caudal epidural injection: a case report of a rare complication of epidural injections. Spine 28:E209–E211, 2002.

79. Tuel SM, Meythaler JM, Cross LL: Cushing's syndrome from epidural methylprednisolone. Pain 40:81–84, 1990.

80. Trattner A, Hodak E, David M, et al: Kaposi's sarcoma with visceral involvement after intraarticular and epidural injections of corticosteroids. J Am Acad Dermatol 28:890–894, 1993.

81. Simon DL, Kunz RD, German JD, et al: Allergic or pseudoallergic reaction following epidural steroid deposition and skin testing. Reg Anesth 14:253–255, 1989.

82. Kay J, Findling JW, Raff H: Epidural triamcinolone suppresses the pituitary–adrenal axis in human subjects. Anesth Analg 79:501–505, 1994.

83. Sandberg DI, Lavyne MH: Symptomatic spinal epidural lipomatosis after local epidural corticosteroid injections: Case report. Neurosurgery 45:162–165, 1999.

84. McCullen GM, Spurling GR, Webster JS: Epidural lipomatosis complicating lumbar steroid injections. J Spinal Disord 12:526–529, 1999.

85. Abram SE, O'Connor JC: Risk of complications following epidural steroid injections. Reg Anesth 21:149–162, 1996.

86. Gutknecht DR: Chemical meningitis following epidural injections of corticosteroids [letter]. Am J Med 82:570, 1987.

87. Nelson DA: Intraspinal therapy using methylprednisolone acetate: Twenty-three years of clinical controversy. Spine 18:278–286, 1993.

88. MacKinnon SE, Hudson AR, Gentilli R, et al: Peripheral nerve injection injury with steroid agents. Plast Reconstr Surg 69:482–490, 1982.

89. Benzon HT, Gissen AJ, Strichartz GR, et al: The effect of polyethylene glycol on mammalian nerve impulses. Anesth Analg 66:553–559, 1987.

90. Abram SE, Marsala M, Yaksh TL: Analgesic and neurotoxic effects of intrathecal corticosteroids in rats. Anesthesiology 81:1198–1205, 1994.
91. Rowlingson TC: Epidural steroids: Do they have a place in pain management? APS J 3:20–27, 1994.
92. Abram SE: Risk versus benefit of epidural steroids: Let's remain objective. APS J 2:28–30, 1994.
93. Hammonds WD: Epidural steroid injections: An unproven therapy for pain. APS J 3:31–32, 1994.
94. Abram SE: Treatment of lumbosacral radiculopathy with epidural steroids. Anesthesiology 91:1937–1941, 1999.
95. Friedman R, Li V, Mehrotra D, et al: Foraminal injection of a painful sacral nerve root using an epidural catheter: Case report. Reg Anesth Pain Med 27:214–216, 2002.
96. Abram SE, Anderson RA: Using a pain questionnaire to predict response to steroid epidurals. Reg Anesth 5:11–14, 1980.
97. Jamison RN, VadeBoncoeur T, Ferrante FM: Low back pain patients unresponsive to an epidural steroid injection: Identifying predictive factors. Clin J Pain 7:311–317, 1991.

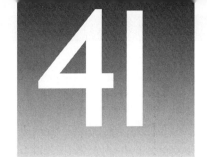

Selective Nerve Root Blocks and Transforaminal Epidural Steroid Injections for Back Pain and Sciatica

Honorio T. Benzon, M.D.

MECHANISM OF RADICULOPATHY AND RATIONALE FOR STEROID INJECTIONS

The rationale for and the results of epidural steroid injections are described in Chapter 40. Briefly, the pain from sciatica is not due to mechanical compression alone, since the presence of herniated discs has been documented in 36% of asymptomatic patients[1] and in 36% of asymptomatic subjects over 60 years of age.[2] Also, the long-term results of discectomy have not been consistently successful. The radiculopathy may be secondary to a combination of factors including chemical irritation of the nerve root, mechanical compression, and vascular compromise. Human discs contain high levels of phospholipase A_2 and the levels of phospholipase A_2 are higher in herniated discs than in normal discs.[3] Phospholipase A_2 is the enzyme responsible for the liberation of arachidonic acid from cell membranes at the site of inflammation. It acts as a catalyst for generating prostaglandins, leukotrienes, platelet-activating factor, and lysophospholipids.[4] Biopsy specimens from noncontained herniated discs have been found to contain higher levels of leukotriene B_4 and thromboxane B_2 than in contained disc herniations.[5] Human disc phospholipase A_2 has been found to be inflammatory.[4,6] The injection of autologous nucleus pulposus into the lumbar epidural space of dogs caused inflammatory changes in the dural sac, spinal cord, and the nerve roots in contrast to the lack of inflammation with saline epidural injection.[7] Finally, the epidural application of autologous nucleus pulposus in pigs, without mechanical nerve root compression, resulted in a pronounced reduction in the nerve conduction velocities in the nerve roots of the cauda equina.[8]

Steroids are anti-inflammatory and their local application relieves inflammatory changes and vascular congestion. The effect of the injected steroid is probably related to inhibition of phospholipase A_2 activity.[9] In a repeat study on the epidural application of autologous nucleus pulposus and decreased conduction velocities in the nerve roots of the cauda equina in pigs the early intravenous injection of high-dose methylprednisolone prevented the reduction in the nerve conduction velocities.[10] Steroids also have a local anesthetic and antinociceptive effect. The local application of methylprednisolone has been shown to block transmission of C fibers but not the A-beta fibers.[11]

EPIDURAL STEROID INJECTIONS

Two review articles published in 1985 and 1986 came up with two different conclusions. Kepes and Duncalf,[12] after a review of spinal and systemic steroids, concluded that these interventions were not effective in relieving backache. Benzon,[13] on the other hand, reviewed epidural steroids only and concluded that the injections were effective in relieving lumbosacral radiculopathy. After a review of the studies, Benzon noted that the indication for epidural steroid injections is nerve root irritation.[13] A meta-analysis of 11 randomized controlled trials involving 907 patients showed the short-term efficacy of epidural steroids in sciatica and that the efficacy was independent of the route of injection.[14] Still, the use of epidural steroids is controversial. Bogduk[15] noted that epidural steroids lack legitimate rationale and lack empirical proof of their efficacy. A study by Carette et al.[16] showed that epidural steroids afforded short-term (3 months) improvement in leg pain and sensory deficits in patients with sciatica due to herniated disc but offered no significant functional benefit and did not reduce the need for surgery. The short-term efficacy of the injections can be clinically useful, however. It provides pain relief during spontaneous resolution of a herniated disc (aggressive conservative management results in partial or complete resolution in 76% of disc herniations[17]), and minimizes opioid dependence and hospitalization.[14]

DIAGNOSTIC NERVE ROOT INJECTIONS

Detailed history and physical examination can localize the level of pathology in the majority of patients with lumbosacral radiculopathy.[18] Elucidation of the etiology of the symptoms requires radiologic tests such as plain radiography, myelography, computerized tomography (CT), and magnetic resonance imaging (MRI). Occasionally, the neurologic examination may be equivocal and the imaging studies may demonstrate nonspecific findings or pathology in more than one level. The abnormality seen on the imaging study may not correlate with the patient's symptoms.[18] Selective nerve root blocks (SNRBs) have been utilized in the evaluation of patients with radicular pain to localize the level of abnormality.[18–20]

SNRBs can be a helpful diagnostic tool. In SNRBs the needle may touch the nerve root responsible for the patient's pain and the patient reports that the elicited pain is concordant with the usual symptom. The elicitation of concordant pain is important in patients with multilevel abnormalities on radiographic imaging. The involved nerve root is identified and the extent of the planned surgery is limited. The surgery may also be obviated if the SNRB does not relieve the patient's pain.

Patients with radicular pain are good candidates for SNRBs if they have the following characteristics:[20,21]

- Minimal or no definite imaging findings.
- Multilevel imaging abnormalities.
- Equivocal neurologic examination findings or a discrepancy between clinical and radiological signs.
- Postoperative patients with unexplainable or complex recurrent pain.
- Patients with combined canal and lateral stenosis. SNRBs may help determine whether nerve root entrapment is the cause of the patient's symptoms necessitating a medial partial facetectomy via an interlaminar approach and avoiding an extensive laminectomy.[20]

Technique of Selective Nerve Root Block: For nerve root injection in the lumbar region, the patient lies either in the lateral[18–20] or prone[21,22] position. In the lateral position the symptomatic side is the upper side. The area is prepared and the site of entry is anesthetized with local anesthetic. The site of needle entry is one hand's breadth lateral to the spinous process[18] or 10 cm lateral to the midline.[19] A 6-inch-long needle is inserted at an angle of 45° relative to the sagittal plane and advanced into the proximal end of the intervertebral foramen. The ideal location of the needle tip is just caudal to the pedicle and just lateral to the line connecting the centers of the pedicles.[18] At this point, the patient may experience a sharp sciatic pain. Dye (1 mL) is injected to outline the nerve root. If the needle is placed too far laterally, the needle may be in the psoas muscle and injection of the dye results in a striated

image. Needles that are placed too medially run the risk of epidural injection.

Local anesthetic (1 mL), usually lidocaine, is injected and the response of the patient is noted. The result is considered positive when the pain that was provoked was similar to the patient's symptom, i.e., concordant pain, and relieved by the local anesthetic injection. The result is negative when the pain is not affected at all and equivocal when the response of the patient is not clear.[18] For therapeutic injections, 0.5 mL betamethasone acetate (Celestone, 6 mg/mL) or 0.5 mL triamcinolone acetonide (Kenalog, 40 mg/mL) in local anesthetic or saline is injected. In the lumbar region methylprednisolone 40 mg may be used instead of the betamethasone or triamcinolone.

Most interventional pain management specialists perform the procedure with the patient in the prone position.[20,21] For the L1 to L4 nerve roots, the C-arm of the fluoroscope is rotated in an ipsilateral oblique angle until the "Scotty dog" appearance comes into view.[21] The C-arm is rotated further until the ventral aspect of the superior articulating process (the ear of the "Scotty dog") is midway between the anterior and posterior borders of the superior end plate of the vertebral body. Note that the superior end plates are superimposed at fluoroscopy. The nerve root passes a few millimeters below the pedicle and the needle tip is positioned in this area. For upper lumbar and lower thoracic SNRBs, Fenton[21] prefers to block the nerve slightly more inferolaterally to the pedicle. This is because the artery of Adamkiewicz enters the neural foramen, in close proximity to the dorsal root ganglion, in the superior or middle portion of the neural foramen.[23] The artery of Adamkiewicz, or arteria radicularis magna, is the main arterial supply to the lower two-thirds of the spinal cord. It enters the spinal canal anywhere from T7 to L4, usually on the left side between T9 and L1 vertebrae.

The L5 nerve root is more difficult to block because the iliac crest may obstruct the pathway of the needle. The path of the needle is a triangular area formed by the superior articulating process of S1, the inferior border of the transverse process of L5, and the iliac crest. The obliquity of the C-arm can be manipulated until the triangle is visualized, the area may be seen with less obliquity.[21] The needle is advanced from a lateral to a medial direction, medial to the iliac crest, until the tip of the needle projects inferior to the pedicle.

The patient lies prone for blockade of the S1 nerve root. The C-arm is in straight anterior–posterior (AP) projection or with 5° to 10° of ipsilateral lateral angulation.[21] The image intensifier, which is above the patient, may have to be angled caudocranially (toward the patient's head) to have a better view of the sacral foramen. The needle is advanced through the posterior sacral foramen until the first sacral root is encountered. Lateral views are taken to ensure that the needle tip is in the caudal epidural space and not inserted too deep into the pelvis.

Thoracic nerve root blocks are difficult to perform. The correct location of the needle tip is inferior and lateral to the pedicle (except in T9 to T12 in which the location of the needle tip is similar to that of lumbar nerve root block), lateral to the medial border of the pedicle so the needle tip does not enter the spinal canal, and medial to the ipsilateral head of the rib and the posteromedial margin of the lung.[21]

For cervical nerve root blocks, the patient is either supine[22] or in the lateral decubitus[21] position and the nerve roots are approached from the anterolateral aspect of the neck. Vital structures such as the carotid sheath and the carotid vessels, vertebral artery, and nerves are located along the pathway of the needle. For these reasons, Fenton recommends the use of CT guidance.[21] When fluoroscopy is used[22] lateral images are obtained and the vertebral bodies counted. While anterior oblique angulation is used initially, lateral images are necessary to guide placement of the needle. The needle is directed medially, ventral to the vertebral artery and dorsal to the pharyngeal structures, until it reaches the sulcus of the cervical transverse process. An AP view is obtained to ascertain that the tip of the needle is along the margin of the vertebra and not pushed too far medially. After careful aspiration, 0.2 to 0.4 mL of dye is injected. The contrast should outline the sulcus on the AP view and appears to silhoutte the ventral aspect of the transverse process on the lateral view.[21] A 1 mL volume of local anesthetic is then injected.

In a prospective study of 134 patients it was found that the distribution of symptom provocation resembled the classic dermatomal maps for cervical nerve roots.[24] However, it was not uncommon that the distribution of the pain was outside the distribution of the classic dermatomal maps. These findings may explain the nondermatomal pain complaints of some patients.

After the procedure, the patients are brought to the recovery room and their vital signs taken. The patients should be checked for the presence of numbness or weakness after the procedure. For this reason, some interventionalists use saline instead of short-acting local anesthetic in their therapeutic injections. Local anesthetics, however, have the added advantage of breaking the cycle of pain and providing lasting relief beyond the duration of their local anesthetic effect. The patients are discharged with an instruction sheet listing the possible side effects and complications and the telephone numbers they are supposed to call in case of an emergency.

Some of the complications include bleeding, infection, puncture of the thecal sac, vagovagal reactions, and allergic reactions to the dye or local anesthetic.[18–22] There is a risk of pneumothorax in the thoracic region and paraplegia secondary to trauma to the artery of Adamkiewicz.[25] As stated, the cervical approach is riskier. Ataxia is a possibility after cervical nerve root blocks. The use of methylprednisolone in cervical nerve root blocks has been advised against. The drug precipitates and embolizes to the brain through a punctured vertebral artery with the precipitant settling on an end cerebral artery and causing a small cerebral infarct. While methylprednisolone can be used in lumbar nerve root blocks, soluble steroids such as triamcinolone or betamethasone are preferred in cervical injections.

Comments: The presence of pain during a SNRB is not a very reliable sign that the needle touched the nerve root sheath. The needle may have irritated sensitive structures such as the joint capsule, periosteum, and annulus fibrosus and may cause referred pain to the leg.[20] The patient may be quite nervous and states that the pain elicited is concordant with the radicular pain even when it is not. The risk of nerve injury is also increased when the nerve root is traumatized. The interventional pain physician should advance the needle slowly, under lateral fluoroscopy, once the tip of the needle is in the intervertebral foramen to minimize trauma to the nerve root. The response of the patient after the diagnostic local anesthetic injection is probably more important in ascertaining the nerve root involved in the patient's pain.

Results of Studies: Several studies showed the applicability of SNRBs.[18–20] In a retrospective study of 62 patients Dooley et al.[18] found four possible responses to the injection, as follows:

1. Patient has concordant pain and the pain is completely relieved for the duration of the local anesthetic.
2. Patient has concordant pain but the pain is not relieved by the local anesthetic.
3. Typical pain is not reproduced on needle insertion but the pain is relieved by the local anesthetic.
4. Pain is not concordant and is not completely relieved by the local anesthetic.

In the study by Dooley et al.[18] most of their patients had response 1 and had good response to surgery. The causes included herniated disc, lateral recess stenosis, central canal stenosis, or pedicular kinking. The patients who had concordant pain but not relieved by the local anesthetic (response 2) either had peripheral neuropathy or multilevel involvement. The patients who did not have concordant pain had other abnormalities such as metastatic carcinoma, multilevel pathology, nerve root cutoff secondary to spinal stenosis, or anomalous nerve roots on surgical exploration.

In another study[19] the nerve root block correctly identified the symptomatic level in 18 of 19 patients. These patients underwent surgery and did well. The authors compared the results of SNRB with radiculography and CT and concluded that SNRB is a more useful test than the two other modalities. Myelography and CT are difficult to interpret after spine surgery[26,27] and cannot identify the offending single nerve root.

TRANSFORAMINAL EPIDURAL STEROID INJECTIONS

The term "selective nerve root block" has been questioned, since volumes as low as 1 to 2 mL typically cover more than one nerve root and false positive results occur since several nerve roots may be unintentionally anesthetized.[28] If the injection is isolated immediately outside the neural foramen, before the rami divides, then it will selectively block the segmental spinal nerve. However, the injection also anesthetizes the dorsal ramus and its innervated structures including the zygapophysial joints.[28] To be selective, the injection is performed extraforaminally and not at the nerve root level. Because of the lack of anatomic selectivity of the nerve blocks, it has been recommended that a more appropriate term is "selective spinal nerve block" or "transforaminal epidural steroid injection."[28]

Transforaminal epidural steroid injections have been proposed to improve the results of the classic interlaminar approach to epidural steroid injections.[29–31] In interlaminar epidural steroid injections the injected drug is deposited mainly in the posterior epidural space (Fig. 41-1). In a study on cervical interlaminar epidural steroid injections ventral epidural spread of the dye was noted in only 28% of the injections.[32] The aim of transforaminal injections is to inject the steroid and diluent in the space between the lateral disc herniation and the nerve root, which is located in the anterior epidural space, and into the affected nerve root. The target area is the posterior annulus and the ventral aspect of the nerve root sleeve.

The transforaminal epidural route was initially described by Derby and colleagues.[30,31] Fluoroscopy is necessary to ascertain the vertebral level of injection, precise placement of the needle,

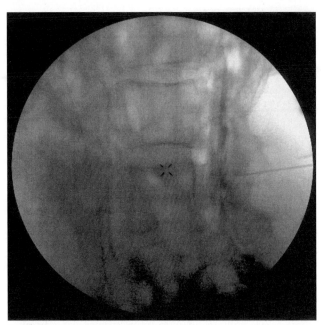

FIGURE 41-1. Spread of the dye in the posterior epidural space in interlaminar epidural injection. There is minimal spread of the dye in the anterior epidural space.

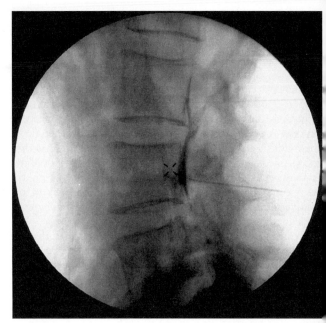

FIGURE 41-2. Lateral fluoroscopic view showing the tip of the needle in the ventral aspect of the intervertebral foramen, just below the pedicle. There is spread of the dye in the anterior epidural space in transforaminal epidural injection.

and document spread of the dye (i.e., medication). In their technique they placed the tip of their needle in the "safe triangle" area. The "safe triangle" is bounded superiorly by the pedicle, medially by the outer margin of the exiting nerve root, and laterally by the lateral border of the vertebral body. Proper needle placement is confirmed by the AP and lateral views. On the AP view the needle is placed just beneath the midportion of the corresponding pedicle. On lateral view the needle is positioned just below the pedicle in the ventral aspect of the intervertebral foramen (Fig. 41-2). Dye (1 to 2 mL) is injected and postinjection fluoroscopy shows the dye outlining the nerve root, entering the intervertebral foramina, and diffusing into the anterior epidural space (Figs. 41-2 and 41-3). At the S1 level, the needle is advanced into the upper outer quadrant of the first sacral foramen.

The site of needle insertion and the distribution of the contrast material has been categorized into the following:[33] (1) type 1, needle tip is below the pedicle at the medial aspect of the foramen, and injection of the dye results in a tubular appearance or outline of the nerve root (intraepineural); (2) type 2, needle tip at the middle of the foramen; nerve root visible as filling defect (extraepineural); and (3) type 3, needle tip at the lateral aspect of the foramen; nerve root is not visible, contrast material has a cloudlike appearance (paraneural). The type 1 injections were noted to be more painful than the type 2 injections. There were no differences in the pain relief, either early or late responses, between the three injections, although there was a trend towards a faster response in the patients who had the type 1 injections.[33]

Prospective Studies on Transforaminal Steroid Injections: There are few prospective studies on transforaminal epidural steroid injections (Table 41-1). Transforaminal epidural steroid injections were found to be effective in patients with herniated disc. Thirty patients, previously

unresponsive to bed rest and nonsteroidal anti-inflammatory agents, had the injections.[29] Immediate relief of symptoms was obtained in 27 patients. Twenty-eight patients were followed for an average of 3.4 years and 22 of them had considerable and sustained relief. The patients' average Low Back Outcome Score improved from 25 (out of 75) before the injection to 54.[29]

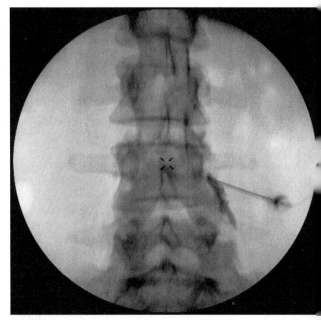

FIGURE 41-3. Anteroposterior fluoroscopic view showing the dye outlining the nerve root and diffusing into the intervertebral foramina into the epidural space.

TABLE 41-1. **PROSPECTIVE STUDIES ON TRANSFORAMINAL EPIDURAL STEROID INJECTIONS**

Type of Study	Diagnosis	Treatments	Follow-up	Result/Success rate	Reference
P, O	HNP	TF ESI	3.4 years (1–10)	78%	29
P, O	HNP	TF ESI	80 weeks (28–144)	75%	34
P, O	SS	TF ESI	12 months	75%	35
P, R,* C, SB	HNP	TF ESI vs. S-TPI	12 months	84% vs. 48%	36
P, R, C, DB	HNP, FS	TF ESI: M/B vs. B	23 months (13–28 months)	Refused surgery: 20/28 (M/B) vs. 9/27 (B)	37
P, R, C, DB	DA	TF ESI: M + B vs. S	12 months	TF M/B: better short-term result	38

* Randomized by patients' choice.
P, prospective; O, outcome; R, randomized; C, controlled; SB, single blind; DB, double blind; HNP, herniated nucleus pulposus; SS, spinal stenosis; FS, foraminal stenosis; DA, disc abnormality (bulging disc, contained herniated disc, extruded disc); TF ESI, transforaminal epidural steroid injection; TPI, trigger point injection; S, saline; M, methylprednisolone; B, bupivacaine.

In an outcome study 52 of 69 patients responded to the transforaminal injections.[34] The patients had lumbar HNP with radiculopathy and their average symptom duration was 22 weeks (4 to 52 weeks). To achieve the results, an average of 1.8 injections were given per patient. It was noted that the patients who had preinjection symptom duration of less than 36 weeks had 79% successful outcome.[34] Another outcome study was performed in patients with degenerative lumbar stenosis who were unresponsive to physical therapy, anti-inflammatory medications, or analgesics.[35] The injection consisted of 12 mg betamethasone and 2 mL of 1% lidocaine with an average of 1.9 injections per patient. Seventy-five percent of 34 patients had greater than 50% reduction in their pain scores, 64% had improved walking tolerance, and 57% had improved standing tolerance at 12 months after injection.[35]

Three prospective randomized studies compared transforaminal epidural steroid injections (TF ESI) with trigger point injections,[36] transforaminal epidural saline,[37] or transforaminal epidural (selective nerve root) bupivacaine.[38] In a study of 48 patients 1.5 mL each of betamethasone acetate (9 mg) and 2% xylocaine were injected in the transforaminal group compared to 3 mL trigger point saline injections in the lumbar paraspinal areas.[36] Although the study was prospective and controlled, the randomization was by patient's choice. The patients were followed at 3 weeks, 6 weeks, 3 months, 6 months, and 12 months. The success rates were statistically different: 84% (21 of 25) for the TF ESI and 48% (11 of 23) for the trigger point injections. The patients' Roland–Morris low back score increased from a mean of 9 to 22 in the transforaminal group compared to an increase from an average score of 10 to 18 in the trigger point group. The finger-to-floor distance decreased from 70 to 20 cm in the TF ESI group compared to 65 to 24 cm in the trigger point group. The improvement in the trigger point saline injection group may have been partly due to the lumbar stabilization program prescribed to all the patients studied. The lumbar stabilization

program consisted of exercises emphasizing hip and hamstring flexibility and abdominal and lumbar paraspinal strengthening.[36]

A randomized, double-blind study compared the efficacy of TF ESI in preventing lumbar spine surgery.[37] The 55 patients studied had radiographic confirmation of nerve root compression secondary to a disc herniation or spinal stenosis and were referred for back surgery. The patients either had SNRBs with bupivacaine–betamethasone or bupivacaine alone. The doses were either 1 mL 0.25% bupivacaine or 1 mL bupivacaine with 1 mL betamethasone (6 mg). Twenty-nine of the original 55 patients, who initially requested surgery before their treatments, decided not to have the operation after the injections. Of the 28 patients who had the betamethasone–bupivacaine injection, 20 decided not to proceed with the operation. This was in contrast to 9 of 27 patients in the bupivacaine group.[37]

A randomized, double-blind trial of 160 patients compared TF ESI with methylprednisolone–bupivacaine combination versus TF ESI with saline.[38] The patients had sciatica secondary to a disc abnormality: a bulge, contained disc herniation, or an extruded disc. The patients who had the steroid injection had better short-term results (immediate results and at 2 and 4 weeks) as evidenced by less leg pain and improved lumbar flexion, straight leg raise, and patient satisfaction. By the 6, 6, and 12 months follow-up, however, no differences were noted in their evaluation outcomes.[38] A subgroup analysis of this trial showed the efficacy of the steroid injection in preventing surgery in contained disc herniations but not in disc extrusions.[39]

Hyaluronidase Added to the Steroid: Defects in fibrinolytic activity have been described in failed back surgery syndrome leading to fibrin deposits and chronic inflammation.[40] This phenomenon led investigators to add hyaluronidase to the steroid and local anesthetic in patients with failed back surgery syndrome.[41,42] The rationale for the addition of hyaluronidase is to facilitate the spread of the injectate through the scar tissue. A retrospective pilot study found that the transforaminal injection of local anesthetic, 1500 u hyaluronidase, and 40 mg methylprednisolone resulted in sustained pain relief in 11 of 20 patients.[41] An open, randomized, nonblinded study[42] compared three solutions: (1) 1 mL bupivacaine 0.5% combined with 1500 u hyaluronidase and 1 mL saline per nerve root sleeve; (2) bupivacaine with 40 mg methylprednisolone; and (3) bupivacaine with methylprednisolone and hyaluronidase. The injections resulted in pain relief at 1 month. The effect, however, decreased at the 3- and 6-month follow-up. There was no statistical difference in the effects between the three combinations. The lack of added benefit from the steroid may be due to the fact the patients had nerve fibrosis (visualized on the MRI and epidurogram) and chronic nerve pathology without acute irritation.

COMPLICATIONS

Spinal injections may cause infectious, cardiovascular, neurologic, and bleeding complications. Exposure to X-ray radiation and adverse, allergic, and anaphylactic reactions to the medications and the dye are added risks. The risks that are specific to SNRBs include trauma to the spinal nerve, intrathecal injection if the needle penetrates the dural root sleeve, or segmental epidural when the medication is injected into the epidural space via the neural foramen. Trauma to the artery of Adamkiewicz may cause paraplegia[28] and trauma to the segmental artery, which travels with the nerve root, may result in segmental cord infarct. Cervical SNRBs are inherently riskier. Spinal cord trauma and vertebral artery injury are added risks. Cortical blindness and neurologic injury from the radiocontrast agent has been described.[43] While methylprednisolone can be used in lumbar selective nerve root injections, its use in cervical SNRBs is not recommended. As previously stated, methylprednisolone precipitates and, if injected through the vertebral artery, may settle in an end-artery in the brain causing a small infarct.

KEY POINTS

- Epidural steroid injections are indicated in patients with lumbosacral radiculopathy. The beneficial effect of the steroids is secondary to its anti-inflammatory effect and specific antinociceptive effect. The anti-inflammatory effect is probably related to inhibition of phospholipase A_2. Local application of methylprednisolone inhibits the transmission of impulses through the C fibers but not in the A-beta fibers.
- Epidural steroids are more effective in patients with acute lumbosacral radiculopathy. Patients with chronic radiculopathy respond to the injections better if they have a symptom-free interval or their new radiculopathy involves a nerve root different from the one involved in their previous radiculopathy.
- Pain during a SNRB is not a reliable sign that the nerve root was touched. Other structures such as the facet joint, periosteum, and annulus fibrosus may have been touched and cause referred pain to the leg.
- In the transforaminal approach the tip of the needle should be placed in the area of the "safe triangle". The "safe triangle" is bounded superiorly by the pedicle and by the outer margin of the exiting nerve root and the border of the vertebral body on either side.
- Compared to the interlaminar approach, better results are expected with the transforaminal approach. In the

transforaminal approach the drug is injected into the anterior epidural space where the herniated disc is located. In the interlaminar approach most of the drug is deposited in the posterior epidural space.
- Prospective, randomized studies showed the transforaminal approach to have better results compared to trigger point injections. Transforaminal injections with bupivacaine–methylprednisolone are better than bupivacaine or saline injections.

REFERENCES

1. Hitselberger WE, Witten RM: Abnormal myelograms in asymptomatic patients. J Neurosurg 28:204–206, 1968.
2. Boden SD, Davis DO, Dina TS, et al: Abnormal magnetic-resonance scans of the lumbar spine in asymptomatic subjects. J Bone Joint Surg 72-A, 403–408, 1990.
3. Saal JS, Franson RC, Dobrow R, et al: High levels of inflammatory phospholipase A_2 activity in lumbar disc herniations. Spine 15:674–678, 1990.
4. Franson RC, Saal JS, Saal JA: Human disc phospholipase A_2 is inflammatory. Spine 17:S129–S132, 1992.
5. Nygaard OP, Mellgren SI, Osterud B: The inflammatory properties of contained and noncontained lumbar disc herniation. Spine 22:2484–2488, 1997.
6. Olmarker K, Blomquist J, Stromberg J, et al: Inflammatogenic properties of nucleus pulposus. Spine 20:665–669, 1995.
7. McCarron RF, Wimpee MW, Hudkins PG, et al: The inflammatory effect of nucleus pulposus: A possible element in the pathogenesis of low back pain. Spine 12:760–764, 1987.
8. Olmarker K, Rydevik B, Nordborg C: Autologous nucleus pulposus induces neurophysiologic and histologic changes in porcine equine nerve roots. Spine 18:1425–1432, 1993.
9. Lee HM, Weinstein JN, Meller ST, et al: The role of steroids and their effects on phospholiapse A_2: An animal model of radiculopathy. Spine 23:1191–1196, 1998.
10. Olmarker K, Byrod G, Cornefjord M: Effects of methylprednisolone on nucleus pulposus-induced nerve root injury. Spine 19:1803–1808, 1994.
11. Johansson A, Hao J, Sjolund B: Local corticosteroid application blocks transmission in normal nociceptive C-fibres. Acta Anaesthesiol Scand 34:3353–3358, 1990.
12. Kepes ER, Duncalf D: Treatment of backache with spinal injections of local anesthetics, spinal, and systemic steroids. A review. Pain 22:33–47, 1985.
13. Benzon HT: Epidural steroid injections for low back pain and lumbosacral radiculopathy. Pain 24:277–295, 1986.
14. Watts RW, Silagy CA: A meta-analysis on the efficacy of epidural corticosteroids in the treatment of sciatica. Anaesth Intens Care 23:464–569, 1995.
15. Bogduk N: Epidural steroids. Spine 20:845–848, 1995.
16. Carette S, Leclaire R. Marcoux S, et al: Epidural corticosteroid injections for sciatica due to herniated nucleus pulposus. N Engl J Med 336:1634–1640, 1997.
17. Bush K, Cowan N, Katz D, et al: The natural history of sciatica associated with disc pathology. A prospective study with clinical and independent radiological follow-up. Spine 17:1205–1212, 1992.
18. Dooley JF, McBroom RJ, Taguchi T, Macnab I: Nerve root infiltration in the diagnosis of radicular pain. Spine 13:79–83, 1988.
19. Stanley D, McLaren MI, Euinton HA, Getty CJM: A prospective study of nerve root infiltration in the diagnosis of sciatica. A comparison with radiculography, computed tomography, and operative findings. Spine 15:540–543, 1990.
20. Akkerveeken PFV: The diagnostic value of nerve root sheath infiltration. Acta Orthop Scand 64S: 61–63, 1993.

21. Fenton DS, Czervionke LF: Selective nerve root block. *In* Fenton DS, Czervionke LF (eds): Image-Guided Spine Intervention. WB Saunders, Philadelphia, 2003, pp 73–98.

22. Raj PP, Lou L, Erdine S, Staats PS: Radiographic Imaging for Regional Anesthesia and Pain Management. Churchill Livingstone, New York, 2003, pp 61–65.

23. Alleyne CH, Cawley CM, Shengelaia GG, et al: Microsurgical anatomy of the artery of Adamkiewicz and its segmental artery. J Neurosurg 89:791–795, 1998.

24. Slipman CW, Plastaras CT, Palmitier RA, et al: Symptom provocation of fluoroscopically guided cervical nerve root stimulation. Are dynatomal maps identical to dermatomal maps? Spine 23:2235–2242, 1998.

25. Windsor RE, Falco FJE: Paraplegia following selective nerve root blocks. Int Spinal Inject Soc Newsletter 4:53, 2001

26. Irstam L: Differential diagnosis of recurrent lumbar disc herniation and post-operative deformation by myelography. Spine 9:759–763, 1984.

27. Teplick JG, Haskin ME: Computed tomography of the post-operative lumbar spine. AJR 141:865–884, 1983.

28. Furman MB: Is it really possible to do a selective nerve root block? Pain 85:526, 2000.

29. Weiner BK, Fraser RD: Foraminal injection for lateral disc herniation. J Bone Joint Surg (Br) 79:804–807, 1997.

30. Derby R, Bogduk N, Kine G: Precision percutaneous blocking procedures for localizing spinal pain: 2. The lumbar neuraxial compartment. Pain Digest 3:175–188, 1993.

31. Derby R, Kine G, Saal JA, et al: Response to steroid and duration of radicular pain as predictors of surgical outcome. Spine 17:S176–S183, 1992.

32. Stojanovic MP, Vu TN, Caneris O, et al: The role of fluoroscopy in cervical epidural steroid injections. Spine 27:509–514, 2002.

33. Pfirrmann CWA, Oberholzer PA, Zanettei M, et al: Selective nerve root blocks for the treatment of sciatica: Evaluation of injection site and effectiveness – A study with patients and cadavers. Radiology 221:704–711, 2001.

34. Lutz GE, Vad VB, Wisneski RJ: Fluoroscopic transforaminal lumbar epidural steroids: An outcome study. Arch Phys Med Rehabil 79:1362–1366, 1998.

35. Botwin KP, Gruber RD, Bouchlass CG, et al: Fluoroscopically guided lumbar transforaminal epidural steroid injections in degenerative lumbar stenosis. An outcome study. Am J Phys Med Rehabil 81:898–905, 2002.

36. Vad VB, Bhat AL, Lutz GE, Cammisa F: Transforaminal epidural steroid injections in lumbosacral radiculopathy: A prospective randomized study. Spine 27:11–15, 2002.

37. Riew RK, Yin Y, Gilula L, et al: The effect of nerve-root injections on the need for operative treatment of lumbar radicular pain: A prospective, randomized, controlled, double-blind study. J Bone Joint Surg (Am) 82:1589–1593, 2000.

38. Karppinen J, Malmivaara A, Kurulanti M, et al: Periradicular infiltration for sciatica: A randomized controlled trial. Spine 26:1059–1067, 2001.

39. Karppinen J, Ohinmaa A, Malmivaara A, et al: Cost effectiveness of periradicular infiltration for sciatica. Subgroup analysis of a randomized controlled trial. Spine 26:2587–2595, 2001.

40. Pountin G, Keegan A, Jayson M: Impaired fibrinolytic activity in defined chronic back pain syndromes. Spine 12:83–86, 1987.

41. Devulder J: Transforaminal nerve root sleeve injection with corticosteroids, hyaluronidase, and local anesthetic in the failed back surgery syndrome. J Spinal Disorders 11:151–154, 1998.

42. Devulder J, Deene P, De Laat M, et al: Nerve root sleeve injections in patients with failed back surgery syndrome: A comparison of three solutions. Clin J Pain 15:132–135, 1999.

43. McMillan MR, Crumpton C: Cortical blindness and neurologic injury complicating cervical transforaminal injection for cervical radiculopathy. Anesthesiology 99:509–511, 2003.

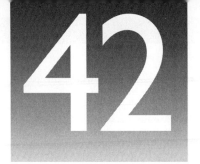

42

Facet Syndrome: Facet Joint Injections and Facet Nerve Blocks

**Rebecca Rallo Clemans, M.D., and
Honorio T. Benzon, M.D.**

ANATOMY OF THE LUMBAR FACET JOINT

The zygapophyseal (facet) joints are true synovial joints, which connect adjacent vertebrae posteriorly. The synovial membrane of the joint contains a rich supply of blood vessels and nerves. The capsule of the facet joint blends with the ligamentum flavum medially and superiorly, preventing the capsule from protruding into the spinal foramen or between the articular processes of the joint.

Each vertebra has a superior and an inferior articular process. The superior articular process of the facet joint originates from the vertebra below the joint, faces posteriorly, and forms the lateral border of the facet joint. The inferior articular process of the facet joint originates from the vertebra above the joint, faces anteriorly, and forms the medial border of the joint. A bony prominence on the superior articular process is called the mammillary process. A prominence on the transverse process, called the accessory process, is connected to the mammillary process by the mammillary-accessory ligament. This ligament forms a tunnel on the superomedial aspect of the transverse process.

The dorsal primary ramus of the spinal nerve gives off its medial and lateral branches at about the level of the intervertebral disc. The lateral branch passes into the longissimus and iliocostalis muscles of the back. The medial branch runs caudally and rostrally, lying against bone, through the tunnel formed by the mammillary-accessory ligament. The medial branch supplies the facet joint: it gives off a proximal zygapophyseal branch, which ascends through the soft tissue to innervate the joint from its caudal aspect. It then continues distally as the medial descending branch to innervate the superior and medial aspects of the facet joint below (Fig. 42-1). It can be seen from this arrangement that the facet joint receives innervation from the spinal nerve (i.e., the medial branch of the dorsal primary ramus) that exits through its adjacent intervertebral foramen and from the spinal nerve above it.

LUMBAR FACET SYNDROME

In 1911 Goldthwait recognized lumbar zygapophysial joints as a potential source of back pain. In 1933 Ghormly introduced the term "lumbar facet syndrome" to describe a typical pattern of back pain.[1] Certain features have been noted to occur in the computed tomographic scans of patients with facet syndrome. These include facet joint asymmetries, joint space narrowing, subchondral sclerosis, erosions, and facet hypertrophy.

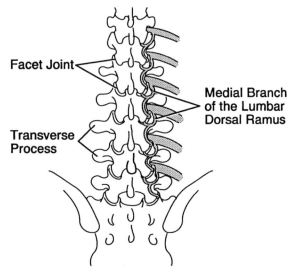

FIGURE 42-1. Innervation of the facet joint (see text for details).

However, the presence of abnormal findings in the joint on radiographic or computed tomographic studies does not imply that they are the cause of the patient's back pain.

Experimental studies on normal volunteers suggest that facet joints are capable of producing characteristic patterns of pain. Hirsch and others performed provocative tests, by infiltrating the facet joints with saline and recording volunteers' symptoms.[1,2] More recently, several authors have investigated the relationship between clinical features of facet pain and pain distribution during the course of diagnostic facet blocks. The results of most studies have shown there is no consistent pattern of pain during facet injection.[1] The correlation of physical examination to facet-related pain is not clear but most accept certain signs and symptoms to diagnose facet syndrome.

Symptoms of facet arthropathy include:

- Hip and buttock pain.
- Cramping lower extremity pain, usually not lower than the knee.
- Low back stiffness, especially in the morning.
- Pain commonly aggravated by prolonged sitting or standing.

Signs of lumbar facet arthropathy are:

- Paraspinal tenderness, worse over the affected joint.
- Pain with movements that stresses the joint, i.e., hyper-extension, lateral rotation, and side bending.
- Hip, buttock, or back pain on straight leg raising.
- Absence of signs of nerve root irritation.

In pure facet syndromes there are no signs and symptoms of nerve root irritation. There are no paresthesias, no radicular leg pain, no sensory deficits, no leg muscle weakness, no pain on flexion of the back, and there is very little limitation of straight leg raising.

LUMBAR FACET JOINT INJECTIONS

Indications: Lumbar facet joint injections are performed for therapeutic and diagnostic reasons. The patients have lumbar facet syndrome, based on the previously described criteria, not controlled by adequate rest, nonsteroidal anti-inflammatory drugs, and physical therapy. These patients do not have radiologic evidence of disc herniation, spinal stenosis, or foraminal nerve root impingement. Jackson et al. found that physical findings of normal gait, absence of muscle spasm, and pain on extension of the back correlated well with pain relief after facet joint injections.[3] Helbig and Lee proposed a scorecard to predict the probability of pain relief from facet joint injections (Table 42-1).[4] All patients with a score of 60 or higher had 100% prolonged response from a facet joint injection. A score of 40 points or higher predicted 78% prolonged response. It should be noted that the therapeutic role of facet injections remains controversial and has not been validated in acute or chronic low back pain. Most acute low back pain episodes improve within 3 weeks; therefore, injections should be limited to those who have failed conservative management for 4 to 6 weeks.[5]

Most studies have found that facet injections provide temporary relief. The current recommendations suggest the primary role of facet injection (intra-articular or medial branch block) to be diagnostic. These procedures may facilitate the

TABLE 42-1. HELBIG AND LEE SCORECARD FOR PROBABILITY OF PAIN RELIEF WITH FACET JOINT INJECTIONS

Back pain associated with groin or thigh pain	+30 points
Reproduction of pain with extension-rotation	+30 points
Well-localized paraspinal tenderness	+20 points
Significant corresponding radiographic changes	+20 points
Pain below the knee	–10 points
TOTAL	100 points

From Helbig T, Lee CK: The lumbar facet syndrome. Spine 13:61, 1988.

diagnosis of facet syndrome and help predict if the patient would benefit from more permanent measures, such as facet rhizotomy.

Diagnostic facet joint block, either with intra-articular injection or medial branch block, is reproducible.[6] Most accept these blocks as the standard for diagnosis of zygapophyseal joint pain;[5] however, spillover and false positive results may occur. Therefore, when diagnosing facet syndrome, some consider the gold standard to be the demonstration of longer-term relief of back pain after denervation procedure and prior short-term relief with diagnostic block (either joint injection or medial branch block). Because of the high false positive results from a single diagnostic block, it is necessary to show positive response from diagnostic block as well as long-term relief from therapeutic rhizotomy before facet syndrome can be reliably diagnosed.[7]

Technique: If no localizing signs are evident, the recommended sites of injection are the L4–5 and L5–S1 facet joints (ipsilateral for unilateral back pain or bilateral injections for bilateral pain) as these are most commonly affected.[5,8] The technique is simple and can be done as an outpatient procedure. The procedure is done under fluoroscopic guidance. The patient is placed prone with a pillow underneath the abdomen. After the back is prepared and draped, the desired joint is visualized under fluoroscopy. The fluoroscope beam is rotated obliquely 10° to 40° to get the best image of the joint space. The lumbar facets are situated so that the superior aspect of the joint is further anterior than the inferior aspect of the joint.[9] A 22-gauge spinal needle is inserted into the joint (Fig. 42-2). A mixture of a local anesthetic agent (1 to 2 mL), either lidocaine or bupivacaine, and 20 to 40 mg of methylprednisolone acetate (Depo-Medrol) is injected into each of the designated facet joints.

Outcome Studies: Lilius and co-workers studied 109 patients and compared results of three treatments: (1) cortisone (80 mg of methylprednisolone acetate) plus local anesthetic (6 mL of bupivacaine) injected into each of two facet joints; (2) cortisone plus local anesthetic injected pericapsularly around the two

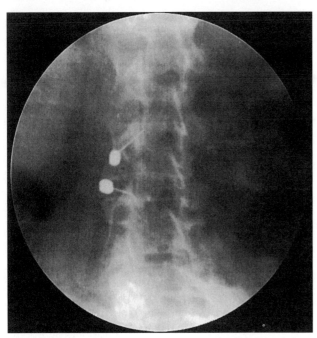

FIGURE 42-2. X-ray showing needles in the facet joints.

joints; and (3) 8 mL of saline injected into the two joints.[10] Their selection criteria included back pain localized to one side, tenderness and muscle spasm over the facet joint, pain radiating to the posterior thigh, and negative straight leg raising. Although there was significant improvement in pain relief (36% had continued pain relief at 3 months), in work attendance, and in disability scores, improvement was independent of the type of treatment given. Although the study was randomized and controlled, it was flawed by the excessive volume injected. This large amount may extravasate from or break the joint capsule (the capacity of the joint is 1 to 2 mL) and would likely produce a high false positive result.

Another study is that of Carette and colleagues.[11] In phase I of the study 2 mL of 1% lidocaine was injected into the L4–5 and L5–S1 facet joints of patients with back pain. Patients with more than 50% relief were enrolled in phase II of the study. In phase II methylprednisolone (20 mg of methylprednisolone acetate mixed with 1 mL of isotonic saline) was injected into the L4–5 and L5–S1 facet joints of patients in the treatment group, whereas the control group received placebo (2 mL of isotonic saline). Follow-up evaluations were performed at 1, 3, and 6 months after injection. Evaluation criteria included relief of pain, functional status, and improvement in movements of the spine. At 1 month postinjection, 20 (42%) of the methylprednisolone group had substantial pain reduction compared to 16 (33%) of the saline group. This difference was not statistically significant.[11] At 6 months postinjection, 46% of the patients in the methylprednisolone group reported improvement, less pain, less physical disability, and greater improvement in spine movement compared with 15% in the placebo group. These differences were reduced when concurrent interventions (epidural steroid injections, antidepressant medications, and physical therapy) were taken into account, to 31% in the methylprednisolone group vs. 13% in the placebo group.

The study by Carette and colleagues did not have strict selection criteria; any patient with low back pain was eligible for inclusion in phase I of their study. Most importantly, they did not control for the concurrent treatments of their patients which were employed almost twice as frequently in the methylprednisolone group. Their conclusion that intra-articular steroid injections in facet joints "have very little efficacy in patients with low back pain" awaits additional randomized studies.[5,11]

Although facet joint injections are routinely used, no study to date has fulfilled the following criteria: prospective, randomized, controlled, with strict selection criteria, and strict adherence to guidelines (e.g., restriction of other treatments) during the administration of the study.

MEDIAL BRANCH BLOCKS

For diagnostic and therapeutic purposes there appears to be no significant difference between facet joint injection and medial branch blocks.[12] Marks et al. compared the effects of intra-articular injection vs. medial branch blocks and concluded that these blocks may be of equal value as diagnostic tests, but neither is a satisfactory treatment for chronic low back pain.[12] Some authors have proposed lumbar medial branch nerve blocks to be a more accurate tool to diagnose lumbar facet syndrome[6] and to predict the success of denervation of the joints by radiofrequency ablation.

To perform the block, the patient is placed prone on the fluoroscopy table and a slight oblique view obtained. A spinal needle is inserted approximately 5 cm from midline and directed obliquely down the X-ray beam. At levels L1–4 the medial branch block is done by targeting the junction of the upper

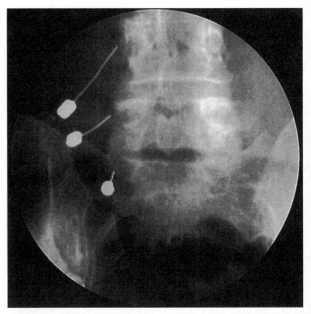

FIGURE 42-3. X-ray showing needles at the junction of the transverse process and the superior articular process of the facet joint. The lowest needle is at the ala of the sacrum along the course of the facet nerve, on its way to the L5–S1 facet joint. The needle positions are acceptable for diagnostic blocks with local anesthetic. For radiofrequency facet denervation, an oblique view should be obtained to confirm the needle position at the leading edge of the superior and medial border of the transverse process.

border of the transverse process and the superior articular process (Fig. 42-3). This is done at two levels for each joint in question (e.g., for the L4–5 joint, the junction of the superior articular process and transverse process of L4 and L5 would be targeted). The L5 posterior primary ramus is blocked in the groove between the ala of the sacrum and the superior articular process of S1.[9] For completeness, if the L5–S1 joint is targeted, the block should be performed at the transverse process of L5; the junction of the ala of the sacrum and the superior articular process of S1; and the S1 nerve should also be blocked.[9] For diagnostic purposes a small amount of local anesthetic is used (0.5 to 1 cm³) to avoid unwanted spread of the injectate. If the block is being done for therapeutic reasons larger volumes may be used.

RADIOFREQUENCY PROCEDURES

Prior to considering ablation, a thorough history and physical examination should be obtained and radiographic studies reviewed. Because of the nonspecific symptoms and lack of radiographic confirmation, diagnostic facet blocks (either medial branch blocks or injection of local anesthetic into the joint) should precede all radiofrequency (RF) facet denervation.[8] Patients who exhibit consistent relief from the medial branch block or facet injection but whose relief is temporary should be considered for a RF ablation of the facet nerve.

RF lesion technology has been developing since the 1950s. Rees, by surgically cutting the medial branch nerves supplying the suspected joint, first demonstrated denervation of the facet joint in 1971. Shealy modified the technique using percutaneous RF to destroy the nerve.[13] The modern RF system includes temperature display, impedance monitor, stimulator, and lesion generator. The RF generator is the source of voltage to the active (lesion) electrode. When the reference (dispersive) electrode is placed on the patient's body a circuit is completed. This establishes lines of an electric field within the patient's body between the two electrodes. The RF voltage generates an electric field in space around the exposed electrode tip. In this way the tissue surrounding the tip is heated but not the tip itself.[14] At the low frequencies used for this procedure (<1 MHz), the mechanism for tissue heating is primarily ionic.[14] Essentially, the electric field oscillates with the alternating RF current causing movement of ions in the tissue. Heat is produced by friction, or resistive energy loss caused by the motion from the ionic current.[14]

Cell death occurs by thermal coagulation necrosis, a result of tissue heating. Cellular homeostasis is maintained at temperatures up to approximately 40°C. When temperatures are elevated to hyperthermic range (42 to 45°C), cells become more susceptible to damage. When temperatures between 60 and 100°C are reached there is near instantaneous induction of protein coagulation. This causes irreversible damage of cytosolic and mitochondrial enzymes, as well as nucleic acid–histone protein complexes.[14] Recently the mechanism of action of RF has been debated. The formation of heat is not the only occurrence during RF treatment. The tissue surrounding the electrode is exposed to an electric field and it may be this exposure that causes changes in gene expression in the affected tissue.[15]

Quantifiable, reproducible lesions can be made from one patient to another by selecting the appropriate temperature and electrode tip size.[14] Temperature is the fundamental determinant of lesion size and must be monitored. The RF current heats the tissue, which, in turn, heats the electrode tip. In this way monitoring the tip temperature allows continuous tissue temperature measurement.[9]

Reports differ as to which nerve fibers are affected by RF lesions. Some investigators[16,17] found a selective effect of heat on small myelinated and unmyelinated nerve fibers. Smith et al. studied effects on peripheral nerves after exposure to RF lesions at different temperatures for different time intervals and found uniform destruction of both small and large fibers.[18]

Pulsed radiofrequency (PRF) is a non-neurodestructive technique, which removes the complications of heat lesioning. In PRF high-frequency current is applied in bursts of 20 ms with a silent time of 480 ms at temperatures not exceeding 42°C, allowing the elimination of heat.[19,20] The method of PRF is based on the concept that the production of heat is only a byproduct of RF treatment and that the clinical effect is due to tissue exposure to the electromagnetic field itself. Thus, an RF lesion can be accomplished without high temperatures.[15] It has been postulated that PRF modulates pain-processing mechanisms at the dorsal root ganglion, dorsal horn, and molecular levels. Another possibility is that the high-frequency component of the PRF signal may be important to the induction of long-term depression in the spinal cord.[21] A third explanation is that PRF works in a similar manner to transcutaneous nerve stimulation, activating both spinal and supraspinal mechanisms, which reduce pain perception.[21] The precise mode of action is unknown at this time.[22]

RF lesioning in the treatment of pain is still a subject of debate. For indications in which heat carries a potential risk or is contraindicated (such as peripheral nerves or in neuropathic pain),[23] the use of PRF is preferred.[24] As for the medial branch nerves, controlled studies are available and support the effectiveness of heat lesions.[20] PRF for lumbar facet rhizotomy appears to be of shorter duration (approximately 4 months) compared to thermal RF (up to 1 year). Thermal RF also denervates the multifidus muscle which would eliminate most of the muscular component of lumbar facet syndrome.[20] Therefore, it is recommended that the traditional thermal RF technique performed in lumbar facet syndrome should not be changed until further studies have been completed.[15,20]

Technique: The patient is positioned prone and the C-arm is positioned in a slightly oblique position. The medial branch nerve is found at the junction of the superior edge of the transverse process and the lateral aspect of the superior articular process at L1–4. The L5 dorsal ramus is found at the junction of the ala of the sacrum and articular process of S1 (this is the first of the typical targets for facet rhizotomy). The second and third common targets are the superior and medial aspects of the transverse processes at L5 and L4. A 22-gauge cannula with a 5 mm active tip is introduced at each entry point and advanced under fluoroscopic guidance until contact is made with bone. The stylet of the cannula is then replaced with a RF probe. The electrical impedance should be checked, as this is a good method for measuring the integrity of the system.

Electrical stimulation at 50 Hz should produce sensory stimulation at less than 1 V if the cannula is placed correctly. Stimulation at 2 Hz should evoke contraction of ipsilateral paraspinal muscles (the multifidus muscles) but not cause contractions in the appropriate limb musculature below 2.5 V. This indicates a safe but effective distance between electrode tip and anterior ramus.[9,25] Once the electrode tip is suitably positioned, 1 cm³ of local anesthetic is injected. A lesion is then made at each site, starting at 80°C for 90 seconds.

Nerve regeneration and pain recurrence after months to a few years is to be expected.[25] Studies have shown RF ablation to be a safe, simple, and reliable method of temporarily relieving pain originating in facet joints.

Outcome Studies: The results from RF facet denervation vary greatly. Most studies report 45% to 80% success rate.[8] North et al. did a retrospective review of the prognostic factors for response to facet joint rhizotomy and found that at 2 years 42% of patients with successful diagnostic facet block had clinical improvement vs. 13% of patients who did not have the denervation procedure.[13] This suggests that rhizotomy is a worthwhile procedure that may produce long-term results.

Van Kleef et al.[26] conducted a randomized, controlled, double-blind trial of the effect of RF lumbar zygapophysial joint denervation for chronic low back pain. After demonstrating at least 50% reduction in pain relief after medial branch blocks, patients were eligible to participate in a double-blind randomized trial. Patients in group I were treated with a 60 second RF lesion of 80°C of the medial branch of the posterior primary ramus on one or both sides. In group II electrodes were introduced but no RF lesion was made. Success was defined as at least 50% pain reduction on global perceived effect and at least a 2-point reduction on the visual analogue scale (VAS). Assessment was conducted at 3, 6, and 12 months after the procedure. The numbers of successes in the sham group at the 3-, 6-, and 12-month assessment periods were 4, 3, and 2 out of 16 patients. The corresponding numbers in the lesion group were 9, 7, and 7 out of 15 patients. This study also showed a reduction in the intake of analgesics and improvement in disability scores.[26]

CERVICAL FACET SYNDROME

The symptoms of cervical facet syndrome include the following:[27,28]

- Neck pain.
- Headache.
- Shoulder pain.
- Suprascapular pain.
- Scapula pain.
- Upper arm pain.

The physical findings may include the following:[27]

- Decreased range of motion of the neck.
- Pain on dorsiflexion.
- Decreased discomfort with forward flexion.
- Tenderness over the affected joint.

The selection of the affected cervical facet joint is difficult and is based primarily on the distribution of the pain (Table 42-2).[29,30]

CERVICAL FACET INJECTIONS

Cervical intra-articular corticosteroid injections have not been shown to be beneficial as a therapeutic treatment.[31] However, cervical facet blocks can be helpful in identifying patients with

TABLE 42-2. DISTRIBUTION OF PAIN OF CERVICAL FACET JOINT ORIGIN

Joint	Distribution
C2–3	Occiput and cervical spine
C3–4	Neck
C4–5	Lateral aspect of the nape of the neck (Dory) and shoulder (Wedel and Wilson)
C5–6	Arm (Wedel and Wilson)
C6–7	Shoulder or upper dorsum as far down as the scapula (Dory)

Adapted from Dory DA: Arthrography of the cervical facet joints. Radiology 148:379, 1983; Wedel DJ, Wilson PR: Cervical facet arthrography. Reg Anesth 10:7, 1985.

cervical facet syndrome. These patients may then be considered for more permanent treatments such as rhizotomy.[32]

Joint Injection: The anatomy of the cervical facets is quite different from that of the lumbar facets. The atlanto-occipital (C0–1) and atlantoaxial joints (C1–2) are innervated by C1 and C2 ventral rami. Therefore the only interventional procedure for these joints is intra-articular injection.[9]

Cervical facet joints can be injected with the patient prone or supine. A lateral and an anteroposterior fluoroscopic view of the appropriate facet joint are obtained. The area is prepared and draped and a 22-gauge spinal needle is advanced under fluoroscopic control (lateral view) into the joint capsule. It must be emphasized that the insertion of the needle should be done carefully and the direction of the needle rechecked by serial fluoroscopy. Once the needle is in the joint, an anteroposterior view is taken to make sure that the needle is not inserted too deep inside the joint. Triamcinolone diacetate (20 to 40 mg) in 0.5 to 1 mL saline or local anesthetic (e.g., 0.5% lidocaine) is injected into each joint. Note that methylprednisolone is not recommended for cervical facet joint injections. The drug precipitates and its unintentional injection into the vertebral artery and into the brain may have serious consequences (e.g., cerebral embolism).

Outcome Studies: Barnsley and co-workers[31] looked into the efficacy of cervical facet joint injections. Patients enrolled in their study had previously responded to facet nerve blocks. The therapeutic part of the study was conducted in a double-blind fashion, with either 1 mL (5.7 mg) of betamethasone or 1 mL of 0.5% bupivacaine injected into the affected joint. They found that patients' pain was substantially reduced initially but returned to its usual level after 1 to 2 days. The median time for return to 50% of the preinjection level of pain was the same in both groups (3 to 3.5 days). Their conclusion was that intra-articular betamethasone is not an effective treatment of cervical facet pain.[31] The study of Barnsley et al. lacked a true control (placebo) group. However, this study has been the basis for criticism of cervical facet joint injections for therapeutic purposes and the reason that performance of a "series" of joint injections has been questioned.[8]

MEDIAL BRANCH BLOCKS

Medial branch blocks assist in the diagnosis of cervical facet joint pain. They may also be used, with varying results, in therapeutic efforts to treat head and neck pain. The C2–3 facet joint is innervated mainly by the third occipital nerve (medial branch of the C3 dorsal ramus) with an inconsistent contribution from the greater occipital nerve (one of five branches off the C2 dorsal ramus). The innervation of this joint is complex but most support the thought that blocking the third occipital nerve at the C3 articular pillar effectively denervates the joint.[9] Cervical facets from C3 to T1 are supplied by medial branches of the dorsal rami above and at the same level as the joint (e.g., C3–4 is innervated by the C3 and C4 medial branch nerves).[9]

Some authors suggest the patient be positioned laterally with the side to be blocked uppermost. Others perform the procedure with the patient in the prone position, to minimize spinal cord trauma, or the supine position for better patient comfort and easier access to the airway if the patient becomes too sedated. It should be noted that it is difficult to perform blockade below C5 with the patient in the supine position because the patient's shoulder blocks visualization of, and access to, the area.

The area is prepared and draped. Under fluoroscopic guidance a 22-gauge spinal needle is inserted. Again, it should be emphasized that insertion of the needle should be done carefully and serial fluoroscopy views be taken during advancement of the needle to ascertain the depth and correct direction of the needle. For each level from C3 to T1, the needle is advanced to the central part of the projection of the articular pillar, as seen on the lateral view. The target area on the anteroposterior view is the central part ("waist") of the articular pillar (Fig. 42-4). Once the needle position is confirmed and aspiration is negative, 0.5 to 1 mL of local anesthetic is injected.[33]

Some studies found medial branch blocks at C2–3 to be ineffective, likely due to malposition and technical difficulty of needle placement at this level.[34] Using fluoroscopic guidance, the needle is advanced using a posterolateral approach until it contacts the C2–3 facet joint. The target points are three injections: placed vertically over the joint line, immediately above the inferior articular facet surface of C2, and immediately below the superior articular facet surface of C3.[33] At each of the sites 0.5 mL of local anesthetic is injected.

Outcome Studies: Lord et al. showed comparative blocks done with two local anesthetics of different duration and with saline.[7] A positive result was diagnosed in patients that had relief for a time period that corresponded to the local anesthetic used. The specificity of a positive result using this method was 85% in diagnosing facet joint pain but only 54% sensitivity. This number of false negative results can be improved by including all patients with reproducible relief irrespective of the duration. Using this method, sensitivity increased to 100% but specificity decreased to 65%.

Medial branch blocks, rather than intra-articular injections, have been recommended in the cervical area. Some of the reasons include: technical difficulty of intra-articular blocks; medial branch blocks target the nerve, with the endpoint being articular pillar while intra-articular injections have an increased risk

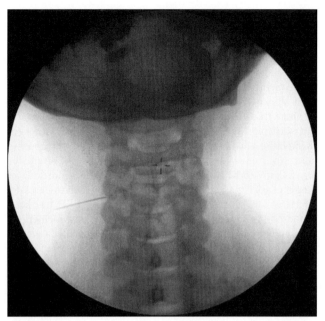

FIGURE 42-4. Anteroposterior view showing correct placement of the needle in cervical medial branch block. Note that the tip of the needle is at the "waist" of the articular pillar.

of advancing the needle into hazardous structures (vertebral artery, epidural space, dural sac).

Radiofrequency: The probe should ideally be placed parallel to the nerve to have a wider area of denervation. To facilitate this, some recommend the patient to be in the prone position. Two skin entry points are used, one directly anteroposterior and the second angled 30° and cephalad. A direct anteroposterior approach can be painful to the patient since the paraspinal muscles are traversed during the insertion of the needle.

A 10 cm 22-gauge electrode with a 4 mm exposed tip is introduced percutaneously, under fluoroscopic guidance to contact each of the two nerves supplying the painful joint. For each nerve the electrode is introduced twice in order to reach the nerve over the anterolateral aspect of the pillar. At each location 2 to 3 lesions should be made: at the target point and 1 mm cephalad and 1 mm caudad from the ideal target point to accommodate possible variation in the course of the nerve.[32]

Outcome Studies: Some randomized, double-blinded trials have shown longer duration of pain relief in the active lesion groups.[8] Lord et al. studied patients with chronic cervical facet pain confirmed by double-blind, placebo-controlled local anesthetic medial branch block. Patients were randomized to have either cervical rhizotomy or a sham procedure. This study demonstrated that median time before return of 50% of the preoperative pain was 263 days in the treatment group and 8 days in the placebo group.[32]

Another study by Sapir et al. showed a statistically significant decrease in VAS in patients who had cervical medial branch neurotomy after failing conservative therapy. Patients had a decrease in VAS of 5.7 after study and at 1 year VAS remained 4.6 below baseline.[27]

CONCLUSION

Facet syndrome is a difficult diagnosis to make due to inconsistent signs and symptoms. Presently there are no pathognomonic, radiographic, historical, or physical examination findings that conclusively diagnose facet pain. Diagnostic blocks have been shown to be a reliable tool in diagnosis and may help facilitate treatment for this problem. Medial branch blocks and intra-articular injections have not had reproducible success in therapeutic treatment but are most valuable in diagnosing facet syndrome. Choosing candidates wisely is important for any therapy to be successful. With the use of diagnostic facet blocks to select patients, rhizotomy has been shown to be a safe, effective, long-term treatment for facet pain. PRF has been proposed as a superior technique in treatment of some peripheral nerve pain syndromes. However, for medial branch neurotomy, heat lesions have been shown to be effective in controlled studies. Therefore, thermal RF continues to be the recommended treatment for zygapophyseal joint pain.

KEY POINTS

- The medial branch is a branch of the dorsal primary ramus of the spinal nerve. The medial branch gives off a proximal zygapophyseal branch which innervates the joint from its caudal aspect. It then continues distally as the medial descending branch to innervate the superior and medial aspects of the facet joint below. It can be seen that the facet joint receives innervation from the spinal nerve (i.e., the medial branch of the dorsal primary ramus) that exits through its adjacent intervertebral foramen and from the spinal nerve above it.
- The symptoms of facet arthropathy include: (1) hip and buttock pain; (2) cramping lower extremity pain, usually above the knee; (3) low back stiffness, especially in the morning; and (4) pain commonly aggravated by prolonged sitting or standing.
- The signs of lumbar facet arthropathy include: (1) paraspinal tenderness, worse over the affected joint; (2) pain with movements that stresses the joint, i.e., hyperextension, lateral rotation, and side bending; (3) hip, buttock, or back pain on straight leg raising; and (4) absence of signs of nerve root irritation.
- Most studies have found that facet injections provide temporary relief. The current recommendations suggest the primary role of facet injections (intra-articular or medial branch block) to be diagnostic. Some consider the gold standard to be the demonstration of short-term relief with diagnostic block (either joint injection or medial branch block) followed by long-term relief after facet denervation as diagnostic of facet syndrome.
- Although facet joint injections are routinely used, there has been no prospective, randomized, controlled study that included strict selection criteria and strict adherence to guidelines (e.g., restriction of other treatments) during the administration of the study.
- The selection of the affected cervical facet joint is difficult and selection is based primarily on the distribution of the pain (see Table 42-2).
- Studies showed the efficacy of cervical facet nerve rhizotomy, after diagnostic local anesthetic blocks, in cervical facet syndrome.
- PRF is a new RF technique that is not neurodestructive. Studies showed its promise in peripheral lesions. The duration of relief in patients who had lumbar facet rhizotomy is shorter after PRF than after thermal RF.

REFERENCES

1. Cho J, Park YG, Chung SS: Percutaneous radiofrequecncy lumbar facet rhizotomy in mechanical low back pain syndrome. Steriotact Funct Neurosurg 68:212–217, 1997.
2. Hirsch C, Ingelmark VE, Miller N: The anatomic basis for low back pain: Studies on the presence of sensory endings in ligamentous capsular and intervertebral disc structures in the human lumbar spine. Acta Orthop Scand 33:1–17, 1963.
3. Jackson RP, Jacobs RR, Montesano PX: Facet joint injection in low back pain: A prospective statistical study. Spine 13:966, 1988.
4. Helbig T, Lee CK: The lumbar facet syndrome. Spine 13:61, 1988.
5. Dreyfuss PH, Dreyer SJ, Stanley JA: Contemporary concepts in spine care lumbar zygapophysial (facet) joint injections. Spine 20:2040–2047, 1995.
6. Saal JS: General principles of diagnostic testing as related to painful lumbar spine disorders. Spine 27:2538–2545, 2002.
7. Lord SM, Barnsley L, Bogduk N: The utility of comparative local anesthetic blocks versus placebo-controlled blocks for the diagnosis of cervical zygapophysial joint pain. Clin J Pain 11:208–213, 1995.
8. Whitworth L, Feler C: Application of spinal ablative techniques for the treatment of benign chronic painful conditions: History, methods and outcomes. Spine 27:2607–2612, 2002.
9. Gray D, Zahid B, Warfield C: Facet block and neurolysis. In Waldman SD (ed): Interventional Pain Management, ed 2. WB Saunders, New York, 2001, pp 446–483.
10. Lilius G, Laasonen EM, Myllynen P, et al: Lumbar facet joint syndrome: A randomized clinical trial. J Bone Joint Surg (Br) 71:681, 1989.
11. Carette S, Marcoux S, Truchon R, et al: A controlled trial of corticosteroid injections into the facet joints for chronic low back pain. New Engl J Med 325:1002–1007, 1991.
12. Marks FC, Houston T, Thulbourne T: Facet joint injection and facet nerve block: Randomized comparison in 86 patients with chronic low back pain. Pain 49:325–328, 1992.
13. North R, Han M, Zahurak M, Kidd D: Radiofrequency lumbar facet denervation: Analysis of prognostic factors. Pain 57:77–83, 1994.
14. Goldberg S, Dupuy D: Image-guided radiofrequency tumor ablation: Challenges and opportunities – Part I. J Vascular Interven Radiol 12:1021–1032, 2001.
15. Sluijter M, Racz G: Technical aspects of radiofrequency. Pain Practice 2:195–200, 2002.
16. van Kleef M, Liem L, Lousberg R, et al: Radiofrequency lesion adjacent to the dorsal root ganglion for cervicobrachial pain: A prospective double blind randomized study. Neurosurgery 38:1127–1132, 1996.
17. Letcher FS, Goldring S: The effect of radiofrequency current and heat on peripheral nerve action potential in the cat. J Neurosurg 22:42–47, 1986.
18. Smith HP, McWhorter JM, Challa VR: Radiofrequency neurolysis in a clinical model. Neuropathological correlation. J Neurosurg 55:246–253, 1981.
19. Van Zunder J, Brabant S, Van de Kelft E, Van Buyetn JP: Pulsed radiofrequency treatment of the Gasserian ganglion in patients with idiopathic trigeminal neuralgia. Pain 104:449–452, 2003.
20. Mikeladze G, Espinal R, Finnegan R, et al: Pulsed radiofrequency application in treatment of chronic zygapophyseal joint pain. Spine J 3:360–362, 2003.

21. Munglani R: The longer term effect of pulsed radiofrequency for neuropathic pain. Pain 80:437–439, 1999.

22. Kuthuru MR, Kabbara AI, Boswell MV: Pulsed radiofrequency ablation of frontal and supraorbital nerves for postherpetic neuralgia: A case report. Reg Anesth Pain Med 28:A56, 2003.

23. Sluijter ME: The role of radiofrequency in failed back surgery patients. Curr Rev Pain 4:49–53, 2000.

24. Cohen SP, Foster A: Pulsed radiofrequency as a treatment for groin pain and orchialgia. Urology 61:645–649, 2003.

25. Tzaan W, Tasker R: Percutaneous radiofrequency facet rhizotomy – Experience with 118 procedures and reappraisal of its value. Can J Neurol Sci 27:125–130, 2000.

26. van Kleef M, Barendse GA, Kessels A, et al: Randomized trial of radiofrequency lumbar facet denervation for chronic low back pain. Spine 24:1937–1942, 1999.

27. Sapir DA, Gorup JM: Radiofrequency medial branch neurotomy in litigant and nonlitigant patients with cervical whiplash: A prospective study. Spine 26:e268–e273, 2001.

28. Sei F, Kiyoshige O, Masahiro S, et al: Referred pain distribution of the cervical zygapophyseal joints and cervical dorsal rami. Pain 68:79–83, 1996.

29. Dory DA: Arthrography of the cervical facet joints. Radiology 148:379, 1983.

30. Wedel DJ, Wilson PR: Cervical facet arthrography. Reg Anesth 10:7, 1985.

31. Barnsley L, Lord S, Wallis B, Bogduk N: Lack of effect of intra-articular corticosteroids for chronic pain in the cervical zygapophyseal joints. New Engl J Med 330:1047–1050, 1994.

32. Lord SM, Barnsley L, Wallis B, et al: Percutaneous radiofrequency neurotomy for chronic cervical zygapophyseal-joint pain. New Engl J Med 335:1721–1726, 1996.

33. Barnsley L, Bogduk N: Medial branch blocks are specific for the diagnosis of cervical zygapophyseal joint pain. Reg Anesth 18:343–350, 1993.

34. Lord SM, Barnsley L, Bogduk N: Percutaneous radiofrequency neurotomy in the treatment of cervical zygapophysial joint pain: A caution. Neurosurgery 36:732–739, 1995.

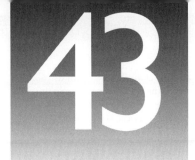

Pain Originating from the Buttock: Sacroiliac Joint Dysfunction and Piriformis Syndrome

Honorio T. Benzon, M.D.

ANATOMY OF THE SACROILIAC JOINT

The sacroiliac joint is considered a diarthrodial joint since it contains synovial fluid, the articulating bones have ligamentous connections, the outer fibrous joint capsule has an inner synovial lining, and the cartilaginous surfaces allow motion to occur.[1] The sacral side of the joint is thicker and made up of hyaline cartilage while the iliac side is made up of thin fibrocartilage, the tissue looks like fibrous cartilage but biochemically consists mostly of type II collagen typical of hyaline cartilage. (Type I collagen is found in fibrocartilage while type II collagen is found in hyaline cartilage.) The adult joint has an irregular and coarse surface and these irregularities increase with age, reflecting the stresses and strains to which the joint is exposed.[2] The ridges and depressions provide a significantly higher coefficient of friction than any other human joint.[1] The irregular contour of the joint contributes to the stability of the sacroiliac joint; it facilitates vertical load bearing but limits movement of the joint. The function of the joint is to transmit or dissipate the loading of the upper trunk to the lower extremities.

The presence of accessory or "axial" sacroiliac joints has been reported.[3] The incidence of its occurrence is between 8% and 40% and more prevalent in males. Accessory joints are located at the level of the sacral crest, at the first and sacral foramina, on the ilium at the medial surface of the posterior superior iliac spine, and on the sacral tuberosity. These accessory joints undergo pathologic changes such as arthritis and ankylosis and may contribute to sacroiliac joint dysfunction. Since the innervation of these joints is not known, the pain referral patterns from pathologic involvement of these joints are also not known.

Ligaments are located anterior and posterior to the joint. These include the anterior sacroiliac ligament that traverses the ilium to the sacrum, the interosseous ligaments, and the posterior sacroiliac ligament that traverses the posterior iliac ridge to the sacrum. The interosseous sacroiliac joint ligament is responsible for the stability of the joint. The sacrotuberous ligament, which is superficial to the posterior sacroiliac ligament, has multiple muscle attachments (e.g., gluteus maximus, piriformis, long head of the biceps femoris). These multiple muscle attachments provide a potential for activities such as walking, sitting, and standing to stress the sacroiliac joint.[1]

The sacroiliac joint has a wide range of segmental innervation. Posteriorly, the joint is innervated by the lateral branches of the posterior primary ramus of the L4 to S3 nerve roots. The anterior innervation is from L2 to S2. The nerve supply of the joint is variable and the extensive innervation accounts for the multiple manifestations and variable referred pain patterns of sacroiliac joint pain.[4] The blood supply of the joint comes from the anastomosis between the median sacral artery and the lateral sacral branches from the internal iliac artery.

Degenerative changes occur within the joint. These affect the iliac side by the third decade of life and the sacral side by the fifth decade of life. These changes affect men more than women. There is increased mobility of the sacroiliac joint during pregnancy and this may be related to the hormone relaxin. Relaxin is produced by the corpus luteum. It decreases the strength and rigidity of collagen and alters the ground substance by decreasing the viscosity and increasing the water content. These changes result in the relaxation of the ligaments.

SACROILIAC JOINT DYSFUNCTION

The pathologic conditions affecting the sacroiliac joint include infectious, inflammatory, degenerative, traumatic, metabolic, tumor, and iatrogenic conditions, and sacroiliac joint syndrome. Sacroiliac joint dysfunction is pain from a sacroiliac joint that has no demonstrable lesion and is presumed to have some type of biochemical abnormality that causes the pain.[5] It is diagnosed by detecting abnormalities on physical examination.

In patients with low back pain, the incidence of sacroiliac joint dysfunction ranges from 13% to 30%. The pain can be dull, sharp, or aching in character. A common initiating event is a history of lifting a heavy object while in a twisted position or misstep off a curb.[1] The pain is aggravated by sitting, bending, or riding in a car and is relieved by walking or standing. There is no numbness, weakness, paresthesia, or dysesthesia. The pain is usually located in the posterior sacroiliac joint and medial buttock with some referral to a distal area. The pain may be referred to the groin, posterior thigh, and occasionally below the knee.[4] Pain in sacroiliac joint dysfunction does not originate in the lumbar area as in facet syndrome and rarely radiates below the knee as in a herniated disc.

The pain referral maps from injection of the sacroiliac joint have been investigated.[6] Fortin et al. injected the sacroiliac joint in asymptomatic volunteers and noted the pain referral patterns on injection. The sensation was felt directly around the injection site and the surrounding gluteal area. The subsequent injection of lidocaine resulted in sensory changes localized to the medial buttock inferior to the posterior superior iliac spine, lateral aspect of the buttock extending to the superior aspect of the greater trochanter, and further extension into the superior lateral thigh.[6] They compiled these pain patterns into one composite pattern which included the area common to all the volunteers: an area approximately 3 cm × 10 cm just inferior to the posterior superior iliac spine. In a subsequent study, the investigators determined the applicability of the pain referral map as a screening tool in sacroiliac joint dysfunction.[7] Patients with pain patterns similar to the composite pain pattern were selected. The patients with pain diagrams consistent with sacroiliac joint pain had a positive provocative response on injection of their sacroiliac joint. Bupivacaine 0.75% was injected into the sacroiliac joint after injection of the dye and the analgesic response of the patients were noted. The responses of the patients were extremely variable: 14 of the 16 patients had an improvement while 2 had exacerbation of their pain. Two patients had complete relief of their pain and 10 of the 16 patients had at least 50% reduction of their symptoms.[7] Fortin attributed the variable referral patterns of the patients to the multiple nerve root innervation of the sacroiliac joint.

The pain referral patterns of sacroiliac joint dysfunction, the validity of pain provocation on injection, and the response of patients to sacroiliac joint injection were investigated by Schwarzer et al.[8] Forty-three patients with chronic low back pain below L5–S1 were studied. The character and distribution of the pain during injection of the contrast medium and the response to subsequent injection of 2% lidocaine were noted. Seventeen of the 43 patients had exact reproduction of their pain on injection, and 13 patients obtained definite pain relief after the local anesthetic injection. There was an association, but not a significant statistical correlation, between the provocation of pain on injection of the contrast medium and relief of pain after the injection of lidocaine. Failure to reproduce pain and provocation of pain dissimilar to the pain of the patient were predictive of failure to relieve pain. There was a correlation between ventral capsular tears of the joint and relief of pain after the local anesthetic injection. From their results, they concluded that the provocation test, i.e., reproduction of pain upon distending the joint, does not apply to the sacroiliac joint. The reproduction of the exact pain occurred in patients who obtained pain relief upon blocking the joint and also in those who did not obtain relief.

The distinguishing feature of the pain patterns of the patients with sacroiliac joint pain was the presence of groin pain.[8] Radiation of pain below the knee was present in the patients with and without sacroiliac joint dysfunction. Another feature noted in patients with sacroiliac joint dysfunction is the lack of pain above the level of the L5 vertebra.[5] From the studies of Fortin, Schwarzer, and from textbooks one can make a composite of the pain diagram from sacroiliac joint dysfunction. The pain from sacroiliac joint dysfunction is located in the superior medial quadrant of the buttock, inferior to the posterior superior iliac spine, the lateral buttock with radiation to the greater trochanter and upper lateral thigh,[6] and in the groin[8] (Fig. 43-1). There may be radiation below the knee.[4,8] As stated, there is usually no pain above the level of L5.[5] The absence of pain above L5 was considered to be a distinguishing feature of sacroiliac joint syndrome.[5] Note that the typical location of pain from a facet joint syndrome is pain from the

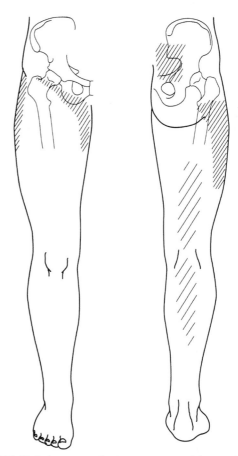

FIGURE 43-1. Location of pain in a patient with sacroiliac joint syndrome.

low back radiating to the posterior thigh to the knee while the pain from a herniated disc usually extends to the leg and foot.

In summary, the pain in sacroiliac joint dysfunction is associated with the following characteristics:

- Location: superior medial quadrant of the buttock, inferior to the posterior superior iliac spine; no pain above the level of L5 vertebra.[5]
- Referred to the greater trochanter, groin, and upper lateral thigh. Less often to the posterior thigh; less often below the knee (posterior leg).
- Aggravated by bending, sitting, and riding.
- Relieved by walking or standing.

The physical examination of a patient with sacroiliac joint syndrome usually reveals tenderness over the posterior aspect of the joint and over the sacral sulcus. Usually, there are no neurological symptoms. The multiple and confusing presentation of sacroiliac joint dysfunction requires the presence of physical examination findings to confirm the diagnosis of sacroiliac joint dysfunction. The following are the commonly used tests to stress the joint and confirm the presence of sacroiliac joint dysfunction.[1,4,9,10]

Faber Patrick test (left sacroiliac joint dysfunction) (Fig. 43-2):

- Patient is supine.
- Left leg, near the ankle, is placed in front of the right thigh above the knee. The physician places one hand over the right iliac crest while the other hand pushes over the medial aspect of the left knee.
- Positive test: pain over sacroiliac joint region (also back, buttock, groin).[4]
- Comment: Test stresses sacroiliac and hip joint.

Gaenslen's test (left sacroiliac joint dysfunction) (Fig. 43-3):

- Patient is supine.
- Left lower thigh and leg hang over the examination table. The examiner flexes right hip and right knee (i.e., hip joint is maximally flexed). The examiner presses downward over the left thigh (hip joint is hyperextended).
- Positive test: pain in the left sacroiliac joint.[10]

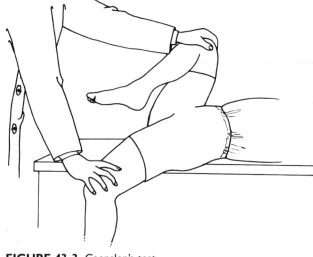

FIGURE 43-3. Gaenslen's test.

- Comments: Test stresses both sacroiliac joints simultaneously by counter-rotation at the extreme range of motion of the joint.[4] Test also stresses the hip joint and stretches the femoral nerve (examiner should ensure the absence of hip pathology or conditions affecting the femoral nerve to diagnose sacroiliac joint syndrome).[4]

Yeoman's test,[4] also called extension test[10] (Fig. 43-4):

- Patient is prone.
- Examiner places one hand above the anterior aspect of the knee and elevates it slightly, the other hand presses downward over the crest of the ilium.[10]
- Positive test: pain over the posterior sacroiliac joint.
- Comments: The hip is extended and the ipsilateral ilium is rotated.[4] Test stresses the sacroiliac joint; it also extends the lumbar spine and stresses the femoral nerve. Most specific and reliable test.[10]

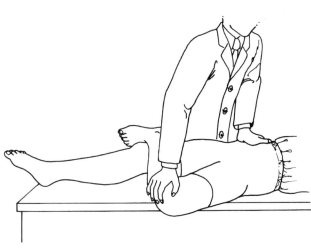

FIGURE 43-2. Faber Patrick test.

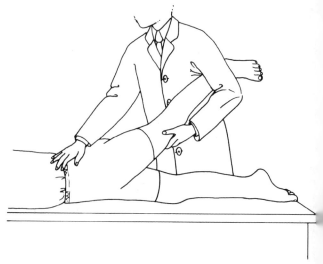

FIGURE 43-4. Yeoman's test (also called extension test).

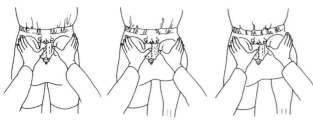

Normal Gillet Test   Abnormal Gillet Test

FIGURE 43-5. Gillet's test.

Gillet's test (Fig. 43-5):

- Patient is standing.
- One of the examiner's thumbs is placed on the second sacral spinous process, the other thumb is placed on the posterior superior iliac spine (PSIS).
- Normal sacroiliac joint: when the patient maximally flexes the hip, the PSIS moves inferior to the S2 spinous process.

Dysfunctional or fixed sacroiliac joint: PSIS remains at the level of the S2 spinous process or moves superior to the sacrum.

Sacroiliac shear test (Fig. 43-6):

- Patient is prone.
- Palm of the examiner's hand is placed over the posterior iliac wing. Shear thrust is directed inferiorly producing a shearing force across the sacroiliac joint.
- Positive test: pain in dysfunctional sacroiliac joint.

Standing flexion test:[9]

- Patient stands with the feet positioned 12 inches apart.
- Examiner sits behind the patient with his thumbs directly beneath the PSIS.
- Patient bends forward as far as possible, knees kept extended.
- Extent of cephalad movement of PSIS is noted.
- Normal joint: each PSIS moves in equal amount in cranial direction.
- Dysfunctional joint: unequal motion of the joints; the joint that moves first and furthest is dysfunctional.

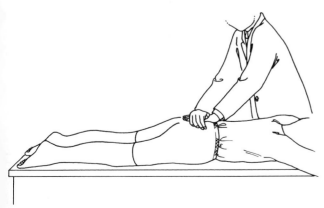

FIGURE 43-6. Sacroiliac shear test.

Seated flexion test:[9]

- Patient seated on a chair, both feet flat on floor.
- Knees flexed at 90° and legs adducted.
- Examiner is behind the patient with thumbs directly under the PSIS.
- Patient bends forward as far as possible.
- Normal joint: each PSIS moves slightly cephalad in equal amount.
- Positive test: PSIS in dysfunctional joint moves more superiorly than the other.

The presence of false positive screening tests was evaluated in 101 patients. The screening tests evaluated were the Gillet test, standing flexion test, and the seated flexion test.[9] The investigators found that 20% of asymptomatic patients had positive findings in one or more of these tests. In another study[5] the same group of investigators tried to identify a single sacroiliac joint test or ensemble of tests that are useful in identifying sacroiliac joint dysfunction. They found no historical feature, and none of the 12 screening tests that they evaluated, and no ensemble of the 12 tests demonstrated worthwhile diagnostic value.[5] No aggravating or relieving factors were of value in diagnosing sacroiliac joint pain. Tenderness over the sacral sulcus, pain over the sacroiliac joint, buttock pain, and the patient pointing to the PSIS as the main source of pain showed better sensitivity than the other tests evaluated.

It is quite obvious then that screening provocative tests do not rule in sacroiliac joint dysfunction nor do they completely rule out other causes of pain (see qualifying comments in the description of the tests). The tests are of added value in confirming the diagnosis of sacroiliac joint syndrome when the history and symptoms are suggestive of sacroiliac joint problem and other causes of the patient's pain have been eliminated.

The diagnosis of sacroiliac joint dysfunction can be presumed based on the history, symptoms, and positive screening tests (some experts require three positive screening tests to confirm sacroiliac joint dysfunction). Radiographic evaluation of the joint rarely adds value. While provocation of pain on injection of the sacroiliac joint is not a suitable criterion of sacroiliac joint dysfunction, a diagnostic local anesthetic block of the joint is considered to be the standard criterion for sacroiliac joint pain.[8]

TECHNIQUE OF SACROILIAC JOINT INJECTION

Fluoroscopy guidance is recommended during injection of the sacroiliac joint. The older technique of injection involves the insertion of three 22-gauge spinal needles into the inferior, middle, and superior aspects of the joint.[1] The needle is inserted in a medial to lateral direction. Newer techniques involve the insertion of a single needle in the inferior aspect of the joint.[8,11] The patient is prone, the fluoroscopy is perpendicular to the table, and the inferior aspect of the joint is marked. The tube is angled 20° to 25° caudad (the image intensifier is above the patient and positioned obliquely towards the patient's head).[11,12] This maneuver projects the posteroinferior portion of the joint in a caudal direction and the anterior joint space in a cephalad direction. Note on the fluoroscopic view that the medial line of the joint (or the "medial joint" if there appears to be two joints on the anteroposterior view) represents

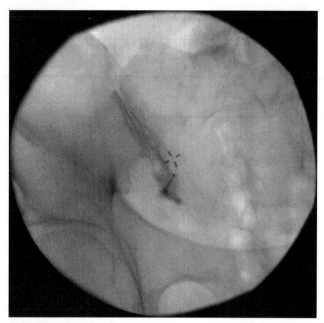

FIGURE 43-7. Fluoroscopic image of the sacroiliac joint after injection of the radiopaque dye.

the posteroinferior portion of the joint while the anterior aspect of the joint is represented by the "lateral joint".[12] After skin infiltration, a 22-gauge, 3.5 cm spinal needle is inserted 1 to 3 cm below the inferior margin of the joint and directed into the inferior aspect of the joint. The needle is advanced through the capsule and ligaments of the joints; angling the needle tip laterally may aid in advancing the needle through the natural course of the sacroiliac joint. Contrast (1 mL) is injected and the joint is outlined (Fig. 43-7). The pain response of the patient to the injection of contrast is noted as either "no pain," "unfamiliar pain," or "similar pain" in comparison to the pain complaint.[8] After the joint is outlined, 1 mL of lidocaine or bupivacaine with steroid (6 mg betamethasone or 40 to 60 mg methylprednisolone) is injected. A greater than 75% reduction of pain over the sacroiliac joint is considered to be a "definite response."[8] The complications of the procedure include bleeding, infection, transient lower extremity weakness, and transient difficulty in voiding.[12] The transient weakness of the lower extremity is secondary to partial block of the sciatic nerve that is located just anterior to the piriformis muscle that is at the same depth as the inferior aspect of the sacroiliac joint. Blockade of the sciatic nerve may be due to extravasation of the local anesthetic or to improper placement of the needle.

TREATMENTS OF SACROILIAC JOINT SYNDROME

The treatments of sacroiliac joint syndrome include exercise, joint mobilization, joint manipulation, or joint injections to restore the balance between joint motion and normal function of the overlying muscle.[14] A 2-week regimen of anti-inflammatory medication is recommended. A range-of-motion exercise program promotes trunk and hip flexibility and stretch of the hamstring muscles. Side posture manipulation of the PSIS and the inferior sacroiliac joint mobilize a stiff sacroiliac joint.[14]

Joint mobilization followed by an exercise program may prevent recurrence of sacroiliac joint syndrome.

The injection of local anesthetic and steroid into the subligamentous portion of the joint has been described previously. Immediate relief is usually seen in 50% to 80% of the patients and 90% have relief within 12 hours.[11,13] Follow-up of the patients who had the injection showed satisfactory relief for 9 months in 81% of 72 patients[14] or good pain relief that lasted 10 ± 5 months.[15]

RADIOFREQUENCY DENERVATION OF THE SACROILIAC JOINT AND LATERAL BRANCH BLOCKS

Radiofrequency (RF) denervation of the sacroiliac joint has been reported to be effective in reducing the pain from sacroiliac joint syndrome. In a retrospective study Ferrante et al. reviewed their results in 33 consecutive patients with sacroiliac joint syndrome who had the treatment.[16] They initially performed a diagnostic injection of bupivacaine and betamethasone under fluoroscopy. The patients who obtained relief were offered RF denervation of the joint. A bipolar system was created by their use of two RF probes. The first RF probe was inserted at the inferior margin of the joint and a second RF probe was placed more cephalad, at a distance of less than 1 cm from the first probe. Lesions were created in the joint when the RF probe was heated to 90°C for 90 seconds. Successive probes were placed less than 1 cm cephalad from the last probe that was placed and multiple lesions were created in a repetitive "leapfrog" manner as high in the joint as possible, creating a "strip lesion" in the posterior joint.[16] They performed a total of 50 sacroiliac joint denervations in the 33 patients. Twelve of the 33 patients (36%) reported at least a 50% decrease in visual analogue pain scores for at least 6 months (the investigators' criteria for success). It should be noted that it can be difficult to place a series of RF probes along the length of the joint because of the overlying iliac bone. The technique described also creates a lesion in the posterior sacroiliac joint and none in the anterior aspect of the joint.

Another retrospective study showed the efficacy of lateral branch blocks in the treatment of sacroiliac joint pain.[17] Eighteen patients with sacroiliac joint pain had nerve blocks of the L4–L5 primary dorsal rami and S1–S3 lateral branches innervating the sacroiliac joint (see Fig. 43-8). Thirteen of the 18 patients obtained greater than or equal to 50% relief, and 2 of the 13 patients had relief that lasted several months. Nine of the 13 patients underwent RF lesioning (80°C for 90 seconds) of the nerves. Eight of the 9 patients who had the RF denervation experienced greater than 50% relief that persisted for at least 9 months.[17] The significance of the study was questioned in view of the multiple innervation of the sacroiliac joint.[18]

PIRIFORMIS SYNDROME

Piriformis syndrome is an uncommon and often undiagnosed etiology of buttock and leg pain.[19–22] In this section the following topics are discussed: (1) the anatomy of the piriformis muscle and anatomical abnormalities that cause piriformis syndrome;[23,24] (2) etiologies of the syndrome; (3) signs and symptoms of the syndrome; and (4) treatments of the syndrome.[25–28]

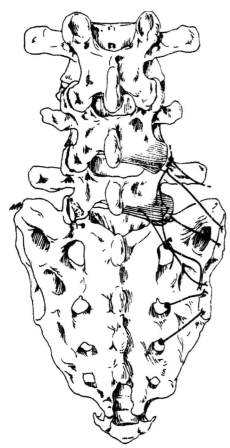

FIGURE 43-8. Innervation of the posterior sacroiliac joint region. A descending branch of the L4 primary ramus innervates the L5–S1 facet joint and the sacroiliac joint. The L5 and S1 primary rami also innervate the L5–S1 facet joint and the sacroiliac joint. Finally, the S2 and S3 sacral nerves innervate the sacroiliac joint. (From Paris SV: Anatomy as related to function and pain. Symposium on Evaluation and Care of Lumbar Spine Problems. Orthop Clin North Am 14:475, 1983.)

Anatomy of the Piriformis Muscle and the Sciatic Nerve:

The piriformis muscle originates from the anterior surface of the S2–S4 sacral vertebrae, the capsule of the sacroiliac joint, and the gluteal surface of the ilium near the posterior surface of the iliac spine.[22,23] It runs laterally through the greater sciatic foramen, becomes tendinous, and inserts into the piriformis fossa at the medial aspect of the greater trochanter of the femur. The piriformis muscle is innervated by the branches of L5, S1, and S2 spinal nerves. The sciatic nerve, posterior femoral cutaneous nerve, gluteal nerves, and the gluteal vessels pass below the piriformis muscle.

Six possible anatomical relationships occur between the sciatic nerve and the piriformis muscle:[19,29,30]

- The sciatic nerve passes below the piriformis muscle.
- A divided nerve passes through and below the muscle.
- A divided nerve passes through and above the muscle.
- A divided nerve passes above and below the muscle.
- An undivided nerve passes through the piriformis.
- An undivided nerve passes above the muscle.

In 120 cadaver dissections Beason and Anson[29] found that the most common arrangement was the undivided nerve passing below the piriformis muscle (84%) followed by the divisions of the sciatic nerve between and below the muscle (12%). This finding was confirmed by Pecina.[30] Pecina also noted the relation between high-level divisions of the sciatic nerve, i.e., in the pelvis, and the common peroneal nerve passing through the piriformis muscle. In a recent study it was found that both components of the sciatic nerve passed below the piriformis muscle in 98.5% (65 of 66 dissections) of the specimens studied.[31] In one specimen the muscle was split: the tibial component of the sciatic nerve passed below the piriformis muscle while the common peroneal nerve passed through the muscle.

Anomalies of the piriformis muscle and the sciatic nerve can cause sciatica. A case report described a patient whose sciatica was relieved after the lower head of the bipartite piriformis muscle was surgically cut.[23] Another patient had a fascial constricting band around the sciatic nerve and a piriformis muscle lying anterior to the nerve.[24] Resection of the fibrous band and the piriformis muscle restored the normal relationship of the muscle and the nerve and relieved the patient's hip and buttock pain and sciatica. Several authors suggested entrapment of the sciatic nerve by the piriformis muscle and recommended surgical release of the muscle and its fascia as treatments for the piriformis syndrome.[32–34]

Pathophysiology, Signs and Symptoms, and Treatment: Piriformis syndrome was a term first coined by Robinson[35] and comprises 5% to 6% of patients referred for the treatment of back and leg pain.[19,36] Etiologies of the syndrome include trauma to the pelvis or buttock,[19,37] hypertrophy of the piriformis muscle,[23,26,27] anatomic abnormalities of the piriformis muscle or the sciatic nerve,[23,24] differences in leg lengths (a minimum of half an inch difference in leg lengths),[22] and piriformis myositis.[38] A history of trauma is usually elicited in approximately 50% of the cases:[36] the trauma is usually not dramatic and may occur several months before the initial symptoms. It may occur after total hip replacement surgery[34] or laminectomy.[32] The scar tissue after laminectomy impinges on the nerve roots and "shortens" the sciatic nerve rendering it prone to repeated tension and trauma by the piriformis muscle.[32] Some investigators consider piriformis syndrome to be a form of myofascial pain syndrome.[28]

Trauma to the buttock leads to inflammation and spasm of the muscle.[36] Inflammatory substances such as prostaglandin, histamine, bradykinin, and serotonin are released from the inflamed muscle and may irritate the sciatic nerve resulting in pain–spasm–inflammation–irritation cycle.[31,40] The stretched, spastic, and inflamed piriformis muscle may compress the sciatic nerve between the muscle and the pelvis,[24,35] with the compression occurring between the tendinous portion of the muscle and the bony pelvis.[22] In patients where the piriformis muscle is anterior to the sciatic nerve the compression of the nerve occurs between the superior border of the piriformis and the superior margin of the greater sciatic foramen.[24] Patients with entrapment of the sciatic nerve may have neurologic deficits and abnormalities in their electrodiagnostic studies.[23]

The differential diagnoses of piriformis syndrome include the causes of low back pain and sciatica. In contrast to herniated disc or foraminal stenosis, the patient with piriformis syndrome usually does not have neurologic deficits.[36] Facet syndrome, sacroiliac joint dysfunction, trochanteric bursitis, myofascial pain syndrome, pelvic tumor, endometriosis, and conditions irritating the sciatic nerve should be considered in the differential diagnoses of piriformis syndrome. These conditions can be ruled out by complete medical history and physical examination.[19] Diagnosis of piriformis syndrome is usually arrived at after exclusion of these possibilities.[31] Isolated involvement of the piriformis muscle is uncommon and usually occurs as a part of soft tissue injuries resulting from rotation and/or flexion movements of the hip and torso.[20] Most patients with piriformis syndrome show the concomitant presence of other causes of back and leg pain.[31]

According to Parziale et al.[19] the following are the six cardinal features of the syndrome:

- History of trauma to the sacroiliac and gluteal region.
- Pain in the region of the sacroiliac joint, greater sciatic notch, and piriformis muscle, extending down the leg and causing difficulty in walking.
- Acute exacerbation of pain by stooping or lifting and moderately relieved by traction.
- Palpable, sausage-shaped mass over the piriformis muscle, which is tender to palpation.
- Positive Laseque sign.
- Possible gluteal atrophy.

Patients with piriformis syndrome usually complain of buttock pain with or without radiation to the ipsilateral leg.[19] The buttock pain usually extends from the sacrum to the greater trochanter.[19,20,23] Pain in the lower back is rare,[4] although some patients have varying degrees of paralumbar pain.[19] Gluteal pain radiating to the ipsilateral leg is present if the piriformis muscle irritates the sciatic nerve.[27] The pain may radiate to the posterior thigh down to the knee if there is involvement of the posterior cutaneous nerve of the thigh.[20,22] The pain is usually aggravated by prolonged sitting, as in driving or biking, or when getting up from a sitting position.[19,20] Pain occurs with bowel movements due to proximity of the piriformis muscle to the lateral pelvic wall and is worse after sitting on hard surfaces. Female patients may complain of dyspareunia.[19] There may be a history of limp and the patient may drag the affected leg on the affected side.[34] Numbness in the foot may occur when the sciatic nerve is compressed by the piriformis muscle.[22]

Physical examination of the patient may reveal a pelvic tilt, uneven scapulas,[22] or tenderness in the buttock from the medial edge of the greater sciatic foramen to the greater trochanter.[19] A spindle-shaped mass may be felt in the buttock and there may be piriformis tenderness on rectal and pelvic examinations.[19,20] The pain is aggravated by hip flexion, adduction, and internal rotation. Neurological signs are usually negative.[19] The straight leg test may be normal or limited, with leg numbness, when the sciatic nerve is irritated. The following physical examination signs help in confirming the presence of piriformis syndrome:

- Pace sign: pain and weakness on resisted abduction of the hip while the patient is seated, i.e., the hip is flexed.[34,36]
- Laseque sign: pain on voluntary flexion, adduction, and internal rotation of the hip.[35,40]
- Freiberg sign: pain on forced internal rotation of the extended thigh[41] is due to stretching of the piriformis muscle and pressure on the sciatic nerve at the sacrospinous ligament.

The Laseque and Freiberg signs are better understood when one realizes that the function of the piriformis muscle is to abduct the flexed thigh[20,42] and externally rotate the hip joint when the thigh is extended at the hip joint.

The diagnosis of piriformis syndrome is made mostly on clinical grounds.[33,34] Recent publications showed the value of electromyography (EMG), computed tomography (CT), and magnetic resonance imaging (MRI). EMG may detect myopathic and neuropathic changes including a delay in the H-reflex with the affected leg in a flexed, adducted, and internally rotated (FAIR) position as compared with the same H-reflex in the normal anatomic position.[43] A three standard deviation prolongation of the H-reflex has recently been recommended as the physiological criterion for piriformis syndrome. This EMG finding suggests entrapment of the nerve by the hip abductor and external rotator, i.e., the piriformis muscle, under which it passes. MRI confirms the enlarged piriformis muscle[40] while CT of the soft tissues of the pelvis may show an enlarged piriformis muscle[40] or abnormal uptake by the muscle.[44]

The treatments of piriformis syndrome include physical therapy combined with the use of anti-inflammatory drugs, analgesics, and muscle relaxants to reduce inflammation, spasm, and pain.[19,20,45] Physical therapy involves stretching of the piriformis muscle with flexion, adduction, and internal rotation of the hip[19,20] followed by pressure applied to the piriformis muscle. Strengthening of the hip abductors is added to the regimen when the symptoms improve.[19] Abnormal biomechanics caused by posture, pelvic obliquities, and leg-length inequalities are corrected.[19] Ultrasound treatments help reduce the pain.[22,46] Vapocoolant spray with soft-tissue stretch of the area has also been recommended.[47]

Patients who do not respond to the above conservative therapy are candidates for local anesthetic and steroid injections. Previous injections were made at the focal point of pain and irritability deep in the belly of the muscle,[36] at the medial aspect of the muscle,[19,20] or at the lateral aspect[48] where firm compression of the sciatic nerve occurs.[24] Caudal steroid and local anesthetic injections have been found to be effective. In caudal injections the injected solution diffuses along the nerve root sleeves and the proximal part of the sciatic nerve and blocks the nerves that innervate the piriformis muscle.[49]

Surgery may be entertained in recalcitrant cases or when there is documented anatomic abnormality of the piriformis muscle. The muscle may be excised, divided, or thinned.[19,20,33,50,51] The obturator internus, gemelli, and quadratus femoris muscles share common insertions with the piriformis muscle and compensate for the loss of piriformis muscle function.[19,35]

Techniques of Piriformis Muscle and Perisciatic Nerve Injections: Initially, piriformis injections were made blindly.[19,20,36] Newer techniques involve identification of the piriformis muscle with a muscle EMG[27] or with the use of CT guidance.[28] In the technique of Fishman et al.[27] fluoroscopy and EMG are utilized to identify the piriformis muscle. The patient is in the prone position and the expected position of the piriformis muscle is identified using the greater trochanter of the femur and lateral border of the sacrum and the sacroiliac joint as landmarks. Correct needle placement is confirmed with muscle EMG and injection of contrast media. The steroid is then injected into the piriformis muscle. Although successful in identifying the piriformis muscle, the technique utilizes a muscle EMG that is not readily available in most pain management centers.

Another technique is the perisciatic injection of Hanania and Kitain.[25,26] In their technique the patient is in the lateral or semiprone position with the nondependent hip and knee flexed and the dependent extremity straight. The sciatic nerve is located with a nerve stimulator, the needle is withdrawn a few centimeters, and then 40 mg methylprednisolone in 5 to 10 mL dilute local anesthetic is injected. Fluoroscopy was not utilized in their technique. Hanania and Kitain described 6 patients who were previously unresponsive or partially responsive to blind piriformis muscle injections or epidural steroid injections. Their patients had relief of their pain for up to 18 months.

A newer technique involves the use of CT guidance.[28] In this technique the position of the muscle is identified and insertion of the needle is guided by the CT. Local anesthetic (2 mL 0.5% bupivacaine) is injected into the muscle followed by the injection of 100 units of botulinum toxin type A (BTX-A). The unavailability of CT equipment in most pain treatment centers limits a wider application of this technique.

A technique was described wherein the lower border of the sacroiliac joint was used as the landmark (Fig. 43-9).[31] The patient is prone and the lower border of the sacroiliac joint, greater sciatic foramen, and the head of the femur are identified by fluoroscopy. The area is prepared and draped, and anesthetized with local anesthetic. A 15 cm insulated needle connected to a nerve stimulator is inserted at 1.5 ± 0.8 cm (range: 0.5 to 3 cm) lateral and 1.2 ± 0.6 cm (range: 0.5 to 2 cm) caudal to the lower border of the sacroiliac joint. The needle is advanced perpendicularly until a motor evoked response of the sciatic nerve is obtained at a depth of 9.2 ± 1.5 cm (range: 7.5 to 13 cm). The evoked motor response of the foot can be inversion, eversion, dorsiflexion, or plantar flexion.[52] The needle is pulled back 0.3 to 0.6 cm, to avoid intraneural injection, and 40 to 60 mg methylprednisolone in 5 to 6 mL saline is injected. The needle is pulled back another 0.5 to 0.7 cm to

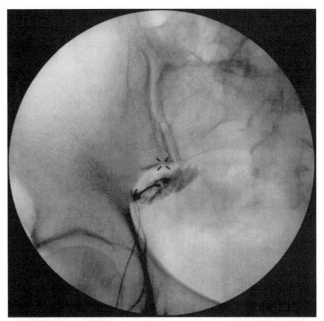

FIGURE 43-10. Fluoroscopic image of the insulated needle in the piriformis muscle with the muscle being outlined by the injected radiopaque dye.

place the tip of the needle at the belly of the piriformis muscle. Radiopaque dye (2 to 3 mL) is injected and the muscle is outlined (Fig. 43-10). Methylprednisolone (40 to 60 mg) in 6 to 8 mL local anesthetic is injected into the muscle.

Steroid can be injected into the piriformis muscle to reduce the swelling and/or spasm of the muscle.[31] Injection of steroid perisciatically is recommended whether there are signs of sciatic nerve entrapment or not, since there is probably some inflammation of the nerve in cases of piriformis syndrome. Steroids are anti-inflammatory and the topical administration of methylprednisolone has been shown to specifically block nociceptive fiber transmission.[53,54] Saline or very dilute local anesthetic is the preferred diluent for the perisciatic injection to minimize motor blockade. For the piriformis muscle injection, local anesthetic (and steroid) is used to relax the piriformis muscle and break the cycle of pain and spasm. Injection of the local anesthetic into the belly of the muscle is important to avoid leakage of the local anesthetic into the sciatic nerve and cause sensory and motor blockade of the leg and foot. Leakage of the injectate can be avoided by pulling the needle back at least 1 cm after the sciatic nerve is stimulated.[31]

Botulinum toxin may be injected into the muscle if the patient has transient response to the steroid and local anesthetic injection. Botulinum toxin blocks the release of acetylcholine at the neuromuscular junction[55] resulting in the prolonged relaxation of the muscle. Recovery of the muscle depends on neuromuscular sprouting and re-innervation of the muscle that takes several weeks to months. Botulinum injections have been employed in the treatment of myofascial pain syndrome,[56,57] piriformis syndrome,[28] and focal dystonias such as blepharospasm, spasmodic torticollis, spasmodic dysphonia, or hemifacial spasm.[55,56] Doses of the botulinum toxin are 100 mouse units for BTX-A (Botox)[28] in 4 mL bupivacaine and 5,000 to 10,00 units for botulinum toxin type B (Myobloc).[58]

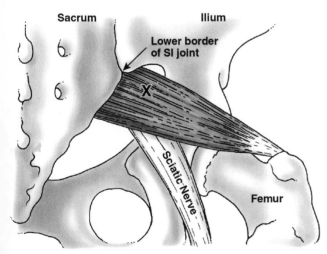

FIGURE 43-9. Posterior view of the sacrum, ilium, and greater trochanter of the femur, illustrating the course of the piriformis muscle, sciatic nerve, and the site of injection (marked "X"). (Reprinted with permission from Benzon HT, Katz JA, Benzon HA, et al: Anesthesiology 98:1442–1448, 2003.)

The reported complications of botulinum toxin injection include brachial plexopathy,[59,60] polyradiculoneuritis,[61] and local psoriasiform dermatitis.[62] If botulinum toxin is used, extreme caution should be observed in avoiding the injection or leakage of the botulinum toxin into the sciatic nerve.

A randomized study compared BTX-A with methylprednisolone in patients with "myofascial piriformis pain."[28] Thirty days after the injection the patients in both groups showed marked reduction in their pain scores with no significant difference between the two groups. The patients who had botulinum injection, however, had significantly lower pain scores at 60 days after the injection.[28] In our clinical experience, some of our patients had sustained relief for up to 3 months with the local anesthetic–steroid injections. The relatively prolonged relief in some of our patients and that of Hanania's[28] may be due to the concomitant perisciatic injection of the steroid. The combined perisciatic and piriformis muscle injections may break the cycle of pain and spasm better than the piriformis muscle injection alone.

KEY POINTS

- Pain from sacroiliac joint dysfunction is usually located in the superior medial quadrant of the buttock, inferior to the superior iliac spine. Usually, there is no pain above the L5 vertebra. The pain may be referred to the ipsilateral greater trochanter, groin, and upper lateral thigh. The pain is aggravated by bending, sitting, or riding.

- The useful physical examination tests for sacroiliac joint dysfunction include the Faber Patrick, Gaenslen's, Yeoman's, Gillet's, and sacroiliac shear tests. Asymptomatic patients may respond positively to these tests since these are not specific for sacroiliac joint syndrome. The physician should integrate the history and physical examination findings in diagnosing sacroiliac joint syndrome.

- A diagnostic local anesthetic block is considered to be the criterion for sacroiliac joint pain. The sacroiliac joint can be approached through its inferior aspect.

- The treatments of sacroiliac joint syndrome include anti-inflammatory medications, exercise, joint mobilization/manipulation, and joint injection. Patients may have pain relief up to 10 months after injection of the symptomatic sacroiliac joint. The role of nerve blocks and radiofrequency rhizotomy has not been firmly established.

- The pain of piriformis syndrome is located in the buttock and radiates to the ipsilateral hip. It may radiate to the leg in an L5–S1 distribution if the sciatic nerve is compromised.

- The physical examination signs to confirm piriformis syndrome include the Pace, Laseque, and Freiberg signs.

- The piriformis muscle can be outlined and injected with the aid of a nerve stimulator and fluoroscopy. The sciatic nerve is identified first, steroid is injected perisciatically, and the needle is pulled back into the belly of the piriformis muscle. Local anesthetic and steroid is injected into the muscle. Some patients have relief up to 3 months after the injection. If the relief is transient and the diagnosis of piriformis syndrome is established, botulinum toxin may be injected into the muscle.

REFERENCES

1. Mooney V: Understanding, examining for, and treating sacroiliac pain. J Musculo Med 10:37–49, 1993.
2. Walker JM: The sacroiliac joint: A critical review. Phys Ther 72:903–916, 1992.
3. Ehara S, El-Koury GY, Bergman RA: The accessory sacroiliac joint: A common anatomic variant. AJR 150:857–859, 1988.
4. Bernard TN, Cassidy JD: The sacroiliac joint syndrome. In Frymoyer JW (ed): The Adult Spine. Raven Press, New York, 1991, pp 2107–2130.
5. Dreyfuss P, Michaelson M, Pauza K, et al: The value of medical history and physical examination in diagnosing sacroiliac joint pain. Spine 21:2594–2602, 1996.
6. Fortin DO, Dwyer AP, West S, Pier J: Sacroiliac joint: Pain referral maps upon applying a new injection/arthrography technique: I. Asymptomatic volunteers. Spine 19:1475–1482, 1994.
7. Fortin JD, Aprill CN, Ponthieux B, Pier J: Sacroiliac joint: Pain referral maps upon applying a new injection/arthrography technique: II. Clinical evaluation. Spine 19:1483–1489, 1994.
8. Schwarzer AC, Aprill AN, Bogduk N: The sacroiliac joint in chronic low back pain. Spine 20:31–37, 1995.
9. Dreyfuss P, Dreyer S, Griffin J, et al: Positive screening tests in asymptomatic adults. Spine 19:1138–1143, 1994.
10. Kirkaldy-Willis WH, Burton CV: Managing Low Back Pain, ed 3. Churchill-Livingstone, New York, 1999, pp 121–148.
11. Dussault RG, Kaplan PE, Anderson MW: Fluoroscopy-guided sacroiliac joint injections. Radiology 214:273–277, 2000.
12. Fenton DS, Czervionke LF: Image-Guided Spine Intervention. WB Saunders, Philadelphia, 2003, pp 127–139.
13. Pulisetti D, Ebraheim NA: CT-guided sacroiliac joint injections. J Spinal Disord 12:310–312, 1999.
14. Bernard TN, Kirkaldy-Willis WH: Recognizing specific characteristics of nonspecific low back pain. Clin Orthop 217:266–280, 1987.
15. Bollow M, Braun J, Taupitz M, et al: CT-guided intraarticular corticosteroid injection into the sacroiliac joints in patients with spondyloarthropathy: Indications and follow-up with contrast enhanced MRI. J Comput Assist Tomogr 20:512–521, 1996.
16. Ferrante FM, King LF, Roche EA, et al: Radiofrequency sacroiliac joint denervation for sacroiliac joint syndrome. Reg Anesth Pain Med 26:137–142, 2001.
17. Cohen SP, Abdi S: Lateral branch blocks as a treatment for sacroiliac joint pain: A pilot study. Reg Anesth Pain Med 28:113–119, 2003.
18. Manchikanti L, Boswell MV, Singh V, Hansen HC: Sacroiliac joint pain: Should physicians be blocking lateral branches, medial branches, dorsal rami, or ventral rami? Reg Anesth Pain Med 28:488–489, 2003.
19. Parziale JR, Hudgins TH, Fishman LM: The piriformis syndrome. Am J Orthop 25:819–823, 1996.
20. Barton PM: Piriformis syndrome: A rational approach to management. Pain 47:345–352, 1991.
21. Durrani Z, Winnie AP: Piriformis syndrome: An undiagnosed cause of sciatica. J Pain Symptom Manage 6:374–379, 1991.
22. Hallin RP: Sciatic pain and the piriformis muscle. Postgrad Med 74:69–72, 1983.
23. Chen WS: Bipartite piriformis muscle: An unusual cause of sciatic nerve entrapment. Pain 58:269–272, 1994.
24. Sayson SC, Ducey JP, Maybrey JB, et al: Sciatic entrapment neuropathy associated with an anomalous piriformis muscle. Pain 59:149–152, 1994.
25. Hanania M: New technique for piriformis muscle injection using a nerve stimulator [letter]. Reg Anesth Pain Med 22:200–202, 1997.
26. Hanania M, Kitain E: Perisciatic injection of steroid for the treatment of sciatica due to piriformis syndrome. Reg Anesth Pain Med 23:223–228, 1998.
27. Fishman SM, Caneris OA, Bandman TB, et al: Injection of the piriformis muscle by fluoroscopic and electromyographic guidance. Reg Anesth Pain Med 23:554–559, 1998.

28. Porta M: A comparative trial of botulinum toxin type A and methylprednisolone for the treatment of myofascial pain syndrome and pain from chronic muscle spasm. Pain 85:101–105, 2000.

29. Beason LE, Anson BJ: The relation of the sciatic nerve and its subdivisions to the piriformis muscle. Anat Record 70:1–5, 1937.

30. Pecina M: Contribution to the etiological explanation of the piriformis syndrome. Acta Anat 105:181–187, 1979.

31. Benzon HT, Katz JA, Benzon HA, Iqbal MS: Piriformis syndrome: Anatomic considerations, a new injection technique, and a review of the literature. Anesthesiology 98:1442–1448, 2003.

32. Mizuguchi T: Division of the piriformis muscle for the treatment of sciatica: Postlaminectomy syndrome and osteoarthritis of the spine. Arch Surg 111:719–722, 1976.

33. Solheim LF, Siewers P, Paus B: The pyriformis muscle syndrome: Sciatic nerve entrapment treated with section of the piriformis muscle. Acta Orthop Scand 52:73–75, 1981.

34. Cameron HU, Noftal F: The piriformis syndrome. Can J Surg 31:210, 1988.

35. Robinson D: Piriformis syndrome in relation to sciatic pain. Am J Surg 73:355–358, 1947.

36. Pace JB, Nagle D: Piriformis syndrome. West J Med 124:435–439, 1976.

37. Thiele GH: Coccydynia and pain in the superior gluteal region. JAMA 109:1271–1275, 1937.

38. Chen WS: Sciatica due to piriformis pyomyositis. J Bone Joint Surg 74A:1546–1548, 1992.

39. Lynn B: Cutaneous hyperalgesia. Br Med Bull 33:103–108, 1977.

40. Jankiewicz JT, Hennrikus WL, Houkom JA: The appearance of the piriformis muscle in computed tomography and magnetic resonance imaging: A case report and review of the literature. Clin Orthop 262:205–209, 1991.

41. Freiberg AH: Sciatic pain and its relief by operations on muscle and fascia. Arch Surg 34:337–350, 1937.

42. Wyant GM: Chronic pain syndromes and their treatment: III. The piriformis syndrome. Can Anaesth Soc J 26:305–308, 1979.

43. Fishman LM, Zybert PA: Electrophysiologic evidence of piriformis syndrome. Arch Phys Med Rehabil 73:359–364, 1992.

44. Karl RD, Yedinak MA, Hartshorne MF, et al: Scintigraphic appearance of the piriformis muscle syndrome. Clin Nucl Med 10:361–363, 1985.

45. Rich B, McKeag D: When sciatica is not disk disease. Phys Sports Med 20:105–115, 1992.

46. Steiner C, Staubs, Gannon M, Buhlinger C: Piriformis syndrome. Pathogenesis, diagnosis and treatment. J Am Osteopath Assoc 87:318–323, 1987.

47. Simons D, Travell J: Myofascial origins of low back pain. Postgrad Med 73:99–108, 1983.

48. Kirkaldy-Willis WH, Hill RJ: A more precise diagnosis for low back pain. Spine 4:102–109, 1979.

49. Mullin V: Caudal steroid injection for treatment of piriformis syndrome. Anesth Analg 71:705–707, 1990.

50. Vandertop WP, Bosma MJ: The piriformis syndrome. A case report. J Bone Joint Surg 73A:1095–1117, 1991.

51. Hughes SS, Goldtsein MN, Hichs DG, Pellegrini VD: Extrapelvic compression of the sciatic nerve. J Bone Joint Surg 74A:1553–1559, 1992.

52. Benzon HT, Kim C, Benzon HP, et al: Correlation between evoked motor response of the sciatic nerve and sensory blockade. Anesthesiology 87:547–552, 1997.

53. Devor M, Govrin-Lippman R, Raber P: Corticosteroids suppress ectopic neural discharge originating in experimental neuromas. Pain 22:127–137, 1985.

54. Johannsson A, Hao J, Sjolund B: Local corticosteroid application blocks transmission in normal nociceptive C-fibers. Acta Anaesthesiol Scand 34:335–338, 1990.

55. Jankovic T, Brin MF: Therapeutic uses of botulinum toxin. N Engl J Med 324:1186–1193, 1991.

56. Cheshire WP, Abashian SW, Mann JD: Botulinum toxin in the treatment of myofascial pain syndrome. Pain 59:65–69, 1994.

57. Wheeler AH, Goolkasian P, Gretz SS: A randomized, double-blind, prospective pilot study of botulinum toxin injection for refractory, unilateral, cervicothoracic, paraspinal, myofascial pain syndrome. Spine 23:1662–1667, 1998.

58. Fishman LM: Myobloc in the treatment of piriformis syndrome. A dose-finding study. Presented at the American Pain Society Annual Meeting, Baltimore, MD, March 2002.

59. Glanzman RL, Gelb DJ, Drury I, et al: Brachial plexopathy after botulinum toxin injections. Neurology 40:1143, 1990.

60. Sampaio C, Castro-Caldas A, Sales-Luis ML, et al: Brachial plexopathy after botulinum toxin administration for cervical dystonia [letter]. J Neurol Neurosurg Psychiatry 56:220, 1993.

61. Haug BA, Dressler D, Prange HW: Polyradiculoneuritis following botulinum toxin therapy. J Neurol 237:62–63, 1990.

62. Bowden JB, Rapini RP: Psoriasiform eruption following intramuscular botulinum A toxin. Cutis 50:415–416, 1992.

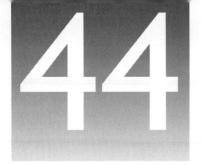

Myofascial Pain Syndrome

Robert E. Molloy, M.D.

Myofascial pain (MP) is local and referred pain that arises from myofascial trigger points. Trigger points (TPs) are localized, very sensitive areas in skeletal muscle that contain palpable, taut bands of muscle. They are painful to palpation, reproduce the patient's pain, and are associated with referred pain.[1] MP is frequently present in acute or chronic regional musculoskeletal pain disorders, with or without other pain generators. When it becomes chronic, it tends to generalize, but it remains distinct from fibromyalgia. It is a treatable condition that responds to physical and injection techniques, if associated conditions and postural/ergonomic factors are also addressed. TPs are identified in 21% to 30% of patients seen with regional pain in orthopedic or general medical clinics, but in more than 85% of patients referred to specialty pain management clinics.[2] MP is most frequently found in the head, neck, shoulders, extremities, and low back; the condition is more prevalent in women than men.[3] Myofascial TPs are often associated with chronic head and neck pain as seen with temporomandibular joint disorders, neck pain after whiplash injury, cervicogenic headache, and tension-type headache.[4] TPs are classified as active or latent. Active TPs are identified in patients with a regional pain complaint as described below. Latent TPs may be identified in asymptomatic patients by their local tenderness to palpation, perhaps associated with diminished range of motion, but not associated with spontaneous pain. Latent TPs have been identified in the shoulder girdle muscles in 45% to 55% of healthy young adults.[5] MP occurs frequently after trauma, e.g., whiplash injury, and after surgery. For example, a TP was identified in the scapular region in 67% of patients with persistent post-thoracotomy pain syndrome, a condition generally attributed to intercostal neuropathic pain.[6]

DIAGNOSIS

MP may present following obvious injury, repetitive trauma, or without obvious cause. There may be associated peripheral somatic pain generators. Patients experience localized or regional deep, aching discomfort of variable intensity. TPs occur in characteristic locations in each muscle, and the pattern of referred somatic pain is predictable and therefore useful in locating the offending TP.[1] Associated symptoms may include autonomic dysfunction, various neurological symptoms, and limitations of functional ability. Abnormal posture and occupational body mechanics may be identified as perpetuating factors.

Therefore, careful musculoskeletal examination seeks to identify postural, mechanical, orthopedic, or neurological abnormalities that may contribute to MP. Active TPs should be sought in suspected skeletal muscle by gentle palpation across and perpendicular to the muscle fibers. TPs are detected by identification of taut muscle bands and production of severe pain which is characteristic of the patient's complaint. Classic referred pain and involuntary muscle contraction or a jump sign may also be elicited. The presence of referred pain may be an unreliable sign that is not useful clinically.[7] Pain relief may occur after muscle stretching or local injection. The ability to reliably detect TPs varies with examiner training, experience, and accessibility of the involved muscle. After extensive training, a group of four blinded observers reliably identified the precise location of the primary latent TP in the upper trapezius; and even two examiners could exceed a criterion reliability threshold of 80%.[8]

MP may be diagnosed upon finding spontaneous local/regional pain, attributable to a specific skeletal muscle site; palpation of a taut muscle band and exquisite localized tenderness along the taut band in this muscle; and evidence of incomplete relaxation/limited range of motion of the muscle. However, there are no established, widely accepted diagnostic criteria for MP syndrome.

Differential diagnosis should include the following: arthritis including facet syndrome, discogenic pain syndromes, radiculopathy, neuropathy, bursitis, tendonitis, referred visceral pain, infectious and autoimmune disorders, abnormal body mechanics, metabolic/endocrine disease including hypothyroidism, psychiatric disorders including depression, and fibromyalgia. MP may occur with or without these other conditions and peripheral pain generators.[2] The Beck Depression Inventory and the Taylor Manifest Anxiety Scale were used to evaluate

102 patients with unilateral MP in the upper trapezius. There was evidence of depression in 22.9% of patients, while high anxiety scores were present in 89.3% of the patients.[9]

PATHOPHYSIOLOGY

MP syndrome and muscle TPs remain controversial. The etiology and mechanism has not been established. It appears that peripheral nociception occurs along with central sensitization and an autonomic component. Simons et al. propose that the primary abnormality is pathologic increase in acetylcholine release by abnormal motor endplates at rest in muscle TPs; and they have demonstrated more frequent endplate noise in myofascial TPs than adjacent muscle outside the TP.[10] Needle examination recordings from TPs show low-voltage spontaneous activity and activity resembling endplate spikes.[11] This endplate noise is characteristic but not diagnostic of myofascial TPs. Increased acetylcholine release may lead to sustained depolarization of the postjunctional membrane and sustained muscle contraction. Sustained maximal shortening of the sarcomere in the region of the motor endplate has been demonstrated in canine and human TPs.[12] Chronic sarcomere shortening may cause localized alterations in energy consumption and perfusion that produce ischemia, and it may contribute to increased resting tension in the taut muscle band. Muscle ischemia elicits the release of vasoactive substances that sensitize afferent nociceptors, leading to increased tenderness to palpation. Chronic MP may create central sensitization, referred pain to adjacent spinal levels, and persistent pain at the spinal cord and brain levels.[2] Vasoactive mediators also tend to further increase acetylcholine release and create a positive feedback loop for MP. Psychological stress and the sympathetic nervous system may perpetuate MP. Endplate potential spike activity in TPs increased with experimental psychological stress.[13] Alpha block with phentolamine or phenoxybenzamine inhibited endplate noise and spike activity in a human study.[14]

TREATMENT: MECHANICAL

The goal of treatment is to educate and empower patients to understand and manage the symptoms of MP and to regain and maintain normal function with as much independence as possible.

It is believed that repetitive microtrauma and occupational myofascial injury lead to muscle shortening and pain. Correction of postural and ergonomic abnormalities therefore is a standard component of patient management, although not well supported by clinical studies. Postural training with behavior therapy accelerated return of full mouth opening in patients treated for oral MP, but with only minor outcome differences.[15] Various stress management interventions have been recommended but not well studied for MP. A study of chronic oral and masticatory muscle pain compared four single treatments: relaxation, physical therapy, transcutaneous electrical nerve stimulation (TENS), and dental splinting. The response was good but similar in all four treatment groups.[16] Acupuncture treatment at points relevant to myofascial neck pain was more effective than treatment with either nonsteroidal anti-inflammatory drugs (NSAIDs) or acupuncture at distant sites.[17] Melzack et al. found a close (71%) correlation between TPs and acupuncture points for pain.[18] The value of massage therapy to supplement exercise for MP has not been demonstrated. Ultrasound does not offer added benefit to combined exercise and massage in treatment of MP.[19]

EXERCISE AND INJECTION THERAPY

Stretching exercises are the cornerstone of all treatment approaches for MP. Slow, sustained muscle stretch aims to restore normal muscle length and activity. This is combined with lightly loaded daily physical activity until patients demonstrate improved pain and range of motion. Topical cold application may be used to facilitate muscle stretch. Previously, a vapocoolant spray was commonly used as part of a spray and stretch technique for passive muscle stretching; and it was recommended in Travell's classic textbook.[20] A home program of ischemic compression followed by sustained stretch was as effective and sometimes superior to an active range of motion program in a well-designed, controlled study.[21] A critical in-depth review of the treatment literature supported the use of therapeutic exercise for low back, neck, and knee pain.[22] After the initial goals of stretching exercise are reached, patients may add a graded stabilization and muscle strengthening program to further improve functional status. An aerobic exercise component is included to maintain muscle and cardiovascular fitness.

Trigger point injections (TPIs) have been used to supplement stretching exercises in the management of MP. They are best suited for initiation of treatment in patients intolerant of physical therapy (PT) and when focused on a difficult area of persistent MP identified by the therapist. A series of TPIs is most likely to be effective when added to an ongoing program of PT and immediately followed by a therapy session using manual myofascial release techniques. The goal of TPI is to facilitate progress in PT and ultimately to support patient success in a program of home stretching exercise.[2] The goal of patient empowerment to self-manage their MP is preferred to creating dependence on repeated TPIs over an extended period. Patient response to a series of TPIs should be documented in the record based upon follow-up evaluation supplemented by feedback from the therapist.

There are many techniques for TPI, and the superiority of any one approach has not been demonstrated. The injected medications may include local anesthetics, steroids, botulinum toxin, or no drug in the case of dry needling. Procaine, lidocaine, bupivacaine, corticosteroids, saline, and sterile water have been employed and evaluated. Injection pain and postinjection soreness vary with the drugs employed, but no difference in efficacy has been demonstrated. Bupivacaine is associated with increased injection pain and greater myotoxicity.[23] Injection pain is diminished when lidocaine or mepivacaine are diluted with water to a concentration of 0.2% to 0.25%.[24] Injections of sterile water alone are more painful than similar injections of normal saline with identical clinical outcomes.[25] The intensity and duration of postinjection soreness is greater after dry needling than after injection of dilute lidocaine.[26] In a systematic review of 23 randomized controlled trials (RCTs) using injection therapies for MP Cummings and White conclude that the drug employed does not alter the outcome or offer any therapeutic benefit over dry needling.[27] They attributed the effect of TPIs to the needle or placebo, not to an active drug or the physical effects of the solution injected. Various injection techniques have been described employing a slow search for the TP, a fast in–fast out technique, superficial dry needling vs. deep TPI, neurogenically evoked muscle twitches, and more thorough injection after initial block. A study comparing TPIs with a dry needle vs. 0.5% lidocaine showed that elicitation of a local twitch response during injection was the best indicator of a successful procedure.[26] Injection of botulinum toxin type A appears to be an increasingly popular but very expensive treatment for TPs in MP. Botox A inhibits muscle contraction by inhibiting release of acetylcholine at the motor endplate, resulting in sustained relaxation of muscles. Results of three RCTs are promising but mixed. Cheshire et al. found improved physical examination and 30% pain reduction after Botox A compared to saline, and the benefit lasted for 5 to 6 weeks.[28] Porta found greater improvement in symptoms after Botox A than steroid injection at 30 and 60 days after TPI combined with PT. The difference was statistically significant at 60 days, but not at 30 days.[29] Wheeler et al. were not able to find a statistically significant benefit for botulinum toxin injection compared to saline for refractory unilateral cervicothoracic paraspinal MP.[30] Cummings and White recommend the technique of TPI that is safest and most comfortable for the patient, in the absence of demonstrated superiority of any particular method.[27]

PHARMACOLOGIC TREATMENT

Stretching exercise, mechanical techniques, and TPIs are often supplemented with medications, although few RCTs have been published on drug therapy for MP. Data from trials in patients with low back pain, arthritis, tension headaches, and fibromyalgia have been used to guide therapy of MP with NSAIDs, tramadol, or antidepressants. Amitriptyline therapy of chronic tension-type headache, when it is effective, also reduces pericranial myofascial tenderness, without altering pain threshold at distant sites.[31] This suggests peripheral and/or spinal actions to reduce pain transmission. The alpha$_2$-adrenergic agonist and muscle relaxant tizanidine provided analgesia in an open-labeled study of patients with MP and fibromyalgia, but no RCTs have been published.[32]

CONCURRENT MANAGEMENT

When patients fail to respond as anticipated to corrections in postural and ergonomic factors, a comprehensive physical exercise program, supplemental TPIs, and pharmacologic therapy, the physician should of course consider other options. Search for a contributing psychological component and for other undiagnosed pain generators should be included in the comprehensive management of these patients. Interventions to address associated high levels of anxiety should be considered to supplement the selected stress management techniques.[9] Myofascial TPs may be associated with other underlying pain sources. For example, lumbar and gluteal MP may be associated with discogenic, ligamentous, facet joint, or sacroiliac joint pathology. Focused treatment of these pain generators may be necessary to produce prolonged pain relief. Undiagnosed visceral pathology may be present, e.g., thoracic TPs and pancreatic cancer. Persistent pain after an initial positive response should prompt a search for other sources of pain.

TABLE 44-1. COMPARISONS OF TWO PAIN SYNDROMES: MYOFASCIAL PAIN AND FIBROMYALGIA

Syndrome	Myofascial Pain Syndrome	Fibromyalgia Syndrome
Pain location	Local or regional	Widespread, in an axial site and in 3 of 4 body quadrants
Diagnostic finding	Trigger points within taut muscle band	Tender points; no palpable abnormality
Associated findings	Referred pain; local twitch response	Diffuse allodynia and hyperalgesia
Location	Trigger points within taut band in belly of muscle	Tender points in muscle, muscle–tendon junctions, bursae, or fat pad
Duration	Acute or chronic	Chronic, more than 3 months
Associated findings	Decreased range of motion; abnormal posture, body mechanics, and ergonomics	Insomnia, fatigue, distress, psychological disturbances, dysautonomia, deconditioning
Pathophysiology	Increased endplate acetylcholine release; sustained sarcomere contraction	Central sensitization; alpha–delta nonrestorative sleep pattern
Primary treatment	Stretching exercise	Multidisciplinary; pharmacologic therapy
Additional treatment	Trigger point injections; improve posture, body mechanics, ergonomics	Aerobic exercise; patient education; cognitive-behavioral therapy; multiple symptom control

OUTCOME

There are few studies of functional outcome in MP. Hanten et al. demonstrated the efficacy of PT in a controlled study referred to above.[21] In a study of pain and disability in patients with chronic low back pain Cassisi and colleagues reported that patients with myofascial low back pain had similar or somewhat worse outcomes than those with a disc herniation.[33] Roth and associates evaluated patient knowledge and satisfaction in chronic MP. MP patients tend to have inaccurate beliefs about their pain symptoms, and they express dissatisfaction with physician efforts to treat their pain and to educate them about the syndrome.[34] Heikkila et al. demonstrated moderate sustained benefit from a multidisciplinary program for patients with MP and whiplash injury.[35] These patients had improved coping skills, increased life satisfaction, and decreased sick time. Factors associated with failure to respond to treatment that included TPI were identified by logistic regression analysis. Only lack of employment due to pain at the start of treatment, prolonged duration of pain, and change in social activity were independently associated with poor treatment outcome.[36]

MP is a common finding in patients with regional musculoskeletal pain. Its etiology remains unknown. It may occur due to trauma, postural, or ergonomic factors, or in combination with other underlying pain generators. The existence of this syndrome has been questioned, and development of widely accepted diagnostic criteria for MP will facilitate future research and progress in management of MP. This syndrome has often been compared to fibromyalgia. This is illustrated in Table 44-1.

KEY POINTS

- MP is present in a significant proportion of patients presenting to chronic pain clinics. The clinician should look for this condition even when other sources of chronic pain have been identified in patients with persistent local or regional pain.
- Detection of active myofascial TPs requires identification by palpation of a taut muscle band associated with either an involuntary contraction (jump sign) or reproduction of the patient's usual pain symptoms.
- There appears to be a pathologic increase in the release of acetylcholine by abnormal endplates occurring in muscle TPs.
- The primary therapeutic intervention for MP is physical therapy. The cornerstone of this treatment is stretching exercise, designed to restore muscle length and activity.
- TPI is recommended to supplement and facilitate progress in physical therapy. The most efficacious technique for TPI has not been identified. The drug employed does not alter the outcome or offer any therapeutic benefit over dry needling; however, it may influence injection pain and postinjection soreness.
- The duration of pain relief is extended when botulinum toxin type A is utilized for TPI.

REFERENCES

1. Simons DG, Travell JG, Simons LS: Myofascial Pain and Dysfunction: The Trigger Point Manual. Vol I: Upper Half of Body, ed 2. Williams & Wilkins, Baltimore, 1999.
2. Borg-Stein J, Simons DG: Myofascial pain. Arch Phys Med Rehabil 83(Suppl 1):S40–S47, 2002.
3. Han SC, Harrison P: Myofascial pain syndrome and trigger point management. Reg Anesth 22:89–101, 1997.
4. Freund B, Schwartz M: Post-traumatic myofascial pain of the head and neck. Curr Pain Headache Rep 6:361–369, 2002.
5. Sola E, Bonica JJ: Myofascial pain syndromes. In Bonica JJ (ed): The Management of Pain, ed 2. Lea & Febiger, Philadelphia, 1990, pp 352–367.
6. Hamada H, Moriwaki K, Shiroyama K, et al: Myofascial pain in patients with postthoracotomy pain syndrome. Reg Anesth Pain Med 25:302–305, 2000.
7. Njoo KH, Van der Does E: The occurrence and inter-rater reliability of myofascial trigger points in the quadratus lumborum and gluteus medius: A prospective study in non-specific low back pain and controls in general medicine. Pain 58:317–323, 1994.
8. Sciotti VM, Mittak VL, DiMarco L, et al: Clinical precision of myofascial trigger point location in the trapezius muscle. Pain 93:259–266, 2001.
9. Esenyel M, Caglar N, Aldemir T: Treatment of myofascial pain. Am J Phys Med Rehabil 79:48–52, 2000.
10. Simons DG, Hong DZ, Simons LS: Endplate potentials are common to midfiber myofascial trigger points. Am J Phys Med Rehabil 81:212–222, 2002.
11. Rivner MH: The neurophysiology of myofascial pain syndrome. Curr Pain Headache Rep 5:432–440, 2001.
12. Simons DG, Stolov WC: Microscopic features and transient contraction of palpable bands in canine muscle. Am J Phys Med 55:65–88, 1976.
13. McNulty WH, Gevirtz RN, Hubbard DR, et al: Needle electromyographic evaluation of trigger point response to a psychological stressor. Psychophysiology 31:313–316, 1994.
14. Hubbard DR: Chronic and recurrent muscle pain: Pathophysiology and treatment, and review of pharmacological studies. J Musculoskeletal Pain 4:123–143, 1996.
15. Komiyama O, Kawara M, Arai M, et al: Posture correction as part of behavior therapy in treatment of myofascial pain with limited opening. J Oral Rehabil 26:428–435, 1999.
16. Crockett DJ, Foreman ME, Alden L, et al: A comparison of treatment modes in the management of myofascial pain dysfunction syndrome. Biofeedback Self Regul 11:279–291, 1986.
17. Birch S, Jamison RN: Controlled trial of Japanese acupuncture for chronic myofascial neck pain: Assessment of specific and nonspecific effects of treatment. Clin J Pain 14:248–255, 1998.
18. Melzack R, Stillwell DM, Fox EJ: Trigger points and acupuncture points for pain: Correlations and implications. Pain 3:3–23, 1977.
19. Gam AN, Warming S, Larsen LH, et al: Treatment of myofascial trigger points with ultrasound combined with massage and exercise: A randomized controlled trial. Pain 77:73–79, 1998.
20. Travell JG, Simons DG: Myofascial Pain and Dysfunction: The Trigger Point Manual, vol I. Williams & Wilkins, Baltimore, 1983.
21. Hanten WP, Olson WL, Butts NL, et al: Effectiveness of a home program of ischemic pressure followed by sustained stretch for treatment of myofascial trigger points. Phys Ther 80:97–1003, 2000.
22. Rothstein JM: Current, critical in-depth reviews of treatment literature by the Philadelphia panel for evidence-based clinical practice. Phys Ther 81:1620–1773, 2001.
23. Krishnan SK, Benzon HT, Siddiqui T, et al: Pain on intramuscular injection of bupivacaine, ropivacaine, with and without dexamethasone. Reg Anesth Pain Med 25:615–619, 2000.
24. Iwama H, Ohmori S, Kaneko T, et al: Water-diluted local anesthetic for trigger-point injection in chronic myofascial pain syndrome: Evaluation of types of local anesthetic and concentrations in water. Reg Anesth Pain Med 26:333–336, 2001.

25. Wreje U, Brorsson B: A multicenter randomized controlled trial of injections of sterile water and saline for chronic myofascial pain syndromes. Pain 61:441–444, 1995.

26. Hong C-Z: Lidocaine injection versus dry needling to myofascial trigger point: the importance of the local twitch response. Am J Phys Med Rehabil 73:256–263, 1994.

27. Cummings TM, White AR: Needling therapies in the management of myofascial trigger point pain: A systematic review. Arch Phys Ther 82:986–992, 2001.

28. Cheshire WP, Abashian SW, Mann JD: Botulinum toxin in the treatment of myofascial pain syndrome. Pain 59:65–69, 1994.

29. Porta M: A comparative trial of botulinum toxin type A and methylprednisolone for the treatment of myofascial pain syndrome and pain from chronic muscle spasm. Pain 85:101–105, 2000.

30. Wheeler AH, Goolkasian P, Gretz SS: A randomized, double-blind, prospective pilot study of botulinum toxin for refractory, unilateral, cervicothoracic, paraspinal, myofascial pain syndrome. Spine 23:1662–1666, 1998.

31. Bendtsen L, Jensen R: Amitriptyline reduces myofascial tenderness in patients with chronic tension-type headache. Cephalalgia 20:603–610, 2000.

32. Barkhuizen A: Rational and targeted pharmacologic treatment of fibromyalgia. Rheum Dis Clin North Am 28:261–290, 2002.

33. Cassisi JE, Sypert GW, Lagana L, et al: Pain, disability, and psychological functioning in chronic low back pain subgroups: Myofascial versus herniated disk syndrome. Neurosurgery 33:379–385, 1993.

34. Roth RS, Horowitz K, Bachman JE: Chronic myofascial pain: Knowledge of diagnosis and satisfaction with treatment. Arch Phys Med Rehabil 79:966–970, 1998.

35. Heikkila H, Heikkila E, Eisemann M: Predictive factors for the outcome of a multidisciplinary pain rehabilitation programme on sick-leave and life satisfaction in patients with whiplash trauma and other myofascial pain: A follow-up study. Clin Rehabil 12:487–496, 1998.

36. Hopwood MB, Abram SE: Factors associated with failure of trigger point injections. Clin J Pain 10:227–234, 1994.

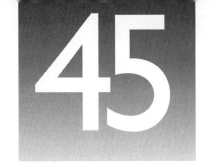

Fibromyalgia

Robert E. Molloy, M.D.

Fibromyalgia (FM) is a prevalent musculoskeletal pain disorder characterized by diffuse pain and abnormal soft tissue tenderness. Associated symptoms include widespread pain at multiple tender points (at the muscle–tendon junction and in muscles, bursae, and fat pads), reduced pain threshold, fatigue, sleep disturbances, morning stiffness, depression, anxiety, psychological distress, subjective swelling, irritable bowel syndrome, headaches, and paresthesias. The etiology and pathophysiology of FM have not been delineated, and effective treatment approaches have not been identified. This syndrome has often been compared to myofascial pain. This comparison is illustrated in Table 44-1.

The syndrome was first described in the 1800s and it has been known by many names. It is a common disorder in countries worldwide, affecting all socioeconomic, ethnic, and racial groups.[1] The prevalence is between 0.5% and 5% of the population. The syndrome is most frequently seen in women between the ages of 20 and 50 years, and the gender ratio is 10:1 favoring women. Some authors claim that Western compensation systems have fostered an epidemic of FM. There is no evidence of an increasing incidence of FM, and current data show no association between FM prevalence and compensation.[2]

DIAGNOSIS

The diagnosis of FM is based on clinical findings. The American College of Rheumatology established the diagnostic criteria for FM in 1990, with a predicted sensitivity of 88% and a specificity of 81%.[3] The criteria are:

1. Chronic widespread pain (CWP), of at least 3 months' duration, present above and below the diaphragm, on both sides of the body, plus axial pain.
2. Painful tender points (TPs) in at least 11 out of 18 characteristic locations (Fig. 45-1). TPs are defined by mild or greater pain after palpation with an approximate force of 4 kg/cm^2 (thumb pressure such that the nail bed starts to blanch) at these sites:

- Bilateral occiput, at the suboccipital muscle insertion.
- Bilateral low cervical, at anterior aspect of intertransverse spaces between C5 and C7.
- Bilateral trapezius, at midpoint of the upper border.
- Bilateral supraspinatus, at its origin above scapular spine near the border.
- Bilateral second rib, just lateral to the costochondral junctions on upper surface.
- Bilateral lateral epicondyle, 2 cm distal to the epicondyle.
- Bilateral gluteal, at the upper outer quadrant of the buttock.
- Bilateral greater trochanter, posterior to the trochanter.
- Bilateral knee, medial fat pad proximal to the joint line.

Only about 20% of individuals in the population with CWP also have 11/18 tender points; these individuals are more likely to be female and have higher levels of psychological distress. While there is no clear diagnosis for these people, it is likely that they have pain that is primarily central rather than peripheral in nature.[4] The 18 selected TPs represent only about 3% of the more than 600 muscles in the body, each of which might theoretically contain a TP. Yunus[5] has classified FM patients into five clinical groups, based upon their predominant symptoms:

- Predominant pain and fatigue.
- Predominant anxiety, stress, and depression.
- Predominant multiple sites of pain complaints and tender points.
- Predominant numbness and swollen feeling.
- Associated features, irritable bowel syndrome, and headaches.

Turk et al.[6] also classified FM patients, based on psychosocial and behavioral factors using the multidimensional pain inventory (MPI), into three subgroups:

- Dysfunctional (DYS): high pain levels, functional limitation, and affective distress.

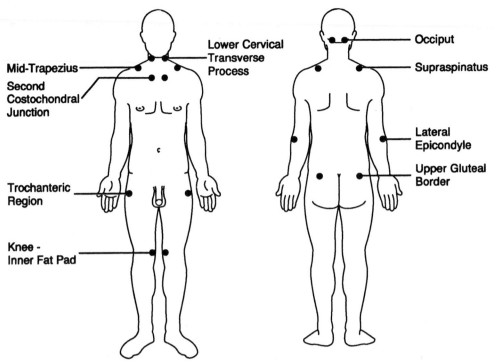

FIGURE 45-1. Characteristic location of 18 painful tender points used for diagnosis of fibromyalgia.

- Interpersonally Distressed (ID): similar to DYS with low levels of support from the partner.
- Adaptive Copers (AC): low levels of pain, distress, and disability.

There was no difference in physical findings between groups, but response to a standard rehabilitation program varied by subgroup. The DYS group improved in all categories, while the ID patients failed to respond to treatment. The AC group showed little change, possibly due to a ceiling effect.[7]

Evaluation of patients with CWP requires a targeted musculoskeletal history and physical examination. The widespread pain is primarily axial and diffuse, but it may affect any region. It may be described as sharp, aching, cramping, dull, or burning; and the severity of pain varies over time. Pain drawings may best assess the widespread nature of the pain. The severity of pain, fatigue, and insomnia are best evaluated with simple verbal rating scores, e.g., 0 to 10. Poor sleep is an important symptom that correlates with fatigue and predicts intensity of pain the next day. Roizenblatt et al. reported that FM patients with phasic alpha sleep reported more pain and TPs following disturbed sleep.[8] Two other important symptoms characteristic of FM are subjective swollen feeling without objective joint swelling and paresthesia without objective neurologic findings.[9] They may reflect heightened sensory perception due to central sensitization. FM symptoms are often aggravated by cold humid weather, interrupted sleep, repeated injury, mental stress, and inactivity. FM symptoms tend to improve with warm dry climate, rest, modest activity, good sleep, and relaxation.[9] FM is associated with many similar conditions, including irritable bowel syndrome (in 30% to 50%), tension headaches, migraine headaches, temporomandibular dysfunction, myofascial pain syndrome, chronic fatigue syndrome, restless legs syndrome

(in one-third), multiple chemical sensitivity, and post-traumatic stress disorder. These conditions may all represent examples based upon central sensitization. Several other diseases may be associated with and aggravate symptoms of FM: systemic lupus, rheumatoid arthritis, Sjogren's syndrome, osteoarthritis, spinal stenosis, neuropathy, hypothyroidism, and growth hormone deficiency (in about one-third of patients).

Underlying psychological symptoms and behavioral adaptations may trigger or aggravate FM symptoms. Screening evaluation for depression, anxiety, stress, and poor coping skills helps select FM patients for whom psychological evaluation or cognitive-behavioral therapy would be appropriate.

PATHOPHYSIOLOGY

The cause of FM remains unclear. Theories have been proposed based upon findings in FM patients. There is a strong association between FM and *sleep disturbance*. Normal sleep involves four nondream stages (non-REM sleep) alternating with a dream stage (REM sleep). Many FM patients exhibit an alpha–delta EEG pattern, which may explain why they do not get into the restorative stages 3 and 4 of non-REM sleep.[1,10] This is due to alpha wave (7.5 to 11 Hz) intrusion during delta wave (0.5 to 2 Hz) sleep. The experimental induction of alpha–delta sleep in healthy individuals has been reported to induce symptoms suggestive of FM, such as muscle aching, stiffness, and tenderness.[11] Nonrestorative sleep often leads to increased pain and fatigue, and pharmacologic correction of the sleep abnormality may improve both symptoms.

FM is often associated with diseases that have an autoimmune basis, such as rheumatoid arthritis and systemic lupus, suggesting a possible *immune system alteration*. No consistent link or pathological evidence has been found. An *endocrine abnormality* has also been proposed. Diminished responsiveness of the hypothalamic–pituitary system has been reported.[12] One-third of a group of FM patients were found to be growth hormone deficient.[13] There is no consistent correlation with hypothyroidism, although it may aggravate symptoms in FM. Hormonal abnormalities appear to be minor, limited to subgroups of patients, and to have a central rather than peripheral origin.[14] An underlying *psychological disturbance* has also been considered. About 30% of FM patients have clinical depression, and a much larger proportion have symptoms of psychological distress.[15]

Muscle pathology is another possible mechanism of FM. There have been no consistent histological findings, although there have been reports of muscle abnormalities of membranes, mitochondria, and fiber type, and an attempt to correlate these structural findings with biochemical abnormalities and defective energy production.[16] The most common findings are changes consistent with disuse or deconditioning. There seems to be an agreement that the pathophysiology is primarily within the central nervous system (CNS) rather than peripheral in FM.[17,18]

Abnormal central neurophysiology resulting in widespread pain seems to be the most accepted pathologic mechanism in FM. Pain perception in FM is due to central sensitization, defined as generalized, heightened pain sensitivity due to pathological nociceptive processing within the CNS.[19,20] There are presumably different levels of central sensitization, which may explain the variable experience of pain in FM patients. Elevations in cerebrospinal fluid levels of substance P and nerve growth factor, neuropeptides that enhance nociceptive neurotransmission, have been reported in FM patients. Activation of *N*-methyl-D-aspartate (NMDA) receptors plays an important part in central sensitization. There is good experimental evidence that blocking NMDA receptors diminishes pain in FM. Infusion of ketamine, an NMDA antagonist, abolished pain for an extended period.[21] Addition of moderate doses of dextromethorphan, a weak NMDA receptor antagonist, to a stable dose of tramadol provided improved analgesia in FM patients, although often with unacceptable central side effects.[22]

MANAGEMENT

The goals of patient management include accurate diagnosis; patient education and empowerment; symptom control for pain, fatigue, and sleep; management of associated psychological, endocrine, and autonomic disorders; treatment of any peripheral pain generators; and improved physical conditioning and function.

PATIENT EDUCATION

The components of a FM educational program have been summarized by Bennett.[23] Key components would include:

- Validate the patient's symptoms and explain nature of FM syndrome.
- Emphasize nondestructive and treatable nature of FM symptoms.
- Set realistic goals: improving function without complete symptom eradication.
- Discuss all treatment options and enlist patient in selection of plan.

- Stress importance of gentle, life-long aerobic exercise and pacing activity.
- Educate patient on principles of sleep hygiene.
- Teach coping skills: meditation and relaxation techniques.
- Improve patient assertiveness and active role in FM management plan.
- Refer patients to educational resources, including on-line self-help material.

NONPHARMACOLOGIC PATIENT MANAGEMENT

The value of patient education in FM was assessed in three randomized controlled trials (RCTs) that compared education programs to wait list or no treatment controls. The experimental groups were significantly better than controls at the end of treatment, and the benefit was sustained for 3 to 12 months after treatment.[24] Cognitive-behavioral strategies teach patients how their thoughts and behaviors influence symptoms, how they can potentially control their symptoms, and specific cognitive and behavioral management skills. Six of seven studies, including five RCTs, have demonstrated patient improvements. These included significant changes in tender points, pain scores, coping scores, or pain behaviors. These trials suggest cognitive-behavioral therapy is beneficial to patients with FM.[24]

EXERCISE THERAPY

FM patients are deconditioned and therefore good candidates for rehabilitative physical therapy. A carefully planned individual exercise program is required, because a too rigorous program may be deleterious for FM patients. There is convincing evidence that aerobic exercise produces significant benefits for patients with FM. The most frequently positive outcome variables were improvements in pain scores and tender points. Busch et al. reviewed 16 RCTs of exercise for FM patients. In seven high-quality studies supervised aerobic exercise training had beneficial effects on aerobic performance, pain scores, and tender point pain pressure thresholds. Strength training may also have had benefits on some FM symptoms.[25] Sim and Adams also performed a systematic review of RCTs of nondrug interventions in FM which included exercise, education, relaxation, cognitive-behavioral therapy, acupuncture, and hydrotherapy. Significant differences were present in 17 of 24 studies. There was not strong evidence to support any single intervention, but moderate support existed for aerobic exercise.[26] There are studies that suggest a positive benefit from both acupuncture and biofeedback in FM.[24]

PHARMACOLOGIC TREATMENT OF PAIN AND ASSOCIATED SYMPTOMS

Pharmacologic therapy is often the mainstay of treatment for patients with FM. Multiple agents may be used to address various symptoms associated with this diagnosis (see Table 45-1). The general principles of drug treatment outlined in Table 45-2 may serve as helpful guidelines in managing these patients. FM patients frequently use nonsteroidal anti-inflammatory drugs (NSAIDs) or acetaminophen. These analgesic agents ideally play a role in addressing peripheral pain generators that have been identified. Most drug therapy aims to address the primary

TABLE 45-1. PHARMACOLOGIC THERAPY

Symptoms Amenable to Pharmacologic Therapy
Pain (acetaminophen, NSAIDs, tramadol, TCAs, NMDA blockers)
Sleep disturbances (antihistamines, sedatives, muscle relaxants; restless leg treatments)
Mood disturbances (antidepressants: TCAs, venlafaxine)
Fatigue (SSRIs and 5-HT$_3$ antagonists, stimulants)
Associated disorders (irritable bowel syndrome, migraine headaches, TMJ disorders)
Peripheral pain generators (TPs, bursitis, tendonitis, arthritis, trauma, neuropathic pain)

Data from Barkhuizen.[30]

pathology which appears to be pain due to central sensitization. Tricyclic antidepressants (TCAs) have been the most common drug treatment for FM. A meta-analysis of antidepressant therapy for FM analyzed 13 RCTs. The overall odds ratio for improvement with therapy was 4.2. Antidepressants improved

TABLE 45-2. PHARMACOLOGIC THERAPY

Pharmacologic Treatment Principles
Emphasize that the goal is to improve function and quality of life
A realistic goal of treatment is to palliate, not abolish, symptoms
Start at extremely low initial doses of drugs
Use very slow incremental dose increases
Cyclical use of insomnia medications may help avoid habituation
Frequently review medications used; employ tapering to document continued efficacy
Periodic drug holidays may confirm utility and increase the efficacy of drug therapy
Limit number of drugs by focus on relief of the primary symptoms, tolerable side effects

Data from Barkhuizen.[30]

sleep, fatigue, pain, and well-being in that order; but they did not improve tender points. Four patients needed to be treated for one patient to experience symptom improvement.[27]

The selective serotonin reuptake inhibitors (SSRIs) have less impressive analgesic effects in FM, but they may be helpful for emotional components and mood disorders that are commonly present. A combination of fluoxetine and amitriptyline was superior to either agent alone for FM symptoms, independent of any change in the Beck depression inventory.[28] The serotonin-norepinephrine dual reuptake inhibitors (SNRIs) are quite similar to TCAs in sharing these two mechanisms of action, but they are devoid of activity at other receptor systems. This may improve on side-effect profile and increase patient tolerance when compared to TCAs. Venlafaxine primarily affects the 5-HT system at low doses, with NE effects apparent at higher doses. In an open clinical trial of venlafaxine, 6 of 11 patients had at least 50% relief of FM symptoms.[29] There have been no clinical trials, but there is anecdotal evidence that tizanidine, an alpha$_2$-adrenergic agonist and muscle relaxant with antinociceptive and antispasmodic actions, has been used effectively for FM-related pain and for sleep disturbance.[30]

Low-dose (started at 5 to 10 mg) TCA therapy at bedtime has been the most common sleep therapy for FM patients with sleep disturbance. Cyclobenzaprine, a TCA-analogue muscle relaxant, also had positive effects on sleep and evening fatigue in FM patients.[31] For patients intolerant of TCAs, short-acting imidazopyridine hypnotics (zolpidem and zaleplon) have been beneficial for many FM patients; unlike benzodiazepines, they do not interfere with stage 3 and stage 4 sleep, or with memory.[32] Alternatively, over-the-counter antihistamines are frequently used in cyclical fashion with prescribed hypnotics. Γ-Hydroxybutyrate was used in a 1-month sleep study; it resulted in increased slow wave sleep, and improved fatigue and pain.[30] The most common sleep disorder in FM patients is restless leg syndrome, characterized by crawling sensations of the legs and an uncontrollable urge to stretch. Treatment with L-dopa/carbidopa at dinner or with clonazepam at bedtime may be effective. Other dopamine agonists (pergolide, pramixepole, and tolixepole) and bedtime methadone have also been effective.[30] Sedative drugs should be avoided in patients with untreated sleep apnea.

Fatigue is often resistant to drug therapy in FM patients. Anecdotal reports suggest SSRI drugs improve symptoms of fatigue in FM. The 5-HT$_3$ antagonist tropisetron has also proven beneficial in FM-related fatigue.[33] Modafinal, a nonamphetamine drug used in narcolepsy, has not been studied in FM patients. Psychiatric syndromes in FM patients should be managed by mental health professionals. Other associated or related syndromes should also be appropriately treated in these patients.

The primary goals of treatment for patients with FM are palliation of symptoms combined with improved physical and emotional well-being. Evaluation of response to treatment over time may employ multiple tools, including pain scores and similar scores for other symptoms, pain drawings, measurements of physical performance, and self-assessment questionnaires. Bennett[23] recommends use of the Fibromyalgia Impact Questionnaire (FIQ), which assesses quality of life and the various problems associated with FM.[34]

KEY POINTS

- The diagnosis of FM depends on two criteria. The first is CWP, present for over 3 months. There must be axial pain and additional painful sites in 3 of 4 body quadrants. The second requirement is the presence of TPs on examination in at least 11 of 18 characteristic predetermined sites.

- A TP is defined by mild or greater pain after palpation with thumb pressure sufficient to produce initial blanching of the nail bed.
- The pathologic basis of FM is primarily altered central neurophysiology rather than a peripheral process. Central sensitization resulting in widespread pain perception is the most commonly accepted mechanism of FM. NMDA receptor antagonists diminish the symptoms of FM.
- The presence of interrupted sleep is an important symptom that correlates with fatigue and predicts intensity of pain the following day.
- TCAs improve sleep, fatigue, pain, and well-being in patients with FM. They are often effective at very low doses.
- FM patients are often deconditioned. There is convincing evidence that aerobic exercise produces significant benefits for these patients; very suggestive evidence also supports the use of cognitive-behavioral therapy.

REFERENCES

1. Parziale JR, Chen JJ: Fibromyalgia. Med Health RI 79:188–192, 1996.
2. White KP, Harth M: Classification, epidemiology, and natural history of fibromyalgia. Curr Pain Headache Rep 5:320–329, 2001.
3. Wolfe F, Smythe HA, Yunus MB, et al: The American College of Rheumatology 1990 criteria for classification of fibromyalgia: Report of the Multicenter Criteria Committee. Arthritis Rheum 33:160–172, 1990.
4. Clauw DJ, Crofford LJ: Chronic widespread pain and fibromyalgia: What we know, and what we need to know. Best Pract Res Clin Rheumatol 17:685–701, 2003.
5. Yunus MB, Aldag JC: The underlying constructs of fibromyalgia syndrome by factor analysis. Arthritis Rheum 39:S275, 1996.
6. Turk DC, Okifuji A, Sinclair JD, et al: Pain, disability, and physical functioning in subgroups of fibromyalgia patients. J Rheumatol 23:1255–1262, 1996.
7. Turk DC, Okifuji A, Sinclair JD, et al: Differential responses by psychosocial subgroups of fibromyalgia syndrome patients to an interdisciplinary treatment. Arthritis Care Res 111:397–404, 1998.
8. Roizenblatt S, Moldofsky H, Beneddito-Silva AA, et al: Alpha sleep characteristics in fibromyalgia. Arthritis Rheum 1:222–230, 2001.
9. Yunus MB: A comprehensive medical evaluation of patients with fibromyalgia syndrome. Rheum Dis Clin N Am 28:201–217, 2002.
10. Drewes AM, Gade K, Nielsen KD, et al: Clustering of sleep electroencephalographic patterns in patients with the fibromyalgia syndrome. Br J Rheumatol 34:1151–1156, 1995.
11. Moldofsky H, Scarisbrick P: Induction of neurasthenic musculoskeletal pain syndrome by selective sleep deprivation. Psychosom Med 38:35–44, 1976.
12. Crofford LJ, Pillemer SR, Kalogeras KT, et al: Hypothalamic–pituitary–adrenal axis perturbations in patients with fibromyalgia. Arthritis Rheum 37:1583–1592, 1994.
13. Bennett RM, Clark SC, Walczyk J: A randomized, double-blind, placebo-controlled study of growth hormone in the treatment of fibromyalgia. Am J Med 104:227–231, 1998.
14. Geenen R, Jacobs JW, Bijlsma JW: Evaluation and management of endocrine dysfunction in fibromyalgia. Rheum Dis Clin North Am 28:389–404, 2002.
15. Okifuji A, Turk DC, Sherman JJ: Evaluation of the relationship between depression and fibromyalgia syndrome: Why aren't all patients depressed? J Rheumatol 27:212–219, 2000.
16. Park JH, Niermann KJ, Olsen NJ: Evidence for metabolic abnormalities in the muscles of patients with fibromyalgia. Curr Rheumatol Rep 2:131–140, 2000.
17. Olsen NJ, Park JH: Skeletal muscle abnormalities in patients with fibromyalgia. Am J Med Sci 315:351–358, 1998.
18. Simms RW: Fibromyalgia is not a muscle disorder. Am J Med Sci 315:346–350, 1998.
19. Bennet RM: Emerging concepts in the neurobiology of chronic pain: Evidence of abnormal sensory processing in fibromyalgia. Mayo Clin Proc 74:385–398, 1999.
20. Staud R, Vierck CJ, Cannon RL: Abnormal sensitization and temporal summation of second pain (wind-up) in patients with fibromyalgia syndrome. Pain 91:165–175, 2001.
21. Sorenson J, Bengtsson A, Backmann A, et al: Pain analysis in patients with fibromyalgia: Effects of intravenous morphine, lidocaine, and ketamine. Scand J Rheumatol 24: 360–365, 1995.
22. Clark SR, Bennett RM: Supplemental dextromethorphan in the treatment of fibromyalgia: A double-blind, placebo controlled study of efficacy and side effects. Arthritis Rheum 43:333, 2000.
23. Bennett RM: The rational management of fibromyalgia patients. Rheum Dis Clin North Am 28:181–199, 2002.
24. Burckhardt CS: Nonpharmacologic management strategies in fibromyalgia. Rheum Dis Clin North Am 28:291–304, 2002.
25. Busch A, Schacter CL, Peloso PM: Exercise for treating fibromyalgia syndrome. Cochrane Database Syst Rev 3:CD003786, 2002.
26. Sim J, Adams N: Systematic review of randomized controlled trials of nonpharmacological interventions for fibromyalgia. Clin J Pain 18:324–326, 2002.
27. O'Malley PG, Balden E, Tomkins G, et al: Treatment of fibromyalgia with antidepressants: A meta-analysis. J Gen Intern Med 15:659–666, 2000.
28. Goldenberg D, Mayskiy M, Mossey C, et al: A randomized, double-blind, crossover trial of fluoxetine and amitriptyline in the treatment of fibromyalgia. Arthritis Rheum 39:1852–1859, 1996.
29. Dwight MM, Arnold LM, O'Brien H, et al: An open clinical trial of venlafaxine treatment of fibromyalgia. Psychosomatics 39:14–17, 1998.
30. Barkhuizen A: Rational and targeted pharmacologic treatment of fibromyalgia. Rheum Dis Clin North Am 28:261–290, 2002.
31. Reynolds WJ, Moldofsky H, Saskin P, et al: The effects of cyclobenzaprine on sleep physiology and symptoms in patients with fibromyalgia. J Rheumatol 18:452–454, 1991.
32. Depoortere H, Zirkovic B, Lloyd KG, et al: Zolpidem, a novel nonbenzodiazepine hypnotic: Neuropharmacological and behavioral effects. J Pharmacol Exp Ther 237:649–658, 1986.
33. Haus U, Varga B, Stratz T, et al: Oral treatment of fibromyalgia with tropisetron given over 28 days: Influence on functional and vegetative symptoms, psychometric parameters, and pain. Scand J Rheumatol Suppl 13:55–58, 2000.
34. Burckhardt CS, Clark SR, Bennett RM: The fibromyalgia impact questionnaire: Development and validation. J Rheumatol 18:728–733, 1991.

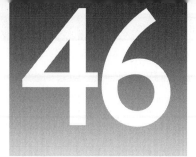

Complex Regional Pain Syndromes: Terminology and Pathophysiology

Theodore S. Grabow, M.D.,
Anthony H. Guarino, M.D., and
Srinivasa N. Raja, M.D.

Silas Weir Mitchell first used the term *causalgia* to describe the chronic pain syndrome observed in Unionist soldiers in the American Civil War who suffered from traumatic nerve injuries. It was almost half a century after the original description of the syndrome before the sympathetic nervous system was implicated in causalgic pain by the French surgeon Rene Leriche. The term *reflex sympathetic dystrophy* (RSD) was introduced first by Evans in the middle of the 20th century. Over subsequent years, the terms reflex sympathetic dystrophy and causalgia have been used in many different and confusing ways. A variety of terms (Table 46-1) have been applied to these syndromes that have similar clinical features resulting in an ambiguous literature which has complicated our understanding of the basic pathophysiology of the disease. In addition, a sympathetic component could not be identified by clinical presentation, diagnostic testing, or therapeutic response to neural blockade in many individuals with the diagnosis of RSD.

In 1993 a panel of experts formulated a consensus opinion that the terms RSD and causalgia had lost their usefulness as a clinical designation and had become a default diagnosis for patients with varying degrees of neuropathic pain and/or resistance to traditional therapeutic strategies. Consequently, a new nomenclature was suggested and subsequently adopted by the International Association for the Study of Pain (IASP) in their *Classification of Chronic Pain*. Despite the new taxonomy, several aspects of the disease continue to generate considerable controversy.[1]

The new term that was introduced to describe all chronic pain states that previously would have been diagnosed as RSD or causalgia-like syndromes was CRPS: complex regional pain syndrome.[2] *Complex* indicates the varied and dynamic nature of the clinical presentation not only within a single individual

over time but also between individuals with apparently similar disorders. *Regional* denotes the distribution of the symptoms that are typically nondermatomal and often with signs and symptoms beyond the region of the original injury. *Pain* is out of proportion to the inciting events. *Syndrome* describes the constellation of symptoms and signs that can be characterized as a distinct entity. Since the contribution of the sympathetic nervous system in CRPS was not constant across patients, the term "sympathetic" was avoided in the revised definition. Thus, CRPS describes a variety of chronic pain states that usually follows a traumatic event, is typically regional and distal in the distribution of pain and sensory changes, exceeds in duration and magnitude the clinical course of the inciting event, has a variable clinical course over time, and often results in significant impairment of motor function.

CRPS type I (RSD) is defined as a syndrome that develops after an initiating noxious event that may or may not be associated with a period of immobilization. Continuous pain often is associated with hyperalgesia and allodynia. Hyperalgesia refers to the perception of exaggerated or increased pain to a normally painful stimulus. Allodynia refers to the perception of pain to an otherwise innocuous stimulus such as light touch. The symptoms are not limited to the territory of a single peripheral nerve and are disproportionate to the inciting event. There is or has been evidence of edema, skin blood flow abnormality, or abnormal sudomotor activity in the painful region since the inciting event. The diagnosis is excluded by the existence of conditions that would otherwise account for the degree of pain and dysfunction. CRPS type II (causalgia) differs from CRPS type I by the presence of a known injury to a peripheral nerve.

In certain patients with CRPS pain depends on sympathetic activity in the affected area. The term "sympathetically maintained

TABLE 46-1. TERMS USED FOR RSD AND CAUSALGIC SYNDROMES

Acute atrophy of the bone
Algodystrophy
Algoneurodystrophy
Causalgia
Chronic traumatic edema
Postinfarctional sclerodactyly
Post-traumatic algodystrophy
Post-traumatic dystrophy
Post-traumatic osteoporosis
Post-traumatic spreading neuralgia
Post-traumatic sympathetic dystrophy
Pseudodystrophy
Reflex neurovascular dystrophy
Reflex sympathetic dystrophy
Shoulder hand syndrome
Sudeck's atrophy
Sympathalgia
Traumatic angiospasm
Traumatic vasospasm

sympathetically mediated pain and the other may not. To differentiate the sympathetic component, one can perform a selective sympathetic block (see Ch. 80, Peripheral Sympathetic Blocks). It is important to understand that the SMP/SIP terminology is an operational definition where the chronic pain syndrome is categorized according to the response to selective sympathetic blockade. Defining a sympathetic component to CRPS is useful from a clinical perspective, since treatment is influenced accordingly.

Many components may contribute to the overall clinical picture of CRPS: sympathetic, sensory, autonomic, inflammatory, motor, and psychological phenomena (Fig. 46-1). Individuals may have varying degrees of each of these aspects which constitutes each person's unique pain experience. In addition, clinical observations indicate that CRPS is a dynamic entity. The different components contributing to a patient's pain can vary with time; the sympathetic efferents may contribute the majority of a patient's pain on one day and on another occasion may contribute only a small proportion of the overall pain. A patient can have CRPS without any sympathetic contribution to the pain.

The sensory symptoms and signs in CRPS are spontaneous pain, hyperpathia, allodynia, and hyperalgesia. Hyperpathia refers to pain elicited by a noxious stimulus that is delayed in onset but outlasts the stimulus duration and spreads beyond the site of the stimulus. Allodynia may result from a cold breeze, touching or brushing of the skin, or movement of the affected joint. Other associated clinical phenomena include

pain" (SMP) describes that aspect of the pain that is relieved by blockade of the efferent sympathetic nervous system. This can be accomplished by local anesthetic blockade of sympathetic ganglia (e.g., stellate ganglion or lumbar sympathetic ganglion) or by pharmacological antagonism of alpha-1 adrenoceptors. In contrast, "sympathetically independent pain" (SIP) refers to that aspect of pain that is not alleviated by sympathetic blockade. The evidence supporting the role of the sympathetic nervous system in chronic pain states including CRPS has been reviewed by Baron and colleagues.[3] Clinically, a patient with CRPS may present with SMP or SIP, or part of his/her chronic pain syndrome may be SMP and part of it may be SIP. There is no definitive way to diagnose SMP on the basis of signs, symptoms, or clinical history. Two patients may have similar clinical presentations and one patient could have

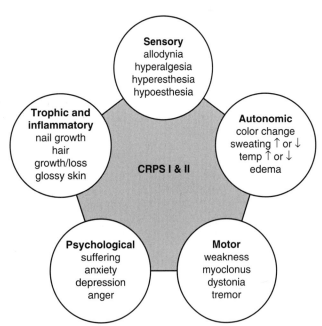

FIGURE 46-1. The principal clinical components of CRPS types I and II. The magnitude of each component as depicted should not be construed as reflecting quantitative relationships. The multidisciplinary approach to the management of CRPS should therefore take into consideration all elements of the syndrome. (Adapted from Boas RA: Complex regional pain syndromes: Symptoms, signs, and differential diagnosis. In Janig W, Stanton-Hicks M (eds): Reflex Sympathetic Dystrophy: A Reappraisal. IASP Press, Seattle, 1996, p. 88.)

changes in skin color, skin temperature, sweating, motor function, and structure of superficial and deep tissues (trophic changes). The syndrome predominantly occurs in the extremities and typically does not follow a dermatomal or peripheral nerve distribution. Patients with CRPS may also have associated psychological and psychiatric disturbances. It is generally agreed that these are consequences rather than causes of the disorder.[4,5]

Historically, RSD was considered to progress through different stages. The stages were described based on the duration of the disease and/or certain clinical characteristics. The consensus of the panel that introduced the new terminology was that staging or grading of CRPS based on clinical presentation had little utility from a descriptive, diagnostic, or treatment standpoint. In fact, there is little scientific evidence that such stages actually exist.

NEURAL MECHANISMS UNDERLYING CRPS: A HYPOTHESIS

The exact pathophysiology of CRPS is unclear. However, recent clinical and experimental studies in animal models of neuropathic pain have shed considerable light on the plastic changes in the peripheral and central nervous system that may contribute to the mechanisms of persistent pain.[6,7] A schema of the hypothesis on the mechanisms leading to CRPS is shown in Fig. 46-2. An initial injury activates nociceptors and results in signals along nociceptive pathways from the periphery to the spinal cord. The input of signals in nociceptive neurons to the spinal cord leads to alterations in spinal modulatory mechanisms resulting in sensitization of central pain signaling neurons. The sensitized dorsal horn neurons could then be activated by low-threshold mechanoreceptive afferents leading to the clinical phenomenon of allodynia. Simultaneously, antidromic excitation produces neurogenic inflammation (vasodilation, increased capillary permeability, and release of inflammatory mediators) which further sensitizes peripheral nociceptors.

An important question is what maintains the state of central hyperexcitability, i.e., sensitization. Unlike inflammatory pain states where hyperalgesia subsides after local healing of tissues, why does the pain persist in CRPS? It is postulated that the persistence of the central state of hyperexcitability is dependent on continued input from the periphery along nociceptive pathways. Painful input may be the result of several possible mechanisms: ectopic activity that develops in neuromas at the site of a nerve injury, ectopic generators in the dorsal root ganglia, or functional coupling between sensory afferent and sympathetic efferent fibers.

Sympathetic–sensory interactions leading to increased activity in nociceptive neurons may be the result of development of alpha-adrenergic receptor sensitivity in nociceptors such that nociceptors are activated by norepinephrine released by tonic activity in sympathetic efferent fibers. Abnormalities in sweating and vasomotor tone led some earlier investigators to postulate an increased sympathetic efferent activity in SMP. However, several recent experimental and clinical studies have confirmed that there is no evidence for an increase in sympathetic drive. In fact regional norepinephrine release in the affected limb is less than that in the unaffected limb of patients with CRPS.

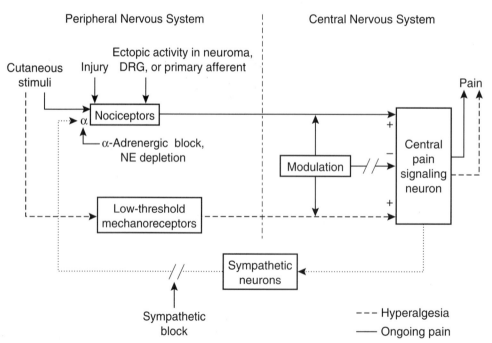

FIGURE 46-2. Model for sympathetically maintained pain. In SMP nociceptors develop adrenergic sensitivity such that the release of norepinephrine by the sympathetic efferent fibers produces activity in the nociceptors. This activity maintains the central nervous system in a sensitized state. Pain to light touch is signaled by activity in low-threshold mechanoreceptors in the presence of an enhanced sensitivity of the central pain-signaling neurons. Local anesthetic blockade of the sympathetic neurons or a peripheral adrenergic block (phentolamine infusion) will eliminate this ongoing activity in the nociceptors and thus lead to reversal of the central sensitized state.

The concept of SMP has generated considerable debate over the last decade. Skeptics were concerned that SMP could only be demonstrated as a consequence of pharmacological treatment such as sympathetic block, alpha-adrenoceptor antagonism, or injection of norepinephrine. Recently two independent laboratories examined the effect of the natural physiological stimulation of the sympathetic nervous system on spontaneous pain and hyperalgesia. Drummond and colleagues demonstrated that sympathetic arousal increased pain and vasoconstriction in the affected extremity of patients with CRPS types I and II.[8] Similarly, Baron and colleagues demonstrated that sympathetic activation increased spontaneous pain and spatial distribution of mechanical hyperalgesia in patients with CRPS type I who were characterized as having SMP by pharmacological tests.[9] These two investigations were the first to demonstrate that physiological activation of the sympathetic nervous system can modulate the pain experience in humans through the release of endogenous norepinephrine from sympathetic nerve endings under physiological conditions. These findings provide the most convincing evidence in support of the concept of SMP in humans.

One potential goal of therapy is identifying the site where the painful input is generated in order to block the signals from reaching the central nervous system such that the pathological process is interrupted. Such a maneuver may allow the central pain signaling neurons to reset themselves to a state of normal excitability. Considerable research is being conducted to determine the pharmacological mechanisms for the sensitization of central neurons in an attempt to interrupt or reverse this process.

OTHER MECHANISMS (INFLAMMATION)

Animal models of nerve injury have provided the foundations for our mechanistic understanding of CRPS type II. Elucidation of the underlying mechanisms of CRPS type I has been more difficult. Nevertheless, clinicians currently utilize preclinical evidence from animal models of inflammatory pain. The rationale for this assumption is derived from clinical experience and scientific investigation suggesting underlying inflammation at least during the acute phase of CRPS. Evidence supporting a regional inflammatory response has been reviewed elsewhere, but includes increased capillary permeability, increased oxidative stress and impaired oxygen metabolism, increased systemic levels of inflammatory mediators, and therapeutic response to corticosteroids.[10] In addition, experimental tissue acidosis leads to increased pain predominantly in the muscles and to a lesser extent in the skin of the affected limb of patients with CRPS. Several investigators have concluded that the clinical presentation may reflect neurogenic rather than humorally mediated inflammation.[11] Neurogenic inflammation is the activity-dependent, primary sensory afferent-mediated, central and peripheral release of neuropeptides which ultimately results in vasodilation and plasma extravasation in the affected region. Recently higher levels of proinflammatory mediators have been detected locally in the affected limbs of patients with CRPS which also suggests involvement of humorally mediated inflammation.[12] Finally, there is preliminary evidence that part of the immunological dysfunction may have a genetic basis. For example, there may be an association between patients with CRPS and the human leukocyte antigen (HLA) system of the major histocompatibility complex (MHC).

REFERENCES

1. Stanton-Hicks M: Complex regional pain syndrome (Type I, RSD; Type II, causalgia): Controversies. Clin J Pain 16:S33–S40, 2000.
2. Stanton-Hicks M, Janig W, Hassenbusch S, et al: Reflex sympathetic dystrophy: Changing concepts and taxonomy. Pain 63:127–133, 1995.
3. Baron R, Levine JD, Fields HL: Causalgia and reflex sympathetic dystrophy: Does the sympathetic nervous system contribute to the generation of pain? Muscle Nerve 22:678–695, 1999.
4. Bruehl S, Carlson CR: Predisposing psychological factors in the development of reflex sympathetic dystrophy. A review of the empiric evidence. Clin J Pain 8:287–299, 1992.
5. Lynch ME: Psychological aspects of reflex sympathetic dystrophy: A review of the adult and paediatric literature. Pain 49:337–347, 1992.
6. Janig W, Baron R: Complex regional pain syndrome is a disease of the central nervous system. Clin Auton Res 12:150–164, 2002.
7. Wasner G, Schattschneider J, Binder A, et al: Complex regional pain syndrome – Diagnostic, mechanisms, CNS involvement and therapy. Spinal Cord 41:61–75, 2003.
8. Drummond PD, Finch PM, Skipworth S, et al: Pain increases during sympathetic arousal in patients with complex regional pain syndrome. Neurology 57:1296–1303, 2001.
9. Baron R, Schattschneider J, Binder A, et al: Relation between sympathetic vasoconstrictor activity and pain and hyperalgesia in complex regional pain syndromes: A case–control study. Lancet 359:1655–1660, 2002.
10. Goris RJA: Reflex sympathetic dystrophy: Model of a severe regional inflammatory response syndrome. World J Surg 22: 197–202, 1998.
11. Birklein F, Schmelz M, Schifter S, et al: The important role of neuropeptides in complex regional pain syndrome. Neurology 57:2179–2184, 2001.
12. Huygen FJ, De Bruijn AG, De Bruin MT, et al: Evidence for local inflammation in complex regional pain syndrome type 1. Mediators Inflamm 11:47–51, 2002.

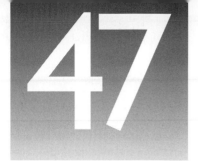

Complex Regional Pain Syndromes: Diagnosis and Treatment

Theodore S. Grabow, M.D.,

Anthony H. Guarino, M.D., and

Srinivasa N. Raja, M.D.

The diagnosis of complex regional pain syndrome (CRPS) is based exclusively on the characteristic clinical features. CRPS type II differs from CRPS type I in that the former is the result of a nerve injury. In this chapter the clinical features of CRPS are expounded and tests that will help in the differential diagnosis of CRPS are discussed. In addition, the various treatment options are described.

DIFFERENTIAL DIAGNOSIS

Many other disease processes may appear as CRPS and include the following: unrecognized local pathology (e.g., fracture, strain, sprain), traumatic vasospasm, cellulitis, lymphedema, Raynaud's disease, thromboangiitis obliterans, erythromelalgia, and deep vein thrombosis. Other neuropathic pain states such as entrapment syndromes, occupational overuse syndromes, and diabetic neuropathy may share some common clinical features of CRPS. It is important to confirm a diagnosis before pursuing treatments that could potentially harm the patient or delay appropriate care.

DIAGNOSTIC ALGORITHM

The current diagnosis of CRPS is based on the recommendations published by the International Association for the Study of Pain (IASP) in 1994 (Table 47-1). Despite the efforts of the IASP, many clinicians are unfamiliar with the modern taxonomy and the majority of recently published studies do not utilize the diagnostic criteria proposed by the IASP. For example, in a review of 92 publications from 1996 to 2000 Reinders and colleagues demonstrated that only 35 (38%) studies utilized *pain* in the diagnostic criterion and only 4 (15%) publications

satisfied all the IASP diagnostic criteria.[1] In a similar review of studies from 1980 to 2000 van de Beek and colleagues reported that only 43% (10 of 23) of studies used the actual term *CRPS* since the publication of the IASP diagnostic criteria.[2] In addition, of these studies, only 30% (3 of 10) utilized the exact criteria published by the IASP. In fact, 30% of studies allowed the diagnosis of CRPS without the presence of sensory features.

The original diagnostic criteria were not empirically validated before introduction. Despite having high diagnostic sensitivity (0.98), the criteria had only moderate diagnostic specificity (0.36) in distinguishing CRPS from other chronic pain conditions. The lack of mechanism-based specificity in the proposed diagnostic criteria has detracted somewhat from their universal acceptance by the scientific community. To improve the diagnostic accuracy, modifications were added to the original criteria to improve disease recognition for research purposes.[3,4] Factor analysis has demonstrated that there are distinct subgroups of symptoms that tend to coexist (e.g., sensory, vasomotor, sudomotor–edema, and motor–trophic subgroups). The first three of these four subgroups reflect indices that are included in the original IASP diagnostic criteria. It is uncertain whether the inclusion of the fourth subgroup, which contains signs of motor and trophic dysfunction, will improve diagnostic accuracy. However, the positive and negative predictive value of the proposed research diagnostic criteria can be maximized across all prevalence rates by including at least two signs and all four symptom categories of these four subgroups.

Unfortunately, historical constructs of disease still persist in the literature today. This lack of uniformity in criteria for diagnosis raises a critical question regarding the external validity of the majority of studies to date. Only the continual use of

TABLE 47-1. IASP DIAGNOSTIC CRITERIA FOR CRPS TYPES I AND II

CRPS type I
1. The presence of an initiating noxious event, or a cause of immobilization
2. Continuing pain, allodynia, or hyperalgesia with which the pain is disproportionate to any inciting event
3. Evidence at some time of edema, changes in skin blood flow, or abnormal sudomotor activity in the region of the pain
4. This diagnosis is excluded by the existence of conditions that would otherwise account for the degree of pain and dysfunction

Note: Criteria 2–4 must be satisfied

CRPS type II
1. The presence of continuing pain, allodynia, or hyperalgesia after a nerve injury, not necessarily limited to the distribution of the injured nerve
2. Evidence at some time of edema, changes in skin blood flow, or abnormal sudomotor activity in the region of the pain
3. This diagnosis is excluded by the existence of conditions that would otherwise account for the degree of pain and dysfunction

Note: All three criteria must be satisfied

---

uniform diagnostic criteria will ensure that CRPS is a homogenous disease entity such that future medical decisions based on the results of present scientific investigation will be meaningful.

EPIDEMIOLOGY

Epidemiological studies show that the peak incidence of CRPS is around the age of 50 years. Until the mid-1980s it was thought that CRPS did not occur in children or adolescents. However, more recent observations indicate that reflex sympathetic dystrophy (RSD) and causalgia also occur in children. Several predisposing factors have been considered as potential risk factors for the development of CRPS.

Genetic Predisposition: Women with certain human leukocyte antigen (HLA) profiles seem to be predisposed to develop refractory CRPS. Similarly, some patients with CRPS have a greater frequency of certain HLA alleles compared to the general population. These alleles are located within or near the major histocompatibility complex (MHC) region of the short arm of chromosome 6.[5] Non-HLA alleles may also be involved. For example, certain patients with CRPS have a greater chance of being homozygous for the angiotensin converting enzyme (ACE) gene deletion on chromosome 17. Other studies report a familial tendency for CRPS.

Disuse: Recent experimentation has demonstrated that immobility of an extremity can produce all of the signs and symptoms of CRPS including pain. Prolonged immobilization leads to sensory and motor changes and may be associated with permanent alteration in central neuronal functioning.

Psychological Factors: There is no scientific evidence that certain personality traits or psychological factors predispose to the development of CRPS. However, stressful life events may be associated with the development of symptoms and inadequate coping mechanisms may influence the severity of symptoms. In general, chronic pain patients frequently have associated comorbid psychiatric disease such as affective disorders like major depression, substance abuse disorders, somatoform disorders, and anxiety disorders.[6] Comorbid psychiatric disease can have a negative impact on pain, coping, and functional status.

CLINICAL CHARACTERISTICS OF CRPS

Spontaneous Pain: CRPS is experienced typically as a spontaneous pain in an extremity. This pain usually follows tissue injury to an extremity, but characteristically is disproportionate in severity, duration, and extent to that expected from the clinical course of the initial injury. CRPS has been reported after central nervous system (CNS) injuries, and following visceral or psychological disorders. Although uncommon, case reports suggest that a similar regional pain syndrome can occur in the trunk and face. The common descriptors used by patients with CRPS are burning pain, constant ache, throbbing, deep pressure, or shooting pains. Blumberg and Janig described an orthostatic component to the pain with pain decreasing when the limb is elevated and pain increasing when the limb is lowered.[7] Consequently, patients prefer to keep their affected extremity elevated above the level of the heart.

Allodynia and Hyperalgesia: The majority of patients with CRPS have altered cutaneous sensation that presents as allodynia or hyperalgesia.[8] Patients often exhibit guarding behavior to prevent contact with external objects. Alternatively, patients may wrap the extremity to avoid the stimulation of a cold breeze. It is not uncommon for patients to present in summer wearing gloves or in winter wearing shorts. One striking clinical feature of sympathetically maintained pain (SMP) is hyperalgesia to cold stimuli. Frost and co-workers observed that hyperalgesia to mechanical stimuli was similar in patients with SMP and sympathetically independent pain (SIP) who had chronic pain syndromes due to traumatic nerve or soft tissue injury.[9] However, all patients with SMP had hyperalgesia to cooling stimuli, whereas <40% of SIP patients had hyperalgesia to cooling. Thus, hyperalgesia to cooling stimuli is a sensitive but not specific test for SMP in patients with CRPS.

Tissue Swelling and Edema: Patients usually describe swelling of the extremity although it may not be evident at the time of patient visit to the clinic. One potential reason for swelling may be dependent edema secondary to disuse of the extremity. The swelling may lead to the characteristic shiny appearance of the skin in some patients.

Temperature and Color Changes: A history of temperature and color changes in the affected extremity is obtained from almost all patients. Although traditionally it has been described that the limb is warmer in the early stages of the disease and colder in the later stages, these observations have not been consistent. Patients often describe the limb as mottled with dark, bluish, or pale white discoloration. Sometimes the limb is described as being hot and red.

Sudomotor and Vasomotor Symptoms: Sweating abnormalities have been reported to be frequent in patients with CRPS. Usually, sweating is increased in the affected region, but sometimes the skin in the affected region may be dry and scaly. The presence of a cold or warm limb is considered to be a sign of altered vascular regulation.

Motor Changes: Distal tremors, dystonia, weakness, reduced movement, and joint stiffness are observed in some patients with CRPS. These motor disturbances can result in marked functional limitation. It is unclear whether these motor symptoms are part of the clinical presentation of the disease or a result of protection of the painful limb and the consequence of disuse. Juottonen and co-workers have demonstrated that patients with CRPS type I have impairment of central sensorimotor integration.[10] Schattschneider and co-workers have demonstrated that motor deficits may be secondary to abnormal integration of visual and sensory inputs to the parietal cortex.[11]

Trophic Changes: Alterations in skin, nail, and hair growth are often observed in patients who have severe allodynia to mechanical stimulation. Osteoporosis may be evident in patients with severe pain and guarding. The demineralization of small bones, particularly in a periarticular distribution, is considered to be characteristic of this disease. Atrophic shiny skin, muscle wasting, and joint stiffness are observed in a subset of patients with CRPS.

Pattern and Spread: Sensory impairments frequently extend beyond the affected area and may involve quadratic or hemilateral regions of the body. Maleka and colleagues demonstrated three patterns of spread in CRPS type I: contiguous spread, dissociated (noncontiguous) spread, or mirror-image spread.[12] Independent spread suggests that some individuals have a generalized susceptibility for the condition. In addition, spread to contralateral or spatially remote regions suggests dysfunction within the CNS.[13]

Stages: Historical understanding suggested that untreated CRPS will progress through three distinct stages. Stage I resembles acute inflammation and the affected extremity is painful to touch, warm, vasodilated, and edematous. Stage II is associated with worsening pain and vasomotor dysfunction, motor abnormalities, and dystrophic changes. The hallmark of stage III is atrophy, continued motor impairment, and possible diminution of sensory disturbance. However, current understanding refutes the notion of progressively worsening stages of disease. In fact, many patients with CRPS do not progressively worsen through these stages but rather stabilize or improve with time. A recent study by Bruehl and colleagues utilized cluster analysis, a statistical method of pattern recognition, and concluded that sequential stages of CRPS do not exist in patients who have received previous treatment.[14] Rather, these authors concluded that there may be three distinct subtypes of CRPS: subtype 1 is a relatively limited syndrome with predominantly vasomotor signs; subtype 2 is a relatively limited syndrome with predominantly sensory abnormalities; and subtype 3 is the florid syndrome with predominance of motor/trophic change.

Patients with SMP and SIP often report similar symptoms and may have similar clinical examination. Clinically, it is difficult to predict which patient with CRPS will have SMP or SIP based on the clinical presentation alone. Hence it may be beneficial to perform selective blockade of sympathetic function to determine the component of the pain syndrome that is sympathetically mediated. Recent systematic reviews have questioned the efficacy of therapies designed specifically for this purpose.[15,16] Nevertheless, these pharmacological tests are often used to aid the diagnosis of autonomic dysfunction particularly when more extensive or costly tests are unavailable.

DIAGNOSTIC TESTS

SMP, by definition, is eliminated by blockade of sympathetic efferent innervation of the painful area. Thus, one can assess the sympathetic component by blocking the sympathetic ganglia supplying the area of pain. It is the efferent sympathetic fibers and not the afferent (visceral sensory) sympathetic fibers that account for SMP as evidenced by aggravation or rekindling of pain with exogenous administration of norepinephrine intradermally. Areas of SMP have been shown to have a normal or decreased sympathetic outflow indicating that the pain is not a result of increased sympathetic activity.

Local Anesthetic Sympathetic Blocks: The traditional sympatholytic test is local anesthetic sympathetic ganglion block. Local anesthetic is administered typically in the region of the stellate ganglion or the lumbar paravertebral sympathetic ganglia for upper and lower extremity pains, respectively. However, the results of local anesthetic sympathetic blocks need to be interpreted with caution: (1) It is important to know whether the sympathetic blockade is complete, especially in patients who do not experience significant pain relief. The efficacy of sympathetic blockade can be objectively assessed by evaluating the effects on sympathetic, sudomotor, and vasoconstrictor function on skin blood flow, skin temperature, and skin resistance. (2) In patients who have pain relief from local anesthetic sympathetic blockade it is important to do a careful sensory examination, since local anesthetic can directly spread to nearby nerve roots, resulting in a somatic nerve block that may have significant effects on the patient's pain. (3) Depending on the total dose of local anesthetic used, pain relief may be due to systemic uptake of the local anesthetic. (4) The invasive procedure might have a significant placebo effect. (5) Local anesthetic sympathetic blockade does not only block sympathetic efferent fibers, but also visceral sensory afferent fibers traveling in the sympathetic chain.

Regional Intravenous Blockade: Clinicians have used regional intravenous blockade with guanethidine for the diagnosis of SMP. The effects of guanethidine are assumed to be related to its action on the noradrenergic system. Guanethidine is taken up by noradrenergic varicosities of postganglionic sympathetic axons and depletes norepinephrine from its stores. This can lead to short-term excitation of nociceptors which is manifested as increased pain during the test. Guanethidine then prevents further release of noradrenaline from depleted postganglionic axons for up to 1 or 2 days. However, review of randomized controlled trials (RCTs) have failed to demonstrate the efficacy of guanethidine for patients with CRPS. In fact, Livingstone and Atkins demonstrated that guanethidine block may actually delay the resolution of vasomotor instability in patients with CRPS.[17]

Quantitative Sensory Testing and Autonomic Testing: Since pain induced by cooling stimuli is a characteristic feature of SMP, quantitative sensory testing is helpful to aid in the diagnosis of SMP. Quantitative sensory testing demonstrates increase in warm perception thresholds and decrease of cold pain thresholds in patients with CRPS types I and II. Quantitative sudomotor axon reflex test (QSART) demonstrates unilateral disturbance (increase in sweating) in sudomotor function in patients with acute CRPS.

Skin Temperature Measurements: CRPS can be distinguished from other diseases associated with extremity pain by the maximal skin temperature difference that occurs during the thermoregulatory cycle. Studies indicate that the temperature differences in CRPS are dynamic and are influenced by environmental conditions and thermoregulatory load. Wasner and colleagues demonstrated that skin temperature asymmetry in combination with maximal side differences greater than 2.2°C result in a sensitivity of 76% and specificity of 93% in the diagnosis of CRPS.[18]

Skin Blood Flow Measurements: In acute CRPS there is an increase in total skin blood flow to the affected extremity likely due to neurogenic inflammation and decreased sympathetic vasoconstrictor activity. This impairment in sympathetic vasoconstrictor activity likely is mediated by a central mechanism. In chronic CRPS total skin blood flow is decreased in the affected extremity. Sympathetic activity is still impaired but secondary changes in the periphery such as denervation supersensitivity to circulating catecholamines produces vasoconstriction and cold skin. Tests of skin blood flow or sympathetic vasoconstrictor activity may be useful in reinforcing the diagnosis of CRPS.

X-Ray and Bone Scan: Increased periarticular uptake in a three-phase bone scan and demineralization on fine-detail radiography have been used by some clinicians to reinforce the diagnosis in the subacute (<1 year) and chronic stages of disease, respectively. However, the use of these tests has been questioned since they cannot distinguish patients with CRPS from those with other post-traumatic syndromes in general.

Phentolamine Infusion Test: This test was introduced independently by two groups of investigators as an additional test for SMP that could minimize expectation bias and placebo responses. The test involves intravenous injection of phentolamine, an alpha-adrenoceptor antagonist, to determine the presence or absence of SMP (see Table 47-2).

TREATMENT OF CRPS

A scientifically validated cure for CRPS does not exist. Accordingly, therapy has been directed at managing the signs and symptoms of disease. As a consequence, several diverse therapeutic strategies have been proposed. Since the disease is chronic in nature, most experts agree that a multidisciplinary approach is required. This approach generally involves concurrent administration of pharmaco-, physio-, and psychotherapeutic modalities.[19]

TABLE 47-2. **PROTOCOL FOR PHENTOLAMINE INFUSION**

Patient preparation	Informed written consent is obtained. A standardized set of directions is read to the patient; the patient is told that pain may increase, decrease, or stay the same, and that the results will help guide future treatments. The patient is placed in supine position. Electrocardiography, blood pressure, heart rate, and skin temperature are monitored. An intravenous line is established. A baseline pain level is established (pain score must be above 4 on a 10-point visual analog scale).
Saline pretreatment	Lactated Ringer's solution is administered at 600 mL/hr throughout the test. Sensory testing is done every 5 min for at least 30 min or until a stable pain rating is achieved,* if pain level is not stable, the test is deferred.
Phentolamine infusion	Propranolol 1–2 mg is administered intravenously. An infusion of phentolamine (1 mg/kg) is given over a 10-min period in single-blinded fashion (no clues provided to the patient on time of initiation of drug infusion). Sensory testing is continued every 5 min during phentolamine infusion
Post-phentolamine testing	Sensory testing is continued for 15–30 min. Electrocardiography, blood pressure, heart rate, and skin temperature monitoring are continued for 30 min or longer, depending on stability of vital signs and presence or absence of orthostatic hypotension.

*Sensory testing is done for ongoing pain at rest and for stimulus-evoked pain (mechanical, cold) if applicable.

Pharmacological Strategies: There are several pharmacological therapies with diverse mechanisms of action that have been advocated for treatment of CRPS. Most of these therapies are based on the premise that CRPS is either a neuropathic or inflammatory pain process. Therapies that have been shown to

TABLE 47-3. **DEMONSTRATED EFFECTIVE THERAPIES FOR CRPS BASED ON CONTROLLED TRIALS**

Drug	Route of Administration	Proposed Mechanism of Action
Prednisone	Oral	Anti-inflammatory and neuronal membrane stabilizer
Vitamin C		Antioxidant
Alendronate	Intravenous	Osteoclast inhibitor
Bretylium		Autonomic ganglion blocker
Ketansarin		Serotonin and alpha-adrenoceptor antagonist
Phentolamine		Alpha-1-adrenoceptor antagonist
Lidocaine		Sodium channel blocker
DMSO	Topical	Free radical scavenger
Calcitonin	Intranasal	Osteoclast inhibitor
Clonidine	Epidural	Alpha-2-adrenoceptor agonist
Baclofen	Intrathecal	GABA-B receptor agonist

DMSO, dimethyl sulfoxide; GABA, gamma-aminobutyric acid.

be effective by RCTs for CRPS are listed in Table 47-3. In addition to these therapies, most clinicians utilize medications that have been shown to be effective in treating neuropathic pain in general. These drugs include but are not limited to anticonvulsant and tricyclic antidepressant medications. In addition, opioids are used frequently despite reports of variable efficacy for neuropathic pain.

Physical Therapy: To date, there has been one randomized, controlled study which demonstrates the short-term efficacy of physical therapy for patients with CRPS.[20] Nevertheless, most authorities recognize that physical therapy modalities are necessary for functional restoration and vocational rehabilitation for patients with CRPS.

Psychological Approach: The efficacy of cognitive behavioral therapy (CBT) modalities for chronic pain disorders has been established in the literature for years. Nevertheless, the specific use of CBT for adult patients with CRPS has not been studied to date in a RCT. Despite this fact, most clinicians utilize CBT modalities or recommend formal psychiatric evaluation for patients who have CRPS longer than 3 months. As previously stated, patients with CRPS have a significant amount of psychological dysfunction. However, no personality trait predisposes to the development of CRPS. Rather, the psychological dysfunction is a reflection of the disease itself and not much different from the psychological dysfunction that accompanies other chronic pain syndromes.

Spinal Cord Stimulation: In a single RCT patients who received physical therapy with spinal cord stimulation received better pain relief than patients who received physical therapy alone.[21] The mechanism of analgesia of spinal cord stimulation in patients with CRPS is unknown. However, patients with CRPS who have had prior sympathectomy also receive pain relief with spinal cord stimulation.

Neuraxial Infusion Therapy: A single RCT demonstrated the efficacy of epidural clonidine for patients with CRPS.

Furthermore, a more recent RCT demonstrated the efficacy of intrathecal baclofen in reducing dystonia in patients with CRPS.[22] To date, the majority of reports describing the effectiveness of intrathecal medication for patients with CRPS have been descriptive case reports or case series.

Neuroablation Strategies: Surgical sympathectomy, chemical sympathectomy, and radiofrequency ablation have been used for treatment of sympathetically mediated pain in patients with CRPS. Unfortunately, some patients develop postsympathectomy neuralgia after these procedures. This phenomenon likely is related to denervation supersensitivity of peripheral alpha-adrenergic receptors.

CRPS AND PEDIATRICS

In general, the signs and symptoms of CRPS in children and adolescents are similar to those in adults. In addition, much of the epidemiology, diagnosis, and treatments are the same. For example, there is a gender predisposition for females (~3:1) as in the adult literature. Special tests such as plain radiographs, bone scans, sympathetic nerve blocks, and nerve conduction studies have been used to reinforce the diagnosis. Focal abnormalities in peripheral sympathetic nervous system function have been demonstrated by sympathetic skin response and laser Doppler flowmetry. Symptom migration or spread of disease has been reported. A high percentage of children with CRPS are diagnosed with psychological dysfunction. Delays in diagnosis are common and many patients receive inappropriate therapy which may be counterproductive (such as limb immobilization). Medications such as nonsteroidal anti-inflammatory drugs (NSAIDs), anticonvulsants, tricyclic antidepressants, and opioids are prescribed based on treatments for neuropathic pain in the adult literature. Finally, the response to sympathetic block is variable: some patients demonstrate dramatic relief to a single block whereas others fail to respond at all.

However, there are a few differences between the pediatric and adult literature. For example, childhood CRPS often affects the lower extremity rather than the upper extremity. Sensory, motor, and autonomic disturbances are the main features. Trophic changes occur but are observed less commonly. An antecedent history of trauma or surgery is determined less frequently. Recurrence rate is higher (~30%) compared to adults (~10%). Conservative treatments such as transcutaneous electrical nerve stimulation (TENS), physical therapy, or CBT modalities tend to be effective. Of note, the effectiveness of physical therapy and CBT for CRPS in children has been demonstrated by a single RCT.[23] CRPS in childhood has a higher likelihood of recovery (better prognosis), although refractory cases resulting in significant disability have been reported. Interventional approaches are rarely needed but include sympathetic blocks, epidural catheters, spinal cord stimulation, and surgical sympathectomy. Familial issues need to be addressed since parental enmeshment and familial dysfunction are observed often in this chronic pain population.

REFERENCES

1. Reinders MF, Geertzen JH, Dijkstra PU: Complex regional pain syndrome type I: Use of the International Association for the Study of Pain diagnostic criteria defined in 1994. Clin J Pain 18:207–215, 2002.
2. van de Beek WJ, Schwartzman RJ, van Nes SI, et al: Diagnostic criteria used in studies of reflex sympathetic dystrophy. Neurology 58:522–526, 2002.
3. Harden RN, Bruehl S, Galer BS, et al: Complex regional pain syndrome: Are the IASP diagnostic criteria valid and sufficiently comprehensive? Pain 83:211–219, 1999.
4. Bruehl S, Harden RN, Galer BS, et al: External validation of IASP diagnostic criteria for Complex Regional Pain Syndrome and proposed research diagnostic criteria. International Association for the Study of Pain. Pain 81:147–154, 1999.
5. Mailis A, Wade JA: Genetic considerations in CRPS. In Harden RN, Baron R, Janig W (eds): Complex Regional Pain Syndrome. IASP Press, Seattle, 2001, pp 227–238.
6. Fishbain DA: Approaches to treatment decisions for psychiatric comorbidity in the management of the chronic pain patient. Med Clin North Am 83:737–760, 1999.
7. Blumberg H, Janig W: Clinical manifestations of reflex sympathetic dystrophy and sympathetically maintained pain. In Wall PD, Melzack R (eds): Textbook of Pain. Churchill Livingstone, London, 1994, pp 685–697.
8. Birklein F, Riedl B, Sieweke N, et al: Neurological findings in complex regional pain syndromes – Analysis of 145 cases. Acta Neurol Scand 101:262–269, 2000.
9. Frost SA, Raja SN, Campbell JN, et al: Does hyperalgesia to cooling stimuli characterize patients with sympathetically maintained pain (reflex sympathetic dystrophy)? In Dubner R, Gebhart GF, Bond MR (eds): Proc 5th World Congress on Pain. Elsevier, Amsterdam, 1988, pp 151–156.
10. Juottonen K, Gockel M, Silen T, et al: Altered central sensorimotor processing in patients with complex regional pain syndrome. Pain 98:315–323, 2002.
11. Schattschneider J, Wenzelburger GD, Baron R: Kinematic analysis of the upper extremity in CRPS. In Harden RN, Baron R, Janig W (eds): Complex Regional Pain Syndrome. IASP Press, Seattle, 2001, pp 119–128.
12. Maleki J, LeBel AA, Bennett GJ, et al: Patterns of spread in complex regional pain syndrome, type I (reflex sympathetic dystrophy). Pain 88:259–266, 2000.
13. Rommel O, Gehling M, Dertwinkel R, et al: Hemisensory impairment in patients with complex regional pain syndrome. Pain 80:95–101, 1999.
14. Bruehl S, Harden RN, Galer BS, et al: Complex regional pain syndrome: Are there distinct subtypes and sequential stages of the syndrome? Pain 95:119–124, 2002.
15. Perez RS, Kwakkel G, Zuurmond WW, et al: Treatment of reflex sympathetic dystrophy (CRPS type 1): A research synthesis of 21 randomized clinical trials. J Pain Symptom Manage 21: 511–526, 2001.
16. Cepeda MS, Lau J, Carr DB: Defining the therapeutic role of local anesthetic sympathetic blockade in complex regional pain syndrome: A narrative and systematic review. Clin J Pain 18: 216–233, 2002.
17. Livingstone JA, Atkins RM: Intravenous regional guanethidine blockade in the treatment of post-traumatic complex regional pain syndrome type I (algodystrophy) of the hand. J Bone Joint Surg Br 84:380–386, 2002.
18. Wasner G, Schattschneider J, Baron R: Skin temperature side differences – A diagnostic tool for CRPS? Pain 98:19–26, 2002.
19. Raja SN, Grabow TS: Complex regional pain syndrome I (reflex sympathetic dystrophy). Anesthesiology 96:1254–1260, 2002.
20. Oerlemans HM, Oostendorp RA, de Boo T, et al: Pain and reduced mobility in complex regional pain syndrome I: Outcome of a prospective randomized controlled clinical trial of adjuvant physical therapy versus occupational therapy. Pain 83:77–83, 1999.
21. Kemler MA, Barendse GA, van Kleef M, et al: Spinal cord stimulation in patients with chronic reflex sympathetic dystrophy. N Engl J Med 343:618–624, 2000.
22. van Hilten BJ, van de Beek WJ, Hoff JI, et al: Intrathecal baclofen for the treatment of dystonia in patients with reflex sympathetic dystrophy. N Engl J Med 343:625–630, 2000.
23. Lee BH, Scharff L, Sethna NF, et al: Physical therapy and cognitive-behavioral treatment for complex regional pain syndromes. J Pediatrics 141:135–140, 2002.

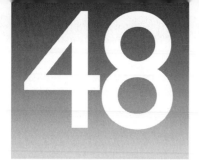

Herpes Zoster and Postherpetic Neuralgia

Robert H. Dworkin, Ph.D., and
Kenneth E. Schmader, M.D.

The objective of this chapter is to provide an overview of the epidemiology, natural history, pathophysiology, treatment, and prevention of herpes zoster and postherpetic neuralgia. Herpes zoster ("shingles") is a viral infection that is accompanied by acute pain in the majority of patients. The pain associated with herpes zoster does not resolve in a substantial number of patients, and postherpetic neuralgia (PHN) is diagnosed when herpes zoster pain persists. The results of research on PHN—a chronic peripheral neuropathic pain syndrome—have added greatly to knowledge of the pathophysiology and treatment of neuropathic pain.

HERPES ZOSTER

Epidemiology: Following a primary chicken pox infection, the varicella-zoster virus (VZV) establishes latency in sensory ganglia throughout the nervous system. Herpes zoster is the reactivation of the virus and its spread from a single dorsal root or cranial nerve ganglion to the corresponding dermatome and neural tissue of the same segment.[1,2] Herpes zoster has the highest incidence of all neurological diseases, occurring annually in approximately 500,000 people in the USA, during the lifetimes of as much as 20% to 30% of the population, and in as many as 50% of those living until 85 years of age.[1,3–6] The likelihood of recurrent zoster, however, is reported to be 5% or less,[1,5] and the true incidence may even be lower because a portion of these cases may have been zosteriform recurrent herpes simplex infections.

A fundamental epidemiological feature of zoster is a marked increase in incidence with aging.[7] For example, Hope-Simpson[1] documented an incidence of 0.74 per 1,000 person-years in children under 10 years old, 2.5 per 1,000 person-years in adults aged 20 to 50 years, and 7.8 per 1,000 person-years in those older than 60 years.

The incidence of herpes zoster is also significantly increased in patients with suppressed cell-mediated immunity—including human immunodeficiency virus infection, acquired immunodeficiency syndrome, certain cancers, organ transplants

(especially bone marrow transplant), immune-mediated diseases, and immunosuppressive treatments—compared to immunocompetent individuals.[7]

Zoster epidemiology is ultimately determined by the transmission and spread of VZV in populations. The most important condition in the spread of VZV is the primary chicken pox infection but latent and reactivated VZV infections also play important roles in maintaining VZV infection in populations.[8] Latently infected elderly adults and immunosuppressed patients are important reservoirs of virus because VZV is more likely to reactivate in these groups. When zoster occurs, VZV can be transmitted during the vesicular phase of the rash and cause primary infection when there is contact with a seronegative individual. A zoster exposure with a seropositive, latently infected individual may result in a subclinical reinfection and boost of humoral and cellular VZV immunity but it is unlikely to cause varicella or herpes zoster.[8]

Natural History: The presentation of pain in herpes zoster is variable. In the majority of patients a prodrome of dermatomal pain precedes the appearance of the characteristic unilateral rash.[9–11] This prodrome begins several days before rash onset in almost all cases, but a series of patients with prodromal pain preceding the appearance of the rash by 7 to more than 100 days has been reported.[12] Thoracic dermatomes are the most commonly affected sites in herpes zoster and account for 50% to 70% of all cases; cranial (especially the ophthalmic division of the trigeminal nerve), cervical, and lumbar dermatomes each account for 10% to 20% of cases, and sacral dermatomes are affected in 2% to 8% of cases.[7,13] The rash becomes vesicular after several days, then forms a crust, and loss of all scabs usually occurs within 2 to 4 weeks.

Pain in the affected dermatome accompanies the rash in most patients. Those who did not have a painful prodrome typically begin to experience pain at rash onset or shortly afterwards (see Fig. 48-1). This acute herpes zoster pain gradually resolves before or shortly after rash healing in most cases. Severe acute pain in herpes zoster interferes with patients' abilities to

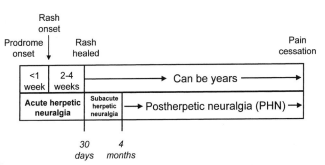

FIGURE 48-1. Timeline of pain experienced by herpes zoster patients.

TABLE 48-1. **SUMMARY ESTIMATES FROM MAJOR PLACEBO-CONTROLLED ANTIVIRAL TRIALS OF THE PERCENTAGES OF HERPES ZOSTER PATIENTS ≥50 YEARS WITH PAIN AT MONTHLY INTERVALS AFTER RASH ONSET**

Days After Rash Onset	Patients With Pain (%)	
	Placebo	Antiviral
30	68	49–57
60	61	50
90	49–54	25–35
120	46	29
150	42	26
180	35–40	15–26

Adapted from Dworkin RH, Schmader KE: The epidemiology and natural history of herpes zoster and postherpetic neuralgia. *In* Watson CPN, AA Gershon AA (eds): Herpes Zoster and Postherpetic Neuralgia, ed 2. Elsevier, New York, 2001, pp 39–64.

carry out normal activities of daily living and is, not surprisingly, associated with greater use of analgesic medications.[14]

Dermatomal pain without a rash, referred to as *zoster sine herpete*, has also been described, and the finding of VZV DNA in the cerebrospinal fluid of patients with prolonged radicular pain and no rash provides evidence of this syndrome.[15]

In addition to acute pain, the morbidity of herpes zoster includes neurological disorders and ophthalmological, cutaneous, and visceral complications. The types of neurological complications include motor neuropathy, cranial polyneuritis, transverse myelitis, meningoencephalitis, and cerebral angiitis and stroke after ophthalmic zoster.[7,16] Ophthalmological complications have been described in 2% to 6% of zoster cases, including keratitis, uveitis, iridocyclitis, panophthalmitis, and glaucoma.[7,16] Elderly and especially immunosuppressed patients are at greater risk for most of the complications of herpes zoster.

Treatment: Treatment of herpes zoster patients with the antiviral agents acyclovir, famciclovir, and valacyclovir inhibits viral replication and has been shown to reduce the duration of viral shedding, hasten rash healing, and decrease the severity and duration of acute pain.[2,17,18] As discussed below, however, the most important complication of herpes zoster in immunocompetent patients is chronic pain, which despite recent treatment advances can be refractory not only to first-line treatment but also to all other therapies. The prevention of PHN is therefore a very important clinical goal. By inhibiting viral replication, antiviral therapy limits the degree of neural damage caused by zoster, and such damage likely contributes prominently to the development of PHN. The results of randomized controlled trials and meta-analyses have demonstrated that antiviral therapy in herpes zoster significantly reduces the risk of prolonged pain (see Table 48-1).[2,17–19] Although the results of each of these studies taken singly can be challenged, the consistency of the findings provides strong support for the use of antiviral agents in the treatment of herpes zoster. Antiviral therapy can be recommended in herpes zoster patients who are older, have moderate or severe rash, have moderate or severe pain, have ophthalmic involvement, or are immunocompromised.[2,17]

Although the reduction in the risk of PHN that accompanies antiviral therapy in herpes zoster patients is both statistically and clinically significant, antiviral therapy does not prevent PHN in all patients. As can be seen from Table 48-1, approximately 20% of patients over the age of 50 years continue to have pain 6 months after their rash despite antiviral treatment beginning within 72 hours of rash onset.[19] How then can the risk of chronic pain be further reduced, beyond that currently achieved by antiviral therapy? Although it is possible that new antivirals with greater efficacy will be developed, a different strategy for preventing PHN is to supplement antiviral treatment. Unfortunately, the results of a number of studies that have examined the long-term benefits of corticosteroids, tricyclic antidepressants, and nerve blocks in herpes zoster patients are either equivocal or in need of replication.[20–23] Peripheral, sympathetic, and epidural nerve blocks with local anesthetics and/or corticosteroids appear to relieve acute pain in patients with herpes zoster, but their role in preventing PHN is uncertain because of the absence of randomized placebo-controlled trials.[22,23] Nevertheless, it can be predicted that combining antiviral therapy with effective relief of acute pain in herpes zoster will further lessen the risk of PHN beyond that achieved by antiviral therapy alone.[24,25] The basis for this hypothesis is provided by the well-replicated relationship between acute pain severity and PHN and by recent research on the pathophysiology of PHN (see below). However, even if there were no benefit with respect to the later development of PHN, the effective relief of acute pain in patients with herpes zoster is clearly a very desirable treatment goal in itself.

Prevention: A live, attenuated varicella vaccine is effective in protecting against varicella and its complications, and the incidence of varicella has been substantially reduced in regions where the vaccine is accepted.[26,27] Because the vaccine virus may be less likely to establish latency and reactivate than wild-type VZV, it is possible that the incidence of herpes zoster will decline as vaccinated children become older adults and adults who are latently infected with wild-type VZV die. This idea is supported by the observation that herpes zoster was less frequent in leukemic children who received the vaccine than in leukemic children with a past history of varicella.[28]

Currently, most individuals are latently infected with wild-type VZV and at risk for herpes zoster. As discussed above, a fundamental feature of herpes zoster is the marked increase in its incidence with aging, a consequence of the decline in VZV-specific cell-mediated immunity that occurs with aging. Administration of a live, attenuated varicella-zoster vaccine to older adults who have not had herpes zoster resulted in increases in mean anti-VZV antibody levels and VZV-specific cell-mediated immunity to levels comparable to those found in individuals with a history of zoster. The results of ongoing clinical trials will determine whether herpes zoster is attenuated by administration of a varicella-zoster vaccine to older adults.[29,30] If vaccination is efficacious and vaccine use becomes widespread in older adults, the incidence of both herpes zoster and PHN may decrease.

POSTHERPETIC NEURALGIA

Epidemiology and Natural History: A variety of definitions of PHN have been used by clinicians and investigators, ranging from any pain persisting after rash healing to pain that has persisted at least 6 months after rash onset.[31] The results of recent studies, however, suggest that the pain associated with herpes zoster has three phases: an acute herpetic neuralgia that accompanies the rash and lasts for approximately 30 days after rash onset, a subacute herpetic neuralgia that lasts from 30 to 120 days after rash onset, and PHN, defined as pain that persists for at least 120 days after rash onset (see Fig. 48-1).[32–34] Although this provides a validated definition for research on PHN, it is probably unnecessary to distinguish between subacute herpetic neuralgia and PHN when treating patients with pain persisting after rash healing.

Because the proportion of herpes zoster patients with pain declines with time, estimates of the percentage of patients who develop PHN depend on its definition. In different clinic and community studies 9% to 34% of adult zoster patients were reported to develop PHN defined variously as pain persisting after rash healing or for at least several months after rash onset.[13,31] There have been no systematic attempts to investigate the prevalence of PHN, and estimates of the number of cases have ranged from 500,000 to 1 million in the USA.[35,36]

PHN is a chronic pain syndrome that can last for years and cause substantial suffering and reduction in quality of life. As is true of other chronic pain syndromes, patients develop depression and other types of psychological distress as well as physical, occupational, and social disability as a consequence of their unremitting pain.[37–39]

There is evidence that pain in PHN can be discontinuous, with pain-free intervals of varying durations occurring.[40] Indeed, PHN can develop even in herpes zoster patients who have not had acute pain.[41]

The quality of pain in PHN compared to herpes zoster has been examined in several studies.[42–44] Sharp, stabbing pain was found to be more common in patients with zoster than in patients with PHN, whereas burning pain was more common in PHN patients and much less likely to be reported by patients with zoster. The investigators noted that the word tender was chosen by both groups of patients to describe allodynia (i.e., pain in response to a stimulus that does not normally provoke pain). These adjectives reflect the three different types of pain that have been distinguished in research on PHN: a steady throbbing or burning pain, an intermittent sharp or shooting pain, and allodynia.

A considerable number of recent studies have investigated risk factors for PHN. Older age is the most well-established risk factor for PHN, and until recently it was the only characteristic of herpes zoster patients that had been associated with an increased likelihood of developing PHN.[13] For example, as early as 50 years ago it was reported that persisting pain was infrequent in herpes zoster patients under 40 years of age, but that the proportion of patients with pain lasting 1 year or more approached 50% in those over the age of 70 years.[45]

There are now a considerable number of independent studies that have reported that patients with more severe acute pain are at greater risk for PHN.[13,34,46] As noted above, the majority of herpes zoster patients have a painful prodrome before their rash appears, and several studies have found that these patients have a greater risk of PHN than patients who did not have a prodrome.[13,34] Greater severity and duration of the herpes zoster rash is another risk factor for the development of PHN that has been identified in multiple studies.[13,34,46]

Because they have been replicated by independent groups of investigators in multiple studies, older age, greater acute pain severity, presence of a prodrome, and greater rash severity can be considered established risk factors for PHN. However, there are a number of other putative risk factors for PHN that have not been consistently replicated by independent groups of investigators. These include greater sensory abnormalities in the affected dermatome, generalized subclinical sensory deficits, diabetes, more pronounced cell-mediated and humoral immune responses, magnetic resonance imaging (MRI) brainstem and cervical cord abnormalities, electromyography (EMG) motor abnormalities, psychological distress, and fever.[13] The results of a number of studies have been inconsistent with respect to whether there are sex differences in the risk of PHN; when significant differences occur, women have been found to have a greater risk than men.[13,34] Patients with trigeminal and ophthalmic zoster have been reported to have an increased risk of PHN in some studies, but this has not been found consistently and when it has been reported the effect appears to be modest.[13]

Pathophysiology: Except for age and psychosocial factors, the risk factors for PHN that have been identified can all be considered concomitants of a more severe infection. More severe zoster infections are accompanied by greater neural damage, and it has been proposed that this neural damage contributes prominently to the development of PHN.[47] However, the nature of this damage and the specific mechanisms by which it causes the persisting pain of PHN remain unclear. What limited knowledge there is of the pathophysiology of PHN derives from studies of neuropathology, sensory dysfunction, and pharmacologic response. At the present time, there is considerable agreement that different peripheral and central mechanisms contribute to PHN, and that the qualitatively different types of pain that characterize PHN probably have different underlying mechanisms. This suggests that there may be pathophysiologically distinct subgroups of patients with PHN or that more than one mechanism may be involved in individual patients or both.[48,49]

Watson and colleagues[50] have conducted an elegant series of postmortem studies of patients who were suffering from

PHN at the time of death and of patients with a history of herpes zoster whose pain did not persist beyond rash healing. In these studies dorsal horn atrophy and pathological changes in the sensory ganglion were found on the affected side (and not on the unaffected side) in patients with PHN, but not in patients with a history of herpes zoster whose pain did not persist. In a more recent set of studies using punch skin biopsy, reductions in epidermal nerve fiber density were found in the affected dermatome but not on the contralateral unaffected side in patients with PHN.[51,52] Notably, in both the postmortem studies and the punch skin biopsy studies, the pathological features were characteristic of only the affected side in patients with PHN and were not found in patients with a history of zoster whose pain did not persist.

Rowbotham and co-workers[48,49] have conducted an important series of studies of sensory dysfunction and pharmacologic response that address the pathophysiology of PHN. PHN patients with prominent allodynia were found to have relatively normal sensory function as assessed by thermal thresholds and were also more likely to report pain relief following local anesthetic infiltration with lidocaine than patients with primarily constant pain. Rowbotham and Fields conclude that at least two different mechanisms may contribute to PHN, and propose that the mechanism of allodynia in PHN is abnormal activity in preserved primary afferent nociceptors that have been damaged by VZV but that remain in continuity with their central targets. Activity in these "irritable" nociceptors may initiate and then maintain a state of central sensitization in which input from large-fiber afferents that respond to nonpainful mechanical stimuli causes allodynia.

As opposed to patients with prominent allodynia, PHN patients with predominantly continuous pain were found to have sensory loss in the areas where they have the most pain. This suggests that continuous pain in PHN is caused by a different mechanism from allodynia, possibly involving central structural and functional changes accompanying deafferentation. These may include a structural reorganization of the spinal cord that involves abnormal synaptic connections, as well as functional abnormalities resulting from deafferentation involving hyperexcitability of dorsal horn neurons.

Treatment: Since publication of the first randomized controlled trials in the early 1980s, tricyclic antidepressants (TCAs) have been considered the first-line treatment for patients with PHN.[53] The efficacy of gabapentin, lidocaine patch 5%, tramadol, and opioid analgesics has now also been demonstrated by the results of randomized controlled trials in patients with PHN. These five medications provide an evidence-based approach for the treatment of PHN that was not available until very recently.[25,54]

The initial choice of these medications should be guided by adverse event profiles, potential for drug interactions, and patient comorbidities and treatment preferences, especially because there are no replicated data demonstrating superior effectiveness of one drug over another. In general, gabapentin, lidocaine patch 5%, and tramadol can be considered first-line treatments for PHN, whereas opioid analgesics and TCAs are more typically second-line treatments because they generally require greater caution in the often elderly patient with PHN.

GABAPENTIN: Patients with PHN have been treated with anticonvulsant medications for many years. Gabapentin, a second-generation antiepileptic drug, was associated with a statistically significant reduction in daily pain ratings as well as improvements in sleep, mood, and quality of life at daily dosages of 1,800 to 3,600 mg in two large clinical trials.[55,56] Side effects of gabapentin include somnolence, dizziness, and (less often) mild peripheral edema, which requires monitoring and possibly dosage adjustment but usually not treatment discontinuation. Gabapentin may cause or exacerbate gait and balance problems and cognitive impairment in the elderly. Dosage adjustment is necessary in patients with renal insufficiency, but its generally excellent tolerability, safety, and lack of drug interactions distinguish gabapentin from the other oral medications used in the treatment of PHN.

To reduce side effects and increase patient compliance with treatment, gabapentin should be initiated at low dosages—100 to 300 mg in a single dose at bedtime or 100 mg three times daily—and then titrated by 100 mg three times daily as tolerated. Because of variability in gabapentin absorption, the final dosage should be determined either by complete pain relief, which is rare, or by unacceptable side effects that do not resolve over a few weeks.

LIDOCAINE PATCH 5%: There are two published, double-blind, vehicle-controlled, randomized trials of lidocaine patch 5% in PHN.[57,58] In these studies PHN patients with allodynia obtained statistically significant greater pain relief with lidocaine patch 5% compared with vehicle-control patches containing no lidocaine. Lidocaine patch 5% is a topical preparation that has excellent safety and tolerability, and the only side effects involve mild skin reactions (e.g., erythema, rash). Systemic absorption is minimal but must be considered in patients receiving oral Class I antiarrythmic drugs such as mexiletine.

Treatment with the lidocaine patch 5% consists of the application of a maximum of three patches daily for a maximum of 12 hours applied directly to the area of maximal PHN pain and allodynia, which typically overlaps the affected dermatome. Lidocaine patch 5% is not approved for patients with herpes zoster, and it should not be used in patients with open lesions because the available formulation is not sterile. Importantly, whether the patient obtains satisfactory relief from lidocaine patch 5% will usually be apparent within two weeks and time-consuming dose escalation is not required.

OPIOID ANALGESICS: The efficacy of opioid analgesics in patients with PHN was first demonstrated in a double-blind study comparing intravenous morphine with placebo.[59] By providing evidence that PHN pain could be temporarily relieved by infusions of opioid analgesics, the results of this study suggested that longer-term oral treatment might also be efficacious. In two double-blind, placebo-controlled, randomized trials of oral opioid analgesics in PHN, controlled-release oxycodone titrated to a maximum dosage of 60 mg daily provided statistically significant benefits on pain, disability, and allodynia[60] and controlled-release morphine titrated to a maximum dosage of 240 mg daily provided statistically significant benefits on pain and sleep but not on physical functioning and mood.[61]

The most common side effects of opioid analgesics are constipation, sedation, and nausea, and cognitive impairment and problems with mobility can occur in elderly patients. Opioid analgesics must be used very cautiously in patients with a history of substance abuse or suicide, and accidental death or suicide can occur with overdose. Patients treated with opioid analgesics may develop analgesic tolerance (i.e., a reduction in analgesic benefit over time), although a stable dosage can often be achieved. All patients will develop physical dependence (i.e., withdrawal symptoms develop with abrupt discontinuation or rapid dose reduction), and must be advised that they should not abruptly discontinue their medication. The risk that substance abuse will develop in patients who do not have a history of substance abuse is not known but thought to be low in the generally elderly patient with PHN.

There are numerous short- and long-acting opioid analgesics available, and treatment can begin with a short-acting medication at morphine oral equianalgesic dosages of 5 to 15 mg every 4 hours as needed. After 1 to 2 weeks of treatment, the total daily dosage can be converted to an equianalgesic dosage of one of the available long-acting opioid analgesics (i.e., controlled-release morphine, controlled-release oxycodone, transdermal fentanyl, levorphanol, and methadone) while the patient continues taking the short-acting medication on an as-needed basis. With careful titration and monitoring, there is no maximum dosage of opioid analgesics, but evaluation by a pain specialist may be considered when morphine equianalgesic dosages exceeding 120 mg daily are contemplated.

TRAMADOL: Tramadol is a norepinephrine and serotonin reuptake inhibitor with a major metabolite that is a mu-opioid agonist. There is one published, double-blind, placebo-controlled, randomized clinical trial of tramadol in PHN,[62] and its results are consistent with studies of other chronic neuropathic pain syndromes.[54] Tramadol was titrated to a maximum dosage of 400 mg daily, and significantly relieved pain and reduced use of rescue medication compared to placebo. The side effects of tramadol include dizziness, nausea, constipation, somnolence, and orthostatic hypotension. These occur more frequently when the dosage is escalated rapidly and with concurrent administration of other drugs with similar side-effect profiles. There is an increased risk of seizures in patients treated with tramadol who have a history of seizures or who are also receiving antidepressants, opioids, or other drugs that can reduce the seizure threshold. Serotonin syndrome may occur if tramadol is used concurrently with other serotonergic medications, especially selective serotonin reuptake inhibitors (SSRIs) and monoamine oxidase inhibitors. Tramadol may cause or exacerbate cognitive impairment in the elderly, and dosage adjustment is necessary in patients with renal or hepatic disease. Abuse of tramadol is thought to be rare but has been observed.

To decrease the likelihood of side effects, tramadol should be initiated at low dosages—50 mg once or twice daily—and then titrated every 3 to 7 days by 50 to 100 mg daily in divided doses as tolerated. The maximum dosage of tramadol is 100 mg 4 times daily; in patients over 75 years of age the maximum dosage of tramadol is 300 mg daily in divided doses.

TRICYCLIC ANTIDEPRESSANTS: An apt summary of studies of the efficacy of TCAs is provided by the title of an article reviewing the relevant literature: "Thirteen consecutive well-designed randomized trials show that antidepressants reduce pain in diabetic neuropathy and postherpetic neuralgia."[53] Amitriptyline is clinically the most widely used TCA in PHN because it is the TCA that has been most extensively studied in PHN and other neuropathic pain syndromes. However, amitriptyline is poorly tolerated and contraindicated in elderly patients.[63,64] In one of the very few randomized, double-blind trials that have compared two different treatments in PHN patients, nortriptyline demonstrated equivalent efficacy to amitriptyline but was better tolerated.[65] Based on the results of this study, nortriptyline should now be considered the preferred TCA for the treatment of PHN; desipramine may be used in patients who experience excessive sedation with nortriptyline.

Despite the efficacy of TCAs in the treatment of PHN, their cardiac toxicity[66] and side-effect profile require considerable caution when treating the older patient. Dry mouth is the most common side effect, and constipation, sweating, dizziness, disturbed vision, and drowsiness also occur frequently. All TCAs must be used very cautiously in patients with a history of cardiovascular disease, glaucoma, urinary retention, and autonomic neuropathy, and a screening ECG to check for cardiac conduction abnormalities is recommended before beginning TCA treatment, especially in patients over 40 years of age. TCAs must be used cautiously when there is a risk of suicide or accidental death from overdose, and TCAs may cause balance problems and cognitive impairment in the elderly. TCAs can block the effects of certain antihypertensive drugs and interact with drugs metabolized by P450 2D6 (e.g., cimetidine, Type 1C antiarrythmics). Because all SSRIs inhibit P450 D26, caution is necessary in the concomitant administration of TCAs and SSRIs to prevent toxic TCA plasma concentrations.

To decrease side effects, all TCAs should be initiated at low dosages—10 to 25 mg in a single dose at bedtime—and should then be slowly titrated as tolerated. It is often claimed that the analgesic effect of TCAs occurs at lower dosages than their antidepressant effect, but there is no controlled evidence of this. Consequently, TCAs should be titrated to dosages of at least 75 to 150 mg daily. For titration above 100 to 150 mg daily, blood levels and the EKG should be monitored. Irrespective of the TCA chosen, it is imperative that patients understand the rationale for treatment, specifically, that TCAs have an analgesic effect that has been demonstrated to be independent of their antidepressant effect.

SEQUENTIAL AND COMBINATION PHARMACOLOGIC TREATMENT: There have been few clinical trials in which medications have been directly compared with one another in patients with PHN.[61,65] Such comparisons would not only make it possible to determine directly whether treatments vary in their efficacy, safety, and tolerability, but when conducted in the same patients, would also make it possible to evaluate the extent to which treatment response to one medication predicts response to another. For example, treatment responses to opioid analgesics and TCAs were uncorrelated in a recent three-period placebo-controlled crossover trial, which suggests that when patients have not responded to one of these types of medication, they may still respond to the other.[61]

The randomized controlled trials of the above treatments for PHN all examined the efficacy of a single medication vs. placebo (or a comparison drug), but combination therapy is the norm in the clinical setting. Unfortunately, there are no data regarding the additive or synergistic benefits of combination treatment and it is not known which patients are most likely to benefit from what combinations. Disadvantages of combination therapy include an increased risk of side effects as the number of medications is increased and the difficulty determining which medication is responsible for which side effects.

BEYOND FIRST- AND SECOND-LINE TREATMENT:

A considerable percentage of PHN patients will not respond to medications when used alone and in combination. For these patients, there is a large number of alternative treatments that deserve consideration and referral to a pain management center should be contemplated, sooner rather than later.[67] Invasive treatments may be considered when patients have failed to obtain adequate relief from other treatment approaches. These include sympathetic nerve blocks, which may provide temporary relief in patients with PHN but typically do not provide longer-lasting benefits.[22,67] Based on a review of 77 patients, it was reported that stellate ganglion blocks provided "good" pain relief in 50% of PHN patients who had pain for less than 1 year but in only 25% of patients who had pain for more than 1 year.[68] Similar data have also been presented by Winnie and Hartwell,[69] comparing sympathetic nerve blocks done within 2 months of the onset of zoster with blocks done more than 2 months after onset. Unfortunately, both of these studies were uncontrolled, making it impossible to distinguish greater efficacy of earlier treatment from the natural history of pain resolution in herpes zoster and PHN.

A recent study examining intrathecal administration of methylprednisolone[70] in patients with PHN has received considerable attention because of the dramatic benefits that were described. However, intrathecal administration of methylprednisolone is not approved by the US Food and Drug Administration (FDA) and the well-known risks of intrathecal steroids include neurological complications and adhesive arachnoiditis.

An uncontrolled study of spinal cord stimulation in 28 patients with PHN demonstrated long-term benefits in 82%, including pain relief and improvements in daily functioning.[71] The authors reported that spontaneous improvement was ruled out by recurrence of pain following inactivation of the spinal cord stimulator. Confirmation of the benefits of spinal cord stimulation in patients with PHN will require use of adequate control groups.

It is important to conclude by emphasizing that the medications and invasive treatments that are currently available are rarely associated with the complete relief of PHN and evidence of their beneficial effects on quality of life is limited. Medical and invasive management of the patient with PHN should therefore be considered components of a more comprehensive treatment approach, which may include various nonpharmacologic treatments such as psychological counseling.[72]

KEY POINTS

- Herpes zoster (shingles) is caused by reactivation of the VZV, which establishes latency in sensory ganglia after primary infection (chicken pox).
- The characteristic unilateral dermatomal vesicular rash of herpes zoster heals within 2 to 4 weeks and is accompanied by pain in the majority of patients.
- Older age is associated with an increased risk of herpes zoster because of an age-associated decline in VZV-specific cell-mediated immunity.

- Antiviral therapy with acyclovir, famciclovir, or valacyclovir in patients with herpes zoster inhibits viral replication and has been shown to reduce the duration of viral shedding, hasten rash healing, and decrease the duration of pain.
- Peripheral, sympathetic, and epidural nerve blocks with local anesthetics and/or corticosteroids appear to relieve acute pain in patients with herpes zoster, but their role in preventing PHN is uncertain because of the absence of randomized placebo-controlled trials.
- PHN refers to pain that continues after healing of the herpes zoster rash. This peripheral neuropathic pain syndrome causes substantial distress and disability and can last for years.
- Well-established risk factors for PHN in patients with herpes zoster include older age, more intense acute pain, more severe rash, and a prodrome of dermatomal pain before the rash appears.
- It is likely that different peripheral and central mechanisms contribute to PHN, and that the qualitatively different types of pain that characterize PHN have different underlying mechanisms.
- The efficacy of gabapentin, lidocaine patch 5%, tramadol, TCAs, and opioid analgesics has been demonstrated by the results of randomized controlled trials in patients with PHN, and these medications provide an evidence-based approach to treatment.

REFERENCES

1. Hope-Simpson RE: The nature of herpes zoster: A long-term study and a new hypothesis. Proc R Soc Med 58:9–20, 1965.
2. Gnann JW Jr, Whitley RJ: Herpes zoster. N Engl J Med 347:340–346, 2002.
3. Hope-Simpson RE: Postherpetic neuralgia. J R Coll Gen Pract 25:571–575, 1975.
4. Kurtzke JF: Neuroepidemiology. Ann Neurol 16:265–277, 1984.
5. Donahue JG, Choo PW, Manson JE, Platt R: The incidence of herpes zoster. Arch Intern Med 155:1605–1609, 1995.
6. Brisson M, Edmunds WJ, Law B, et al: Epidemiology of varicella zoster virus infection in Canada and the United Kingdom. Epidemiol Infect 127:305–314, 2001.
7. Schmader K: Epidemiology of herpes zoster. In Arvin AM, Gershon AA (eds): Varicella-Zoster Virus: Virology and Clinical Management. Cambridge University Press, Cambridge, 2000, pp 220–245.
8. Arvin AM: Varicella-zoster virus. In Fields BN, Knipe DM, Howley PM, et al (eds): Fields Virology, ed 3. Lippincott-Raven, Philadelphia, 1996, pp 2547–2587.
9. Haanpää M, Laippala P, Nurmikko T: Pain and somatosensory dysfunction in acute herpes zoster. Clin J Pain 15:78–84, 1999.
10. Haanpää M, Laippala P, Nurmikko T: Allodynia and pinprick hypesthesia in acute herpes zoster, and the development of postherpetic neuralgia. J Pain Symptom Manage 20:50–58, 2000.
11. Dworkin RH, Nagasako EM, Johnson RW, et al: Acute pain in herpes zoster: The famciclovir database project. Pain 94:113–119, 2001.
12. Gilden DH, Dueland AN, Cohrs R, et al: Preherpetic neuralgia. Neurology 41:1215–1218, 1991.
13. Dworkin RH, Schmader KE: Epidemiology and natural history of herpes zoster and postherpetic neuralgia. In Watson CPN, Gershon AA (eds): Herpes Zoster and Postherpetic Neuralgia, ed 2. Elsevier, New York, 2001, pp 39–64.
14. Lydick E, Epstein R, Himmelberger D, et al: Herpes zoster and quality of life: A self-limited disease with severe impact. Neurology 45(Suppl 8):S52–S53, 1995.

15. Gilden DH, Wright RR, Schneck SA, et al: Zoster sine herpete, a clinical variant. Ann Neurol 35, 530–533, 1994.

16. Galil K, Choo PW, Donahue JG, et al: The sequelae of herpes zoster. Arch Intern Med 157:1209–1213, 1997.

17. Kost RG, Straus SE: Postherpetic neuralgia: Pathogenesis, treatment, and prevention. N Engl J Med 335:32–42, 1996.

18. Whitley RJ: Herpes zoster: Natural history, diagnosis and therapy. In Watson CPN, Gershon AA (eds): Herpes Zoster and Postherpetic Neuralgia, ed 2. Elsevier, New York, 2001, pp 65–78.

19. Tyring SK, Beutner KR, Tucker BA, et al: Antiviral therapy for herpes zoster: Randomized, controlled clinical trial of valacyclovir and famciclovir therapy in immunocompetent patients 50 years and older. Arch Fam Med 9:863–869, 2000.

20. Whitley RJ, Weiss H, Gnann JW Jr, et al: Acyclovir with and without prednisone for the treatment of herpes zoster: A randomized, placebo-controlled trial. Ann Intern Med 125:376–383, 1996.

21. Bowsher D: The effects of pre-emptive treatment of postherpetic neuralgia with amitriptyline: A randomized, double-blind, placebo-controlled trial. J Pain Symptom Manage 13:327–331, 1997.

22. Wu CL, Marsh A, Dworkin RH: The role of sympathetic nerve blocks in herpes zoster and postherpetic neuralgia. Pain 87:121–129, 2000.

23. Opstelten W, Van Wijck AJM, Stolker RJ: Interventions to prevent postherpetic neuralgia: Cutaneous and percutaneous techniques. Pain 107:202–206, 2004.

24. Dworkin RH, Perkins FM, Nagasako EM: Prospects for the prevention of postherpetic neuralgia in herpes zoster patients. Clin J Pain 16(Suppl):S90–S100, 2000.

25. Dworkin RH, Schmader KE: Treatment and prevention of postherpetic neuralgia. Clin Infect Dis 36:877–882, 2003.

26. Gershon AA: Live-attenuated varicella vaccine. Infect Dis Clin North Am 15:65–81, 2001.

27. Seward JF, Watson BM, Peterson CL, et al: Varicella disease after introduction of varicella vaccine in the United States, 1995–2000. JAMA 287:606–611, 2002.

28. Hardy IB, Gershon AA, Steinberg S, et al: The incidence of zoster after immunization with live attenuated varicella vaccine: A study in children with leukemia. N Engl J Med 325:1545–1550, 1991.

29. Oxman M: Immunization to reduce the frequency and severity of herpes zoster and its complications. Neurology 45(Suppl 8):S41–S46, 1995.

30. Levin MJ: Use of varicella vaccines to prevent herpes zoster in older individuals. Arch Virol Suppl 17:151–160, 2001.

31. Dworkin RH, Portenoy RK: Pain and its persistence in herpes zoster. Pain 67:241–251, 1996.

32. Dworkin RH, Portenoy RK: Proposed classification of herpes zoster pain. Lancet 343:1648, 1994.

33. Desmond RA, Weiss HL, Arani RB, et al: Clinical applications for change-point analysis of herpes zoster pain. J Pain Symptom Manage 23:510–516, 2002.

34. Jung BF, Johnson RW, Griffin DRJ, et al: Risk factors for postherpetic neuralgia in patients with herpes zoster. Neurology 62:1545–1551, 2004.

35. Bennett GJ: Neuropathic pain: An overview. In Borsook D (ed): Molecular Neurobiology of Pain. IASP Press, Seattle, 1997, pp 109–113.

36. Bowsher D: The lifetime occurrence of herpes zoster and prevalence of postherpetic neuralgia: A retrospective survey in an elderly population. Eur J Pain 3:335–342, 1999.

37. Schmader K: Postherpetic neuralgia in immunocompetent elderly people. Vaccine 16:1768–1770, 1998.

38. Schmader K: Herpes zoster in older adults. Clin Infect Dis 32:1481–1486, 2001.

39. Davies L, Cossins L, Bowsher D, et al: The cost of treatment for post-herpetic neuralgia in the UK. PharmacoEconomics 6:142–148, 1994.

40. Watson CPN, Watt VR, Chipman M, et al: The prognosis with post-herpetic neuralgia. Pain 46:195–199, 1991.

41. Huff JC, Drucker JL, Clemmer A, et al: Effect of oral acyclovir on pain resolution in herpes zoster: A reanalysis. J Med Virol Suppl 1:93–96, 1993.

42. Bhala BB, Ramamoorthy C, Bowsher D, et al: Shingles and postherpetic neuralgia. Clin J Pain 4:169–174, 1988.

43. Bowsher D: Sensory change in postherpetic neuralgia. In Watson CPN (ed): Herpes Zoster and Postherpetic Neuralgia. Elsevier, Amsterdam, 1993, pp 97–107.

44. Bowsher D: Acute herpes zoster and postherpetic neuralgia: Effects of acyclovir and outcome of treatment with amitriptyline. Br J Gen Pract 42:244–246, 1992.

45. De Moragas JM, Kierland RR: The outcome of patients with herpes zoster. Arch Dermatol 75:193–196, 1957.

46. Whitley RJ, Weiss HL, Soong SJ, et al: Herpes zoster: Risk categories for persistent pain. J Infect Dis 179:9–15, 1999.

47. Bennett GJ: Hypotheses on the pathogenesis of herpes zoster-associated pain. Ann Neurol 35(Suppl):S38–S41, 1994.

48. Fields HL, Rowbotham M, Baron R: Postherpetic neuralgia: Irritable nociceptors and deafferentation. Neurobiol Dis 5:209–227, 1998.

49. Rowbotham MC, Petersen KL, Fields HL: Is postherpetic neuralgia more than one disorder? Pain Forum 7:231–237, 1998.

50. Watson CPN, Deck JH, Morshead C, et al: Post-herpetic neuralgia: Further post-mortem studies of cases with and without pain. Pain 44:105–117, 1991.

51. Rowbotham MC, Yosipovitch G, Connolly MK, et al: Cutaneous innervation density in the allodynic form of postherpetic neuralgia. Neurobiol Dis 3:205–214, 1996.

52. Oaklander AL: The density of remaining nerve endings in human skin with and without postherpetic neuralgia after shingles. Pain 92:139–145, 2001.

53. Max MB: Thirteen consecutive well-designed randomized trials show that antidepressants reduce pain in diabetic neuropathy and postherpetic neuralgia. Pain Forum 4:248–253, 1995.

54. Dworkin RH, Backonja M, Rowbotham MC, et al: Advances in neuropathic pain: Diagnosis, mechanisms, and treatment recommendations. Arch Neurol 60:1524–1534, 2003.

55. Rowbotham MC, Harden N, Stacey B, et al: Gabapentin for the treatment of postherpetic neuralgia: A randomized controlled trial. JAMA 280:1837–1842, 1998.

56. Rice ASC, Maton S, Postherpetic Neuralgia Study Group: Gabapentin in postherpetic neuralgia: A randomised, double blind, placebo controlled study. Pain 94:215–224, 2001.

57. Rowbotham MC, Davies PS, Verkempinck C, et al: Lidocaine patch: Double-blind controlled study of a new treatment method for post-herpetic neuralgia. Pain 65:39–44, 1996.

58. Galer BS, Rowbotham MC, Perander J, et al: Topical lidocaine patch relieves postherpetic neuralgia more effectively than a vehicle topical patch: Results of an enriched enrollment study. Pain 80:533–538, 1999.

59. Rowbotham MC, Reisner-Keller L, Fields HL: Both intravenous lidocaine and morphine reduce the pain of postherpetic neuralgia. Neurology 41:1024–1028, 1991.

60. Watson CPN, Babul N: Efficacy of oxycodone in neuropathic pain: A randomized trial in postherpetic neuralgia. Neurology 50:1837–1841, 1998.

61. Raja SN, Haythornthwaite JA, Pappagallo M, et al: Opioids versus antidepressants in postherpetic neuralgia: A randomized, placebo-controlled trial. Neurology 59:1015–1021, 2002.

62. Boureau F, Legallicier P, Kabir-Ahmadi M: Tramadol in post-herpetic neuralgia: A randomized, double-blind, placebo-controlled trial. Pain 104:323–331, 2003.

63. Aparasu RR, Sitzman SJ: Inappropriate prescribing for elderly outpatients. Am J Health System Pharm 56:433–439, 1999.

64. Mort JR, Aparasu RR: Prescribing of psychotropics in the elderly: Why is it so often inappropriate? CNS Drugs 16:99–109, 2002.

65. Watson CPN, Vernich L, Chipman M, et al: Nortriptyline versus amitriptyline in postherpetic neuralgia: A randomized trial. Neurology 51:1166–1171, 1998.

66. Roose SP, Laghrissi-Thode F, Kennedy JS, et al: Comparison of paroxetine and nortriptyline in depressed patients with ischemic heart disease. JAMA 279:287–291, 1998.

67. Kanazi GE, Johnson RW, Dworkin RH: Treatment of postherpetic neuralgia: An update. Drugs 59:1113–1126, 2000.

68. Milligan NS, Nash TP: Treatment of post-herpetic neuralgia: A review of 77 consecutive cases. Pain 23:381–386, 1985.

69. Winnie AP, Hartwell PW: Relationship between time of treatment of acute herpes zoster with sympathetic blockade and prevention of postherpetic neuralgia: Clinical support for a new theory of the mechanism by which sympathetic blockade provides therapeutic benefit. Reg Anesthesia 18:277–282, 1993.

70. Kotani N, Kushikata T, Hashimoto H, et al: Intrathecal methylprednisolone for intractable postherpetic neuralgia. N Engl J Med 343:1514–1519, 2000.

71. Harke H, Gretenkort P, Ladleif HU, et al: Spinal cord stimulation in postherpetic neuralgia and in acute herpes zoster pain. Anesth Analg 94:694–700, 2002.

72. Turk DC, Gatchel RJ (eds): Psychological Approaches to Pain Management: A Practitioner's Handbook, ed 2. Guilford Press, New York, 2002.

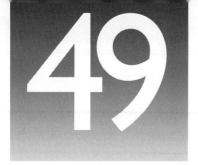

Phantom Pain

Srinivasa N. Raja, M.D., and
Honorio T. Benzon, M.D.

Amputation of the limb can lead to painful and nonpainful sequelae such as phantom sensation, telescoping, stump pain, and phantom pain. Although the phenomena of abnormal sensations and pain in amputated limbs have been reported earlier by several physicians, Weir Mitchell is generally credited with coining the term "phantom limb" to describe the symptoms he observed in American Civil War soldiers. These phenomena occur in the majority of patients after limb amputation, although the nature, frequency, intensity, and duration of symptoms may vary considerably.[1–3] Postamputation pains often delay rehabilitation, limit the use of prosthetic devices, and have a profound influence on the quality of life of the amputee.

PHANTOM SENSATION

Phantom sensations are nonpainful sensations usually occurring after a traumatic or surgical amputation that is perceived as emanating from the missing body part. Phantom sensations are common after surgery with an incidence of 90% during the first 6 months after surgery. A third of the patients experience phantom sensations within 24 hours after their surgery.[4] Excision of a body part, however, is not essential for phantom sensation. Phantom sensation of the arm has been reported after avulsion of the brachial plexus without amputation of the limb.[5] Excision of other body parts such as tongue, bladder, rectum, breast, and genitalia may also present with phantom sensations.[5,6]

Nonpainful phantom sensation may have various manifestations including kinetic sensations, and kinesthetic and exteroceptive perceptions.[7] Kinetic sensations are exemplified by perception of movements in the amputated body region, such as flexion/extension of the toes. Kinesthetic perceptions are characterized by distorted representations in size or position of the missing body part, e.g., the perception that the hand or foot is twisted. Exteroceptive perceptions include paresthesia, tingling, touch, pressure, itching, heat, cold, and wetness.[5,6] Complete paraplegic and quadriplegic patients also have phantom sensation.[5,6] Phantom sensations are commonly experienced

in the distal portion of the limbs—hands and feet—possibly due to the rich innervation of these regions and the disproportionately large cortical representation of these regions in the homunculus.

TELESCOPING

Phantom limbs are also associated with a phenomenon called "telescoping": the perception of progressive shortening of the phantom body part resulting in the sensation that the distal part of the limb is becoming more proximal.[4] At the start of the phenomenon, the phantom sensation usually feels so real that the patient may actually reach for objects or attempt to ambulate with a phantom limb.[5] However, with time phantom sensations of the distal extremities may change and become less distinct so that the patient may feel a hand close to the stump, but not feel the forearm or distal arm. This phenomenon is common and occurs in about two-thirds of limb amputees.

PHANTOM PAIN

Phantom pain is the perception of a painful, unpleasant sensation in the distribution of the missing or deafferented body part. Phantom limb pain has been reported to occur in about two-thirds of postamputation patients in the first 6 months after surgery, and about 60% of patients still had significant phantom pain 2 years after surgery.[8] The overall incidence of phantom pain several years after surgery has been reported to be as high as 85%.[6,8] The pain can vary in character, duration, frequency, and intensity. It can present as sharp, dull, burning, squeezing, cramping, shooting, or as a shock-like electrical sensation.[6] Patients may occasionally complain of intermittent tremors or painful muscle spasms in the stump associated with paroxysms of phantom pain.

In a prospective study by Jensen and colleagues of 58 patients undergoing limb amputation phantom pain changed in presentation within the first 6 months after amputation. The characteristic of the phantom pain changed from a mainly exteroceptive-like pain (knifelike or sticking), localized in the entire limb or at least involving proximal parts of the lost limb, to a mainly proprioceptive type of pain (squeezing or burning) localized in the distal parts of the amputated limb.[8] Forty-seven percent of patients had phantom pain within 24 hours after the amputation and 83% within the first 4 days. The study also showed that the frequency, duration, and severity of the phantom pain decreased during the first 6 months, and then the characteristics of the phantom pain did not change significantly thereafter. Sometimes, phantom pain can resolve spontaneously with or without treatment. However, it seems that phantom pain persisting 6 months after the amputation is difficult to treat.[6]

The incidence of phantom pain seems to be independent of the patient's age, sex, previous health status, and cause of amputation.[6,8] One factor that increases the incidence of phantom pain after amputation is the presence of pain in the limb before the amputation.[4,8,9] In a prospective study of 56 patients who had amputation of a lower limb Nikolajsen and colleagues noted that the presence of preamputation pain significantly increased the incidence of stump pain and phantom pain after 1 week and the incidence of phantom pain after 3 months.[9] Approximately 42% of the patients reported that their phantom pain resembled the pain they had experienced at the time of amputation.[9]

STUMP PAIN

Stump pain or *residual limb pain* is pain localized to the residual body part following amputation. Longitudinal studies report that the incidence of stump pain more than 2 years after amputation is about 20%. Surveys of veterans suggested a higher incidence of pain (56%) in the residual limb and a more recent survey reported a 74% incidence.[10] Stump pain is usually secondary to local pathologic processes in the region of the stump, such as infection, lesions of the skin, soft tissue or bone, or local ischemia. However, various etiologies of stump pain have been identified: postoperative nociceptive, neurogenic, prosthogenic, arthrogenic, ischemic, referred, sympathetically maintained, or abnormal stump tissue.[6] Stump pain can be superficial (localized to the scar region of the incision), felt deep in the distal stump, or encompass the whole residual limb. Stump pain can be differentiated from phantom pain because the most common reasons for stump pain are bony spurs or an ill-fitting prosthesis which can cause pressure on the skin leading to decubitus ulcers and infection, or cause traction or pressure on a neuroma.[6] Stump pain can be managed by careful evaluation of the stump and proper fitting prosthesis. Arthrogenic and referred stump pains are usually secondary to abnormal gait resulting in excessive stress on adjacent joints or on lumbosacral vertebrae resulting in discogenic disease and radicular symptoms.

PHANTOM PHENOMENA AFTER MASTECTOMY

Phantom sensations are felt by 15% to 64% of patients who had mastectomy, the average incidence is 30%.[11] Most of these phantom sensations are felt intermittently, occurring once every 2 or 4 weeks. The incidence of phantom pain after mastectomy appears to be lower than after limb amputation: it ranges from 0% to 44% with an average of 20%.[11] The lower incidence may be related to missing kinesthesis of the breast[11,12] and the small cortical representation of the breast.[13] The onset of phantom sensation and/or pain occurs within 3 months of surgery, with most occurring within 1 month after surgery. The phantom pain is localized in the entire breast or in the nipple. The relationship between preamputation pain and phantom pain appears to be less after mastectomy than after limb amputation. In fact, preamputation pain has a stronger relationship with phantom sensations than with phantom pain. There is, however, a striking similarity in the location and character of the pain before and after mastectomy,[11] a phenomenon seen after other amputations.[14] The relationship between phantom pain and preamputation pain is more significant within the first month after mastectomy.

THEORETICAL MECHANISMS

The proposed mechanisms for phantom sensation and phantom pain are unclear and controversial. Although phantom pain and sensations may coexist, they may not share the same mechanism because the relief of one is not always associated with the relief of the other.[6] It has been reported that the phantom sensation disappears after a parietal cortical lesion but phantom pain remains.[9] Several lines of evidence suggest that the phantom phenomenon is the result of interactions between altered peripheral, spinal, and supraspinal mechanisms. The demonstration of spontaneous neuronal activity in the proximal end of cut nerves,[15] the presence of stump pathology in some patients with phantom pain, and the relief of phantom pain after the injection of local anesthetic into the painful stump have all been considered as supportive evidences of peripheral mechanisms of phantom pain.[4,15] Peripheral nerve damage during an amputation initiates axonal regeneration creating an area of hyperexcitability known as a neuroma. Afferent fibers in a neuroma develop ectopic activity, mechanical sensitivity, and chemosensitivity to catecholamines. These physiological changes may lead to spontaneous pain and explain the increased pain caused by emotional distress or exposure to cold that may result in increased sympathetic discharge and circulating catecholamines. However, there is evidence against a purely peripheral mechanism for phantom phenomena. Total spinal anesthesia, cordotomy, and cordectomy have all failed to relieve phantom pain and in some cases spinal anesthesia can result in the development or rekindling of phantom pain that had subsided.[16,17]

There is reason to think that a spinal cord mechanism explains phantom phenomena. Peripheral nerve injury leads to deafferentation—removal of afferent input to the dorsal column of the spinal cord—causing structural, neurochemical, and physiologic changes in the central nervous system neurons. These changes result in functional alterations, plasticity, in central neurons that lead to spontaneous pain signals which are transmitted centrally. Peripheral sensory input at the level of the spinal cord also has inhibitory effects on the transmission of pain centrally. The changes in the dorsal horn and the loss of afferent input lead to decreased impulses from the brainstem reticular areas which normally have inhibitory effects on sensory transmission.[16] Therefore, the absence of inhibitory effects of sensory input from the missing peripheral body part causes increased autonomous activity of the dorsal horn neurons, in effect becoming "sensory epileptic discharges."[6,8] The spinal cord mechanism is supported by the fact that anticonvulsants

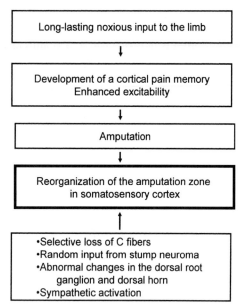

FIGURE 49-1. Schematic of factors involved in the mechanisms of phantom limb pain. (From Flor H: Phantom-limb pain: Characteristics, causes, and treatment. Lancet Neurol 1:182–189, 2002.)

and lesions placed in the substantia gelatinosa are effective in treating phantom pain.[12]

A proposed supraspinal mechanism to explain phantom pain is the neuromatrix theory proposed by Melzack.[5,18] The neuromatrix consists of a network of neurons that extends throughout the brain. The repeated cyclical processing of peripheral nerve impulses in the neuromatrix imparts a characteristic pattern, a neurosignature, according to Melzack. Therefore, a person may have the sensation that a body part is present even in the absence of peripheral input. In the absence of modulating input from the limbs, the neuromatrix produces abnormal signature patterns which are interpreted as painful sensation.[5,18] In phantom limb pain the patterns produced are transduced in the neural hub as a hot or burning sensation. The cramping muscle pain may be due to messages from the action-neuromodule to move the muscles of the absent limb.[5]

Several studies on the structural and functional changes in the architecture of the somatosensory cortex after upper limb amputation have provided new insights into the mechanisms of phantom pain.[2] Ramachandran and co-workers[19] reported that in upper limb amputees sensations in the phantom limb could be elicited by brushing the face. Imaging studies have shown a shift of the mouth representation in the somatosensory cortex to the hand region (cortical reorganization) in upper limb amputees.[20] There was a good correlation between the magnitude of the shift of the mouth representation into the zone that previously represented the amputated hand and arm and the intensity of the phantom limb pain. A schematic of the factors thought to be relevant in the development of phantom pain is shown in Fig. 49-1.

TREATMENT

Amputation of a limb affects not only the physical functioning of the individual but may also have significant psychological, social, and societal consequences. Hence, early and appropriate management of amputees is critical. Surveys suggest that lasting relief from prescribed medications occurs in less than 10% of patients. However, few controlled clinical trials are available to guide the practitioner in the optimal management of post-amputation pains and most therapies are empirical based on their effectiveness in other neuropathic pain states. A systematic search of the literature between 1966 and 1999 identified only 12 controlled trials.[21] Earlier trials focused on the treatment of established stump or phantom pain, but more recent strategies have examined the potential beneficial effects of preventive strategies.

Controlled Trials of Preoperative and Early Postoperative Interventions: Eight studies examined the treatment of acute phantom pain with preoperative, intraoperative, or early (<2 weeks) postoperative interventions such as epidural anesthesia, regional nerve blocks, intravenous calcitonin, and transcutaneous electrical nerve stimulation (TENS).[21] Follow-up periods ranged from 6 months to 2 years. The incidence of phantom pain in the control group ranged from a low of 27% at 12 months to a high of 78%. The role of preoperative epidural anesthesia is unclear with conflicting results from three studies. Perineural and intraneural bupivacaine blocks of the sciatic or posterior tibial nerves in the perioperative periods resulted in short-term pain relief but no significant long-term benefits. Intravenous calcitonin and TENS similarly resulted in reduced phantom pain in the early postoperative period but the long-term effects are uncertain.

Controlled Trials of Late Postoperative Interventions: Four studies examined the treatment of chronic phantom pain (36 days to 46 years) with interventions such as TENS, Farabloc (a metal threaded sock), ketamine infusion, and vibratory stimulation. These studies showed a modest reduction in the intensity of phantom pain, but the duration of follow-up was short-term.

Stump Pain: The first step in the management of stump pain is to identify a specific etiology for the pain that can be the target for developing treatment strategy. The stump should be carefully examined for a localized tender spot where a Tinel's sign can be elicited suggestive of a neuroma. The stump should also be examined for ulcers, potential sites of inflammation or bony abnormalities, evidence of ischemia, or recurrence in the case of malignancy. Consultation with an experienced prosthetist for rectifying an ill-fitting prosthesis is often helpful, as patients may experience exaggeration of their phantom sensation or have increased pain from use of the prosthetic limb. This may result from pressure from the prosthesis at a site of a neuroma. In addition, change in gait and altered body mechanics may result in musculoskeletal pain. Rehabilitation therapy to correct gait and postural compensations that result in arthritic or referred pain may be useful.

Reports suggest that TENS may be beneficial in 25% to 50% of patients with stump pain. Medication management will depend on whether the pain is suspected to be of somatic or neuropathic mechanisms. In the former cases, nonsteroidal anti-inflammatory drugs (NSAIDs), cyclooxygenase-2 (COX-2) antagonists, and/or opioids may be indicated. Neuropathic pain resulting from neuromas should be treated with adjuvant analgesics such as tricyclic antidepressants (e.g., nortriptyline) and anticonvulsants (e.g., gabapentin).

Surgical therapies are indicated only when a specific rectifiable pathology is identified. Protruding bone, bony exostosis, wound infection, and poorly healed wounds are clear indications for surgery.[3] A neuroma under constant pressure or near a joint resulting in repeated traction may be treated by excision of the neuroma and repositioning the nerve end in bone or muscle. Selective nerve blocks of peripheral nerves may be useful as a prognostic indicator of the success of excision of the neuroma.[22] Dorsal root entry zone (DREZ) lesioning has not been effective in patients with isolated stump pain. Dorsal column stimulation was reported to be effective in 52% of patients early on but declined to 39% of patients with good relief after 5 years.[23]

Phantom Pain: In the case of surgical amputations, education and counseling of the patient on the consequences of amputation, the rehabilitation process, and the prosthetic options should be initiated in the preamputation phase. Phantom pain has been suggested to be more likely in amputees who had severe pain before or immediately after the amputation. This observation along with the preclinical studies suggesting a beneficial effect of blocking the nociceptive input to the central nervous system is the basis for the use of preemptive epidural or peripheral nerve blocks. Bach et al. showed that epidural bupivacaine, with or without morphine, when given for 72 hours before amputation decreased the incidence of phantom limb pain.[24] The incidences of phantom pain at 1 week, 6 months, and 1 year in the epidural group were 27%, 0%, and 0%, respectively. These incidences were significantly less than the corresponding incidences of 64%, 38%, and 27% in the control group.[24] Subsequent controlled trials have failed to replicate this finding.[9]

Numerous treatment approaches have been attempted for phantom pain. These include a wide variety of medications, physical therapy, psychological interventions, cognitive behavioral therapies, complementary and alternative therapies, neurostimulation, and ablative procedures at various sites in the peripheral and central nervous systems. No one therapy has been uniformly effective and there is a lack of controlled trials examining the effectiveness of these different therapies.

Numerous medical treatments have been proposed, but controlled trials have only been done with opioids, calcitonin, and ketamine, all of which are effective in reducing phantom pain. Other commonly used medications are the anticonvulsants and the antidepressants.[6,16] Other drugs include beta-blockers, neuroleptic agents, mexiletine, and capsaicin. Combined treatment with anticonvulsants and antidepressants is the usual regimen, treating both the lancinating pain and the burning pain components of phantom limb pain.[16] Gabapentin, carbamazepine, clonazepam, and valproic acid are anticonvulsants that have been used. For cramping pain, stump movement disorders, or flexor spasticity, baclofen or clonazepam may be effective.[16] Opioid therapy has been shown to provide short-term relief of stump and phantom pains,[25,26] but the efficacy of long-term opioid usage needs further investigation.

Various physical modalities such as ultrasound, vibration, TENS, and acupuncture offer temporary relief with no significant long-term benefits.[6,27] These therapies rely on the gate control theory of pain transmission which proposes that stimulation of large nerve fibers closes the gate and inhibits the transmission of pain centrally.

Surgical interventions have not been shown to be of significant benefit in phantom pain.[6] Spinal cord stimulation has been recommended to replace the loss of afferent input to the dorsal column and enhance the descending inhibition of pain transmission. However, the results with dorsal column stimulation have not been uniform.[28,29] The same results have been found with DREZ lesions. While the procedure showed promise as treatment for avulsion injuries, its long-term effects on phantom pain have been fair, at best.[30]

Psychological interventions for phantom pain include hypnosis, biofeedback, cognitive and behavioral therapies, and support groups.[31,32] These interventions may facilitate adaptation to a change in body image, adaptation to chronic pain, and relief of grief and anger.[33] Another behaviorally oriented approach, using a mirror placed in a box, has been suggested as a means of reversing the cortical reorganization that occurs in amputees. Psychological preparation, treatment of the patient's pain, and educational efforts during the preamputation and postamputation periods can be very helpful. These include psychologically preparing patients for amputation, preparing for a change in their body image, introduction to the use of a prosthesis, information on the care and treatment of the stump, and explanation of the rehabilitation process.[6]

REFERENCES

1. Weinstein SM: Phantom limb pain and related disorders. Neurol Clin 16:919–936, 1998.
2. Flor H: Phantom-limb pain: Characteristics, causes, and treatment. Lancet Neurol 1:182–189, 2002.
3. Wellons JC, Gorecki JP, Friedman AH: Stump, phantom, and avulsion pain. *In* Burchiel K (ed): Surgical Management of Pain. Thieme, New York, 2002, pp 422–442.
4. Jensen TS, Krebs B, Nielsen J, Rasmussen P: Phantom limb, phantom pain and stump pain in amputees during the first 6 months following limb amputation. Pain 17:243–256, 1983.
5. Melzack R: Labat lecture. Phantom limbs. Reg Anesth 14:208–211, 1989.
6. Davis RW: Phantom sensation, phantom pain, and stump pain. Arch Phys Med Rehabil 74:79–91, 1993.
7. Tasker RR: Chronic pain syndromes of the central nervous system, phantom and stump pain. *In* North RB, Levy RM (eds): Neurosurgical Management of Pain. Springer-Verlag, New York, 1997, pp 100–105.
8. Jensen TS, Krebs B, Nielsen J, Rasmussen P: Immediate and long-term phantom limb pain in amputees: Incidence, clinical characteristics and relationship to pre-amputation limb pain. Pain 21:267–278, 1985.
9. Nikolajsen L, Ilkjaer S, Kroner K, et al: The influence of pre-amputation pain on postamputation stump and phantom pain. Pain 72:393–405, 1997.
10. Ehde DM, Czerniecki JM, Smith DG, et al: Chronic phantom sensations, phantom pain, residual limb pain, and other regional pain after lower limb amputation. Arch Phys Med Rehabil 81:1039–1044, 2000.
11. Rothemund Y, Grusser SM, Liebeskind U, et al: Phantom phenomena in mastectomized patients and their relation to chronic and acute pre-mastectomy pain. Pain 107:140–146, 2004.
12. Kroner K, Krebs B, Skov J, Jorgensen HS: Immediate and long-term phantom breast syndrome after mastectomy: Incidence, clinical characteristics and relationship to pre-mastectomy pain. Pain 36:327–334, 1989.
13. Itomi K, Kakigi R, Maeda K, Hoshiyama M: Dermatome versus homunculus: Detailed topography of the primary somatosensory cortex following trunk stimulation. Clin Neurophysiol 111:405–412, 2000.

14. Grusser SM, Winter C, Schaefer M, et al: Perceptual phenomena after unilateral arm amputation: A pre-post-surgical comparison. Neurosci Lett 302:13–16, 2001.

15. Carlen PL, Wall PD, Nadvorna H, Steinbach T: Phantom limbs and related phenomena in recent traumatic amputations. Neurology 28:211–217, 1978.

16. Iacono RP, Linford J, Sandyk R: Pain management after lower extremity amputation. Neurosurgery 20:496–500, 1987.

17. Murphy JP, Anandaciva S: Phantom limb pain and spinal anaesthesia. Anaesthesia 39:188, 1984.

18. Melzack R: Phantom limbs and the concept of a neuromatrix. TINS 13:88–92, 1990.

19. Ramachandran VS, Rogers-Ramachandran D, Stewart M: Perceptual correlates of massive cortical reorganization. Science 258:1159–1160, 1992.

20. Flor H, Elbert T, Knecht S, et al: Phantom-limb pain as a perceptual correlate of cortical reorganization following arm amputation. Nature 375:482–484, 1995.

21. Halbert J, Crotty M, Cameron ID: Evidence for the optimal management of acute and chronic phantom pain: A systematic review. Clin J Pain 18:84–92, 2002.

22. Burchiel KJ, Ochoa JL: Surgical management of post-traumatic neuropathic pain. Neurosurg Clin North Am 2:117–126, 1991.

23. Krainick JU, Thoden U, Riechert T: Pain reduction in amputees by long-term spinal cord stimulation. Long-term follow-up study over 5 years. J Neurosurg 52:346–350, 1980.

24. Bach S, Noreng MF, Tjellden NU: Phantom limb pain in amputees during the first 12 months following limb amputation, after preoperative lumbar epidural blockade. Pain 33:297–301, 1988.

25. Wu CL, Tella P, Staats PS, et al: Analgesic effects of intravenous lidocaine and morphine on postamputation pain: A randomized double-blind, active placebo-controlled, crossover trial. Anesthesiology 96:841–848, 2002.

26. Huse E, Larbig W, Flor H, Birbaumer N: The effect of opioids on phantom limb pain and cortical reorganization. Pain 90:47–55, 2001.

27. Lundeberg T: Relief of pain from a phantom limb by peripheral stimulation. J Neurol 232:79–82, 1985.

28. Wester K: Dorsal column stimulation in pain treatment. Acta Neurol Scand 75:151–155, 1987.

29. Kumar K, Nath R, Wyant GM: Treatment of chronic pain by epidural spinal cord stimulation: A 10-year experience. J Neurosurg 75:402–407, 1991.

30. Saris SC, Iacono RP, Nashold BS, Jr: Dorsal root entry zone lesions for post-amputation pain. J Neurosurg 62:72–76, 1985.

31. Sherman RA, Sherman CJ, Bruno GM: Psychological factors influencing chronic phantom limb pain: An analysis of the literature. Pain 28:285–295, 1987.

32. Siegel EF: Control of phantom limb pain by hypnosis. Am J Clin Hypn 21:285–286, 1979.

33. Arena JG, Sherman RA, Bruno GM, Smith JD: The relationship between situational stress and phantom limb pain: Cross-lagged correlational data from six month pain logs. J Psychosom Res 34:71–77, 1990.

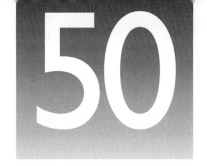

Central Pain States

Muthukumar Vaidyaraman, M.B.B.S.,
and Srinivasa N. Raja, M.D.

Central pain states result when lesions or diseases affect pain pathways within the brain and/or spinal cord. The International Association for the Study of Pain (IASP) defines *central pain* as regional pain usually associated with abnormal sensitivity to temperature and to noxious stimulation. Approximately two-thirds of patients with spinal cord injury (SCI) experience chronic pain that significantly affects their quality of life. Central pain states are often refractory to presently available treatment modalities. In this chapter we discuss the clinical presentations, pathophysiology, and therapeutic options for central pain of brain and spinal cord origin.

CAUSES OF CENTRAL PAIN

The leading cause of central pain originating in the brain is stroke. Poststroke pain affects 2% to 8% of stroke victims, or approximately 30,000 patients in the USA alone.[1] In 1906 two French neurologists first described this poststroke "thalamic pain syndrome," also known as the "Dejerine–Roussy syndrome" in

their honor. The first postmortem studies of Dejerine–Roussy syndrome revealed that many of its victims had extrathalamic lesions, and modern imaging methods have confirmed and extended these findings. These pain-generating lesions extend from the first synapse of the dorsal horn, or trigeminal nuclei, to the cerebral cortex. The predominant etiology is vascular in origin, accounting for 90% of brain central pain (supratentorial 78% and infratentorial 12%; Fig. 50-1). Extrathalamic sites are involved in 50% to 75% of cases.[1–3] Chronic poststroke pain more commonly occurs in the presence of right-sided thalamic lesions.[4]

Central pain of spinal origin is predominantly the result of trauma (Fig. 50-1). However, pain can also result from spinal cord tumors and demyelinating lesions. The incidence is reported to vary from 34% to 94% in patients with SCI[5,6] and 29% to 75% in multiple sclerosis patients.[6]

Central pain is also prevalent in patients with chronic degenerative diseases of the central nervous system (CNS). For example, almost 10% of patients with Parkinson's disease may

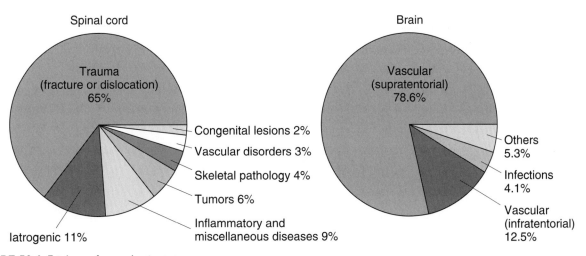

FIGURE 50-1. Etiology of central pain states.

TABLE 50-1. TAXONOMY OF SPINAL CORD INJURY PAIN

Broad Type (Tier One)	Broad System (Tier Two)	Specific Structures and Pathology (Tier Three)
Nociceptive	Musculoskeletal	Bone, joint, muscle trauma or inflammation Mechanical instability Muscle spasm Secondary overuse syndromes
	Visceral	Renal calculus, bowel dysfunction, sphincter dysfunction, etc. Dysreflexic headache
Neuropathic	Above-level	Compressive mononeuropathies Complex regional pain syndromes
	At-level	Nerve root compression (including cauda equina) Syringomyelia Spinal cord trauma/ischemia Dual level cord and root trauma
	Below-level	Spinal cord trauma/ischemia

From Siddall PJ, Yezierski RP, Loeser JD: Pain Following Spinal Cord Injury: Clinical Features, Prevalence and Taxonomy. IASP Press, Seattle, 2000.

have sensory complications, including pain;[7] and epilepsy can manifest as painful seizures. Also, in contrast to most pathologic processes affecting the CNS, clinicians cannot predict the development of central pain based on the location of a lesion. Many central pain patients maintain their ability to sense touch, vibration, and joint movements. This supports the belief that the central pain involves the spinothalamic tract and its thalamocortical projections. The highest prevalence of central pain is reported in cases of lesions in the spinal cord, medulla, and ventroposterior part of the thalamus.

TAXONOMY

The IASP established a task force recently to classify the pain states resulting from a SCI. The taxonomy suggested by the SCI Pain Task Force is shown in Table 50-1.[8] SCI pain is broadly divided into *nociceptive* and *neuropathic* with subclassification into second and third tiers based on the anatomical structures involved, the site of pain, and the etiology. Nociceptive pain may be musculoskeletal or visceral in nature. The former may be secondary to overuse of certain parts of the body to compensate for regions of paresis or result from secondary changes in bone or joints. Neuropathic pain is usually seen in areas of sensory abnormalities. Neuropathic pain has been subdivided on the basis of region, into *at-level* (radicular or central), *above-level*, and *below-level* pain to indicate the presumed site of the lesion responsible for pain generation.[9] Following SCI, it is reported that 91% of patients have pain 2 weeks after injury. This decreased to 64% at 6 months. Neuropathic, at-level pain was present in 38% at 2 weeks and remained the same at 6 months. Neuropathic below-level pain occurred in 14% of subjects at 2 weeks and increased to 19% at 6 months. The distribution and the anatomic location of the pain in relation to the site of injury and sensory deficits in patients with complete and incomplete spinal cord lesions are shown in Fig. 50-2. The pain can be spontaneous or stimulus evoked. Recent longitudinal

studies indicate that at-level pain has an early onset while the below-level pain develops months to years after the spinal injury.[10]

CLINICAL PRESENTATIONS

The neuropathic component of central pain is often reported starting days to weeks after the CNS lesion and presents as a steady dysesthesia or neuralgia, and may also have an evoked component. The quality of the pain may be burning, aching, shooting, pricking, and tingling. The discomfort is generally constant but may wax and wane and often has a deep and/or a superficial component. In a minority of patients

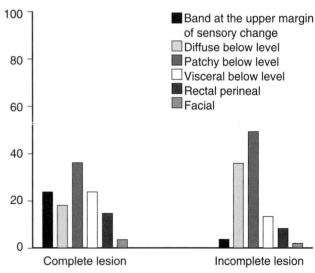

FIGURE 50-2. Distribution of the location of steady pain relative to the site of lesion in complete and incomplete spinal cord lesions.

the pain is intermittent and daily. Nonpainful tactile, thermal, vibratory, auditory, visual, olfactory, and visceral stimuli can provoke or exacerbate spontaneous pain. Anxiety and/or fear can also exacerbate symptoms. Some patients with central pain exhibit the most striking symptoms seen in clinical practice. Patients with classic Dejerine–Roussy syndrome have a rapidly regressing hemiparesis and a sensory deficit to touch, temperature, and pain. Allodynia, hyperalgesia, and spontaneous severe paroxysmal pain on the hemiparetic side also often occur. These patients can exhibit hemiataxia, hemiastereognosia, and choreoathetoid movements. Patients with central pain may have any or all of these features, depending on the location of the underlying lesion. Organic signs on sensory examination of patients with thalamic lesions include the so-called thalamic midline split for sensory loss and pain. The fact that central pain of any cause is accompanied by delayed hyperalgesia supports the hypothesis of a polysynaptic response. Pain intensity for brainstem and suprathalamic lesions are moderate in intensity averaging 61 and 50 mm, respectively (on a 100 mm visual analogue scale), while pain in thalamic lesions can be severe (average = 79 mm).[11] Several scales exist that are useful for evaluating this pain; for example, its sensory and affective features can be evaluated with the McGill Pain Questionnaire, and psychologic aspects can be evaluated using the Minnesota Multiphasic Personality Inventory (MMPI).

Patients with a history of spontaneous or evoked dysesthesia, hyperesthesia, or paresthesia should undergo specific but simple bedside testing. Sensory testing in the region where the pain is localized usually shows a paradoxic hypoalgesia (decreased sensitivity to painful stimulus). The region where the patient feels the pain often has decreased sensitivity to thermal stimuli, especially to cold. In fact, the intensity of the pain seems to be related to the magnitude of thermal sensibility loss. Testing for disturbed temperature sensation can be accomplished with a cold metal instrument, ice, or ethyl chloride spray. Touch can be tested with cotton wool. The pinprick sensation is tested using the contralateral side as a control. Chronic poststroke pain patients have an intact vibration sensation. Patients may exhibit *mitempfindung* (*with sympathy*), a phenomenon in which stimulation in one area of the body results in a simultaneous sense of the provoked sensation in another part of the body. These patients may also experience alloesthesia, in which a sensory stimulus on one side of the body is perceived on the other side. A subset of patients who experience burning pain lose the sensation of cold, warmth, and sharpness. In another subgroup of patients who experience shooting/pricking/aching pain, tactile allodynia is predominant. Although some disturbance of sensory function is almost always present on physical examination, clinical findings are few or subtle in many patients. Thus, a definite diagnosis might require a detailed neurologic examination. Quantitative sensory testing might reveal side-to-side asymmetries in cooling, warmth, and heat-pain sensation thresholds.

Testing for autonomic dysfunction may be important in patients with SCI. Lesions above the sixth thoracic level (splanchnic outflow) are often associated with autonomic dysreflexia. The dysreflexia is characterized by sudden dramatic increases in blood pressure, heart rate, and headache after sensory input such as a full bladder. Complications may include seizures and cerebral hemorrhage.

PATHOPHYSIOLOGIC MECHANISMS

Central pain states likely result from pathophysiologic changes caused by irritation of, or damage to, central pain pathways. The possible pathophysiologic mechanisms that cause and maintain central pain are complex and not well understood (for a recent review see Finnerup and Jensen[12]). Injury to the CNS may result in anatomic, neurochemical, inflammatory, and excitotoxic changes that result in a sensitized and hyperexcitable CNS. Three general mechanisms are considered to be involved in the mechanisms of central pain:

Maladaptive reorganization. Injury to the central neurons or pathways may result in Wallerian degeneration. The latter could trigger plastic changes characterized by abnormal synaptic reorganization, and altered processing in the forebrain of nociceptive and/or innocuous input. When this occurs, presynaptic neurons display spontaneous discharges. The up- or down-regulation of receptors may explain the delay in symptom onset.[13]

Denervation supersensitivity. The loss of innervation from injury to the CNS leads to overactivity among central pain-signaling neurons, such as those in the thalamus or dorsal horn. An argument against this hypothesis is that if denervation leads to supersensitivity of nerve impulses, it would respond to pharmacotherapy that depresses the CNS.

Neurochemical changes. Several neurotransmitters, such as glutamate, gamma-aminobutyric acid (GABA), norepinephrine, serotonin, histamine, and acetylcholine, are involved in the processing of noxious input along the pain pathway. The shift in firing from a rhythmic burst to a single spike is determined by noradrenergic, serotonergic, and cholinergic input to the reticular and relay cells of the thalamus. Similarly, excitatory amino acids such as glutamate are released in the region of SCI and may lead to neuronal hyperexcitability. At the spinal cord level, substance P and cholecystokinin (CCK) might play an additional role by influencing the voltage-gated sodium and calcium channels. Potassium channels play a critical role in setting the resting membrane potential and controlling the excitability of neurons. A K^+ channel, the M channel that regulates the excitability of central and peripheral neurons, is also considered to play a role in neuropathic pain states.[14]

Hypotheses specific to central pain of cerebral origin include:

Disinhibition of nociceptive input. It is postulated that the injury to central neurons diminishes the negative feedback control that is normally associated in the processing of pain sensations. Craig and co-workers showed that, under normal conditions, the cool-sensitive pathway in the spinothalamic tract (STT) might suppress the forebrain's response to nociceptive STT activity.[15] Damage to this pathway may thus explain some of the phenomena seen in a central pain state. They hypothesize that, for central pain to occur, a lateral lamina I spinothalamocortical pathway lesion must be sufficiently large to produce contralateral sensory symptoms. This assumes that central pain is a release phenomenon resulting from the disruption of the normal integrative controls of sensory processing. The disruption of thermal sensibility results in a loss of the cold-induced inhibition of pain, with a resultant disinhibition of cold-evoked burning pain. Craig and co-workers suggested that the ventromedial posterior (VMPo) nucleus of the thalamus plays a critical role. Investigations in monkey, however, strongly support the existence of a spinothalamocortical pathway from lamina I and the deep layers of the dorsal horn to the contralateral ventral posterior lateral (VPL) nucleus, which extends to area 1 of the S1 somatosensory cortex. A similar pathway might activate neurons of the SII cortex because direct projections connect the VPL and VPI (inferior) to SII and SI to SII.[16]

Maladaptive reorganization. In the dorsal and lateral aspects the thalamus is surrounded by reticular cells, which are innervated by corticothalamic axons and secrete GABA that, in turn, inhibits thalamic relay cells. The reticular cells and relay cells display a bursting pattern when hyperpolarized, and a single spike activity when depolarized. Deafferentated cells can generate intrinsic bursting activity,[17] and bursting can be transmitted to the relay cells. In positron emission tomography (PET) scans with fluorodeoxyglucose (FDG) tracer deafferentation is associated with decreased metabolic activity. Metabolic activity can also decrease in painful states that arise outside of the CNS. Hence, changes with PET scanning are not specific for central poststroke pain (CPSP). Lenz et al. have shown that bursting can signal pain activity.[18,19] However, whether this abnormal bursting is due to a loss of afferent input or to increased activity at *N*-methyl-D-aspartate (NMDA) receptors

is not known. Jeanmonod's group has reported considerable success in treating central pain with iatrogenic medial thalamic lesions, targeting the bursting cells that are the presumed pain generators.[20] These results should, however, be interpreted with caution as it is unclear if the abnormal bursting activity is the primary event or a secondary manifestation of a CNS lesion occurring elsewhere. Current evidence points to the posterior inferior part of the VPI as the critical target for the thalamic lesions that cause central pain.[11,21]

Postlesion imbalance between facilitatory and inhibitory neural pathways and chaotic neural activity in the deafferentated circuits. Lesions in the spinothalamocortical pathways can cause ectopic discharges in various neurons of the spinal cord and brain. Such ectopic neuronal discharges create an illusion of noxious input because of the imbalance between the lateral (inhibitory) and medial (excitatory) STT. This might explain why pain occurs more often in patients with partial lesions than in those with complete cord and thalamic injuries. It appears that severe CNS lesions, with total destruction of ascending sensory systems, do not lead to a central pain syndrome and that mild, moderate, or severe disruption of the

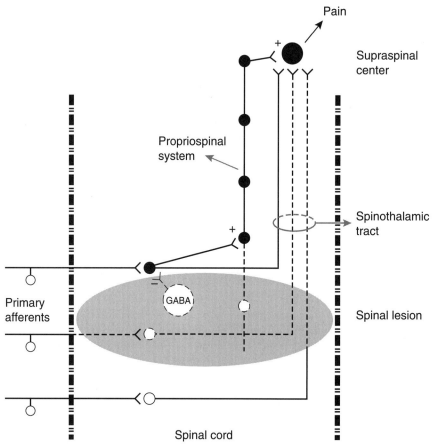

FIGURE 50-3. Proposed mechanism of central pain in spinal cord injury. Input from primary afferents can be distorted by two mechanisms. The spinothalamic tract projection neurons from below the spinal injury may be lesioned and give rise to deafferentation hyperexcitability in higher-order neurons including the thalamus. Second-order neurons in the dorsal horn at the rostral end of the spinal lesion may become hyperexcitable as a consequence of excitotoxic changes and disinhibition from damaged GABA-ergic neurons at the level of injury. Abnormal input from these second-order neurons in the rostral end of the spinal cord lesion may propagate via the propriospinal system to the deafferented thalamic neurons resulting in pain referred to areas below injury level. (From Finnerup NB, Jensen TS: Spinal cord injury pain – Mechanisms and treatment. Eur J Neurol 11:73–82, 2004.)

anterolateral ascending system, with partial or complete preservation of the dorsal column/medial lemniscus functions, is most frequently associated with central pain syndrome. Furthermore, even during remission, dysesthesias and pain could be triggered by additional afferent input to the large fiber/dorsal column/medial lemniscus system and, once established, might not be abolished by additional deafferentation.

Hypotheses specific to central pain of spinal cord origin are summarized in Fig. 50-3. Central pain in SCI may result from a combination of deafferentation-induced plastic changes in supraspinal areas along with abnormal input from a pain generator in the spinal cord. The changes in the CNS may include *neuronal hyperexcitability*. In SCI, NMDA receptor activation might trigger the intracellular cascade leading to the up-regulation of neuronal activity/excitability that results in spontaneous and evoked neuronal hyperactivity/hyperexcitability and causes abnormal pain perception. Changes in voltage-sensitive sodium channels can also contribute to changes in nerve membrane excitability. Other important mechanisms might be a loss of endogenous inhibition, including reduced GABAergic, opioid, and monoaminergic inhibition. Wide dynamic range (WDR) neuronal hypersensitivity in excitotoxic or ischemic SCI models reveals changes similar to central sensitization following peripheral nerve injury. Analogous to epilepsy, SCI causes one neuronal population to generate hyperactivity and another to respond to this chaotic activity. It appears that a critical threshold in the size of this population must be reached before a patient will experience spontaneous pain.[5,22]

Sensory stimuli act on neural systems that have been modified by previous inputs, the "memory" of which significantly influences pain behavior. The fact that a memory is not activated by the development of a lesion might explain the long delay in the onset of central pain in some patients. The long-term potentiation that is important for this memory might be mediated by NMDA receptors and their influence on calcium conductance.[23,24]

Thus, central pain frequently develops weeks or months after development of the lesion and is associated with sensory changes involving the spinothalamic pathways, especially changes in temperature perception. The increased availability of functional brain imaging has helped facilitate the investigation of the pathophysiology underlying central pain states. Available evidence suggests that a spinothalamic pathway lesion is necessary, but not necessarily sufficient, for the development of central pain. STT deficits are seen in more than 50% of stroke patients who do not develop central pain.

EXPERIMENTAL MODELS OF CENTRAL PAIN SECONDARY TO SPINAL CORD INJURY

Interesting insights about the mechanisms of central pain following SCI and the potential effects of drugs on pain behavior have been gained from experimental models in the rat. The Stockholm group led by Wiesenfeld-Hallin developed a model of photochemically induced spinal cord ischemia[25,26] while Yezierski et al. developed a model of excitotoxic SCI.[5,27] Rats with lesions involving both white and gray matter develop instantaneous morphine-resistant tactile allodynia, which responds to the systemic GABA-B agonist baclofen, and can be prevented by pretreatment with the NMDA antagonist MK 801. Intrathecal morphine and clonidine reduced the allodynia. Injections of a CCK-B antagonist decreased allodynia.

TREATMENT OPTIONS

An important aspect of treating patients with central pain is to define and continuously review the goals of treatment. It needs to be emphasized to patients that complete cessation of pain may not be achieved. Hence, the goal of therapy is to improve function and reduce pain without creating intolerable side effects. In addition, including treatment strategies for each of the multiple components of the central pain syndrome is of paramount importance. Thus, a patient's anxiety, fear, depression, and any suicidal ideation should also be treated. The options available for managing central pain include pharmacotherapy, behavioral therapy, physical therapy, neuro-modulation, other interventional therapies, and ablative neurosurgery.

Pharmacotherapy: The pharmacologic approach is based on a strategy of stepwise combination therapy. The mainstay of this therapy is antidepressants that possibly act by modulating the thalamic burst firing activity via its actions on locus coeruleus noradrenergic neurons and the serotoninergic cells in the dorsal raphe.[28] Amitriptyline is effective in central post-stroke control.[11] Amitriptyline's benefit derives, in part, from its ability to prevent reuptake of noradrenaline and serotonin. Tricyclic antidepressants (TCAs) should be titrated to 50 to 100 mg/day. Insufficient plasma levels at this dose might indicate the need for higher doses. A pilot study showed no statistically significant benefit when 39 patients received amitriptyline to prevent the development of pain after a thalamic stroke.[29] Similarly, findings in a controlled trial failed to support the use of amitriptyline in the treatment of chronic central pain of spinal cord origin.[30] However, a combination of a TCA (e.g., amitriptyline), clonazepam, a benzodiazepine, and a nonsteroidal anti-inflammatory drug (NSAID) is reportedly a good regimen to control the common, steady, burning, dysesthetic component of this syndrome.[31] For spinal cord central pain, the NMDA antagonist ketamine and the mu-opioid agonist alfentanil[32] reportedly reduce spontaneous and evoked components.

Antiepileptic drugs (AEDs) are useful for the neuralgic component. A controlled study[11] showed no benefit of using carbamazepine to treat central pain, but the study nonresponders did not have a neuralgic component to their pain. The newer AEDs seem to act at multiple receptor types. In a controlled study pain scores decreased from 7 to 5 in patients with poststroke pain who were given 200 mg/day of lamotrigine.[33] In patients with incomplete SCI lamotrigine titrated to 400 mg/day significantly reduced pain at or below the injury level. Patients with brush-evoked allodynia and wind-up-like pain in the area of maximal pain were more likely to have a beneficial effect with lamotrigine than patients without these evoked pains. This trial, however, showed no significant effect of lamotrigine on spontaneous and evoked pain in patients with complete SCI.[34] In a controlled trial gabapentin significantly decreased unpleasant sensations and caused a trend toward a decrease in pain intensity and burning sensation in the SCI population.[35] Chiou-Tan and colleagues found mexiletine of no use in the treatment of central pain states of spinal cord origin.[36]

Opioid administration may benefit some patients, although it is not first-line therapy. Patients who respond to a trial of opioid infusion may be prescribed long-acting opioids, such as the slow-release formulations or the transdermal preparation. In a controlled study the reduction in the intensity of neuropathic pain was significantly greater during treatment with a high dose (0.75 mg) than it was with lower doses of the mu-agonist levorphanol. Patients with central pain after stroke, however, were the least likely to report benefit.[37] Another controlled trial revealed that intravenous (IV) morphine induces analgesic effects on some components of central neuropathic pain syndromes, but only a minority of patients may benefit from long-term opioid treatment.[38] Morphine significantly reduced the intensity of brush-induced allodynia, but had no effect on other evoked pains (i.e., static mechanical and thermal allodynia/hyperalgesia).

The efficacy of systemic lidocaine (5 mg/kg IV over 30 minutes) was evaluated in a double-blind, placebo-controlled, crossover trial on spontaneous and evoked pains (allodynia and hyperalgesia) in 16 patients with chronic post-stroke ($n = 6$) or SCI ($n = 10$) pain.[39] Systemic lidocaine induced a significant and selective reduction of several components of pain caused by CNS injuries. The observed preferential antihyperalgesic and antiallodynic effects of lidocaine suggest a selective central action on the mechanisms underlying these evoked pains. Canavero and colleagues found IV propofol (0.2 mg/kg) useful in the treatment of brain central pain, but not for other neuropathic pain states.[40] IV sodium pentothal (50 to 225 mg) also reduces brain central pain.

Behavioral Therapy: Activities that promote general mental activity, including distraction techniques and physical therapy, seem to play a role in reducing the pain in central pain states. Peripheral sensory input and activation of fronto-orbital brain areas inhibit specific and nonspecific pain pathways. Based on an examination of a series of case reports, Haythornthwaite and colleagues suggest that biofeedback, hypnosis, and cognitive-behavioral interventions all have a beneficial impact on neuropathic pain.[41]

Physical Therapy: Physiotherapy may be beneficial, but treatments such as acupuncture, ultrasound, and massage are not effective for long-term treatment of central pain states. Transcutaneous electrical nerve stimulation (TENS) provides long-term benefits to patients with central poststroke pain and those with incomplete SCI.[11,42]

Neuromodulation: Optimal therapies for chronic pain states often need a multidisciplinary approach. This is also true for central pain states. A careful psychosocial evaluation is essential prior to initiating any invasive therapy. Spinal cord stimulation (SCS) must be the first surgical procedure considered for spinal cord central pain because it is simple and reversible.

Patient selection is critical. Dorsal columns should be functional above the level of injury to produce paresthesia. Patients with anesthesia dolorosa (pain in an anesthetic area) and patients with incomplete lesions are poor candidates. Patients who experience more than 50% pain relief during trial stimulation are potential candidates for an implant. Although Pagni and Nashold concluded that SCS is disappointing for central pain, it does help reduce the steady dysesthetic component. For treatment failure, deep brain stimulation (DBS) of the tactile relay nucleus of the thalamus or the lemniscal radiations offers hope. Data from Bendok and Levy suggest that paresthesia-producing DBS alleviates steady neuropathic pain.[43] Periventricular/periaqueductal gray (PVG/PAG) DBS is appropriate for nociceptive pain.

For brain origin central pain, data from Tasker and colleagues show that brain stimulation relieves the steady dysesthetic component in 53% of patients and the evoked component in 25% of patients, but offers no help for the neuralgic component.[44] The neuralgic component is the component responsive to ablative neurosurgery. SCS is of no benefit for brain-origin central pain, although patients might report relief during a trial. Paresthesia-producing DBS and motor cortex stimulation are appropriate for the steady component of the pain. For those with allodynia or hyperpathia, PVG/PAG DBS seems to be beneficial.

Stimulating the motor cortex offers a new target for the neuromodulation of central pain. Yamamoto and colleagues concluded that patients whose pain was diminished by thiamylal and ketamine, but not by morphine, respond best to motor cortex stimulation.[45] Canavero and colleagues concluded that motor cortex stimulation controls spontaneous and evoked pain, but not the nonpainful paresthesias. Patients who might respond well to motor cortex stimulation also respond to transcranial magnetic stimulation and to a GABA agonist (e.g., propofol).

Other Interventional Therapies: Baclofen, a GABA agonist, has antinociceptive effects, and its intrathecal administration reduces allodynic responses in animal models of neurogenic central pain. A pilot study found that intrathecal baclofen suppresses central pain of spinal cord origin.

A report by Taira and colleagues suggests that intrathecal baclofen may be an option to consider for central pain states. In their study in addition to reducing spasticity, it reduced spinal cord-origin central pain by 64%.[46] Canavero and colleagues reported that infusing propofol (0.2 mg/kg) IV, a GABA agonist, relieved both the evoked and the spontaneous components of central pain.[40] If the IV propofol test is positive, then patients might benefit from intrathecal baclofen and intrathecal midazolam. Similarly, patients who respond to an IV opioid trial followed by long-acting oral opioids and demonstrate improved functional status, not just pain relief, may be considered for intrathecal opioids with or without adjuvant clonidine and bupivacaine. For SCI, a controlled study found that intrathecal morphine and clonidine relieved neuropathic at-level pain (this includes three dermatomes adjacent to the level of SCI). The fact that the responders did not achieve pain relief through systemic administration suggests a local spinal cord-mediated effect.[47] The role of intrathecal ziconotide, now known as PRIALT, an N-type calcium channel blocker, is promising but remains to be confirmed by controlled trials.

Ablative Neurosurgery: Ablative neurosurgery plays a role in the treatment of the neuralgic component of central pain. Percutaneous radiofrequency dorsal rhizotomy is an option for monoradicular pain syndromes. Ablative surgery includes cordotomy, cordectomy, and dorsal root entry zone (DREZ) lesioning. The goal of cordotomy and cordectomy is interruption of STTs. Cordectomy, the simplest destructive procedure, benefits patients with complete lesions. It is not acceptable to most patients because it obviates their hope for eventual restoration of spinal cord function. Percutaneous/open cordotomy achieves the same results as cordectomy and is offered to patients with incomplete lesions, but carries the risk of aggravating bladder dysfunction and inducing ipsilateral limb paresis. DREZ is equally effective for the neuralgic and the evoked elements of spinal-origin central pain. Nashold and colleagues found this procedure most useful for the relief of end-zone pain (pain starting at the level of injury and extending distally). Pain extending diffusely, often sacrally distributed, and remotely distributed pain, described as phantom or diffuse burning pain, do not respond well to DREZ. Although the procedure preserves the hope for future spinal cord function and avoids risk of limb paresis, it can interfere with residual bladder function and requires a laminectomy and considerable skill. Studies on using DREZ to treat central neuropathic pain in patients with traumatic SCI indicate promising results in selected patients, but the strength of the evidence is poor in terms of study design, outcome measures, and reports on the severity of adverse effects, patient selection criteria, and patient description.

In the past surgeons attempted to relieve central pain of cerebral origin with cordotomy, trigeminal DREZ, medial thalamotomy, and mesencephalic tractotomy. Of these, only mesencephalic tractotomy is encouraging. Destructive procedures on the cerebral cortex are of historic note only.

FUTURE DIRECTIONS

Ongoing research is likely to shed light on the role of the therapies under investigation for central pain states. A number of drugs such as ketamine, lamotrigine, agmantine, cannabinoid receptor agonists, and CCK receptor antagonists are under investigation.[48,49]

KEY POINTS

- Central pain states are common sequelae of SCI and stroke. Documentation of abnormal temperature perception in the affected region is critical to the diagnosis.
- Pathophysiology is not fully understood but includes disinhibition of nociceptive input, denervation supersensitivity, and maladaptive reorganization.
- Involvement of the spinothalamocortical pathway is strongly supported by animal models, but the precise pathway in humans is unknown.
- Neurochemical studies suggest the involvement of glutaminergic, GABA-ergic, noradrenergic, serotonergic, histaminergic, and cholinergic input to the thalamus.
- The three components of central pain (steady dysesthetic, intermittent neuralgic, and evoked) must all be treated. In central pain of brain origin steady and evoked components predominate, while in central pain of spinal cord origin steady and neuralgic components predominate.
- A multidisciplinary approach is recommended, and, because poorly controlled central pain carries a high suicide risk, psychosocial support is crucial.
- Pharmacotherapy should begin with a TCA, especially amitriptyline for brain-origin central pain.
- Membrane stabilizers, especially lamotrigine, should be considered for combination with TCAs as a second step.
- The steady dysesthetic component may be addressed by neuromodulation.
- Select patients may benefit from intrathecal therapies with GABA agonists and opioids.

- Intermittent neuralgic and evoked components may be addressed by ablative neurosurgery with its attendant risks.
- Experience from neuromodulation suggests that central pain of brain origin can be reversible. Evidence also suggests that central pain may diminish in some patients over a period of years.

REFERENCES

1. Andersen G, Vestergaard K, Ingeman-Nielsen M, Jensen TS: Incidence of central post-stroke pain. Pain 61:187–193, 1995.
2. Bowsher D, Leijon G, Thuomas KA: Central poststroke pain: Correlation of MRI with clinical pain characteristics and sensory abnormalities. Neurology 51:1352–1358, 1998.
3. Lewis-Jones G, Smith T, Bowsher D, Leijon G: MRI imaging in 36 cases of central post stroke pain. Pain 5:278, 1990.
4. Nasreddine ZS, Saver JL: Pain after thalamic stroke: Right diencephalic predominance and clinical features in 180 patients. Neurology 48:1196–1199, 1997.
5. Yezierski RP: Pain following spinal cord injury: The clinical problem and experimental studies. Pain 68:185–194, 1996.
6. Rintala DH, Loubser PG, Castro J, et al: Chronic pain in a community-based sample of men with spinal cord injury: Prevalence, severity, and relationship with impairment, disability, handicap, and subjective well-being. Arch Phys Med Rehabil 79:604–614, 1998.
7. Koller WC: Sensory symptoms in Parkinson's disease. Neurology 34:957–959, 1984.
8. Siddall PJ, Yezierski RP, Loeser JD: Pain Following Spinal Cord Injury: Clinical Features, Prevalence and Taxonomy. IASP Press, Seattle, 2000.
9. Siddall PJ, Taylor DA, Cousins MJ: Classification of pain following spinal cord injury. Spinal Cord 35:69–75, 1997.
10. Siddall PJ, McClelland JM, Rutkowski SB, Cousins MJ: A longitudinal study of the prevalence and characteristics of pain in the first 5 years following spinal cord injury. Pain 103:249–257, 2003.
11. Leijon G, Boivie J, Johansson I: Central post-stroke pain – Neurological symptoms and pain characteristics. Pain 36: 13–25, 1989.
12. Finnerup NB, Jensen TS: Spinal cord injury pain – Mechanisms and treatment. Eur J Neurol 11:73–82, 2004.
13. Bowsher D: Pathophysiology of postherpetic neuralgia: Towards a rational treatment. Neurology 45:S56–S57, 1995.
14. Kornhuber J, Maler M, Wiltfang J, et al: [Neuronal potassium channel opening with flupirtine]. Fortschr Neurol Psychiatr 67:466–475, 1999.
15. Craig AD, Reiman EM, Evans A, Bushnell MC: Functional imaging of an illusion of pain. Nature 384:258–260, 1996.
16. Willis WD, Jr., Zhang X, Honda CN, Giesler GJ, Jr.: A critical review of the role of the proposed VMpo nucleus in pain. J Pain 3:79–94, 2002.
17. Sherman SM, Koch C: Synaptic organization of the brain. In Sheperd GM (ed): Thalamus. Oxford University Press, Oxford, 1990, pp 246–278.
18. Lenz FA, Seike M, Lin YC, et al: Neurons in the area of human thalamic nucleus ventralis caudalis respond to painful heat stimuli. Brain Res 623:235–240, 1993.
19. Lenz FA, Dougherty PM: Neurons in the human thalamic somatosensory nucleus (ventralis caudalis) respond to innocuous cool and mechanical stimuli. J Neurophysiol 79:2227–2230, 1998.
20. Jeanmonod D, Magnin M, Morel A: Thalamus and neurogenic pain: Physiological, anatomical and clinical data. Neuroreport 4:475–478, 1993.
21. Clifford DB, Trotter JL: Pain in multiple sclerosis. Arch Neurol 41:1270–1272, 1984.

22. Yezierski RP: Pain following SCI: Pathophysiology and central mechanisms. *In* Sandkuhler J, Brown B, Gebhart GF (eds): Progress in Brain Research. Elsevier, Amsterdam, 2000, pp 429–449.

23. Bear MF, Malenka RC: Synaptic plasticity: LTP and LTD. Curr Opin Neurobiol 4:389–399, 1994.

24. Lenz FA, Tasker RR, Dostrovsky JO: Abnormal single unit activity and response to stimulation in the presumed ventrocaudal nucleus of patients with central pain. *In* Dubner R, Gebhart GF, Bond MR (eds): Pain Research and Clinical Management. Elsevier, Amsterdam, 1988, pp 157–164.

25. Hao J-X, Xu X-J, Aldskogius H, et al: The excitatory amino acid receptor antagonist MK-801 prevents the hypersensitivity induced by spinal cord ischemia in the rat. Exper Neurol 113:182–191, 1991.

26. Xu XJ, Hao JX, Seiger A, et al: Chronic pain-related behaviors in spinally injured rats: Evidence for functional alterations of the endogenous cholecystokinin and opioid systems. Pain 56:271–277, 1994.

27. Yezierski RP, Liu S, Ruenes GL, et al: Excitotoxic spinal cord injury: Behavioral and morphological characteristics of a central pain model. Pain 75:141–155, 1998.

28. Pape HC, McCormick DA: Noradrenaline and serotonin selectively modulate thalamic burst firing by enhancing a hyperpolarization-activated cation current. Nature 340:715–718, 1989.

29. Lampl C, Yazdi K, Roper C: Amitriptyline in the prophylaxis of central poststroke pain. Preliminary results of 39 patients in a placebo-controlled, long-term study. Stroke 33:3030–3032, 2002.

30. Cardenas DD, Warms CA, Turner JA, et al: Efficacy of amitriptyline for relief of pain in spinal cord injury: Results of a randomized controlled trial. Pain 96:365–373, 2002.

31. Fenollosa P, Pallares J, Cervera J, et al: Chronic pain in the spinal cord injured: statistical approach and pharmacological treatment. Paraplegia 31:722–729, 1993.

32. Eide PK, Stubhaug A, Stenehjem AE: Central dysesthesia pain after traumatic spinal cord injury is dependent on N-methyl-D-aspartate receptor activation. Neurosurgery 37:1080–1087, 1995.

33. Vestergaard K, Andersen G, Gottrup H, et al: Lamotrigine for central poststroke pain: A randomized controlled trial. Neurology 56:184–190, 2001.

34. Finnerup NB, Sindrup SH, Bach FW, et al: Lamotrigine in spinal cord injury pain: A randomized controlled trial. Pain 96:375–383, 2002.

35. Tai Q, Kirshblum S, Chen B, et al: Gabapentin in the treatment of neuropathic pain after spinal cord injury: A prospective, randomized, double-blind, crossover trial. J Spinal Cord Med 25:100–105, 2002.

36. Chiou-Tan FY, Tuel SM, Johnson JC, et al: Effect of mexiletine on spinal cord injury dysesthetic pain. Am J Phys Med Rehabil 75:84–87, 1996.

37. Rowbotham MC, Twilling L, Davies PS, et al: Oral opioid therapy for chronic peripheral and central neuropathic pain. N Engl J Med 348:1223–1232, 2003.

38. Attal N, Guirimand F, Brasseur L, et al: Effects of IV morphine in central pain – A randomized placebo-controlled study. Neurology 58:554–563, 2002.

39. Herman RM, D'Luzansky SC, Ippolito R: Intrathecal baclofen suppresses central pain in patients with spinal lesions. A pilot study. Clin J Pain 8:338–345, 1992.

40. Canavero S, Bonicalzi V: Therapeutic extradural cortical stimulation for central and neuropathic pain: A review. Clin J Pain 18:48–55, 2002.

41. Haythornthwaite JA, Benrud-Larson LM: Psychological aspects of neuropathic pain. Clin J Pain 16:S101–S105, 2000.

42. Eriksson MB, Sjolund BH, Nielzen S: Long term results of peripheral conditioning stimulation as an analgesic measure in chronic pain. Pain 6:335–347, 1979.

43. Bendok B, Levy RM: Brain stimulation for persistent pain management. *In* Gildenberg PL, Tasker RR (eds): Textbook of Stereotactic and Functional Neurosurgery. McGraw-Hill, New York, 1998, pp 1539–1546.

44. Tasker RR: Central pain states. *In* Loeser JD (ed): Bonica's Management of Pain. Lippincott Williams and Wilkins, Philadelphia, 2001, pp 433–453.

45. Yamamoto T, Katayama Y, Hirayama T, Tsubokawa T: Pharmacological classification of central post-stroke pain: Comparison with the results of chronic motor cortex stimulation therapy. Pain 72:5–12, 1997.

46. Taira T, Kawamura H, Tanikawa T, et al: A new approach to control central deafferentation pain: Spinal intrathecal baclofen. Stereotact Funct Neurosurg 65:101–105, 1995.

47. Siddall PJ, Molloy AR, Walker S, et al: The efficacy of intrathecal morphine and clonidine in the treatment of pain after spinal cord injury. Anesth Analg 91:1493–1498, 2000.

48. Fairbanks CA, Schreiber KL, Brewer KL, et al: Agmatine reverses pain induced by inflammation, neuropathy, and spinal cord injury. Proc Natl Acad Sci USA 97:10584–10589, 2000.

49. Wade DT, Robson P, House H, et al: A preliminary controlled study to determine whether whole-plant cannabis extracts can improve intractable neurogenic symptoms. Clin Rehabil 17:21–29, 2003.

Pelvic Pain

Sunil J. Panchal, M.D.

Chronic pelvic pain (CPP) is a common problem for women and may lead to a significant impairment in the ability to lead a productive life. It has been estimated that approximately 10% of visits to gynecologists are related to complaints of CPP.[1] Numerous causes are theorized for this condition, impeding the development of a widely accepted specific definition at this time. However, CPP is distinguished from acute pelvic pain by the nature of the progression of complaints. Acute pelvic pain develops over the course of days with a rapid onset and usually is caused by infection, torsion, or rupture of visceral structures. The events causing acute pelvic pain can also result in CPP.

Causes for CPP include endometriosis, dysmenorrhea, dyspareunia, mononeuropathies, myofascial pain, vulvitis, cystitis, and sympathetically maintained pain. Many patients have no known or suspected organic pathology for their discomfort; this results in a diagnosis of pelvic pain of unknown etiology. Other terms include pelvic congestion, pelvic fibrosis, pelvic neurodystonia, pelvalgia, and irritable uterus syndrome. Confounding factors include a high incidence of physical and/or sexual abuse (30% to 50%) in this patient population, underscoring the need for a multidisciplinary approach.[2]

EPIDEMIOLOGY

It is estimated that overall risk for the development of CPP is 5% for the general population of women, and the risk increases to 20% in those with a previous diagnosis of pelvic inflammatory disease.[3] Women in their reproductive years had a 14.7% rate of CPP.[4]

The estimated percentage of new referrals to gynecology clinics for CPP is approximately 10%. These patients are estimated to undergo up to 20% of hysterectomies and 40% of laparoscopies in the general population.[5,6] Some 30% to 50% of patients with CPP are classified as having "chronic pelvic pain without obvious pathology." This difficulty in determining a diagnosis is underscored by the high incidence of hysterectomy without pelvic pain relief (about 25%).[7]

Laparoscopy of patients with CPP reveals endometriosis in one-third of patients, adhesions in one-third, and no apparent pathology in the remaining third, but laparoscopy also reveals significant pathology in other women who do not complain of pain.[8] This makes diagnosis difficult in the CPP population.

ASSOCIATION OF PELVIC PAIN AND ABUSE

An accurate history of sexual or physical abuse is often difficult to obtain, and this fact has resulted in controversy regarding studies finding a high correlation of such histories with CPP. Some studies report a 50% or higher incidence of abuse in patients with CPP.

Comparison of patients with a history of abuse vs. nonabused control subjects reveals a higher incidence of unexplained gastrointestinal and pelvic symptoms, psychiatric diagnoses, and surgical procedures. Therefore, the physician should always be concerned about a history of abuse in patients who do not respond well to pharmacologic interventions or diagnostic blockade.

ETIOLOGY

Pain in the pelvic region can originate from the following:

- Pelvic viscera: uterus, ovaries, bladder, urethra, rectum, sigmoid, or descending colon.
- Somatic structures: skin, vulva, clitoris, vaginal canal.
- Musculoskeletal and ligamentous structures.
- Spinal lesions or gastrointestinal or urologic conditions (referred pain).

Acute pelvic pain may originate from ectopic pregnancy, ruptured ovarian cyst, pelvic abscess, ureteral stone, urinary tract infection, or cystitis. CPP may be caused by ectopic endometrial tissue, infection, neoplasm, trauma, postsurgical changes, or somatization disorder.

HISTORY

The taking of a history from a patient with pelvic pain should be thorough and detailed and should include the following:

- Pattern of onset
- Inciting event
- Quality (e.g., burning, aching, dull, sharp, cramping)
- Severity
- Duration and progression of complaints
- Constant or intermittent nature
- Exacerbating factors (e.g., position, eating, urination, defecation, Valsalva maneuver)
- Alleviating factors
- Efficacy and toxicity of previous medications
- Association with menstrual cycle
- Incontinence
- Pregnancy
- Sexual activity
- Sudden weight loss or gain
- Breast or endocrinologic difficulties
- Family history of ovarian, uterine, or breast cancer

A comprehensive assessment often demonstrates associations that make diagnosis simpler for the physician. These associations are discussed under specific syndromes later in this chapter.

PHYSICAL EXAMINATION

A thorough physical examination is critical. A complete neurologic examination should be performed to identify any cause of neural injury, possibly from the central nervous system, or injury to peripheral innervation. Allodynia, hyperesthesia, or hyperalgesia may indicate injury to the pudendal nerve, intercostal nerve, ilioinguinal nerve, iliohypogastric nerve, genitofemoral nerve, or a nerve root (T10–L2, S2–4). Examination of surgical scars may indicate nerve entrapment or a possible neuroma formation. Abdominal examination is useful to localize the source of pain and to determine whether there are any objective signs of an acute process (i.e., rebound tenderness). Finally, a bimanual pelvic examination in the presence of a nurse should be performed. Cervical tenderness may indicate infection. The existence of anatomic abnormalities of the uterus or adnexa and the presence of any trigger points in the musculature must be determined. All findings should be discussed with the referring gynecologist to assess any progression of complaints.

DIAGNOSTIC STUDIES

Diagnostic studies are tools to assist in making a diagnosis and should always be used as an adjunct to the history and physical examination, not as a substitute. Infection, bleeding, and inflammatory processes should be assessed by checking a complete blood count, urinalysis, urine and cervical cultures, and erythrocyte sedimentation rate. A determination of the level of the B subunit of human chorionic gonadotropin should be performed in fertile women for the possibility of ectopic pregnancy. Computed tomography or ultrasound help in evaluating a possible mass lesion, free fluid, or free air (e.g., hemorrhage, perforated viscus).

Diagnostic neural blockade is an invaluable tool if used appropriately. Diagnostic blockade indicates whether a particular neural structure is a pathway for nociception for the patient's complaints. Blockade of the pudendal nerve, intercostal nerves, ilioinguinal nerves, iliohypogastric nerve, genitofemoral nerve, spinal nerve root, or trigger point should provide relief if pain originates from the somatic structures. Blockade of visceral afferent fibers can be achieved by superior hypogastric nerve block or ganglion impar block, resulting in relief for pain originating from the uterus, bladder, ovaries, testicles, sigmoid colon, descending colon, or rectum. The physician utilizing diagnostic blocks must always perform a neurologic examination after the intervention to determine whether the targeted nerve was successfully blocked and whether there was any inadvertent blockade of other neural structures before arriving at a conclusion. Differential epidural and intrathecal blocks cannot selectively block specific fiber classes (A-beta vs. A-delta vs. C fibers) and should no longer be used for diagnosis.[9] A neuraxial sensory block may help to differentiate a central pain syndrome, however. Diagnostic laparoscopy is a safe, effective, and well-accepted tool to detect or confirm endometriosis, adhesions, ovarian cyst, ectopic pregnancy, and uterine malformations. As previously discussed, findings during laparoscopy do not necessarily correlate with the presence or absence of pelvic pain.

GENERAL CONCEPTS OF VISCERAL PAIN APPLIED TO PELVIC PAIN

Visceral pain refers to pain mediated by the soft organs in the thorax, abdomen, and pelvis. It is usually described as dull and vague in location and radiates away from the affected organ. It frequently is associated with hyperalgesia (or spasm) of the overlying somatic tissues. Its poor localization is probably caused by the small number of visceral afferents, which subserve a wide anatomic area and then converge in the spinal cord at the same site at which somatic structures converge. Only 2% to 15% of afferents in the spinal cord (7% in the thoracic region) arise from the viscera.[10] These visceral afferents synapse on second-order neurons at the same level of the spinal cord as somatic afferents. Specifically, visceral afferents terminate in laminae I and V of the dorsal horn, with significant ramification occurring in lamina I both rostrally and caudally, therefore achieving wide receptive fields.[11] This *viscerosomatic convergence* (visceral innervation that converges terminally in the spinal cord at the same level as overlying somatic structures) is what makes it difficult for the patient to distinguish accurately between visceral and somatic origins for the pain and explains the commonly described phenomena of referred pain to the mandible or left upper extremity during myocardial ischemia and referred pain to the shoulder from diaphragmatic irritation. Accordingly, it is difficult to diagnose accurately visceral pain problems on the basis of the pain complaint. In a review of 64 patients with abdominal pain only 15% had an accurate diagnosis.[12]

Visceral pain can be induced by

- Abnormal distention and contraction of the hollow visceral walls.
- Rapid stretching of the capsules of hollow visceral organs.
- Formation and accumulation of algogenic substances.
- Ischemia of visceral musculature.

- Direct action of chemical stimuli on compromised mucosa.
- Traction or compression of ligaments, vessels, or mesenteries.[13]

Notably, the viscera generally are not sensitive to heat or cutting stimuli.

Anatomically, the majority of visceral afferents run with sympathetic fibers via the celiac and other plexi; travel through the sympathetic chain on their way to the dorsal root ganglion, where the cell bodies for these fibers reside; and terminate in the dorsal horn laminae I and V. Vagal afferent neurons project viscerotopically to the nucleus of the solitary tract in the medulla oblongata. Functionally, there exist three general classes of visceral afferents. There are low-threshold mechanosensitive afferents that respond to distention and contraction and other stimuli; specific chemosensitive afferents (probably vagal); and high-threshold mechanosensitive afferents.[11] This separation of function was investigated in the cat model, with identification of ischemia-sensitive C fiber afferents. Graded distention of the gastrointestinal tract demonstrated that ischemia-insensitive C fibers had a low threshold in response to distention (13 ±5 mmHg) with a plateau of discharge frequency. This contrasted sharply with ischemia-sensitive C fibers, which had a high threshold (86 ± 12 mmHg) and a larger peak response to distention in the noxious range (60 to 180 mmHg).[14] Visceral afferents can be sensitized, and hyperalgesia may ensue. This has been demonstrated experimentally in rats by applying intracolonic acetic acid to create visceral inflammation, with subsequent sensitization recorded in both low- and high-threshold mechanosensitive afferents.[15] This phenomenon has also been observed in patients with irritable bowel syndrome, who reported pain at significantly lower volumes of colonic balloon distention than did control subjects.[16] Therefore, visceral afferents may undergo a change in function similar to those of somatic nociceptors.[17]

ENDOMETRIOSIS

Endometriosis is defined as the presence of endometrial tissue outside the uterus. It has a prevalence of approximately 7% among women of reproductive age. Ectopic sites include the peritoneum, uterosacral ligaments, fallopian tubes, round and broad ligaments, and, most commonly, the ovaries.[18] This ectopic spread may be caused by retrograde menstruation or by lymphatic *or* hematogenic spread. Pain may result from prostaglandin release, distention, nerve irritation, or tissue irritation by menstrual products. Pain is typically cyclical, increasing during menstruation and subsiding a few days after its completion. Patients complain of pelvic pain, dysmenorrhea, and dyspareunia, which often resolve with menopause or oophorectomy. Diagnosis requires visualization of lesions during laparoscopy or laparotomy.

Treatment options are based on evidence correlating pain and size of endometrial implants with plasma estrogen levels. After considering the patient's age and reproductive desires, the options include hormonal manipulation (usually a 6-month trial, with a response rate of approximately two-thirds) and surgery (controversial). Hormonal manipulation may consist of reduction of estrogen (leuprolide acetate; Lupron), reduction of pituitary gonadotropin production (danazol), gonadotropin-releasing hormone analogues, or use of low-dose oral contraceptives.[19] Surgical options are removal of endometrial implants (resection, laser, thermal probes), total abdominal hysterectomy for severe endometriosis (ovaries may be preserved if they are disease free), and presacral neurectomy. Laparoscopic approach to presacral neurectomy has been gaining in popularity, and a prospective, 1-year observational study utilizing phenol in 15 patients demonstrated a 73% reduction in analgesic use, improved sexual function, but also an increase in constipation.[20] A prospective, randomized, double-blind trial evaluating presacral neurectomy in 141 women with severe dysmenorrhea who underwent laparoscopy reported results after 1 year. While both groups had lower frequency and severity of dysmenorrhea, dyspareunia, and CPP compared to baseline, the neurectomy group had significantly lower values for pain intensity compared to the controls.[21]

INFECTION

Infection is often a cause of CPP and may predispose patients to infertility. Infection of the uterus is called endometritis; it is associated with events facilitating entrance of bacteria via the cervix, such as dilation and curettage, term pregnancy, or spontaneous abortion. Infection by normal vaginal flora or a sexually transmitted organism usually results in crampy suprapubic pain and uterine tenderness. Other findings include foul-smelling discharge, bleeding, urinary frequency, low-grade fever, and leukocytosis. Gram staining and cultures should be performed, followed by appropriate antibiotic treatment. Urinalysis may help distinguish this condition from cystitis.

Pelvic inflammatory disease (PID) is an infection involving the pelvic organs and nearby supportive structures. PID is associated with loss of cervical integrity, multiple sexual partners, sex with an infected person, and use of intrauterine devices (IUDs), especially the Dalkon shield. *Neisseria gonorrhoeae* and *Chlamydia trachomatis* are the most common causative organisms. Gonorrhea produces severe postmenstrual pain, whereas chlamydia is usually asymptomatic. Findings include dyspareunia, dysuria, generalized abdominal and pelvic pain, rebound tenderness, pain with cervical manipulation, nausea, and diarrhea. Cultures and antibiotic treatment are essential. Approximately 50% of patients with PID develop CPP, and 30% become infertile.

OTHER CAUSES OF UTERINE PAIN

Primary dysmenorrhea is pain associated with menstruation that has no other identifiable cause. It is present in 50% of adult women and is severe in 15% of women. Patients have increased levels of prostaglandins in endometrium and menstrual products. Treatment includes nonsteroidal anti-inflammatory drugs (NSAIDs), oral contraceptives to reduce menstrual flow, and calcium-channel blockers or B_2-agonists to reduce uterine contractility.

Secondary dysmenorrhea is pain associated with menstruation that is caused by fibroids, adenomyosis, or an IUD. It commonly occurs in patients in their late thirties or forties. Patients may have heavy, irregular bleeding and anemia. Sharp, sudden exacerbation may indicate fibroid degeneration and ischemia. Fibroid resection or removal of the IUD may be successful. Hysterectomy is appropriate for heavy bleeding, severe pain, or ureteral compression, but in more than 25% of cases this fails to relieve pain.

PELVIC CONGESTION

Observations of absent venodilation with exacerbation of pain from administered vasoactive compounds support a theory of pelvic venous congestion as a cause of CPP.[22] It has been proposed that venous stasis and reflux in dilated ovarian varices causes pelvic pain, especially with prolonged standing. Further observations include reduced pain in patients with venographic evidence of diminished congestion from hormonal therapy.[23]

Proponents of this theory claim associated findings that include uterine enlargement, thickened endometrium, and polycystic ovaries and have advocated ovarian vein ligation, bilateral venous embolization, and hysterectomy. To date, this diagnosis remains controversial because the literature lacks good documentation. A case series of 6 patients treated with ovarian vein embolization showed improvement in 5 patients, and suggests a minimally invasive method to achieve this goal.[24]

PELVIC ADHESIONS

The idea that adhesions are a cause for unexplained pelvic pain remains controversial. Laparoscopies in patients with CPP demonstrate a prevalence of 30% to 50%, with prior pelvic surgery as a predictor of presence of adhesions.[25] Because adhesions are found during laparoscopy in many patients without CPP, the correlation is tenuous. One randomized trial suggested successful outcome in women with CPP who underwent adhesiolysis for dense, vascularized adhesions, especially if they involved the gastrointestinal tract, but this treatment was not very effective for moderate adhesions.[26] One recent study supported the concept of adhesions as a source for nociception. In this study adhesions removed from patients underwent histologic, immunohistochemical, and ultrastructural analysis. Nerve fibers were identified in all of the adhesions including those that express calcitonin gene-related peptide, as well as substance P.[27]

OVARIAN REMNANT SYNDROME

Ovarian remnant should be included in the differential diagnosis for patients with CPP after bilateral oophorectomy. Increased levels of follicle-stimulating hormone and luteinizing hormone in women of reproductive age are suggestive of this syndrome. An adnexal mass that is palpable or imaged by ultrasound is also supportive. Surgical resection is the recommended treatment.[28]

CANCER PAIN

Carcinoma of pelvic structures may elicit pain due to distention of a hollow viscus, pressure or traction of sensitive tissues, obstruction, inflammation, necrosis, or direct invasion of neural elements. Pain is often diffuse and may radiate to the lower back or rectum.

Treatment of pain from pelvic neoplasms includes surgical resection or debulking when technically feasible, chemotherapy, or radiation therapy. This is supplemented with systemic pharmacologic agents such as NSAIDs, tricyclic antidepressants, and opioids. Anticonvulsants are added for neuropathic symptoms.

If inadequate analgesia or intolerance of side effects occurs, intraspinal drug delivery or neurolytic techniques may be attempted. Previous economic analyses suggested if life expectancy is 3 months or less, an externalized epidural catheter is appropriate after evaluation for spinal metastases. Longer life expectancy would indicate use of an implanted intrathecal pump. However, since predictions of life expectancy have a poor correlation with actual outcome, the selection should be based on the patient's condition, patient's desire, and physician judgment. Drugs approved for use in implanted pumps by the US Food and Drug Administration include only morphine and baclofen, but reports exist of successful use of other opioids, local anesthetics, and clonidine in various combinations.

NEURAL BLOCKS AND CONSIDERATION FOR NEUROLYSIS

General principles for neural blocks include the diagnostic value of local anesthetic injection, and many physicians have observed improved pain in response to a series of local anesthetic injections (with or without steroids) in patients with chronic neuropathic nonmalignant pain. The mechanism of this seeming reversal of adverse neuroplastic changes is unknown. Once the nociceptive pathways have been identified, neurolysis may be of long-term benefit. Complications from neurolysis include possible neuroma formation, deafferentation pain, permanent motor or sensory deficits, orthostatic hypotension, diarrhea, sexual dysfunction, and bowel or bladder incontinence. Risk of neuroma formation varies with choice of technique. Neuroma formation is more likely with surgical or radiofrequency ablation than with alcohol, phenol, or cryolysis, because cutting or burning destroys the neural sheath.[29] Neuritis is another risk, but it occurs rarely with neurolysis of sympathetic nerves or visceral afferents.

Peripheral Nerve Blocks: These blocks are valuable for neuropathic pain or neuroma of somatic nerves of the pelvic skin, muscles, and bone. Neurolysis should be cautiously considered for severe nonmalignant pain that is refractory to conservative measures.

Superior Hypogastric Nerve Block (Presacral Nerve): Surgical presacral neurectomy has a long history of success for relief of pain of pelvic visceral structures by an open approach, and more recently via the laparoscope.

A percutaneous technique to block the superior hypogastric plexus has been described for treatment of pelvic cancer pain. The plexus is located anterior to the L5 vertebral body and sacrum at the bifurcation of the common iliac vessels. The visceral afferents that travel through this plexus have their cell bodies located in the dorsal root ganglia from T10 to L2. Blockade of the superior hypogastric plexus has been reported to decrease pelvic pain by 70% in patients with cervical, prostate, or testicular cancer.[30] No complications were reported. This can be performed by a bilateral posterior approach with fluoroscopy or by a single-needle anterior approach with computed tomography guidance (Figs. 51-1 and 51-2). The use of a percutaneous catheter to allow frequent injection has been reported in the treatment of nonmalignant pelvic visceral pain with good success, but prospective trials are needed.[31,32]

Ganglion Impar (Ganglion of Walther) Block: The ganglion impar is the termination of the paired paravertebral sympathetic chains. This terminal end is a single ganglion

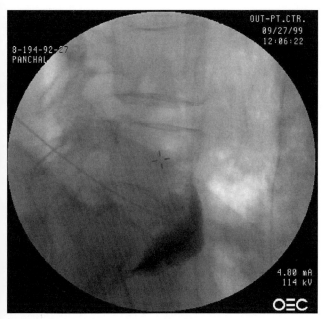

FIGURE 51-1. Lateral view of the needle placement and contrast dye spread during a superior hypogastric plexus block.

located anterior to the sacrococcygeal junction. Blockade of this structure has been introduced within the last decade to manage intractable perineal cancer pain involving the sympathetic nervous system.

Sympathetically mediated perineal pain usually is poorly localized and has components of burning and urgency. Ganglion impar block and neurolysis has been reported to achieve 70% to 100% pain relief for perineal pain caused by cancer of the cervix, colon, bladder, rectum, or endometrium.[33] The procedure is performed with the patient in the lateral decubitus position with a single, bent needle inserted just superior to the anus and advanced to the sacrococcygeal ligament, or by inserting a needle directly through the sacrococcygeal ligament. The position is confirmed with injection of contrast medium under fluoroscopy. Local anesthetic or neurolytic solution is then injected, usually with a volume of 4 to 6 mL. No complications have been reported to date.

Neuromodulation: While the use of sacral root neurostimulation has been mostly used in the treatment of voiding dysfunction, it has been noted to also reduce pelvic visceral pain. Limited case series have demonstrated significant reduction of pain over a follow-up period of 14 to 19 months in patients with interstitial cystitis as well as CPP.[34,35] These reports involve the use of transforaminal S3 and S4 stimulation, but there is also an emerging experience with the use of traditional spinal cord stimulation devices placed in a retrograde fashion to achieve the same goals.

Intrathecal and Epidural Block and Neurolysis: Intractable pelvic cancer pain with somatic involvement may be alleviated by destruction of the appropriate somatic sensory fibers. Intrathecal neurolysis is preferred for unilateral pain and carries a reduced risk of motor fiber destruction. In patients who have undergone a urinary diversion and colostomy epidural or saddle block neurolysis is an effective means of achieving effective pain relief, but the risk of incontinence or lower extremity paresis is high.

Neurosurgical Ablative Techniques: *Percutaneous cordotomy* provides unilateral relief only. *Bilateral cordotomy* is rarely performed and carries a significant risk of fatal sleep apnea (Ondine's curse). *Midline myeletomy* is very invasive; it may be successful for bilateral pain, but the results have been unpredictable. A computed tomography-guided percutaneous punctuate midline myelotomy has been reported to be effective, and has improved safety, but a larger number of patients is required before firm conclusions can be made about its merits.[36]

COMPLEMENTARY AND ALTERNATIVE MEDICINE (CAM) FOR CPP

There are limited studies done in a high-quality manner evaluating CAM techniques for the treatment of CPP. True blinding has often been a limiting factor in performing these studies. For example, a randomized, double-blind study evaluating a static magnetic field for CPP demonstrated statistically significant improvements in disability scores as well as global impression scores; but the investigator reported that the blinding efficacy was compromised by patients testing the magnetic field with metallic objects.[37] Systematic reviews of randomized controlled trials have concluded that overall there is no evidence to suggest that spinal manipulation is effective in the treatment of primary and secondary dysmenorrhea. Vitamin B1 is shown to be an effective treatment for dysmenorrhea taken at 100 mg daily based on only one large randomized controlled trial. Magnesium appears to be a promising treatment for dysmenorrhea, but it is unclear what dose should be used for magnesium therapy due to variations in the included trials. Overall there is insufficient evidence to recommend the use of any of the other herbal and dietary therapies for the treatment of primary or secondary dysmenorrhea.[38,39]

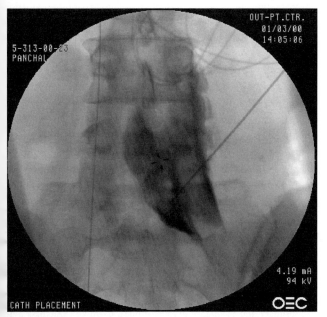

FIGURE 51-2. Anteroposterior view of the needle placement and dye spread for a superior hypogastric plexus block.

CONCLUSION

Pelvic pain has often been difficult to diagnose and treat, resulting in frustrated patients with little support from family and friends. A thorough multidisciplinary assessment is critical, with appropriate use of diagnostic studies and nerve blocks. Application of visceral pain studies involving the gastrointestinal tract supports concepts of sensitization of the pelvic viscera. This further supports use of tricyclic antidepressants, anticonvulsants, and opioids in patients with otherwise undetectable pathology. Nerve blocks, spinal cord stimulators, and implantable pumps are also appropriate in carefully selected candidates. Neurolytic techniques have been reported for general diagnoses of CPP, but most experts advocate restriction of these procedures for pain of oncologic origin.

REFERENCES

1. Reiter RC, Gambone JC: Demographic and historic variable in women with idiopathic chronic pelvic pain. Obstet Gynecol 75:428–432, 1990.
2. Toomey TC, Hernandez JT, Gitelman OF, et al: Relationship of sexual and physical abuse to pain and psychological assessment variables in chronic pelvic pain patients. Pain 53:105–109, 1993.
3. Ryder RM: Chronic pelvic pain. Am Family Physician 54: 2225–2232, 1996.
4. Mathias SD, Kupperman M, Liberman RF, et al: Chronic pelvic pain: Prevalence, health related quality of life, and economic correlates. Obstet Gynecol 87:321–327, 1996.
5. Lee NC, Dicker RC, Rubin GL, et al: Confirmation of the pre-operative diagnosis of hysterectomy. Am J Obstet Gynecol 150: 283–287, 1984.
6. Peterson HB, Hulka JF, Phillips JM: American Association of Gynecologic Laparoscopists' 1988 membership survey on operative laparoscopy. J Reprod Med 35:587–589, 1990.
7. Stovall TG, Ling FW, Crawford DA: Hysterectomy for chronic pelvic pain of presumed uterine etiology. Obstet Gynecol 75: 676–679, 1990.
8. Stout AL, Steege JF, Dodson WC, et al: Relationship of laparoscopic findings to self-report of pelvic pain. Am J Obstet Gynecol 164:73–79, 1991.
9. Hogan QH, Abrams SE: Neural blockade for diagnosis and prognosis: A review. Anesthesiology 86:216–241, 1997.
10. Cervero F, Connel LA: Distribution of the somatic and visceral primary afferents of the thoracic spinal cord of the cat. J Comp Neurol 230:88–98, 1984.
11. Janig W: Neurobiology of visceral afferent neurons: Neuroanatomy, functions, organ regulations and sensations [review]. Biol Psychol 42:29–51, 1996.
12. Sarfeh IS: Abdominal pain of unknown etiology. Am J Surg 132:22–25, 1976.
13. Docherty RH: Visceral pain. In Raj P (ed): Pain Medicine: A Comprehensive Review. Mosby-Year Book St Louis, 1996, pp 430–438.
14. Pan HL, Longhurst JC: Ischaemia-sensitive sympathetic afferents innervating the gastrointestinal tract function as nociceptors in casts. J Physiol (Lond) 492:841–850, 1996.
15. Sengupta JN, Su X, Gebhart GF: Kappa, but not mu or delta, opioids attenuate responses to distension of afferent fibers innervating the rat colon. Gastroenterology 111:968–980, 1996.
16. Ritchie J: Pain from distension of the pelvic colon by inflating a balloon in the irritable colon syndrome. Gut 14:125–132, 1973.
17. Panchal SJ, Staats PS: Visceral pain: From physiology to clinical practice. J Back Musculoskeletal Rehabil 9:233–246, 1997.
18. Johnson JG: Gynecologic pain: Locating its source. Pain Manage May/June:143–152, 1990.
19. Baxter N, Black J, Duffy S: The effect of a gonadotrophin-releasing hormone analogue as first-line management in cyclical pelvic pain. J Obstet Gynaecol 24:64–66, 2004.
20. Soysal ME, Soysal S, Gurses E, et al: Laparoscopic presacral neurolysis for endometriosis-related pelvic pain. Hum Reprod 18:588–592, 2003.
21. Zullo F, Palomba S, Zupi E, et al: Effectiveness of presacral neurectomy in women with severe dysmenorrheal caused by endometriosis who were treated with laparoscopic conservative surgery: A 1 year prospective randomized double-blind controlled trial. Am J Obstet Gynecol 189:5–10, 2003.
22. Stones RW, Thomas DC, Beard RW: Suprasensitivity to calcitonin gene-related peptide but not vasoactive intestinal peptide in women with chronic pelvic pain. Clin Auton Res 2:343–348, 1992.
23. Reginald PW, Adams J, Franks S, et al: Medroxyprogesterone acetate in the treatment of pelvic pain due to venous congestion. Br J Obstet Gynaecol 96:1148–1152, 1989.
24. Bachar GN, Belenky A, Greif F, et al: Initial experience with ovarian vein embolization for the treatment of chronic pelvic pain syndrome. Isr Med Assoc J 5:843–846, 2003.
25. Stovall TG, Elder RF, Ling FW: Predictors of pelvic adhesions. J Reprod Med 34:345–348, 1989.
26. Peters AAN, Trimbos-Kemper GCM, Admiraal C, et al: A randomized clinical trial on the benefit of adhesiolysis in patients with intraperitoneal adhesions and chronic pelvic pain. Br J Obstet Gynaecol 99:59–62, 1992.
27. Sulaiman H, Gabella G, Davis C, et al: Presence and distribution of sensory nerve fibers in human peritoneal adhesions. Ann Surg. 234:256–261, 2001.
28. Webb MJ: Ovarian remnant syndrome. Aust N Z J Obstet Gynaecol 29:433–435, 1989.
29. Panchal SJ: The rationale and efficacy of zygapophyseal blocks and denervation techniques for low back pain. J Back Musculoskeletal Rehabil 12:151–163, 2000.
30. Plancarte R, Ahescha C, Patt RB, et al: Superior hypogastric plexus block for pelvic cancer pain. Anesthesiology 73:236, 1990.
31. Panchal SJ: Continuous superior hypogastric plexus block in the treatment of chronic orchalgia. Abstract presented at 1999 World Congress of Pain.
32. Panchal SJ, Gurbuxani G: A novel treatment for chronic pelvic pain utilizing repeated injections of bupivacaine via superior hypogastric plexus catheter. Abstract presented at 2002 World Congress of Pain.
33. Kames LD, Rapkin AJ, Naliboff BD, et al: Effectiveness of an interdisciplinary pain management program for treatment of chronic pelvic pain. Pain 41:41–46, 1990.
34. Comiter CV: Sacral neuromodulation for the symptomatic treatment of refractory interstitial cystitis: A prospective study. J Urol 169:1369–1373, 2003.
35. Siegel S, Paszkiewicz E, Kirkpatrick C, et al: Sacral nerve stimulation in patients with chronic intractable pelvic pain. J Urol 166:1742–1745, 2001.
36. Vilela FO, Araujo MR, Florencio RS, et al: CT-guided percutaneous punctate midline myelotomy for the treatment of intractable visceral pain: A technical note. Stereotact Funct Neurosurg 77:177–182, 2001.
37. Brown CS, Ling FW, Wan JY, et al: Efficacy of static magnetic field therapy in chronic pelvic pain: Double-blind pilot study. Am J Obstet Gynecol 187:1581–1587, 2002.
38. Proctor ML, Hing W, Johnson TC, Murphy PA. Spinal manipulation for primary and secondary dysmenorrhoea. Cochrane Database Syst Rev 4:CD002119, 2001.
39. Wilson ML, Murphy PA: Herbal and dietary therapies for primary and secondary dysmenorrhoea. Cochrane Database Syst Rev 3:CD002124, 2001.

Sickle Cell Anemia

Robert E. Molloy, M.D.

Sickle cell anemia is a genetic disorder of hemoglobin synthesis that follows classic Mendelian inheritance. The sickle gene is inherited homozygously from both parents. The sickle mutation is the result of a single base change (GAT → GTT) in the sixth codon of exon 1 of the beta-globulin gene responsible for synthesis of the beta chain polypeptide.[1] Normal hemoglobin A (HbA) is formed by two alpha chains and two beta chains. Hemoglobin S (HbS) differs from normal adult HbA by the substitution of valine for glutamic acid at the sixth position on the beta chain. This replacement leads to interaction between the hydrophilic valine residue and other hydrophilic regions on adjacent hemoglobin molecules.

EPIDEMIOLOGY

The condition is more common in East Africa, the Mediterranean, and parts of southern Asia and the Middle East. The gene involved seems to offer some protection against malaria in the heterozygous form (sickle trait). The incidence of sickle cell anemia in the black American population is 0.15%.[2] Disease severity is highly variable. Pain is the most common manifestation of sickle cell disease (SCD) after the age of 2 years, and painful crises occur most frequently between the ages of 20 and 40 years. The median life expectancy of patients with sickle cell anemia was only 14.3 years in the early 1970s. This had risen to 42 years for men and to 48 years for women in the 1990s.[3]

PATHOPHYSIOLOGY

Molecules of HbS tend to stack or polymerize under deoxygenated conditions (i.e., partial pressure of oxygen < 40 mmHg); this is the fundamental molecular event that underlies the many manifestations of SCD.[4] Repeated deoxygenation and prolonged hypoxia result in cellular membrane damage, cellular dehydration, and formation of deformed, sickled cells. The membrane of sickled cells is sticky and adheres to endothelial cells. The eventual formation of irreversibly sickled cells leads

to vascular occlusion, which is the single most important pathophysiologic process leading to the acute complications of SCD. Microvascular occlusion leads progressively to tissue hypoxia, further sickling, and the start of a vicious cycle that result in tissue infarction, the release of inflammatory mediators, and acute pain.[4] White blood cells elaborate the cytokines interleukin-1 (IL-1), tumor necrosis factor (TNF), and IL-6, which upregulate various cellular adhesion molecules on endothelial cells. As a result, endothelial cells bind sickle cells, platelets, and neutrophils, and the coagulation system is activated.[4] Further HbS polymerization, red blood cell sickling, sickle cell adhesion to endothelium, fibrin deposition, and microvascular occlusion follow.

CLINICAL PRESENTATION

Ischemic tissue damage most commonly occurs in the spleen, bones, and joints; it also affects the chest, abdomen, and extremities. Repeated vascular occlusive events occur that can result in acute pain crises, acute chest syndrome, stroke, priapism, and splenic sequestration. Abdominal pain can mimic other surgical causes of acute abdomen. Acute chest syndrome, with hypoxemia and hypoventilation, may occur, but pneumonia and pulmonary embolus should be considered and ruled out. Autoinfarction of the spleen results in functional hyposplenism by the age of 7 years. This results in a marked increase in the risk of Gram-positive bacterial infections. Patients also have chronic hemolytic anemia, employing maximal erythropoiesis to maintain resting Hb levels. They also experience poor growth, reduced fertility, pigment gallstone formation, and chronic cholecystitis. Aseptic necrosis of the humeral or femoral head and compression fractures from chronic vertebral bone infarction may occur. Chronic painful leg ulcers are also common.[5]

The natural history of sickle cell anemia is characterized by frequent and unpredictable painful vasoocclusive crises. The frequency of crises is variable, averaging 0.8 per patient-year. However, 1% of patients have more than six episodes each year, while some patients experience none.[6] This may skew the perception of health care workers, who see the most difficult cases repetitively, about the natural history of most SCD patients. Patients with higher levels of HbF, which inhibits HbS polymerization, and those with lower hemoglobin levels, and thus lower blood viscosity, both experience fewer painful crises. Patients with more than three acute crises per year are at increased risk for early death, and some develop a chronic pain syndrome.[6] Although painful crisis may be precipitated by nocturnal hypoxemia, dehydration, alcohol intake, hypothermia, stress, menstruation, and bacterial or viral infection, there is often no clear etiologic factor.[7] The pain typically affects two to three sites simultaneously; the most common areas are the lumbar spine, femur, knee, sternum, and abdomen. Fever is present in about 50% of acute crises, but an infectious cause is not usually confirmed. This is believed to represent a painful crisis-associated acute inflammatory syndrome.

MANAGEMENT OF SICKLE CELL CRISIS

Because of the variability in frequency and intensity of pain in sickle cell patients, this disease remains a challenge to manage clinically. In the normal patient acute pain is often accompanied by signs of tachycardia, hypertension, diaphoresis, and pupillary dilatation. These signs are helpful in objectively assessing or substantiating a patient's subjective level of pain. However, when pain becomes chronic, as in the most severe forms of SCD, objective autonomic signs are often absent. Common pain behaviors were studied in sickle cell patients and included guarding, bracing, rubbing, grimacing, and sighing. Of these, guarding was the most observed behavior, and it was highly correlated with the physician's rating of the pain.[5]

The mainstays of management of the acute pain crisis are analgesia, hydration, rest, and search for an infectious focus. Broad-spectrum antibiotics, with coverage of potential streptococcal infection, are often used in the presence of fever, until the results of cultures are available. Blood transfusion is employed only in the presence of acute chest syndrome, stroke, or a pain crisis that is either refractory to therapy or rapidly relapses. The goal of exchange transfusion has been to increase or maintain the Hb level at 10 gm% and to decrease the level of HbS to <30%. An endpoint of <50% has been used to prevent recurrence after stroke.[8] There are no controlled studies to select the appropriate target HbS level for treatment of acute crisis.[9] A trial of high-dose methylprednisolone for 24 hours was designed to combat the inflammatory component. The duration and total dose of opioid analgesic therapy was significantly reduced.[10] However, rebound attacks were frequent, and long-term complications of steroid therapy have limited the use of this option.

Almost 90% of painful episodes are managed at home with fluids and oral analgesics.[11] Home treatment is advantageous because the patient remains in familiar surroundings and has support from family, facilitating an early return to activities of daily living. Episodes of crisis may last minutes to weeks; and both severity and location of pain may vary over time. Younger children tend to have limb pain, while adolescents often suffer from abdominal pain. The few crises that require hospital treatment are often severe, hospital staff may underestimate the severity of pain, and the resultant pain control is often inadequate. Sickle cell crisis pain is one of the most severe forms of acute pain. The average pain score during observed crisis was 9.5 on a 10 cm visual analogue scale.[12] Physicians may hesitate to administer large doses of opioids because of concerns about overdose and drug dependence. From a demographic viewpoint, SCD patients might be expected to be at high risk for drug abuse problems because of their social and economic environment. The limited evidence about the incidence of problem drug use among SCD patients suggests that addiction is reported rarely in descriptive studies.[13] When more attention has been given to drug-seeking behavior, dependence, and addiction, drug-related problems were identified in about to 7% to 9% of patients.[14,15] The most important risk factor for drug addiction among patients treated for chronic or episodic pain is a history of drug abuse that predates their current illness. This concern has limited application to the SCD population with the experience of lifelong pain. However, past experiences of undertreatment for severe acute pain may predispose these patients to develop pseudoaddiction, drug-seeking behavior, drug misuse, and development of a chronic pain syndrome.[4]

OPIOID THERAPY

There is consensus in the USA that opioid analgesics are required to treat a severe painful crisis. Aggressive intravenous opioid administration is indicated in the emergency department. Morphine is the initial drug of choice. Large doses, given at frequent intervals, titrated to effect, may provide adequate pain control within 4 to 6 hours. These patients may be discharged home with a 1- to 2-week supply of oral sustained-release morphine. Patients who do not obtain satisfactory relief are admitted to the hospital.[16]

Patients with persistent moderate to severe pain are hospitalized for intravenous hydration, parenteral opioids, and treatment of any underlying cause. The choice of opioid and route of administration vary from institution to institution. The primary goal of opioid administration is to provide a constant level of analgesia and avoid the extremes of pain and sedation. Meperidine appears to have been the most frequently selected opioid despite its considerable potential for side effects and limitation as an analgesic. In a comparison of meperidine with morphine in children lethargy, constipation, pruritis, and wheezing were more common with morphine; dizziness was less common.[17] The pharmacokinetics of meperidine have been shown to be abnormal in sickle cell patients, with unexpectedly low peak blood levels observed compared to surgical patients.[18]

Normeperidine is a renally excreted active metabolite of meperidine with a half-life of 18 hours. It can accumulate in patients with borderline or compromised renal function who receive frequent or high doses of meperidine. Normeperidine toxicity manifests as tremors, agitation, multifocal myoclonus, and seizures. Nine of 21 centers treating SCD in the USA reported problems with meperidine-associated seizures in a survey.[19] The risk of seizures is the main reason that meperidine is no longer recommended for treatment of pain in SCD. Other opioids, such as morphine, hydromorphone, and methadone, are at least as effective.

Opioid requirements of patients with sickle cell crisis are high because of the severe nature of vasoocclusive episodes and the predictable development of tolerance to opioids from previous use.[16] Regardless of the requirements, rapid titration to effect is necessary. The intravenous (IV) route is always preferred once it is established, although intermittent intramuscular administration has previously been the most popular route. A loading dose followed by a continuous IV infusion may be employed with frequent rate titration.[16] The use of patient-controlled analgesia (PCA) is increasingly popular. PCA has several advantages. First, in an era of cost containment and managed care, PCA allows a more effective use of nursing resources. Second, PCA offers a better pharmacokinetic profile, avoiding high peaks and low troughs of plasma concentrations. Third, patients feel more in control of their care, which may add a psychological benefit beyond analgesia.[20] A prospective randomized controlled trial (RCT) of IV morphine PCA compared to an aggressive schedule of intermittent IV bolus morphine demonstrated equivalent efficacy and safety.[20] The main disadvantage of PCA was long set-up time. One problem with fixed-dose IV bolus vs. PCA is the variability in pharmacokinetics. A recent pediatric study of SCD patients demonstrated a 10-fold range of morphine clearances.[21] A background infusion and demand PCA dosing may be necessary initially, with gradual tapering of the infusion as the patient's pain is controlled. Frequent recording of pain scores is essential to document efficacy and safety of analgesic administration. In general, studies comparing PCA and intermittent or fixed-schedule IV injections have not demonstrated consistent differences in total drug dose, length of hospital stay, or pain scores. The same conclusion applies to studies comparing continuous IV infusions to intermittent bolus injections.[13] There is a suggestion that use of continuous infusions may provide effective analgesia but increase the risk of overdose.

Patients may be given a 1- to 2-week supply of oral sustained-release opioid (morphine or oxycodone) and an immediate-release rescue drug at the time of discharge from the hospital.[16] This type of regimen has been reported to decrease opioid use and admissions in two small studies. However, the possibility that patients were induced to transfer to another institution, by introduction of the new treatment protocol, was suggested in a subsequent report.[16,22]

Nonopioid analgesics like acetaminophen and nonsteroidal anti-inflammatory drugs (NSAIDs) may play a useful role, particularly for less severe episodes of pain. The risks of NSAID therapy must be considered when there is a history of peptic ulcer disease, and particularly when renal function has been impaired by SCD. Tricyclic antidepressant therapy has a limited role for initial sickle crisis management, but may be an effective adjuvant for supplemental analgesia over a longer time frame.[23]

Epidural analgesia has been used effectively to manage acute sickle cell crisis. Children who were previously unresponsive to conventional therapy, including IV meperidine, had immediate and continuous relief of SCD pain after an epidural local anesthetic infusion lasting for 1.5 to 5 days.[24]

NONPHARMACOLOGIC PAIN MANAGEMENT

Self-hypnosis, biofeedback, acupuncture, and transcutaneous electrical nerve stimulation (TENS) have all been used to manage pain in SCD. The results in anecdotal reports have been mixed but generally encouraging. No significant benefits have been confirmed in RCTs.[25] These nondrug methods have the potential to reduce reliance on conventional analgesia and to promote greater individual autonomy in pain management for some patients.

Behavioral and interpersonal factors may influence patient response to the above analgesic techniques. Young adult men seem to require more frequent medical therapy for SCD. This phenomenon peaks for men in their twenties and decreases to the same level as women patients by the age of 35 years.[3] Evidence about cognitive and behavioral strategies for coping with pain appears to show an effect on the outcome of acute episodes rather than on their incidence. Negative thoughts about pain and passive coping strategies do not predict an increase in painful episodes; however, they correlate with more pain, more hospitalizations, and more distress when these episodes occur.[26]

Interpersonal factors can contribute to unsuccessful pain management in SCD. It is strongly recommended that medical staff take patient reports of pain seriously and respond to them as a high priority. Patients report dissatisfaction with their treatment in the emergency room, with the attitudes of medical staff about possible drug addiction in young male patients, and with physicians' negative reactions when patients ask questions about their care.[27] The risk that effective pain management will be compromised by poor relationships between patients and medical staff is greatest for the minority of SCD patients who most frequently require hospital treatment for pain management. These patients have frequent severe pain episodes; cope poorly with pain; are less well adjusted psychologically; and present challenges to the attitudes and skills of hospital medical staff.[13] Many of these patients may meet the criteria for drug misuse or dependence. The most important factor influencing the outcome of painful crises is the quality of cognitive and behavioral coping strategies. The main barrier to better clinical outcome may be poor interpersonal relationships and between patients and hospital medical staff.

LONG-TERM MANAGEMENT STRATEGIES FOR SCD

Routine supportive care for patients with SCD should include the following:[1]

- Education about SCD, its inheritance, and genetic counseling.
- Compliance with regular follow-up medical care.
- Avoidance of situations that exert an adverse effect on SCD.
- Education about rights and responsibilities as a patient when dealing with health care providers, hospitals, and employers.
- Participation in local support groups.

Prophylactic measures against pediatric infection may include:

- Prophylactic oral penicillin for infants and young children.
- Vaccinations recommended for pneumococcus, hemophilus influenza type B, and hepatitis type B.

SPECIFIC TREATMENTS FOR SCD

The potential to provide curative treatment for selected children with SCD is encouraging. It is not clear how to select patients most likely to benefit from this therapy. Attempted curative treatments have involved the use of transplantation therapy in selected children. Bone marrow transplantation has been provided for over 100 patients with SCD. More than 90% of the initial patients survived, 70% to 85% had event-free survival, and 15% experienced graft rejection.[28,29] Umbilical cord blood transfusion from related and unrelated donors has been successful in a few cases.[30–32]

Preventative treatments have been designed to ameliorate the symptoms of SCD. The primary approach has been to prevent the polymerization of HbS with drugs that increase production of HbF. Higher levels of HbF have a beneficial effect on painful crises in sickle cell anemia. Hydroxyurea monotherapy has been the least toxic and most effective therapy to increase the level of HbF in humans.[33,34] Hydroxyurea is a cell cycle-specific cytotoxic agent that inhibits ribonucleotide reductase. The mechanism by which it increases HbF production is not known. Long-term therapy, with maximally tolerated doses, has increased HbF by an average of about 15%. In a RCT hydroxyurea resulted in significant reductions in painful crises, acute chest syndrome, and transfusions.[34] Additional drugs and novel treatments are being developed to improve future patient management.

KEY POINTS

- Polymerization of HbS molecules under deoxygenated conditions is the fundamental molecular event that underlies the manifestations of SCD. Formation of irreversibly sickled cells leads to vascular occlusion, the most important pathologic process leading to acute complications of SCD.

- Repeated vascular occlusive events lead to ischemic tissue damage and acute pain. The frequency of painful crises averages 0.8 per patient-year; however, 1% of patients have more than 6 crises each year. Painful crises occur most frequently between the ages of 20 and 40 years, requiring greater medical therapy in male patients in this age range.

- The mainstays of management for acute pain crises are analgesia, hydration, rest, and search for an infectious source. Almost 90% of crises are managed at home with fluids and analgesics. However, opioids are required to manage a severe painful crisis.

- Cognitive and behavioral coping strategies are the most important factors influencing the outcome of a painful crisis but do not alter the frequency of these events.

REFERENCES

1. Ballas SA: Sickle cell anemia: Progress in pathogenesis and treatment. Drugs 62:1143–1172, 2002.
2. Platt O, Dover G: Sickle cell disease. *In* Nathan D, Oski F (eds): Hematology of Infancy and Childhood, ed 4. WB Saunders, Philadelphia, 1993, p 732.
3. Platt OS, Thorington BD, Brambilla DJ, et al: Pain in sickle cell disease: Rates and risk factors. N Engl J Med 325:11–16, 1991.
4. Vijay V, Cavenagh JD, Yate P: The anaesthetist's role in acute sickle cell crisis. Br J Anaesth 80:820–828, 1998.
5. Gil KM, Phillips G, Abrams MR, et al: Observation of pain behaviors during episodes of sickle cell disease pain. Clin J Pain 10:128–132, 1994.
6. Platt OS, Brambilla DJ, Rosse WF, et al: Mortality in sickle cell disease. N Engl J Med 330:1639–1644, 1994.
7. Sergeant GR, Ceulaer CD, Lethbridge R, et al: The painful crisis of homozygous sickle cell disease: Clinical features. Br J Haematology 87:586–591, 1994.
8. Cohen AR, Martin MB, Silber JH, et al: A modified transfusion program for prevention of stroke in sickle cell disease. Blood 79:1657–1661, 1992.

9. Ohene-Frempong K: Indications for red cell transfusions in sickle cell disease. Semin Hematol 38(Suppl 1):5–13, 2001.
10. Griffin TC, McIntyre D, Buchanan GR: High-dose methylprednisolone therapy for pain in children and adolescents with sickle cell disease. N Engl J Med 330:733–737, 1994.
11. Shapiro BS, Dinges DF, Orne EC, et al: Home management of sickle cell-related pain in children and adolescents: Natural history and impact on school attendance. Pain 61:139–144, 1995.
12. Ballas SK, Delengowski A: Pain measurement in hospitalized adults with sickle cell painful episodes. Ann Clin Lab Sci 23:358–361, 1993.
13. Elander J, Midence K: A review of evidence about factors affecting quality of pain management in sickle cell disease. Clin J Pain 12:180–193, 1996.
14. Vichinsky EP, Johnson R, Lubin H: Multidisciplinary approach to pain management in SCD. Am J Pediatr Hematol Oncol 4:328–333, 1982.
15. Payne R: Pain management in sickle cell disease: Rationale and techniques. Ann N Y Acad Sci 565:189–206, 1989.
16. Brookoff D, Polomano R: Treating sickle cell pain like cancer pain. Ann Intern Med 116:364–368, 1992.
17. Cole TB, Sprinkle RH, Smith SJ, et al: Intravenous narcotic therapy for children with severe sickle cell pain crisis. Am J Dis Child 140:1255–1259, 1986.
18. Abbuhl S, Jacobson S, Murphy JG, et al: Serum concentration of meperidine in patients with sickle cell crisis. Ann Emerg Med 15:433–438, 1986.
19. Pegelow CH: Survey of pain management therapy provided for children with sickle cell disease. Clin Pediatr 31:211–214, 1992.
20. Gonzalez GR, Bahal N, Hansen LA, et al: Intermittent injection vs. patient-controlled analgesia for sickle cell crisis pain: A comparison of patients in the emergency department. Arch Intern Med 151:1373–1378, 1991.
21. Dampier CD, Setty BN, Logan J, et al: Intravenous morphine pharmacokinetics in paediatric patients with sickle cell disease. J Pediatr 126:461–467, 1995.
22. Ballas SK, Rubin RN, Gabuza TC: Treating sickle cell pain like cancer pain [letter]. Ann Intern Med 117:263, 1992.
23. Sanders DY, Severance HW, Pollack CV: Sickle cell vaso-occlusive pain crisis in adults: Alternative strategies for management in the emergency department. South Med J 85:808–811, 1992.
24. Yaster M, Tobin JR, Billet C, et al: Epidural analgesia in the management of severe vaso-occlusive sickle cell crisis. Pediatrics 93:310–315, 1994.
25. Zeltzer L, Dash J, Holland JP: Hypnotically induced pain control in sickle cell anaemia. Pediatrics 64:533–536, 1979.
26. Gil KM, Williams DA, Thompson RJ, et al: Sickle cell disease in children and adolescents: The relation of child and parent pain coping strategies to adjustment. J Pediatr Psychol 16:643–663, 1991.
27. Shelley B, Kramer KD, Nash KB: Sickle cell mutual assistance groups and the health services delivery system. *In* Nash KB (ed): Psychosocial Aspects of Sickle Cell Disease: Past, Present and Future Directions of Research. Haworth Press, New York, 1994, pp 243–259.
28. Walters MC, Patience M, Leisenring W, et al: Bone marrow transplantation for sickle cell disease. N Engl J Med 335:369–376, 1996.
29. Ballas SK: Sickle Cell Pain: Progress in Pain Research and Management, vol II. IASP Press, Seattle, 1998.
30. Reed W, Woodward P, Walters M, et al: Successful related cord blood transplantation for hemoglobinopathies [abstract no. 1766]. Blood 96(Suppl 1, Pt 1):410a, 2000.
31. Yeager AM, Mahta PS, Adamkiewiez TV, et al: Unrelated placental umbilical cord blood cell (UCBC) transplantation in children

with high risk sickle cell disease (SCD) [abstract no.5536]. Blood 96(Suppl 1, Pt 2):366b, 2000.

32. Gore L, Lane PA, Quinones R, et al: Successful cord blood transplantation for sickle cell anemia from a sibling who is human leukocyte antigen-identical: Implications for comprehensive care. J Pediatr Hematol Oncol 22:437–440, 2000.

33. Charache S, Dover DG, Moore RD, et al: Hydroxyurea: Effects on hemoglobin F production in patients with sickle cell anemia. Blood 79:2555–2565, 1992.

34. Charache S, Terrfin ML, Moore RD, et al: Effect of hydroxyurea on the frequency of painful crises in sickle cell anemia. N Engl J Med 332:1317–1322, 1995.

Diabetic and Other Peripheral Neuropathies

**Jeffrey A. Katz, M.D., and
James P. Rathmell, M.D.**

DEFINITIONS

The term *neuropathy* describes a disturbance of nerve function or structure. Neuropathies arise from many different etiologies and can be painful (e.g., diabetic neuropathy) or painless (e.g., neuropathy of chronic renal failure). Single or multiple peripheral nerves as well as cranial nerves may be involved. Painful neuropathies fall under the broader descriptive category of *neuropathic pain*, or pain arising from abnormalities within the central or peripheral nervous systems. This chapter presents a brief overview of the evaluation of patients with painful peripheral neuropathy, describes an approach to the differential diagnosis of these disorders, and outlines the therapeutic modalities that may be useful in treating patients with neuropathic pain.

CLASSIFICATION

Neuropathic Pains: Because of the many etiologies and manifestations of neuropathic pain, it is helpful to categorize them broadly according to the site of initial injury (Table 53-1).[1] Injury to the nervous system that results in chronic pain can occur anywhere from the peripheral nerve terminal to the cerebral cortex. Despite the differing locations and the myriad of underlying causes for injury, patients with neuropathic pain often share similar symptoms (Table 53-2).[2]

Peripheral Neuropathies: There are numerous potential causes for painful polyneuropathy. They include metabolic derangement, drug toxicity, paraneoplastic processes, vasculitis, and genetic disturbances. It is important to diagnose the underlying etiology in the hope of reversing nerve dysfunction or preventing further nerve damage. A classification of painful neuropathies based on their etiology is shown in Table 53-3.[3]

MECHANISMS OF NEUROPATHIC PAIN

Many of the proposed mechanisms of pain arising from peripheral nerve injury have been summarized in recent reviews.[4,5] These can be generally broken down into peripheral and central mechanisms.

Peripheral: Following trauma to a nerve, sodium channels accumulate in a higher than normal concentration around the area of injury and along the entire axon, resulting in hypersensitivity of the nerve and ectopic foci. This is often the basis for

TABLE 53-1. NEUROPATHIC PAIN SYNDROMES

Peripheral
Painful peripheral polyneuropathies
Focal entrapment/traumatic neuropathies
Postsurgical syndromes
    Phantom pain and stump pain following amputation
    Post-thoracotomy syndrome

Central
Traumatic brachial plexus avulsion
Traumatic spinal cord injury
Ischemic cerebrovascular injury
Syringomyelia
Arachnoiditis

Mixed
Complex regional pain syndromes
    Type I (reflex sympathetic dystrophy)
    Type II (causalgia)
Meningoradiculopathies
Epidural spinal cord compression
Acute herpetic and postherpetic neuralgia

Adapted from Elliott KJ: Taxonomy and mechanisms of neuropathic pain. Semin Neurol 14:195–205, 1994.

TABLE 53-2. THE ABNORMAL SENSATIONS OF NEUROPATHIC PAIN

Spontaneous pain: burning, shooting, lancinating
Paresthesias: abnormal nonpainful sensations that may be spontaneous or evoked (tingling)
Dysesthesias: abnormal pain that may be spontaneous or evoked (unpleasant tingling)
Hyperalgesia: an exaggerated painful response to a normally noxious stimulus
Hyperpathia: an exaggerated painful response evoked by a noxious or non-noxious stimulus
Allodynia: a painful response to a normally non-noxious stimulus (e.g., light touch is perceived as burning pain)

Modified from Pain, Suppl 3: Mersky H (ed): Classification of chronic pain: description of chronic pain syndromes and definition of pain terms, p S1. Copyright (1986), with permission from the International Association for the Study of Pain.

TABLE 53-3. ETIOLOGIES OF PAINFUL PERIPHERAL POLYNEUROPATHY

Metabolic   Diabetes mellitus   Amyloidosis   Multiple myeloma   Hypothyroidism
Nutritional   Beriberi   Alcoholic   Pellagra
Toxic   Isoniazid   Cisplatin   Arsenic   Thallium
Genetic   Fabry's disease   Hereditary sensory neuropathy
Infectious   Acquired immunodeficiency syndrome   Acute inflammatory polyneuropathy

Adapted from Lewis MS, Hill CS, Warfield CA: Medical diseases causing pain. In Raj PP (ed): The Practical Management of Pain. Mosby Year Book, St Louis, 1992, pp 329–342.

the use of sodium channel blockers and membrane stabilizers in neuropathic pain.[4] It has also been suggested that nerve injury can result in the release of neuropeptides which might further cause peripheral sensitization through neurogenic inflammation.[6]

Nerve injury also can result in sprouting of sympathetic fibers into the dorsal root ganglia of the affected nerve, and in partially injured nerves the uninjured fibers may increase expression of alpha-adrenoreceptors. In both of these circumstances, sympathetically mediated pain may occur. This pain may be able to be blocked at least temporarily by the application of sympathetic blocks or by the administration of systemic alpha-adrenoreceptor antagonists (phentolamine).[4]

Another proposed but poorly documented mechanism is that of ephaptic transmission: peripheral nerve injury resulting in "cross-circuiting" of peripheral fibers. In theory, sympathetic efferents would be able to activate nociceptive afferent fibers, explaining spontaneous pain and worsening of pain with activation of the sympathetic nervous system in some patients with neuropathic pain. However, there is little evidence to support this longstanding theory.[7]

Central: The central nervous system (CNS) undergoes changes with peripheral nerve injury. In fact, this mechanism may be a primary one in those conditions where peripheral neuropathy results in reduced input to the CNS (postherpetic neuralgia, diabetic neuropathy). It is frequently stated in the literature that in diabetic neuropathy there is little evidence that peripheral sensitization (as might be seen with increased sodium channels or with ephaptic transmission) occurs: rather the evidence points toward reduced neural input to the CNS occurring as in diabetic neuropathy.[8]

Several potential mechanisms exist for a central contribution to the pain from peripheral neuropathy. Loss of large fiber (A-beta) sensory input could result in a reduction in nonnociceptive sensory input, thereby reducing the effectiveness of the "gate" as proposed by Wall and Melzack.[4] In experimental models of nerve injury opioid and gamma-aminobutyric acid (GABA) receptors (both involved in inhibition of nociceptive transmission in the CNS) are downregulated and the amount of GABA in the dorsal horn is reduced. Another mechanism suggests death of dorsal horn interneurons in lamina II, many of which are involved in inhibition of nociceptive transmission in the dorsal horn, by overexposure to excitatory amino acids (EAA cytotoxicity). Cholecystokinin, involved in opioid receptor inhibition, has also been found to be upregulated in the spinal cord following experimental nerve injury.[4]

The net effect of the above changes in the spinal cord serve to "disinhibit" nociceptive transmission, thereby creating an imbalance of painful over nonpainful impulses. These changes might also explain the relative opioid resistance seen in neuropathic pain.

Another central mechanism that may explain the allodynia seen in some peripheral neuropathies involves A fiber sprouting and A fiber "phenotypic switching".[4] A fibers normally synapse in all lamina of the spinal cord except lamina II where C fiber input predominates. However, following peripheral C fiber nerve injury, A fiber "sprouting" into lamina II is seen to occur, allowing therefore mechanical non-nociceptive input via the peripheral A fibers to trigger second-order pain pathways. A-beta fibers in the dorsal horn also do not normally express substance P (as seen in C fibers), but following peripheral nerve injury they can (the phenotypic switching), again thereby allowing non-nociceptive input to trigger CNS nociceptive transmission.[4]

The above mechanisms are likely far from complete in terms of explaining the changes in the CNS following peripheral nerve injury. It is very likely that significant changes also occur throughout the spinal cord even in levels not directly involved with the peripheral injury, including the contralateral side, midbrain, and cerebral cortex.

The wide variability in how individuals respond to peripheral nerve injury is likely the result of genomic differences. Differences in the ability of A fibers or sympathetic fibers to sprout, the amount of neuropeptides available for release peripherally, the susceptibility of inhibitory interneurons to EAA in the dorsal horn are all likely to be highly variable between patients, possibly explaining why some patients with the same condition (e.g., diabetic neuropathy) may or may not have pain.[4] Animal models demonstrate notable differences between strains in their reaction to peripheral nerve injury and in their responsiveness to analgesics.[9]

EVALUATION OF THE PATIENT WITH NEUROPATHIC PAIN

When a patient presents with signs and symptoms suggestive of neuropathic pain—most notably allodynia—the first useful distinction to be made is the pattern of involvement. Focal lesions of peripheral nerves (mononeuropathies) result from processes that produce localized damage and include nerve entrapment; mechanical injuries; thermal, electrical, or radiation injuries; vascular lesions; and neoplastic or infectious processes. In contrast, polyneuropathies result in a bilaterally symmetric disturbance in function as a result of agents that act diffusely on the peripheral nervous system: toxic substances, deficiency states, metabolic disorders, and immune reactions. The diagnosis of painful polyneuropathy is most often made by history and standard neurologic examination. In some cases ancillary studies may be needed to document the disease process.

History: Pain is often the presenting symptom for polyneuropathy but it rarely presents in the absence of other sensory abnormalities. Many of the terms used to describe these abnormalities are listed in Table 53-2.[2] Paresthesias ("tingling" or "pins and needles" sensations) are particularly common. However, since the characteristics of neuropathic pain are almost always multiple (e.g., varying combinations of burning, stabbing, aching, etc.) they cannot be used as a useful guide to determining the etiology of the neuropathy.[7,10] The location of the pain and other symptoms is frequently the most important piece of historical information.

Neurologic Examination: In the patient suspected of having polyneuropathy the clinician should focus on sensory evaluation. Strength and deep tendon reflexes are preserved in many patients with polyneuropathy. In addition to testing vibration, proprioception, and light touch, the sensory examination should include several special stimuli including light-touch rubbing, ice, single pinprick, and multiple pinpricks. Lightly stroking the affected area with a finger will assess for allodynia (pain provoked by non-noxious stimuli). Ice application will test for both temperature sensation and abnormal sensations such as pain and lingering after-sensations. Single pinprick

testing may elicit a sensory deficit or hyperpathia (an exaggerated response to a normally painful stimulus). Repeated pinprick testing may elicit summation (pain growing more intense with subsequent stimuli) or lingering after sensations, both common findings in polyneuropathy.

Electrodiagnostic Testing: Patients suspected of having polyneuropathy should be considered for electromyography (EMG) and nerve conduction (NCV) studies, which may offer insights into whether the process is a demyelinating (reductions in nerve conduction velocities) or axonal (reductions in the amplitude of evoked responses) neuropathy. However, such differentiation rarely offers any change in therapy when managing neuropathic pain. These tests are best used to demonstrate large fiber involvement, however, and since many painful peripheral neuropathies involve small fibers these tests may be completely normal in patients with painful polyneuropathy.[7]

For this reason quantitative sensory testing (QST) may be useful in the assessment and tracking of painful peripheral neuropathies. While large fibers are assessed through the use of sensory thresholds to vibration, small fibers can be assessed through threshold assessment of heat, painful heat, cold, and painful cold stimuli. On the other hand, thermography has found little role in the assessment, management, or tracking of painful peripheral neuropathies despite much published literature on the method.[11]

DIFFERENTIAL DIAGNOSIS

After assembling the historical information, neurologic examination, and results of electrodiagnostic studies, the underlying etiology will most often already be apparent. Several recent reviews present detailed discussions of diagnosis and management of the patient with painful polyneuropathy.[3,12] A brief description of the clinical features and useful supportive tests for the most common painful polyneuropathies follows.

Metabolic Causes of Peripheral Polyneuropathy: Diabetes: Painful polyneuropathy is most often due to a metabolic disorder, the most common being diabetes mellitus. The reported frequency of neuropathy in patients with diabetes mellitus ranges from 4% to 8% at the time of initial presentation and rises to 15% to 50% after 20 to 25 years of follow-up.[13] Other studies report an incidence of neuropathy (not necessarily painful) of up to 66%, but clearly the likelihood of neuropathy increases with the duration of the disease.[14,15] However, the incidence of painful neuropathy was reported in one study to average about 11.6% in insulin-dependent diabetes mellitus (IDDM) and 32.1% in non-insulin-dependent diabetes mellitus (NIDDM).[16,17]

The cause of diabetic neuropathy has not been determined with certainty.[18] Current hypotheses focus on the possibilities of metabolic and ischemic nerve injury. Pathologic examination of nerves taken from diabetic patients has revealed evidence of microvascular disease supporting the ischemic nerve theory. Metabolic abnormalities include: (1) accumulation of sorbitol in diabetic nerve as excess glucose is converted to sorbitol by the enzyme aldose-reductase, (2) autooxidation of glucose resulting in reactive oxygen molecules, and (3) inappropriate activation of protein kinase C.[19,20] Other theories suggest that impaired nerve regeneration may contribute to the polyneuropathy in diabetes as demonstrated in animal models of nerve injury.[21]

Therapeutic strategies aimed at reducing sorbitol accumulation (aldose-reductase inhibitors) have demonstrated only minor improvements in neuropathy. There is strong evidence, however, that good glycemic control can prevent the appearance and worsening of polyneuropathy in patients with both IDDM[22] and NIDDM.[4] A major trial found that the incidence of neuropathy was reduced by 60% over a 5-year period with aggressive glycemic control.[22]

A practical clinical classification scheme for diabetic neuropathy that divides the neuropathies according to the pattern of distribution of involved nerves is shown in Table 53-4.[5] The most common form of diabetic neuropathy is distal symmetric polyneuropathy. It is predominantly a sensory disturbance. Patients present with gradual onset of paresthesias and pain in the legs and feet. Symptoms begin in the toes and gradually ascend over months to years to involve more proximal levels. The fingertips and hands become involved later, usually when symptoms in the lower extremities have ascended to the knee level. Allodynia (e.g., pain in the feet brought on by even the light pressure of contact with bed sheets) and burning pain are common and are often worse at night. Examination reveals graded distal sensory loss predominantly affecting vibration and position sensation. Reflexes may be diminished or absent. Electrophysiologic testing reveals decrease in the amplitude of evoked responses to a greater degree than reduction in nerve conduction velocities as the neuropathy progresses.[6] This reflects primarily axonal damage rather than demyelination. Severe sensory loss may allow repeated trauma to go unnoticed, resulting in development of foot ulcers and diabetic neuroarthropathy (Charcot's joints). This last condition is critical to identify in the diabetic patient with a unilateral, painful swollen foot.

The syndrome of acute painful diabetic neuropathy may also occur in diabetics.[3,5] This uncommon disorder is characterized by the rapid onset of severe pain in the distal lower extremities characterized by constant burning in the feet, dysesthesiae, allodynia, and lancinating leg pains. Examination reveals little or no sensory loss with preserved reflexes. Electrophysiologic testing reveals decreased amplitude or absent sensory potentials, but may be normal. This type of neuropathy often remits within a year after blood sugars are controlled.

Autonomic neuropathy manifest by abnormalities in tests of autonomic function occurs in 20% to 40% of diabetics.[5] Symptomatic autonomic neuropathy most often occurs as a component of distal symmetric polyneuropathy. Autonomic nervous system abnormalities include postural hypotension, impaired heart rate control (resting tachycardia and fixed heart rate), esophageal dysmotility, gastroparesis, and erectile dysfunction.

Lower extremity proximal motor neuropathy is an uncommon painful disorder associated with diabetes.[5] It is characterized by acute or subacute onset of moderate to marked weakness and wasting of the pelvifemoral muscles accompanied by back, hip, and thigh pain with preserved sensation in the regions of pain. The condition may be painless or accompanied by pain described as a constant, severe, deep ache. Complete recovery occurs in 60% of patients over 12 to 24 months.

Diabetic lumbosacral radiculoplexus neuropathy (DLRPN) is sometimes referred to as diabetic amyotrophy, proximal diabetic neuropathy, diabetic polyradiculopathy, Bruns–Garland syndrome, or diabetic lumbar plexopathy. It usually affects individuals with type 2 diabetes over the age of 50 years, and presents as an asymmetric weakness associated with pain in the legs that appears subacutely and progresses over weeks to months. Although motor function recovery is slow and often incomplete, the pain usually resolves.[23,24] Both microvascular inflammation as well as autoimmune mechanisms have been proposed, with no one clear treatment plan being particularly effective.[25,26] A similar syndrome has been seen in patients without diabetes, with no differences in clinical presentation, physical examination, or nerve biopsy studies.[27]

Diabetic truncal neuropathy involves acute or gradual onset of unilateral pain in the chest or abdomen and may mimic myocardial infarction, intra-abdominal pathology, or spinal disorders.[28] Examination reveals marked allodynia and hyperpathia in the distribution of pain. Truncal neuropathy occurs most often in long-standing diabetics and those over the age of 50 years. EMG typically reveals denervation in the abdominal or intercostal musculature.

Cranial mononeuropathies involving the oculomotor, abducens, trochlear, and facial nerves may occur in diabetic patients.[5] The most common of these is oculomotor neuropathy that is manifest as ophthalmoplegia and ptosis. The eye is deviated laterally and has impaired movement vertically and medially. Pain occurs in 50% of patients and may precede ophthalmoplegia by several days.

Entrapment neuropathies are believed to occur more frequently in patients with diabetes mellitus.[5] Carpal tunnel syndrome is believed to occur more than twice as frequently as in the nondiabetic population. This association must be kept in mind when evaluating the diabetic patient with an isolated peripheral mononeuropathy.

Metabolic Causes of Peripheral Polyneuropathy: Other: Metabolic causes of painful peripheral neuropathy other than diabetes mellitus (and excluding postherpetic neuralgia) are uncommon. Amyloidosis is a disease caused by extracellular deposition of amyloid, a fibrous protein. Amyloidosis can be primary, familial, or associated with other conditions such as multiple myeloma, chronic infectious or inflammatory states, aging, and long-term hemodialysis.

TABLE 53-4. CLASSIFICATION OF NEUROPATHIES ASSOCIATED WITH DIABETES MELLITUS

Generalized polyneuropathies
Distal symmetric polyneuropathy
Acute painful diabetic neuropathy
Autonomic polyneuropathy

Multiple mononeuropathies
Proximal lower extremity motor neuropathy
Truncal neuropathy

Mononeuropathies
Cranial mononeuropathy
Compression mononeuropathy

Adapted from Ross MA: Neuropathies associated with diabetes. Med Clin North Am 77:111–124, 1993.

The biochemical composition of the amyloid protein varies with the associated disease state. Painful peripheral neuropathy in amyloidosis is characterized by deep aching and occasional shooting pains, distal sensory loss, and autonomic and motor involvement.[29] As the neuropathy progresses, all modalities are affected, reflexes are lost, and there is motor involvement. Treatment of neuropathy associated with amyloidosis is aimed at the underlying condition when such is identifiable.

Multiple myeloma is due to malignant plasma cell growth. Painful neuropathy can appear in myeloma with or without amyloid deposition. The neuropathy is extremely variable in severity and rate of progression, ranging from a mild, predominantly sensory neuropathy to a complete tetraplegia.[10] Pain in myeloma often declines with successful treatment using chemotherapy, radiation therapy (especially for isolated plasmacytomas), or plasmapheresis.

Patients with untreated hypothyroidism may also develop painful sensorimotor neuropathy.[10] This uncommon disorder may present with longstanding pain in either the hands or the feet accompanied by weakness in the distal limb musculature. The neuropathy often resolves with successful replacement of thyroid hormone.

Nutritional Causes of Peripheral Polyneuropathy: Thiamine deficiency is seen in alcoholics, chronic dialysis patients, and people on restrictive diets. Thiamine deficiency appears to lead to beriberi, which consists of heart failure, vasodilatation, and peripheral neuropathy. The neuropathy is characterized by hand, foot, and calf pains with allodynia, decreased sensation, and motor involvement.[30] Administration of thiamine may reduce the symptoms of neuropathy, including pain.

The incidence of neuropathy in chronic alcoholism is about 9%.[10] Alcoholic neuropathy is characterized by motor and sensory deficits, often accompanied by pain.[10] The pain consists of aching in the legs or feet with intermittent lancinating pains. The upper limbs are rarely involved. Burning of the soles and allodynia may also occur. Alcoholic neuropathy occurs only after chronic and severe alcohol abuse and is invariably accompanied by severe nutritional deficiency. Pathologically, alcoholic neuropathy cannot be distinguished from beriberi, and both likely result from thiamine deficiency. Treatment consists of abstinence and thiamine supplementation.

Pellagra is caused by niacin deficiency and is rarely seen in the USA.[10] Signs and symptoms include dermatitis, gastrointestinal complaints, neurasthenia, and spinal cord dysfunction. Pellagra is associated with a mixed, painful polyneuropathy similar to that seen with beriberi. A predominant feature of the sensorimotor neuropathy is spontaneous pain in the feet and lower legs, with tenderness of the calf muscles and cutaneous hyperesthesia of the feet. Treatment of pellagra with niacin often results in resolution of all symptoms except the peripheral neuropathy.

Toxic Causes of Peripheral Polyneuropathy: Isoniazid is a frequently used antituberculous drug. Chronic administration in individuals with slow metabolism of the drug (slow acetylators) is associated with the development of painful neuropathy.[3,10] Initial symptoms of distal numbness and tingling paresthesias are later accompanied by pain, which may be felt as a deep ache or burning. The calf muscles are painful and tender, and walking often aggravates symptoms.

Symptoms may be particularly troublesome at night. Prophylactic coadministration of pyridoxine (vitamin B_6) prevents development of neuropathy. Once neuropathy develops, administration of pyridoxine does not have an effect on recovery.

Cisplatin is a chemotherapeutic agent used to treat solid tumors and can lead to a painful, dose-dependent peripheral neuropathy.[31] The earliest manifestations of neuropathy are decreased vibration sense in the toes and loss of ankle jerk reflexes. At larger doses, paresthesias may appear and progress to severe dysesthesias. The neuropathy is reversible, but recovery may take more than a year after discontinuation of cisplatin.

Arsenic is now ingested only rarely in suicide or homicide attempts. It is associated with a painful subacute sensorimotor peripheral neuropathy.[32] Acute ingestion is followed by gastrointestinal symptoms, psychosis, delirium, stupor, and renal failure. Cardiovascular collapse may occur. If the patient survives the initial insult, signs of chronic exposure including skin and nail changes and pancytopenia may appear. Five to ten days after arsenic ingestion, symptoms of neuropathy including aching, burning, tingling, and numbness may appear. Treatment begins with removing further exposure. Recovery from neuropathy may take years. BAL (British antilewisite) may reverse other symptoms of acute arsenic poisoning, but has little effect on recovery from neuropathy.

Thallium is used as an insecticide/rodenticide and in small doses in myocardial perfusion imaging. In many ways, thallium poisoning resembles arsenic toxicity. In the first day, gastrointestinal symptoms and cardiovascular collapse may occur. Within the following week, confusion, psychosis, choreoathetosis, convulsions, and coma may ensue. Alopecia, the hallmark of thallium poisoning, develops weeks after exposure. Nail changes may also occur late. Painful neuropathy may appear within 48 hours of ingestion. Initially there are leg and arm pains and distal paresthesias.[3] In severe cases cranial nerves and the muscles of respiration may be involved. Treatment should include intravenous hydration and diuresis to promote urinary excretion of thallium. Early use of charcoal hemoperfusion may be of benefit. Neurologic function should improve over time, but may be incomplete.

Genetic Causes of Peripheral Polyneuropathy: Fabry's disease is an X-linked recessive disease caused by accumulation of ceramide trihexose in the absence of alpha-galactosidase A. The pain is associated with a length-dependent small-fiber neuropathy that affects most patients in the first three decades of life.[33] This explains why these patients typically present as boys or young men with a painful neuropathy characterized by tender feet and burning in the calves.[34] Abdominal pain may also occur. Other manifestations include multiple angiokeratomas, anhidrosis, renal failure, corneal and lenticular opacities, hypertension, stroke, and myocardial infarction. Although cold perception is typically reduced, cold seems to exacerbate the pain.[33] No specific therapy exists for Fabry's disease. Peripheral neuropathy has been treated with some success using phenytoin and carbamezepine.

Dominantly inherited hereditary sensory neuropathy is insidious in onset and typically appears in the second decade of life or later.[3] There is decreased sensation in the feet and distal legs leaving patients prone to ulcer formation often leading to cellulitis and osteomyelitis. There may be associated peroneal muscle atrophy and hearing loss. Patients often experience intermittent lancinating pains in the shoulder, thigh, leg, and foot. There is no specific treatment for this disorder.

Infectious and Inflammatory Causes of Peripheral Polyneuropathy:

As many as 30% of patients with acquired immunodeficiency syndrome (AIDS) or AIDS-related complex may develop painful neuropathy.[35] Patients report pain in the soles with accompanying paresthesias in the feet. Allodynia may be so severe as to interfere with walking. EMG testing often reveals evidence of denervation. Treatment consists of zidovudine (AZT), tricyclic antidepressants, and anticonvulsants.

Acute inflammatory polyneuropathy (AIP or Guillain–Barré syndrome) is characterized by areflexic motor paralysis.[36] It is often preceded by viral infections with relationships to cytomegalovirus, Epstein–Barr virus, and smallpox/vaccine. Guillain–Barré syndrome may also follow surgery. The onset of symptoms develops over several weeks. Pain is a common early symptom; weakness, usually in the legs, may progress to respiratory failure requiring mechanical ventilation. Sensory symptoms include parasthesias often in the presence of decreased sensation in a glove-stocking distribution. Autonomic dysfunction is also common evidenced by tachycardia and orthostatic hypotension. Pain may occur in up to 72% of patients. The pain is principally an ache, strain, or deep burning sensation in the thigh or buttocks and can be quite severe. While pain in AIP may be severe, it is usually transient. Pain is usually worse at night. Nerve conduction studies and lumbar puncture aid the diagnosis. General therapy for AIP is supportive along with plasmapheresis. Glucocorticoids and other immunosuppressants have not been clearly shown to be helpful. Pain may respond to oral narcotics, quinine, and other drugs typically useful for treating neuropathic pain. Epidural narcotics have also been used successfully in relieving pain associated with Guillain–Barré syndrome.[37]

Neuroma:

Although not considered classically to be a neuropathy, neuromas are a not infrequent cause of pain from peripheral nerve injury. Typically resulting from the complete disruption of a peripheral nerve, the ends of the axons continue to grow. However, anatomical separation of the ends prevents proper realignment. The proximal end may continue to grow around itself in an unorganized bulbous collection of unmyelinated fibers producing a neuroma. Neuromas are far more thermosensitive and mechanosensitive than normal nerve endings, and can produce spontaneous discharges as well. Furthermore, abnormal afferent impulses can result in the dorsal root ganglia following injury to the peripheral nerve.[38]

Idiopathic Small-Fiber Neuropathy:

This condition usually presents with painful feet in patients over the age of 60 years. Although most often classified as idiopathic, autoimmune mechanisms are largely suspected in those cases. While diabetes and the metabolic/genetic causes above can cause small-fiber neuropathy, it can also be present in the absence of those conditions, and this state has been the subject of thorough review.[39] It can be defined as the presence of paresthesias (usually painful) with the absence of significant large-fiber dysfunction (atrophy, loss of vibratory sense, or loss of reflexes). It should be noted that small-fiber neuropathy might not be painful. Diagnosis is often confirmed through tests of autonomic function or quantitative sensory testing.

TREATMENT OF NEUROPATHIC PAIN

There are a wide variety of medications and proposed algorithms that are used in the treatment of neuropathic pain, reflecting the lack of any one highly effective regimen. Proper randomized, double-blind, placebo-controlled studies are largely lacking, and given the inconsistency and variability of most neuropathic conditions and the highly variable genomic contribution between patients, the conclusions from a study of one group of patients with neuropathy will likely not apply to another.

Detailed elsewhere in this book, the mainstay pharmacologic options for peripheral neuropathic pain remains the antidepressants.[4,40,41] Caution must be used with these medications especially with those medications having anticholinergic side effects in patients with autonomic neuropathy. The selective serotonin reuptake inhibitors (SSRIs) may be used, although while paroxitene demonstrated benefit in diabetic neuropathy fluoxitene did not.[19]

Anticonvulsants, including newer agents such as gabapentin, have become a common part of the pharmacotherapy for neuropathic pain and their use is detailed elsewhere in this book.[4] Similarly local anesthetics and antiarrhythmics have also been recognized to suppress ectopic impulses in experimental nerve injury and so their use has also been proposed for peripheral neuropathic pain.[20,42,43]

Sympatholytic Agents:

Sympatholytic agents have been proposed for both the diagnosis and treatment of peripheral neuropathic pain, based on the concept of expression of alpha-adrenoreceptors in damaged peripheral nerves. Analgesic response to intravenous phentolamine infusion may be predictive of response to regional sympathetic ganglion blockade[44] and oral or transdermal sympatholytic agents.[4] The alpha$_2$-adrenergic agonist clonidine has been reported as a useful analgesic in treating neuropathic pain as have anecdotal reports of the oral alpha-adrenergic antagonists prazosin, terazosin, and phenoxybenzamine.[4,20]

Corticosteroids both systemically and by peripheral application have been used based on empirical response. When injected perineurally (but not systemically), corticosteroids reduce the spontaneous ectopic discharge rate seen in nerve injuries and neuromas, probably by a membrane stabilizing effect.[45] They also have been found to have a short-lasting suppressive effect on transmission in normal C fibers, but more recent studies on peripheral nerve injury models in the rat confirm that local application of steroid on the area of injured nerve may produce an analgesic effect by suppression of peripheral ectopic sites.[46]

Use of opioids for the long-term treatment of noncancer pain remains controversial.[47] Opioids are among the most universally effective analgesic agents known, but fear of addiction and tolerance limits their usefulness. Historically, neuropathic pain has been considered "opioid resistant," and evidence exists to support that contention.[48] However, data also exist supporting the concept that opioids are capable of relieving noncancer neuropathic pain.[49] A small series of patients with neuropathic pain who responded to intrathecal morphine has been reported;[50] it is unclear where in the treatment process this option should be considered. The use of opioids in chronic benign pain, including neuropathic pain, is reviewed in detail elsewhere.[51]

Various publications mention other options for approaching patients with pain from peripheral neuropathies, including sympathetic nerve blocks, neurolytic sympathetic blocks, spinal cord stimulation, transcutaneous electrical nerve stimulation (TENS), and deep brain stimulation. As the information in such sources is anecdotal, it is not possible to draw conclusions beyond the fact that these are possible options worth further study.[52,53]

KEY POINTS

- Neuropathic pain arises from disorders of the peripheral nervous system. Although there are many etiologies of peripheral neuropathy, not all of which always produce pain, the most prominent and common is diabetic neuropathy.

- Many mechanisms have been proposed for the pain that occurs in peripheral neuropathic states, but they can be categorized into peripheral and central. Peripheral mechanisms proposed include: formation of ectopic foci, formation of ephapses (unlikely), release of neuropeptides with neurogenic inflammation, and increased expression of alpha adrenoreceptors.

- Central mechanisms of neuropathic pain proposed include: loss of large-fiber pain inhibition, downregulation of opioid and GABA receptors, reduction of GABA release, death of inhibitory interneurons, A fiber sprouting, A fiber phenotypic switching, and cholecystokinin upregulation.

- History and physical examination remain the mainstay in evaluating and following peripheral neuropathic pain. EMG provides evidence of large-fiber changes but rarely will alter therapeutic decisions, while QST may aid in diagnosing subtle aspects of peripheral neuropathy and allow monitoring for scientific study.

- Pain in diabetic neuropathy may have a strong central component, given that evidence supports a reduced sensory input in those patients suffering from pain. There are specific syndromes within the class of painful diabetic neuropathy that have profound components, include rapid onset of symptoms, and significant motor components. It is important in painful diabetic neuropathy not to overlook the development of Charcot's joints, which can also be painful and progress to significant deformity if not addressed.

- The treatment of neuropathic pain typically involves the use of antidepressants, anticonvulsants, and other sodium channel stabilizers. Opioids have been shown to be effective in selected cases, although many are opioid resistant. Sympatholytics and sympathetic blockade may also be useful in selected cases. Treatment remains largely empiric; genomic variation makes any one patient's response to peripheral neuropathy unique and hence responsiveness to therapy will be unpredictable.

REFERENCES

1. Elliott KJ: Taxonomy and mechanisms of neuropathic pain. Semin Neurol 14:195–205, 1994.
2. Mersky H (ed): Classification of chronic pain syndromes and definition of pain terms. Pain Suppl 3:S1, 1996.
3. Lewis MS, Hill CS, Warfield CA: Medical diseases causing pain. *In* Raj PP (ed): The Practical Management of Pain, ed 2. Mosby Year Book, St Louis, 1992, pp 329–342.
4. Woolf CJ, Mannion RJ: Neuropathic pain: Aetiology, symptoms, mechanisms, and management. Lancet 353:1959–1964, 1999.
5. Zimmermann M: Pathobiology of neuropathic pain. Eur J Pharmacol 429:23–37, 2001.
6. Fields HL, Rowbotham MC: Multiple mechanisms of neuropathic pain: A clinical perspective. *In* Gebhart GF, Hammond DL, Jensen TS (eds): Proc 7th World Congress on Pain. IASP Press, Seattle, 1994, pp 437–454.
7. Galer BS: Neuropathic pain of peripheral origin: Advances in pharmacologic treatment. Neurology 45(Suppl 9):S17–S25, 1995.
8. Calcutt NA: Potential mechanisms of neuropathic pain in diabetes. Int Rev Neurobiol 50:205–228, 2002.
9. Devor M, Raber P: Heritability of symptoms in an experimental model of neuropathic pain. Pain 42:51–67, 1990.
10. Vrethem M, Boivie J, Arnqvist H, et al: Painful polyneuropathy in patients with and without diabetes: Clinical, neurophysiologic, and quantitative sensory characteristics. Clin J Pain 18:122–127, 2002.
11. Report of the American Academy of Neurology, Therapeutics and Technology Assessment Subcommittee. Assessment: Thermography in neurologic practice. Neurology 40:523–525, 1990.
12. Galer BS: Painful polyneuropathy: Diagnosis, pathophysiology, and management. Semin Neurol 14:237–246, 1994.
13. Ross MA: Neuropathies associated with diabetes. Med Clin North Am 77:111–124, 1993.
14. Dyck PJ, Kratz KM, Karnes JL, et al: The prevalence by staged severity of various types of diabetic neuropathy, retinopathy, and nephropathy in a population-based cohort: The Rochester diabetic neuropathy study. Neurology 43:817–824, 1993.
15. Partanen J, Niskanen L, Lehtinen J, et al: Natural history of peripheral neuropathy in patients with non-insulin-dependent diabetes mellitus. N Engl J Med 333:89–94, 1995.
16. Zeigler D, Gries FA, Spuler M, Lessmann F: The epidemiology of diabetic neuropathy. J Diabetic Complications 6:49–57, 1992.
17. Partenen J, Niskanen L, Lehtinen J, et al: Natural history of peripheral neuropathy in patients with non-insulin-dependent diabetes mellitus. N Engl J Med 333:89–94, 1995.
18. Thomas PK: Diabetic neuropathy: Models, mechanisms, and mayhem. Can J Neurol Sci 19:1, 1992.
19. Feldman EL, Russell JW, Sullivan KA, Golovoy D: New insights into the pathogenesis of diabetic neuropathy. Curr Opin Neurol 12:553–563, 1999.
20. Verrotti A, Giuva T, Morgese G, Chiarelli F: New trends in the etiopathogenesis of diabetic peripheral neuropathy. J Child Neurol 16:389–394, 2001.
21. Xu G, Sima AAF: Altered immediate early gene expression in injured diabetic nerve: Implications in regeneration. J Neuropathol Exp Neurol 60:972–983, 2001.
22. Diabetes Control and Complications Trial Research Group: The effect of intensive treatment of diabetes on the development and progression of long-term complications in insulin-dependent diabetes mellitus. N Engl J Med 329:977–986, 1993.
23. Bastron JA, Thomas JE: Diabetic polyradiculopathy: clinical and electromyographic findings in 105 patients. Mayo Clin Proc 56:725–732, 1981.
24. Barohn RJ, Sahenk Z, Warmolts JR, Mendell JR: The Bruns–Garland syndrome (diabetic amyotrophy) revisited 100 years later. Arch Neurol 48:1130–1135, 1991.
25. Dyck PJB, Norell JE, Dyck PJ: Microvasculitis and ischemia in diabetic lumbosacral radiculoplexus neuropathy. Neurology 53:2113–2121, 1999.
26. Krendel DA, Zacharias A, Younger DS: Autoimmune diabetic neuropathy. Neurol Clin 15:959–971, 1997.
27. Dyck PJB, Norell JE, Dyck PJ: Non-diabetic lumbosacral radiculoplexus neuropathy: Natural history, outcome and comparison with the diabetic variety. Brain 124:1197–1207, 2001.

28. Harati Y, Niakin E: Diabetic thoracoabdominal neuropathy: A cause for chest and abdominal discomfort. Arch Intern Med 146:1493–1494, 1986.

29. Scadding JW: Peripheral neuropathies. *In* Wall PD and Melzack R (eds): Textbook of Pain. Churchill Livingstone, New York 1992, pp 667–683.

30. Victor M: Polyneuropathy due to nutritional deficiency and alcoholism. *In* Wilson JD, Braunwald E, Isselbacher KJ, et al (eds): Harrison's Principles of Internal Medicine, ed 12. McGraw-Hill, New York, 1991.

31. Mollman JE: Cisplatin neurotoxicity. N Engl J Med 322: 126–127.

32. Windebank AJ. Metal neuropathy. *In* Dyck PJ, Thomas PK, Griffin JH, et al (eds): Peripheral Neuropathy, ed 3. WB Saunders, Philadelphia, 1993, pp 1549–1570.

33. Schiffmann R, Scott LJ: Pathophysiology and assessment of neuropathic pain in Fabry disease. Acta Paediatrica Suppl 91(439):48–52, 2002.

34. Brady RO: Fabry disease. *In* Dyck PJ, Thomas PK, Griffin JH, et al (eds): Peripheral Neuropathy, ed 3. WB Saunders, Philadelphia, 1993, pp 1169–1178.

35. Cornblath DR, McArthur JC, Parry GJG, Griffin JW: Peripheral neuropathies in human immunodeficiency virus infection. *In* Dyck PJ, Thomas PK, Griffin JH, et al (eds): Peripheral Neuropathy, ed 3. WB Saunders, Philadelphia, 1993, pp 1343–1353.

36. Arnason BGW, Solevin B: Acute inflammatory demyelinating polyradiculopathy. *In* Dyck PJ, Thomas PK, Griffin JH, et al (eds): Peripheral Neuropathy, ed 3. WB Saunders, Philadelphia, 1993, pp 1437–1497.

37. Connelly M, Shagrin J, Warfield C: Epidural opioids for the management of pain in a patient with Guillain–Barré syndrome. Anesthesiology 72:381–383, 1990.

38. Hartrick C: Pain due to trauma including sports injuries. *In* Raj P (ed): Practical Management of Pain, ed 2. Mosby Year Book, St Louis, 1992, p 425.

39. Lacomis D: Small-fiber neuropathy. Muscle Nerve 26:173–188, 2002.

40. Hammond DL: Pharmacology of central pain-modulating networks (biogenic amines and non-opioid analgesics). Adv Pain Res Ther 9:499, 1985.

41. Calissi PT, Jaber LA: Peripheral diabetic neuropathy: Current concepts in treatment. Ann Pharmacother 29:769–777, 1995.

42. Devor M, Wall P, Catalan N: Systemic lidocaine silences ectopic neuroma and DRG discharge without blocking nerve conduction. Pain 48:261–268, 1992.

43. Galer B, Harle J, Rowbotham M: Response to intravenous lidocaine infusion predicts subsequent response to oral mexiletine: A prospective study. J Pain Sympt Manage 12:161–167, 1996.

44. Raja SN, Treede RD, Davis KD, Campbell JN: Systemic alpha-adrenergic blockade with phentolamine: A diagnostic test for sympathetically maintained pain. Anesthesiology 74:691–698, 1991.

45. Devor M, Govrin-Lippman R, Raber P: Corticosteroids suppress ectopic neural discharge originating in experimental neuromas. Pain 22:127–137, 1985.

46. Johansson A, Bennett G: Effect of local methylprednisolone on pain in a nerve injury model. Reg Anesth 22:59–65, 1997.

47. Portenoy RK: Chronic opioid therapy for chronic nonmalignant pain: From models to practice. APS J 1:285–288, 1992.

48. Arner S, Meyerson B: Lack of analgesic effect of opioids on neuropathic and idiopathic forms of pain. Pain 33:11–23, 1988.

49. Dellemijn P, Vanneste J: Randomised double-blind active-placebo-controlled crossover trial of intravenous fentanyl in neuropathic pain. Lancet 349:753–758, 1997.

50. Penn RD, Paice JA: Chronic intrathecal morphine for intractable pain. J Neurosurg 67:182–186, 1987.

51. Rathmell JP, Jamison RN: Opioid therapy for chronic noncancer pain. Curr Opin Anesthesiol 9:436–442, 1996.

52. Tasker R, Filho O: Deep brain stimulation for neuropathic pain. Stereotactic Funct Neurosurg 65:122–124, 1995.

53. Kumar K, Toth C, Nath R: Spinal cord stimulation for chronic pain in peripheral neuropathy. Surg Neurol 46:363–369, 1996.

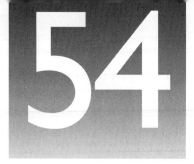

Entrapment Neuropathies

**Michael Minieka, M.D., and
Takashi Nishida, M.D.**

There are a number of anatomic locations where nerves are vulnerable to compression or entrapment. The entrapment syndromes that result have been well described and are a common cause of pain. Table 54-1 lists major nerves, possible anatomical sites of entrapment (shown in Figs. 54-1 and 54-2), and resulting entrapment syndromes with eponyms. We review five of these syndromes in detail: carpal tunnel syndrome, cubital tunnel syndrome, thoracic outlet syndrome, meralgia paresthetica, and tarsal tunnel syndrome.

Patterns of weakness and sensory loss can identify which nerves are injured and localize the site of injury. Provocative maneuvers, which briefly increase pressure at a site of compression, aid diagnosis by recreating or exacerbating symptoms.

When an entrapment neuropathy is clinically suspected, electrodiagnostic testing should be performed to confirm the diagnosis and exclude other neurological disorders. If electrodiagnostic testing suggests that the site of compression or entrapment is not typical, e.g., median nerve compressed in the forearm rather than at the carpal tunnel, then magnetic resonance imaging should be performed to identify the source of compression. Magnetic resonance imaging can miss smaller compressive lesions and, if clinically appropriate, surgical exploration may be necessary.

Electrodiagnostic testing can also provide prognostic information. Electrodiagnositc testing can often differentiate myelin dysfunction from axon damage. When a compressive lesion causes only focal demyelination, the injury is called *neurapraxic*, and carries a better prognosis for quick and complete recovery. If axon loss has occurred, then recovery will be slower and perhaps incomplete.

CARPAL TUNNEL SYNDROME

Carpal tunnel syndrome is the most common and most studied entrapment neuropathy. It may occur in as many as 1 in 1,000 people in the general population, and even more frequently in high-risk groups.

Pathology: The median nerve can be compressed as it passes through the carpal tunnel. The tunnel is at the base of the hand. The carpal, or wrist bones, form the floor of the tunnel and the flexor retinaculum forms the roof. Nine flexor tendons also pass through the tunnel. Due to this crowded arrangement, any tenosynovial proliferation, fluid collection, or arthritic deformity can lead to carpal tunnel syndrome. Pressure in the tunnel increases several fold with wrist extension or flexion. In those with carpal tunnel syndrome, pressures can reach over 100 mmHg in flexion or extension, pressures high enough to impede arterial flow.

Symptoms: Classically, patients report numbness on the palmar surface of the thumb and index, middle, and half the ring finger. However, in practice, reports of numbness often involve only a portion of the median distribution, especially the middle or index finger. Patients are often not aware of the true distribution of numbness and may report that all five fingers are involved. However if patients are specifically asked to observe which fingers are involved they will observe that the fifth finger is spared.

Carpal tunnel syndrome can cause pain. The pain can be both distal and proximal to the site of compression. Patients can report pain in the hand, wrist, elbow, and shoulder. Carpal tunnel syndrome should be considered in any obscure complaint of pain in the arm.

Pain and numbness may increase when the wrist is flexed or extended. For this reason patients often report symptoms at night when they awake after sleeping with their wrists in flexion. Many patients will report needing to shake their hand on waking to relieve their numbness. This is sometimes called the "flick sign." Driving is another common situation in which the wrist may be in flexion for an extended period of time and elicit carpal tunnel syndrome symptoms.

Patients usually do not complain of weakness. They may report dropping things or having difficulty with certain motor activities like doing up buttons or opening a jar. These complaints are probably the result from a combination of mild thenar weakness and sensory loss.

TABLE 54-1. **MAJOR NERVES, POSSIBLE SITES OF ENTRAPMENT, AND RESULTING ENTRAPMENT SYNDROMES WITH EPONYMS**

Nerve	Site of Entrapment	Syndrome
Upper extremity		
Brachial plexus	Anterior and medial scalene muscle Subclavius muscle Pectoralis minor and coracoid process Cervical rib or band, medial antebrachial cutaneous nerve	Anterior scalene syndrome Costoclavicular syndrome Hyperabduction syndrome Thoracic outlet syndrome
Long thoracic		"Rucksack" palsy
Suprascapular	Transverse scapular ligament, scapular notch or foramen Spinoglenoid ligament or notch	
Musculocutaneous	Coracobrachialis muscle Brachial fascia, lateral antebrachial cutaneous nerve	
Axillary	Quadrangular foramen or lateral axillary hiatus (long head of triceps, teres major and minor)	Quadrilateral space syndrome
Radial	Lateral intermuscular septum	"Saturday night" palsy, "honeymooners'" palsy
	Arcade of Frohse (supinator), leash of Henry (brachioradialis, extensor carpi radialis brevis), Monteggia lesion	Supinator syndrome, posterior interosseous syndrome, radial tunnel syndrome, tardy radial palsy, "tennis elbow," "frisbee flinging"
	Superficial branch	Cheiralgia paresthetica, Wartenberg's disease, "hand-cuff" or "wristwatch" neuropathy
Median	Ligament of Struthers (supracondylar process: medial epicondyle)	
	Pronator teres muscle, sublimis bridge (flexor digitorum sublimis), lacertus fibrosis	Pronator syndrome, flexor digitorum sublimis syndrome
	Gantzer's muscle (flexor pollicis longus)	Anterior interosseous syndrome, Kiloh–Nevin syndrome
	Transverse carpal ligament	Carpal tunnel syndrome
	Transverse metacarpal ligament	Intermetacarpal tunnel syndrome, "bowlers' thumb"
Ulnar	Arcade of Struthers (internal brachial ligament, medial head of triceps, medial intermuscular septum)	
	Epicondylo-olecranon ligament, cubital tunnel retinaculum, arcuate ligament of Osborne	Cubital tunnel syndrome
	Humeroulnar aponeurosis (flexor carpi ulnaris)	"Tardy" ulnar palsy

Continued

TABLE 54-1. MAJOR NERVES, POSSIBLE SITES OF ENTRAPMENT, AND RESULTING ENTRAPMENT SYNDROMES WITH EPONYMS—CONT'D

Nerve	Site of Entrapment	Syndrome
	Deep flexor-pronator aponeurosis	
	Guyon's canal (piso-hamate ligament, volar and transverse carpal ligament)	Ulnar tunnel syndrome, "cyclists'" palsy (Radfahrerlahung)
	Deep branch	Piso-hamate hiatus syndrome
	Transverse and oblique heads of adductor pollicis	
Lower extremity		
T2–6 posterior rami		Notalgia paresthetica
L5 spinal	Iliolumbar ligament (fifth lumbar: wing of the ilium)	Lumbosacral tunnel syndrome
Ilioinguinal	Transverse abdominis muscle	
Genitofemoral	Inguinal canal	
Lateral femoral cutaneous	Inguinal ligament at anterior superior iliac spine	Meralgia paresthetica, Roth's meralgy, Bernhardt's syndrome
Femoral	Iliopectineal arch	Iliacus tunnel syndrome
	Hunter's canal (vastus medialis, adductor longus, sartorius), subsartorial canal	
	Infrapatellar branch of saphenous nerve	Gonyalgia paresthetica, "housemaids' knee"
Obturator	Obturator canal	Howship–Romberg syndrome
Sciatic	Pyriformis muscle	Pyriformis syndrome
	Greater and lesser sciatic foramens, sciatic notch, Gibraltar of the gluteus	
Common peroneal	Fibular neck, peroneus longus muscle	"Cross leg" palsy
	Crural fascia, superficial branch	
	Inferior external retinaculum (ligamentum cruciforme)	(Anterior) tarsal tunnel syndrome
Posterior tibial	Canal calcaneen de Richet (ligamentum laciniatum)	(Posterior) tarsal tunnel syndrome
	Medial plantar nerve	"Joggers' foot," abductor hallucis tunnel syndrome
	Medial plantar proper digital nerve	Joplin's neuroma
	Transverse metatarsal ligament	Morton's neuroma (metatarsalgia)

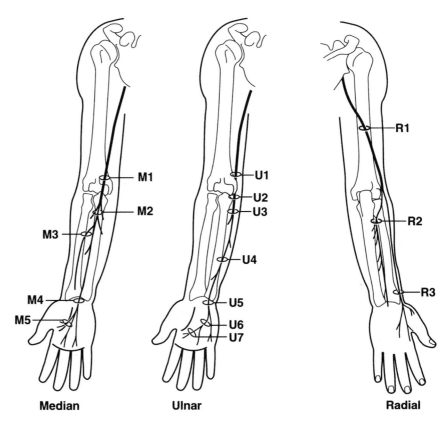

FIGURE 54-1. Sites of possible entrapments of the median, ulnar, and radial nerves (see Table 54-1 for details).

Median **Ulnar** **Radial**

Physical Findings: The median nerve after it exits the carpal tunnel supplies sensation to the palmar surface of the thumb and index, middle, and half the ring finger. It also supplies the dorsal tips of these same fingers. The palmar branch of the median nerve, which supplies sensation to the proximal portion of the palm and thenar eminence, does not go through the carpal tunnel and is therefore spared in carpal tunnel syndrome. Two-point discrimination and pinprick testing will often elicit sensory deficits in parts of the median sensory territory. Often these deficits are only noted when direct comparisons are made with the unaffected hand.

The median nerve after exiting the carpal tunnel innervates a number of intrinsic hand muscles. Those of the thenar eminence, especially the abductor pollicis brevis, are the easiest to test. To test the strength of the abductor pollicis brevis, the patient should place the thumb perpendicular to the plane of the hand and then resist as the examiner attempts to push the thumb into the plane of the hand. In most patient's weakness will only be appreciated when compared to the unaffected hand or flexor pollicis longus muscle of the affected side.

Symptoms can also be provoked by transiently increasing the pressure in the carpal tunnel. Phalen's maneuver increases pressure by putting the patient's wrist in hyperextension or hyperflexion. Tinel's sign involves tapping over the carpal tunnel to elicit brief symptoms. It should be noted that brief symptoms can be elicited in anyone if the tapping is vigorous enough.

Electrodiagnosis: Electrodiagnostic testing is very sensitive for confirming a diagnosis of carpal tunnel syndrome. Some studies report sensitivity as high as 95%. The hallmark of electrodiagnosis is a delay in the distal latency of median nerve conduction. This suggests a conduction delay through the carpal tunnel. Electrodiagnosis is also useful to rule out other disorders with similar symptoms, such as cervical radiculopathy, thoracic outlet syndrome, and diffuse peripheral neuropathy.

Treatment: The first line of treatment for carpal tunnel syndrome is splinting to maintain the wrist in a neutral position and thereby minimize the pressure in the carpal tunnel. Splints should be worn both day and night. Anti-inflammatory treatments including steroid injection benefit some selected patients. Should conservative measures fail, then surgical decompression is indicated.

Risk Factors: Carpal tunnel syndrome is well known as one of the repetitive stress injuries that occur with computer use. Indeed any occupation that requires repeated flexion and extension at the wrist can put an individual at risk for carpal tunnel syndrome. Other risk factors include obesity, arthritis, diabetes, and hypothyroidism.

The shape of the wrist can also be a risk factor for carpal tunnel syndrome. Square wrists, i.e., those whose dorsal–volar distance is close to the medial–lateral distance with a ratio greater than 0.7 are at increased risk for developing carpal tunnel syndrome. Perhaps this is why carpal tunnel syndrome seems to present in several members of a family and in both hands in most individuals.

CUBITAL TUNNEL SYNDROME

Ulnar nerve entrapment at the elbow is the second most common compression neuropathy in the upper extremity.

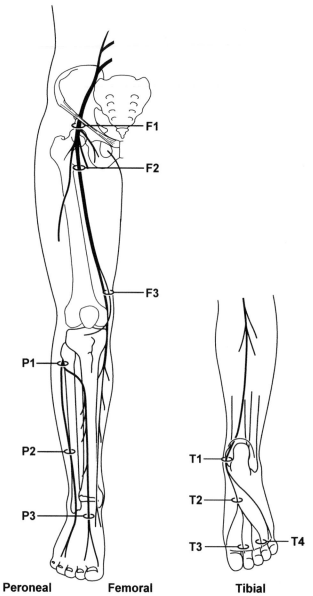

Peroneal   Femoral   Tibial

FIGURE 54-2. Sites of possible entrapments of the peroneal, femoral, and tibial nerves (see Table 54-1 for details).

Pathology: The ulnar nerve is particularly vulnerable to compression as it crosses the elbow and passes through the cubital tunnel. The roof of the cubital tunnel starts with a ligamentous band that stretches from the medial epicondyle to the olecranon of the ulna and then blends into the aponeurosis of the flexor carpi ulnaris muscle (humeroulnar aponeurotic arcade). Compression or impingement of the nerve can occur by a number of mechanisms and it can occur anywhere over several centimeters from the ulnar groove through the cubital tunnel.

When the elbow is flexed, the ulnar nerve is relatively superficial and can be easily compressed. Chronic leaning on a bent elbow can compress the ulnar nerve. An acute blow to a bent elbow can compress the ulnar nerve, as most people have experienced when they have "hit the funny bone." The nerve is also vulnerable to impingement at the elbow, especially if there is a bony deformity or scar formation. Patients with a remote history of supracondylar fracture can develop such a bony

deformity and what has been called "tardy ulnar palsy." The nerve can also be trapped in the cubital tunnel. Pressure in the cubital tunnel increases as the elbow is flexed. In some individuals the ulnar nerve can subluxate over the medial epicondyle with elbow flexion, and be more susceptible to direct trauma.

Symptoms: Intermittent numbness and tingling in the distribution of the ulnar nerve is usually the first symptom of ulnar palsy. Patients can wake up with elbow pain radiating into the fifth digit. There can be cramping and aching in the hypothenar eminence. Symptoms can be exacerbated by flexion of the elbow. Patients may complain about a generalized loss of strength in the hand or loss of dexterity.

Physical Findings: The ulnar nerve supplies sensory fibers to the fifth finger, both palmar and dorsal surfaces, and usually half of the ring finger. Sensory deficits that split the ring finger are classic for an ulnar nerve injury. However, in some individuals the ulnar nerve may supply the whole ring finger and even part of the long finger. In these individuals it may be difficult to distinguish the sensory loss from that of a C8 root lesion. Light touch and two-point discrimination are often more sensitive for detecting ulnar sensory deficits than pinprick or temperature testing.

The ulnar sensory territory ends proximally at about the wrist crease. The ulnar half of the forearm is supplied by the medial antebrachial cutaneous nerve, a branch of the brachial plexus. This area should not be involved in ulnar lesions at the elbow.

Ulnar injury can weaken grasp and pinch strength. However, the easiest muscles to test directly are the first dorsal interosseous and the abductor digiti minimi. The hands are placed on a flat surface and the patient is asked to spread the fingers apart and resist the examiner's attempt to bring the fingers closer together.

Atrophy of the hypothenar eminence and the first dorsal interosseous can often be seen. Clawing of the ring and little finger is common in chronic cases.

Palpation of the ulnar groove and over the cubital tunnel can often elicit tenderness and help to localize the ulnar lesion. Flexion of the elbow beyond 90° can often provoke sensory complaints or pain.

Electrodiagnosis: Electrodiagnostic testing is necessary to confirm a diagnosis and to exclude other causes including brachial plexopathy, cervical radiculopathy, and an ulnar entrapment at the wrist. Nerve conduction studies will usually show slowing across the elbow and sometimes a drop in response amplitude across the elbow. Inching techniques can sometimes localize the site of compression to the ulnar groove or the cubital tunnel.

Treatment: Mild cases of ulnar palsy at the elbow can be successfully treated with an elbow pad to reduce trauma to the nerve or by avoiding prolonged flexion at the elbow. More severe cases may require surgery. The precise site of entrapment will determine the surgical procedure, which can include transposition of the nerve, decompression at the aponeurosis, or even medial epicondylectomy.

Risk Factors: Resting a bent elbow on a hard surface is a behavior that can provoke ulnar palsy. For example, truck drivers can develop a left ulnar palsy from resting their elbow on the window of the truck while driving. Long-distance airline passengers have developed palsies from resting on an armrest. Those confined to bed can develop ulnar palsy when sitting up and resting on their elbows.

Direct trauma including elbow fractures can cause acute ulnar nerve injury. Delayed or tardy ulnar palsies can result from bony deformities that develop after trauma or fracture.

THORACIC OUTLET SYNDROMES

There are many structures that can compress or impinge the brachial plexus as it enters the arm. Vascular structures can also be compressed in the same way. Various positions of the shoulder can also compromise both vascular and neural structures in the thoracic outlet. This has all led to much confusion and disagreement concerning what is called thoracic outlet syndrome. In our opinion it may be better to consider the thoracic outlet as being the site of several syndromes, vascular, neurogenic, and positional, that are not mutually exclusive.

Pathology: Various structures in the thoracic outlet can be the source of compression or impingement. A cervical rib is the most discussed source of compromise in thoracic outlet syndrome, but this may be because it is easily identified by X-ray, where as other structures are not as easily imaged. An anomalous fibrous band from the transverse process of the last cervical vertebra to the first rib is a common cause of impingement. Entrapments by the scalenes, subclavius, and pectoralis minor muscles have all been reported.

Symptoms: The symptoms of thoracic outlet syndromes depend on whether they are primarily vascular or neurologic and can vary with shoulder position.

Neurogenic symptoms include numbness of the medial forearm and ulnar side of the hand. This is usually the first symptom reported. This can be followed by an aching pain, poorly localized in the arm and anterior chest. Certain positions or activities can exacerbate the symptoms, e.g., carrying a heavy briefcase or combing one's hair. Later patients may complain of clumsiness or weakness in the hands and fingers. There may be atrophy of both the thenar and hypothenar eminences.

Coldness, aching muscles, and loss of strength with continued use are typical vascular symptoms. The hand may appear pale or cyanotic with vascular compression.

Anterior flexion of the shoulders can elicit symptoms. For this reason some patients who sleep on their side may wake with symptoms that resolve on repositioning. Abduction and supination of the arm can also elicit symptoms.

Physical Findings: True neurogenic thoracic outlet syndrome initially affects sensation on the ulnar side of the arm and hand. As the syndrome progresses, sensory loss can include the whole hand and arm.

Vascular compression can cause diffuse but subjective sensory deficits. Position changes such as Adson's maneuver can result in both signs, i.e., loss of radial pulse, and increase in symptoms. It should be noted that the diagnostic value of such provocative tests is controversial. For example, even some normals can lose their radial pulse during Adson's maneuver.

True neurogenic thoracic outlet syndrome initially causes weakness of median innervated hand muscles and later ulnar

innervated muscles. Atrophy of both thenar and hypothenar eminences can occur. Vascular compression alone usually does not cause loss of strength. However, arm and hand muscles will easily fatigue with use.

Electrodiagnosis: Early neurogenic thoracic outlet syndrome can present with a normal electrodiagnostic study. One of the first abnormalities seen is a reduction in the amplitude of the medial antebrachial cutaneous sensory response. Later ulnar sensory responses in the hand will be diminished. Needle examination may elicit denervation changes in both median and ulnar innervated hand muscles.

Treatment: Correction of shoulder posture can improve if not completely eliminate the symptoms of thoracic outlet syndrome. Exercises that strengthen the rhomboid and trapezius muscles can improve shoulder posture. Clavicle straps can help maintain correct shoulder posture.

Surgery to open the thoracic outlet was popular during the last century, but its efficacy is controversial. There are indeed some patients who improve with surgery, but selection of appropriate surgical candidates is not clear. The most common surgical procedures are resection of cervical rib and fibrous band, and scalenectomies. Both these procedures carry significant morbidity.

Risk Factors: Activities that promote poor shoulder posture can provoke thoracic outlet syndrome. This is seen in professional musicians who play string instruments, nursing mothers, and computer users, especially on the side that operates the mouse.

Bony deformities from clavicular fracture, cervical ribs, and sloped shoulders all predispose one to thoracic outlet syndrome.

MERALGIA PARESTHETICA

Entrapment of the lateral femoral cutaneous nerve of the thigh has been well described for over 100 years. It is often called meralgia from the Greek *meros* meaning "thigh" and *algo* meaning "pain."

Pathology: The lateral femoral cutaneous nerve of the thigh arises from upper lumbar roots, travels through the pelvis, and exits into the leg at the upper lateral end of the inguinal ligament. The nerve is usually trapped as it passes under or through the inguinal ligament. Blunt trauma to this area can also cause meralgia.

Symptoms: Patients complain of unpleasant sensations and numbness in the lateral thigh. Light touch in the area can be unpleasant. Even clothing touching the area can be unpleasant. Walking, standing, or lying flat can sometimes exacerbate symptoms.

Physical Findings: Findings are completely sensory. Sensory loss usually can be identified in a portion of the distribution of the nerve, i.e., part of the lateral thigh.

Electrodiagnosis: It can be technically difficult to elicit sensory responses from the lateral femoral cutaneous nerve in normal individuals. This makes interpretation of a lost or diminished response suspect. Electrodiagnosis is better suited to ruling out other possible diagnoses such as lumbar radiculopathy.

Treatment: Pain control with medication is the standard treatment. Reduction of risk factors can also be beneficial. Surgical decompression can be difficult because it is not always easy to locate the nerve.

Risk Factors: Obesity, pregnancy, and tight-fitting clothes all increase the risk for meralgia paresthetica.

TARSAL TUNNEL SYNDROME

Here we use the term tarsal tunnel syndrome to describe entrapment of the posterior tibial nerve at the ankle. Some people also use the term to describe entrapment of the peroneal nerve as it enters the foot anteriorly.

Pathology: The tarsal tunnel is formed by the ankle bones and the flexor retinaculum. Through the tunnel passes the posterior tibial nerve, tendons of the foot and toe flexors, and the posterior tibial artery. Increased pressure in the tunnel brings on the syndrome. This can occur from an ankle fracture or sprain, arthritic changes, tenosynovitis, or fluid collection.

Symptoms: The primary complaint is foot pain, often described as burning. Many patients will isolate the burning to the sole of the foot.

Physical Findings: The posterior tibial nerve has three branches: calcaneal, medial plantar, and lateral plantar. Not all the branches may be affected, so some or all of the sole of the foot may lose sensation.

Intrinsic foot muscles can be affected but clinical testing of these muscles can be difficult.

Electrodiagnosis: Nerve conduction studies can reveal both motor and sensory slowing through the tarsal tunnel. The syndrome is usually unilateral so comparisons with the unaffected side make electrodiagnosis easier. Needle examination of intrinsic foot muscles can be misleading. Some 10% to 20% of normal intrinsic foot muscles may demonstrate denervation changes, i.e., fibrillations and positive waves, as a result of direct muscle trauma from walking.

Treatment: Anti-inflammatory medication can be useful in certain cases in which tenosynovitis or arthritis are suspected. Surgical decompression is highly effective.

Risk Factors: Ankle trauma even if remote is common in tarsal tunnel syndrome. Tarsal tunnel is seen in about 5% of patients with rheumatoid arthritis.

KEY POINTS

- When an entrapment neuropathy is clinically suspected, electrodiagnostic testing should be performed to confirm the diagnosis and exclude other neurological diseases.
- In those with carpal tunnel syndrome pressure in the tunnel can reach over 100 mmHg in flexion and extension, pressure high enough to impede arterial flow.
- The ulnar nerve is most vulnerable to impingement at the humeroulnar aponeurotic arcade.
- The thoracic outlet is the site of several syndromes, vascular, neurogenic, and positional, which are not mutually exclusive.
- The diagnostic value of the provocative tests such as Adson's maneuver is controversial.
- There are two types of tarsal tunnel syndrome: entrapment of the deep peroneal nerve at the ankle (anterior) and tibial nerve at the ankle (posterior).

BIBLIOGRAPHY

Dawson DM, Hallett M, Millender LH: Entrapment Neuropathies, ed 2. Little, Brown, Boston/Toronto, 1990.

Logigian EL (ed): Entrapment and Other Focal Neuropathies. Neurol Clin 17(3), 1999.

Rosenbaum RB, Ochoa JL: Carpal Tunnel Syndrome. Butterworth-Heinemann, Stoneham, 1993.

Verghese G (ed): Peripheral Nerve Compressions of the Upper Extremity. Ortho Clin North Am 27(2), 1996.

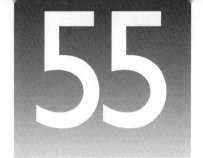

Chronic Pain Management in Children

Santhanam Suresh, M.D., F.A.A.P.

Children experience chronic pain more often than is reported.[1] Children, unlike adults, do not have any associated liabilities including workers' compensation or disability insurance.[2] However, school absenteeism plays a major role in examining and deciding on treatment modalities for children in chronic pain.[3] Family dynamics and the presence of chronic painful conditions in children predispose children to experience pain.

ASSESSMENT OF CHRONIC PAIN

Assessment of chronic pain in childhood requires a biopsychosocial perspective to take into account multiple factors that can influence the child's pain experience. Multidimensional models elaborate various biological, developmental, cognitive, behavioral, affective, social, and situational factors that may shape the child's pain experience, and the pathways by which they exert their effects.[4] Each domain may become a target of assessment and intervention. Several developmentally sensitive, validated instruments are now available to measure the physiological, sensory, affective, and behavioral aspects of children's pain.[4]

Measures for infants and young children necessarily rely on observer reports of behavioral and/or physiological data,[5,6] whereas children of 5 years and older can provide self-reports on one of several validated visual analogue (VAS) or faces scale.[7] The well-documented discordance between an observer's ratings of a child's pain and the child's self-report[8] compel the clinician to consider the child's self-report as the gold standard whenever this can be obtained reliably, usually in children 5 years and older. However, for those children with significant developmental delay and who are nonverbal, McGrath and colleagues have developed scales that rely upon caregiver observations that identify core pain cues in this vulnerable group of children.[4] A majority of the measures developed thus far focus on acute, procedure-related pain. These scales do not capture changes in the behavioral and sensory aspects of pain that may habituate when pain becomes chronic. The systematic evaluation of chronic pain in children, which includes but

moves beyond the sensory aspects of the pain experience, is described below.

Two standardized interviews for school age and adolescent children and their parents provide comprehensive yet practical evaluations of the child's chronic pain: the Children's Comprehensive Pain Questionnaire (CCPQ) and the Varni-Thompson Pediatric Pain Questionnaire (VTPPQ).[9] These interviews separately assess the child and parents' experience of the child's pain problems with open-ended questions, checklists, and quantitative pain rating scales. They also gather information regarding a variety of factors shown to influence the child's pain experience, including the child's developmental level and understanding of their pain,[10,11] pain and medical treatment history, interactions with others in relation to pain complaints[12,13] and painful procedures,[14] affect and behavior,[11,15,16] and the impact of pain on the child's functional abilities, peer relationships, and school and extracurricular activities.[17] Family environment, stresses, and coping,[18] including history of psychiatric[19] and medical problems,[18] particularly chronic pain,[12] are also assessed (Table 55-1).

TABLE 55-1. PEDIATRIC QUESTIONNAIRE COMPONENTS

1. Developmental level
2. Understanding of pain
3. Pain and medical treatment history
4. Interactions with others in relation to pain
5. Affect and behavior
6. Impact of pain on functional abilities
7. Family environment and stresses
8. Coping skills
9. History of psychiatric illness
10. Medical problems

Questionnaires that evaluate the child's coping with chronic pain, the Waldron/Varni Pediatric Pain Coping Inventory[15] and the Pain Coping Questionnaire, provide valuable information for planning behavioral rehabilitation. For example, if the child endorses a catastrophizing coping style, an established risk factor for poor adaptation to chronic pain,[20] then this coping style can become a target of treatment. If a particular domain of the child's pain experience requires assessment in greater depth, such as when a child is exhibiting psychiatric symptoms as well as a pain complaint, more specific inventories can be added to elaborate the assessment (e.g., Child Behavior Checklists (CBCL), Youth Self-Report (YSR), Children's Depression Inventory (CDI), Screen for Child Anxiety Related Emotional Disorders (SCARED)). Sleep is also being investigated as a possible factor in the onset and maintenance of pain problems[21] with some studies finding a relationship between sleep quality and migraine activity in children, while others have not found a relationship between sleep abnormalities in onset of chronic benign pain syndromes such as fibromyalgia. A measure that specifically assesses disability associated with chronic pain in children has been developed to assess headache-related disability.[22] The domains assessed by this scale, including school absences and participation in social and recreational activities, are relevant to all chronic pain conditions in children. Quality of life is also becoming an important focus of assessment and a potential index of treatment progress in children with chronic pain,[23,24] with one study finding the quality of life of children with recurrent headaches similar to that of children with rheumatoid arthritis or cancer.[25]

PSYCHOLOGICAL METHODS IN THE MANAGEMENT OF CHRONIC PAIN

Psychological pain management methods are directed toward increasing the child's and family's understanding of the child's pain and its treatment including factors that may reduce or exacerbate the child's pain, and enhancing their cognitive and behavioral coping skills so that pain-related discomfort and disability are reduced. Three principles guide the use of psychological techniques in the management of chronic pain:

- The first and most important principle is the education of children and their parents about the multidimensional nature of pain and its treatment as it is crucial to the success of behavioral approaches.[26–28] The dualistic categorization of pain as organic or functional especially needs to be avoided. Psychological rehabilitative strategies need to be understood as essential treatment components and not as treatments for pain when no organic basis can be identified or when pain is seen as psychological in origin.[29] Explaining how psychological interventions take advantage of the plasticity of the sensory system involved in the perception of pain and include both psychological and physical strategies to decrease discomfort and disability associated with chronic pain can help parents better appreciate the value of psychological interventions. Without an understanding of the role psychological treatments play in the treatment of pain and the mechanisms by which they may exert their effects, children and parents may refuse such treatments, due to concern that health care providers do not see their pain as "real."
- The second principle involves taking a rehabilitative approach that emphasizes improving the child's and family's ability to cope with the chronic condition. The focus shifts from the narrow goal of pain reduction and broadens to include decreasing pain-related emotional and behavioral disability, and thereby increasing the child's functional status.[30]
- The third principle is the recognition that interventions need to be tailored to the child's individual characteristics, not just to his/her specific pain condition. For example, children's developmental level will determine what types of assessment tools can be used, how they understand their pain, the factors that may shape their pain experience, the coping skills they can use for managing pain, and the most suitable treatment regimen that will fit their needs.

The initial comprehensive assessment of the child's pain guides the treatments chosen. Psychological interventions include a diverse array of techniques that treat chronic pain by modifying children's cognitive, affective, and sensory experience of pain, their behavior in response to pain, and environmental and social factors that influence the child's pain experience. Some techniques deal primarily with altering situational factors that influence pain expression, such as when a family member is encouraged to acknowledge a child's coping behaviors rather than reinforcing a child's pain complaint with attention. Others work more specifically to alter the sensory aspects of the child's pain experience, as in the use of hypnoanalgesia. Techniques aimed at modifying situational factors that exacerbate chronic pain and disabilities include contingency or behavioral management methods, and modification of activity and rest cycles. Problem solving for managing and preventing pain exacerbations or relapses is central to the child and family assuming an active role in managing chronic pain. Cognitive techniques are targeted at modifying children's thoughts about their pain, in particular to increase their sense of predictability and control over their pain and to alter memories about painful experiences,[31] negative cognitions, especially catastrophizing somatic preoccupation, and pain-related rumination.[30] The teaching of active coping strategies whereby pain and pain-related behaviors and cognitions are identified and targeted for self-regulation encourages children to recognize their competence in coping. This sense of self-efficacy has been associated with positive outcomes in multiple pain management studies.[9,15]

Methods for managing sensory as well as psychological aspects of pain include relaxation, breathing and imagery exercises, hypnosis, and distraction techniques such as music, videos, bubble blowing, and pop-up books. It appears that at least one mechanism by which these methods work is that they engage the child's attention. It has further been hypothesized that the extent to which children can redirect their attention away from pain and pain-related concerns will determine the effectiveness of the psychological pain management techniques, although this latter hypothesis requires further empirical validation.

An essential component of any intervention is the ongoing assessment of the child's pain and pain-related functional disability. This assessment will ultimately determine the effectiveness of the strategies chosen, indicate what different interventions may need to be added, and provide concrete evidence of how treatment is progressing. Charting progress with treatment allows the child and family to see positive change when the increments are small, as when a child with complex regional pain syndrome is able to tolerate 10 minutes of activity on an affected limb after only having been able to tolerate only 1 to 2 minutes before treatment was initiated. In contrast to the management of acute pain, the focus in the management of chronic pain is less upon the child's pain ratings than upon the child's functional improvements. The family's help in monitoring the child's progress can encourage their taking an active role in their child's treatment, which in turn can increase their sense of efficacy in dealing with the child's chronic pain. In fact, family involvement in treatment has been shown to produce superior results to usual pediatric care for children with recurrent abdominal pain.[32,33] Not all families are ready to assume an active role, but the behavioral principle of "shaping," whereby the desired behavior is broken down into its component parts and each successive approximation of the desired behavior is reinforced by the pain clinician, can help the child and his/her parents or other carers become more involved in the child's pain management. It is also helpful to screen parents for psychiatric symptoms (e.g., SCL-90-R, Symptom Checklist 90-Revised), disability (e.g., Medical Outcomes Survey, Short Form-36), and to assess family environment with standardized questionnaires (e.g., FACES II, Family Adaptation and Cohesion Scales II) to characterize any parental or family issues that could impede the child's progress with treatment. At times, the parents themselves may need to be referred for either rehabilitation or psychiatric treatment to assist them in their efforts to help their child's rehabilitation. The child's school and other caretakers also need to be included in the treatment team to ensure a consistent approach to the child's pain and disability. For example, if a child's pain management involves strategies to cope with stress and headache pain at school, then the school nurse can prompt the child to use these strategies, rather than defaulting to having parents to pick the child up from school to rest at home.

The complex nature of chronic pain in children creates many challenges to its assessment and treatment, but this same complexity can be exploited to provide optimal methods of pain control and functional rehabilitation. Multidimensional assessment provides the foundation for optimal management of chronic pain in children. Psychological interventions include a diverse array of techniques that treat chronic pain by modifying children's cognitive, affective, and sensory experience of pain, their behavior in response to pain, and environmental and interactional factors that influence the child's pain experience. Medical treatment of a child's chronic pain without addressing the situational, psychological, and interactional factors that may contribute to pain and pain-related disability may result in poorer outcomes. Research that is informed by multidimensional models of pediatric chronic pain can guide investigators in their efforts to identify effective pain treatments, as well as the individual children for whom they work best. Finally, as prevention is the best medicine, to the fullest extent possible the lessons learned about optimal management of pain in children need to be practiced so that the incidence of suffering and disability for children with chronic pain conditions may be reduced.

MANAGEMENT OF CHRONIC PAIN

Chronic pain in children is one of the most ignored and undertreated symptoms of disease. Over the last decade there have been numerous studies in the literature that have addressed pain in children, its measurement, and management.[34–36]

TABLE 55-2. **CHRONIC PAIN IN CHILDREN: COMMON DIAGNOSES**

Neuropathic pain
    Reflex sympathetic dystrophy
    Peripheral nerve injuries
    Postamputation pain
    Deafferentation pain
Headache
Cancer pain
Chest pain
Sickle cell crisis
Recurrent abdominal pain
Back pain

This chapter discusses chronic pain and its management in children. Recurrent or persistent pain is seen in 5% to 10% of children sampled randomly. The most common diagnoses of pediatric pain patients include headache, abdominal pain, chest pain, neuropathic pain, back pain, and cancer pain (Table 55-2).

The diagnosis and management of some of the common chronic pain syndromes that are diagnosed in pediatric patients referred to the chronic pain clinic for management are briefly discussed.

COMPLEX REGIONAL PAIN SYNDROME TYPE I (CRPS-I OR REFLEX SYMPATHETIC DYSTROPHY)

Neuropathic conditions are those that are associated with injury, dysfunction, or altered excitability of portions of the peripheral or central nervous system. CRPS-1 or reflex sympathetic dystrophy (RSD) is defined as "A continuous pain in a portion of an extremity after trauma which may include fracture but does not involve major nerve lesions and is associated with sympathetic hyperactivity." This is often seen with any traumatic injury and presents as pain along with discoloration in a swollen extremity. The incidence of neuropathic pain is greater in teenage girls than in boys.[37] Due to the underdiagnosis of this syndrome in children, the general incidence in pediatric population is less reported than in adults. Although RSD has been reported in a boy of $3\frac{1}{2}$ years of age, it is generally seen in children beyond the age of 9 years and is more frequently seen in girls 11 to 13 years old. RSD is seen in girls of middle-class families, commonly over-achievers who participate in competitive athletic programs. This explanation underscores the psychological contribution to this disease state. Pain often persists despite the absence of ongoing tissue injury or inflammation.

The mechanisms that generate neuropathic pain are varied and complex. Injuries to peripheral nerves may involve crush, transection, compression, demyelination, axonal degeneration, inflammation, ischemia, or other processes. The primary loci of increased irritability following peripheral nerve injury may be at several levels in the nervous system including axonal sprouts or neuroma, the dorsal root ganglia, the dorsal horn of the spinal cord, or sites more rostral in the central nervous system.[38,39] Although neuropathic pain has generally been regarded as psychogenic in children, it is also important to understand that neuropathic pain rarely keeps the subject from harm since it involves erroneous generation of impulses.

Evaluation of Neuropathic Pain

HISTORY: A detailed history of the nature of injury, the type and duration of pain, relieving and aggravating factors, and the dependence on medications is mandatory prior to the evaluation.

PHYSICAL EVALUATION

1. A thorough and systematic neurologic examination should be obtained. A complete evaluation of motor, sensory, cerebellar, cranial nerve, reflex, cognitive, and emotional functioning is important. A concerted effort must be made to rule out the rare but possible malignancy or degenerative disorder.
2. Strength: the strength of the extremity should be evaluated on several occasions.
3. Allodynia: innocuous stimuli like stroking elicit excruciating pain. This is very characteristic of neuropathic pain. Tactile allodynia in the absence of skin problems signifies the presence of neuropathic pain.
4. Hyperalgesia: this means a patient has a decreased threshold to pain. Hyperalgesia to cold is seen more frequently than to warmth. The distribution is generally not restricted to particular dermatomes like an adult and is along a glove and stocking distribution.
5. Nerve conduction studies: these may give some insight into the location and type of nerve injury.[40] However, the use of invasive electromyogram (EMG) may not be acceptable to children.

DIAGNOSIS: Diagnosis is made usually on the basis of symptoms and signs (Table 55-3). A diagnostic test with phentolamine has been used to confirm the diagnosis and to predict the response to a sympathetic blockade.[41]

Treatment of Neuropathic Pain: The management of neuropathic pain can be frustrating for the caregiver, as well as the patient. There is no single therapy that can uniformly provide relief to these patients. Much of the management depends on the response to various clinical measures. The titration of medications is limited by the presence of side effects and complications. One of the main goals is to get the child back to a functional state and back in school. Definitive resolution of the pain is not always possible. Most of the management techniques are extrapolated from work done in adult patients[42] (Table 55-4). It is important to gain the trust of the patients and their parents. Family dynamics are important, because the added burden of familial disharmony or parental abuse can increase the symptoms. There seems to be a greater propensity for "enmeshment" in these families. The algorithm followed by our pain clinic is set out below (Fig. 55-1).[43]

1. Psychological/behavioral therapy. Behavioral measures are extremely useful in the management of neuropathic pain. Family therapy is very helpful for the family to cope with the situation.[44] We generally advocate a consultation with the medical psychologist on their first visit to the pain clinic. We have used a number of techniques including biofeedback, visual guided imagery, and structured counseling regarding coping skills.
2. Physical therapy. This is an integral part of our management of these patients. Transcutaneous electrical nerve stimulation (TENS)[45] is widely used and its efficacy studied in adults as well as children. Good therapeutic benefits with the TENS unit in children with RSD has been reported by Kessler and colleagues. Acupuncture is also helpful in these patients.[46] A dedicated physical therapist who works with our pain management team has been essential.
3. Medical therapy. Most of the work in children is extrapolated from the experience in adults. It is best to start with nonsteroidal anti-inflammatory drugs (NSAIDs) in moderate doses, followed by other medications. There are certain differences between adult and pediatric patients: neuropathic pain may differ in children and in adults in its presenting symptoms; there may be a difference in the response to medication; and there may be unrecognized toxicity to medications.

TABLE 55-3. SYMPTOMS AND CHANGES WITH VARIOUS STAGES OF CRPS-I

Characteristic	Acute	Dystrophic	Atrophic
Pain	Hyperpathic and burning	Hyperpathic	Hyperalgesia
Blood flow	Increased	Decreased	No change
Temperature	Increased	Decreased	No change
Hair and nail growth	Increased	Decreased	Chronic change
Sweating	Decreased	Increased	No change
Edema	None	Brawny edema	Wasted muscles, atrophic skin
Color	Red	Cyanotic	Atrophic

TABLE 55-4. **MANAGEMENT OF NEUROPATHIC PAIN**

Nonpharmacological treatment
Offered to all patients
Hypnosis, biofeedback, visual guided imagery (psychologist)
TENS and physical therapy
Individual and family therapy

Pharmacological therapy
Acetaminophen, NSAIDs
Tricyclic antidepressants, e.g., amitriptyline, nortriptyline,
    doxepin (start low doses 0.1 mg/kg and advance slowly)
Anticonvulsants (carbamazepine, phenytoin, clonazepam),
    systemic local anesthetics (mexiletine, lidocaine)
Opioids (morphine, methadone given orally or intravenously
    or through a regional technique especially in cancer
    patients)

Regional blockades for chronic pain
Epidural, subarachnoid, and sympathetic plexus blockade
Sympathetic blockade for CRPS – Type I
    >8 years under sedation
    <8 years under general anesthesia
    Continuous catheter techniques may be used for
    5 to 7 days
    Epidural and subarachnoid block for cancer patients: left
    in place for longer periods by tunneling subcutaneously
    Neurolytic blockade for cancer

NSAID, nonsteroidal anti-inflammatory drug; RSD, reflex sympathetic dystrophy; TENS, transcutaneous electrical nerve stimulation.

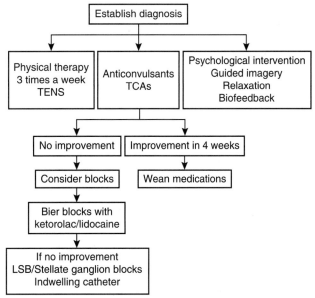

FIGURE 55-1. Algorithm for the management of CRPS-1. (Modified from Suresh S, Wheeler M, Patel A: Case series: IV regional anesthesia with ketorolac and lidocaine: Is it effective for the management of complex regional pain syndrome 1 in children and adolescents? Anesth Analg 96:694–695, 2003.)

TRICYCLIC ANTIDEPRESSANTS: Adults are frequently placed on tricyclic antidepressants (TCAs) for the management of neuropathic pain.[47] Despite the lack of adequate pediatric controlled studies, TCAs are widely prescribed for several forms of neuropathic pain. The choice of agents depends on the side effects. If the patient is unable to sleep at night, amitriptyline may be a good choice. On the other hand, if the patient experiences a lot of anticholinergic side effects like dry mouth and morning sleepiness, an agent such as nortriptyline or desimipramine can be used. A thorough examination of the cardiovascular system is necessary prior to instituting TCA treatment because of associated tachydysrhythmias and other conduction abnormalities of the heart particularly prolonged Q-T syndrome.

ANTICONVULSANTS: Some children seem to benefit from the use of anticonvulsants in the management of neuropathic pain. Gabapentin, carbamazepine, clonazepam, and phenytoin are the most commonly used. Regular monitoring of drug levels, blood counts, and liver function studies are recommended for these patients. Carbamazepine has especially proven to be very useful in neuropathic pain. More recently the use of gabapentin has been shown to be very effective in the management of neuropathic pain.[48,49]

OPIOIDS: Opioids can be helpful in the management of neuropathic pain, especially for cancer-related neuropathic pain. Arner and colleagues have shown that there are several types of neuropathic pain that are resistant to the effects of opioids.[50] They have shown that opioids reduce the emotional aspect of pain, rather than the sensory aspect of pain. It is optimal to titrate the narcotic in a graded fashion in order to optimize the effect. Sedation is a side effect that may be desirable and in some cases may need to be antagonized with the addition of amphetamines.[41,51] For those children with noncancer neuropathic pain, it is desirable to try nonopioid techniques, including behavior modification, prior to starting on large doses of opioids. We prefer using oral opioids like morphine, hydromorphone, methadone, and oxycodone with the doses titrated individually to suit each patient.

SYSTEMIC VASODILATORS: Several patients with RSD have benefited from the use of vasodilators like prazosin, nifedipine, or phenoxybenzamine.[52] Overwhelming adverse effects of orthostatic hypotension often offset the efficacy of this therapy.

SYMPATHETIC BLOCKS: The most common treatment for these syndromes is to provide interruption of the apparent pathologic reflexes by sympathetic blocks. With serial blocks the patient should notice pain relief that increases with each block and prevents the pain from returning to its original level. If no symptomatic relief is obtained after two or three blocks, an alternative approach should be instituted. Concurrent physical therapy is indicated to improve range of motion and improve function.

We prefer intravenous regional Bier blocks for the management of pain in RSD.[43,53] Using mild sedation, and, after venous drainage of the extremity, a tourniquet is placed on the proximal end of the extremity. Intravenous local anesthetic with ketorolac is injected into a distal vein. The tourniquet is kept inflated for about 30 minutes and then slowly released. A single block has provided total pain relief in some patients in our pain clinic.

An alternative approach to the management of the peripheral manifestations of neuropathic pain is to use adrenergic blocking drugs such as guanethidine (not available in the USA) or bretylium as an intravenous regional technique. Occasionally in the patient with upper extremity RSD, a stellate ganglion block may be necessary to alleviate pain. Lumbar sympathetic blocks and epidural blocks with local anesthetics are resorted to if the initial Bier block with local anesthetic and ketorolac is not effective. Several sympathetic blocks at intervals of 1 to 2 weeks may be necessary in order to see improvement in symptoms.

Prognosis: Varni has reported uniform improvement among his series of patients in a prolonged program of physical therapy and inpatient rehabilitation programs.[54] Ashwal et al. in a review conclude that the prognosis of childhood RSD is more favorable than adult RSD.[55] Out of the 55 children that Olsson reported, 33 underwent complete remission with one intravenous regional sympathetic block, 14 were improved, and in 7 the block had no effect. Neuropathic pain can be puzzling and frustrating and requires a strong alliance with the family and the patient. A multidisciplinary approach with an algorithmic management using available techniques can be helpful.

HEADACHES IN CHILDREN

Few physicians discussed headaches in children until 1873 when William Henry Day, a British pediatrician, devoted a chapter to the subject of headaches in his book *Essays on Diseases in Children*.[56] In 1967 Freidman and Harms published much of the available data in the book *Headaches in Children*.[57] These early works have given a lot of impetus to the many subsequent papers dealing with headaches in children. Each year at least 80% of the population will suffer from headaches. However, many child care providers do not think that children have appreciable number of headaches. In a study of 9,000 children in Sweden Bille reported an incidence of 75% of children under the age of 15 reporting headaches.[58] The difficulty for the practitioner arises from the fact that the headache may be functional. A thorough physical examination helps to determine the nature of the headache.

Pathophysiology: A headache is modulated by extracranial as well as intracranial structures (Table 55-5).

Classification: The classification of headaches is based on the presumed location of the abnormality, its origin, its pathophysiology, or the symptom complex with which the patient presents. The International Headache Society has recently updated its classification. By plotting the severity of a headache over time, headaches can be classified into five major categories (Table 55-6).

Evaluation: A thorough questionnaire should be routinely used to evaluate headaches in children. Other specific questions

TABLE 55-5. HEADACHE: PATHOPHYSIOLOGY

Pain sensitive
Extracranial
Skin
Subcutaneous tissue
Muscles
Mucous membrane
Teeth
Larger vessels
Intracranial
Vascular sinuses
Larger veins
Dura surrounding the veins
Dural arteries
Arteries at the base of the brain
Pain insensitive
Brain
Cranium
Most of the dura
Ependyma
Choroid plexus

about neurologic symptoms like ataxia, lethargy, seizures, or visual impairments are asked. Other important medical problems like hypertension, sinusitis, and other emotional disturbances have to be evaluated. A history of a severe headache without a previous history of headache, pain that awakens a child from sleep, headaches associated with straining, change

TABLE 55-6. CLASSIFICATION OF HEADACHES: DIFFERENTIAL DIAGNOSIS

Acute
Systemic illness
Subarachnoid hemorrhage
Trauma
Toxins like lead or carbon monoxide
Electrolyte imbalances
Hypertension
Acute Recurrent Headaches
Migraine
Chronic progressive headaches
Organic brain disease
Ventriculoperitoneal shunt malfunction
Chronic Nonprogressive headaches
Functional in quality
Mixed headaches

TABLE 55-7. **EXAMINATION FOR HEADACHES**

General physical examination
Blood pressure
Careful skin examination for café au lait, adenoma
   sebaceum, hypopigmented lesions, petechiae

Neurological examination
Cranial circumference measurement
Bruit on ausculatation of the cranium
Tenderness in the sinuses or presence of occult trauma
   indicating a battered child
Funduscopic examination: optic atrophy, papilloedema
Cranial nerve examination for the presence of damage
Mental status
Alteration in language skills
Alteration in the gait

Laboratory tests
EEG: very nonspecific
CT scan especially with contrast may be useful in
   determining vascular abnormalities
MRI: best for delineating abnormalities in the sella turcica,
   posterior fossa, and temporal lobes
Lumbar puncture is helpful in determining acute infectious
   causes
Psychological tests to determine if there is a psychological
   basis for the headache

---

in chronic headache patterns, or the presence of a headache with associated symptoms like nausea or vomiting suggests a more pathological origin to the headache and has to be very carefully evaluated (Table 55-7).

We have had particular success with patients with ventriculoperitoneal (VP) shunts with headaches that are not related to a shunt malfunction.

Headaches in Patients with Ventriculoperitoneal Shunts:

Headaches in children are a perplexing problem by itself. We have several patients referred to us by the neurosurgery service for management of headaches not related to shunt malfunctions. The presence of a VP shunt may pose an additional risk to the patient and a diagnostic dilemma for the care provider. These patients are also subjected to emotional and psychological stress associated with chronic illness. Self-esteem and the will to excel academically are also altered to a great degree. The management of these children involves a multidisciplinary approach with the involvement of several specialties including anesthesiology, neurosurgery, neurology, and psychiatry services, and physical therapy. An aggressive approach to managing these children has led to a decrease in operative procedures, school absenteeism, fewer visits to the hospital and increased self-esteem.

We routinely review the patient's clinical status and computed tomography (CT) scans with the neurosurgeons. Once it has been established by the neurosurgical service that the headaches are not related to increased intracranial pressure, we schedule the patient for a visit to the chronic pain clinic. The following information is obtained:

- Neurological status including a complete neurological examination.
- Physical status of the patient (i.e., is the patient actively mobile?).
- Does the headache prevent the child from performing his or her normal activities, e.g., interacting with others, participating in sports, etc.?
- Is there school absenteeism?
- What is the child's interaction with the parents and siblings at home?
- Are there any relieving factors for the headache?
- Has the child been placed on any medications for pain? Has there been any improvement at all in the clinical characteristic of pain?
- When was the last shunt revision? Was the pain any better after the last shunt revision?

Having answered some or all the questions, we then offer various modalities in a step-ladder fashion based on the pain status.

We have treated several patients in our institution who had been debilitated due to headaches and have now resumed normal activity. Most of these children also have musculoskeletal problems. Hence the addition of physical therapy has been shown to increase muscle strength and also help in the recovery of these patients. The intervention of our medical psychologist proficient in pain management has been vital to their recovery. They not only help deal with family dynamics but also help in the management of pain by teaching the patient coping mechanisms, visual guided imagery, and biofeedback techniques.

CANCER PAIN

One of the most challenging issues that is presented to us is the management of cancer pain, especially in the terminally ill patient. The management of pain in cancer patients requires the understanding of normal childhood development and the natural history and treatment of childhood malignancies.[59–62] Pain in a cancer patient can result from:

- **Tumor invasion.** Cancer-related pain can be recognized from knowledge of the natural history of the tumor in question. Bone pain is most common, usually from a metastasis of the tumor to the bone. Other less common, but important, reasons for cancer-related pain include compression of the spinal cord, tumor involvement of the central or the peripheral nervous system, and viscus obstruction.
- **Procedure.** This pain arises from bone marrow aspiration, lumbar puncture, venipuncture, etc. Its optimal management is important for the well-being of the child and family and, in some cases, for the success of the anticancer treatment.
- **Therapy.** The type of tumor and the anticancer therapy that is being administered can predict the magnitude of pain. Most commonly seen problems include mucositis, neuropathy, surgical incisions, corticosteroid-induced bone changes, and gastritis from mucosal damage.

TABLE 55-8. ANALGESIC INTERVENTION FOR CHILDREN WITH CANCER PAIN

Anticancer therapy 　Radiotherapy 　Chemotherapy 　Biologic therapy 　Surgery
Analgesic drugs
Noninvasive techniques 　Transcutaneous nerve stimulation 　Physical therapy 　Hypnosis 　Biofeedback 　Relaxation
Neurosurgical interventions
Regional nerve blocks
Supportive counseling

TABLE 55-9. APPROACHES TO PAIN MANAGEMENT IN TERMINALLY ILL PATIENTS

Pharmacological Opioid analgesics Nonsteroidal analgesics Steroids
Chemotherapy
Psychological Support Distraction Hypnosis
Anesthetic Regional anesthetics 　Indwelling epidural and intrathecal catheters 　Regional blocks
Surgical Neuroablative procedures Tumor debulking to reduce compression
Physical therapy TENS Acupuncture Heat/cooling Exercise

TENS, transcutaneous electrical nerve stimulation.

Evaluation of Cancer Pain: The following are factors in the evaluation of cancer pain:

- Etiology and location of the painful source.
- Qualitative features and intensity of the pain.
- Anticipated course of painful experience, i.e., the nature of clinical spread of the disease.
- Nature and efficacy of recent analgesic therapy.
- Available routes of administration of medication (i.e., central venous access).
- Psychological state of the child and the family.
- Age-appropriate pain assessment.

The World Health Organization has suggested an analgesic step-ladder protocol for the management of pain in cancer patients (Table 55-8).[63]

The analgesic intervention of a child with cancer involves a multidisciplinary approach (Table 55-9). Multiple methods are available, but have to be chosen on the merit of the treatment modality in managing the pain and the effect it has on the child.

PAIN IN TERMINAL ILLNESS

There has recently been a surge in treatment modalities and children have been part of a cure-oriented and technology-based heath care system. Recently, with the involvement of organizations like hospices, the care of terminally ill children has been developed, based on the same philosophy as that of adults.[64] Pain can be a significant problem in children who require terminal care. When some children with a life-threatening illness have a significant setback, there may be no firm criteria to stop treatment and direct palliative care.

Alternative novel methods for providing analgesia have been used by our pain service in children who do not have intravenous access. Nebulized opioids or the use of transdermal delivery systems have been used to offset pain in children with intractable pain.[65,66] The adverse effect associated with long-term use of opioids include tolerance and withdrawal. Careful rotation of opioids along with the judicious use of other adjuvants including N-methyl-D-aspartate (NMDA) receptor antagonists should be considered in their care.

Several approaches to pain management are taken based on the state of the patient, the involvement of the disease process, and the general state of the caregivers. Patient-controlled analgesia (PCA) has been widely used in our institution for home-bound patients with terminal cancer.[67] Smaller, more user-friendly pumps have been devised for easy programming and less frequent changing.[68,69] In patients who do not have venous access we have recommended the use of subcutaneous PCA. A number of other drugs are very useful in the terminally ill child. NSAIDs and steroids are particularly useful in the management of bone pain from metastasis.[70,71] Carbamazepine, gabapentin, and TCAs are useful for the management of neuropathic pain.[72] TCAs can be used for the management of neuropathic pain. Hypnosis, biofeedback, and distraction techniques can be used very effectively in children who are not heavily sedated.[73–75]

A child's view of death is very different from that of an adult. There is a consistent progression of the conceptual aspect of death in children as they grow older. The school age child finally understands the permanence of death. Home care may be very useful for the family to cope with the grief and sorrow. It also allows other siblings to spend some time with a loved one. A home care coordinator should be available for the management of any adverse conditions. Knowing the family helps the coordinator understand the goals of the family. One of the basic tenets of hospice care is to enable the patient to lead a full life, of the best quality, for what time they have remaining. Cooperation between the family and the care giver should allow the child to die with as much dignity as possible. It is the responsibility of the home coordinator to give the care givers enough information on the management of pain.

The combination of various techniques for the management of cancer pain is to enhance the child's motivation and will to lead as normal a life as is allowed by the disease state.

CONCLUSION

Pediatric pain is mostly a hidden problem. No attempt to meet a need is begun until the need has been documented. Careful surveys of children in hospitals or in outpatient settings can yield data on prevalence and severity of pain for both professionals and policy makers. A standard of practice in pediatric pain is needed. With the understanding of pain in children and the presence of available professional help, more children can be helped by chronic pain clinics. A multidisciplinary approach to pain management helps determine the course of action and prognosis of the particular patient. When pediatric pain is severe, most management techniques include potent analgesics or the use of narcotics. There is a lot of resistance to the use of narcotics in children for fear of addiction or the increase in respiratory depression. This may also pose an ethical dilemma to nursing staff.[76] The use of various methods including physical therapy and the services of a good child psychiatry/psychology department can help children cope and overcome persistent pain. Chronic pain can be devastating to a child's morale and has to be treated the same way any other disease is addressed. The key to good continuing care for these children is a multidisciplinary approach with a psychologist, physical therapist, and a pain management specialist.

REFERENCES

1. Cassidy JT: Progress in diagnosing and understanding chronic pain syndromes in children. [Review]. Curr Opin Rheumatol 6:544–546, 1994.
2. Webster BS, Snook SH: The cost of 1989 workers' compensation low back pain claims. Spine 19:1111–1115, 1994.
3. Perquin CW, Hunfeld JA, Hazebroek-Kampschreur AA, et al: Insights in the use of health care services in chronic benign pain in childhood and adolescence. Pain 94:205–213, 2001.
4. Breau LM, McGrath PJ, Camfield C, et al: Preliminary validation of an observational pain checklist for persons with cognitive impairments and inability to communicate verbally. Dev Med Child Neurol 42:609–616, 2000.
5. Stevens BJ, Franck L: Special needs of preterm infants in the management of pain and discomfort. J Obstet Gynecol Neonatal Nurs 24:856–862, 1995.
6. Grunau RE, Holsti L, Whitfield MF, Ling E: Are twitches, startles, and body movements pain indicators in extremely low birth weight infants? Clin J Pain 16:37–45, 2000.
7. Pasero CL, Reed B, McCaffery M: How aging affects pain management. Am J Nurs 98:12–13, 1998.
8. Manne SL, Jacobsen PB, Redd WH: Assessment of acute pediatric pain: Do child self-report, parent ratings, and nurse ratings measure the same phenomenon? Pain 48:45–52, 1992.
9. Thompson KL, Varni JW: A developmental cognitive-biobehavioral approach to pediatric pain assessment. Pain 25:283–296, 1986.
10. Andrews K, Fitzgerald M: Biological barriers to paediatric pain management. Clin J Pain 13:138–143, 1997.
11. McGrath PA: Pain in the pediatric patient: Practical aspects of assessment. Pediatr Ann 24:126–128, 1995.
12. Merlijn VP, Hunfeld JA, van der Wouden JC, et al: Psychosocial factors associated with chronic pain in adolescents. Pain 101:33–43, 2003.
13. Merlijn VP, Hunfeld JA, van der Wouden JC, et al: Shortening a quality of life questionnaire for adolescents with chronic pain and its psychometric qualities. Psychol Rep 90:753–759, 2002.
14. Blount RL, Schaen ER, Cohen LL: Commentary: Current status and future directions in acute pediatric pain assessment and treatment. J Pediatr Psychol 24:150–152, 1999.
15. Varni JW, Jay SM, Massek BJ, et al: Cognitive-behavioral assessment and management of pediatric pain. In Holzman ATD (ed): Pain Management: A Handbook of Psychological Treatment Approaches. Pergamon, New York, 1986, pp 168–192.
16. Masek BJ, Russo DC, Varni JW: Behavioral approaches to the management of chronic pain in children [Review]. Pediatric Clin North Am 31:1113–1131, 1984.
17. Hunfeld JA, Perquin CW, Hazebroek-Kampschreur AA, et al: Physically unexplained chronic pain and its impact on children and their families: The mother's perception. Psychol Psychother 75:251–260, 2002.
18. Reid GJ, Lang BA, McGrath PJ: Primary juvenile fibromyalgia: Psychological adjustment, family functioning, coping, and functional disability. Arthritis Rheum 40:752–760, 1997.
19. Williamson GM, Walters AS, Shaffer DR: Caregiver models of self and others, coping, and depression: Predictors of depression in children with chronic pain. Health Psychol 21:405–410, 2002.
20. Keefe FJ, Bonk V: Psychosocial assessment of pain in patients having rheumatic diseases. Rheum Dis Clin North Am 25:81–103, 1999.
21. Lewin DS, Dahl RE: Importance of sleep in the management of pediatric pain. J Dev Behav Pediatr 20:244–252, 1999.
22. Hershey AD, Powers SW, Bentti AL, et al: Characterization of chronic daily headaches in children in a multidisciplinary headache center. Neurology 56:1032–1037, 2001.
23. Varni JW, Seid M, Smith KT, et al: The PedsQL in pediatric rheumatology: Reliability, validity, and responsiveness of the Pediatric Quality of Life Inventory Generic Core Scales and Rheumatology Module. Arthritis Rheum 46:714–725, 2002.
24. Hunfeld JA, Perquin CW, Duivenvoorden HJ, et al: Chronic pain and its impact on quality of life in adolescents and their families. J Pediatr Psychol 26:145–153, 2001.
25. Powers SW, Mitchell MJ, Byars KC, et al: A pilot study of one-session biofeedback training in pediatric headache. Neurology 56:133, 2001.
26. McGrath PJ, Vair C: Psychological aspects of pain management of the burned child. Child Health Care 13:15–19, 1984.
27. McGrath PJ, Johnson GG: Pain management in children. Can J Anaesth 35:107–110, 1988.
28. Fanurik D, Zeltzer LK, Roberts MC, Blount RL: The relationship between children's coping styles and psychological interventions for cold pressor pain. Pain 53:213–222, 1993.
29. Kuttner L: Managing pain in children. Changing treatment of headaches. Can Fam Physician 39:563–568, 1993.
30. Zeltzer L, Bursch B, Walco G: Pain responsiveness and chronic pain: A psychobiological perspective. J Dev Behav Pediatr 18:413–422, 1997.
31. Chen PP, Ma M, Chan S, Oh TE: Incident reporting in acute pain management. Anaesthesia 53:730–735, 1998.

32. Sanders MR, Rebgetz M, Morrison M, et al: Cognitive-behavioral treatment of recurrent nonspecific abdominal pain in children: An analysis of generalization, maintenance, and side effects. J Consult Clin Psychol 57:294–300, 1989.

33. Sanders MR, Shepherd RW, Cleghorn G, Woolford H: The treatment of recurrent abdominal pain in children: A controlled comparison of cognitive-behavioral family intervention and standard pediatric care. J Consult Clin Psychol 62:306–314, 1994.

34. Anand KJ, Hickey PR: Pain and its effects in the human neonate and fetus [Review]. N Engl J Med 317:1321–1329, 1987.

35. Romej M, Voepel-Lewis T, Merkel SI, et al: Effect of preemptive acetaminophen on postoperative pain scores and oral fluid intake in pediatric tonsillectomy patients. AANA J 64:535–540, 1996.

36. McGrath P, Johnson G, Goodman J: CHEOPS: A behavioral scale for rating postoperative pain in children. Adv Pain Res Ther 9:395–402, 1985.

37. Wilder RT, Berde CB, Wolohan M, et al: Reflex sympathetic dystrophy in children. Clinical characteristics and follow-up of seventy patients. JBJS (Am) 74:910–919, 1992.

38. Stanton-Hicks M: Reflex sympathetic dystrophy: A sympathetically mediated pain syndrome or not? Curr Rev Pain 4:268–275, 2000.

39. Stanton-Hicks M: Complex regional pain syndrome (type I, RSD; type II, causalgia): Controversies. Clin J Pain 16:S33–S40, 2000.

40. Konen A: Measurement of nerve dysfunction in neuropathic pain. Curr Rev Pain 4:388–394, 2000.

41. Arner S: Intravenous phentolamine test: Diagnostic and prognostic use in reflex sympathetic dystrophy. Pain 46:17–22, 1991.

42. Stanton-Hicks M, Baron R, Boas R, et al: Complex regional pain syndromes: Guidelines for therapy [see comments]. Clin J Pain 14:155–166, 1998.

43. Suresh S, Wheeler M, Patel A: Case series: IV regional anesthesia with ketorolac and lidocaine: Is it effective for the management of complex regional pain syndrome 1 in children and adolescents [table]. Anesth Analg 96:694–695, 2003.

44. Brown CR: Pain management. Biofeedback and relaxation therapy. Pract Periodontics Aesthet Dent 9:1068, 1997.

45. Kesler RW, Saulsbury FT, Miller LT, Rowlingson JC: Reflex sympathetic dystrophy in children: Treatment with transcutaneous electric nerve stimulation. Pediatr Ann 82:728–732, 1988.

46. Kemper KJ, Sarah R, Silver-Highfield E, et al: On pins and needles? Pediatric pain patients' experience with acupuncture. Pediatr Ann 105:941–947, 2000.

47. Richlin DM: Nonnarcotic analgesics and tricyclic antidepressants for the treatment of chronic nonmalignant pain. Mt Sinai J Med 58:221–228, 1991.

48. Wheeler DS, Vaux KK, Tam DA: Use of gabapentin in the treatment of childhood reflex sympathetic dystrophy. Pediatr Neurol 22:220–221, 2000.

49. Mellick GA, Mellick LB: Reflex sympathetic dystrophy treated with gabapentin. Arch Phys Med Rehabil 78:98–105, 1997.

50. Arner S, Killander E, Westerberg H: [Poor leadership behind poor pain relief. Medical audit of cancer-related pain treatment]. Lakartidningen 96:33–36, 1999.

51. O'Neill WM: The cognitive and psychomotor effects of opioid drugs in cancer pain management. Cancer Surv 21:67–84, 1994.

52. Paulson RR: Reflex sympathetic dystrophy in a teenaged girl. Postgrad Med 81:66–67, 1987.

53. Connelly NR, Reuben S, Brull SJ: Intravenous regional anesthesia with ketorolac-lidocaine for the management of sympathetically mediated pain. Yale J Biol Med 68:95–99, 1995.

54. Varni JW: Behavioral medicine in hemophilia arthritic pain management: Two case studies. Arch Phys Med Rehabil 62:183–187, 1981.

55. Ashwal S, Tomasi L, Neumann M, Schneider S: Reflex sympathetic dystrophy syndrome in children. Pediatr Neurol 4:38–42, 1988.

56. Day WH: Headaches in children. In Essays on Diseases of Children. J&A Churchill, 1873.

57. Freidman AP, Harms E: Headaches in Children. Charles C Thomas, Springfield, IL, 1967.

58. Bille B: Migraine in school children. Acta Paediatr 51:1–51, 1962.

59. McGrath PJ, Beyer J, Cleeland C, et al: American Academy of Pediatrics report of the subcommittee on assessment and methodologic issues in the management of pain in childhood cancer. Pediatrics 86:814–817, 1990.

60. Brown RE Jr, Schmitz ML, Andelman P: The treatment of pain in children with cancer. J Arkansas Med Soc 90:316–318, 1998.

61. Collins JJ, Grier HE, Kinney HC, Berde CB: Control of severe pain in children with terminal malignancy [see comments]. J Pediatr 126:653–657, 1995.

62. Collins JJ: Intractable pain in children with terminal cancer [Review]. J Palliat Care 12:29–34, 1996.

63. McGrath PA: Development of the World Health Organization guidelines on cancer pain relief and palliative care in children [Review]. J Pain Symptom Manage 12:87–92, 1995.

64. Hollen PJ: Intervention booster: Adding a decision-making module to risk reduction and other health care programs for adolescents. J Pediatric Health Care 12:247–255, 1998.

65. Howe JL: Nebulized morphine for hospice patients. Am J Hosp Palliat Care 12:6, 1995.

66. Collins JJ, Dunkel IJ, Gupta SK, et al: Transdermal fentanyl in children with cancer pain: Feasibility, tolerability, and pharmacokinetic correlates. J Pediatrics 134:319–323, 1999.

67. Dunbar PJ, Buckley P, Gavrin JR, et al: Use of patient-controlled analgesia for pain control for children receiving bone marrow transplant. J Pain Symptom Manage 10:604–611, 1995.

68. Suresh S, Anand KJ: Opioid tolerance in neonates: Mechanisms, diagnosis, assessment, and management [Review]. Semin Perinatol 22:425–433, 1998.

69. Berde CB, et al: Cancer Pain Relief and Palliative Care in Children. WHO Press, Geneva, 1998.

70. Chiang JS: New developments in cancer pain therapy. Acta Anaesthesiol Sin 38:31–36, 2000.

71. Kasai H, Sasaki K, Tsujinaga H, Hoshino T: [Pain management in advanced pediatric cancer patients – A proposal of the two-step analgesic ladder]. Masui 44:885–889, 1995.

72. Rosner H, Rubin L, Kestenbaum A: Gabapentin adjunctive therapy in neuropathic pain states. Clin J Pain 12:56–58, 1996.

73. Montgomery GH, DuHamel KN, Redd WH: A meta-analysis of hypnotically induced analgesia: How effective is hypnosis? Int J Clin Exp Hypn 48:138–153, 2000.

74. Rusy LM, Weisman SJ: Complementary therapies for acute pediatric pain management. Pediatr Clin North Am 47:589–599, 2000.

75. Belgrade MJ: Control of pain in cancer patients. Postgrad Med 85:319, 1989.

76. Siever BA: Pain management and potentially life-shortening analgesia in the terminally ill child: The ethical implications for pediatric nurses. J Pediatr Nurs 9:307–312, 1994.

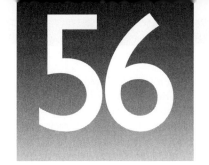

Geriatric Pain

Lowell Davis, D.O.,
Robert E. Molloy, M.D., and
Honorio T. Benzon, M.D.

The definition of geriatric medicine is a concept that is progressively changing. What was old 50 years ago can be considered middle aged today. Geriatric medicine has been defined as a branch of medicine that concerns itself with the aging process: the prevention, diagnosis, and treatment of health care problems in the aged. The US population aged 65 years and older increased by more than 30% from 1994 to 1999.[1] Older Americans constitute the fastest growing segment of the nation's population. At the turn of the millennium, 13.1% of the population were over the age of 65; and by 2030 it is projected that 20% may be over the age of 65.[2] The higher rates of chronic illness and need for assistance with activities of daily living that characterize this frail population may soon overwhelm many health service systems.[3] We are not prepared for the burdens this will place on our health care and financing systems. Approximately 35% of total health care dollars are spent on the geriatric population.[3,4] In developed countries the geriatric patient uses medical services at a rate three to four times higher than the general population, which primarily reflects the increased prevalence of most diseases and physical disabilities among this population.[4] Advances in preventative and curative medicine have increased life expectancy, but, in many cases, living longer means getting sicker. Increased morbidity in the elderly is associated with a higher prevalence of painful conditions.[4]

According to the International Association for the Study of Pain, pain is defined as "an unpleasant sensory and emotional experience associated with actual or potential tissue damage."[5] Pain is now recognized as a complex, multidimensional phenomenon that is sensory, perceptual, and subjective in nature. The terms persistent or chronic pain are used interchangeably in the medical literature. Chronic or persistent pain can be defined as a painful experience that continues for a prolonged period of time, usually greater than six months, and that may or may not be associated with a recognizable disease process. Classifying persistent pain into pathophysiologic terms may help the clinician select therapy and determine prognosis.

Four basic categories that encompass most syndromes can be described:

- *Malignant pain* that arises from the effects of cancer's effects on the body.
- *Nonmalignant pain* includes pain from tissue inflammation, mechanical deformation, ongoing injury, or destruction. Some examples are musculoskeletal pain, visceral, and somatic pain.
- *Neuropathic pain* which results from damage to the peripheral nerves or central nervous system. Examples include diabetic neuropathy, reflex sympathetic dystrophy, phantom limb pain, and central pain syndrome.
- *Psychologically based pain.* Examples include somatoform disorders and conversion reactions.

The prevalence of pain increases with each decade of life.[6] Pain is a common experience for many elderly adults; it has negative consequences for their health, functioning, and quality of life. Pain is one of the most common symptoms reported by the elderly during office visits, but continues to be overlooked by many physicians.[6] The reasons for this under treatment of pain are poorly understood, but physicians and caregivers very often find it difficult to assess the elderly patient's complaints. Only 1% of the medical papers published about pain are related to geriatric pain.[7] Older adults are twice as likely to experience pain in comparison to younger adults. In the community setting, an estimated 25% to 50% of the elderly experience pain. Some 75% to 85% of elderly people in residential settings report pain, with one-third reporting chronic pain.[8,9] Population-based studies also suggest that the prevalence of pain increases with age, although pain reports tend to decrease slightly among the oldest. The prevalence of pain is approximately two-fold higher in those over the age of 60 compared to those under the age of 60.[10]

Population studies indicate that up to 50% of geriatric outpatients and 80% of nursing home residents suffer from chronic pain.[11] A recent survey found that one in five older Americans are taking analgesic medications regularly, and 63% of those had taken prescription pain medications for more than six months. The survey also acknowledged that 45% of patients who take pain medications regularly had seen three or more doctors for pain in the past five years, 79% of whom were primary care physicians.[12] It has also been reported that 71% of nursing home residents had at least one pain complaint, and 51% described pain on a daily basis.[13]

Many epidemiological studies conducted in the community setting have reported that the overall prevalence of pain complaints, including headache, migraine, and low back pain, peaks in middle age and decreases thereafter.[14–16] In contrast, there have been reports of an age-related increase in the prevalence of persistent pain, joint pain, and fibromyalgia.[17] An age-related decrease in the prevalence of pain problems for all sites other than the joints has also been reported.[18]

ASSESSMENT OF PERSISTENT PAIN

The approach to medical care of the elderly requires a perspective different from that of younger generations. A thorough pain history is essential for management of the older patient. The spectrum of complaints, manifestations of distress, and differential diagnoses are often different in the elderly which make this a very challenging process.[19] Older patients often present with multiple medical problems, many of which are irreversible; and cure-oriented physicians are especially vulnerable to frequent disappointments.[20] Accurate assessment will help to identify the underlying source and associated physiologic pain mechanisms and to select the most effective treatment to maximize patient outcome. The following are examples of some geriatric symptoms and conditions:[20]

- Dementia
- Inappropriate prescribing of medications
- Incontinence
- Depression
- Delirium
- Iatrogenesis, including consequences of hospitalization and bed rest
- Falls
- Osteoporosis
- Alterations in the special senses including hearing and vision impairment
- Failure to thrive
- Immobility and gait disturbances
- Pressure ulcers
- Sleep disorders
- Nonspecific presentation of disease

It is important to have knowledge of diseases and disorders that are more common or have particular features in older people. Caregivers should have at least "broad" knowledge of the pathophysiology, presenting signs and symptoms, differential diagnosis, and initial diagnostic evaluation for common diseases in older people, including:[21]

- Rheumatological diseases (e.g., osteoarthritis, rheumatoid arthritis, temporal arteritis/polymyalgia rheumatica)
- Genitourological diseases (e.g., benign prostatic hyperplasia, sexual dysfunction)

- Neurological diseases (e.g., Parkinson's disease, stroke and transient ischemic attack, dizziness/syncope)
- Cardiovascular diseases (e.g., congestive heart failure, atrial fibrillation, valvular heart disease); hypertension (diastolic and systolic)
- Endocrinological diseases (e.g., type II diabetes mellitus, hyperosmolar nonketotic coma, hyper- and hypothyroidism, Paget's disease of the bone)
- Cancer of various organs, including breast, lung, colon, prostate, and hematologic malignancies
- Infections, including: pneumonia, tuberculosis, and urinary tract infection
- Renal diseases (e.g., fluid and electrolyte disturbances)
- Gastroenterological disorders (e.g., constipation, malnutrition, diverticulitis, diverticulosis)
- Psychiatric diseases (e.g., depression)
- Others, such as fractures, amyloidosis

Age differences in the experience of chronic pain remain unclear. Evidence regarding age differences in postoperative pain levels is equivocal. Although several studies have suggested that elderly patients report lower pain intensity than younger patients, others have found that age is not related to postoperative pain intensity.[22,23] A serious barrier to progress in the field of pain and aging arises from the lack of data regarding the psychometric properties of pain scales for use with the elderly.[24] Pain is an undertreated and often undiagnosed problem amongst the geriatric population.[25] It has been known to decrease function, increase agitation, increase emotional distress, and possibly increase the risk of mortality.[26,27] Moreover, inadequate assessment tools and procedures often compromise adequate pain treatment, particularly in the institutional setting.[28] Thorough pain assessment requires careful, detailed communication between the patient and the caregiver. Pain assessment should include observation of physical function and range of motion; determining the degree of anxiety and depression present; and assessment of coping skills and pain-related fears. A multidisciplinary team should be incorporated when diagnosing and treating chronic pain. This team should consist of a pain specialist, physical therapist, and a psychologist or psychiatrist.

A publication of the American Geriatrics Society Panel on Persistent Pain in Older Persons is germane to this topic. The specific recommendations for the assessment of pain in the elderly are as follows:[29]

I.   On initial presentation or admission of any older person to any health care service, a healthcare professional should assess the patient for evidence of persistent pain.
II. Any persistent pain that has an impact on physical function, psychological function, or other aspects of quality of life should be recognized as a significant problem.
III. All patients with persistent pain that may affect physical function, psychosocial function, or other aspects of quality of life should undergo a comprehensive pain assessment, with the goal of identifying all potentially remedial factors.
     A. History
         1. Initial evaluation of present pain complaint should include characteristics, such as intensity, character, frequency, location, duration, and precipitating and relieving factors.

2. Initial evaluation should include a description of pain in relation to impairments in physical and social function.

3. Initial evaluation should include a thorough analgesic history, including current and previously used prescription medications, over the counter medications, complementary or alternative remedies, and alcohol use or abuse. Effectiveness and side effects of medications should be recorded.

4. The patient's attitudes and beliefs regarding pain and its management, as well as knowledge of pain management strategies, should be assessed.

5. Effectiveness of past pain-relieving treatments should be determined.

6. The patient's satisfaction with current pain treatment or health should be determined and concerns should be identified.

B. Physical examination
   1. Physical examination should include careful examination of reported pain sites, common sites for pain referral, and common sites of pain in older adults.
   2. Physical examination should focus on the musculoskeletal system. Practitioners skilled in musculoskeletal examination should be considered for consultation.
   3. Physical examination should focus on the neurologic system.
   4. Initial assessment should include observation of physical function.

C. Comprehensive pain assessment should include results of pertinent laboratory and other diagnostic tests.

D. Initial assessment should include evaluation of psychologic function, including mood, self-efficacy, pain-coping skills, helplessness, and pain-related fears.

E. Initial assessment should include evaluation of social support, caregivers, family relationships, work history, cultural environment, spirituality, and healthcare accessibility.

F. Cognitive function should be evaluated for new of worsening confusion.

G. For the older adult who is cognitively intact or has mild to moderate dementia, the practitioner should attempt to assess pain by directly querying the patient.
   1. Quantitative estimates of pain based on clinical impressions or surrogate reports should not be used as a substitute for self-report unless the patient is unable to communicate reliably his or her pain.
   2. A variety of terms synonymous with pain should be used to screen older patients.
   3. A quantitative assessment of pain should be recorded by the use of a standard pain scale that is sensitive to cognitive, language, and sensory impairments. A variety of verbal descriptor scales, pain thermometers, numeric rating scales, and facial pain scales have acceptable validity and are acceptable for many older adults.
   4. The use of a multidimensional pain instrument that evaluates pain in relation to other domains should be considered.
   5. Elderly persons with limited attention span or impaired cognition should receive repeated instructions and be given adequate time to respond. Assessment may be done in several steps, requiring assistance from family or caregivers.
   6. Patients should be queried about symptoms and signs that may indicate pain, including recent changes in activities and functional status.
   7. Patients can also be asked about their worst pain experience over the past week.
   8. With mild to moderate cognitive impairment, assessment questions should be framed in the present tense because patients are likely to have impaired recall.

IV. For the older adult with moderate to severe dementia or the older adult who is nonverbal, the practitioner should attempt to assess pain via direct observation or history from caregivers.
   A. Patients should be observed for evidence of pain-related behaviors during movement.
   B. Unusual behavior in a patient with severe dementia should trigger assessment for pain as a potential cause.

V. The risks and benefits of various assessments and treatment options should be discussed with patients and families, with consideration for patient and family preferences in the design of any assessment or treatment strategy.

VI. Patients with persistent pain should be reassessed regularly for improvements, deterioration, or complications.
   A. The use of a pain log or diary with regular entries of pain intensity, medication use, mood, response to treatment, and associated activities should be considered.
   B. The same quantitative pain assessment scales should be used for initial and follow-up assessments.
   C. Reassessment should include evaluation of analgesic and nonpharmacologic interventions, side effects, and compliance issues.
   D. Reassessment should consider patient preference in assessment and treatment revisions.

Psychometric Tools: A variety of standardized instruments and self-report tools exist to assess pain. Results of these are helpful in documenting and communicating pain experiences. Some psychometric tools may be more reliable than others, depending upon the patient's impairment. Most pain assessment instruments are either one-dimensional measures that may focus on pain intensity, or multidimensional measures of the pain experience. An example of the multidimensional scale is the McGill Pain Questionnaire (MPQ). It provides a more comprehensive picture of the pain. It assesses the sensory, affective, evaluative, temporal, and miscellaneous qualities of pain. A comprehensive pain assessment should include both types of measures, as each samples an important part of the overall experience.[23]

One-dimensional scales consist of a single item that usually relates to pain intensity alone. The most widely used one-dimensional measure is the visual analogue scale (VAS), a 10 cm line, the ends of which are anchored with descriptors of the extremes of pain intensity such as "no pain" and "worst pain possible".[30] Other examples of one-dimensional pain scales include the Verbal Descriptor Scale (VDS), the Numerical Rating Scale, and the pain thermometer. Most of these scales are easy to perform and are usually easy to administer.

In some studies increasing age has been associated with a higher frequency of incorrect responses to the VAS.[31] However, in a sample of elderly pain patients it was found that the error rate in the use of several different measures of pain intensity was comparable to that reported in the general population.[32,33] Although scores on all of the intensity scales used in this study were highly correlated, the mean scores were significantly different, indicating inconsistencies in the intensity of pain reported by the elderly in response to different tools. This difference was due mostly to the horizontal VAS, suggesting that a vertical orientation may be more appropriate for the elderly. Interestingly, 40% of this sample felt that the VDS was the easiest to use and described their pain best.[23] Although preliminary, these data suggest that intensity scales, especially the VDS, may be used effectively in the assessment of pain in the elderly.

The MPQ is the most widely used multidimensional pain inventory scale.[34] The assessment tool is made up of 20 categories of adjectives that describe the qualities of pain. Subjects are asked to endorse those words that describe their feelings and sensations at that moment. There is much evidence for the validity, reliability, and discriminative abilities of the MPQ when used with younger adults. However, it has been suggested that the MPQ may be too complex and time-consuming for the elderly.[34] Older patients may have difficulty understanding some of the pain descriptors and may be overwhelmed by the large number of choices.[34] Furthermore, a short form of the MPQ (SF-MPQ), made up of 15 descriptors drawn from the MPQ, is less complicated and may also be appropriate for use with the elderly.[33] Patients indicate to what extent from "none" to "severe" each of the descriptors applies to their pain. Pain intensity is measured on a VAS. There is evidence for the validity and reliability of this version of the MPQ, administered as the SF-MPQ, to geriatric pain patients.[34]

Cognitively Impaired Patients: About 5% of those over 65 years and 20% of those over 80 years suffer from dementia.[35] In nursing homes the prevalence of pain and dementia are high, ranging from 45% to 84% for pain and from 40% to 78% for dementia.[36] Pain, a subjective complaint, as stated above, is a complex phenomenon. Although the patient's report is the most accurate method for measuring pain, patients with very advanced dementia cannot convey the experience of pain verbally.[36] These patients are therefore at risk for undetected and untreated pain. The reliability and validity of facial expressions and vocalizations as markers of pain in nonverbal, severely demented patients remain poorly defined. However, some studies suggest that facial expressions correlate with intensity of pain.[37] Because of the cognitive changes that occur with aging, it may be difficult to assess the quality and intensity of pain in this group. The elderly have multiple medical problems and multiple complaints, which make adequate assessments of pain difficult and confusing for the practitioner. Even with appropriate assessment, this group of patients may, because of memory problems or confusion, present with special treatment issues. They may not understand directions for taking medications, may forget these directions, or may forget to take their medications altogether.

The first step when evaluating elderly patients for pain is determining their level of cognitive and verbal function.[38] This information can be obtained by using assessment tools such as the Mini Mental Status Questionnaire or the Short Mental

TABLE 56-1. COMMON PAIN BEHAVIORS IN COGNITIVELY IMPAIRED ELDERLY PERSONS

Facial expressions
Frown; sad, frightened face
Grimace, wrinkled forehead, tightened eyes
Distorted expression; rapid blinking

Verbalizations, vocalizations
Sighing, moaning, groaning, grunting
Calling out, asking for help
Noisy breathing; verbally abusive

Body movements
Rigid, tense body posture; guarding, fidgeting
Pacing, rocking; restricted movement
Gait or mobility changes

Changes in interpersonal interactions
Aggressive, combative, resisting care
Decreased social interactions, withdrawn
Socially inappropriate, disruptive

Changes in activity patterns or routines
Refuses food, appetite change
Sleep, rest pattern changes
Sudden cessation of common routines

Mental status changes
Crying, tears
Increased confusion
Irritability or distress

From AGS Panel on Persistent Pain in Older Persons: Management of persistent pain in older persons. J Am Geriatr Soc 50:S205–S224, 2002.

Status Questionnaire. Often, family and caregivers become the most important source of information, which presents another set of problems in validity and reliability when assessing pain.[39] Even though there are a wide variety of psychometric tools available to assess pain, few studies have tested these tools across levels of cognitive impairment among an elderly population. Table 56-1 gives a description of common pain behaviors seen in cognitively impaired elderly patients.

PHYSIOLOGIC CHANGES IN GERIATRICS

Effective pain management in geriatrics presupposes understanding the physiology of aging and its effects on the clinical aspects of analgesic interventions. As life expectancy increases, knowledge of the physiological mechanisms associated with the normal aging process assumes greater importance, so that quality of life can be sustained.[40]

The physiologic changes of aging have many effects on elderly patients' health and functional status. Aging is characterized by impairment in the function of the many regulatory processes that provide functional integration between cells and organs. The overall process is one of gradual decrements in structure and function, but it is not uniform throughout all organ systems. No organ system is immune to the process of aging, but some systems are much more resistant than others. Maintaining physiological function or "health" in an aging population will help to reduce the burden on the existing medical systems as older individuals consume medical services. The effects of the aging process on various organ systems do not usually affect function in the normal state; however, during periods of stress (such as with a surgical procedure or illness), the elderly patient may not be able to meet the increased metabolic demand.

Cardiovascular System: With aging there are changes in the cardiovascular system, which result in alterations in cardiovascular physiology. The changes in cardiovascular physiology must be differentiated from the effects of pathology, such as coronary artery disease, that occur with increasing frequency as age increases. Age-related changes occur in everyone, but not necessarily at the same rate, therefore accounting for the difference seen in some people between chronologic age and physiologic age.[41] Changes in the cardiovascular system associated with aging are a decrease in elasticity and an increase in stiffness of the arterial system.[42] This results in increased afterload on the left ventricle, an increase in systolic blood pressure, and left ventricular hypertrophy, as well as other changes in the left ventricular wall that prolong relaxation of the left ventricle in diastole. Cardiac index decreases approximately 1% per year after the age of 30 years. Therefore, any medications that are given intravenously may have a slower circulation time and a longer onset to effect.[43,44]

Central Nervous System (CNS): Age-related neurodegenerative conditions are characterized by neuronal death and degeneration that lead to a progressive functional decline. It is not uncommon to find gradual cognitive decline with aging. The CNS and peripheral nervous system begin to deteriorate as early as 50 years of age, although in many individuals this process does not occur until they are in their seventies or eighties.

Dementia is a general term used to describe significant decline in two or more areas of cognitive functioning. It is the most common cause of mental decline in old age. Of those who suffer from dementia, most have Alzheimer's disease (AD), which affects an estimated 4 million people in the USA.[45] Vascular dementia is the second most common cause of progressive dementia, accounting for 15% to 25% of all dementias. Epidemiologic projections estimate that by 2040 approximately 14 million Americans will suffer from AD.[46] The pain and anguish of the disorder also afflicts many more caregivers and relatives, who must cope with the patient's progressive and irreversible decline in cognition, functioning, and behavior. Both caregivers and patients may misinterpret initial symptoms of AD for normal age-related cognitive losses, and physicians may not recognize early signs or may misdiagnose them. Dementia and aging are not synonymous. As people age they usually experience memory changes such as slowing in information processing, but these kinds of changes are benign. By contrast, dementia is progressive and disabling and not an inherent aspect of aging.

Parkinson's disease (PD), which is more commonly seen in the geriatric patient, is a neurodegenerative disorder associated with the loss of dopaminergic neurons in the substantia nigra. The decline of dopamine leads to motor dysfunction manifested as tremor, rigidity, and bradykinesia. The pharmacological treatment of choice for the past 30 years has been the dopamine precursor levodopa. Pain is a common yet rarely identified component in these patients.[47] As many as half of all patients with PD can experience pain related to their disease. Pain can develop from complications of the disease itself as well as primary sensory pain syndromes. The most common cause of pain in PD is limb rigidity, usually occurring in the lower limbs.[48] This condition has the tendency to be misdiagnosed as radicular type symptoms. The treatment should be focused on optimizing antiparkinson drugs. Dystonic posturing of the face, arm, jaw, neck, and leg can also occur. Improvement in the dystonic symptoms is best achieved by raising the drug dose to the appropriate level. Botulinum toxin type A (Botox) can also be used to treat dystonias.[49] Other conditions that can be present in patients with PD are restless leg syndrome, decreased intestinal motility leading to gastrointestinal (GI) upset, and orthostatic hypotension which can often cause headaches.[50] Primary pain, which can be diffuse in PD, is described as a vague overall sensation of tension, discomfort, or paresthesia that may improve with motion. The cause of the sensory symptoms is unknown, but some evidence suggests that the basal ganglia may modify sensory information.[51]

PHARMACOKINETICS

Pharmacokinetic principles determine the relationship between dose of the drug administered and the concentration of drug at the receptor site. Aging causes physiological changes that alter the pharmacokinetics and pharmacodynamics of analgesics, narrowing their therapeutic index and increasing the risk of toxicity and drug–drug interactions.[52] The contributions of disease and drug therapy are considered because age-related physiologic changes may be most important in the frail elderly patient with multiple chronic disorders and polypharmacy. Physiologic changes may include altered absorption, distribution, and changes in the renal and hepatic system leading to changes in metabolism and elimination. These changes can result in longer duration of activity and altered concentration for many drugs including analgesics. This can lead to increased incidence of drug toxicity and adverse reactions.

Absorption: Various anatomic and physiologic changes that occur with normal aging can affect drug absorption. The absorption of most drugs from the GI tract is a passive process that can be influenced by several factors. Age-related changes in absorption include increase in gastric pH, and decreases in GI motility, splanchnic blood flow, and the mucosal surface of the small intestine.[53–56] In most cases, however, absorption proceeds by passive diffusion in the small intestine; and these age-related factors are not sufficient to influence overall absorption. Conditions that occur more commonly in the aged population such as various types of malabsorptive states, partial resection of the small bowel, and the concomitant administration of several drugs have been shown to decrease drug absorption.[57] Examples of drugs influencing absorption include antacids which may interfere with the absorption of oral antibiotics, digoxin, and phenytoin; laxatives and antimicrobial agents which may affect the rate and/or extent of absorption; and antidepressants which affect bowel motility, therefore affecting the absorption of other drugs.[58]

Distribution: The duration that a particular drug exerts its effect in a patient depends on the volume of distribution (Vd) of the drug, the metabolism of the drug, the clearance of the drug, or some combination of these factors, all of which change with aging. The half-life of a drug is directly proportional to the Vd and is inversely proportional to clearance of the drug. The Vd of a particular drug is determined by the patient's body composition and the degree of plasma protein binding. Distribution is the reversible transfer of drug from one location to another within the body. Body composition, plasma protein binding, and organ blood flow play roles in drug distribution. In the elderly a decline in lean muscle mass by approximately 10% to 20% and in total body water by approximately 25% to 30%, and an increase in the percentage of adipose tissue help explain the decrease in Vd seen in this population.[59] Whether these changes are truly age related is unclear; one report has indicated that the percentage of body fat does not increase significantly after the age of 40 years, except as the result of weight gain alone.[60]

Physiochemical properties of drugs, whether hydrophilic or lipophilic, are important when age-related changes in body composition are present. Lipid-soluble drugs such as opioids, benzodiazepines, and barbiturates have an increased Vd. When combined with decreases in certain components of metabolism, there may be a substantial increase in their biologic half-life and increased serum levels. Water-soluble drugs such as lidocaine have a reduced Vd, hence increased serum levels after a standard loading dose. Changes in Vd will affect the amount of drug needed for a loading dose or the time needed to achieve steady state. Drugs with a large Vd take a longer time to reach steady state and a higher loading dose is required.

While many drugs are bound to plasma proteins, this characteristic becomes important only when the degree of binding exceeds 90%, with no more than 10% of the drug unbound and pharmacologically active. The major factors influencing protein binding include protein concentrations, concurrent disease and drugs, and nutritional status. Basic drugs, such as lidocaine, propranolol, and imipramine, have a higher binding affinity for alpha1-acid glycoprotein, which increases in response to inflammatory disease. The concentration of alpha1-acid glycoprotein appears to increase with age; as a result there may be potential for an increase in the protein binding of basic drugs in the elderly person and a reduction in the amount of free, pharmacologically active drug.[61] Acidic drugs such as naproxen, phenytoin, warfarin, and meperidine bind primarily to albumin, which may decrease slightly in the healthy elderly patient. This would lead to a greater free fraction of the drug, therefore increasing the drug's effect. In the elderly patient with poor nutritional status and chronic medical issues the relatively larger declines in albumin concentration may result in clinically important increases in unbound drug concentration.

Metabolism: The rate of metabolism of drugs is influenced by nutrition, other drugs, disease, smoking, serum albumin, hepatic function, and age. There is a 1% annual reduction in hepatic blood flow after the age of 25 and a 1% annual decrease in liver mass. Phase I metabolism (hydrolysis, oxidation, reduction), primarily oxidation, declines with age.[62] Phase II metabolism (conjugation) is relatively unaffected by age.[63]

Aging is associated with morphological changes in human liver, such as decrease in size, attributable to decreased activity of different enzyme systems and hepatic blood flow. Hepatic drug metabolism is mainly mediated by the cytochrome P450 system, but it can also be influenced by concomitant drug therapy, comorbid conditions, nutritional status, gender, and genetics. Drugs that are enzyme inducers or inhibitors can increase or decrease the metabolism of other drugs.

Elimination: Renal function can be easily compromised in the elderly. The glomerular filtration process is reduced with increasing age; this is characterized by reductions in kidney size, in the number of nephrons, in the number of functioning glomeruli, and in renal blood flow. Glomerular filtration rate (GFR) falls approximately 1mL/minute each year after the age of 40. Serum creatinine is also decreased with age because of reduction in muscle mass and an associated decrease in creatinine synthesis. It is important to remember that "normal" BUN and creatinine values do not mean normal renal function in the elderly. Clearance (Cl) is the single best measure to describe the ability of the body or an organ system to remove drug. Its value is unaltered by changes in other pharmacokinetic parameters. Clearance is the primary determinant of steady-state drug levels, with chronic use of any dose of a drug.

PHARMACODYNAMICS

Changes occur in end organ responsiveness to medications with aging. Pharmacodynamic changes (the effect of the drug on its target site) in the elderly may be due to changes in receptor affinity or number, or to altered translation of a receptor-initiated cellular response into a biochemical reaction. The action of drugs affecting the CNS (benzodiazepines, anesthetics, metoclopramide, narcotics) and the cardiovascular system (beta-blockers, calcium channel blockers, diuretics) is frequently altered in older adults.[40]

Treatment of Pain

It is well documented that pain is under treated in the elderly.[8] Inadequate treatment of pain may have additional serious consequences on the health status of the elderly. A noted complication of unrelieved pain is loss of function; this may result in complications of immobility and in heavier reliance on others to perform necessary activities of daily living (ADL). Additionally, elderly patients who experience unrelieved pain are more likely to be affected by depression and anxiety. Pain, loss of function, depression, and anxiety then contribute to growing social isolation, loss of appetite, poor nutrition, more nonrestorative sleep, and increased risk of deteriorating health.[64,65] Quality of life is significantly impaired when pain is not treated.

Recent advances in pain research provide the scientific rationale for using new, improved methods of treatment. These include better and more effective use of standard drug therapy, the development of new drugs, the use of novel methods and routes of drug administration, and the use of selective anesthetic and neurosurgical approaches to pain control. Greater reductions in pain and improvements in functional capacity are usually obtained by combining pharmacologic and nonpharmacologic treatments.[66,67] This can also decrease the incidence of drug–drug interaction and side effects. The success of treatment should be measured by improvement in pain intensity as well as physical, psychosocial, and cognitive function. Effective pain management may have an impact on any or all of these functional domains and, therefore, substantially improve the patient's functional capacity.

Pharmacologic Treatment of Pain: Analgesic agents are effective in the elderly and constitute the most common approach to pain treatment.[29] The safe and effective use of analgesic drugs in the elderly requires a thorough understanding of the mechanism of action and potential negative effects of the particular drug. Older patients are generally more susceptible to adverse drug reactions. Therefore, the physician has to balance the risks and benefits of the drugs prescribed.[68] It is well documented that the elderly are more likely to develop adverse reactions to pharmacological treatments for pain and that these reactions occur at much lower dosages than those seen in younger patients. Drug regimens should be started at the lowest anticipated therapeutic dose and titrated to effect, keeping in mind the half-lives of the drugs prescribed. Routine follow-up visits should include evaluation of clinical, functional, cognitive, and social circumstances.

When prescribing analgesics in the geriatric patient it is useful to follow the World Health Organization (WHO) analgesic ladder, which was originally developed as a guide for the management of cancer pain.[69] This protocol advocates using a tiered system whereby less potent drugs are used first so that the patient is made comfortable with minimal side effects. The use of this system can decrease overall complication rates. The first-tier drugs include nonopioids such as nonsteroidal anti-inflammatory drugs (NSAIDs), acetaminophen, tricyclic antidepressants, and tramadol. The second-tier medications include the "weak" opioids, such as combination drugs with acetaminophen and codeine, oxycodone, or hydrocodone. The third-tier medications include all other opioids including short- and long-acting agents. The American Geriatric Society published clinical practice guidelines for therapy of persistent pain in the elderly. Specific recommendations for pharmacological therapy are summarized below.[29]

Nonopioid Analgesics: Acetaminophen and NSAIDs are the most commonly used first-line analgesic therapies for management of pain.[70] Acetaminophen is an appropriate and relatively safe first-line drug of choice for mild to moderate pain, with few known side effects. It does not produce gastric bleeding and other potential bleeding complications as does aspirin or NSAIDs; however, it can be associated with increased risk of hepatic toxicity, with daily doses greater than 4,000 mg, and renal disease with long-term use. Acetaminophen, partly because it is used so frequently, is the number one cause of accidental drug poisoning. In patients with renal or hepatic disease it is recommended to decrease the dosage by 50% to 75%. A study done by Bradley and colleagues showed that acetaminophen (4,000 mg/day) resulted in analgesia similar to that of ibuprofen, administered at analgesic dose (1,200 mg/day) or at an anti-inflammatory dose (2,400 mg/day), to patients with chronic osteoarthritis of the knee.[71] Thus, acetaminophen may be the preferred choice for patients without substantial inflammation because of its lower side-effect profile.

NSAIDs include several different chemical entities, all of which inhibit cyclooxygenase (COX), an essential group of enzymes in the biosynthesis of prostaglandins. These agents act peripherally on the nervous system, affecting pain receptors, nerve conduction, and inflammatory conditions that can stimulate pain. All NSAIDs appear to be similarly efficacious with regard to their analgesic and anti-inflammatory actions. The analgesic activity of NSAIDs is limited by a ceiling effect. The ceiling effect represents a level beyond which increasing the dose of the analgesic agent does not further increase analgesia but can lead to greater side effects.

While mediation of the inflammatory response is considered a major determinant of the therapeutic effect of NSAIDs, the inhibition of prostaglandins causes toxicity in multiple organs. Renal insufficiency and disruption of GI mucosa are two prominent adverse effects of nonselective NSAID use. Although only a minority of patients using NSAIDs appear to develop serious GI problems, because of widespread usage it is estimated that there are at least 16,500 NSAID-related deaths each year in the USA among patients with degenerative and rheumatoid arthritis.[72] Toxicity related to NSAID use represents the 15th most common cause of death in the USA.[73] Geriatric patients appear to be at increased risk for developing GI problems associated with NSAID use, with 3% to 4% of patients aged 60 years or older developing GI bleeding, compared to 1% of the general population.[74] The increased risk of NSAID toxicity in older adults has been attributed to more frequent use and higher consumption of NSAIDs, existence of additional illnesses such as atrial fibrillation, and concomitant use of medications such as diuretics and anticoagulants, which may potentially lead to adverse drug–drug interactions. Age-related changes in prostaglandin physiology in certain organ systems may also predispose older adults to NSAID-related adverse events. The natural decrease in GI prostaglandin levels in older patients may lead to greater mucosal fragility. Studies of renal physiology show some evidence of age-related prostaglandin changes that might support the relationship between age and increased risk of NSAID toxicity. NSAIDs interact with other commonly prescribed medications. They can increase the serum concentration of digoxin and attenuate the effects of beta-adrenergic blockers, ACE inhibitors, and thiazides. The nephrotoxic effects of triamterene are also potentiated by the use of NSAIDs.[75] However, recommendations for NSAID use and prophylaxis should not be based on the patient's age, but rather on relevant comorbid conditions such as peptic ulcer history, edematous states, or concurrent medication use.

In terms of GI morbidity and antiplatelet effects, COX-2-selective drugs appear to be safer than nonselective COX inhibitors. The efficacy of COX-2-selective inhibitors in relieving chronic pain from osteoarthritis and rheumatoid arthritis is comparable to that of nonselective NSAIDs. However, the occurrence of GI complications may be less frequent in patients who receive COX-2-selective inhibitors than in patients receiving nonselective NSAIDs.[76] Thus, the use of COX-2-selective inhibitors for the management of chronic pain in the elderly may reduce overall costs and provide an alternative with an improved safety profile compared with nonselective NSAIDs.

Opioid Analgesics: For pain that is not adequately controlled by first-line analgesics, chronic opioid therapy should be considered. Opioids are the most potent analgesics. They have a higher analgesic potency and a wider range of indications than any of the other currently available medications for pain control. The use of opioid analgesics for persistent noncancer pain is becoming more acceptable, but potential drug abuse continues to be of major concern. Opioids provide a treatment option for the management of pain in elderly patients when pain control under standard management is poor. However, various therapeutic difficulties are encountered in the heterogeneous elderly population; these include increased risk of adverse effects, multiple comorbid conditions, and polypharmacy. Lower initial opioid dosage, prolonged dosage intervals, and slower dosage titrations are advisable because of the alterations in pharmacokinetics and pharmacodynamics. Kidney function should be tightly monitored, and the use of laxatives must be encouraged. Randomized clinical studies of opioids in musculoskeletal pain have increasingly extended the scientific basis for their use.

Opioids also demonstrate an analgesic effect following local peripheral application. Transdermal fentanyl is a slow-release, cutaneous preparation that has a low adverse-effect profile. In a study comparing transdermal fentanyl and sustained-release morphine patients reported less nausea and sedation during the day and night with transdermal fentanyl patch. However, patients reported less sleep disturbance with sustained-release morphine.[77] In another study patients receiving transdermal fentanyl were significantly more satisfied than the group that received oral morphine.[78] This method of drug administration can lead to greater compliance and a more convenient way of administering analgesic medications. Breakthrough pain should not be overlooked when using the transdermal patch. A short-acting opioid should also be included in the regimen for these episodes.

Two opioid analgesics that have been recently reviewed for use in the geriatric population, for patients with persistent mild to moderate pain, are tramadol and methadone. The mechanism of action of tramadol is by both opioid receptor stimulation and inhibition of norepinephrine and serotonin reuptake. Its efficacy in mild to moderate pain associated with osteoarthritis, low back pain, and diabetic neuropathy has been reviewed.[79,80] The efficacy and safety of tramadol appear to be similar to equianalgesic doses of codeine and hydrocodone. There has been renewed interest in the use of methadone, a mu opioid receptor agonist, due to its effectiveness with neuropathic pain, slow development of opioid tolerance, and relatively low cost.[81] It has a long and variable half-life, which makes this drug difficult to titrate. Plasma concentrations continue to rise toward steady state for days or weeks after analgesia has been obtained.

Side effects of the opioid analgesics should be considered when administering them to the geriatric population. Respiratory depression, sedation, confusion, depression, constipation, nausea, vomiting, and urinary retention are some of the common side effects seen with opioid administration. Geriatric patients have less reserve than the average adult; therefore titration is very important. In the majority of patients, pharmacological tolerance develops to all of the common side effects, except constipation, within 1 to 2 weeks. Preventative treatment for constipation, to promote normal bowel function, should be initiated at the beginning of the opioid trial. This can be accomplished with increased daily fluids and dietary fibers, supplemented with stool softening agents and laxatives. Nausea and vomiting may be experienced in opioid-naive patients who are placed on a short course of an opioid agent. If nausea and/or vomiting persist, simply changing the opioid or the route of administration, or adding an antiemetic, may resolve the problem. Like nausea, drowsiness that occurs when initiating an opioid will usually dissipate after the first week or so. Persistent somnolence may be managed by maintaining adequate hydration and renal clearance, changing to a sustained-release product to minimize peak effects, changing the opioid drug, changing the route of administration, or adding a psychostimulant such as methylphenidate HCl (Ritalin) or dextroamphetamine (Dexedrine).

Adjuvant Agents: Adjuvant analgesics are drugs used to enhance the analgesic efficacy of opioids, treat concurrent symptoms that exacerbate pain, and/or provide independent analgesia for specific types of pain. Adjuvant agents may be used in all stages of the analgesic ladder. These drugs are most beneficial in neuropathic pain states and mixed nociceptive–neuropathic pain syndromes.

Anticonvulsants such as carbamazepine, phenytoin, and gabapentin are used either alone or in addition to opioids and other analgesics, to manage neuropathic pain. Anticonvulsants have been particularly advocated for neuropathic pain with a shooting or lancinating quality (such as trigeminal neuralgia or nerve root compression). Gabapentin appears to have a better adverse-effect profile and to provide similar efficacy for treating painful diabetic neuropathy and postherpetic neuralgia.[82] The most common adverse events are mild to moderate dizziness and somnolence. These side effects are often transient and occur during the titration phase.[83]

Tricyclic antidepressants are particularly useful in the management of neuropathic pain. They have innate analgesic properties and are effective through mechanisms that include enhanced inhibitory modulation of nociceptive impulses at the level of the dorsal horn. Cognitive impairment, sedation, and orthostatic hypotension are common side effects that may limit use of antidepressants in the elderly.[84] The newer selective serotonin reuptake inhibitors (SSRIs) have, comparatively, only serotonin-receptor-mediated side effects. These agents have not been thoroughly studied in the treatment of chronic pain. Moreover, because SSRIs have an impact on reuptake in only one monoamine system, it is plausible that they may be less efficacious than the tricyclic antidepressants in treating chronic pain.[85]

Nonpharmacological Strategies: A variety of nonpharmacologic interventions, used alone or combined with drug therapy, have been shown to be effective in treating pain in the geriatric patient.[29] A physical activity program, designed to meet individual patient needs and preferences, should be considered for all older patients. Severely impaired patients require supervised rehabilitation therapy, while healthy elderly patients should be referred to a group exercise program. Older patients should perform exercises that improve flexibility, strength, and endurance. Patient education programs are important in treatment of chronic pain. These should include training in self-help techniques that allow patients to better understand, manage, and cope with chronic pain.[29] Formal training in cognitive-behavioral therapies may be helpful for older patients with persistent pain. Other techniques (heat, cold, massage, manipulation, acupuncture, and transcutaneous electrical nerve stimulation) often provide temporary relief; and they can be used as adjunctive therapy.[29]

Interventional Pain Management Techniques: Older patients may be candidates for injection therapies. Myofascial pain is a frequent finding in pain treatment clinics. Trigger point injection may be a low-risk and very good option for treatment of myofascial pain, provided that it is combined with a home exercise program. Older patients often suffer from back pain due to degenerative disc and joint processes. Epidural steroid injection, using interlaminar, translaminar, or caudal catheter techniques, may be indicated for relief of radicular pain associated with spinal pathology. Potential complications from systemic effects of injected steroids must be anticipated and managed in these patients; these may include infection, hypertension, hyperglycemia, heart failure, and adrenal suppression. Nevertheless, the procedure has an impressive safety record, and it should be offered when indications for injection are present. Degenerative joint disease in the elderly may involve the sacroiliac and spinal facet joints. Injection of these joints, and interruption of their innervation with local anesthetic or rhizotomy procedures, may be effective in carefully selected patients. Older patients may also benefit significantly from vertebroplasty for relief of intractable pain due to spinal compression fracture or from neurolytic blocks for cancer pain. Interventional techniques are considered in other chapters in this book. These therapies should not be withheld solely because of patient age. However, it is particularly important that a complete and accurate assessment precedes interventional pain management procedures. The implications of concurrent medical, emotional, social, and physical limitations must be considered. When interventional procedures are clearly indicated, they should be offered to elderly patients. It is important that reasonable expectations for treatment outcome be conveyed to patients, using understandable terms, when obtaining informed consent after discussion of the benefits and risks of procedures. It is ideal, and may often be necessary, to include family members in these discussions. When elderly patients live alone, and have very limited interaction with friends or relatives, it can be challenging to provide for safe transportation and aftercare for these patients.

KEY POINTS

- One-dimensional pain scales may be used effectively in the assessment of pain in older patients, especially the Verbal Descriptor Scale, which appears to be easy to use and to best describe their pain.
- The first step when evaluating elderly patients for pain is determining their level of cognitive and verbal function.
- Under treatment of pain has been documented in the elderly. Unrelieved pain then leads to immobility, loss of function, anxiety, depression, social isolation, loss of appetite, and poor sleep.
- The elderly are more likely to develop adverse reactions to pharmacological treatments for pain and at much lower dosages than those seen in younger patients. Drug regimens should be started at the lowest anticipated therapeutic dose and titrated to effect.
- The use of COX-2-selective inhibitors for the management of chronic pain in the elderly may reduce serious GI bleeding and overall costs, thus providing an alternative with an improved safety profile compared with non-selective NSAIDs.

REFERENCES

1. NIH News Release. Dramatic Decline in Disability Continues for Older Americans. National Institute of Aging, May 2001.
2. US Bureau of the Census: Statistical Abstract of the United States, 1990, ed 110. US Government Printing Office, Washington, DC, 1990.
3. Desai MM, Zhang P: Surveillance for morbidity and mortality among older adults – United States, 1995–1996. MMWR CDC Surveill Summ 48:7–25, 1999.
4. Federal Interagency Forum on Aging Related Stats. Older Americans 2000: Key indicators of well being. Undated Detailed Tables 25–30.
5. Merskey H, Bogduk N: Classification of Chronic Pain, IASP Task Force on Taxonomy. IASP Press, Seattle, 1994.
6. Ferrell BA: Overview of aging and pain. *In* Ferrell BR, Ferrell BA (eds): Pain in the Elderly. IASP Press, Seattle, 1996, pp 1–10.
7. Helme RD, Gibson SJ: Pain in older people. *In* Crombie IK, Croft PR, Linton SJ, et al (eds): Epidemiology of Pain. IASP Press, Seattle, 1999.
8. Ferrell BA: Pain management in elderly people. J Am Geriatr Soc 39:64–73, 1991.
9. Gaston-Johansson F, Johansson F, Johansson C: Pain in the elderly: Prevalence, attitudes and assessment. Ann Long Term Care 7:190–196, 1999.
10. Melding PS: Is there such a thing as geriatric pain? Pain 46:119, 1991.
11. Crook J, Rideout E, Browne G: The prevalence of pain complaints in the general population. Pain 18:299–314, 1984.
12. The management of chronic pain in older persons. AGS Panel on Chronic Pain in Older Persons. American Geriatric Society. Geriatrics 53(Suppl 3):S8–S24, 1998.
13. Manton KG: Chronic morbidity and disability in the US elderly populations. *In* Mostofsky DI, Lomranz J (eds): Handbook of Pain and Aging. Plenum Press, New York, 1997, pp 37–67.
14. Andersson HI, Ejilertsson G, Leden I, at al: Chronic pain in a geographically defined population: Studies of differences in age, gender, social class and pain localization. Clin J Pain 9:174–182, 1993.
15. Lipton RB, Pfeffer D, Newman LC, et al: Headaches in the elderly. J Pain Sympt Manage 8:87–97, 1993.
16. Wright D, Barrow S, Fisher AD, et al: Influence of physical, psychological and behavioral factors on consultations for back pain. Br J Rheumatol 34:156–161, 1995.
17. Badley EM, Tennan A: Changing profile of joint disorders with age: Findings from a postal survey of the population of Calderdale, West Yorkshire, United Kingdom. Ann Rheum Dis 51:366–371, 1992.
18. Sternbach RA: Survey of pain in the United States: The Nuprin pain report. Clin J Pain 2:49–53, 1986.
19. Herr KA, Garand L: Assessment and measurement of pain in older adults. Clin Geriatric Med 17:457–478, 2001.
20. Ardery G: Assessing and managing acute pain in older adults: A reserve base to guide practice. Medsurg Nursing 12:7–18, 2003.
21. Flahaerty E: Assessing pain in older adults. Director 8:101–130, 2000.
22. Gagliese L, Katz J: Age differences in postoperative pain are scale dependent: A comparison of measures of pain intensity and quality in younger and older surgical patients. Pain 103:11–20, 2003.
23. Harkins SW, Price DD: Assessment of pain in the elderly. *In* Turk DC, Melzack R (eds): Handbook of Pain Assessment. Guilford Press, New York, 1992, pp 315–331.
24. Melzack R, Katz J: The McGill Pain Questionnaire: Appraisal and current status. *In* Turk DC, Melzack R (eds): Handbook of Pain Assessment. Guilford Press, New York, 1992, pp 152–168.
25. Stein WM: Pain management in the elderly: Pain in the nursing home. Clin Geriatr Med 17:575–594, 2001.

26. Geda YE, Rummans TA: Pain: Cause of agitation in elderly individuals with dementia. Am J Psychiatry 156:1662–1663, 1999.

27. Rakowski W, Mor V: The association of physical activity with mortality among older adults in the longitudinal study of aging (1984–1988). J Gerontol 47:M122–M129, 1992.

28. Weisman DE, Matson S: Pain assessment and management in the long-term care setting. Theor Med Bioeth 20:31–43, 1999.

29. AGS Panel on Persistent Pain in Older Persons: Management of persistent pain in older persons. J Am Geriatr Soc 50:S205–S224, 2002.

30. Huskisson EC: Visual analogue scales. In Melzack R (ed): Pain Measurement and Assessment. Raven Press, New York, 1983, pp 33–37.

31. Jensen MP: Validity of self-report and observation measures. In Jensen TS, Turner JA, Wiesenfeld-Hallin Z (eds): Proc 8th World Congress on Pain. IASP Press, Seattle, 1997, pp 637–662.

32. Feldt KS, Ryden MB, Miles S: Treatment of pain in cognitively impaired compared with cognitively intact older patients with hip-fracture. J Am Geriatr Soc 46:1079–1085, 1998.

33. Herr KA, Mobity PR: Comparison of selected pain assessment tools for use with the elderly. Appl Nursing Res 6:39–46, 1993.

34. Melzack R, Katz J: The McGill Pain Questionnaire: Appraisal and current status. In Turk DC, Melzack R (eds): Handbook of Pain Assessment. Guilford Press, New York, 2001, pp 35–52.

35. Blair KA: Aging: Physiological aspects and clinical implications. ANCP 15:14–28, 1990.

36. Manz BD, Moisier R, Nusser MA: Pain assessment in the cognitively impaired and unimpaired elderly. ASPMN 1:106–115, 2000.

37. Chibnall JT: Pain assessment in cognitively impaired and unimpaired older adults: A comparison of four scales. Pain 92: 173–186, 2001.

38. Manfrei PL, Breuer B: Pain assessment in elderly patients with severe dementia. J Pain Symptom Manage 25:48–52, 2003.

39. Hurley AC: Evaluation of pain in cognitively impaired individuals. J Am Geriatr Soc 4:1607–1611, 2000.

40. Mangoni A, Jackson SHD: Age-related changes in pharmacokinetics and pharmacodynamics: Basic principles and practical applications. Br J Pharmacol 57:6–14, 2004.

41. Brandfonbrener M, Landowne M, Shock N: Changes in cardiac output with age. Circulation 12:557–566, 1955.

42. Cheitlin MD: Cardiovascular physiology-changes with aging. Am J Geriatr Cardiol 12:9–11, 2003.

43. Evans TI: The physiological basis of geriatric general anesthesia. Anesth Intensive Care 1:319, 1973.

44. Lakatta EG: Cardiovascular aging research: the next horizons. J Am Geriatr Soc 47:613–625, 1999.

45. Bachman R: Incidence of dementia and probable Alzheimer's disease in a general population. Neurology 43:115–119, 1998.

46. United States General Accounting Office: Report of the Secretary of Health and Human Services: Alzheimer's disease estimates of prevalence in the US. US Government Printing Office, Washington, DC, 1998.

47. Waseem S, Gwinn-Hardy K: Pain in Parkinson's disease: Common yet seldom recognized symptom is treatable. Postgrad Med 110:33–40, 46, 2001.

48. Goetz CG, Tanner CM, Levy M: Pain in Parkinson's disease. Mov Disord 1:45–49, 1986.

49. Pacchetti C, Albani G, Martignoni E: "Off" painful dystonia in Parkinson's disease treated with botulinum toxin. Mov Disord 10:333–336, 1995.

50. Bleasdale-Barr KM, Mathias CJ: Neck and other muscle pains in autonomic failure: Their association with orthostatic hypotension. J R Soc Med 91:355–359, 1998.

51. Chudler EH, Dong WK: The role of the basal ganglia in nociception and pain. Pain 60:3–38, 1995.

52. Davis MP, Srivastava M: Demographics, assessment and management of pain in the elderly. Drugs Aging 20:23–57, 2003.

53. Evans MA, Triggs EJ, Cheung M, et al: Gastric emptying rate in the elderly: Implications for drug therapy. J Am Geriatr Soc 29:201–205, 1981.

54. Bender A: The effect of increasing age on the distribution of peripheral blood flow in man. J Am Geriatr Soc 16:192–198, 1965.

55. Warren PM, Pepperman MA, Montgomery RD: Age changes in small-intestinal mucosa. Lancet 14:849–850, 1978.

56. Corazza GR, Frazzoni M, Gatto MR, et al: Ageing and small-bowel mucosa: A morphometric study. Gerontology 32:60–65, 1986.

57. Husebye E, Engedal K: The patterns of motility are maintained in the human small intestine throughout the process of aging. Scand J Gastroenterol 27:397–404, 1992.

58. Gainsborough N, Maskrey VL, Nelson ML, et al: The association of age with gastric emptying. Age Ageing 22:37–40, 1993.

59. Fulop T Jr, Worum I, Csongor J, et al: Body composition in elderly people: I. Determination of body composition by multiisotope method and the elimination kinetics of these isotopes in healthy elderly subjects. Gerontology 31:6–14, 1985.

60. Mayersohn M: Special pharmacokinetic considerations in the elderly. In Evans WE, Schentag JJ, Jusko WJ (eds): Applied Pharmacokinetics, ed 2. Applied Therapeutics, Spokane, WA, 1986, pp 229–293.

61. Gunasekera JBL, Lee DR, Jones L, et al: Does albumin fall with increasing age in the absence of disease? Age Ageing 25(Suppl 1): 29, 1996.

62. O'Malley K, Crooks J, Duke E, et al: Effect of age and sex on drug metabolism. BMJ 3:607–609, 1971.

63. Wynne HA, Cope LH, Herd B, et al: The association of age and frailty with paracetamol conjugation in man. Age Ageing 19: 419–424, 1990.

64. Magni G, Marchetti M, Moreschi C: Chronic musculoskeletal pain and depressive symptoms in the national health and nutrition examination: Epidemiologic follow-up study. Pain 53:163–168, 1993.

65. Herr K, Mobily P: Depression and the experience of chronic back pain: A study of related variables and age differences. Clin J Pain 9:104–114, 1993.

66. Jacox A, Carr DB, Payne R: Management of Cancer Pain. Clinical Practice Guidelines No. 9, AHCPR Publication No. 94-0592. Agency for Health Care Policy and Research, Rockville, MD, US Department of Health and Human Services, Public Health Service, 1994.

67. Ferrell BR: Patient education and non-drug interventions. In Ferrell BR, Ferrell BA (eds): Pain in the Elderly. IASP Press, Seattle, 1996, pp 35–44.

68. Gurwitz JH, Avorn J: The ambiguous relation between aging and adverse drug reactions. Ann Intern Med 114:956–966, 1991.

69. Cancer Pain Relief and Palliative Care: Report of a WHO expert committee, World Health Organization Technical Report Series, 804. World Health Organization, Geneva, 1990.

70. Cooner E, Amorosi S: The Study of Pain in Older Americans. Louis Harris & Associates, New York, 1997.

71. Bradley JD, Brandt KD, Katz BP, et al: Comparison of an anti-inflammatory dose of ibuprofen, an analgesic dose of ibuprofen, and acetaminophen in the treatment of patients with osteoarthritis of the knee. N Engl J Med 325:87–91, 1991.

72. Singh G, Triadafilopoulos G: Epidemiology of NSAID induced gastrointestinal complications. J Rheumatol 26(Suppl 56): 18–24, 1999.

73. Wolfe MM, Lichtenstein DR, Singh G: Gastrointestinal toxicity of nonsteroidal antiinflammatory drugs. N Engl J Med 340: 1888–1899, 1999.

74. Greenberger NJ: Update in gastroenterology. Ann Intern Med 127:827–834, 1997.

75. Chutka DS, Evans JM, et al: Drug prescribing for elderly patients. Mayo Clin Proc 70:685–693, 1995.

76. McAdam BF, Catella-Lawson F, Mardini IA, et al: Systemic biosynthesis of prostacyclin by cyclooxygenase (COX)-2: The human pharmacology of a selective inhibitor of COX 2. Proc Natl Acad Sci USA 96:272–277, 1999.
77. Ahmedzai S, Brooks D: Transdermal fentanyl versus sustained release oral morphine in cancer pain: Preference, efficacy, and quality of life. J Pain Symptom Manage 13:254–261, 1997.
78. Payne R, Mathias SD, Pasta DJ, et al: Quality of life and cancer pain: Satisfaction and side effects with transdermal fentanyl versus oral morphine. J Clin Oncol 16:1588–1593, 1998.
79. Fleischmann RM, Cadwell JR, Roth SH, et al: Tramadol for the treatment of joint pain associated with osteoarthritis: A randomized, double-blinded, placebo controlled trial. Curr Ther Res Clin Exp 62:113–128, 2001.
80. Schnitzer TJ, Gray WL, Paster RZ, et al: Efficacy of tramadol in treatment of chronic low back pain. J Rheumatol 27:772–778, 2000.
81. Ripamonti C, Dickerson ED: Strategies for cancer pain in the new millennium. Drugs 61:955–977, 2001.
82. Ahmad M, Goucke CR: Management strategies for the treatment of neuropathic pain in the elderly. Drugs Aging 19:929–945, 2002.
83. Serpell MG: Gabapentin in neuropathic pain syndromes: A randomized, double-blind, placebo-controlled trial. Pain 103:227, 2003.
84. Reisner L: Antidepressants for chronic neuropathic pain. Curr Pain Headache Rep 7:24–33, 2003.
85. Barkin RL, Fawcett J: The management challenges of chronic pain: The role of antidepressants. Am J Ther 7:31–47, 2000.

Spinal Cord Stimulation

**Mikhail Fukshansky, M.D., and
Allen W. Burton, M.D.**

Spinal cord stimulation (SCS) describes the use of pulsed electrical energy near the spinal cord to control pain.[1] This technique was first applied in the intrathecal space and finally in the epidural space as described by Shealy in 1967.[2] At present most commonly used neurostimulation involves the implantation of leads in the epidural space to transmit this pulsed energy across the spinal cord or near the desired nerve roots. This chapter concentrates on this modality: spinal cord stimulation, sometimes called dorsal column stimulation. This technique has notable analgesic properties for neuropathic pain states, anginal pain, and peripheral ischemic pain. The same technology can be applied in deep brain stimulation, cortical brain stimulation, and peripheral nerve stimulation.[3–5] These techniques are mainly in the realm of the neurosurgeon.

MECHANISM OF ACTION

Neurostimulation began shortly after Melzack and Wall proposed the gate control theory in 1965.[6] This theory proposed that painful peripheral stimuli carried by C fibers and lightly myelinated A-delta fibers terminated at the substantia gelatinosa of the dorsal horn (the gate). Large myelinated A-beta fibers responsible for touch and vibratory sensation also terminated at "the gate" in the dorsal horn. It was hypothesized that their input could be manipulated to "close the gate" to the transmission of painful stimuli. As an application of the gate control theory, Shealy implanted the first spinal cord stimulator device for the treatment of chronic pain.[2] This technique was noted to control pain, and has undergone numerous technical and clinical refinements in the ensuing years. Although the gate theory was initially proposed as the mechanism of action, the underlying neurophysiologic mechanisms are not clearly understood.

The neurophysiologic mechanisms of action of spinal cord stimulation are not completely understood; however, recent research has given us insight into effects occurring at the local and supraspinal levels, and through dorsal horn interneuron and neurochemical mechanisms.[7,8] Linderoth and others have noted that the mechanism of analgesia when SCS is applied in neuropathic pain states may be very different from those involved in analgesia due to limb ischemia or angina. Experimental evidence points to SCS having a beneficial effect at the dorsal horn level by favorably altering the local neurochemistry in that zone thereby suppressing the hyperexcitability of the wide dynamic range interneurons. Specifically, there is some evidence for increased levels of gamma-aminobutyric acid (GABA) release, serotonin, and perhaps suppression of levels of some excitatory amino acids including glutamate and aspartate. In the case of ischemic pain analgesia seems to be obtained through restoration of a favorable oxygen supply and demand balance—perhaps through a favorable alteration of sympathetic tone.

TECHNICAL CONSIDERATIONS

SCS is a technically challenging interventional/surgical pain management technique. It involves the careful placement of an electrode array (leads) in the epidural space, a trial period, anchoring the lead(s), positioning and implantation of the pulse generator or radiofrequency (RF) receiver, and the tunneling and connection of the connecting wires. The authors advocate a collaborative effort between a surgeon and anesthesiologist for optimal success with neurostimulation.

Electrodes are of two types: catheter or percutaneous versus paddle or surgical (Fig. 57-1). These electrodes are connected to an implanted pulse generator (IPG) or an RF unit (Fig. 57-2). Currently two companies, Medtronic Inc. and American Neuromodulation Systems Inc., make neurostimulation equipment (see Appendix). Interested readers are directed to these companies for further specific information on the equipment.

A stimulator trial may be accomplished in two ways: "straight percutaneous" or "implanted lead." In both trial methods, under fluoroscopy and sterile conditions, a lead is introduced into the epidural space with the standard epidural needle placement (Fig. 57-3). The lead is steered under fluoroscopic imaging into the posterior paramedian epidural space up to the

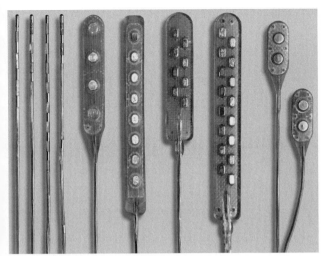

FIGURE 57-1. Neurostimulator leads: (left to right) percutaneous type to paddle type. (Courtesy of ANS Inc.)

desired anatomic location. Trial stimulation is undertaken to attempt to "cover" the painful area with an electrically induced paresthesia. After the painful area is "captured" either with one or two leads, the two techniques diverge.

In the straight percutaneous trial the needle is withdrawn; an anchoring suture placed into the skin, and a sterile dressing is applied. When the patient returns after a trial of several days the dressing is removed, the suture clipped, and the lead removed and discarded *regardless* of the success of the trial. When the patient returns for implant, a new lead is placed in the location of the trial lead and connected to an implanted IPG.

In the implanted lead trial after successful positioning of the trial lead(s), local anesthetic is infiltrated around the needle(s) and an incision is made, cutting down to the supraspinous fascia to anchor the leads securely using nonabsorbable suture (Fig. 57-4). Then a temporary extension piece is tunneled away from the back incision and out through the skin. This exiting piece is secured to the skin using a suture, antibiotic ointment, and a sterile dressing. If the trial is successful, at the time of implant the back incision is opened up, the percutaneous lead is cut, pulled out through the skin site, and discarded. The permanent lead(s) that were used for the trial are hooked to new extension(s) and tunneled to an implanted IPG.

The implanted lead method has the advantages of saving the cost of new electrodes at implant and ensuring that the implanted lead position matches the trial lead position. Advantages of the percutaneous lead approach include avoiding the costs of two trips to the operating room (even for an unsuccessful trial to remove the anchored trial lead), avoiding an incision and postoperative pain during the trial, which may confuse trial interpretation by the patient, and the percutaneous temporary extension is a risk for infection. The percutaneous extension must be anchored and meticulously dressed or the risk of infection may be higher than with the straight percutaneous technique.[9] Most consider 50% or more pain relief to be indicative of a successful trial, although the ultimate decision also should include other factors such as activity level and medication intake. To paraphrase, some combination of pain relief, increased activity level, and decreased medication intake is indicative of a favorable trial.

A trial with paddle-type electrodes requires the implanted lead approach—with the significant addition of a laminotomy to slip the flat plate electrode into the epidural space. Some physicians trial the patient with the straight percutaneous approach and if successful will send the patient to a neurosurgeon for a paddle-type implant. The authors' preference is to do a straight percutaneous trial, with an implant using nonpaddle-type electrodes.

The IPG/RF unit is generally implanted in the lower abdominal area or in the posterior superior gluteal area (Fig. 57-5). It should be in a location the patient can access with their dominant hand for adjustment of their settings with the patient-held remote control unit. The decision to use a fully implantable IPG or an RF unit depends on several considerations. If the patient's pain pattern requires the use of many anode/cathode settings with high power settings during the trial, consideration of an RF unit should be given. The IPG battery life will largely depend on the power settings utilized, but the newer IPG units (Synergy or Genesis XP) will generally last several years at average power settings.

PATIENT SELECTION

Appropriate patients for neurostimulation implant must meet the following criterion: the patient has a diagnosis amenable to this therapy (i.e., neuropathic pain syndromes), the patient has failed conservative therapy, significant psychological issues have been ruled out, and a trial has demonstrated pain relief.[10] However, pure neuropathic pain syndromes are relatively less common than the mixed nociceptive/neuropathic disorders including failed back surgery syndrome (FBSS) (Fig. 57-6). Also, many patients with chronic pain will have some depressive symptomatology, but psychological screening can be extremely helpful to avoid implanting patients with major psychological disorders. An interesting study by Olson and colleagues revealed a high correlation between many items on a complex psychological testing battery and favorable response to trial stimulation.[11] This is to say that overall mood state is an important predictor of outcomes.

A careful trial period is advocated to avoid the failed implant. Trials of different lengths have been advocated; the risks of a longer trial are mainly infection, whereas the risks of too short a trial are misreading success. The authors utilize a 5- to 7-day trial with the use of oral antibiotics. We encourage the patient to be as active as possible in their usual environment, with the exception of limiting bending/twisting movements. In spite of advances in the understanding of diagnosis which respond to neurostimulation, increased understanding of and improved psychological screening, and improved multi-lead systems, clinical failures of implanted neurostimulator devices remain too common and pain practitioners must critically evaluate their own outcomes and adhere to strict selection criterion outlined above.

COMPLICATIONS

Complications with SCS range from simple, easily correctable problems, such as lack of appropriate paresthesia coverage, to devastating complications, such as paralysis, nerve injury, and death. Prior to the implantation of the trial lead, an educational session should occur with the patient and significant family members. This meeting should include a discussion of possible risks and complications. In the postoperative period

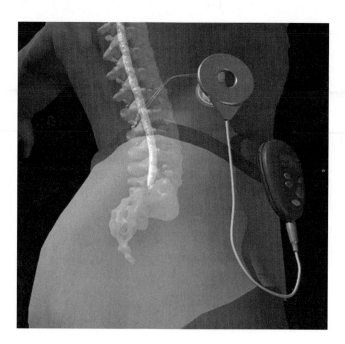

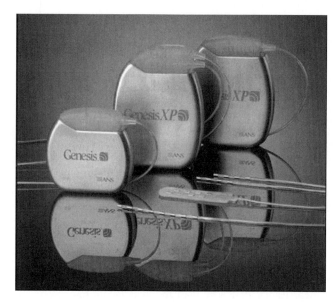

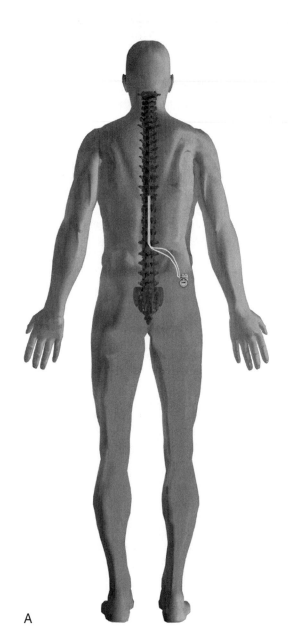

A

B

C

FIGURE 57-2. *A,* Schematic view of an implanted pulse generator system. (Courtesy of Medtronic Inc.) *B,* Schematic view of an implanted radiofrequency spinal cord stimulation system. (Courtesy of ANS Inc.) *C,* Representative implanted pulse generator neurostimulation units with leads. (Courtesy of ANS Inc.)

the caregiver should be involved in identifying problems and alerting the health care team.

North and colleagues reported their experience in 320 consecutive patients treated with SCS between 1972 and 1990.[12] A 5% rate of subcutaneous infection was seen and is consistent with the literature. The predominant complication consisted of lead migration or breakage. This remains the "Achilles' heel" of neurostimulation. In an earlier series bipolar leads required electrode revision in 23% of patients. The revision rate for patients with multichannel devices was 16%. Failure of the electrode lead was observed in 13% of patients and steadily declined

over the course of the study. When analyzed by implant type (single-channel percutaneous, single-channel laminectomy, and multichannel), the lead migration rate for multichannel devices was approximately 7%. Analysis of hardware reliability for 298 permanent implants showed that technical failures (particularly electrode migration and malposition) and clinical failures had become significantly less common as implants had evolved into programmable, "multichannel" devices.

More recent studies by Barolat et al. and May et al. reported lead revision rates due to lead migration of 4.5% and 13.6% and breakage of 0% and 13.6%, respectively.[13,14] Infections occurred

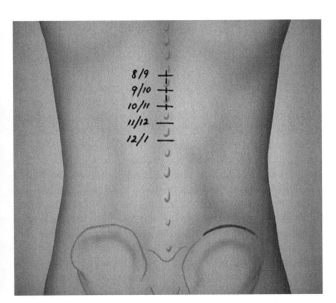

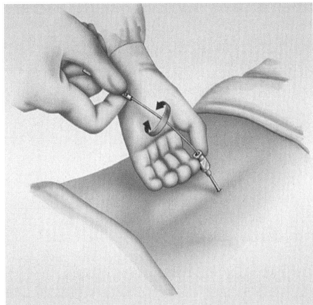

A

B

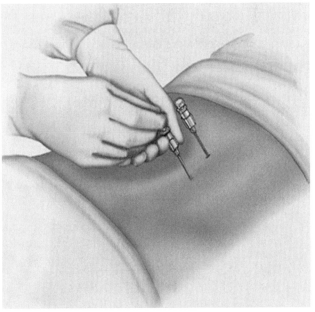

C

FIGURE 57-3. *A,* Percutaneous lead placement: marking the interspinous level. *B,* Percutaneous lead insertion. *C,* Dual lead trial. (Courtesy of Medtronic Inc.)

in 7% and 2.5% of cases, respectively. No serious complications were seen in either study. These studies are representative of the complication rate of neurostimulation therapy.

Infections range from simple infections at the surface of the wound to epidural abscess. The patient should be instructed on wound care and recognition of signs and symptoms indicative of infection. Many superficial infections can be treated with oral antibiotics or simple surgical exploration and irrigation. At the authors' center, the standard includes prophylactic intraoperative antibiotics and oral coverage postoperatively for 10 days.

If infection reaches the tissues involving the devices, in most cases the implant should be removed. In such cases one should

have a high index of suspicion for an epidural abscess. Abscess of the epidural space can lead to paralysis and death if not identified quickly and treated aggressively. In the case of temporary epidural catheters (somewhat analogous to a percutaneous stimulator trial) Sarubbi and Vasquez discovered only 20 well-described cases.[15] The mean age of these 22 patients was 49.9 years, the median duration of epidural catheter use was 3 days, and the median time to onset of clinical symptoms after catheter placement was 5 days. The majority of patients (63.6%) had major neurological deficits, and 22.7% also had concomitant meningitis. *Staphylococcus aureus* was the predominant pathogen. Despite antibiotic therapy and drainage

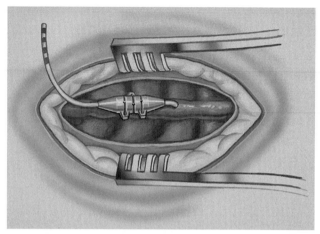

FIGURE 57-4. Anchoring the lead. (Courtesy of Medtronic Inc.)

procedures, 38% of the patients continued to have neurological deficits. These unusual but serious complications of temporary epidural catheter use require efficient and accurate diagnostic evaluation and treatment, as the consequences of delayed therapy can be substantial. Schuchard and Clauson reported an infection with Pasturella during an implanted lead trial, which required explanting the system.[16] One of the present authors (A.B.) has experienced one similar case with *S. aureus* requiring explant of the entire system (unpublished).

PROGRAMMING

There are four basic parameters in neurostimulation, which may be adjusted to create stimulation paresthesias in the painful areas thereby mitigating the patient's pain (Fig. 57-7). They are: amplitude, pulse width, rate, and electrode selection.[17]

Amplitude is the intensity or strength of the stimulation measured in volts (V). The voltage may be set from 0 to 10 V, with lower settings typically used over peripheral nerves and with paddle-type electrodes. Pulse width is a measure in microseconds (μs) of the duration of a pulse. Pulse width is usually set between 100 and 400 μs. A larger pulse width will typically give the patient a broader coverage. Rate is measured in hertz (Hz) or cycles per second, between 20 and 120 Hz. At lower rates the patient feels more of a thumping, whereas at higher Hz, the feeling is more of a buzzing. Electrode selection is a complex topic that has been the subject of some research by Barolat and colleagues who provided mapping data of coverage patterns based on lead location in 106 patients.[18] The primary target is the cathode ("−"), with electrons flowing from the cathode(s) "−" to the anode(s) "+." Most patients' stimulators are programmed with electrode selection changed until the patient obtains anatomic coverage, then the pulse width and rate are adjusted for maximal comfort. The patient is left with full control of turning the stimulation off and on, and the voltage up and down to comfort.

The authors use an analogy of a stereo to discuss programming with patients. Amplitude is the "volume control," the pulse width is "how many speakers are on mono versus surround sound," and the rate is the "bass or treble control." The lowest acceptable settings on all parameters are generally used to conserve battery life. Other programming modes that save battery life include a cycling mode during which the stimulator cycles full on/off at patient-determined intervals (minutes, seconds, or hours). The patients' programming may change over time and reprogramming needs are common. Both neurostimulator manufacturing companies are very helpful to clinicians with patient reprogramming assistance. Many busy pain practices designate a stimulator nurse to handle patient reprogramming needs.

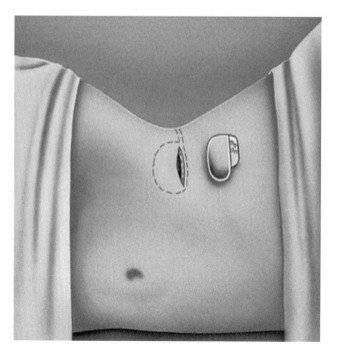

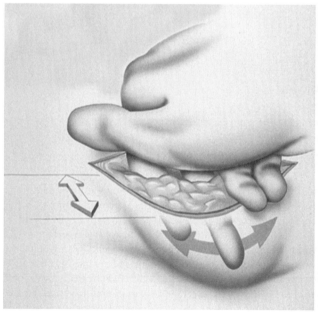

A

B

FIGURE 57-5. *A, B,* Permanent implant: pulse generator internalization. (Courtesy of Medtronic Inc.)

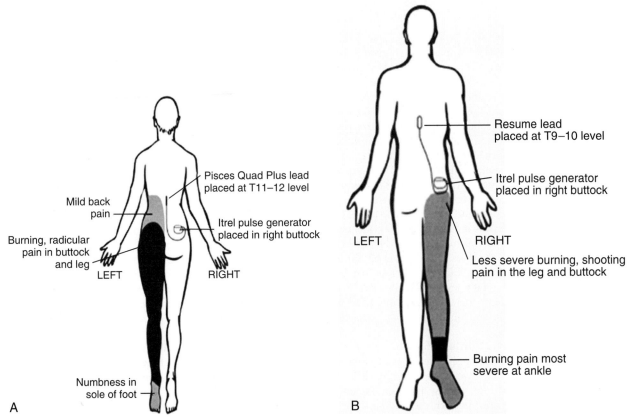

FIGURE 57-6. A, B, Ideal candidates: failed back surgery syndrome/complex regional pain syndrome. Note the radicular versus axial pain pattern. (Courtesy of Medtronic Inc.)

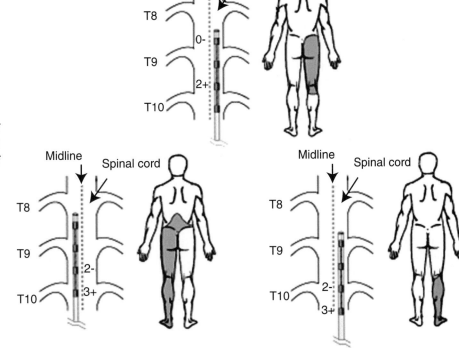

FIGURE 57-7. Typical patterns of coverage using different anodal and cathode combinations. (Courtesy of Medtronic Inc.)

OUTCOMES

The most common use for SCS in the USA is in FBSS, whereas in Europe peripheral ischemia is the predominate indication. With respect to clinical outcomes it makes sense to subdivide the outcomes based on diagnosis. In a review of the available SCS literature most evidence falls within the level IV (limited) or level V (indeterminate) categories due to the invasiveness of the modality and inability to provide blinded treatment. Recognition must also be given to the time frame within which a study was performed due to rapidly evolving SCS technology. Basic science knowledge, implantation techniques, lead placement locations, contact array designs, and programming capabilities have changed dramatically from the time of the first implants. These improvements have led to decreased morbidity and much greater probability of obtaining adequate paresthesia coverage with subsequent improved outcomes.[19] Thus, even a level II review study such as the one by Turner et al. with FBSS patients from 1966 to 1994 reported less positive outcomes than Barolat's level IV FBSS study in 2001.[20,21] The authors believe this represents the effect of improving technology.

Failed back surgery syndrome: There has been one recent prospective, randomized study. North et al. selected 50 patients as candidates for repeat laminectomy. All the patients had undergone previous surgery, and were excluded from randomization if they presented with severe spinal canal stenosis, extremely large disc fragments, a major neurological deficit such as foot drop, or radiographic evidence of gross instability. In addition, patients were excluded for untreated dependency on narcotic analgesics or benzodiazepines, major psychiatric comorbidity, the presence of any significant or disabling chronic pain problem, or a chief complaint of low back pain exceeding lower extremity pain. Crossover between groups was permitted. The 6-month follow-up report included 27 patients. At this point, they became eligible for crossover. Of the 15 patients who had undergone re-operation, 67% (10 patients) crossed over to SCS. Of the 12 who had undergone SCS, 17% (2 patients) opted for crossover to re-operation. Additionally, of the 19 patients who reached their 6-month follow-up assessment after re-operation, 42% (8 patients) opted for SCS outside the study. For 90% of the patients, long-term (3-year follow-up) evaluation has shown that SCS continues to be more effective than re-operation, with significantly better outcomes by standard measures and significantly lower rates of crossover to the alternative procedure. Additionally, patients randomized to re-operation used significantly more opioids than those randomized to SCS. Other measures assessing activities of daily living and work status did not differ significantly. The preliminary results have been published in abstract format, but the definitive study has yet to be published.[22]

Two recent, prospective case series have been done. The first, by Barolat et al., examined the outcomes of patients with intractable low back pain treated with epidural SCS utilizing paddle electrodes and an RF stimulator.[23] In four centers 44 patients were implanted and followed with the visual analogue scale (VAS), the Oswestry Disability Questionnaire, the Sickness Impact Profile (SIP), and a patient satisfaction rating scale. All patients had back and leg pain, and all had at least one previous back surgery, with most (83%) having 2 or more back surgeries, and 51% having had a spinal fusion. Data were collected at baseline, at 6 months, 12 months, and 2 years.

All patients showed a reported mean decrease in their 10-point VAS scores compared to baseline. The majority of patients reported fair to excellent pain relief in both the low back and legs. At 6 months, 91.6% of the patients reported fair to excellent relief in the legs and 82.7% of the patients reported fair to excellent relief in the low back. At 1 year, 88.2% of the patients reported fair to excellent relief in the legs and 68.8% of the patients reported fair to excellent relief in the low back. Significant improvement in function and quality of life was found at both the 6-month and 1-year follow-ups using the Oswestry and SIP, respectively. The majority of patients reported that the procedure was worthwhile (92% at 6 months, 88% at 1 year). The authors concluded that SCS proved beneficial at 1 year for the treatment of patients with chronic low back and leg pain.

The second multicenter prospective case series was published by Burchiel et al. in 1996.[24] The study included 182 patients with a permanent system after a percutaneous trial. Patient evaluation of pain and functional levels was performed before and 3, 6, and 12 months after implantation. Complications, medication usage, and work status also were monitored. A 1-year follow-up evaluation was available for 70 patients. All pain and quality-of-life measures showed statistically significant improvement, whereas medication usage and work status did not significantly improve during the treatment year. Complications requiring surgical interventions were experienced by 17% (12 of 70) of the patients.

There have been two systematic review articles on neurostimulation. Turner et al. completed a meta-analysis from the articles related to the treatment of FBSS by SCS from 1966 to 1994.[25] They reviewed 39 studies that met the inclusion criteria. The mean follow-up period was 16 months with a range of 1 to 45 months. Pain relief exceeding 50% was experienced by 59% of patients with a range of 15% to 100%. Complications occurred in 42% of patients, with 30% of patients experiencing one or more stimulator-related complications. However, all the studies were case control investigations. Based on this review, the authors concluded that there was insufficient evidence from the literature for drawing conclusions about the effectiveness of SCS relative to no treatment or other treatments, or about the effects of SCS on patient work status, functional disability, and medication use.

The second study by North and Wetzel consisted of a review of case control studies and two prospective control studies.[26] They concluded that if a patient reports a reduction in pain of at least 50% during a trial, as determined by standard rating methods, and demonstrates improved or stable analgesic requirements and activity levels, significant benefit may be realized from a permanent implant. The authors concluded that the bulk of the literature appears to support a role for SCS (in neuropathic pain syndromes) but cautioned that the quality of the existing literature was marginal and consisted largely of case series.

Complex Regional Pain Syndrome (CRPS): Research of high quality regarding SCS and CRPS is limited, but existing data are overwhelmingly positive in terms of pain reduction, quality of life, analgesic usage, and function.

Kemler and colleagues published a prospective, randomized, comparative trial to compare SCS versus conservative therapy for CRPS.[27] Patients with a 6 month history of CRPS of the upper extremities were randomized to undergo trial SCS (and implant if successful) plus physiotherapy versus physiotherapy alone. In this study 36 patients were assigned to receive a standardized physical therapy program together with SCS, whereas 18 patients were assigned to receive therapy alone. In 24 of the 36 patients randomized to SCS, along with physical therapy, the trial was successful, and permanent implantation was performed. At a 6-month follow-up assessment, the patients in the SCS group had a significantly greater reduction in pain, and a significantly higher percentage was graded as much improved for the global perceived effect. However, there were no clinically significant improvements in functional status. The authors concluded that in the short term SCS reduces pain and improves the quality of life for patients with CRPS involving the upper extremities.

Several important case series have been published on the use of neurostimulation in the treatment of CRPS. Calvillo et al. reported a series of 36 patients with advanced stages of CRPS (at least 2 years' duration) who had undergone successful SCS trial (>50% reduction of pain).[28] They were treated with either SCS or peripheral nerve stimulation, and in some cases with both modalities. Thirty six months after implantation the reported pain measured on VAS was an average of 53% better; this change was statistically significant. Analgesic consumption decreased in the majority of patients. Some 41% of patients had returned to work on a modified duty. The authors concluded that in late stages of CRPS neurostimulation (with SCS or peripheral nerve stimulation) is a reasonable option when alternative therapies have failed.

Another case series reported by Oakley and Weiner is remarkable in that it utilized a sophisticated battery of outcome tools to evaluate treatment response in CRPS using SCS.[29] The study followed 19 patients and analyzed the results from the McGill Pain Rating Index, the SIP, Oswestry Disability Profile, Beck Depression Inventory, and VAS. Nineteen patients were reported as a subgroup enrolled at two centers participating in a multicenter study of efficacy/outcomes of SCS. Specific preimplant and postimplant tests to measure outcome were administered. Statistically significant improvement in the SIP physical and psychosocial subscales was documented. The McGill Pain Rating Index words chosen and sensory subscale also improved significantly as did VAS scores. The Beck Depression Inventory trended toward significant improvement. All patients received at least partial relief and benefit from their device, with 30% receiving full relief. Eighty percent of the patients obtained at least 50% pain relief through the use of their stimulators. The average pain relief was 61%. The authors concluded that patients with CRPS benefit significantly from the use of SCS, based on average follow-up of 7.9 months.

A literature review by Stanton-Hicks of SCS for CRPS consisted of seven case series. These studies ranged in size from 6 to 24 patients. Results were noted as "good to excellent" in greater than 72% of patients over a time period of 8 to 40 months. The review concluded that SCS has proven to be a powerful tool in the management of patients with CRPS.[30]

A retrospective, three-year, multicenter study of 101 patients by Bennett et al. evaluated the effectiveness of SCS applied to CRPS type I and compared the effectiveness of octapolar vs. quadrapolar systems, as well as high-frequency and multiprogram parameters.[31] VAS was significantly decreased in the group using the dual-octapolar system with reductions in overall VAS approaching 70%. Of the dual-octapolar group, 74.8% used multiple arrays to maximize paresthesia coverage. VAS reduction in the group using quadrapolar systems approached 50%; 86.3% of quadrapolar systems and 97.2% of dual-octapolar systems continued to be utilized. Overall satisfaction with stimulation was 91% in the dual-octapolar group and 70% in the quadrapolar group ($p < 0.05$). The authors concluded that SCS is effective in the management of chronic pain associated with CRPS I and that use of dual-octapolar systems with multiple-array programming capabilities appeared to increase the paresthesia coverage and, thus, further reduce pain. High-frequency stimulation (>250 Hz) was found to be essential in obtaining adequate analgesia in 15% of the patients using dual-octapolar systems (this frequency level was not available to those with quadrapolar systems).

Peripheral Ischemia and Angina: Cook et al. reported in 1976 that SCS effectively relieved pain associated with peripheral ischemia.[32] This result has been repeated and noted to have particular efficacy in conditions associated with vasospasm such as Raynaud's disease.[33] Many studies have shown impressive efficacy of SCS to treat intractable angina.[34] Reported success rates are consistently greater than 80% and these indications, already widely utilized outside of the USA, are certain to expand within the USA.

COST EFFECTIVENESS

Cost effectiveness of SCS (in the treatment of chronic back pain) was evaluated by Kumar and colleagues in 2002.[35] They prospectively followed 104 patients with FBSS. Of the 104 patients, 60 were implanted with a spinal cord stimulator using a standard selection criterion. Both groups were monitored over a period of 5 years. The stimulation group annual cost was $29,000 versus $38,000 in the control group. The authors found 15% return to work in the stimulation group versus 0% in the control group. The higher costs in the nonstimulator group were in the categories of medications, emergency center visits, X-rays, and ongoing physician visits.

Bell and North performed an analysis of the medical costs of SCS therapy in the treatment of patients with FBSS.[36] The medical costs of SCS therapy were compared with an alternative regimen of surgeries and other interventions. Externally powered (external) and fully internalized (internal) SCS systems were considered separately. No value was placed on pain relief or improvements in the quality of life that successful SCS therapy can generate. The authors concluded that by reducing the demand for medical care by FBSS patients, SCS therapy could lower medical costs and found that, on average, SCS therapy pays for itself within 5.5 years. For those patients for whom SCS therapy is clinically efficacious, the therapy pays for itself within 2.1 years.

Kemler and Furnee performed a similar study but looked at "chronic reflex sympathetic dystrophy (RSD)" using outcomes and costs of care before and after the start of treatment.[37] This essentially is an economic analysis of the Kemler RSD outcomes paper. Fifty-four patients with chronic RSD were randomized to receive either SCS together with physical therapy (SCS + PT; $n = 36$) or physical therapy alone (PT; $n = 18$). Twenty-four SCS + PT patients responded positively to trial stimulation and underwent SCS implantation. During 12 months of follow-up, costs (routine RSD costs, SCS costs, out-of-pocket costs) and effects (pain relief by VAS, health-related quality of life (HRQL) improvement by EQ-5D) were assessed in both groups. Analyses were carried out up to 1 year and up to the expected time of death. SCS was both more effective and less costly than the standard treatment protocol. As a result of high initial costs of SCS, in the first year the treatment per patient is $4,000 more than control therapy. However, in the lifetime analysis SCS per patient is $60,000 cheaper than control therapy. In addition, at 12 months, SCS resulted in pain relief (SCS + PT (−2.7) vs. PT (0.4) ($p < 0.001$)) and improved HRQL (SCS + PT (0.22) vs. PT (0.03) ($p = 0.004$)). The authors found SCS to be both more effective and less expensive as compared with the standard treatment protocol for chronic RSD.

PERIPHERAL, CORTICAL, AND DEEP BRAIN STIMULATION

Although this chapter concentrates on the technique of SCS, it must be noted that neurostimulation can successfully be utilized at other locations in the peripheral and central nervous systems to provide analgesia.

Peripheral nerve stimulation was introduced by Wall, Sweet, and others in the mid-1960s.[38] This technique has shown efficacy for peripheral nerve injury pain syndromes as well as CRPS, with the use of a carefully implanted paddle lead utilizing a fascial graft to help anchor the lead without traumatizing the nerve.[39]

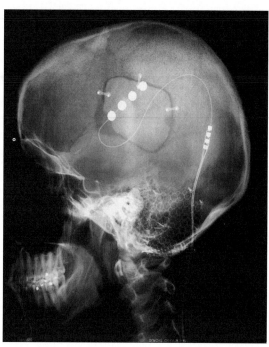

FIGURE 57-8. Radiograph of motor cortex stimulation. (Courtesy of Ali Rezai, M.D., Cleveland Clinic Foundation.)

Motor cortex and deep brain stimulation are techniques that have been explored to treat highly refractory neuropathic pain syndromes including central pain, deafferentation syndromes, trigeminal neuralgia, and others (Fig. 57-8).[40] Deep brain stimulation has become a widely used technique for movement

TABLE 57-1. PRINCIPLES OF NEUROSTIMULATION

SCS mechanism of action is not completely understood but influences multiple components and levels within the central nervous system with both interneuron and neurochemical mechanisms.
SCS therapy is effective for many neuropathic pain conditions. Stimulation-evoked paresthesia must be experienced in the entire painful area. No consistent evidence exists for the efficacy of neurostimulation in primary nociceptive pain conditions.
Stimulation should be applied with low intensity, just suprathreshold for the activation of the low-threshold, large-diameter fibers, and should be of nonpainful intensity. To be effective SCS must be applied continuously (or in cycles) for at least 20 minutes prior to the onset of analgesia. This analgesia develops slowly and typically lasts several hours after cessation of the stimulation.
SCS has demonstrated clinical and cost effectiveness in FBSS and CRPS. Clinical effectiveness has also been shown in peripheral ischemia and angina.
Multicontact, multiprogram systems improve outcomes and reduce the incidence of surgical revisions. Insulated, paddle-type electrodes *probably* decrease the incidence of lead breakage, prolong battery life, and show early superiority in quality of paresthesia coverage and analgesia in FBSS as compared to permanent percutaneous electrodes.
Serious complications are exceedingly rare but can be devastating. Meticulous care must be taken during implantation to minimize procedural complications. The most frequent complications are wound infections (approximately 5%) and lead breakage or migration (approximately 13% each for permanent percutaneous leads and 3% to 6% each for paddle leads).

CRPS, complex regional pain syndrome; FBSS, failed back surgery syndrome; SCC, spinal cord stimulation.
Modified from Linderoth B, Meyerson BA: Spinal cord stimulation: Mechanisms of action. *In* Burchiel K (ed): Surgical Management of Pain. Theime Medical, New York, 2002, pp 505–526.

disorders, and much less so for painful indications, although there have been many case reports of utility in treating highly refractory central pain syndromes.[41]

CONCLUSIONS

SCS is an invasive, interventional surgical procedure. Linderoth and Meyerson have written some principles of neurostimulation that are cornerstones of SCS theory and practice (Table 57-1).[42] The difficulty of randomized clinical trials in such situations is well recognized. Based on the present evidence with two randomized trials, one prospective trial, and multiple retrospective trials, the evidence for SCS in properly selected populations with neuropathic pain states is moderate. Clearly, this technique should be reserved for patients who have failed more conservative therapies. With appropriate selection and careful attention to technical issues, the clinical results are overwhelmingly positive.

KEY POINTS

- The pain practitioner must have a thorough grasp of spinal fluoroscopic anatomy and basic surgical techniques prior to introducing neurostimulation into their practice. One must understand the "marriage" of the implanted pain device and select patients carefully.
- Neurostimulation mechanisms of analgesia are poorly understood, but neurostimulation probably works via interneuronal and neurochemical mechanisms. It is one of the few nonpharmacologic techniques available to help patients with severe chronic neuropathic pain.
- Neurostimulation is effective for many neuropathic pain conditions with the caveat that stimulation-evoked paresthesias must be experienced in the painful area. Basic programming skills take some years to refine, but the device companies can be very helpful in this training. Having a trained physician extender practice programmer can be very effective in a practice with numerous stimulation patients.
- Neurostimulation has demonstrated clinical and cost-effectiveness in FBSS patients, CRPS patients, peripheral ischemia patients, and angina patients.
- Multicontact, multielectrode systems improve outcomes and reduce the need for surgical revisions. Paddle-type electrodes may provide superior coverage at lower power settings in some patients.
- The "Achilles' heel" of the implanted neurostimulation system is lead migration. One should consider working with a surgeon to assist in anchoring leads into place for optimal outcome until very familiar and comfortable with the techniques.
- Serious complications are rare, but can be devastating. Complete informed consent must be obtained before trial or implant.
- With these caveats in mind, the clinician may use this elegant, effective modality judiciously to help patients with refractory, severe, neuropathic pain states.

APPENDIX

Medtronic Inc., 710 Medtronic Parkway, Minneapolis, MN 55432-5604, USA; 763-514-5604; www.medtronic.com.

American Neuromodulation Systems Inc., 6501 Windcrest Dr, Ste 100, Plano, TX 75024, USA; 800-727-7846; www.ans-medical.com.

REFERENCES

1. Kumar K, Nath R, Wyant GM: Treatment of chronic pain by epidural spinal cord stimulation: A 10-year experience. J Neurosurg 5:402–407, 1991.
2. Shealy CN, Mortimer JT, Resnick J: Electrical inhibition of pain by stimulation of the dorsal columns: Preliminary reports. J Int Anesth Res Soc 46:489–491, 1967.
3. Kumar K, Toth C, Nath RK: Deep brain stimulation for intractable pain: A 15-year experience. Neurosurgery 40:736–746, 1997.
4. Nguyen JP, Lefaucher JP, Le Guerinel C, et al: Motor cortex stimulation in the treatment of central and neuropathic pain. Arch Med Res 31:263–265, 2000.
5. Campbell JN, Long DM: Stimulation of the peripheral nervous system for pain control. J Neurosurg 45:692–699, 1976.
6. Melzack R, Wall PD: Pain mechanisms: A new theory. Science 150:971–979, 1965.
7. Oakley J, Prager J: Spinal cord stimulation: Mechanism of action. Spine 22:2574–2583, 2002.
8. Linderoth B, Foreman R: Physiology of spinal cord stimulation: Review and update. Neuromodulation 3:150–164, 1999.
9. May MS, Banks C, Thomson SJ: A retrospective, long-term, third party follow-up of patients considered for spinal cord stimulation. Neuromodulation 3:137–144, 2002.
10. Burchiel KJ, Anderson VC, Wilson BJ, et al: Prognostic factors of spinal cord stimulation for chronic back and leg pain. Neurosurgery 36:1101–1111, 1995.
11. Olson KA, Bedder MD, Anderson VC, et al: Psychological variables associated with outcome of spinal cord stimulation trials. Neuromodulation 1:6–13, 1998.
12. North RB, Kidd DH, Zahurak M, et al: Spinal cord stimulation for chronic, intractable pain: Two decades' experience. Neurosurgery 32:384–395, 1993.
13. Barolat G, Oakley J, Law J, et al: Epidural spinal cord stimulation with a multiple electrode paddle lead is effective in treating low back pain. Neuromodulation 2:59–66, 2001.
14. May MS, Banks C, Thomson SJ: A retrospective, long-term, third party follow-up of patients considered for spinal cord stimulation. Neuromodulation 3:137–144, 2002.
15. Sarubbi F, Vasquez J: Spinal epidural abscess associated with the use of temporary epidural catheters: Report of two cases and review. Clin Infect Dis 25:1155–1158, 1997.
16. Schuchard M, Clauson W: An interesting and heretofore unreported infection of a spinal cord stimulator: Smitten by a kitten revisited. Neuromodulation 4:67–71, 2001.
17. Alfano S, Darwin J, Picullel B: Programming principles. *In* Spinal Cord Stimulation: Patient Management Guidelines for Clinicians. Medtronic Inc., Minneapolis, MN, 2001, pp 27–33.
18. Barolat G, Massaro F, He J, et al: Mapping of sensory responses to epidural stimulation of the intraspinal neural structures in man. J Neurosurg 78:233–239, 1993.
19. North RB, Kidd DH, Zahurak M, et al: Spinal cord stimulation for chronic, intractable pain: Experience over two decades. Neurosurgery 32:384–394, 1993.
20. Turner JA, Loeser JD, Bell KG: Spinal cord stimulation for chronic low back pain: A systematic literature synthesis. Neurosurgery 37:1088–1095; discussion 1095–1096, 1995.
21. Barolat G, Oakley J, Law J, et al: Epidural spinal cord stimulation with a multiple electrode paddle lead is effective in treating low back pain. Neuromodulation 2:59–66, 2001.
22. North RB, Kidd DH, Piantadosi S: Spinal cord stimulation versus reoperation for failed back surgery syndrome: A prospective, randomized study design. Acta Neurochir Suppl (Wien) 64:106–108, 1995.

23. Barolat G, Oakley J, Law J, et al: Epidural spinal cord stimulation with a multiple electrode paddle lead is effective in treating low back pain. Neuromodulation 2:59–66, 2001.

24. Burchiel KJ, Anderson VC, Brown FD, et al: Prospective, multicenter study of spinal cord stimulation for the relief of chronic back and extremity pain. Spine 21:2786–2794, 1996.

25. Turner JA, Loeser JD, Bell KG: Spinal cord stimulation for chronic low back pain: A systematic literature synthesis. Neurosurgery 37:1088–1095, 1995.

26. North R, Wetzel T: Spinal cord stimulation for chronic pain of spinal origin. Spine 22:2584–2591, 2002.

27. Kemler MA, Barendse GA, van Kleef M, et al: Spinal cord stimulation in patients with chronic reflex sympathetic dystrophy. N Engl J Med 343:618–624, 2000.

28. Calvillo O, Racz G, Didie J, et al: Neuroaugmentation in the treatment of complex regional pain syndrome of the upper extremity. Acta Orthopeadica Belgica 1:57–63, 1998.

29. Oakley J, Weiner R: Spinal cord stimulation for complex regional pain syndrome: A prospective study of 19 patients at two centers. Neuromodulation 1:47–50, 1999.

30. Stanton-Hicks M: Spinal cord stimulation for the management of complex regional pain syndromes. Neuromodulation 3:193–201, 1999.

31. Bennett D, Alo K, Oakley J, et al: Spinal cord stimulation for complex regional pain syndrome I (RSD): A retrospective multicenter experience from 1995–1998 of 101 patients. Neuromodulation 3:202–210, 1999.

32. Cook AW, Oygar A, Baggenstos P, et al: Vascular disease of extremities: Electrical stimulation of spinal cord and posterior roots. N Y State J Med 76:366–368, 1976.

33. Broseta J, Barbera J, De Vera JA: Spinal cord stimulation in peripheral arterial disease. J Neurosurg 64:71–80, 1986.

34. Eliasson T, Augustinsson LE, Mannheimer C: Spinal cord stimulation in severe angina pectoris – Presentation of current studies, indications, and clinical experience. Pain 65:169–179, 1996.

35. Kumar K, Malik S, Demeria D: Treatment of chronic pain with spinal cord stimulation versus alternative therapies: Cost-effectiveness analysis. Neurosurgery 51:106–115, 2002.

36. Bell G, North R: Cost-effectiveness analysis of spinal cord stimulation in treatment of failed back surgery syndrome. J Pain Symptom Manage 13:285–296, 1997.

37. Kemler M, Furnee C: Economic evaluation of spinal cord stimulation for chronic reflex sympathetic dystrophy. Neurology 59:1203–1209, 2002.

38. Wall PD, Sweet WH: Temporary abolition of pain in man. Science 155:108–109, 1967.

39. Hassenbusch SJ, Stanton-Hicks M, Shoppa D: Long-term results of peripheral nerve stimulation for reflex sympathetic dystrophy. J Neurosurg 84:415–423, 1996.

40. Tsubokawa T, Katayama Y, Yamamoto T, et al: Chronic motor cortex stimulation in patients with thalamic pain. J Neurosurg 78:393–401, 1993.

41. Limousin P, Krack P, Pollack P, et al: Electrical stimulation of the subthalamic nucleus in advanced Parkinson's disease. N Engl J Med 339:1105–1111, 1998.

42. Linderoth B, Meyerson BA: Spinal cord stimulation: Mechanisms of action. In Burchiel K (ed): Surgical Management of Pain. Theime Medical, New York, 2002, pp 505–526.

Implanted Drug Delivery Systems for the Control of Chronic Pain

Kenji Muro, M.D., and
Robert M. Levy, M.D., Ph.D.

Oral, parenteral, and transdermal narcotics are extremely effective analgesic agents; however, systemic administration may cause significant side effects (Table 58-1) and long-term use in sufficient doses may result in tolerance and increased potential for addiction. Thus, the control of chronic pain with systemic narcotics is often accompanied by a marked reduction in the quality of life.

The discovery of opiate receptors in the substantia gelatinosa of the spinal cord first led to the recognition of opioids

TABLE 58-1. SIDE EFFECTS FROM SYSTEMIC ADMINISTRATION OF ORAL, PARENTERAL, AND TRANSDERMAL NARCOTICS

Central nervous system effects of opiates
Analgesia
Mydriasis
Euphoria or dysphoria
Nausea and vomiting
Sedation
Confusion
Cough reflex depression
Respiratory depression
Peripheral effects of opiates
Decreased gastrointestinal tract motility
Constipation
Urinary retention
Histamine release
Pruritis
Increased biliary duct pressure

having a spinal, as well as supraspinal, analgesic action. Fields and Basbaum[1] in the USA and Besson in France subsequently elucidated and described the descending pain inhibition system. This pathway begins with projections from the frontal cortex and hypothalamus to the periaqueductal gray (PAG) of the midbrain. The next projection goes to the dorsal pons and the rostroventral medulla, through the dorsolateral funiculus, to terminate in the substantia gelatinosa of the spinal cord dorsal horn. These efferent projections inhibit the second-order ascending nociceptive neurons, blocking pain transmission. Understanding this spinal level antinociceptive mechanism led to the first trials of direct intraspinal administration of opioids, with morphine administered epidurally[2] and intrathecally[3] for the treatment of cancer pain.[4] Since the discovery of opiate receptors in the substantia gelatinosa in 1976 to 1990, spinal opioids have been used in over 120,000 patients.[5]

Intraspinal pharmacotherapy for pain largely restricts drug effects to regions associated with the source of noxious input. Systemic side effects are essentially eliminated, and a much higher local analgesic concentration is achieved at its site of action, even at comparatively lower doses. Morphine is particularly well suited for this application, due to its hydrophilicity and resulting slow absorption from the cerebrospinal fluid (CSF). As a result, analgesia from intrathecal morphine not uncommonly lasts up to 24 hours.[3]

At the spinal level of antinociceptive processing, opiates presynaptically diminish primary afferent terminal excitability and inhibit substance P release. Postsynaptically, opiates act to suppress excitatory amino acid–evoked excitatory postsynaptic potentials (EPSP) in dorsal horn neurons. There are at least five opioid receptor subclasses, three of which (mu, delta, and kappa) are thought to mediate antinociception. Morphine, D-alanine-D-leucine enkephalin (DADLE), and dynorphin, respectively, are the prototype agonists for these receptor subclasses.

The discovery of multiple receptor systems involved in nociceptive transmission and modulation has allowed the testing and application of other receptor selective drugs (Table 58-2). Among the non-narcotic agents, alpha-adrenergic agonists are the most widely used receptor agonists for intraspinal pain pharmacotherapy. Alpha-adrenergic receptors exist in the substantia gelatinosa of the spinal cord, situated on both pre- and postsynaptic terminals of small primary afferents. They appear to mediate antinociception by indirectly decreasing the release of substance P. These agents have the particular advantage over opiates of little or no effect on respiratory centers, thus eliminating the possibility of respiratory depression. Another potential advantage of adrenergic agents is their efficacy in the management of neuropathic pain states; there is both experimental[6] and clinical[7–9] supporting evidence in the literature. Within this category, clonidine has been recently approved for instraspinal use and tizanidine has been tested in clinical trials.

While other agents, such as gamma-aminobutyric acid B (GABA-B) agonists, ziconotide, calcitonin, and somatostatin[10] and its analogue octreotide, have been investigated clinically, narcotics, local anesthetics, and adrenergic agonists are most often used clinically. At the present time, however, morphine and clonidine are the only agents approved by the United States Food and Drug Administration (FDA) for intraspinal analgesic use.

PATIENT SELECTION

To achieve optimal results, proper patient selection is crucial. The clinician must weigh several patient factors to indicate or contraindicate intraspinal analgesic treatment (Table 58-3).

Failure of Maximal Medical Therapy: If a noninvasive treatment program provides satisfactory pain relief without intolerable side effects, then intraspinal drug administration is not necessary. Therefore, patients should fail a multidisciplinary pain treatment program, including anti-inflammatory agents, tricyclic antidepressants, non-narcotic analgesics, and long-term systemic narcotics. Other therapies include physical and psychological therapies. Should these therapies be effective and well tolerated, intraspinal drug administration is not indicated. On the other hand, it is important to recognize early the failure of medical therapy in these patients. Hence, patients on increasing oral, transdermal, or intravenous doses of morphine who have already been treated with anti-inflammatory and tricyclic analgesics should be referred for trial of intraspinal drug administration to limit their suffering and their exposure to extremely high narcotic doses.

Favorable Psychosocial Evaluation: While most investigators highlight the importance of a favorable psychosocial

TABLE 58-2. SOME INTRASPINALLY ADMINISTERED DRUGS IN THE TREATMENT OF INTRACTABLE PAIN

| **Opiates** |
| Morphine |
| Hydromorphone |
| Fentanyl |
| Sufentanyl |
| Dynorphin |
| Beta-endorphin |
| D-ala-D-leu-enkephalin |
| Methadone |
| Meperidine |
| **Alpha-adrenoceptor agonists** |
| Clonidine |
| Tizanidine |
| **GABA B agonists** |
| Baclofen |
| **Naturally occurring peptides and their analogues** |
| Somatostatin |
| Octreotide |
| Vapreotide |
| Calcitonin |
| **Local anesthetics** |
| Bupivacaine |
| Ropivacaine |
| Tetracaine |
| **NMDA agonists** |
| Ketamine |
| **Other agents** |
| Ziconotide (SNX111) |
| Midazolam |
| Neostigmine |
| Aspirin |
| Droperidol |
| Gabapentin |

GABA, gamma-aminobutyric acid; NMDA, N-methyl-D-aspartate.

TABLE 58-3. INDICATIONS AND CONTRAINDICATIONS FOR CHRONIC INTRASPINAL ANALGESIC ADMINISTRATION

| **Indications** |
| Chronic pain with known pathophysiology |
| Sensitivity of the pain to the agent to be infused |
| Failure of maximal medical therapy |
| Favorable psychosocial evaluation |
| Favorable response to trial of intraspinal analgesic agents |
| **Contraindications** |
| Intercurrent systemic infection |
| Uncorrectable bleeding diathesis |
| Allergy to agent to be infused |
| Failure of a trial of intraspinal analgesic agents |

evaluation in the screening for potential implant candidates, the specific variables, their quantization, and their treatment are not widely agreed upon. As part of this analysis, most advocate evaluating both the patient and their support system. Clearly, acute psychotic illnesses and severe, untreated depression need diagnosis and treatment prior to surgical consideration. Other psychological issues are less clearly accepted as reasons to delay or contraindicate surgery. For example, a behavioral abnormality may affect a patient's ability to judge adequately their degree of pain or pain relief. Deficiencies in social support systems may leave the patient without someone to aid them in the event of a pain-related emergency or in the maintenance of the drug administration system (either drug administration or transfer of the patient for refilling of the drug administration device).

Absence of Systemic Infection:
The consequences of infection involving the drug administration system range from the need to remove the entire system and thus eliminate, at least for some time, this option for pain control, to the potentially life-threatening complication of meningitis. Therefore, any local infection at the surgical site or any systemic infection contraindicates the implantation of drug administration devices. Furthermore, the use of peri- and postoperative prophylactic antibiotics is recommended.

Absence of Clotting Disorders:
Coagulopathic states, not uncommon among patients harboring a malignancy, present an obstacle to surgery. Not only can the surgery be made more difficult by the hemorrhage, but it also can be complicated by the development of subcutaneous, epidural, or intradural hematomas. All efforts should be made to reverse clotting disorders; significant uncorrectable coagulation disorders contraindicate the implantation of drug infusion systems.

Absence of Drug Allergy:
Allergy to the analgesic agent to be infused obviously and absolutely contraindicates its use. With the advent of multiple intrathecal analgesic agents, however, this should become a less frequent reason to abandon this mode of therapy. Nonallergic reaction to the infused agent, such as urinary retention or pruritis, usually occurs in the acute period after exposure to the drug and may resolve with time or respond to specific treatment. This therefore does not represent absolute contraindications to chronic drug infusion.

Absence of Obstruction of CSF Flow:
Obstruction of CSF flow has been identified as a relative contraindication to intraspinal drug delivery, depending on the size, location, and cause of the obstruction. In our experience this has not been a significant problem and patients derive excellent drug benefits despite an obstruction. More important than the presence of an obstruction to CSF flow is the patient's favorable response to the intraspinal drug trial administered at the level where permanent catheter implantation is intended.

Life Expectancy Greater Than Three Months:
While the expected length of life is not a contraindication to the use of intraspinal drug administration, it does influence the method of drug administration. Percutaneous epidural catheter attached to external pump, internalized passive catheter with reservoir requiring percutaneous bolus drug administration, patient-activated

mechanical system, constant rate infusion pump, and programmable infusion pump are all viable options. The choice among these approaches, based upon ambulatory status and life expectancy, is discussed below.

Favorable Response to an Intraspinal Narcotic Trial:
Not all patients suffering from chronic pain syndromes will benefit from intraspinal narcotics. The pain relief in response to acute intraspinal analgesic agents is generally regarded as an excellent indicator of long-term efficacy.[11] The inability to achieve pain relief after such a trial is a contraindication to implantation.

Careful preoperative candidate screening for indwelling drug administration systems can help exclude those who will not benefit from this technology and predict efficacy in others. Unfortunately, bias on the part of both the treating physician and the patient can inappropriately skew the results of subjective or improperly controlled trials. This may lead to drug administration system implantation in patients who will not benefit from chronic intrathecal narcotics.

Several approaches to the trial of intrathecal narcotics have been described, including single versus multiple injections, administration via lumbar puncture versus indwelling catheter, epidural versus intrathecal routes, and bolus versus continuous infusion of the drug. Testing with a single intraspinal dose of an active agent raises the possibility that the strong desire of the physician and other health care personnel to help, and the patient's desperation to find some relief from their intractable pain, will lead to a significant placebo response. This may occur in at least 30% of cases. Attempts to control patient bias by blinded testing of both morphine and saline still does not account for the bias of the care team. Furthermore, the conclusions arrived from preimplantation drug trials are often based upon subjective criteria. This subjectivity can have a negative impact on the validity and reliability of these screening protocols. We have thus developed a quantitative, crossover, double-blind trial for the preimplantation screening of candidates for chronic drug infusion therapy for the control of intractable pain. Application of this protocol has resulted in the elimination of approximately 30% of potential implant candidates. Of those patients with a successful screening trial, approximately 70% have achieved good to excellent long-term pain relief. This screening paradigm appears to be both reliable and easily applied.[12]

ROUTE OF ADMINISTRATION

While no study has directly compared the relative efficacy of epidural versus intrathecal administration to control intractable pain, observations made by comparing the results of previous studies employing both routes are outlined below (Table 58-4).

The equianalgesic epidural dose is roughly 10 times that of an intrathecal dose.[13] As 80% to 90% of an epidural injection is systemically absorbed, this larger dose requirement may lead to greater systemic side effects, including constipation and urinary retention. These higher doses further increase the probability of developing narcotic tolerance. Also, there is maximum morphine solubility in saline of approximately 55 mg/mL and pump reservoirs are of limited size; therefore, the higher dose requirement with epidural infusion to reach equivalent subarachnoid concentration necessitates refilling

TABLE 58-4. INTRATHECAL VERSUS EPIDURAL ADMINISTRATION

	Advantages	Disadvantages
Intrathecal	Lower dosage requirement (10 times more potent than epidural dose) Less systemic effect No dural fibrosis at tip of catheter Possible to sample spinal fluid for culture diagnosis and drug levels	Increased risk of neural injury Increased risk of spinal headaches Increased risk of supraspinal distribution
Epidural	Reduced risk of respiratory depression Reduced risk of spinal headache Reduced risk of neural injury	Greater dose requirement Higher systemic effect Dural fibrosis possible Question of increased tolerance Limited reservoir volume

the reservoir on a more frequent basis. In addition, epidural catheter placement has known complication of dural scarring, resulting in catheter failure due to occlusion, kinking, or displacement.

Although it avoids these complications, intrathecal drug administration carries the disadvantages of potential CSF leak and postdural spinal headaches, respiratory depression due to supraspinal redistribution of narcotic, and meningeal infection or neural injury.

Thus, the major advantage of epidural administration is the theoretically lower risk of serious complication, although this is remarkably uncommon. In addition, epidural catheters can be placed at virtually any level, making it potentially more useful for the treatment of upper body pain. Anderson and colleagues, however, have reported excellent results treating pain of the trunk, neck, and even the head with lumbar intrathecal morphine administration.[14] The advantages of the intrathecal route, including the lower drug dosage requirements leading to increased intervals between pump refills, the lower risk of catheter failure, and the infrequent occurrence of potential complications, suggest this is the preferred route for intraspinal drug delivery.

DRUG DELIVERY SYSTEM

Despite the popularity of implantable drug pumps, there are a number of different methods to accomplish intraspinal drug delivery. These systems include percutaneous epidural catheter attached to external pump, internalized passive catheter and reservoir requiring percutaneous drug administration, patient-activated mechanical system, constant rate infusion pump, and programmable infusion pump. In the light of the significant expense of drug pumps and the surgery required for their implantation, the choice of drug administration system should be made with careful consideration of the benefits of bolus versus continuous drug infusion and the patient's general medical status, ambulatory status, and estimated life expectancy.

Several investigators have explored the question of continuous versus bolus infusion. Continuous spinal infusion results in lower peak CSF morphine concentrations and corresponding lower plasma levels than bolus administration, while providing stable steady-state levels at the spinal site of action. It has been suggested that continuous infusion may result in a reduced rate of opioid receptor tachyphylaxis[15] and decrease the risk of producing delayed respiratory depression.[16] Clinical studies, however, have not clearly confirmed the superiority of continuous over bolus intraspinal drug infusion.

Given there is no consistent evidence showing whether continuous or bolus administration is clinically more effective, the choice of drug delivery device should be based on the patient's ambulatory status, general health, and estimated length of life. Thus, for patients with short life expectancy of days to weeks, especially those who are bed-bound, a percutaneously implanted tunneled epidural catheter attached to an external drug pump is a viable, inexpensive option. While the risk of infection increases over time, these catheters can be maintained for several weeks to months without complication. Over time, however, the total cost of renting the external drug pump along with the required nursing and pharmacy services makes this option quite costly. Careful tunneling of the catheter and rigorous hygiene of the catheter and its dressing will help ensure infusion system durability.

For patients with limited life expectancy who are ambulatory, an implanted reservoir system attached to an intraspinal catheter is an attractive option. An intraspinal catheter is tunneled subcutaneously and connected to a reservoir placed in the anterior or anterolateral chest wall. Implanting the reservoir over the lower ribs allows easy localization and stabilization during drug administration. There are subcutaneous reservoirs manufactured specifically for this application; they are rated to withstand hundreds of punctures, while other familiar reservoirs, such as the Ommaya reservoir, are rated only for several dozen punctures. These reservoir systems require daily percutaneous access and are associated with discomfort and increased risk of infection. They do, however, allow the patient unencumbered activity during the day and can be accessed for either bolus administration or for continuous infusion by attachment to an external pump.

Mechanical patient-controlled indwelling drug administration systems are a third option for intraspinal drug therapy. Unfortunately, at present these devices are in clinical trials and are only available for implantation outside of the USA. One such device consists of an implanted drug reservoir and an intraspinal catheter, both of which are connected to a subcutaneously placed patient activated control system. This panel consists of two silastic chambers; depression of the first chamber allows for drug delivery while the second chamber is depressed. A maximum dose per unit time results, determined by the fixed interval required for refilling the drug delivery chamber. This is the functional equivalent to the patient lock-out times programmed into external patient-controlled analgesia pumps.

Two major types of implanted drug pumps are currently marketed. The device marketed by Infusaid consists of a drug-filled bellows compressed by pressurized freon gas with its outflow regulated by a high-resistance valve. The infused solution is then delivered at a fixed rate; dose changes are made by changing the solution concentration. Thus, there is some increased cost and patient discomfort when dose changes are indicated. Furthermore, changes in temperature and atmospheric pressure subject these devices to small variations in drug delivery rates.

Somewhat more expensive is the programmable, electronic drug pump. This pump can be programmed transcutaneously and sophisticated drug dose regimens can be instituted. Dose changes can be made with noninvasive reprogramming. Since these pumps are battery operated, they require surgical replacement when the batteries expire; under average conditions, this is about every 4 years. Both implanted pump types need to be refilled every 1 to 2 months, depending on the rate of drug delivery.

While carefully controlled studies are lacking, several models have been explored to determine the relative costs of these drug administration systems over time. In general, it appears that for patients whose life expectancy and intraspinal drug use will exceed 3 months, it is cost effective to choose a fully implanted drug pump, while for patients with shorter life expectancy a percutaneous catheter or implanted reservoir may be more reasonable.[15,17] Kumar and colleagues[18] recently published their work demonstrating the cost effectiveness of intrathecal drug therapy for the management of failed back syndrome. Of the 67 patients in this study, 23 underwent implantation of a programmable drug delivery pump while 44 patients continued with conventional pain therapy. During the 5-year follow-up period, the actual costs of care related to failed back syndrome were tabulated. Although the intrathecal drug therapy group incurred a high initial cost due to equipment needs, at 28 months follow-up the cumulative cost of conventional medical therapy exceeded intrathecal drug therapy. In the light of current health care reform and the demands for greater cost containment in medicine, these issues must be considered in every patient who is deemed a candidate for intraspinal analgesic therapy.

RESULTS

Opioids: Morphine is the most studied intrathecal drug for the management of refractory chronic pain of both malignant and nonmalignant origin. Several publications on the efficacy of intraspinally administered morphine are reported; most are case reports and retrospective studies, with few prospective studies (Table 58-5).[19–23] While some investigators initially reported poor results,[15,17] others have found significant success. Early data suggest an efficacy of roughly 80% in the setting of cancer pain; prospective trials confirm this efficacy. Auld and co-workers reported two studies of intraspinal narcotics for the treatment of nonmalignant pain; in the first report 21 of 32 patients demonstrated adequate relief,[24] while in the second study 14 of 20 patients obtained satisfactory pain relief with intraspinal morphine.[7] With results from recent prospective trials, the reported efficacy for nonmalignant pain states remains variable, with the range between 25% and 57.5%.

At the present time the data concerning intraspinal morphine for pain secondary to cancer appear to be compelling and

TABLE 58-5. **A COMPARISON OF PROSPECTIVE STUDIES ON INTRASPINALLY ADMINISTERED MORPHINE**

Authors	Number of Patients	Route	Efficacy
Anderson et al., 1999	22	Intrathecal	11 patients with >25% reduction in nonmalignant pain after 24 months
Kumar et al., 2001	16	Intrathecal	57.5% reduction in pain, best results in deafferentation and mixed pain
Smith et al., 2002	143	Intrathecal	60 of 71 (84.5%) with cancer pain achieved clinical success ($p = 0.05$)
Rauck et al., 2003	119	Intrathecal	Overall success in 83%, 90%, 85%, and 91% at months 1, 2, 3, and 4 for cancer pain
Deer et al., 2004	136	Intrathecal	Oswestry Low Back Pain Disability Scale improved by 47% for patients with low back pain; >31% for patients with leg pain

consistent, with a success rate of approximately 80%. Data concerning its use in the setting of nonmalignant pain are less clear. While intraspinal morphine may provide pain relief in carefully selected patients with intractable benign pain, further work needs to be done before this should be considered a regular part of the neurosurgical armamentarium.

Hydromorphone is a potent opioid with increasing intraspinal use to treat cancer and nonmalignant pain. It is approximately five times more potent than morphine, theoretically translating to longer periods of time between pump refills; the most common indication for using hydromorphone appears to be inadequate pain control or intolerable side effects with morphine. Although there are no prospective controlled trials evaluating the efficacy and toxicity of hydromorphone, the side-effect profile appears similar to or better than morphine.[19] Anecdotally, and also in a recent retrospective study evaluating the efficacy of hydromorphone to treat nonmalignant pain,[25] 37 patients who failed treatment with intrathecal morphine had improvement in their pain scores when switched to hydromorphone.

The most widely recognized side effects of intraspinal narcotics include urinary retention, pruritis, and, rarely, delayed respiratory depression. Respiratory depression is most often seen in the opioid-naive patient and results from supraspinal redistribution of the drug; this side effect is both dose dependent and naloxone reversible. Other potential side effects include a decrease in sexual libido and decreased testosterone levels in men.[26]

Clinical experience has demonstrated the occurrence of increased narcotic requirement to maintain a similar degree of pain control in a significant fraction of patients. While this may reflect the development of tolerance at the receptor level, in many cases this apparent tolerance results from a change in the status of the patient's disease. For example, in the setting of pain secondary to a malignancy, tumor progression may involve new areas of pain, invade more pain-sensitive structures, or change the nature of the pain from predominantly nociceptive to neuropathic. Furthermore, changes in the patient's psychosocial status may result in the decreased ability to cope, resulting in perceived increase in the degree of pain.

Several strategies have been advanced to manage such situations. First, simply increasing the drug dose may re-achieve excellent long-term pain control. When this fails, or when the drug dose is escalated to levels that are felt to be potentially problematic, some authors suggest temporarily using systemic analgesics while the pump is turned off for a period of several days to a few weeks, a so called "drug holiday." If the decreased efficacy of intraspinal narcotics is due to receptor tolerance, this "drug holiday" often results in the down regulation of the opioid receptor and a return of efficacy when intraspinal narcotics are reinstituted.

Another strategy is the use of narcotics active at other opioid receptor subclasses. Like mu receptor agonists, delta receptor agonists appear to work through a G-protein system to hyperpolarize the neuronal membrane through an increase in potassium conductance and thus inhibit neuronal activity. Kappa receptor agonists appear to function differently than mu or delta receptor agonists. These agents appear to activate a different G-protein mechanism which blocks calcium entry through a voltage-dependent calcium channel. Investigators have had some success with delta receptor agonists or those with mixed receptor subclass activity.

A final strategy is the concomitant administration of low-dose local anesthetics with the narcotic. The combination of morphine and a local anesthetic has been successfully tried and seems to provide equivalent pain relief while decreasing opiate requirement. Bupivacaine is an amide class local anesthetic whose role in the management of nonmalignant pain, specifically neuropathic pain, has increased. There is extensive experience on its efficacy when delivered epidurally to manage postoperative and obstetrical pain. In this use, it was also noted that bupivacaine, in combination with an opioid, reduces the opioid dose without compromising pain control. Hassenbusch and co-workers[27] reported good results lasting over 1 year in 4 of 7 patients whose pain was not of malignant origin using an epidural infusion of morphine sulfate combined with bupivacaine (MS-MARC). While satisfactory results were achieved, care should be exercised in interpreting the outcome. In this study a high concentration of epidural morphine was used; 80% to 90% of this high dose is likely to have been systemically absorbed and would result in systemic levels of morphine similar to oral administration. Du Pen and co-workers[28] examined the efficacy of epidural MS-MARC in a series of 68 patients who found no relief from epidural opioids alone. Sixty-one patients (90%) were considered treatment successes with chronic bupivacaine infusion. Sjoberg and colleagues[29] reported the long-term results of intrathecal MS-MARC administration in 52 "refractory" cancer patients. They assessed the quality of analgesia as adequate in 2, good in 12, very good in 31, and excellent in 7. Side effects of bupivacaine in this study included transient paraesthesias, motor blockade, and gait impairment. In two prospective studies[19,30] patients who failed intrathecal therapy with morphine or hydromorphone benefited from the addition of bupivacaine. There is one randomized, double-blind trial of 24 patients with chronic nonmalignant pain in which the addition of bupivacaine to morphine or hydromorphone improved the patients' quality of life, but did not seem to have a significant effect on pain scores.[31]

Adrenergic Agonists: Eisenach and co-workers[32] used epidural clonidine to treat 9 patients with intractable cancer pain tolerant to instraspinal opioids. Patients received between 100 and 1000 µg per day; clonidine produced analgesia lasting more than 6 hours but also decreased blood pressure by more than 30%. Hypotension was treatable with intravenous ephedrine. Clonidine also decreased heart rate by 10% to 30% and produced transient sedation at higher doses. There were no opioid-like side effects of respiratory depression, pruritis, or nausea. Several other studies have reported similar results. In a prospective, randomized trial of adding epidural clonidine to intrathecal morphine in 85 patients with cancer pain[33] analgesia was achieved more commonly in the clonidine group (45% vs. 21%), especially among patients with a component of neuropathic pain. A recent prospective cohort study[9] of 10 patients with neuropathic pain treated with the combination of intrathecal morphine and clonidine resulted in a 70% to 100% reduction in pain. Furthermore, 4 of 8 patients with concomitant non-neuropathic pain also benefited from the addition of clonidine. In a phase I/II study[8] 59% of the cohort were considered long-term success with a mean follow-up of 16.7 months. As a result of a recent multicenter trial, intraspinal clonidine for the treatment of chronic pain has been approved by the FDA.

In contrast to clonidine, the alpha-2-adrenergic agonist tizanidine does not appear to induce hypotension. This agent has been demonstrated to be an effective analgesic agent when administered intrathecally in experimental[6] paradigms. Tizanidine appears to be particularly useful in the treatment of narcotic insensitive neuropathic pain syndromes.

Ziconotide: Ziconotide, also known as SNX-111, is a novel 25-amino-acid peptide isolated from a marine snail venom. It is a highly selective N-type voltage-sensitive calcium channel antagonist, which is found at the presynaptic nerve terminals in the spinal dorsal horn. Putative mechanism of action in the production of pain control is by blocking neurotransmitter release at the primary afferent nerve terminal. There are no data on the long-term use of ziconotide; however, early experience[34] of intrathecal ziconotide with 3 patients showed numerous side effects, including nystagmus, dysmetria, ataxia, sedation, agitation, hallucinations, and coma. Ellis et al.[35] reported their experience in 643 patients receiving intrathecal ziconotide for chronic, severe pain with favorable response (50% for failed back pain and 58% for back pain). A recent randomized, blinded trial among patients with cancer or AIDS[36] showed intrathecal ziconotide resulted in 52.9% moderate to complete pain relief (vs. 17.5% placebo).

The flexibility of the intrathecal drug administration system has allowed advancement of the clinical practice of pain management ahead of scientific data. Currently, opioids, nonmorphine opioids, nonopioids, and combinations of these drugs are being delivered intraspinally. Often, this occurs without solid clinical data. Clearly, the ability to help patients in pain is enhanced by the current technology; however, more controlled trials are needed to establish efficacy, long-term toxicity, and compatibility of these agents.

COMPLICATIONS

Although implanted drug delivery systems offer a unique method of pain control in selected patients, they are not without significant complication. The risk of infection is common to all drug delivery devices. Percutaneous catheters and implanted reservoirs appear particularly susceptible to infection because of their communication with the skin or frequent access through the skin. Infection may involve the surgical wound or the subcutaneous region surrounding the hardware. This is effectively treated by removal of all implanted hardware and the administration of appropriate intravenous antibiotics; cure is seldom accomplished without hardware externalization. Reimplanting the drug delivery system is usually delayed for 3 months after completion of antibiotic therapy.

Infusion of contaminated drug solution is of great concern as this may lead to a potentially life-threatening meningitis. The risk of this complication can be limited by the use of an in-line bacteriostatic filter; unfortunately, not all systems allow for or provide such filters. Early recognition and treatment of meningitis is critical.

Erosion of the hardware through the skin is a less common complication, and may occur especially in cachectic, poorly nourished patients. This risk can be limited by placing the implant in a deep pocket, by ensuring the hardware does not lie directly under the incision, and by performing a meticulous multilayer closure.

The most frequently observed complication involves failure of the system itself. Pump failures are uniquely uncommon but may occur, particularly with the complex electronics of programmable pumps. Catheter problems, however, are most common, reported in up to 25% of patients. These include kinking, obstruction, disconnection, or shearing of the catheter. There are several techniques to limit the risk of catheter failure and include the use of fluoroscopy during catheter placement to confirm the absence of loops, partial kinks or malposition in a dural nerve root sheath. Observation of CSF flow during each stage of implantation helps detect catheter obstruction during surgery. The paraspinous approach limits the sharp angle of the catheter as it enters and exits the interspinous ligament and guards against shearing at these sites. Securing the catheter with a purse string suture as it exits the interspinous ligament, and again with a silastic fixation device, also helps prevent CSF leak and migration of the catheter out of the subarachnoid space. A loop of catheter distal to this point relieves strain on the catheter and prevents catheter migration or dislocation. Finally, dissection of a small space above the fascia in which the catheter comfortably rests will help prevent kinking when the wound is closed.

Despite great care during catheter implantation, these problems may still occur. Patients with drug delivery system failure usually present with increased pain or with subcutaneous infusate accumulation. Initial evaluation includes the comparison of the expected and true residual volume in the pump reservoir; a significant disparity warrants further investigation. Plain radiologic evaluation of the entire system may reveal catheter disconnection and may also demonstrate kinking or migration of the catheter from the subarachnoid space. Occasionally, the instillation and attempted intrathecal delivery of iodinated contrast material via the pump may be helpful in differentiating between catheter or pump failure. Quantitative nuclear medicine studies may also be helpful; the pump can be filled with dilute solutions of radioactive material and the delivery of these materials can be followed over time. Even these diagnostic tests may be equivocal, requiring surgical exploration and revision of the pump and/or catheter. With such a rigorous approach, virtually all such mechanical problems can be corrected and pain relief restored.

Another problem common to all implanted drug delivery systems is the potential for overdose. With an externalized system, this may result from improper setting of the external drug pump or improper dilution of the infusate by the pharmacy. Great care must be used to ensure appropriate drug concentration and delivery. Far more insidious can be the incorrect reprogramming of indwelling drug pumps, as these errors are potentially subtle and not immediately recognized. Such drug overdoses resulting from programming errors or incorrect infusate concentrations have occurred.

A further risk is created by the presence, in some pumps, of a side port intended for bolus drug injection or for testing catheter patency. There are two reported deaths resulting from accidental access of this side port rather than the refill port, resulting in the entire refill volume of the drug infusing into the CSF. Modifications have recently been made to prevent access to the bolus port by needles intended for pump refilling; nonetheless, great care must be exercised to avoid this potentially life-threatening complication.

FUTURE DIRECTIONS

While tremendous progress has been made in the use of intraspinal analgesics for the treatment of intractable pain, there are several areas that need to be addressed before the technique is more widely accepted and can be of broader clinical use. First, while its efficacy in the treatment of pain secondary to malignancy appears clear, the use of intraspinal drug administration for pain of nonmalignant origin remains to be elucidated. Properly controlled, large-scale trials are lacking; until such evidence is available, use in this setting should be considered investigational.

Second, patient selection criteria need to be better defined and validated. In particular, the psychosocial evaluation and specific pain states responsive to this intervention need better characterization. In the light of the cost and modest invasiveness of this approach, great attention must be paid to refining the patient selection criteria to ensure a good chance of successful pain relief.

Finally, and perhaps most significantly, further development in analgesic pharmacology needs to be applied to intraspinal drug therapy. While there are currently dozens of available analgesic agents for oral or parenteral use capitalizing on the complex neurochemistry of pain transmission and modulation pathways, there are but two agents available for intraspinal use. With the development of newer and more specific agents, and with the utilization of agents active at a number of receptor systems involved in pain perception, intraspinal drug administration may help limit the suffering of many more people with otherwise intractable pain.

REFERENCES

1. Basbaum AI, Clanton CH, Fields HL: Opiate and stimulus-produced analgesia: Functional anatomy of a medullospinal pathway. Proc Natl Acad Sci 73:4685–4688, 1976.
2. Behar M, Magora F, Olshwang D, Davidson JT: Epidural morphine in treatment of pain. Lancet 1:527, 1979.
3. Wang JK, Nauss LE, Thomas JE: Pain relief by intrathecally applied morphine in man. Anesthesiology 50:149–151, 1979.
4. Matsuki A: Nothing new under the sun – A Japanese pioneer in the clinical use of intrathecal morphine [editorial]. Anesthesiology 58:289–290, 1983.
5. Waldman SD, Yaksh TL: Historical overview and future horizons. J Pain Symptom Manage 5:1, 1990.
6. Leiphart JW, Dills CW, Zikel OM, et al: A comparison of intrathecally administered narcotic and nonnarcotic analgesics in experimental chronic neuropathic pain. J Neurosurg 82:595–599, 1995.
7. Auld AW, Murdoch DM, O'Laughlin KA: Intraspinal narcotic analgesia: Pain management in the failed laminectomy syndrome. Spine 12:953–954, 1987.
8. Hassenbusch SJ, Gunes S, Wachsman S, et al: Intrathecal clonidine in the treatment of intractable pain: A phase I/II study. Pain Med 3:85–91, 2002.
9. Uhle EI, Becker R, Gatscher S, et al: Continuous intrathecal clonidine administration for the treatment of neuropathic pain. Stereotact Funct Neurosurg 75:167–175, 2000.
10. Kloke M: Somatostatin and neoplastic pain. In Recent Results in Cancer Research, vol 129. Spriner-Verlag, Berlin, 1993.
11. Onofrio BM, Yaksh TL, Arnold PG: Continuous low dose intrathecal morphine administration in the treatment of chronic pain of malignant origin. Mayo Clin Proc 56:516–520, 1981.
12. Levy RM: Quantitative crossover double blind trial paradigm for patient screening for chronic intraspinal narcotic administration. Neurosurg Focus 2:2.1–2.4, 1997.
13. Arner S, Arner B: Differential effects of epidural morphine analgesia. Acta Anaesthesiol Scand 28:535–539, 1984.
14. Anderson PE, Cohen JI, Everts EC, et al: Intrathecal narcotics for relief of pain from head and neck cancer. Arch Otolaryngol Head Neck Surg 117:1277–1280, 1991.
15. Coombs DW: Intraspinal analgesic infusion by implanted pump. Ann N Y Acad Sci 531:108–122, 1988.
16. Brazenor GA: Long term intrathecal administration of morphine: A comparison of bolus injection via reservoir with continuous infusion by implanted pump. Neurosurgery 21:484–491, 1987.
17. Krames ES, Gershow J, Glassberg A, et al: Continuous infusion of spinally administered narcotics for the relief of pain due to malignant disorders. Cancer 56:696–702, 1985.
18. Kumar K, Hunter G, Demeria DD: Treatment of chronic pain by using intrathecal drug therapy compared with conventional pain therapies: A cost-effectiveness analysis. J Neurosurg 97:803–810, 2002.
19. Anderson VC, Burchiel KJ: A prospective study of long-term intrathecal morphine in the management of chronic nonmalignant pain. Neurosurgery 44:289–300, 1999.
20. Deer T, Chapple I, Classen A, et al: Intrathecal drug delivery for treatment of chronic low back pain: Report for the National Outcomes Registry for Low Back Pain. Pain Med 5:6–13, 2004.
21. Kumar K, Kelly M, Pirlot T: Continuous intrathecal morphine treatment for chronic pain of nonmalignant etiology: Long-term benefits and efficacy. Surg Neurol 55:79–86, 2001.
22. Rauck RL, Charry D, Boyer MF, et al: Long-term intrathecal opioid therapy using a patient-activated implanted delivery system for the treatment of refractory cancer pain. J Pain 4:441–447, 2003.
23. Smith TJ, Staats PS, Deer T, et al: Randomized clinical trial of an implantable drug delivery system compared with comprehensive medical management for refractory cancer pain: Impact on pain, drug-related toxicity, and survival. J Clin Oncol 20:4040–4049, 2002.
24. Auld AW, Maki-Jokela A, Murdoch DM: Intraspinal narcotic analgesia in the treatment of chronic pain. Spine 10:778–781, 1985.
25. Anderson VC, Cooke B, Burchiel K: Intrathecal hydromorphone for chronic nonmalignant pain: A retrospective study. Pain Med 2:287–297, 2001.
26. Paice JA, Penn RD, Ryan WG: Altered sexual function and decreased testosterone in patients receiving intraspinal opioids. J Pain Symptom Manage 9:126–131, 1994.
27. Hassenbusch SJ, Stanton-Hicks MD, Soukap J, et al: Sufentanil citrate and morphine/bupivicaine as alternative agents in chronic epidural infusions for intractable non-cancer pain. Neurosurgery 29:76–82, 1991.
28. Du Pen SL, Kharasch ED, Williams A, et al: Chronic epidural bupivicaine–opioid infusion in intractable cancer pain. Pain 49:293–300, 1992.
29. Sjoberg M, Appeloren L, Einarsson S, et al: Long term intrathecal morphine and bupivicaine in 'refractory' cancer pain. Results from the first series of 52 patients. Acta Anaesthol Scand 35:30–43, 1991.
30. Van Dongen RT, Crul BJ, van Egmond J: Intrathecal coadministration of bupivicaine diminishes morphine dose progression during long-term intrathecal infusion in cancer patients. Clinc J Pain 15: 66–172, 1999.
31. Mironer YE, Haasis JC, Chapple I, et al: Efficacy and safety of intrathecal opioid/bupivacaine mixture in chronic nonmalignant pain: A double blind, randomized, crossover, multicenter study

by the National Forum of Independent Pain Clinicians (NFIPC). Neuromodulation 5:208–213, 2002.

32. Eisenach JC, Rauck RL, Buzzaneli, Lysak SZ: Epidural clonidine analgesia for intractable cancer pain: Phase I. Anesthesiology 71:647–652, 1989.

33. Eisenach JC, Du Pen S, Dubois M, et al: Epidural clonidine analgesia for intractable cancer pain. The Epidural Clonidine Study Group. Pain 61:391–399, 1995.

34. Penn RD, Paice JA: Adverse effects associated with the intrathecal administration of ziconotide. Pain 85:291–296, 2000.

35. Ellis D, Henderson R, Royal M, et al: Efficacy of intrathecal ziconotide in patients with chronic, severe pain. J Pain 4(Suppl 1): 54, 2003 (abstract 812).

36. Staats PS, Yearwood T, Charapata SG, et al: Intrathecal ziconotide in the treatment of refractory pain in patients with cancer or AIDS: A controlled clinical trial. JAMA 291:63–70, 2004.

Lumbar Discography

Ali Shaibani, M.D., and
Honorio T. Benzon, M.D.

In the evaluation of lumbar discogenic pain, discography is currently the only diagnostic technique that directly correlates the patient's symptoms with disc morphology and anatomy. Discography entails the injection of radiographic contrast into the nucleus of an intervertebral disc, with simultaneous recording of the patient's symptoms and documentation of discal anatomy.

HISTORY

In 1940 Lindblom, a radiologist in Sweden, was the first physician to inject contrast material (red lead) into cadaveric discs, and he published his findings in 1948.[1] Hirsch in 1948 reported 16 cases of lumbar discography. Wise and Wieford performed the first discography in the USA in 1950. In the 1950s and 1960s several investigators raised concerns over the safety of discography after reports of discitis, meningitis, arachnoiditis, intrathecal hemorrhage, postdural puncture headache, and damage to the disc.[2–4] A later study by Hirsch,[5] wherein the patients were operated on after a discography, showed the lack of injury to the disc after a discography.

During the last few years there has been a significant resurgence in the performance of discography. This is probably related to an improved understanding of discogenic pain and improvements in the technique, resulting in a low incidence of complications, as well as the publication of studies showing the value of discography in cases where other diagnostic tests are equivocal. When performed by an experienced operator, and for the evaluation of discogenic pain, discography is felt by many to yield valuable diagnostic information not provided by other diagnostic techniques. Axial computed tomography (CT) scanning is done after discography[6] to show crisp, cross-sectional detail of the internal structure of the nucleus or the presence of fissures in the annulus fibrosus.

DISCOGENIC PAIN

Lumbar discography is only indicated in the work-up and diagnosis of suspected discogenic pain. To understand the current theoretical mechanisms underlying discogenic pain, one must have a solid understanding of the structural anatomy of, and neural supply to, the intervertebral disc.

The disc is sandwiched between the cartilaginous endplates of the vertebrae above and below. It is composed of an outer layer, the annulus fibrosus, and an inner core, the nucleus pulposus. The annulus fibrosus is composed of concentric lamellae of fibrocartilage, running obliquely from one vertebra to the other. It inserts, via Sharpey's fibers, into the periosteum at the margin of the endplates. The lamellae are thinner and less numerous posteriorly, leading to more tears posteriorly. The normal annulus is of low signal in T1- and T2-weighted magnetic resonance imaging (MRI). The nucleus pulposus is made of a complex of collagen, proteoglycans, and water. It has a high signal on T2-weighted MRI and a low signal on T1-weighted MRI. It has an intranuclear cleft made of collagen and reticular fiber (Fig. 59-1). The nucleus functions as a shock absorber during axial loading, and like a semifluid ball bearing during flexion, extension, lateral bending, and rotation.

The neural supply to the intervertebral disc includes branches of the sinuvertebral (Luschka's) nerves that innervate the outer third of the posterior annulus and posterior longitudinal ligament. Branches of the gray rami communicantes (sympathetic plexus) innervate the outer third of the lateral annulus while branches of the lumbar ventral rami innervate the outer third of the ventral annulus. Neurotransmitters involved in nociception have been detected in the annulus and posterior longitudinal ligament.[7]

The theories on the mechanisms of discogenic pain include the following: (1) annular tears extending into the outer third of the annulus irritate the neural supply; (2) ingrowth of granulation tissue (as a reparative response) into the annular tear which contains nerve endings and can be the source of discogenic pain; and (3) the irritant nature of the nucleus pulposus.

The primary symptoms of discogenic pain are low back pain with frequent extension into the gluteal regions. The pain can extend into the anterior and/or the posterior thighs, and less frequently below to the calves or ankles. The low back and/or gluteal components of the pain are almost invariably the main symptom and complaint. Any thigh component, if present, is

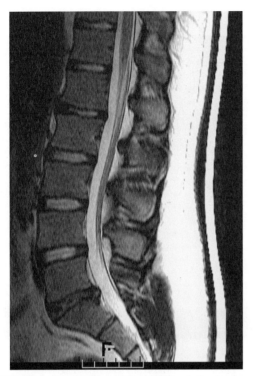

FIGURE 59-1. Sagittal T2-weighted MRI of the lumbar spine, demonstrating a normal appearance of the discs from T12–L1 to L4–5, and disc degeneration at L5–S1. The normal nucleus pulposus demonstrates high T2 signal, with the thick low-signal bands of the anterior and posterior annulus anterior and posterior to it. The internuclear band (cleft) of collagen is seen as a thin dark line in the center of the nucleus.

significantly less in severity. The patient has intolerance of cumulative axial loading, such as the inability to stand for long periods due to pain. Symptoms usually worsen with back flexion, as in prolonged sitting. The symptoms are nonradicular, and there is no associated weakness or abnormality of the reflexes.[8]

IMAGING CORRELATES OF DISCOGENIC PAIN

The primary noninvasive diagnostic imaging modality is MRI. MRI provides the best noninvasive evaluation of the intervertebral disc, with information on the presence of annular degeneration/tear, degree of hydration of the nucleus pulposus, and the degree of height loss of the disc (the primary sign of disc degeneration).

Annular tears, either full-thickness or near-full-thickness tears, are very well depicted on T2 sagittal images as foci of high signal called the "high intensity zone" (HIZ)[9] (Fig. 59-2). The most sensitive sequence for depicting an annular tear is probably the postcontrast T1 since there is enhancement of the granulation tissue that is invariably present as a result of the reparative response (Fig. 59-3). In a patient with the clinical symptoms of discogenic pain the presence of an annular tear on MRI (HIZ) is associated with a high likelihood of a concordant pain response with discography.[9] Several studies correlated the presence of HIZ and the likelihood of concordant discography.[9–11] Schellhas et al.[9] demonstrated a positive predictive value of 87% while Lam et al.[10] showed a sensitivity of 81%, a specificity of 79%, and a positive predictive value of 87%. Not all discs with HIZs or annular tears are symptomatic. At least 13% of HIZs detected on MRI occur in patients with no symptoms of discogenic pain.[9] It should be

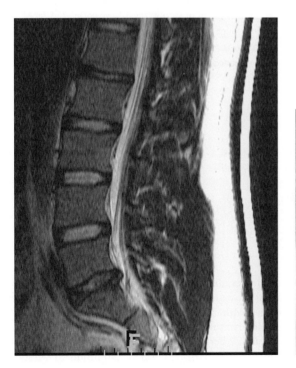

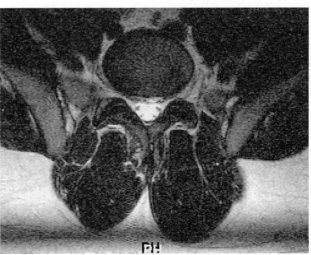

A   B

FIGURE 59-2. Sagittal (*A*) and axial (*B*) T2-weighted MRI of the lumbar spine, demonstrating disc degeneration at the L5–S1 level with a "high-intensity zone" in the posterior annulus corresponding to a posterior annular tear.

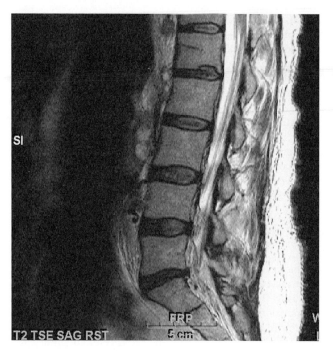

A

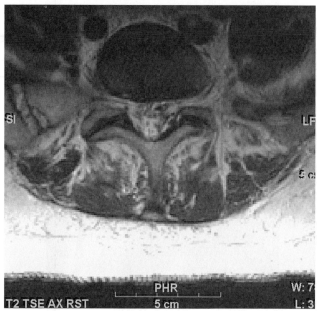

B

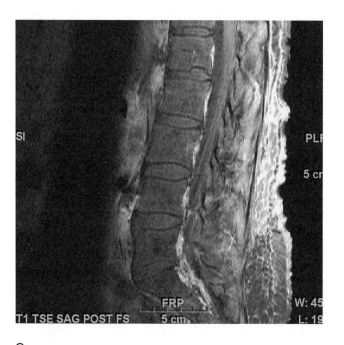

C

FIGURE 59-3. Sagittal T2-weighted *(A)*, axial T2-weighted *(B)*, and sagittal postcontrast T1-weighted *(C)* fat-saturated MRI through the lumbar spine demonstrating a focal "high-intensity zone" (posterior annular tear) at the L5–S1 level with enhancement after contrast.

noted, however, that a morphologically normal disc on MRI is not going to be the source of discogenic pain.[12]

INDICATIONS FOR LUMBAR DISCOGRAPHY

As previously stated, discography should only be used in the evaluation of discogenic pain. Guyer and Ohnmeiss[13] in their review on lumbar discography included the following indications for lumbar discography in patients with probable discogenic pain:

- Further evaluation of demonstrably abnormal discs to help assess the extent of abnormality or correlation of the abnormality with the clinical symptoms. Such symptoms may include recurrent pain from a previously operated disc and lateral disc herniation.
- Patients with persistent, severe symptoms in whom other diagnostic tests have failed to reveal clear confirmation of a suspected disc as the source of pain.
- Assessment of patients who have failed to respond to surgical intervention to determine if there is painful pseudarthrosis

or a symptomatic disc in a posteriorly fused segment and to help evaluate possible recurrent disc herniation.

- Assessment of discs before fusion to determine if the discs within the proposed fusion segment are symptomatic and to determine if discs adjacent to this segment are normal.
- Assessment of candidates for minimally invasive surgical intervention to confirm a contained disc herniation or to investigate dye distribution pattern before chemonucleolysis or percutaneous procedures.

An additional indication is the evaluation of discs above a prior fusion, in patients with recurrent symptoms suggestive of discogenic pain after a spinal fusion. This phenomenon is due to the known accelerated degeneration of discs adjacent to (usually above) a fused segment.

CONTROVERSY ON THE USE OF DISCOGRAPHY

The controversy regarding the use of discography as a diagnostic test has primarily revolved around its usefulness as the primary diagnostic test in the evaluation of discogenic pain. Discography has been considered to be more sensitive for the diagnosis of anatomical abnormalities than plain radiography, myelography, or MRI. Proponents stated that discography is the diagnostic test of choice for low back pain wherein there is a physiological endpoint relevant to the patient's complaint. Critics, however, consider discography to be oversensitive. Critics have noted that concordant pain is possible in patients with back pain from a nonspinal source[14] and that morphological features do not correlate with clinical complaints. Holt reported a 37% false positive result in asymptomatic subjects.[15] However, it has been pointed out that Holt's subjects had no previous symptoms and that his technique in 1968 was different from the technique being performed today including the use of nonirritating contrast material, accuracy of needle placement, and CT confirmation of the integrity of the disc and the injection site.[16] Another study showed a 40% false positive rate in asymptomatic subjects.[17] The morphological appearance of the disc does not always correlate with the result of the pain provocation on discography.[13] There does not appear to be a correlation between the location of the pain and the location of the annular tear.[18] Finally, MRI, which shows fine details of the disc, is noninvasive and less painful than discography. For these reasons, Resnick et al.[14] recommended MRI as the primary diagnostic modality in the evaluation of low back pain. Our opinion about the previous studies is that the use of discography in asymptomatic patients is not an appropriate way of testing the method. As mentioned above, a large proportion of the population has asymptomatic annular tears. Discography with consequent significant increase in intradiscal pressure usually produces pain, although nonconcordant, in these discs.

Resnick et al.[14] recommended the following for the diagnosis of painful degenerative lumbar disc disease:

- MRI is the recommended diagnostic modality for the management of low back pain.
- The presence of concordant pain response (pain that is identical or very similar to the patient's pain) as well as morphological changes is required for the definition of a positive finding on discography.

- Discography should not be performed as a stand-alone test for treatment decisions in patients with low back pain.
- Discography should be reserved for cases in which MRI findings are equivocal, especially at levels adjacent to clearly pathological levels.
- Patients who have back pain on discography but without MRI or radiological findings of disc degeneration should not be considered for any type of surgical intervention.
- It is recommended that psychological evaluation be performed in patients with positive discography finding and equivocal findings on MRI or plain radiography.

Contraindications to discography include the following:

- Pregnancy.
- Systemic infection, or localized infection at skin access site.
- Severe known allergy to contrast or the medications used. This is a relative contraindication, as patients can be premedicated, or tested with sterile saline, or a mix of gadolinium and sterile saline.
- Severe spinal stenosis at the level being tested.
- Coagulopathy.
- Lack of access to the disc.

OUR APPROACH TO THE USE OF LUMBAR DISCOGRAPHY

In our practice we subscribe to the recommendations proposed by Resnick et al.[14] If a patient presents with symptoms suggestive of discogenic pain, the first diagnostic test obtained is MRI of the lumbar spine. The spine is fully assessed with special emphasis on the presence or absence of annular degeneration or tears. If the lumbar discs are entirely normal on MRI, we discard the possibility of discogenic pain, and will not perform discography. On the other hand, if annular degeneration and especially a focal annular tear are present, then discography is performed. We also select a morphologically normal disc on MRI as the control level.

Pre-procedure Patient Interview: The pre-procedure interview with the patient is invaluable, and at least as important as performing the procedure itself. It allows the discographer to develop a rapport with the patient and obtain a detailed understanding of the characteristics and distribution of the patient's pain. We usually employ a pain diagram (such as the Brief Pain Inventory or the McGill Melzack Pain Questionnaire) allowing the patient to draw the pain distribution and use descriptors for the pain.[19] This further aids the discographer in gaining a solid understanding of the patient's symptoms. It also helps to confirm whether or not the symptoms are in keeping with the characteristics previously described for discogenic pain. During this interview the discographer gives the patient a thorough explanation of the procedure and describes the patient's paramount role in communicating the symptoms during the test.

Medications and Contrast Used
- Omnipaque, a contrast agent labeled as safe for intrathecal use.
- Ancef: 1 dose intravenously in the holding room, and powder to mix with Omnipaque.
- Clindamycin: if patient has allergy to penicillin or cephalosporin.
- Midazolam, 1 to 2 mg intravenously.

- Fentanyl, 50 to 100 μg.
- Lidocaine: local anesthetics are used liberally through the soft tissues but not injected adjacent to the annulus.

Equipment

- Good-quality fluoroscopy: biplane fluoroscopy is preferable but not necessary.
- Needles: coaxial system, 20-gauge guide, 25-gauge coaxial; 22 gauge without guide.
- Optional: manometer.

Procedure

- If the pain is more pronounced on one side, approach from contralateral side.
- Patient in prone position.
- Profile the disc space/endplate.
- Rotate the image intensifier obliquely to place the facet joints just dorsal to the midpoint of the disc.
- Advance the guide needle under flouroscopic guidance to the edge of the annulus.
- Advance the coaxial needle into the center (central third) of the disc.

Discography: The posterolateral extraspinal approach[20] is the preferred approach. The patient is usually in the prone position,[20] although some authors prefer the lateral decubitus position.[21] The site of needle entry is chosen by fluoroscopic guidance and not by arbitrary measurement from the spine (midline) of the patient.[20] The asymptomatic side is the preferred side of injection; this is to prevent confusion from reflux of the dye through the needle tract with pathological conditions. The C-arm of the fluoroscope is slowly rotated to the oblique position until the superior articular facet of the subjacent vertebra projects just posterior to the midpoint of the disc (Fig. 59-4). The needle entry site is placed just anterior to the facet joint. With this view, the site of entry for the L3–L4 and

L4–L5 discs is 8 to 10 cm from the midline. The site of entry for the L5–S1 disc is usually 1 cm lateral and proximal to the L4–L5 entry point.[21] The skin is prepared aseptically and draped. After a skin wheal, the needle is inserted into the center of the disc.

A lot of physicians prefer the double-needle technique to decrease the incidence of discitis. In this technique an 18- or 20-gauge needle is advanced to the edge of the annulus and a 22- or 25-gauge needle is inserted through the larger guide needle into the center of the disc. Positioning of the coaxial needle is very important, and care must be taken to place the tip within the central third of the disc if at all possible.[22] The position of the needle is confirmed in both true anteroposterior and lateral planes (Fig. 59-5). A total of 0.5 to 2 mL of water-soluble radiopaque contrast is injected. The normal disc accepts 0.5 to 1.5 mL of solution with a firm endpoint during injection. The volume, resistance, pain response, and radiographic appearance are noted. Anteroposterior and lateral radiographic images of the disc are taken at the point of maximal injection. The patient's symptoms are recorded during injection, and preferably at their maximal level. A sensation of pressure or fullness is considered a normal response.[21] Injection is stopped when resistance is encountered and no more fluid could be injected without placing inordinate pressure on the syringe. A large volume of contrast can be injected if the disc is degenerated or there is a fissure extending through the outer annular wall. Low resistance is associated with a tear through the outer annulus.[23]

Preferably, a very light sedation is used to better assess the response of the patient. The patient's response can be noted as no pain, atypical pain, or familiar/concordant pain.[21] Guyer and Ohnmeiss[23] recommended classifying the patient's response as:

- No pain or pressure only.
- Pain dissimilar to clinical symptoms.
- Pain similar to clinical symptoms.
- Exact reproduction of symptoms.

The pain may be secondary to increased intradiscal pressure stretching the nerve endings within the annulus.[24,25] Biochemical or neurochemical stimulation may occur.[26] Finally, discography may increase the pressure at the endplates or the pressure may be transmitted to the vertebral body the endplate increasing the intraosseous pressure and causing pain.[27] The pain from an injection of a normal disc has been attributed to transfer of the increased pressure to an adjacent abnormal and symptomatic disc or to psychologic factors.

The pain must be an exact reproduction of the patient's symptoms to be called "concordant pain." A "positive discogram" or "concordant discogram," as defined by Walsh et al.[28] and accepted by clinicians, requires morphological abnormalities to be present along with the provocation of pain that was identical or very similar to the patient's complaint of back pain. A morphological abnormality in the disc may or may not be associated with the production of concordant pain. Abnormal morphological features on discography are considered to be too nonspecific to be useful clinically.

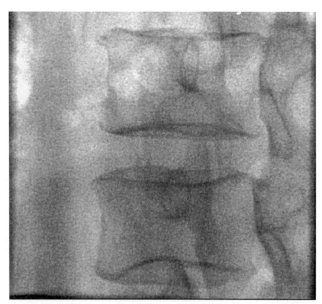

FIGURE 59-4. Optimal obliquity for a lumbar discogram. The disc space has been outlined sharply, and the facet joint is just dorsal to the midpoint of the disc.

Helpful Tips

- Always test a normal disc (as identified on MRI) as a control level.

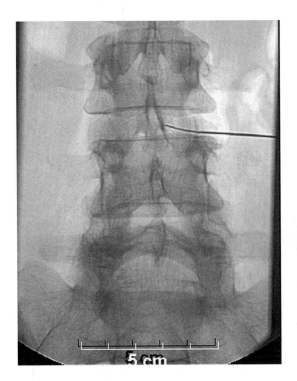

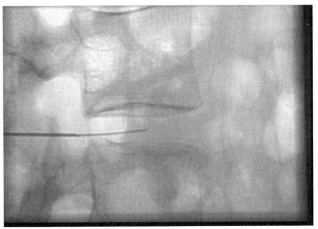

A   B

FIGURE 59-5. Anteroposterior (A) and lateral (B) radiographic views showing optimal positioning of the needle tip in the center of the disc.

- During the procedure, specific information such as the level being tested, or the timing of the injection, should not be conveyed to the patient. This maintains as much objectivity as possible.
- Meticulous recording of the patient's symptoms during the procedure is paramount.
- Look for secondary signs of pain during the injection such as visible grimacing, tears, etc.
- If the initial injection of the disc produces symptoms that are equivocal, the disc can be reinjected after waiting for 8 to 10 minutes. In these cases we often engage the patient in conversation, and perform the injection during this distracting maneuver.
- Anteroposterior and lateral radiographs are obtained with maximal filling of the nucleus pulposus during contrast injection.
- If the oblique approach to the L5–S1 disc space is not possible, it may be reached via a transthecal approach in some patients. This must be performed with great care and while using a small needle (22 or preferably 25 gauge). The patient must be told of the possibility of a dural puncture headache.

Characteristics of Concordant Pain

- The location/distribution of the elicited pain is the same as the pain for which the patient saw his or her doctor.
- The quality of the elicited pain is the same.
- The *intensity* of the pain may be *worse* than the patient's usual pain because of the sudden intentional increase in the intradiscal pressure.
- Injection of a morphologically normal disc is either asymptomatic or may cause mild pressure in the midline at the level of the disc.

- Injection of a morphologically *abnormal* disc *not responsible* for the patient's symptoms will often produce pain that is *discordant*.

Imaging Evaluation: The nucleogram is considered normal when the contrast material occupies the nucleus in a characteristic unilocular, bilocular, collar button, or biscuit-shaped pattern[21] (Fig. 59-6). The nucleogram is abnormal when the contrast material extends beyond the confines of the nucleus through the annulus fibrosus. The contrast may extravasate into the epidural space, nerve root sheath, or into the vertebral body (Figs. 59-7–59-9).

POST-DISCOGRAPHY CT

There is no rival for CT discography in the assessment of the ability of the annulus to hold liquid under pressure,[13] although less frequently MRI discography can also be performed. In a study of patients with back pain Bernard[21] showed that discography followed by CT scanning provided additional useful information in 234 of 250 (94%) patients. The additional information included another painful or abnormal motion segment not suspected by the other tests, the determination of the type of disc herniation, evaluation of a previously operated spine, determination of the source of pain when the abnormality seen in the other tests was equivocal, and in defining surgical options. Not infrequently, especially in patients who have a radicular component of pain, postdiscogram CT scans can demonstrate a focal disc protrusion or extrusion not previously depicted. CT discography shows crisp cross-sectional detail of the internal structure of the nucleus and the presence of fissures in the annulus.

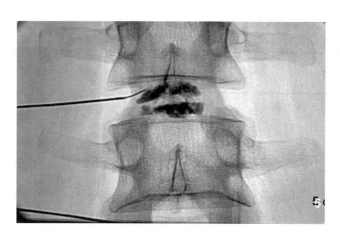
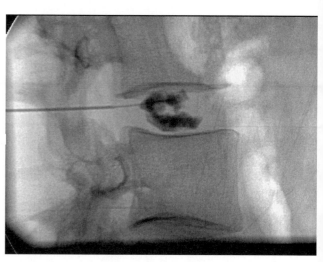

A   B

FIGURE 59-6. Anteroposterior (A) and lateral (B) views of the discographic appearance of a normal disc. The internuclear cleft is clearly seen.

CT should be performed within 4 hours after discography. The normal disc on the CT discogram shows the contrast to be contained symmetrically with the region of the nucleus pulposus.[21] Abnormal CT discograms include the presence of radial fissures, annular enhancement, contrast-enhanced disc protrusions, or epidural collection of contrast material. Bernard[21] concluded that CT scanning after lumbar discography has proven valuable in two areas. CT discography has provided additional insight into the pathogenesis of lumbar disc disease and is useful in the identification of symptomatic disc disease. Classification schemes have been developed for describing the disc morphology.[29,30]

PATTERNS OF DISC PROTRUSION

Acute herniated nucleus pulposus usually affect young and the middle-aged people. The nucleus usually has degenerated and undergone fibrosis in the older population making acute herniations less likely to occur. Herniations are usually central or posterolateral. In a bulging disc the annulus fibers weaken or

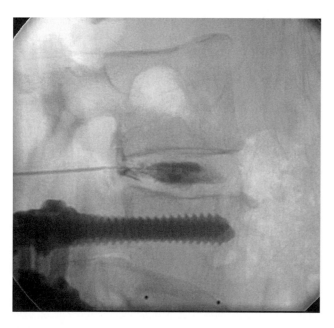
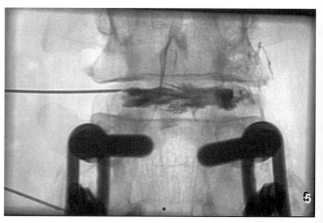

A   B

FIGURE 59-7. Lateral (A) and anteroposterior (B) views of a discogram above a fusion, demonstrating a full-thickness posterior annular tear. This disc did not produce concordant pain.

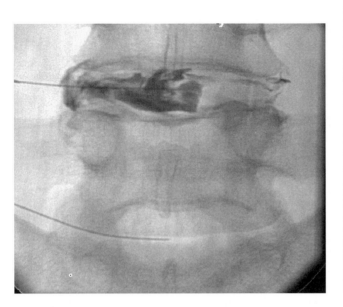

A

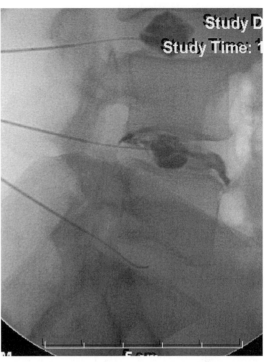

B

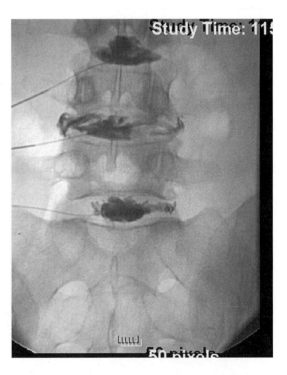

C

FIGURE 59-8. Anteroposterior (A), lateral (B), and demagnified antero-posterior (C) views of a left posterolateral annular tear with concordant pain.

are thinner and the disc is characterized by a smooth, broad, and expanding posterior disc contour. Annular tears usually precede herniated discs, and may be the result of an acute trauma or a degenerative phenomenon. Annular tears create a channel for migration of the nucleus pulposus. Protrusion connotes the presence of nuclear material in the annular tear.

In protruded disc herniations the nucleus is contained by the outer annular fibers or posterior longitudinal ligament. Protruded disc herniations are contained when the contrast does not leak into the epidural space during injection.[21] When there is a full-thickness tear in the annulus and the contrast leaks in the epidural space then the protrusion in noncontained.

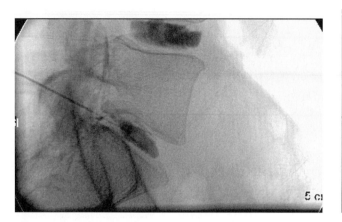

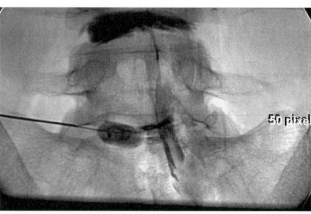

A

B

FIGURE 59-9. Lateral (*A*) and anteroposterior (*B*) views of a full-thickness posterior annular tear at L5–S1 with extravasation of contrast into the epidural space.

When the herniated nuclear material has extended through a complete annular tear but maintains contiguity with the parent disc, extrusion is present. A herniated disc can be a subligamentous extrusion where the extruded nuclear material is contained by the intact posterior longitudinal ligament or a transligamentous extrusion wherein the extruded disc dissects through the posterior longitudinal ligament. There is abnormality in the contour of the disc and the extruded material appears as a hyperintense nuclear signal on MRI. The disc has an irregular margin in transligamentous extrusions. Disc extrusions are identified discographically by a spongy endpoint during injection, extravasation of contrast into the epidural space, and there is usually reproduction of the patient's pain.[21] Contrast fills the disc fragment on CT discography. Finally, a free fragment means that the disc fragment is separate from the parent disc whether the fragment is contained by the posterior longitudinal ligament or not (Fig. 59-10).

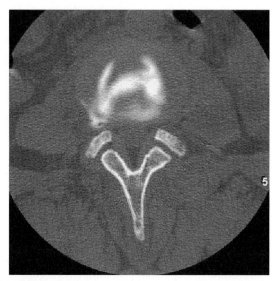

FIGURE 59-10. Postdiscogram CT showing an unsuspected right foraminal disc protrusion.

MANOMETRIC DISCOGRAPHY

Nachemson performed several studies on intradiscal pressure in the 1960s and 1970s using a polyethylene-covered disc pressure needle. Apparently, the apparatus was cumbersome to assemble and calibrate and exhibited poor dynamic characteristics.[31] There is controversy as to whether manometric studies should be performed during discography. Derby et al.[32] correlated the intradiscal pressure, the onset of pain, and the possible cause of the discogenic pain (see Table 59-1). In their study patients with highly sensitive (chemical) discs achieved significantly better long-term results with interbody/combined fusion than with intertransverse fusion.

COMPLICATIONS OF DISCOGRAPHY

Potential complications of discography include the following:

- Bleeding: usually not a concern, although serious epidural or retroperitoneal hemorrhage rarely occurs.
- Drug or contrast allergies.
- Inadvertent or intentional puncture of the thecal sac with possible spinal headache.
- Infection: epidural abscess, discitis, osteomyelitis.

The most dreaded complication is discitis. The incidence is 2% to 3% for the single-needle technique and 0.7% incidence for the double-injection technique.[33,34] Schellhas reported 6 confirmed cases of discitis in over 40,000 injected discs.[30] The patients often do have a worsening of their usual symptoms for 3 to 4 days following the discography.

CONCLUSION

Discography and CT scanning after discography are very useful diagnostic procedures in the evaluation of patients with suspected discogenic pain, for determining the type of disc herniation, for defining surgical options, for evaluating the significance of equivocal abnormalities, and in assessing previously operated spines.[20]

TABLE 59-1. **DISCOGRAPHIC DIAGNOSTIC CATEGORIES**

Disc Classification	Intradiscal Pressure at Pain Provocation	Pain Severity	Pain Type	Ruling
Chemical	Immediate onset of familiar pain occurring as <1 mL of contrast is visualized reaching the outer annulus,* or pain provocation at <15 psi (103.5 kPa) above opening pressure	≥6/10	Concordant	Positive
Mechanical	Between 15 and 50 psi (104.5–344.7 kPa) (above opening pressure)	≥6/10	Concordant	Positive (but other pain generators may be present; further investigation may be warranted)
Indeterminate	Between 51 and 90 psi (346.2–620.5 kPa)	≥6/10	Concordant	Further investigation warranted
Normal	>90 psi (620.5 kPa)	No pain		Negative

*Typically contrast will be visualized reaching the outer annulus at <10 psi above opening pressure. Consequently, a disc generating familiar/concordant pain as contrast is visualized reaching the outer annulus may be deemed chemically sensitive as defined within the context of the study.
From Derby R, Howard M, Grant JM, et al: The ability of pressure-controlled discography to predict surgical and nonsurgical outcomes. Spine 24:364–371, 1999.

REFERENCES

1. Linblom K: Diagnostic puncture of intervertebral disks in sciatica. Acta Orthop Scand 13:375–377, 1948.
2. Goldie I: Intervertebral disc changes after discography. Acta Chir Scand 113:438–439, 1957.
3. Collis JS, Gardner WJ: Lumbar discography: Analysis of 1000 cases. J Neurosurg 19:452–461, 1962.
4. Massie WK, Stevens DB: A critical evaluation of discography. J Bone Joint Surg (Am) 49:1243–1244, 1967.
5. Hirsch C: An attempt to diagnose the level of a disc lesion clinically by disc puncture. Acta Orthop Scand 18:132–140, 1948.
6. Videman T, Malmivaara S, Mooney V: The value of the axial view in assessing discograms: An experimental study with cadavers. Spine 12:299–304, 1987.
7. Bogduk N: The innervation of the lumbar spine. Spine 8:286–293, 1983.
8. Tehranzadeh J: Discography 2000. Radiol Clin North Am 36:463–495, 1998.
9. Schellhas KP, Pollei SR, Gundry CR, Heithoff KB: Lumbar disc high-intensity zone. Correlation of magnetic resonance imaging and discography. Spine 21:79–86, 1996.
10. Lam KS, Carlin D, Mulholland RC: Lumbar disc high-intensity zone: The value and significance of provocative discography in the determination of the discogenic pain source. Eur Spine J 9:36–41, 2000.
11. Smith BM, Hurwitz EL, Solsberg D, et al: Interobserver reliability of detecting lumbar intervertebral disc high-intensity zone on magnetic resonance imaging and association of high-intensity zone with pain and annular disruption. Spine 23:2074–2080, 1998.
12. Weishaupt D, Zanetti M, Hodler J, et al: Painful lumbar disc derangement: Relevance of endplate abnormalities at MR imaging. Radiology 218:420–427, 2001.
13. Guyer RD, Ohnmeiss DD: Contemporary concepts in spine care. Lumbar discography. Position statement from the North American Spine Society Diagnostic and Therapeutic Committee. Spine 20:2048–2059, 1995.
14. Resnick DK, Malone DG, Ryken TC: Guidelines for the use of discography for the diagnosis of painful degenerative lumbar disc disease. Neurosurg Focus 13:E1–E6, 2002.
15. Holt EP: The question of lumbar discography. J Bone Joint Surg (Am) 50:720–726, 1968.
16. Simmons JW, April CN, Dwyer AP, Brodsky AE: A reassessment of Holt's data on "The question of lumbar discography." Clin Orthop 237:120–124, 1988.
17. Caragee EJ, Alamin TF, Miller J, Grafe M: Provocative discography in volunteer subjects with mild persistent low back pain. Spine J 2:25–34, 2002.
18. Slipman CW, Patel RK, Zhanag L, et al: Side of symptomatic annular tear and site of low back pain: Is there a correlation? Spine 26:E165–E169, 2001.
19. Ohnmeiss DD, Vanharanta H, Ekholm J: Relationship of pain drawings to invasive tests assessing intervertebral disc pathology. Eur Spine J 8:126–131, 1999.
20. Mink JH: Imaging evaluation of the candidate for percutaneous lumbar discectomy. Clin Orthop Rel Res 238:83–91, 1989.
21. Bernard TN: Lumbar discography followed by computed tomography. Refining the diagnosis of low back pain. Spine 15:690–707, 1990.
22. Urasaki T, Muro T, Ito S, et al: Consistency of lumbar discograms of the same disc obtained twice at a 2-week interval: Influence of needle tip position. J Orthop Sci 3:243–251, 1998.
23. Guyer RD, Ohnmeiss DD: Lumbar discography. Spine J 3(Suppl 3):11S–27S, 2003.
24. Gunzburg R, Parkinson R, Moore R, et al: A cadaveric study comparing discography, magnetic resonance imaging, histology, and mechanical behavior of the human lumbar disc. Spine 17:417–426, 1992.

25. Wiley JJ, Mcnab I, Wortzman G: Lumbar discography and its clinical application. Can J Surg 11:280–289, 1968.

26. Weinstein J, Claverie W, Gibson S: The pain of discography. Spine 13:1344–1348, 1988.

27. Heggenesss MH, Doherty BJ: Discography causes end plate deflection. Spine 18:1050–1053, 1993.

28. Walsh TR, Weinstein JN, Spratt KF, et al: Lumbar discography in normal subjects. A controlled, prospective study. J Bone Joint Surg (Am) 72:1081–1088, 1990.

29. Sachs BL, Vanharanta H, Spivey MA, et al: Dallas discogram description: A new classification of CT/discography in low-back disorders. Spine 12:287–298, 1987.

30. Schellhas KP: Discography. *In* Mathis JM (ed): Image-guided Spine Interventions. Springer Verlag, New York, 2004, pp 94–120.

31. Sato K, Kikuchi S, Yonezawa T: In vivo intradiscal pressure measurement in healthy individuals and in patients with ongoing back problems. Spine 24:2468–2474, 1999.

32. Derby R, Howard MW, Grant JM, et al: The ability of pressure-controlled discography to predict surgical and nonsurgical outcomes. Spine 24:364–371, 1999.

33. Fraser RD, Osti OL, Vernon-Roberts B: Discitis after discography. J Bone Joint Surg (Br) 69:31–35, 1987.

34. Osti OL, Fraser RD, Vernon-Roberts B: Discitis after discography: The role of prophylactic antibiotics. J Bone Joint Surg (Br) 72: 271–274, 1990.

60

Intradiscal Techniques: Intradiscal Electrothermal Therapy and Nucleoplasty

David R. Walega, M.D.

INTRADISCAL ELECTROTHERMAL THERAPY

Intradiscal electrothermal therapy (IDET) was developed by Saal and Saal in the late 1990s as a treatment for chronic low back pain caused by intervertebral disc derangement or disease. It has long been postulated that annular disruption can be a source of low back pain. In normal disc anatomy nociceptive fibers innervate only the outer third of the disc annulus, but as shown in important in vitro and in vivo studies, nerve and blood vessel in-growth into deeper layers of the annulus is correlated with high expression of substance P and clinically severe discogenic low back pain.[1,2]

It is widely accepted that 30% to 50% of all cases of low back pain are due to internal disc disruption (IDD).[3] IDD is defined as a "biochemical, biophysical, and morphologic disruption of the nucleus pulposis and annulus fibrosis of the disc,"[3] typically characterized by radial or circumferential fissures extending from the nucleus pulposis into the outer third of the posterior or posterolateral annulus. The presence of fissures or tears within the annulus can create a chronic inflammatory response as well as mechanical stresses in the intervertebral disc, resulting in neoinnervation and disc sensitization. Figure 60-1 demonstrates a normal appearing disc on postdiscogram axial computed tomography (CT) images. Figure 60-2 shows a similar axial CT image that demonstrates a clinically significant annular tear in a patient with IDD and discogenic low back pain amenable to IDET. Note the abnormal dye spread into the outer third of the annulus. The complete diagnostic criteria for IDD are listed in Table 60-1.

Traditionally, discogenic low back pain, or pain from IDD has been treated with conservative care: activity modification, rest, opiate and nonopiate analgesic medication, physical therapy, steroid spine injections, chiropractic care, manual therapy, acupuncture, and other modalities. Surgical arthrodesis has been a generally accepted treatment for discogenic low back pain unresponsive to conservative treatments. Significant variability in outcome following arthrodesis is noted in the literature.[4] Problems encountered with surgical arthrodesis include infection, pseudarthrosis, adjacent segmental instability, and other perioperative complications.

IDET is a minimally invasive technique currently used to treat highly selected patients with chronic low back pain from IDD. It is contraindicated for use in the cervical or thoracic

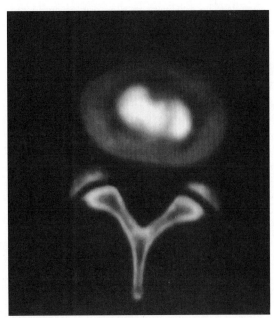

FIGURE 60-1. Axial CT image of a normal L4–5 intervertebral disc following discography. Note the contrast material held tightly within the nucleus pulposis.

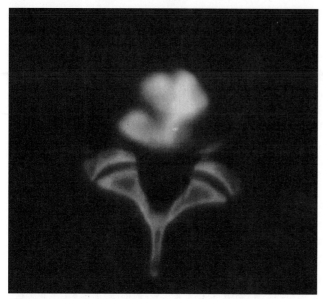

FIGURE 60-2. Axial CT image of an abnormal L4–5 intervertebral disc following discography. Note the extension of contrast material through a right posterior fissure with slight circumferential spread into the right posterolateral annulus. This is a grade 3 tear. There is no extension of contrast into the epidural space.

spine. IDET was developed on the premise that thermal heating of a disc annulus will result in collagen fiber contraction and neurolysis of nociceptors within the painful or sensitized disc.[5] The actual mechanism of action of IDET continues to foment significant debate.

Sluiter initially studied the effect of radiofrequency lesioning on nociceptors in the disc annulus in 800 patients and reported variable relief of pain.[6] It was these early data that indicated that radiofrequency heat delivery to the annulus could result in

TABLE 60-1. INTERNAL DISC DISRUPTION DIAGNOSTIC CRITERIA

Disc stimulation is positive at low pressures (<50 psi)
Disc stimulation produces pain of intensity >6/10 on visual analogue scale
Disc stimulation reproduces concordant pain
Computed tomography discography shows a grade 3 or greater annular tear (tear extends into the outer third of annulus) (See Figs. 60-1 and 60-2)
Control disc stimulation is negative at one and preferably two adjacent levels

From Karasek M, Bogduk N: Intradiscal electrothermal annuloplasty: Percutaneous treatment of chronic discogenic low back pain. Tech Reg Anesth Pain Manage 5:130–135, 2001.

inactivation of nociceptors in the annulus of a painful intervertebral disc. Unfortunately, the relatively small lesion size of conventional radiofrequency needles limited the efficacy of this technique. Hayashi et al. showed contraction of collagen fibers when exposed to temperatures greater than 65°C during laser therapy of shoulder joint capsules.[7]

IDET uses a thermal resistive catheter placed intradiscally at the site of a radial or circumferential annular fissure, to deliver radiofrequency energy to the posterior or posterolateral intervertebral disc in its entirety. This radiofrequency energy is converted into conductive heat which results in a thermal lesion of the disc annulus.[8] Temperatures at or above 65°C result in consistent shrinkage of collagen fibers.[5,9] Heat-labile hydrogen bonds cause the triple helix of the collagen molecule to unwind and transition into a less organized, random, contracted state. Subsequent to thermal treatment, fibroblast activity is increased and new, more stable and stiffer collagen is formed.[10] In addition, temperatures above 45°C are known to cause neurolysis. Thus, IDET is thought to cause mechanical modulation of disc material, as well as thermal neurolysis of nociceptive fibers within a painful disc.

Technique: The IDET procedure is performed percutaneously, similar to standard disc puncture techniques like discography. After diagnostic criteria for IDD and selection criteria for IDET have been met, informed consent for the procedure is obtained. Parenteral antibiotics are typically delivered to the patient pre-procedurally as a standard of care. Anteroposterior (AP) and lateral fluoroscopic guidance is used with the patient positioned prone on a radiolucent table under strict sterile conditions. The procedure can be performed in a fluoroscopy suite or sterile operating room. Table 60-2 lists a technique algorithm for IDET.

Local anesthesia is used to anesthetize the skin, subcutaneous tissues, and periosteum at the level at which the IDET will be performed. Minimal intravenous anesthesia is used to ensure patient comfort. Typically, 1 to 2 mg midazolam with/without 50 to 100 μg fentanyl is sufficient to sedate patients undergoing IDET. Heavy sedation or general anesthesia is contraindicated. Patients must remain awake and coherent enough to respond to commands and accurately report feelings of dysesthesias or radicular pain during needle placement, catheter placement, and heating protocol.

Using an extrapedicular approach, a 17-gauge, 6-inch introducer needle is placed into the disc to be treated. Needle entry into the disc is performed similar to conventional lumbar discography: ventral to the superior articular process of the zygophyseal joint at the level IDET is to be performed (Fig. 60-3). Fluoroscopic guidance is crucial to avoid trauma to the traversing nerve roots, and precisely position the needle tip half-way between the superior and inferior endplates of the adjacent vertebral bodies, in addition to being just anterior to the midpoint of the disc on lateral projection. There is no general agreement as to which side of the disc the introducer needle should be placed: some authors recommend entering the disc on the side contralateral the fissure to be lesioned, while other authors recommend the opposite.[11]

The thermal resistive catheter is then navigated meticulously to the posterior or posterolateral annulus to the site of the previously diagnosed fissure or tear, as seen in Figs. 60-4 and 60-5. CT discography results must be available to plan appropriately the positioning of the catheter for optimal

TABLE 60-2. **TECHNIQUE ALGORITHM FOR INTRADISCAL ELECTROTHERMAL THERAPY (IDET)**

Obtain informed consent from patient
Parenteral prophylactic antibiotic delivery
Sterile preparation and drape
Identify level to be treated with fluoroscope
Anesthetize skin/tissues, administer light intravenous sedation as needed
Confirm status of equipment/functioning IDET catheter, generator
Place introducer needle into disc to be treated (Fig. 60-3)
Place IDET catheter, confirm intradiscal placement with fluoroscopy (Figs. 60-4, 60-5)
Heating protocol
Remove IDET catheter
Administer intradiscal antibiotics
Remove introducer
Apply dressing to site
Recover patient
Place patient in corset/back brace
Follow up, activity restrictions, etc.

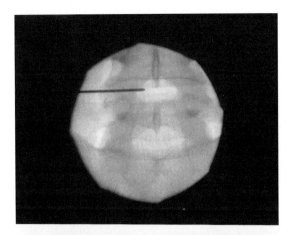

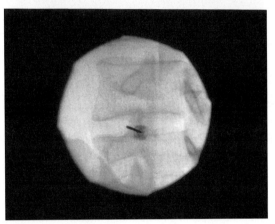

FIGURE 60-3. Anteroposterior and oblique fluoroscopic views of introducer needle placement via a left extrapedicular approach into the L4–5 disc. Note how the introducer needle "hugs" the superior articular process on the oblique image, preventing potential for nerve root injury.

lesioning. Karaseck and Bogduk report that meticulous positioning of the catheter will improve postprocedural results.[3]

The catheter is then heated to a maximum temperature of 85 to 90°C for a total of 16.5 minutes, via a heating protocol set forth by Saal and Saal.[5] A maximum temperature of 90°C for 4 minutes is recommended. The avascular disc acts as a heat sink, allowing the disc to retain this delivered heat, and effect collagen conformation distant to the catheter, without causing nerve root or spinal cord damage. The countercurrent blood flow in the epidural and perineural vessels appears to have a neuroprotective effect, preventing heat from building up within or near neural tissue when the catheter is appropriately placed intradiscally. A single heating treatment is performed at each disc level to be treated.

Most patients experience their typical low back pain reproduced during the heating protocol, often with vague aching into the buttocks or legs. This must be differentiated from true radicular pain, specifically if these symptoms are severe and occur early in the heating cycle (65 to 80°C). If true radicular pain occurs during the heating protocol, the catheter must be removed and/or repositioned.

Catheter kinking has been known to occur, as has catheter breakage. When breakage occurs, it is typically at the connection of the catheter to the catheter hub, but it can occur along the body of the catheter from damaged incurred at the introducer needle tip. Kinking of the catheter can occur when the tip becomes lodged within a radial fissure or circumferential tear. The catheter should be withdrawn under these circumstances, and the introducer needle moved anteriorly or posteriorly prior to reinsertion of the catheter. If a catheter is severely bent or kinked it should be discarded and replaced. If removal of the catheter from the introducer needle is met with resistance, the introducer and catheter should be removed en bloc and then replaced separately. If the catheter cannot be navigated successfully across the length of a fissure, the introducer needle can be removed, placed via a contralateral extrapedicular technique, with reattempts at optimal catheter placement. Another alternative salvage maneuver, the "pig tail" technique, is described by Navani and Tsiridis.[12]

Only the most distal portion of the catheter is able to transmit heat. This length is demarcated by radiopaque markers on

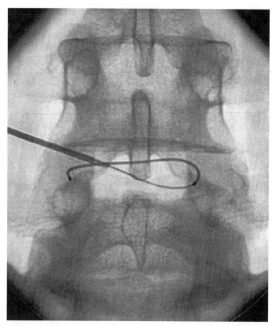

FIGURE 60-4. Anteroposterior fluoroscopic view of IDET catheter placed into an L4–5 intervertebral disc. Note the radiopaque markers on the catheter, delineating the thermal conductive portion of the device.

the catheter that is easily visualized with fluoroscopy (Figs. 60-4 and 60-5). If this length of catheter makes contact with the introducer needle during the heating protocol, there is potential to cause thermal injury to the tissues immediately surrounding the introducer needle, including the exiting nerve root, paravertetral muscles, and skin. On occasion, the introducer needle will need to be retracted to the most outer portion of the annulus, while keeping the catheter in place intradiscally.

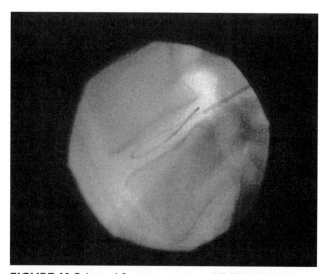

FIGURE 60-5. Lateral fluoroscopic view of IDET catheter placed into an L4–5 intervertebral disc. The lateral projection is used to confirm that the catheter has not been erroneously placed into the spinal canal or into a foramen. Note that the introducer needle has been pulled back into the outer annulus to prevent heating of the introducer needle.

Following the heating protocol, the catheter is removed from the patient, and 2 to 20 mg cefazolin is typically injected into the disc for prophylaxis against disc infection.[8] Gentamycin or another alternative method of prophylaxis should be used in those allergic or sensitive to cephalosporins. The introducer needle is then removed, and the patient is moved to a recovery/observation area and then discharged home with activity restrictions (see Table 60-3).

Complications: In the initial studies of patient outcome Saal and Saal reported no complications in any IDET patient, and specifically mentioned "no nerve injuries, no infections, and no neurologic deficits" in their study population.[8] There is one case of cauda equina syndrome following IDET that was reported in the literature,[13] but this case was clearly the result of catheter placement within the spinal canal, instead of intradiscally, prior to any heating of tissue. The only other reported complications in the literature are a case of verterbral osteonecrosis several months following IDET in a 28-year-old male,[14] and a large disc herniation in a 152-kg, 29-year-old male soldier following IDET.[15]

Results: Saal and Saal presented their initial data of 25 consecutive IDET patients in 1998.[16] All patients experienced low

TABLE 60-3. POSTOPERATIVE GUIDELINES FOR INTRADISCAL ELECTROTHERMAL THERAPY (IDET) PATIENTS

Wear a lumbar corset/back brace for 6–8 weeks after IDET
Limit sitting to 30–40 minutes at a time for the first 6 weeks
Perform sedentary activity at 1–3 weeks after the procedure, but excessive sitting (>30 minutes) is to be avoided
Driving is prohibited for the first 5 days, then only 20–30 minutes at a time for the first 6 weeks
Riding as a passenger is acceptable for up to 45 minutes in a comfortable seat
Lifting limit is 10 pounds for the first 6 weeks
Walk 20 minutes daily after the first week; advance to 20 minutes twice daily as tolerated
Do stretching exercises for legs (gently) after first week
No swimming in the first 6 weeks
Resume graded activity on a graded program, with attention to back care, commencing at approximately 8 weeks as tolerated, supervised by a physical therapist or physiatrist if required

From Saal JA, Saal JS: Intradiscal electrothermal therapy for the treatment of chronic discogenic low back pain. Op Tech Orthop 10:271–281, 2000.

back pain for greater than 6 months and underwent discography following a failed trial of 6 months of conservative care. Some 80% of patients who underwent IDET in this study experienced clinical improvement, described as a 2-point decrease in visual analogue scale (VAS) score. In addition, 72% of patients demonstrated functional improvement or reduction/discontinuance of analgesic use. Less than 20% of patients that underwent IDET had no improvement in their pain.

This initial work was met with great skepticism given the nonrandomized, uncontrolled study design, as well as the fact that the investigators were also the developers of the IDET technology. Despite this skepticism and lack of controlled, prospective, randomized studies to support the use of this technology, IDET was brought to the marketplace in the late 1990s and was performed on extensive patient populations with mixed, and sometimes disappointing results.

Saal and Saal published 2-year follow-up data of 62 IDET patients.[8] This study group was comprised of consecutive patients from a pool of 1,116 patients who did not respond to 6 months of conservative nonsurgical therapy and all underwent pre-IDET discography. Of the 62 patients who underwent IDET, 4 were lost to follow-up at 1 year.

All patients were subjected to the same inclusion and exclusion criteria, and were specifically excluded from IDET if they had prior spine surgery at symptomatic levels, specific inflammatory arthritides, or nonspinal causes of low back pain. All patients underwent the same thermal catheter protocol, and postprocedure care which included graduated physical exercise for 5 to 6 months. Outcome measures included VAS, sitting tolerance, and a SF-36 assessed at 6, 12, and 24 months and then compared to pretreatment values.

At 24 months, Saal and Saal reported that mean post-IDET VAS was 3.41 as compared to 6.57 preprocedurally.[8] Fifty percent of patients experienced a 4-point reduction in VAS, and 71% experienced a 2-point reduction in VAS. There was no statistical difference in outcome between one-level ($n = 30$) and two-level cases ($n = 21$) of IDET. Patients showed statistically significant improvements in sitting tolerance and SF-36 scores, specifically between the 1-year and 2-year observation points. Some 78% of the patients had improvements of at least 7 points on SF-36 scores. The IDET patients at 2-year follow-up showed a significant improvement in quality of life as compared to pretreatment values. There was no difference between the "private pay" patients and the workers' compensation patients. Return to work occurred in 97% of private pay patients and 83% of workers' compensation patients respectively. Saal and Saal further argued that, alone, natural history of back pain could not account for the improvement seen in the IDET-treated patients at 2-year follow-up. No IDET patient in this study experienced a complication.

This study was criticized for its lack of randomization and lack of a control group with which to compare IDET results, and accusations of investigator bias continue to plague the results.

Bogduk and Karasek published a 2-year follow-up study[17] of patients who had undergone IDET, and included a comparison group of "untreated" patients with discogenic low back pain. True randomization did not occur in this study, as the comparison "untreated" group was comprised of patients who met selection criteria for IDET but were subsequently denied treatment by an insurance carrier.

A total of 150 consecutive patients were enrolled in the study based on clinical criteria for discogenic low back pain.

All patients had low back pain for at least 3 months. Provocative discography and postinjection CT scanning was performed in 110 patients. Based on discography results, 53 patients were diagnosed with IDD, demonstrated disc height at the affected level to be 80% or more of normal height, and were identified as IDET candidates. The procedure was performed in 36 patients, using thermal catheter temperatures of 90, 85, or 80°C, depending on patient tolerance of the procedure. The remaining 17 patients were denied the procedure by their respective insurance carriers and thus comprised a comparison group. The comparison group was referred for multidisciplinary rehabilitation (physical therapy, exercise, and counseling). The IDET group underwent "graded reactivation" for up to 4 months following IDET. This included back bracing and progressive exercise, with limitation of lumbar flexion and rotation in the postprocedure phase. The comparison group was referred out for physical therapy and/or behavioral therapy, but did not have close follow-up care with the investigators.

VAS for pain, work status, and opiate use were used as outcome measures in both groups, and followed for a period of 24 months when possible. At 3-month follow-up, the VAS in the treatment group dropped from a pretreatment mean of 8.0 to a post-treatment mean of 3.4, whereas the mean VAS score in the control group remained unchanged.[17] At 24 months, 57% of the IDET group had at least 50% relief of pain, and 20% were completely pain free. In contrast, the comparison group at 12 and 24 months demonstrated no significant improvements from baseline. Fifty-four percent of IDET patients exhibited profound and durable improvement in pain scores at 24 months. Forty-six percent of IDET patients had an initial good response but experienced a relapse in pain scores by 24 months. In assessing function and disability, the authors showed that "patients who achieved a VAS at 2 years of 4 or who achieved greater than 50% reduction of their pain returned to work," regardless of compensation/insurance status.[17]

This study nicely documented the natural history of IDET response in a tightly selected treatment group with minimal operator variability with regard to the technical aspects of the IDET procedure and postprocedure care. However, inferences with regard to the nontreated comparison group are tenuous, given the lack of true randomization to the non-IDET group, and the inherent biases of a comparison group created by "rejection" by a third party. However, the incidence of complete and durable pain relief in 20% of the treatment population remains extremely promising. The authors comment that their favorable results may have been related to "(catheter) placement…purposely as close as possible to any circumferential fissure, and…as far as possible into the outer annulus opposite a radial fissure."[17]

Lee and Cooper conducted a prospective, nonrandomized study of IDET in a group of 62 patients with chronic low back pain of moderate to severe intensity of duration greater than 6 months. Fifty-one of 62 patients (82%) were available for a minimum follow-up of 24 months. Each patient underwent provocative discography and post injection CT scanning prior to IDET. Strict inclusion and exclusion criteria for lumbar discogenic pain were followed; however, prior lumbar spine surgery was not a contraindication to IDET in this study. A total of 70 levels were treated with IDET in 51 patients.[18] The most common level treated in this group was L4–5

(37/70). Thirty-two patients underwent single-level IDET versus 19 patients who underwent multilevel treatment.[18] There was a statistically significant improvement in low back visual numeric pain score of 3.2 ($p < 0.001$) in patients who underwent IDET. Patients who had a history of prior microdiscectomy and subsequently underwent IDET ($n = 4$) responded favorably with a mean decrease in pain scores of 6.3 ($p < 0.05$). In addition, there was no difference in outcome between patients with workers' compensation/no-fault insurance versus patients with traditional third-party insurance coverage.[18]

These investigators opine that prior discectomy is not an immediate contraindication to IDET, and that this particular subset of patients significantly improved following IDET. Again, this study was nonrandomized and had no placebo control group for comparison, but had an extended follow-up period.

Derby et al. presented outcome data of a 1-year pilot study of 32 patients who underwent IDET for intractable discogenic low back pain.[19] Seven of these patients had undergone prior spine surgery. Inclusion criteria were similar to the studies mentioned previously, but disc manometry was also performed at the time of discography, and no more than two symptomatic levels were treated with IDET in any patient. In addition, IDET catheter placement was assessed as fair, good, or excellent during the study, with varying heating protocols from 75 to 150°C.

Outcome was assessed with a Roland–Morris Disability Questionnaire (RM), VAS, NASS Low Back Pain Outcome Assessment Instrument Patient Satisfaction Index (PSI), and general activity questionnaire. Outcomes were assessed at 6 and 12 months.

There was no significant difference in outcomes at 6 and 12 months.[19] The average drop in VAS was 1.84. Sixty-three percent of patients reported a favorable outcome, and 25% reported no change. Seventy-five percent of patients with low-pressure discs on manometry reported a favorable outcome. Over 50% of patients reported improvements in activity level. No patients experienced a complication. Patients did not undergo extensive physical rehabilitation following IDET. Again, this was a nonrandomized and noncontrolled study of highly selected patients for IDET, but the data indicate that patients with low-pressure discs have a more favorable outcome of pain relief following IDET.

A randomized, placebo-controlled trial of IDET was performed by Pauza et al. in an ambitious prospective study.[20] Uncompensated volunteers for this study were screened via telephone, of which 264 were eligible for discography. Patients were excluded from the study if they had prior spine surgery, a radicular pattern of pain, extruded intervertebral disc, spinal stenosis, scoliosis, narcotic usage >100 mg of morphine equivalent/day, or if they had workers' compensation issues, personal injury, application for disability, or active litigation involving pain.

A total of 64 patients were candidates for randomization after clinical examination, psychological testing, discography, and postinjection CT scanning. Patients were randomized to IDET or sham procedure in a blinded fashion, and all patients in both groups had the IDET introducer needle introduced into the annulus of the affected disc(s). Randomization took place at the time of introducer needle placement. The IDET group underwent standard heating of the IDET probe to 90°C, and the sham group experienced the same "visual and auditory environment" as the treatment group.[20] Following these procedures, both groups underwent postprocedural back bracing and a graded physical rehabilitation program, and were evaluated by blinded investigators. Follow-up was maintained for 12 months.

There were 32 patients in the IDET group, 24 controls, and 8 drop-outs due to various causes. Pain and disability were assessed using VAS scores, Oswestry testing, and the SF-36 and follow-up lasted 12 months. Approximately 40% of patients treated with IDET experienced 50% or more pain relief, but 50% of patients experienced no notable improvement. Some 6% of the IDET group showed worsening of pain by VAS on follow-up, while 33% of the control group showed similar deterioration. Only 21% of the IDET group experienced >80% relief of pain, while only 4% of the control group showed similar levels of improvement in pain. Function remained the same in both groups, even when pain levels improved. The investigators theorize that one reason for the limited categorical benefit was due to a "healthy patient effect": "improvements are difficult to demonstrate statistically if a large proportion of patients are not particularly disabled at inception."[3] Patients in this study with low physical function levels and high disability scores improved significantly with IDET. One patient in the placebo group experienced complete relief of pain.

In this rigorous study, despite the technical and ethical difficulties and dubious nature of "sham" treatment, it is clear that the efficacy of IDET cannot purely be attributed to placebo effect. The investigators concluded that although "IDET is not uniformly successful, [it] provides worthwhile relief of otherwise intractable back pain…"[20] It appears that nonspecific factors are a major determinant in IDET outcome. This study is commended for being the only known placebo-controlled trial for a surgical procedure used for discogenic low back pain.[20]

Although the true efficacy of IDET is not clearly elucidated, all of the cited studies show a clinical benefit of the procedure, and no complications occurred in any of the study patients outlined previously. Several studies show that IDET is not universally successful,[17] nor are the results consistently reproducible in all study groups. The reasons are not entirely clear.

The mechanism of action for IDET remains controversial and several current theories are listed in Table 60-4. Most

TABLE 60-4. POSSIBLE MECHANISMS OF ACTION FOR INTRADISCAL ELECTROTHERMAL THERAPY

Alteration in spinal segment mechanics via collagen modification
Thermal nociceptive fiber destruction
Biochemical mediation of inflammation
Stimulation of outer annulus healing process
Cauterization of vascular in-growth
Induced healing of annular tears

From Derby R: Intradiscal electrothermal annuloplasty: Current concepts. Pain Physician 6:383–385, 2003.

TABLE 60-5. SELECTION CRITERIA INTRADISCAL ELECTROTHERMAL THERAPY

Chronic, intrusive low back pain for greater than 3 months
Failure to achieve adequate improvement with comprehensive nonoperative treatment
No red-flag condition
No medical contraindications
No neurologic deficit
Normal straight leg raise
Nondiagnostic magnetic resonance imaging scan
No evidence for segmental instability, spondylolisthesis at target level
No irreversible psychological barriers to recovery
Motivated patient with realistic expectations of outcome
No greater than 75% loss of disc height
Criteria for internal disc disruption satisfied

From Karasek M, Bogduk N: Intradiscal electrothermal annuloplasty: Percutaneous treatment of chronic discogenic low back pain. Tech Reg Anesth Pain Manage 5:130–135, 2001.

investigators agree that large-scale, multicenter controlled studies of IDET may be more successful in delineating the true mechanism of action for IDET, and may also elucidate factors that predict outcome and explain poor outcome when it occurs. Despite Pauza et al.'s rigorous study of IDET, these answers to the IDET question were not entirely clear. Requiring limited annular disruption and/or an intact annulus may improve outcomes.[21] Bogduk and Karasek selected patients for IDET that had no more than two quadrants of disruption on CT discography in their study[17] and appeared to have very favorable outcomes. All investigators have recommended strict selection criteria for IDET (see Table 60-5).

In general, IDET is a minimally invasive technique that shows significant promise in treating the pain of IDD or discogenic low back pain, with minimal risk of complication when performed by experienced practitioners. Derby states that strict inclusion criteria, specifically "less than 30% disc height decrease without obesity may afford [approximately] 2.5 mean VAS improvement with 'as much or somewhat better pain' in >50% of patients."[21] As compared to open surgical procedures like fusion, IDET is minimally invasive and avoids the inherent perioperative risks of lumbar spine fusion. A summary of study results is given in Table 60-6.

NUCLEOPLASTY

Nucleoplasty is an increasingly popular method of percutaneous disc decompression (PDD) developed in 2000 for selected patients with persistent radicular pain due to small, contained herniated lumbar discs or contained disc bulges, unresponsive to conservative, nonsurgical therapy. PDD is based on the principle that decreases in volume within an enclosed space will result in a disproportionately higher drop in pressure. Other methods of PDD used in the past include chymopapain nucleolysis, percutaneous manual nucleotomy, nucleotomy via nucleotome use, and thermal vaporization via laser.[22]

Nucleoplasty uses radiofrequency energy delivered through a percutaneous electrode to create a voltage gradient within the intervertebral disc. A plasma field is then created between an electrode tip within the disc and the surrounding nucleus pulposis. This intradiscal transmission of energy excites the surrounding tissues, causing molecular bonds of the nucleous pulposis to break, vaporizing disc material into low molecular weight gases (hydrogen, oxygen, carbon dioxide) which then exit the percutaneous needle.[22] Thus, a small volume of the nucleous pulposis is removed, creating a dramatic decrease in intradiscal pressure. Decreased annular wall stress allows the

TABLE 60-6. SUMMARY OF INTRADISCAL ELECTROTHERMAL THERAPY (IDET) STUDY RESULTS

Author	Year published	No. in IDET group	Follow-up period (months)	Controlled?	Randomized?	Favorable Outcome (%)
Saal and Saal[8]	2000	62	24	No	No	72
Bogduk and Karasek[17]	2002	36	24	No	No	60 (23%) complete relief
Lee et al.[18]	2003	51	24	No	No	63
Derby et al.[19]	2000	32	12	No	No	63
Pauza et al.[20]	2004	32	12	Yes	Yes	40

intact annulus to retract from irritated neural tissue, thereby providing pain relief.[23]

In contrast to IDET, nucleoplasty creates a lower temperature range of heat, typically 40 to 70°C, and because the plasma field is created within the central portion of the disc, the risk of thermal injury of surrounding neural structures is theoretically lower.

Technique: Nucleoplasty is performed in a similar manner to other intradiscal techniques like discography and IDET. After appropriate selection (see Table 60-7), preparation of the patient, and informed consent, an introducer needle is placed in the disc to be treated under fluoroscopic guidance via an extrapedicular approach, with needle placement ventral to the superior articular process. This procedure is accomplished successfully with local anesthesia and minimal intravenous sedation. Again, it is recommended that patients be awake and coherent during this procedure, able to report paresthesias, dysesthesias, or any other untoward sensation.

The needle is advanced to the interface between the annulus fibrosis and the nucleus pulposis in the posterolateral disc, ipsilateral to the patient's symptoms of radicular pain. A nucleoplasty electrode is then placed through the introducer needle and advanced across the disc space to the adjacent annulus in the anterior portion of the disc. Tissue ablation and coagulation is performed with each "pass" across the nucleus, creating a channel within the disc. After making six channels within the disc, a total of 1 cm³ of intradiscal volume is vaporized, with a significant decrease in intradiscal pressure.[23]

Following disc vaporization, intradiscal delivery of antibiotics is recommended, similar to those doses recommended by Saal and Saal.[8] Back bracing is not required following this procedure, nor is a protracted course of physical therapy. Patients are typically able to resume normal activities within 1 to 2 weeks of the procedure.

Results: To date, there are no published studies of placebo-controlled randomized trials of nucleoplasty. Singh et al.[22]

TABLE 60-7. CONTRAINDICATIONS TO NUCLEOPLASTY

Greater than 1/3 loss of disc height
Herniation >1/3 sagittal diameter of spinal canal
Nonqualifying provocative discography
Complete annular disruption
Free fragment
Disc extrusion
Spinal stenosis
Spinal instability
Tumor, infection, fracture

published a prospective outcome analysis of 67 patients who underwent nucleoplasty for low back and/or leg pain due to a contained disc herniation who had failed conservative, nonsurgical therapy. All patients underwent provocative discography with a negative control disc. Following a standard nucleoplasty technique, patient activity was limited for the following 2 weeks, and all patients were counseled by a physical therapist regarding proper body mechanics. Outcome measures included VAS and functional status. At 12 months, 80% of patients had improvements in pain, 56% had >50% relief of pain, and approximately 60% had improvements in functional status. Indices were comparably more favorable at 3-month follow-up.

Sharps and Issac[24] reported another prospective analysis of 49 patients with back and/or leg pain due to focal lumbar disc protrusion who had failed to improve with 6 weeks of conservative nonsurgical therapy. Exceptions were made if "pain was functionally incapacitating and refractory to the use of oral narcotics." All patients underwent discography prior to nucleoplasty, and returned to sedentary work activity 3 to 4 days after surgery. VAS, narcotic use, return to work, and patient satisfaction were measured at 1, 3, 6, and 12 months. Success, rated as a 2 or more point drop in VAS, was found in 79% in the study group. At 12 months, the mean VAS was 4.3 versus a preprocedure mean baseline of 7.9. No complications were found at any point in follow-up.

OTHER METHODS OF PERCUTANEOUS DISC DECOMPRESSION

PDD can also be accomplished with a pecutaneous disc probe. This device is placed similarly to the nuceoplasty electrode. In contrast to nucleoplasty and IDET, however, the probe mechanically removes approximately 1 cm³ of disc material without radiofrequency energy or thermal heat. Disc material collects within a collection hub on this disposable device, and can be used for measurement purposes or can be sent for pathologic analysis, when indicated.

Again, limited inference can be made on the basis of the prospective studies outlined previously. A randomized case-controlled study of long-term outcomes will be helpful in developing more stringent and reliable selection criteria for this minimally invasive technique.

REFERENCES

1. Freemont A, Peacock T, Goupille P, et al: Nerve in-growth into diseased intervertebral disc in chronic low back pain. Lancet 350:178–181, 1997.
2. Coppes M, Marani E, Thomeer R, Groen G: Innervation of painful discs. Spine 22:2342–2349, 1997.
3. Karasek M, Bogduk N: Intradiscal electrothermal annuloplasty: Percutaneous treatment of chronic discogenic low back pain. Tech Reg Anesth Pain Manage 5:130–135, 2001.
4. Wetzel T, McNally T, Phillips F: Intradiscal electricothermal therapy used to manage chronic discogenic low back pain. Spine 27:2621–2626, 2002.
5. Saal JA, Saal JS: Intradiscal electrothermal therapy for the treatment of chronic discogenic low back pain. Clin Sports Med 21:167–187, 2002.
6. Sluijter M: The use of radiofrequency lesions for pain relief in failed back patients. Int Disability Studies 10:37–43, 1988.
7. Hayashi K, Tabit G, Vailas A: The effect of nonablative laser energy on joint capsular properties: An in vitro histologic and

biochemical study using a rabbit model. Am J Sports Med 24:640–646, 1996.

8. Saal JA, Saal JS: Intradiscal electrothermal treatment for chronic discogenic low back pain: Prospective outcome study with a minimum 2-year follow-up. Spine 27:966–974, 2000.

9. Heary R: Intradiscal electrothermal annuloplasty: The IDET procedure. J Spinal Disord 14:353–360, 2001.

10. Narvani A, Tsiridis E, Wilson L: High intensity zone, intradiscal electrothermal therapy, and magnetic resonance imaging. J Spinal Disord Techniques 16:130–136, 2003.

11. Karaseck M, Bogduk N: Twelve month follow up of a controlled trial of intradiscal thermal annuloplasty for back pain due to internal disc disruption. Spine 25:2601–2607, 2000.

12. Navani A, Tsiridis E: "Pig tail" technique in intradiscal electrothermal therapy. J Spine Disord Techniques 16:280–284, 2003.

13. Hsia A, Isaac K, Katz J: Cauda equina syndrome from intradiscal electrothermal therapy. Neurology 55:320–322, 2000.

14. Djurasovic M, Glassman S, Dimar J, Johnson J: Vertebral osteonecrosis associated with the use of intradiscal electrothermal therapy: A case report. Spine 27:325–328, 2002.

15. Cohen S, Larkin T, Polly D: A giant herniated disc following intradiscal electrothermal therapy. J Spinal Disord Techniques 15:537–541, 2002.

16. Saal JA, Saal JS: Thermal characteristics of lumbar discs: Evaluation of a novel approach to targeted intradiscal thermal therapy. Presented at the 13th Annual Meeting of the North American Spine Society, San Francisco, CA, 23–28 October 1998.

17. Bogduk N, Karasek M: Two year follow up of a controlled trial of intradiscal electrothermal anuloplasty for chronic low back pain resulting from internal disc disruption. Spine 2:343–350, 2002.

18. Lee M, Cooper G, Lutz C, Hong H: Intradiscal electrothermal therapy (IDET) for treatment of chronic lumbar discogenic pain: A minimum 2-year clinical outcome study. Pain Physician 6:443–448, 2003.

19. Derby R, Bjorn E, Yung C, et al:. Intradiscal electrothermal annuloplasty (IDET): A novel approach for treating chronic discogenic back pain. Neuromodulation 3:82–88, 2000.

20. Pauza K, Howell S, Dreyfuss P, et al: A randomized, placebo-controlled trial of intradiscal electrothermal therapy (IDET) for the treatment of discogenic low back pain. Spine 4:27–35, 2004.

21. Derby R: Intradiscal electrothermal annuloplasty: Current concepts. Pain Physician 6:383–385, 2003.

22. Singh V, Piryani C, Liao K, Nieschulz S: Percutaneous disc decompression using Coblation (nucleoplasty) in the treatment of chronic discogenic pain. Pain Physician 5:250–259, 2002.

23. Chen Y, Lee S, Chen D: Intradiscal pressure study of percutaneous disc decompression with nucleoplasty in human cadavers. Spine 28:661–665, 2003.

24. Sharps L, Issac Z: Percutaneous disc decompression using nucleoplasty. Pain Physician 5:121–126, 2002.

61

Osteoporosis and Percutaneous Vertebroplasty

John C. Liu, M.D., and
Bernard R. Bendok, M.D.

Bone is a connective tissue that is responsible for hematopoiesis, mechanical and structural support, and mineral storage of inorganic salts and organic material. Bone is constantly broken down and architecturally rebuilt to provide optimal mechanical support for its various functions. If bone turnover, the breakdown and formation of new bone, is unbalanced then progression of bone loss develops. However, peak bone mass is achieved at 35 years of age and is in decline thereafter; thus, bone loss is expected in adulthood and consequently in old age. Although various other factors also contribute to progressive bone loss, an increase in bone resorption and a decrease in new bone formation are the hallmarks of osteoporosis.

Osteoporosis, the most common debilitating metabolic bone disease, is marked by a reduction in bone mass per unit volume with normal bone chemical composition, decreased skeletal function, progressive spinal deformity, and vulnerability to fractures. Also dubbed "porous bone disease" or "brittle bone disease," osteoporosis is a universal disease with a common language of improper bone remodeling posing an array of complications.

Spine surgery concerns in osteoporotic patients are abundant. Decreased bone mass density (BMD) provides the foundation for numerous intra- and postoperative complications. Proper surgical approach and instrumentation constructs and application must be selected to cater to the spine's altered state.

Osteoporosis increases the risk for fracture leading to discomfort and pain often difficult to manage. Vertebral fractures often provide excruciating pain and ensuing deformity. Thorough knowledge of diagnosis and therapeutic treatment is imperative to manage an osteoporotic spine. Although avenues exist that aid in the prevention and conservative treatment of the disease, percutaneous vertebroplasty and recently kyphoplasty are innovative procedures that offer immediate vertebral pain relief and restoration of vertebral height where applicable to combat the effects of vertebral compression fractures.

PREVALENCE

Metabolic diseases of the skeletal system are either congenital or secondary in nature. The primary effect on bone in lieu of osteoporosis is a decrease in bone mass due to improper bone remodeling. As is often the case, the disease tends to affect more women than men, as women possess 10% to 25% less total bone mass at maturity. Moreover, osteoporosis has a high predilection to occur in Caucasian and Asian women than any other race with a high risk of developing an osteoporotic fracture due to low bone mineral density.[1-3] In the USA 35% of women over the age of 65 years and 15% of Caucasian postmenopausal women are osteoporotic.[4] In the USA this debilitating disease amasses 1 million individuals with fractures per year with $14 billion spent for treatment.[5] Hip and vertebral fractures occur in women at a rate of 250,000 and 500,000 yearly, respectively, and an additional 250,000 fractures are experienced by men yearly.[6,7] Vertebral fractures in women increase as menopause approaches and with old age with a ratio of 2:1 for that of women compared to men.[8]

BONE BIOLOGY

Bone is the grand architect of the human body providing structure, stability, protection, and movement via muscular assistance. The primary structure of bone is distinguished by cortical bone, also known as compact bone, and trabecular bone, otherwise called cancellous or spongy bone. Trabecular bone has many interconnecting cavities consisting of red bone marrow forming red blood cells and yellow bone marrow composed of fat cells. Conversely, cortical bone is generally on the surface and is characterized by its dense composition without cavities. The extent of trabecular and cortical bone varies depending on the location of bone. Bone is composed of osteoprogenitor cells, osteoblasts, osteocytes, osteoclasts, neurovascular cells of external origin, bone surface lining cells, and an array of inorganic and organic constituents. Furthermore, two types of bone are evident: primary and secondary. Primary or woven bone first appears in early embryonic development characterized by its low mineral content, higher abundance of osteocytes, and increased presence of collagen fibers. Although primary bone still remains in adulthood, as is evident at cranial bone sutures, tooth sockets, and tendon insertions, secondary bone is primarily present. Secondary or lamellar bone consists of parallel collagenous fibrils know as lamellae.

The bone matrix is the extracellular mineralized component of bone which contains 10% to 20% water[9] and inorganic and organic constituents that account for 65% to 70% and 30% to 35% of its dry weight, respectively.[9,10] Proportions of hydrated and dry weight of bone vary with age, location, sex, and metabolic prowess. Furthermore, an immature or demineralized bone matrix in the process of bone formation is referred to as an osteoid.

The inorganic constituents or bone crystals are electrodense and become more abundant with age while water content decreases. Bone crystals are small with large surfaces and are interconnected with narrow gaps containing water and organic macromolecules. The majority of bone ions are calcium, phosphate, hydroxy, and carbonate. However, citrate, copper, boron, aluminum, sodium, magnesium, potassium, chloride, iron, zinc, lead, strontium, silicon, and fluoride are also present in smaller amounts. The main mineral formed by bone crystals is hydroxyapatite ($Ca_{10}(PO_4)_6(OH)_2$). About 99% of the body's calcium deposit is harvested by bone which is found in hydroxyapatite and provides a constant interchange between calcium reserve in the bone and that in the periphery. Calcified bone matrix prohibits diffusion of metabolites into peripheral tissue. However, canaculi are utilized for transporting material between blood vessels and osteocytes. Various group II ions, such as lead, radium, and strontium, are bone-seeking cations and could replace calcium posing hazardous toxic effects to bone marrow's hematopoietic tissue.

The bone matrix is also composed of organic constituents. Type I collagen is the most abundant material in the organic bone matrix that provides strength and mineral deposition primarily of hydroxyapatite. Collagen present in bone is synthesized from osteoblasts and forms strong covalent cross-links with enlarged fibrillar transverse spacings that inorganic minerals inhabit. The collagen is located within the inner and outer bone and forms parallel fibers in secondary lamellar bone.

Less abundant organic constituents are also present. Growth factors, such as proteases and protease inhibitors produced by osteoblasts, also make up the organic matrix. Sialoproteins, osteoporotin, and thrombospondin are responsible for bone-cell adhesion and are also found in the organic matrix. Glycoproteins, such as sparc/osteonectin and osteocalcin, are also present in the organic matrix with biglycan and decorin proteoglycans.

Osteoblasts and osteoclasts are the main bone cells integral in bone remodeling. According to Frost in 1964 osteoclasts are multinucleated cells responsible for bone resorption and osteoblasts are bone-forming cells.[11] Bone cells possess a plasticity that provides remodeling capabilities in response to bone cell-derived growth factors, local factors, and varying degrees of stress that induce osteogenesis.[10,12,13] Parathyroid hormone (PTH), 1,25-dihydroxyvitamin, prostaglandins E2, and interleukin (IL-1) are some of the hormones and local factors that influence bone turnover. Therefore, these factors stimulate the activation of osteoclasts which further require osteoblast and osteoclast precursors for a fully operable osteoclast.

Osteoprotegerin ligand (OPGL), osteoclast differentiating factor (ODF), and RANK or TRACE ligands alter the molecular surface of osteoblast precursors allowing interaction with osteoclast precursors. As a result, osteoprogenitor cells, derived from pluripotential stem cells, are thoroughly involved in intramembranous and endochondral bone formation by proliferating and differentiating into osteoblasts. Osteoblasts further proliferate and develop into osteocytes that remain in primary or secondary bone. Osteocytes and osteoblasts can therefore "revert to osteoprogenitor" cells to adapt to changing conditions.

Bone resorption begins once complete osteoclast differentiation is accomplished. Osteoclasts then form erosive cavities at the bone surface priming migration of mononuclear cells to occupy that area. Of these cells, osteoblasts arise and over a process of 3 to 4 weeks fill the cavities made by the osteoclasts. In the young adult bone resorption equals bone formation. With age, osteoblast activity decreases priming and increases bone resorption. The resorptive activity seems to increase with age due to prevention of cell apoptosis by interleukins and tumor necrosis factor as is noted in postmenopausal women who are estrogen deficient. If cavities still remain, trabecular or cancellous bone weakens. If widespread bone resorption is present and progresses, trabecular bone becomes more perforated allowing limited surface for new bone to build upon. Since bone turnover is dependent upon surface area, trabecular bone is largely targeted. Therefore, vertebrae in postmenopausal women are more susceptible to decreased bone mass and ensuing fracture because of their abundant cancellous bone.

OSTEOPOROTIC FRACTURES

Also dubbed "porous bone disease" or "brittle bone disease," osteoporosis is associated with increased risk of fractures. Fractures are more prone to occur at the hip, ribs, wrists, and vertebrae. In 1990 it was estimated that 1.66 million osteoporotic individuals worldwide suffered hip fractures. An increased risk of mortality exists among osteoporotic patients who experience a hip fracture with 25% of patients dying in the first year.[14–19] Of those who survive, 50% are unable to resume their previous independent lifestyle.[20] Such complications as pneumonia, blood clots in the lungs, and heart failure contribute to the complications of an osteoporotic hip fracture. Vertebral compression fractures (VCFs) can decrease height by up to 15 cm and result in kyphotic deformity called "dowagers' hump." VCFs in women result in 15% higher mortality compared to women with no disruption.[21] Furthermore, VCFs increase with age affecting 40% of women in their eighties.[22]

VCFs occur due to the inability for the osteoporotic vertebra to sustain internal stresses applied from vertebral load from daily life or from minor or major traumatic events. Trabecular bone is largely responsible for the majority of the axial forces and inherited extra-axial stress and strains. With the cascade of osteoporotic effects and aging, the architecture of trabecular bone becomes altered, characterized with increased spaces, thinness, disorientation, and weakened connectivity. Although trabecular bone network maintains both horizontal and vertical framework, decrease in density and loss of structural strength compromise the vertebra's mechanical prowess, integrity, and spinal column stability predisposing it to trabecular buckling. Therefore, alteration of trabecular bone as seen in osteoporotic individuals and with age is accompanied with a decrease in bone density[23–26] and a propensity for fracture.[27,28]

Diagnosis of vertebral fracture is difficult to assess compared to peripheral fractures. Decrease in height and vertebral deformities are indications of vertebral fractures. According to Cooper et al., 16% of vertebral fractures are diagnosed radiographically when initial investigation was for another problem.[8] VCFs maintain an axis of rotation at the middle column. As a result, anterior column disruption is seen with intact middle and posterior columns. Since the neural arch remains intact, neurologic deficits are not as common. Bioconcave VCFs manifest as a central vertebral deformity as a crush fracture involves anterior, posterior, and central aspects. Wedge fractures are the most common VCFs, affecting anterior elements more often than posterior. Whatever the morphology VCFs adopt, fractures occur more often at the thoracolumbar and mid-thoracic region.[8,29,30] The tendency of VCFs to occur at these regions could possibly be attributed to alterations of stiffness from thoracic spine to the more mobile lumbar region and transitory curvature from kyphosis to lordosis.

Multiple VCFs develop a hyperkyphotic or "dowagers' hump" at the thoracic level with a stooped posture decreasing abdominal and thoracic cavities. Multiple lumbar VCFs further increase lordosis creating a protruding abdomen. Decrease in axial height is a result of reduction of intervertebral and vertebral loss of height. Also, developed stooped posture progresses to the point where ribs rest on the iliac crest with circumferential pachydermal skin folds developing at the pelvis and ribs. As this posture becomes more severe, eating is difficult and the patient eats less feeling full and bloated. The cauda equina or spinal cord related symptoms are uncommon and are secondary to other conditions, such as Paget's disease, lymphoma, primary or metastatic bone tumors, myeloma, and infection.[31] When awakening, the abdomen appears normal only to distend throughout the day. Nonrestorative sleep or trouble getting to sleep is often the case with patients. Lifestyle changes occur, such as difficulty driving a car, getting dressed, fear of large crowds, and depression develops. Self-esteem is also compromised as a result of a socially unacceptable body image.[32] After a second vertebral fracture, women report high levels of anxiety due to fear of future recurrences[33,34] and accompanying stress.[35,36] With time progression and continued osteoporotic problems, signs of depression develop in women.[34,37] Social support and social roles are affected by decreased function and progressed disease related problems of osteoporotic VCFs and deformity.

Most VCFs are asymptomatic with unknown origin of injury. Nonetheless, pain could occur abruptly. Initially, pain is acute lasting 2 to 3 months comprising of deep back pain with or without unilateral or bilateral radiculopathy and/or segmental costal nerve symptoms and paravertebral muscle spasms. Spinal movement is restricted with flexion primarily decreased. Pain is experienced when standing from a seated position, bending, lifting, and prolonged seating and standing. Walk is sluggish, but normal gait continues. Coughing, sneezing, and bowel exertion exacerbate pain. A succession of VCFs could follow the first initial fracture with discontinued pain between each period of disruption or continually present. However, cluster VCFs have a string of fractures with severe and persistent pain. Pain is relieved by recumbent positioning and bed rest.

DIAGNOSIS

Osteoporosis, as noted by Riggs and Melton, is categorized into two types.[20] Type I osteoporosis, also known as postmenopausal osteoporosis, occurs at a ratio of 6:1 of females to males between 51 and 65 years, primarily involves trabecular bone, presents no calcium deficiency, estrogen deficiency is present, and associated vertebral and Colles fractures are prevalent; whereas type II osteoporosis or senile osteoporosis occurs in twice as many women as men of 75 years or older, involves cortical bone, is related to calcium intake, and is void of estrogen deficiency. Moreover, fractures of type II osteoporosis entail the pelvis, hip, proximal tibia, and proximal humerus. Also, decrease in vitamin D and increased PTH activity and impaired bone formation are indicated in type II osteoporosis. Type I osteoporosis risk factors are low calcium intake, low weight-bearing regime, cigarette smoking, and excessive alcohol consumption.

Iatrogenic osteoporosis greatly affects trabecular bone and BMD depending upon the dose and duration of therapy. Corticosteroid-induced osteoporosis affects bone loss within the first 6 to 12 months of use. Corticosteroids increase urinary excretion of calcium and interfere with gastrointestinal absorption of calcium. These events reduce serum calcium levels and influence the parathyroid hormone to compensate for the loss by stimulating osteoclasts to increase bone resorption in an effort to increase serum calcium levels. On the other hand, BMD is reduced progressing to osteoporosis and fractures. Furthermore, corticosteroids inhibit osteoblasts, which in turn decrease bone formation and reduce the release of gonadal hormones. As a loop diuretic, Furosemide increases renal calcium excretion and decreases serum calcium levels. Thyroid supplements suppress the production of TSH and decrease BMD. Also, anticonvulsants enhance the hepatic degradation of calcium, vitamin D, and vitamin D receptors. Heparin inhibits osteoblast formation and stimulates osteoclasts. Antacids containing aluminum interact with gastrointestinal calcium and decrease calcium absorption. Hyperparathyroidism can be increased with an increase of PTH as a result of lithium use. In addition, cytotoxic agents could also inhibit bone remodeling.

The best indication of osteoporosis is low bone mass. However, a slew of secondary causes that affect bone mass must be excluded before rendering a diagnosis of primary, idiopathic, or iatrogenic osteoporosis. Such secondary causes include Paget's disease, osteomalacia hypogonadism, malabsorption syndrome, primary hyperparathyroidism, multiple myeloma, and hyperthyroidism. Prolonged drug therapy could also affect bone mass. Medication has been shown to affect bone mass as well as age, gender, early menopause, genetics, and race further contributing to the risk of developing osteoporosis. Moreover, inadequate nutrition, smoking, excessive alcohol consumption, and sedentary lifestyle lower BMD and increase fracture risk.[7]

Medical evaluation requires thorough investigation of family and medical history as well as physical and gynecological assessment. As is often the case, secondary causes or coexisting diseases may be the catalyst for or exacerbate bone loss. In order to eliminate extraneous factors and properly develop a therapeutic regime various measures are required. A complete blood cell count, serum chemistry group, and a urinalysis including a pH count should be carried out. Further tests should be undertaken if the physician has reason to suspect other underlying causes. These tests include thyrotropin, a 24-hour urinary calcium excretion, erythrocyte sedimentation rate, parathyroid hormone and 25-hydroxyvitamin D concentrations, dexamethasone suppression, acid–base studies, serum or urine protein electrophoresis, bone biopsy and/or bone marrow examination, and an undecalcified iliac bone biopsy.

Radiographic assessment in diagnosing osteoporosis is difficult to confirm for a minimum of 30% bone mass loss is necessary for the condition to surface.[4] Osteopenia is a term used to denote visible radiographic changes of decreased bone mass. Osteoporosis is more commonly diagnosed when a fracture occurs and when computed tomography (CT) or bone densitometry measures bone mass and indicates low BMD. Since osteoporosis is a disease characterized by low bone mineral density, dual-energy X-ray absorptiometry (DXA) measures bone density of the axial skeleton, hip, trochanter, wrist, and heel. In 1994 the World Health Organization (WHO) established diagnostic criteria to designate the presence of osteoporosis based on DXA measurements.[38] Normal individuals possess a bone mineral density of 1 standard deviation (SD) of the mean of young adults. Osteopenia is indicated if the SD of bone mineral density is between 1.0 and 2.5 below the mean of a young adult population. If bone mineral density is measured 2.5 or more SDs below the mean of a young adult population then osteoporosis is present. Furthermore, severe osteoporosis is denoted when one or more accompanying fragility fractures is present. Low BMD has been associated with an increased likelihood of developing a fracture.[1-3] Based on these criteria, it is estimated that 38% of white females in their mid-seventies will have osteoporosis and low bone mass will arrest 94% of that population.[39-42]. However, these criteria set forth by the WHO are a measure of the prevalence of osteoporosis and are not intended as a guideline for therapeutic course. An individual assessment of the patient is required that not only measures bone mass, but accounts for risk factors that guide diagnosis and proper treatment modalities.

Radiographic Techniques: A variety of imaging techniques are available for noninvasive assessment of the appendicular and axial skeleton. These techniques facilitate early diagnosis of osteoporosis and provide a baseline for long-term monitoring of the disease. On plain radiographs, certain calibration methods could be employed to measure the cortical thickness of bone at various sites, such as the metacarpal shafts and phalanges of the hand. Although plain radiographic assessment and monitoring of osteoporosis is difficult since 30% of bone mass must be lost for radiographic changes to become evident, the use of bone densitometry allows assessment of cortical and trabecular bone with greater ease, accuracy, precision, low radiation exposure, and reasonable cost.

One of the first techniques utilized to assess peripheral bone mass was radiographic absorptiometry (RA). This technique utilized an aluminum film wedge incorporated on hand X-rays and an optical densitometer to assess the presence of bone loss. In the 1960s single-photon absorptiometry (SPA) was introduced and widely used to measure wrist and heel BMD until the advent of single X-ray absorptiometry (SXA). Although these methods provided some insight into BMD, the presence of composition and variable thickness in soft tissue in such areas as the hip, spine, and the whole body in general ushered in dual-photon absorptiometry (DPA) in the 1980s. However, in 1987 DXA was established affording improved spatial resolution, more precision, and decreased examining time. Equipped with a C-arm, DXA assessment allows for anteroposterior and lateral evaluation of the spine's trabecular and cortical bone with the patient in a supine position. Peripheral DXA (pDXA)

is also available assessing BMD at the heel and proximal and distal forearm. Recently an innovative method called instant vertebral assessment (IVD) revealed existing vertebral deformities that could contribute to the risk of fracture which affect the modality of treatment.

A CT scanner implementing low doses could perform quantitative computed tomography (QCT) images primarily to determine vertebral trabecular bone density. Through QCT, three-dimensional images of the volumetric density of trabecular bone and metabolic activity can be ascertained providing discriminatory criteria between osteoporosis disease progression, aging, therapy, and fracture. Moreover, peripheral QCT (pQCT) scanners have been developed that also operate with reasonable precision and accuracy. However, a portable and low-cost method of monitoring BMD and the risk of fracture has been designed called quantitative ultrasound (QUS). Ultrasound transmission velocity or broadband ultrasound attenuation is measured by QUS at the toes, heel, knee, tibia, and fingers.

PREVENTION AND CONSERVATIVE TREATMENT

Antiresorptive therapy and preventative measures are essential considerations in managing and preventing osteoporotic manifestations. An attempt to slow bone loss is of utmost concern. Bone mass is ever changing with peak levels obtained in the mid-thirties. Since more women are osteoporotic and are at greater risk for developing osteoporosis than men, various factors are at play accounting for the variable rates in bone loss. Women lose 3% to 7% of BMD around the onset of menopause followed by a 1% to 2% decline yearly in the postmenopausal period. Men also lose bone with age, but at similar levels as postmenopausal women. Yet men seem to continue to increase cortical surface by gaining cortical bone through periosteal deposition until the age of 75 years.[24,41] Nevertheless, numerous factors must be considered before administering an appropriate regime of preventative and therapeutic measures to combat osteoporosis.

Calcium and Vitamin D: The use of calcium in preventing and reestablishing bone mass for osteoporotic conditions has often been met with incredulity. However, proper calcium intake in childhood could establish optimal peak bone mass in adulthood and decrease the risk of fracture. Obviously, age dictates appropriate calcium intake. Children below 10 years of age require 700 mg of calcium intake daily, whereas 1,300 mg of calcium daily are essential for ages 10 to 25 to provide the foundation for peak bone mass. Particular attention must be directed towards teenaged girls who have a propensity for improper calcium intake.[43] Afterwards, adults sustain adequate calcium concentrations with 800 mg a day. Furthermore, daily calcium intake must be increased for pregnant women to 1,500 mg and 2,000 mg during lactation. Also, caffeine, alcohol consumption, heparin, tetracycline, furosemide, isoniazid, corticosteroids, drugs detoxified by the P450 hydrolase system, and high-fiber foods containing oxalic acid have a tendency to interfere with the body's calcium retention and absorption.

Premenopausal women lose approximately 0.3% of bone mass yearly and 2% is lost yearly in menopausal women. This rapid succession of bone loss is addressed with an increase of calcium intake to 1,200 mg and 1,500 mg daily for premenopausal and menopausal women, respectively. An increase in calcium slows down or prevents bone loss in pre- and postmenopausal women and has shown an increase in femoral bone mass by 3% to 5% after the first year of use.

Although appropriate calcium can be obtained from a daily calcium-rich diet, supplement intervention offers sufficient substitution and possibly a more reliable route to increase and maintain an appropriate calcium intake. The two most common forms of calcium supplementation are calcium citrate and calcium carbonate. Calcium carbonate increases the risk of kidney stones, not preferred for patients with constipation, requires gastric acidity, and histamine blockers may interfere with its absorption. However, calcium citrate is preferred over calcium carbonate because absorption is easier especially for individuals with increased gastric pH and the risk for kidney stones is decreased. In addition, calcium supplements could cause constipation and hypercalciuric patients should not receive calcium supplementation.

The recommended daily allowance of Vitamin D is 400 to 800 IU daily. Its role in bone deposition and calcium absorption is essential. The most common compound belonging to the vitamin D family is D_3, cholecalciferol. Vitamin D_3 is obtained from the skin as a result of irradiation of 7-dehydrocholesterol by ultraviolet rays from the sun or from food. However, vitamin D_3 is not the active substance that is actively employed in osteoporotic prevention. Vitamin D_3 or cholecalciferol must be converted to 1,25-dihydroxycholecalciferol (1,25-dihydroxyvitamin) and is accomplished with the aid of the liver and kidney. In the kidney cholecalciferol is converted to 25-hydroxycholecalciferol and is later converted to 1,25-dihydroxycholecalciferol by PTH in the proximal tubules in the kidney. In the intestinal epithelium over two days, 1,25-dihydroxycholecalciferol increases calcium-binding proteins located on brush borders that transport calcium ions by facilitated diffusion through the cell membrane and is absorbed and deposited in bone and various other tissues. After removal of 1,25-dihydroxycholecalciferol, calcium-binding proteins remain in the intestine for several weeks. Although individuals usually obtain vitamin D through food and sun exposure, supplemented daily allowances are recommended for those with a vitamin D-deficient diet and whose lifestyles mean they remain indoors. If greater amounts than 800 IU daily are administered, serum and urine calcium levels should be monitored.

Sources of calcium and vitamin D are present in various foods, but supplementation is available. Usually, suitable doses of vitamin D are accompanied with calcium supplements or are present in multivitamins. The combination of calcium and vitamin D should always be utilized when calcitonin or bisphosphonates are implemented. The combination of calcium and vitamin D has been shown to lower the fracture rate, primarily hip fractures.[44,45]

Bisphosphonates: Presently, bisphosphonates are the most influential class of antiresorptive agents implemented for the treatment of metabolic bone diseases encompassing osteoporosis, Paget's disease, hypercalcemia, and tumor-associated osteolysis. These compounds, which possess a low bioavailability with less then 1% absorption when taken orally, target bone mineral due to their high affinity for calcium and inhibit osteoclast function by binding to osteoclast-resorbing cells. The molecular mechanism of action of bisphosphonates involves a nitrogen-containing class that inhibits a rate-limiting step in the cell's mevalonic acid pathway preventing prenylation of GTPase signaling proteins that are crucial for osteoblast function.[46,47] In addition, bisphosphonates have been shown to promote osteoclast apoptosis.[48,49]

Alendronate is the first bisphosphonate approved by the US Food and Drug Administration (FDA) for the treatment of osteoporosis. Although other bisphosphonates, such as clonitrate, pamidronate, risedronate, and tiludronate, are being investigated for osteoporosis treatment,[50] alendronate since the early 1990s has been heralded as improving bone mass quality by increasing forearm, hip (1% to 2% per year), and spine (2% to 3% per year) BMD and reducing the risk of fractures by 50% after the first year.[51–53] In men Orwoll et al. conducted a double-blind study of 244 osteoporotic men over a two-year period and found that alendronate has been shown to reduce the risk of vertebral fractures, increase hip, spine, and total body BMD, and reduce the loss of vertebral height.[54] A DXA value of 0 to 2.0 SD below peak recommends a dosage of 5 mg a day of alendronate for preventative measures; 10 mg a day is preferred as treatment for a SD greater than 2.0. However, alendronate may not be ideal for newly developed fractures, but is recommended for the typical postmenopausal nonfractured patient with accompanied estrogen replacement therapy. Also, a patient with a family history of breast cancer, a normal cardiolipid profile, manageable postmenopausal symptoms, and a history of thrombophlebitis would benefit from alendronate therapy.[55] With prolonged use or improper use the patient may experience esophagitis from oral alendronate. To eliminate the problem, dosage may be reduced or the patient must take the drug in an upright position and remain so for at least a half hour before lying down.

Of the longest used bisphosphonates, etidronate enjoyed success in treating Paget's disease and has been used to treat osteoporosis patients in Canada. Although not approved by the FDA for treatment of osteoporosis in the USA, cyclic etidronate with a dosage of 400 mg daily for 14 days for 2.5 months has been reported to decrease vertebral fractures and increase BMD.[56,57] Also, etidronate has shown effectiveness in patients with long-term glucocorticoid use.[58] The long-term effects of etidronate for treatment of osteoporosis are still debatable and require extensive testing and observation.

Calcitonin: Calcitonin is a large polypeptide secreted by the parafollicular cells or C cells of the thyroid gland. The C cells comprise 0.1% of the thyroid gland. Besides reducing plasma concentration of calcium ions, calcitonin redirects calcium deposition and decreases osteoclast formation and their absorptive properties, thereby preventing osteolytic effects. Originally approved to treat Paget's disease, synthetic calcitonin has been marketed and widely used to decrease osteoclast activity thereby increasing spine bone density and vertebral fracture reduction.[59,60] A subcutaneous injection, approved in 1984, and a nasal spray, approved in 1995, of calcitonin are available with greater acceptance and fewer side effects with the latter. Also, calcitonin provides an analgesic effect by increasing the brain's B-endorphins, decreasing prostaglandin E_2, calcium flux interference, neuromodulator effect, involvement of cholinergic or serotoninergic systems, or direct central nervous system (CNS) receptor effects.[60,61] The nasal spray is available which helps increase the body's calcitonin level through a daily dosage of one spray of 200 IU.

Hormone Replacement Therapy: The role of hormones in the development of osteoporosis has been the catalyst of many studies. Estrogens have been widely utilized owing their conception to laboratory isolation in 1929. In 1941 Fuller Albright reported in *JAMA* the presence of postmenopausal osteoporosis and its clinical manifestations. Between 1942 and 1943 oral estrogens became available and have remained so over the years. Estrogen replacement therapy (ERT) has been indicated for the treatment and prevention of atrophic vaginitis and vasomotor symptoms. Further preventative uses of estrogen include delay of Alzheimer's disease and macular degeneration, coronary heart disease, and tooth decay. Although many uses have been indicated for ERT, eventually it has become utilized for the treatment and prevention of osteoporosis in postmenopausal women by increasing BMD and decreasing the risk of fracture.[62–65] Currently ERT is present with dosage as conjugated equine estrogen, 17B-estradiol, and transdermal estrogen. If initiated within 10 years of menopause, ERT decreases bone loss of the hip and spine,[66,67] and increases BMD in patients 60 years and older.[68] Moreover, the efficacy of ERT in increasing BMD is enhanced when calcium and vitamin D accommodate low-dose estrogen.[69–72]

The precise mechanism of how estrogen functions is not yet well understood, but it is believed that the presence of estrogen inhibits the levels of cytokine activity associated with osteoclast stimulation thus reducing bone resorption.[73] It is possible that estrogen decreases the formation of osteoclasts by lowering the production of osteoclast precursors, IL-1, IL-6, tumor necrosis factor, monocytes, and granulocytes.[74] Moreover, it has been indicated that estrogen is involved in calcium absorption. However, ERT benefits cease when therapy is terminated.[66,75] and use has been shown to increase the risk of breast[62,76] and uterine cancer[77,78] and increases the incidence of venous thromboembolism.[79,80] Due to these effects of estrogen use, a low compliance is observed and as many as 70% of women refuse ERT.[81] As a result, selective estrogen receptor modulators (SERMs) have been developed as an alternative therapeutic method to provide the benefit of estrogen without its many complications for postmenopausal women. SERMs bind to estrogen receptors and depending upon the tissue and type of SERM an agonist or antagonistic effect is seen.

Various SERMs exist including benzothiophenes, benzopyrans, tetrahydronaphthylenes, and triphenylethylene that vary in safety and clinical efficacy. Tamoxifen, a triphenylethylene, is the first SERM and has been widely employed in the treatment and reduction of risk for breast cancer.[46,82] Having antiestrogen effects on the breast, tamoxifen possess estrogen-like effects on the prevention of bone loss and the build-up of BMD in postmenopausal women.[83] However, tamoxifen users are at risk of developing endometrial cancer[46,84] and thromboembolism.[85] Alternatively, raloxifene hydrochloride, a benzothiophene-derived SERM, has prominent skeletal antiresorptive efficacy and estrogen antagonistic effects on breast and uterine tissue for postmenopausal women.[86,87] According to Cummings et al., raloxifene decreases the risk of breast cancer by 76% in postmenopausal osteoporotic women.[16] Furthermore, after a period of 12 to 24 months of raloxifene use by postmenopausal women, BMD has been shown to increase at various sites by 2.5%[88,89] and decrease the risk of vertebral fractures.[90]

Although postmenopausal women enjoy the availability of ERT or selected SERMs to reduce bone turnover, increase BMD, and decrease the risk of fracture, osteoporotic men with hypogonadism or low levels of testosterone due to age are unable to achieve peak bone mass but have the availability of testosterone replacement therapy (TRT). TRT in men is indicated if testosterone deficiency is present,[91] vertebral fracture without established testosterone deficiency,[92] or in the presence of corticosteroid therapy.[93] Studies have shown that 59% to 70% of men with hip fractures had low levels of testosterone.[94,95] Furthermore, an increase of 5% spine BMD in 6 months is noted when testosterone is administered to osteoporotic eugonadal men.[92]

Parathyroid Hormone: The use of PTH and its various peptides and analogues in the treatment and prevention of osteoporosis has been an issue of heated debate and vigorous study. PTH has been employed since the 1920s in connection with its role in bone mass. Four parathyroid glands are present in the human body. Chief cells and oxyphil cells are the main cells of the parathyroid gland with chief cells predominantly secreting PTH. Naturally, PTH is a hormone produced by the body's parathyroid glands instrumental in calcium and phosphate absorption in bone, excretion by the kidneys, intestinal absorption, as well as its interplay with vitamin D.

Synthetic PTH is not FDA approved, but is believed to play a therapeutic role in the treatment and prevention of osteoporosis.[96–102] Rat studies have indicated that continuous administration of PTH increases bone turnover in favor of bone formation. Over a two-week period, PTH-related protein (PTHrP) has been shown to increase bone mass in rats in vivo.[103,104] PTH treatment has been shown to increase cancellous vertebral bone volume at the first lumbar vertebra and fifth caudal vertebra by 67% and 37%, respectively, in ovariectomized rats with an equally impressive increased bone formation of 63.5% and 35.9% at the same locations.[105] Lindsay et al. reported that postmenopausal women on HRT receiving 25 μg subcutaneous injections daily of PTH for three years increased lumbar bone mineral content by 18.9% as opposed to 3% increase in HRT alone of which 50% of the increase was noted in the first year.[106] Furthermore, PTH and HRT therapy increased vertebral area by 5.5% as compared to a 2% increase with HRT alone. Of further interest, an anabolic synergistic or additive strength increasing effect of PTH and growth hormone has also shown promise in ovariectomized osteopenic rats.[107] Moreover, PTHrP (1-36) administered to humans for two weeks has been associated with suppression of bone resorption in postmenopausal women and stimulation of bone formation.[108] Other studies indicate that hPTH (1-34) treatment between 1 and 3 months has a potent effect on increasing lumbar BMD in osteoporotic postmenopausal women[98] and in corticosteroid-induced osteoporosis.[99]

Sodium Fluoride: Initial insight into the role of fluoride on the musculoskeletal system was reported in 1937 by Roholm.[109] His observations of industrial workers exposed to fluoride resulted in tendon and ligament calcification and periosteal new bone formation contingent upon the duration and amount of fluoride exposure. Almost a quarter of a century later, Rich and Ensinck conducted the first clinical experiments with sodium fluoride in an attempt to substantiate Rohom's claims.[110] They concluded that a positive calcium balance was achieved in patients with postmenopausal or steroid-induced osteoporosis including patients with Paget's disease at a dosage of 60 mg daily for 14 weeks or more. In the ensuing years radiographic changes were noted from sodium fluoride use.[111,112]

Sodium fluoride alters bone remodeling by stimulating osteoblast proliferation.[113] Fluoride ions have an affinity for apatite ions and form fluorapatite by replacing the hydroxyl group. Fluorapatite crystals become more stable by being deposited along collagen fibrils, thus establishing more resistance to osteoclastic resorptive activity. A dose of 80 mg daily or more of sodium fluoride could induce osteomalacia by altering bone matrix.[114] Fluoride-induced osteomalacia is not dependent upon vitamin D, vitamin D therapy does not resolve the developed disease, and calcium supplementation may not be sufficient to prevent formation of the disease. Bone formation rates and osteoblast aptitude is impaired after three years of continuous sodium fluoride therapy. However, this alteration is rectified after continued therapy exceeding three years.[115]

Fluoride is commonly found in water, food processed with fluoridated water, toothpaste, and mouthwash. Oral fluoride is absorbed 75% to 90% in the stomach as hydrofluoride. However, absorption decreases with age and various factors, such as aluminum, calcium, and magnesium, reduce fluoride absorption to 20% to 35%.[116–118] Since calcium is utilized in the treatment and prevention of osteoporosis and could interfere with fluoride absorption, it is recommended that these two substances be administered one hour apart. Also, fluoride consumption should be limited in individuals with renal impairment to avoid toxicity.

The effects of sodium fluoride on increasing BMD and decreasing fracture risk remain controversial demanding further controlled studies. However, sodium fluoride at 30 mg daily has been found to increase spinal bone mass with a linear relationship between duration of therapy and bone mass.[119,120] Therapy response is established between 12 to 24 months after initial treatment.[121] However, not all patients benefit from sodium fluoride therapy with 70% of treated patients increasing in bone mass[119,122] and volume.[123]

Various side effects accompany sodium fluoride use. Painful lower extremity syndrome, gastrointestinal discomfort, frank hematemesis, and melena are known complications of sodium fluoride. Symptoms subside after 12 to 48 hours of therapy interruption. Therapy could be restarted 6 to 8 weeks after interruption and side effects are further minimized by taking sodium fluoride with food or calcium.

Exercise: Fracture rate is related to falls, which increase with age. Over 90% of falls result in hip or wrist fracture.[124,125] Some 30% of patients over 65 years suffer at least one fall per year.[126,127] Muscle strength, postural stability, and adequate BMD are factors that prevent falls and subsequent fracture.

Bone remodeling relies a great deal on bone mechanical loading through exercise or daily activity. Bone cellular activity changes in response to loads that fall below or above the threshold by adjusting bone mass and strength to accommodate strain.[128,129] Once loads stop falling outside the threshold, bone remodeling is not required. Yet, changes in BMD are highly correlated with changes in calcium balance. Healthy subjects placed on bed rest lose approximately 0.5% of total body calcium per month and subsequently develop a negative calcium balance.

Muscle mass and strength decrease with age.[130] A decline of muscle fibers, motor units, and metabolic capacity are characteristic of aged muscle.[131] Although decrease in muscle performance is expected with aging, physical activity limits the degree of age-related muscle decline. Strength training increases muscle size, improves aerobic activity, and enhances metabolic rate.

Inactivity and aging results in parallel decline of BMD and muscle mass and strength.[132,133] For example, weight bearing in paralyzed patients with the absence of muscle activity is an ineffective measure for prevention of osteoporosis.[134] The microgravity of space flight is known to reduce BMD and produce a negative calcium balance in astronauts.[135,136] In immobilatory conditions bone loss is localized at the site of immobilization. Therefore, bone strengthening is contingent upon normal muscular forces. However, recovery from bone loss occurs at less of a rate than initial bone loss.[137–140]

Participation in an exercise program improves mobility and balance in an attempt to reduce the rate of falls.[141,142] A proper weight-bearing and strength-training program should be tailored to prevent bone loss. Sports, dancing, and various other exercise routines have been advantageous for balance training. For example, 15 weeks' participation in Tai Chi Quan classes results in a decreased risk of falling.[143,144] However, frail, disabled, and chronically diseased individuals may not have the capacity to tolerate certain strenuous exercise programs.

Various factors related to exercise could influence BMD. Maximum oxygen uptake from cardiorespiratory fitness is a predictor for BMD. Although maximum oxygen uptake is found to relate to femoral and vertebral BMD, the latter is significantly correlated in elderly men and premenopausal women.[145,146] Also, peri- and postmenopausal females who were active in sports during their adolescence display a greater amount of vertebral BMD than women whose youth was sedentary.[147] However, amenorrheic female athletes have lower vertebral BMD than menstruating athletes.[148,149] Furthermore, reduced progestogen levels in female athletes may contribute to reduced BMD.[150]

Modifiable Risk Factors: Various risk factors contributing to osteoporosis are unavoidable. For example, history of fracture, family history, poor health, race, gender, early menopause, genetics, and ethnic background could account for a reduction of BMD and an increased risk for fracture. However, certain risk factors can be modified to reduce the rate of bone loss, increase BMD, and prevent fractures. Elimination of excess alcohol intake, smoking, anticonvulsants, long-acting benzodiazepines, excess thyroid, and prolonged use of glucocorticoids could drastically affect the rate of bone loss. However, if medication is required the minimal effective dosage should be administered with intermittent use and increased nutritional intake, such as calcium and vitamin D, and appropriate exercise to prevent bone demineralization and subsequent fractures. Furthermore, monitoring BMD with bone densitometry measurements every 6 months could prove invaluable to prevent the dire effects of the aforementioned risk factors.

OPERATIVE MANAGEMENT

Spine surgery coupled with severe osteoporotic manifestations is a recipe for intra- and postoperative complications. The vertebral body is rich in trabecular bone and is more susceptible to osteoporotic invasion. Tackling an osteoporotic spine during surgery requires consideration of the biomechanical alterations inherited by the disease and alternative modalities to reduce surgical complications and ascertain beneficial results.

Various factors contribute to poor surgical outcome. For example, pseudoarthrosis, subluxation, fracture risk, and hardware pullout are some of the complications associated with an osteoporotic spine. A simple laminectomy could often result in vertebral collapse. Fusion failure is high as a result of poor bone stock to accommodate instrumentation and should be avoided, especially threaded cage constructs. Intraoperatively, spinal osteoporosis creates difficulty obtaining proper screw placement and achieving adequate bone purchase. As is often the case, alternative sites or alteration in instrumentation is pursued as well as accepting less deformity correction and opting for circumferential fixation. If anterior approach is selected, bicortical bone purchase must be obtained and posterior stabilization is also performed. Moreover, supplement screws with cement, bone stimulator, and bone matrix also prove advantageous. Postoperatively, hardware prominence could be observed, radiographic hardware pullout or loosening, pain, and neurologic deficits may also arise. Radiographically, screws develop a halo effect indicating poor bone-screw incorporation. In such a case, revision surgery is required with additional release to decrease excessive forces and provide more flexibility.

Autogenous bone grafting is commonly utilized in spine surgery offering optimal fusion rates. However, osteoporotic bone possesses poor bone stock for autogenous grafting due to decreased trabeculae and increased fatty marrow content that offer less osteoconductive and osteoinductive factors for proper bone fusion. Alternatively, allograft substrates are utilized to compensate for poor-quality autograft. Then again, although allograft is an appropriate supplement, fusion rates are not as successful as in autograft.[95,151,152]

Pedicle screw implementation has been utilized for many years for spinal stabilization. Pedicle screw pullout strength is correlated with BMD.[153–157] With the presence of osteoporosis, the efficacy of pedicle screws is threatened.[158] Screw augmentation doubles pullout strength. Proper screw hole preparation and implementing larger and longer screws provides a quick fix without the addition of more hardware.[159,160] However, larger screws could increase the risk of pedicle fracture. In lieu of osteoporosis, trabecular bone stock and cortical thickness further contribute to fracture risk in addition to malposition or inappropriate screw size. According to Misenheimer et al., a screw diameter exceeding 80% of the pedicle's outer diameter developed plastic pedicle deformation followed by fracture.[161] Sjostrom et al. also reported that 85% of pedicles expanded with a pedicle size 60% of the outer pedicle diameter.[162] Furthermore, Hirano et al. concluded that a vertebral BMD less than 0.7 g/cm^2 dictates a screw diameter not to exceed 70% of the outer pedicle diameter to prevent fracture.[163] Possible bicortical purchase, polymethylmethacrylate (PMMA)[157] or other bioactive cement,[164] transverse connections,[165] and laminar hooks[154,165,166] accompanying pedicle screws could enhance fixation and decrease osteoporotic-associated complications.

Laminae are considered to possess more cortical bone than trabecular bone compared to other spinous structures;[153] thus, osteoporotic effects are less common or slowly manifested than in other vertebral regions. As a result, laminae are more capable of accommodating greater posterior resistance forces. Likewise, laminae could increase screw stiffness by 50% and could accommodate screw augmentation. Use of laminar hooks allows multiple purchase points and rigid fixation.

Sublaminar wires have also been employed for segmental fixation. This type of fixation is commonly utilized for neuromuscular deformities.[167,168] Nevertheless, sublaminar wiring in an osteoporotic spine is advantageous at thoracic segments because of the unpopular use of laminectomy and pedicle screw fixation at this region, multiple segment fixation dexterity, and tightening capabilities to achieve desired fixation. However, passage of sublaminar wires is often associated with neurologic injury mainly occurring at extreme kyphotic or lordotic segments.[169–173] Axial control is limited in the absence of rod fixation. In addition, junctional kyphosis[174] is a concern when a construct ends proximally with sublaminar wires at a kyphotic segment. Use of proximal hooks and increasing instrumentation past the site of fusion can diminish the probability of such an occurrence.

VCFs have the potential to affect dramatically vertebral integrity by decreasing axial height throughout the spine resulting in possible gross deformity. A thoracic hyperkyphosis or "dowagers' hump" is a physical manifestation that commonly manifests as a result of VCFs. This spinal deformity could be asymptomatic or present with pain, neurologic deficit, pulmonary dysfunction, and physical abnormality. Usually VCFs are treated nonsurgically with bracing, bed rest, analgesics, and often calcitonin. However, immobilization could further contribute to bone demineralization, chronic back pain may exist, neurologic deficit may continue to persist due to spinal or foraminal canal compromise, and gross spinal instability could offset the efficacy of nonsurgical management. In such an osteoporotic kyphotic spine certain stresses are present at various sites dictating various vertebral segment corrections. Multiple segmental fixation is dictated to correct for an osteoporotic kyphotic spine. Sublaminar wiring, hooks, and transpedicular screw fixation are various internal instrumentation utilized to correct for spinal deformity and pain relief secondary to osteoporosis. However, such instrumentation is also accompanied with numerous pitfalls, most importantly poor hardware–bone incorporation and resulting pullout. Recently, various minimally invasive procedures have evolved avoiding internal spinal instrumentation and providing immediate pain relief in treating VCFs.

PERCUTANEOUS VERTEBROPLASTY

Percutaneous vertebroplasty (PV) is a radiographic guided procedure for injection of PMMA bone cement into the vertebral body to relieve pain due to fractured or neoplastic manifestation at the vertebral body (Fig. 61-1). Furthermore, PV provides bone strengthening, offers decompression, increases mobility, decreases analgesic dependency, and ultimately improves the quality of life. Since its inception in 1984 in France by Galibert et al.,[175] PMMA has been used for treatment of giant cell tumors of long bones,[176,177] vertebral hemangiomas,[175,176,178–182] osteolytic metastasis, multiple myelomas, and vertebral collapse due to osteoporotic compression fractures. Although PMMA injection via PV gathered a following, international fame escaped it until it was introduced in the USA in 1988 at the annual meeting of the Radiological Society of North America.[183] Nevertheless, it is a fairly new procedure that has managed to gain a following for its invasive nature. However, PMMA bone cements are not presently approved by the FDA, most health insurance companies in the USA are skeptical of their efficacy, and they attract eager physicians searching to

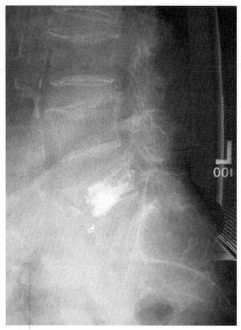

FIGURE 61–1. Lateral X-ray showing barium highlighted polymethylmethacrylate filling the fractured vertebral body spanning the endplates.

expand their repertoire who lack the clinical expertise to rule out alternative appropriate measures to treat the patient. At any rate, understanding the procedure is essential to obtain beneficial outcome and avoid further injury.

Indications for Procedure

VERTEBRAL NEOPLASMS: Osteolytic metastases or myeloma are the main indicators for PV. Multiple myelomas are the most common primary malignant tumors of the bony spine that rarely affect the posterior elements.[184–186] These tumors are rare radiosensitive lesions occurring in 2 to 3 cases per 100,000. Diffuse multiple myeloma presents reoccurring lesions at previously radiated levels and offers poor prognosis. Initially, patients report severe pain and disability and are unresponsive to drug treatment. The disease is usually multifocal in nature and surgical consolidation is not advantageous. In spite of this, single-level lesions are treated with vertebrectomy and strut grafting with some success. Nonetheless, radiation therapy alone or as an adjunct to surgery to address the painful manifestation of malignant lesion offers partial or complete pain relief in 90% of patients. However, this pain relief is delayed 10 to 14 days after initial radiotherapy.[187] Also, initiation of spine strengthening begins 2 to 4 months after initial radiotherapy.[187,188] Thus, delayed reconstruction predisposes the spine to vertebral collapse and ensuing neural compromise. PV offers an alternative route for immediate pain relief, bone strengthening, and mobility. Although PV goes some way to restoring the mechanical integrity of the vertebral body and provides a degree of pain relief, tumor growth is not prevented. Therefore, radiotherapy accompanying PV is appropriate because it does not affect the properties of the bone cement, affects tumor growth, compliments pain relief, and effects spine strengthening.[189]

Hemangiomas are benign bony spine lesions whose detection is dubious due to their asymptomatic disposition. Often, hemangiomas are detected during evaluation of back pain and subsequent routine plain radiographs. Soft tissue extension of the lesion may compress the spinal cord and nerve roots producing neurologic symptoms and even produce epidural hemorrhage.[190,191] If extensive growth of the hemangioma transpires, vertebral integrity may be compensated resulting in fracture with pain associated at the level of the lesion.[192] Hemangioma aggressiveness is indicative upon clinical symptoms and radiological evaluation. Vertebral collapse, neural arch invasion, and soft tissue mass extensions are signs of the aggressive nature of hemangiomas and their candidacy for PV. Furthermore, lymphomas and eosinophilic granulomas are also candidates for PV treatment.

OSTEOPOROTIC VERTEBRAL BODY COLLAPSE: Osteoporotic individuals are susceptible to VCFs due to the low bone mass that inadequately sustains mechanical forces. Some 16% of postmenopausal osteoporotic women experience VCFs.[193] However, 65% of individuals presenting with compression fractures are asymptomatic.[31,194] These fractures lead to decreased height, back pain, neurologic compromise, and disability. Analgesics, bed rest, and external bracing could offer some relief, but conservative therapy may fail and demand alternative intervention. PV is preferred for immediate pain relief and decompression of the neural elements.

Patient Work-up

HISTORY: It is vitally important to evaluate the clinical history of vertebroplasty candidates with standard physical and radiographic examinations. The information sought from these examinations can be used to differentiate the pain of vertebral compression fracture from other common spine disorders such as disc herniation, spinal cord or nerve root compression, or spinal stenosis.

Clinical history evaluation should include a discussion of the event that led to the precipitation of the patient's pain. This will most likely include a description of a minor trauma. The physical examination should demonstrate pain and tenderness corresponding to the region(s) the patient describes, and the degree of pain and tenderness should correlate with the level of fracture deformity. If multiple levels of fracture are thought to be present, then only careful radiographic analysis can accurately target the afflicted levels.

IMAGING: Typical magnetic resonance imaging (MRI) examinations include transverse and sagittal T1- and T2-weighted imaging. Studies have found MRI to be more conclusive than radiography in the evaluation of acute versus chronic compression fractures and is a recommended asset to an initial imaging protocol. MRI allows one to assess canal compromise, R/O tumor, and acuteness of fracture (edema on T2).

Short tau inversion recovery (STIR) is a type of MRI that is used to suppress the hyperintensive image readings of substances such as fatty tissue and cerebrospinal fluid. STIR is the most sensitive imaging sequence for visualizing edema, and fractures with edema are more likely to respond to PV than those without it. STIR is a very sensitive sequence for depicting circumscribed lesions and post-therapy complications, but not suitable for differentiation (Fig. 61-2).

Thin-section (3 mm or less) CT is often used in conjunction with MRI reconstructions in order to derive the most accurate visualization of the target vertebral levels. CT has been cited specifically as the best modality for determining

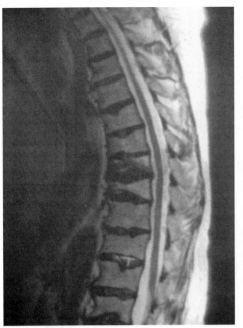 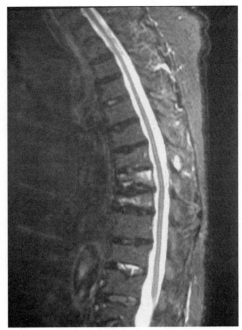

A   B

FIGURE 61–2. Sagittal MRI Spine T2 (*A*) and STIR (*B*) demonstrating compression fractures in the mid thoracic spine. Bone edema is better demonstrated on the STIR image and is ideal for pre-surgery planning.

whether or not a fracture line has extended through the posterior wall of a vertebral body. CT can also see fracture cavities that should be the targets. Aiming the pedicle needle for fracture cavities increases the success rate (Fig. 61-3). One can also assess size and trajectory of pedicles with 3D CT. In addition, certain fracture types may be less amenable to vertebroplasty. This would include a "butterfly" shaped fracture (Fig. 61-4).

A study has shown that increased activity revealed by bone scan imaging in a vertebral compression fracture is strongly indicative of a positive clinical outcome after PV. The study claimed a 90% achievement of pain relief after PV among 28 particularly difficult cases (i.e., multiple fracture levels and/or no localization of pain during physical examination). The investigators attributed their success to bone scan imaging, citing it as a useful tool in guiding therapy related to PV, especially with more challenging cases.

Materials Used: Location of the lesion dictates appropriate surgical instrumentation utilized to acquire appropriate depth and vertebral insertion. A 14- to 15-gauge needle 7 cm in length is utilized for the cervical spine. For the thoracic and lumbar spine a 10- to 11-gauge needle 10 to 15 cm long is implemented. The bone cement is loaded in a 1 to 3 mL Luer-Lok syringe or one of several commercially available injectors.

Bone liquid cement, containing methylmethacrylate (MMA), is contained in a sterile ampule. Bone cement powder containing PMMA and barium sulfate as the radiopaque agent are enclosed in a sterile polyethylene bag. Barium helps to visualize clearly the PMMA during its injection to avoid extravasation of the bone cement beyond the body.

Technique

IMAGING: Appropriate intraoperative imaging is essential to assess properly paravertebral vascularity, needle guidance to avoid neurovascular damage, and correct bone cement placement. Moreover, radiographic assessment is imperative to detect bone leakage and hematoma development because of the inability to assess the patient's neurological level when under general anesthesia. As a response to these concerns, a biplane C-arm fluoroscopy is commonly utilized.

Although fluoroscopy alone is adequate, scapular obstruction could prevent sufficient view of the upper thoracic vertebrae. Nevertheless, a combined CT and fluoroscopy is preferred.[195,196] CT guidance is advantageous for transpedicular needle placement especially for the thoracic spine. Pedicle dimensions are more elaborated with CT and one can avoid pedicle fracture dictating appropriate needle size. Epidural leakage is identified on CT which decreases injury to the spinal cord, ganglion, and nerve root. Also, CT monitoring is employed postinjection to detect bone cement extravasation and development of a hematoma. Fluoroscopy could detect bone cement leakage, but a hematoma on fluoroscopy is radiolucent. Biplane fluoroscopy, if available, can decrease procedural time.

PMMA PREPARATION: MMA is mixed with bone cement powder to achieve a paste or liquid consistency. However, a liquid may leak into the paravertebral tissue and venous leakage could occur in highly vascular regions. The temperature and quantity of the solvent determine the viscosity of the mixture into a liquid or paste consistency. The MMA and barium powder are mixed in a sterile, clean, and dry mixing bowel.[197] The contents are then mixed with MMA liquid for less than 1 minute to obtain a homogenous mixture. The mixture is then allowed

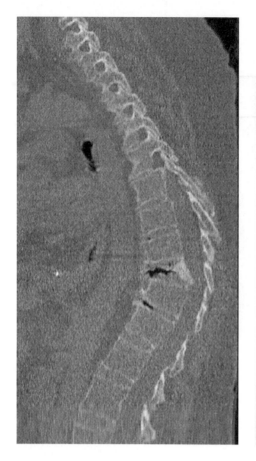

A

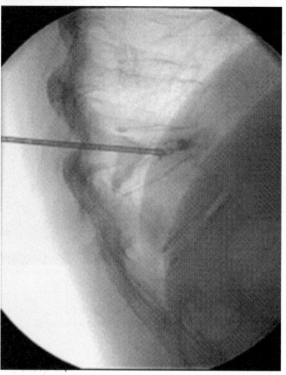

B

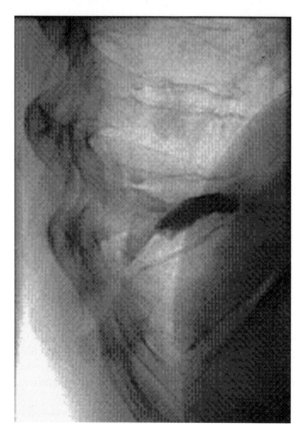

C

FIGURE 61–3. *A,* CT spine sagittal demonstrating space within the vertebral body allowing delivery of bone cement into the cavity. *B* and *C,* Lateral fluoroscopic images showing delivery of bone cement into a fractured cavity.

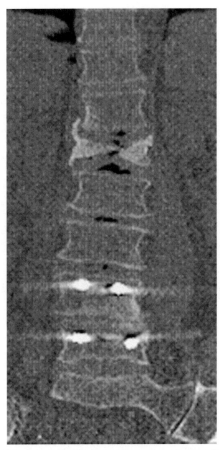

FIGURE 61–4. Coronal CT reconstruction showing "butterfly" compression of vertebral body. Fractures like this would be more difficult to treat with percutaneous vertebroplasty.

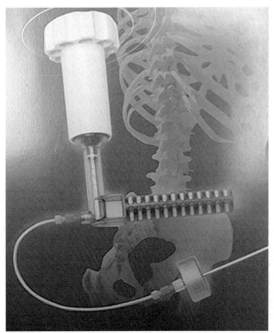

FIGURE 61–5. Pressure injection device allows more controlled delivery of the bone cement during percutaneous vertebroplasty.

anatomical compromise of the pedicle.[198] However, if osteolytic invasion affects the pedicles and poor imaging visualization is present the transpedicular approach is detrimental.

The patient is placed prone on a CT scanner table which facilitates segmental needle guidance by providing segmental images. If desired, a C-arm fluoroscopy could provide lateral

to polymerize to obtain a loose paste-like consistency. This should be loose enough to allow for injection without requiring undo force. Injection equipment is available for applying consistent force during the injection process (Fig. 61-5). This allows for safer introduction of the bone cement and prevents the sudden delivery of a large quantity of bone cement.

VERTEBRAL PUNCTURE APPROACH: Surgical approach is based on location and characteristics of the lesion and extent of vertebral destruction. Moreover, needle size, as was previously noted, is established by the location of the lesion on the spine. The patient is placed in a prone position under general or local anesthesia. However, treating the patient with PV in hyperextension for kyphotic reduction and height restoration is an alternative route.[178] At the cervical spine, an anterolateral approach is preferred with lateral vessel finger manipulation directing the needle between the vessels and the pharyngolarynx. A posterolateral approach is utilized at the thoracic and lumbar levels with preference at the lumbar vertebrae. Although risk of pneumothorax is present at the thoracic level, in general this approach could injure segmental nerves and predispose paravertebral tissue to PMMA leakage. A transpedicular approach reduces paravertebral tissue leakage and decreases risk of segmental nerve injury (Fig. 61-6). Usually, half the vertebral body can be reached via a transpedicular approach without

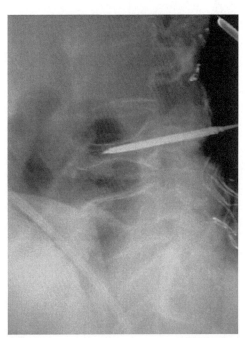

FIGURE 61–6. Lateral X-ray showing transpedicular approach to fractured vertebral body.

viewing to assist in pedicle needle insertion. A biplane fluoroscopy is preferred to allow imaging of two planes of the stylet tip positioning. Whatever the choice of image guidance, the needle is inserted at the level of the lesion.

Venography can be performed before injection of PMMA in order to highlight direct anastomosis of the epidural, central veins, and inferior vena cava. This provides an outline of the venous drainage, delineates vertebral cortex fractures, and confirms needle placement within the bony trabeculae.[199] Furthermore, shunting is avoided from bone to venous structures and epidural space. If needle injection risks compromise as indicated on the venogram, repositioning is immediately performed with gradual injection. However, in the presence of metastatic tumors, injection of contrast media diffuses into the tumoral tissue and stains it causing interference of proper fluoroscopic guidance of needle insertion and PMMA injection. Also, spinal biopsy could be obtained by inserting a biopsy needle into the vertebroplasty needle. Spinal biopsy is recommended for spinal metastases and osteoporotic vertebral body collapse due to metastatic lesion, but is not recommended for angiomas.

Once proper needle placement is obtained crossing the midline, one or multiple injections are performed under pressure to obtain the desired stability. Depending on the extent of the lesion, between 2 and 10 ml of bone cement can be utilized per level avoiding the posterior cortex. Once the cement crosses the midline, adequate stability is usually achieved (Fig. 61-7). However, injection is terminated if leakage occurs

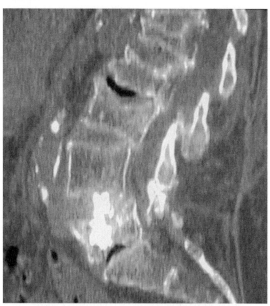

FIGURE 61–8. CT sagittal lumbar spine showing extravasation of methylmethacrylate into the adjoining disc space.

at the foraminal, epidural, or vascular structures to prevent pulmonary embolism and further neural compression. The procedure is also terminated if leakage migrates to the intervertebral disc (Fig. 61-8) or the anterior internal venous plexus that could compress the spinal cord. Furthermore, proper needle placement and removal is essential to avoid proximal needle breakage. Therefore, minimal force must be applied to the needle when inserted and upon removal the needle must be rotated on its axis to avoid adhering to the intravertebral cement.

Postoperative: Immediately following PV procedure a CT scan is administered to determine leakage of the bone cement and hematoma development. Axial loading is avoided for 3 hours to allow settling of the PMMA, the patient is observed overnight, and analgesics and nonsteroidal anti-inflammatory drugs (NSAIDs) are administered for 1 to 2 days depending on the clinical status of the patient. Prophylactics are continued if the patient is immunosuppressive or immunodeficient.

Complications: The complication rate for PV is reported to be between 0% and 65%,[65,175,196,199–201] and varies depending upon the initial indication for the procedure. Vertebral malignant tumors pose the greatest complication of PV followed by vertebral angiomas and osteoporotic lesions. Of primary concern in the cervical spine is to avoid injury to the carotid and jugular vein. Pleural injury and rib fracture with ensuing radicular symptoms in the thoracic region is an ever-present concern. In the thoracic and lumbar spine pedicle disruption by the transpedicular approach could occur with inner cortex disruption and following PMMA leakage into the foramina and spinal canal (Fig. 61-9). Also, proper needle placement is essential to avoid epidural and nerve root injury. Furthermore, accidental bone cement injection into venous structures could result in pulmonary embolism. Nevertheless, needle track leakage

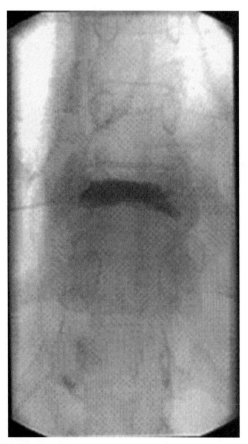

FIGURE 61–7. AP fluoroscopy showing bone cement crossing midline thus providing optimal structural support.

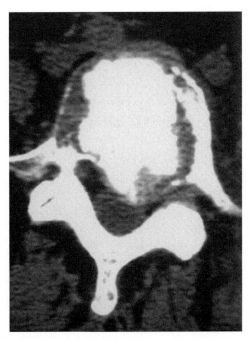

FIGURE 61–9. CT axial lumbar spine shows extravasation of bone cement along soft tissue tumor into the spinal canal.

and leakage from primary cortical hole as a result of secondary injection are complications that could arise regardless of the approach. Although infection could occur regardless of procedure, antibiotic powder mixed within the PMMA bone cement could reduce such a risk.

In 1997 Jensen et al. were the first in the USA to report their experience with PV by treating 29 patients.[199] In their three years of performing PV, two patients who had thoracic vertebral puncture experienced a nondisplaced rib fracture producing limited chest pain. Two patients had cement leakage to the inferior vena cava with pulmonary embolism, and leakage into the lumbar internal venous plexus compressing the thecal sac was noted in one patient. Furthermore, nine patients experienced adjacent disc leakage with no clinical symptoms.

Since 1997 similar findings were reported regarding PV. Cortet et al. reported 13 of 20 (65%) vertebrae treated with PV experienced cement leakage.[201] Leakage was noted in 6 cases in the paravertebral soft tissue, 3 cases in the peridural space seen in only tumoral lesions not osteoporotic vertebral collapse, 3 cases involved adjacent disc infiltration, and 1 venous plexus. Barr et al. noted that 6.4% of patients treated by PV who also had osteoporotic fractures had complications, such as dermatome radicular neuritis, nonbacterial urethritis due to catheter placement, and ulnar fracture possibly not related to the procedure.[178] According to Barr et al., osteoporotic patients with one level treated by PV are predisposed to secondary vertebral fractures due to added mechanical forces posed by the strengthened vertebra.[178] Therefore, Barr et al. advocate prophylaxis to avoid adjacent vertebral fractures following PV. Furthermore, Grados et al. reported long-term observations with a mean follow-up of 48 months for VCFs treated by PV and noted the development of a newly formed vertebral fracture postoperatively in 13 of 25 osteoporotic cases.[202] This study also indicated that the manifestation of the newly formed fractures in the majority of cases occurred near the cemented site.

The chemical effects of PMMA have also been an issue. Thermal reaction due to polymerization generates a certain amount of heat that could potentially harm adjacent neural structures and could be responsible for postoperative transitory radicular pains. However, Wang et al. postulate that ligamentous structures and dural-rich vascularity are insulators and impede heat dissipation.[203]

Outcome: Although leakage of bone cement is of utmost concern, results of PV are encouraging. Debussche-Depriester et al. reported 90% pain relief in myeloma.[204] Jensen et al. noted 90% pain relief within 24 hours in 29 osteoporotic patients with 47 vertebral fractures treated by PV and 2 patients experiencing immediate pain relief.[199] Furthermore, Barr et al. detailed 95% of 38 patients treated by PV to report initial pain relief with similar maintained relief at 18 months follow-up.[178]

KYPHOPLASTY

Kyphoplasty is a variant of vertebroplasty recently introduced in order to overcome some of the limitations of PV. It involves percutaneous introduction of a balloon (Kyphon, Sunnyvale, CA) into the vertebral body through a cannula, which is then inflated in order to reduce the fracture. The cannula is usually inserted through a bipedicular approach (Fig. 61-10). Deflation of the balloon leaves a void between the vertebral endplates, which can then be filled with PMMA that is more viscous than is possible with PV. Technical revisions and improvements continue to be made.[205]

There are several advantages for using kyphoplasty over PV (Table 61-1). In cadaveric models, kyphoplasty results in significant restoration of vertebral body height.[206,207] Although an increase in vertebral height has been seen with vertebroplasty alone,[208] kyphoplasty has shown significantly greater

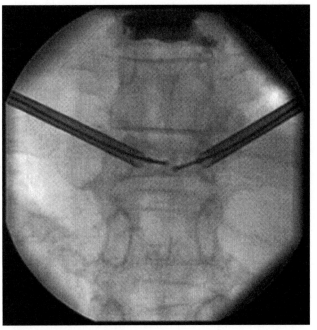

FIGURE 61–10. AP fluoroscopic view of bipedicular insertion of dilating pressure balloons into fractured body.

TABLE 61-1. **ADVANTAGES AND DISADVANTAGES OF VERTEBROPLASTY AND KYPHOPLASTY**

	Advantages	Disadvantages
Vertebroplasty	Lower cost Shorter procedure Decreases pain Increases VB strength Increases VB stability Infrequent clinical sequelae due to cement extravasation May be done through unipedicular approach Often done under local anesthesia	Increased risk of cement extravasation Cannot correct lost VB height Cannot correct sagittal imbalance
Kyphoplasty	Lower extravasation rate than vertebroplasty Lower complication rate than vertebroplasty? Equivalent pain relief Can restore lost vertebral body height Can correct sagittal imbalance Can use more viscous cement Increases vertebral body strength Increases vertebral body stability	Increased cost Increased procedural time Requires general anesthesia Usually requires overnight hospital stay Larger device Requires bipedicular approach

height restoration (97%) compared with vertebroplasty (30%).[206] Both treatments result in increased strength of the vertebral body, but only kyphoplasty restores stiffness.[206] When a similar model was used simulating physiologic load conditions on the vertebral body, the average height restoration by kyphoplasty was 63% and 55% for low and high loads.[209] The vertebral body height was fully restored in 22% of both experimental groups.

Kyphoplasty is associated with a lower rate of cement extravasation due to the high viscosity of the cement and the lower injection pressure. Cadaveric models show decreased leakage of PMMA cement in kyphoplasty compared with vertebroplasty.[206] An in vivo comparison of kyphoplasty with vertebroplasty showed a greater propensity for extravasation of injected contrast with vertebroplasty than with kyphoplasty.[210] The inflatable bone tamp used during kyphoplasty compacts the trabecular bone, which may seal potential paths of cement leakage through bone or veins.[210] Due to these advantages, some authors believe that kyphoplasty should be the standard of care for patients with VCFs who have failed medical management.[211]

Disadvantages include a significantly increased cost, exposure to contrast material, the requirement for general anesthesia, increased procedural time, and overnight hospital stay. There are currently no reported randomized controlled trials comparing kyphoplasty with either vertebroplasty or conservative treatment. Clearly such trials will be needed to determine the true efficacy of this promising technique.

Indications for kyphoplasty (Table 61-2) are generally the same as for vertebroplasty and include painful VCFs due to osteoporosis or osteolytic lesions. In addition, it may be used to prevent the sequelae of immobility and deformity due to VCFs such as decreased lung function, decubitus ulcers, urinary tract infections, and deep vein thromboses.

Although the ideal duration of nonoperative treatment before kyphoplasty has not been established, some authors feel when kyphoplasty is performed within 1 month of the fracture that it is easier to elevate the end plate and restore vertebral body height compared with patients treated months after their fracture.[212] Others believe that the procedure must be performed within 10 days at the most, before impaction of the fracture occurs, in order to correct any deformity that occurs.[213] However, by favoring early intervention, many patients might undergo procedures who would have otherwise experienced improvement with nonoperative care.[214] It is not clear whether these same concerns relate to compression fractures due to osteolytic lesions.

Contraindications (Table 61-3) include pregnancy, uncorrected coagulopathy, active infection, fractured pedicles, young age, contrast allergy, burst fractures, soft tissue tumors, and osteoblastic lesions. It is also contraindicated in patients with pain unrelated to the vertebral collapse.

The technique has been described in detail elsewhere,[215] and a brief description is included here. A bone tamp is inserted into the vertebral body under image guidance. A balloon is

TABLE 61-2. **INDICATIONS FOR KYPHOPLASTY**

Painful or progressive osteoporotic vertebral compression fractures
Painful or progressive osteolytic vertebral compression fractures
Prevent the sequelae of immobility (decubitus ulcers, decreased lung function, DVTs, UTIs)

TABLE 61-3. CONTRAINDICATIONS TO KYPHOPLASTY

Active infection (epidural abscess, sepsis, osteomyelitis, discitis)
Uncorrectable coagulopathy
Pregnancy
Contrast allergy
Pain unrelated to the vertebral collapse
Fractured pedicles
Burst fractures
Young age
Solid tissue or osteoblastic tumors
Vertebra plana (relative)

then inserted through the tamp into the vertebral body and filled with radiocontrast medium for visualization. The endplates are elevated by the balloon, thus reducing the fracture. Two balloons are usually used. The cavity created by the balloons is then filled with thick cement through the cannula under low pressure.

The results for kyphoplasty and pain relief are comparable to vertebroplasty. Some 80% to 100% of patients report decreased pain at some point after the procedure.[211,216–219] Hospital stays average between 1 and 3 days.[211,218,220,221] Improvements are reported in vertebral body height,[215–217,219–221] sagittal deformity,[216,217,219] and functional mobility.[218,220]

In a phase I study of kyphoplasty procedures, Lieberman et al. evaluated 30 patients with vertebral compression fractures, including 6 patients with multiple myeloma.[220] Seventy percent of patients had height restoration after the procedure (Table 61-4). Vertebral height restoration averaged 35% in the total group and 47% in the subset of patients who had some height restoration. They reported significant improvement in 5 of 8 Short Form-36 (SF-36) scales, including bodily pain, physical functioning, vitality, mental health, and social functioning. General health, role physical, and role emotional scores were not significantly improved. The average hospital stay was 1.8 days excluding 1 patient who had a "long stay inpatient

because of premorbid conditions." Several patients were able to mobilize who were previously unable to do so.

Garfin et al. report a 90% symptomatic and functional improvement rate for 340 patients undergoing kyphoplasty.[215] The average anterior height improved from 83% to 99% of predicted. The average midline height went from 76% to 92% of predicted.

Ledlie et al. report a retrospective analysis of 96 patients with 133 vertebral compression fractures who underwent 104 procedures.[221] Six of these patients had metastatic cancer. Some 73% reported their pain was eliminated and 15% reported their pain was reduced. Their mean hospital stay was 2 days. The increase in anterior and midline vertebral body height was 25% and 27%, respectively, after the procedure. These heights remained stable through 1-year follow-up. Ambulatory status also improved after the procedure. Some 31% of patients were initially nonambulatory. Following the procedure, only 5% of patients remained nonambulatory at 1 week. These results were stable over 1 year.

Coumans et al. report their experience with 78 patients who underwent 188 kyphoplasty procedures and were followed for a mean of 18 months.[218] A total of 63 patients had osteoporosis and 15 had multiple myeloma. Their mean hospital stay was 1.2 days. They reported significant improvement in several measures of quality of life. Visual analogue scale (VAS) and the Oswestry disability index scores significantly improved and persisted at 1 year. The patients also reported statistically significant improvements in 7 of 8 categories of the SF-36; physical functioning, bodily pain, vitality, social functioning, role physical, role emotional, and mental health all improved and were stable over 1 year, despite a nonsignificant decrease in their general health.

Theodorou et al. report on 15 patients with 24 vertebral compression fractures due to osteoporosis.[217] A total of 100% of patients experienced pain relief that was stable for the 6- to 8-month follow-up time. The vertebral height improved from 78.6% to 91.5% of the predicted prefracture height. The anterior, midvertebral, and posterior vertebral height improvements averaged 52%, 66%, and 53%. The degree of kyphosis in these patients improved by 62.4%, from 25.5° to 15.6°.

Fourney et al. reported 32 kyphoplasties for patients with painful vertebral body fractures due to cancer.[216] Some 80%

TABLE 61-4. RESULTS OF STUDIES ON KYPHOPLASTY

Author	Predicted Height Before Kyphoplasty (%)	Predicted Height After Kyphoplasty (%)	Lost Height Restored (%)
Lieberman et al. (2001)	66	78	35
Garfin et al. (2001)	Anterior, 83; midline, 76	Anterior, 99; midline, 92	Anterior, 94; midline, 67
Theodorou et al. (2002)	78.6	91.5	Total, 60; anterior, 52; midline, 66; posterior, 53
Ledlie et al. (2003)	Anterior, 66; midline, 65	Anterior, 89; midline, 90	Anterior, 68; midline, 71
Fourney et al. (2003)	Not reported	Not reported	42

of these patients reported their pain was completely relieved or improved. Pain relief remained significant at 1 year. The mean height restored was 42%. The average angle of kyphosis improved 4.1°, from 25.7° pretreatment to 20.5° post-treatment. One patient who underwent kyphoplasty at T11 and vertebroplasty at T12 subsequently required T11–T12 vertebrectomy at 2 months due to progressive disease.

Complications from kyphoplasty appear to be less than with vertebroplasty, likely due to the decreased rate of cement extravasation. Lieberman et al. report a cement extravasation rate was 8.6% with no clinical repercussions.[220] Three patients had a clinically significant complication due to the procedure. One patient had pulmonary edema and a myocardial infarction and two patients suffered rib fractures from patient positioning. Garfin et al. reported a complication rate of 0.7% per fracture and 1.2% per patient.[215] Two patients required decompressive surgery: one for an epidural hematoma after receiving a heparin bolus postoperatively and one after cement was delivered into the spinal canal. One patient in their series developed anterior cord syndrome secondary to a difficult needle insertion. Ledlie et al. had two complications (1.9%), with one patient requiring intubation and another experiencing a pulmonary embolus two weeks after the procedure.[221] Their cement leakage rate was 9%, although none were clinically significant. Coumans et al. reported a complication rate of 8%, including clinically insignificant cement leaks. One patient had a myocardial infarction due to fluid overload and there were five cases of cement extravasation.[218] Several series have reported no complications.[211,216,217]

SUMMARY

Osteoporosis is a worldwide disease affecting millions. The advent and evolution of preventative and therapeutic modalities provide new routes of management of the disease. The effects of VCFs are usually asymptomatic, but threaten the integrity of the vertebral body resulting in decreased height and possible neurologic deficit. PV is a minimally invasive option for painful fractures providing an overall safe, effective, and immediate therapeutic outcome as opposed to the alternative of long-term bracing, bed rest, and chemotherapeutic treatment. However, risk of complications does exist which requires accurate localization of the pain segment, proper needle placement, and intra- and postoperative radiographic monitoring to avoid cement extravasation. Implemented to reduce pain, PV is not intended to substitute for spinal canal and foraminal compromise nor for correction of deformity. As an alternative, kyphoplasty also provides pain relief, and restores vertebral height and decreases the progression of spinal deformity in patients with VCFs. In addition, managing an osteoporotic spine in spine surgery requires an alternative approach from traditional modalities to avoid complications and obtain beneficial outcome.

REFERENCES

1. Courtney AC, Wachtel EF, Myers ER, Hayes WC: Age-related reductions in the strength of the femur tested in a fall-loading configuration. J Bone Joint Surg 77:387–395, 1995.
2. Mosekilde L, Bentzen SM, Ortoft G, Jorgensen J: The predictive value of quantitative computed tomography for vertebral body compressive strength and ash density. Bone 10:465–470, 1989.
3. Spadaro JA, Werner FW, Brenner RA, et al: Cortical and trabecular bone contribute strength to the osteopenic distal radius. J Orthop Res 12:211–218, 1994.
4. World Health Organization: Assessment of fracture risk and its application to screening for postmenopausal osteoporosis: Report of a World Health Organization Study Group. WHO Tech Rep Ser 843:1–129, 1994.
5. Riggs BL, Khosla S, Melton LJ: A unitary model for involutional osteoporosis: Estrogen deficiency causes both Type I and Type II osteoporosis in postmenopausal women and contributes to bone loss in aging men. J Bone Miner Res 13:763–773, 1998.
6. Burger H, de Laet CE, van Daele PL, et al: Risk factors for increased bone loss in an elderly population: The Rotterdam Study. Am J Epidemiol 147:871–879, 1998.
7. Kenny AM, Prestwood KM: Osteoporosis: Pathogenesis, diagnosis, and treatment in older adults. Rheum Dis Clin North Am 26:569–591, 2000.
8. Cooper C, Atkinson EJ, O'Fallon WM, Melton LJ: Incidence of clinically diagnosed vertebral fractures: A population based study in Rochester, Minnesota, 1985–1989. J Bone Miner Res 7:221–277, 1992.
9. Recker RR: Embryology, anatomy, and microstructure of bone. In Coe FL, Favus MJ (eds): Disorders of Bone and Mineral Metabolism. Raven Press, New York, 1992, pp 219–240.
10. Prolo DJ: Biology of bone fusion. Clin Neurosurg 36:135–146, 1988.
11. Frost HM: Dynamics of bone remodeling. In Frost HM (ed): Bone Biodynamics. Little, Brown, Boston, 1964, pp 315–333.
12. Burchardt H: Biology of bone transplantation. Orthop Clin North Am 18:187–196, 1987.
13. Kaufman HH, Jones E: The principles of bony spinal fusion. Neurosurgery 24:264–270, 1989.
14. Browner WS, Pressman AR, Nevitt MC, Cummings SR: Mortality following fractures in older women: The study of osteoporotic fractures. Arch Intern Med 156:1521–1525, 1996.
15. Browner WS, Seeley DG, Vogt TM, Cummings SR: Non-trauma mortality in elderly women with low bone mineral density: Study of Osteoporotic Fractures Research Group. Lancet 338:355–358, 1991.
16. Cummings SR, Kelsey JL, Nevitt MC, O'Dowd KJ: Epidemiology of osteoporosis and osteoporotic fractures. Epidemiol Rev 7:178–208, 1985.
17. Jacobsen SJ, Goldberg J, Miles TP, et al: Race and sex differences in mortality following fracture of the hip. Am J Public Health 82:1147–1150, 1992.
18. Lu-Yao GL, Baron JA, Fisher ES: Treatment and survival among elderly Americans with hip fractures: a population-based study. Am J Public Health 84:1287–1291, 1994.
19. Magaziner J, Simonsick EM, Kashner TM, et al: Survival experience of aged hip fracture patients. Am J Public Health 79:274–278, 1989.
20. Riggs BL, Melton LJ: Involutional osteoporosis. N Engl J Med 9:1005–1010, 1986.
21. Cooper C, Atkinson EJ, Jacobsen SJ, et al: Population-based study of survival after osteoporotic fractures. Am J Epidemiol 137:1001–1005, 1993.
22. Melton LJ, Kan SH, Frye MA, et al: Epidemiology of vertebral fractures in women. Am J Epidemiol 129:1000–1011, 1989.
23. Mosekilde L: Age-related changes in vertebral trabecular bone architecture. Bone 9:247–250, 1988.
24. Mosekilde L, Mosekilde L: Sex differences in age-related changes in vertebral body size, density and biomechanical competence in normal individuals. Bone 11:67–73, 1990.
25. Preteux F, Bergot C, Laval-Jeantet AM: Automatic quantification of vertebral cancellous bone remodeling during aging. Anat Clin 7:203–208, 1985.
26. Snyder BD, Piazza S, Edwards WT, Hayes WC: Role of trabecular morphology in the etiology of age-related vertebral fractures. Calcif Tissue Int 53:S14–S22, 1993.

27. Ross PD, Wasnich RD, Heilbrun LK, Vogel JM: Definition of a spine fracture threshold based upon prospective fracture risk. Bone 8:271–278, 1987.

28. Wasnich RD, Ross PD, Maclean CJ, et al: A prospective study of bone mass measurements and spine fracture incidence. *In* Christiansen C, Johansen JS, Riis BJ (eds): Osteoporosis. Osteopress, Denmark, 1987, pp 377–378.

29. Hedlund LR, Gallagher JC, Meeger C, Stoner S: Change in vertebral shape in spinal osteoporosis. Calcif Tissue Int 44:168–172, 1989.

30. Krolner B, Pors-Nielsen S: Bone mineral content of the lumbar spine in normal and osteoporotic women: Cross-sectional and longitudinal studies. Clin Sci 62:329–336, 1982.

31. Glaser DL, Kaplan FS: Osteoporosis: Definition and clinical presentation. Spine 22(Suppl 24):12S–16S, 1997.

32. Linnel PW, Hermansen SE, Elias MF, et al: Quality of life in osteoporotic women. J Bone Min Res 6(Suppl):S106, 1991.

33. Gold DT, Bales CW, Lyles KW, Drezner MK: Treatment of osteoporosis: The psychological impact of a medical education program on older patients. J Am Geriatr Soc 37:417–422, 1989.

34. Gold DT, Lyles KW, Bales CW, Drezner MK: Teaching patients coping behaviors: An essential part of successful management of osteoporosis. J Bone Miner Res 4:799–801, 1989.

35. Pearlin LI, Menaghan ED, Lieberman MA, Mullan JT: The stress process. J Health Soc Behav 22:337–356, 1981.

36. Roberto KA: Stress and adaptation patterns of older osteoporotic women. Women Health 14:105–119, 1988.

37. Gold DT, Bales CW, Lyles KW, et al: Osteoporosis in late life: Does health locus of control affect psychosocial adaptation. J Am Geriatr Soc 39:670–675, 1991.

38. Assessment of fracture risk and its application to screening for postmenopausal osteoporosis. Report of a World Health Organization Study Group. WHO Tech Rep Ser 843:1–129, 1994.

39. Melton LJ: How many women have osteoporosis now? J Bone Miner Res 10:175–177, 1995.

40. Melton LJ, Riggs BL: Risk factors for injury after a fall. Clin Geriatr Med 1:525–539, 1985.

41. Riggs BL, Melton LJ: The worldwide problem of osteoporosis: Insights afforded by epidemiology. Bone 17(Suppl):505S–511S, 1995.

42. Riggs BL, Wahner HW, Dunn WL, et al: Differential changes in bone mineral density of the appendicular and axial skeleton with aging: Relationship to spinal osteoporosis. J Clin Invest 67:328–335, 1981.

43. Foundation NO: Osteoporosis: Physician's Guide to Prevention and Treatment of Osteoporosis. Excerpta Medica, Belle Mead, NJ, 1998.

44. Chapuy MC, Arlot ME, Duboeuf F, et al: Vitamin D3 and calcium to prevent hip fractures in the elderly woman. N Engl J Med 327:1637–1642, 1992.

45. Dawson-Hughes S, Harris SS, Krall EA, Dallal GE: Effect of calcium and vitamin D supplementation on bone density in men and women 65 years of age and older. N Engl J Med 337:670–676, 1997.

46. Fisher B, Costantino JP, Wickerham DL, et al: Tamoxifen for prevention of breast cancer: Report of the National Surgical Adjuvant Breast and Bowel Project P-1 Study. J Natl Cancer Inst 90:1371–1388, 1998.

47. Rogers MJ, Gordon S, Benford HL, et al: Cellular and molecular mechanisms of action of bisphosphonates. Cancer 88(Suppl 12):2961–2978, 2000.

48. Coxon FP, Benford HL, Russel RGG, Rogers MJ: Protein synthesis is required for caspase activation and induction of apoptosis by bisphosphonate drugs. Mol Pharmacol 54:631–638, 1998.

49. Luckman SP, Coxon FP, Ebetino FH, et al: Heterocycle-containing bisphosphonates cause apoptosis and inhibit bone resorption by preventing protein prenylation: Evidence from structure–activity relationships in J774 macrophages. J Bone Miner Res 13:1668–1678, 1998.

50. Ott SM: Clinical effects of bisphosphonates in involutional osteoporosis. J Bone Miner Res 8(Suppl 2):S597–S606, 1993.

51. Black DM, Cummings SR, Karpf DB, et al: Randomized trial of effect of alendronate on risk fracture in women with existing vertebral fractures. Lancet 348:1535–1541, 1996.

52. Cummings SR, Black DM, Thompson DE, et al: Effect of alendronate on risk of fracture in women with low bone density but without vertebral fractures. JAMA 280:2077–2082, 1998.

53. Lieberman UA, Weiss SR, Broll J, et al: Effect of oral alendronate on bone mineral density and the incidence of fracture in postmenopausal osteoporotic women. N Engl J Med 333:1437–1443, 1995.

54. Orwoll E, et al: Alendronate for the treatment of osteoporosis in men. N Engl J Med 343:604–610, 2000.

55. Lane JM, Bernstein J: Metabolic bone disease of the spine. *In* Herkowitz HN, Garfin SR, Balderston RA, et al (eds): The Spine. WB Saunders, Philadelphia, 1999, pp 1259–1280.

56. Evans WJ, Campbell WW: Sarcopenia and age-related changes in body composition. J Nutr 123:465–468, 1993.

57. Watts NB, Harris ST, Genant HK, et al: Intermittent cyclical etidronate treatment of postmenopausal osteoporosis. N Engl J Med 323:73–79, 1990.

58. Adachi JD, Bensen WG, Brown J, et al: Intermittent etidronate therapy to prevent corticosteroid induced osteoporosis. N Engl J Med 337:382–387, 1997.

59. Overgaard K, Hansen MA, Nielsen VAH, et al: Discontinuous calcitonin treatment of established osteoporosis—effects of withdrawal of treatment. Am J Med 89:1–6, 1990.

60. Silverman SL: Calcitonin. Am J Med Sci 313:13–16, 1997.

61. Lyritis GP, Tsakalakos N, Karachalios T, et al: Analgesic effect of salmon calcitonin in osteoporotic vertebral fractures: A double-blind placebo-controlled clinical study. Calcif Tissue Int 49:369–372, 1991.

62. Collaborative Group on Hormonal Factors in Breast Cancer: Breast cancer and hormone replacement therapy: Collaborative reanalysis of data from 51 epidemiological studies of 52,705 women with breast cancer and 108,411 women without breast cancer. Lancet 350:1047–1059, 1997.

63. Kiel DP, Felson DT, Anderson JJ, et al: Hip fracture and the use of estrogens in postmenopausal women. N Engl J Med 317:1169–1174, 1987.

64. Lindsay R, Tohme JF: Estrogen treatment of patients with established postmenopausal osteoporosis. Obstet Gynecol 76:290–295, 1990.

65. Weill A, Chiras J, Simon J, et al: Spinal metastases: Indications for and results of percutaneous injection of acrylic surgical cement. Radiology 199:241–247, 1996.

66. Cauley JA, Seeley DG, Ensrud K, et al: Estrogen replacement therapy and fractures in older women. Study of Osteoporotic Fractures Research Group. Ann Intern Med 122:9–16, 1995.

67. Lindsay R, Bush TL, Grady D, et al: Therapeutic controversy: Estrogen replacement in menopause. J Clin Endocrinol Metab 81:3829–3838, 1996.

68. Schneider DL, Barrett-Connor EL, Morton DJ: Timing of postmenopausal estrogen for optimal bone mineral density: The Rancho Bernardo Study. JAMA 277:543–547, 1997.

69. Naessen T, Berglund L, Ulmsten U: Bone loss in elderly women by ultralow doses of parenteral 17B estradiol. Am J Obstet Gynecol 177:115–119, 1997.

70. Prestwood KM, Fall PM, Pilbeam CC, et al: Estrogen and calcium have an additive effect on bone turnover in older women. J Bone Miner Res 11(Suppl 1):450, 1996.

71. Prestwood KM, Pilbeam CC, Fall PM, et al: Low dose conjugated estrogen reduces biomechanical markers of bone turnover in older women [abstract]. J Bone Min Res 10(Suppl 1):256, 1995.

72. Reckers RR, Davies KM, Dowd RM, et al: The effect of low-dose continuous estrogen and progesterone therapy with calcium and vitamin D on bone in elderly women: A randomized, controlled trial. Ann Intern Med 130:897–904, 1999.

73. Jilka RL: Cytokines, bone remodeling, and estrogen deficiency. Bone 23:75–81, 1998.

74. Gass MLS: Hormonal replacement therapy. South Med J 92: 1124–1127, 1999.

75. Felson DT, Zhang Y, Hannan MT, et al: The effect of post-menopausal estrogen therapy on bone mineral density in elderly women. N Engl J Med 329:1141–1146, 1993.

76. Colditz GA, Hankinson SE, Hunter DJ, et al: The use of estrogens and progestins and the risk of breast cancer in postmenopausal women. N Engl J Med 332:1589–1593, 1995.

77. Beresford SA, Weiss NS, Voigt LF, Mcknight BS: Risk of endometrial cancer in relation to use of estrogen combined with cyclic progestogen therapy in postmenopausal women. Lancet 349:458–461, 1997.

78. Grady D, Rubin SM, Petitti DB, et al: Hormone therapy to prevent disease and prolong life in postmenopausal women. Ann Intern Med 117:1016–1037, 1992.

79. Daly E, Vessey MP, Hawkins MM, et al: Risk of venous thrombo-embolism in users of hormone replacement therapy. Lancet 348:977–980, 1996.

80. Jick H, Derbey LE, Myers MW, et al: Risk of hospital admission for idiopathic venous thromboembolism among users of post-menopausal estrogens. Lancet 348:981–983, 1996.

81. Ravnikar VA: Compliance with hormone replacement therapy preventative health benefits? Women's Health Issues 2:75–82, 1992.

82. Osborne CK: Tamoxifen in the treatment of breast cancer. N Engl J Med 339:1609–1618, 1998.

83. Love RR, Mazess RB, Barden HS, et al: Effects of tamoxifen on bone mineral density in postmenopausal women with breast cancer. N Engl J Med 326:852–856, 1992.

84. Barakat RR: Tamoxifen and the endometrium. Cancer Treat Res 94:195–207, 1998.

85. Saphner T, Tormey DC, Gray R: Venous and arterial thrombosis in patients who received adjuvant therapy for breast cancer. J Clin Oncol 9:286–294, 1991.

86. Boss SM, Huster WJ, Neild JA, et al: Effects of raloxifene hydrochloride on the endometrium of postmenopausal women. Am J Obstet Gynecol 177:1458–1464, 1997.

87. Khovidhunkit W, Shoback DM: Clinical effects of raloxifene hydrochloride in women. Ann Intern Med 130:431–439, 1999.

88. Delmas PD, Bjarnason NH, Mitlak BH, et al: Effects of raloxifene on bone mineral density, serum cholesterol concentrations, and uterine endometrium in postmenopausal women. N Engl J Med 337:1641–1647, 1997.

89. Lufkin EG, Whitaker MD, Nickelsen T, et al: Treatment of established postmenopausal osteoporosis with raloxifene: A randomized trial. J Bone Miner Res 13:1747–1754, 1998.

90. Ensrud K, Black DM, Recker R, et al: For the MORE study group: The effect of 2 and 3 years of raloxifene on vertebral and non-vertebral fractures in postmenopausal women with osteoporosis. Bone 23:S174(abstract 1105), 1998.

91. Katznelson L, Finkelstein JS, Schoenfeld DA, et al: Increase in bone density and lean body mass during testosterone administration in men with acquired hypogonadism. J Clin Endocrin Metab 81:4358–4365, 1996.

92. Anderson FH, Francis RM, Peaston RT, et al: Androgen supplementation in eugonadal men with osteoporosis: Effects of six months treatment on markers of bone formation and resorption. J Bone Miner Res 12:472–478, 1997.

93. Reid IA, Wattie D, Evans MC, et al: Testosterone therapy in glucocorticoid-treated men. Arch Intern Med 156:1173–1177, 1996.

94. Jackson JA, Riggs MW, Spiekerman AM: Testosterone deficiency as a risk factor for hip fracture in men: A case control study. Am J Med Sci 304:4–8, 1992.

95. Herron LD, Newman MH: The failure of ethylene oxide gas-sterilized freeze-dried bone graft for thoracic and lumbar spinal fusion. Spine 14:496–500, 1990.

96. Finkelstein JS, Arnold AL: Increases in bone mineral density after discontinuation of daily human parathyroid hormone and gonadotrophin-releasing hormone analog administration in women with endometriosis. J Clin Endocrinol Metab 84: 1214–1219, 1999.

97. Finkelstein JS, Klibanski A, Schaefer EH, et al: Parathyroid hormone for the prevention of bone loss induced by estrogen deficiency. N Engl J Med 331:1618–1623, 1994.

98. Hodsman AB, Fraher LJ, Watson PH, et al: A randomized controlled clinical trial to compare the efficacy of cyclical parathyroid hormone versus cyclical parathyroid hormone and sequential calcitonin to improve bone mass in postmenopausal women with osteoporosis. J Clin Endocrinol Metab 82:620–628, 1997.

99. Lane NE, Sanchez S, Modin GW, et al: Parathyroid hormone treatment can reverse corticosteroid-induced osteoporosis. J Clin Invest 102:1627–1633, 1998.

100. Lindsay R, Hodsman A, Genant HK, Bolognese M, Ettinger M: A randomised clinical trial of the 1-84 hpth for treatment of postmenopausal osteoporosis. Bone 23(Suppl):1109, 1998.

101. Lindsay R, Nieves J, Formica C, et al: Randomized clinical trial of the effect of parathyroid hormone on vertebral bone mass and fracture incidence among postmenopausal women with osteoporosis. Lancet 350:550–555 1997.

102. Reeve J: A future role in the management of osteoporosis? J Bone Miner Res 11:440–445, 1996.

103. Hock JM, Fonseca J, Gunness-Hey M, et al: Comparison of the anabolic effects of synthetic parathyroid hormone-related protein (pthrp) 1-34 and PTH 1-34 on bone in rats. Endocrinology 125:2022–2027, 1989.

104. Weir EC, Terwilliger G, Sartori L, Insogna KL: Synthetic parathyroid hormone-like protein (1-74) is anabolic for bone in vivo. Calcif Tissue Int 51:30–34, 1992.

105. Li M, Liang H, Shen Y, Wronski TJ: Parathyroid hormone stimulates cancellous bone formation at skeletal sites regardless of marrow composition in ovariectomized rats. Bone 24:95–100, 1999.

106. Lindsay R, Cosman F, Nieves J, Woelfert L: Does treatment with parathyroid hormone increase vertebral size? [Abstract.] Osteoporosis Int Suppl 2:S206, 2000.

107. Mosekilde L, Tornvig L, Thomsen JS, et al: Parathyroid hormone and growth hormone have additive or synergetic effect when used as intervention treatment in ovariectomized rats with established osteopenia. Bone 26:643–651, 2000.

108. Plotkin H, Gundberg CM, Mitnick M, Stewart AF: Dissociation of bone formation from resorption during two-week treatment with hpthrp(1-36) in humans: Potential as an anabolic therapy for osteoporosis. J Clin Endocrinol Metab 83:2786–2791, 1998.

109. Roholm K: Fluorine Intoxication: A Clinical-Hygienic Study, with a Review of the Literature and Some Experimental Observations. HK Lewis, London, 1937.

110. Rich C, Ensinck J: Effect of sodium fluoride on calcium metabolism of human beings. Nature 191:184–185, 1961.

111. Cohen P, Gardner FH: Induction of subacute skeletal fluorosis in a case of multiple myeloma. N Engl J Med 271:1129–1133, 1964.

112. Largent EJ: The Health Aspects of Fluorine Compounds. Ohio State University Press, Columbus, OH, 1961.

113. Farley JR, Wergedal JE, Baylink DJ: Fluoride directly stimulates proliferation and alkaline phosphatase activity of bone forming cells. Science 222:330–332, 1983.

114. Parfit AM: Osteomalacia and related disorders. In Avioli LV, Krane SM (eds): Metabolic Bone Disease and Clinically Related Disorders. WB Saunders, Philadelphia, 1990, pp 329–396.

115. Lundy MW, Wergedal JE, Teubner E, et al: The effect of prolonged fluoride therapy for osteoporosis: Bone composition and histology. Bone 10:321–327, 1989.

116. Jowsey J, Riggs BL: Effect of concurrent calcium ingestion on intestinal absorption of fluoride. Metabolism 27:971–974, 1978.

117. Shulman ER, Vallejo M: Effect of gastric contents on the bioavailability of fluoride in humans. Pediatr Dent 12:237–240, 1990.

118. Trautner K: Influence of food on relative bioavailability of fluoride in man from Na$_2$FPO$_3$-containing tablets for the treatment of osteoporosis. Int J Clin Pharmacol Ther Toxicol 27:242–249, 1989.

119. Kleerekoper M, Balena R: Fluoride and osteoporosis. Ann Rev Nutr 11:309–324, 1991.

120. Riggs BL, Hodgson SF, O'Fallon WM, et al: Effect of fluoride treatment on the fracture rate in postmenopausal women with osteoporosis. N Engl J Med 322:802–809, 1990.

121. Hodgson AB, Droost DJ: The response of vertebral bone mineral density during the treatment of osteoporosis with sodium fluoride. J Clin Endocrin Metab 69:932–938, 1989.

122. Pak CYC, Sakhaee K, Gallagher C, et al: Attainment of therapeutic fluoride levels in serum without major side effects using a slow-release preparation of sodium fluoride in postmenopausal women. J Bone Miner Res 1:563–571, 1986.

123. Briancon D, Meunier PJ: Treatment of osteoporosis with fluoride, calcium and vitamin D. Orthop Clin North Am 12:629–648, 1981.

124. Grisso JA, Kelsey JL, Strom BL, et al: Risk factors for falls as a cause of hip fracture in women. N Engl J Med 324:1326–1331, 1991.

125. Melton LJ, Chao EYS, Lane JM: Biomechanical aspects of fractures. In Riggs BL, Melton LJ (eds): Osteoporosis: Etiology, Diagnosis, Management. Raven Press, New York, 1988, pp 111–131.

126. Campbell AJ, Borrie MJ, Spears GF: Risk factors for falls in a community-based prospective study of people 70 years and older. J Gerontol 44:112–117, 1989.

127. Tinetti ME, Speechley M, Ginter SF: Risk factors for falls among elderly persons living in the community. N Engl J Med 319:1701–1707, 1988.

128. Frost HM: A new direction for osteoporosis research: A review and proposal. Bone 12:429–437, 1991.

129. Lanyon L: Control of bone architecture by functional load bearing. J Bone Miner Res 7(Suppl):369–375, 1992.

130. Rogers MA, Ebvans WJ: Changes in skeletal muscle with aging: Effects of exercise training. Exerc Sport Sci Rev 21:65–102, 1993.

131. Booth FW, Weeden SH, Tseng BS: Effect of aging on human skeletal muscle and motor function. Med Sci Sports Exerc 26:556–560, 1994.

132. Cohn SH, Vartsky D, Yasumura S, et al: Compartmental body composition based on total-body nitrogen, potassium, and calcium. Am J Physiol 239:524–530, 1980.

133. Evans WJ, Campbell WW: Sarcopenia and age-related changes in body composition. J Nutr 123:465–468, 1993.

134. Plum F, Dunning MF: The effect of therapeutic mobilization on hypercalcuria following poliomyelitis. Arch Intern Med 101:528, 1958.

135. Mack PB, Lachance PA, Vose GP, et al: Bone demineralization of foot and hand of gemini-titan IV, V and VII astronauts during orbital flight. Am J Roentgen Rad Ther Nuc Med 100:503–511, 1967.

136. Rambaut PC, Goode AW: Skeletal changes during space flight. Lancet 2:1050–1052, 1985.

137. Kannus P, Leppala J, Lehto M, et al: A rotator cuff rupture produces permanent osteoporosis in the affected extremity, but not in those with whom shoulder function has returned to normal. J Bone Miner Res 10:1263–1271, 1995.

138. Kannus P, Sievanen H, Jarvinen M, et al: A cruciate ligament injury produces considerable, permanent osteoporosis in the affected knee. J Bone Miner Res 7:1429–1434, 1992.

139. Lane NE, Kaneos AJ, Stover SM, et al: Bone mineral density and turnover following forelimb immobilization and recovery in young adult dogs. Calcif Tissue Int 59:401–406, 1996.

140. Mosekilde L: Age-related changes in vertebral trabecular bone architecture. Bone 9:247–250, 1988.

141. Lord SR, Ward JA, Williams P, et al: The effect of a 12-month exercise trial on balance, strength and falls in older women: A randomized controlled trial. J Am Geriatr Soc 43:1198–1206, 1995.

142. Shumway-Cook A, Gruber W, Baldwin M, et al: The effect of multidimensional exercises on balance, mobility, and fall risk in community-dwelling older adults. Phys Ther 77:46–57, 1997.

143. Wolf SL, Barnhart HX, Ellison GL, et al: The effect of Tai Chi Quan and computerized balance training on postural stability in older subjects. Phys Ther 77:371–381, 1997.

144. Wolf SL, Barnhart HX, Kutner NG, et al: Reducing frailty and falls in older persons: An investigation of tai chi and computerized training. J Am Geriatr Soc 44:489–497, 1996.

145. Bevier WC, Wiswell RA, Pyka G, et al: Relationship of body composition, muscle strength and aerobic capacity to bone mineral density in older men and women. J Bone Miner Res 4:421–432, 1989.

146. Kirk S, Sharp CF, Elbaum N, et al: Effect of long-distance running on bone mass in women. J Bone Miner Res 4:515–522, 1989.

147. Puntilla E, Kroger H, Lakka T, et al: Physical activity in adolescence and bone density in peri- and postmenopausal women: A population-based study. Bone 21:363–367, 1997.

148. Drinkwater B, Nilson K, Chestnut C, et al: Bone mineral content of amenorrheic and eumenorrheic athletes. N Engl J Med 311:277–281, 1984.

149. Marcus R, Cann C, Madvig P, et al: Menstrual function and bone mass in elite women distance runners. Ann Intern Med 102:158–163, 1985.

150. Prior JC, Vigna YM, Schechter MT, et al: Spinal bone loss and ovulatory disturbances. N Engl J Med 323:1221–1227, 1990.

151. An HS, Lynch K, Toth J: Prospective comparison of autograft versus allograft for adult posterolateral spine fusion differences among freeze-dried, frozen, and mixed grafts. J Spinal Disord 8:131–135, 1995.

152. Jorgenson SS, Lowe TG, France J, Sabin J: A prospective analysis of autograft versus allograft in posterolateral lumbar fusion in the same patient. Spine 19:2048–2053, 1994.

153. Coe JD, Warden KE, Herzig MA, Mcafee PC: Influence of bone mineral density on the fixation of the fixation of thoracolumbar implants: A comparative study of transpedicular screws, laminar hooks, and spinous process wires. Spine 15:902–907, 1990

154. Halvorson TL, Kelley LA, Thomas KA, et al: Effects of bone mineral density on pedicle screw fixation. Spine 19:2415–2420, 1994.

155. Okuyama K, Sato K, Abe E, et al: Stability of transpedicle screwing for the osteoporotic spine: An in vitro study of the mechanical stability. Spine 19:2240–2245, 1993.

156. Soshi S, Shiba R, Kondo H, Murota K: An experimental study on transpedicular screw fixation in relation to osteoporosis in the lumbar spine. Spine 16:1335–1341, 1991.

157. Zindrick MR, Wiltse LL, Widell JEH, et al: A biomechanical study of intrapedicular screw fixation in the lumbosacral spine. Clin Orthop 203:99–112, 1986.

158. Yamagata M, Kitahara H, Minami S, et al: Mechanical stability of the pedicle screw fixation systems for the lumbar spine. Spine 17:S51–S54, 1992.

159. Krag MH, Beynnon BD, Pope MH, Decoster TA: Depth of transpedicular vertebral screws into human vertebrae: effect upon screw-vertebra interface strength. J Spinal Disord 1:287–294, 1989.

160. Zdeblick TA, Kunz DN, Cooke ME, McCabe R: Redicle screw pullout strength. Spine 18:1673–1676, 1993.

161. Misenheimer GR, Peek RD, Wiltse LL, et al: Anatomic analysis of pedicle cortical and cancellous diamter as related to screw size. Spine 14:367–372, 1988.

162. Sjostrom L, Jacobsson O, Karlstrom G, et al: CT analysis of pedicles and screw tracts after implant removal in thoracolumbar fractures. J Spinal Research 6:225–231, 1993.

163. Hirano T, Hasegawa K, Washio T, et al: Fracture risk during pedicle screw insertion in osteoporotic spine. J Spinal Disord 11:493–497, 1998.

164. Moore DC, Maitra RS, Farjo LA, et al: Restoration of pedicle screw fixation with an in situ setting calcium phosphate cement. Spine 22:1696–1705, 1997.

165. Ruland CM, Mcafee PC, Warden KE, Cunningham BW: Triangulation of pedicular instrumentation. Spine 16:S270–S276, 1991.

166. Hasegawa K, Hirano T, Hara T, et al: An experimental study of a combination method using pedicle screw and laminar hook for osteoporotic spine. Spine 22:958–962, 1997.

167. Stevens DB, Beard C: Segmental spinal instrumentation for neuromuscular spinal deformity. Clin Orthop 242:164–168, 1989.

168. Wenger DR, Carollo JJ, Wilkerson JA: Biomechanics of scoliosis correction by segmental spinal instrumentation. Spine 7:260–264, 1982.

169. Turner PL, Mason SA, Webb JK: Neurologic complications with segmental spinal instrumentation. Orthop Trans 10:14, 1986.

170. Weber SC, Benson DR: A comparison of segmental fixation and Harrington instrumentation in the management of unstable thoracolumbar spine fractures. Orthop Trans 9:36, 1985.

171. Wilber SR, Thompson SH, Shaffer JW, et al: Postoperative neurological deficits in segmental instrumentation. J Bone Joint Surg 66:1178–1187, 1984.

172. Zindrick MR, Knight G, Bunch W, et al: The depth of penetration of intra-segmental wire in the neural canal at insertion. Orthop Trans 10:6, 1986.

173. Zindrick MR, Knight G, Bunch WH: Factors influencing the penetration of wires into the neural canal during segmental wiring. J Bone Joint Surg 71:742, 1989.

174. Reinhardt P, Bassett GS: Short segmental kyphosis following fusion for Scheuermann's disease. J Spinal Disord 3:162–168, 1990.

175. Galibert P, Deramond H, Rosat P, Le Gars D: Preliminary note on the treatment of vertebral angioma by percutaneous acrylic vertebroplasty. Neurochirurgie 33:166–168, 1987.

176. Laredo JD, Bellaiche L, Hubault A, Deramond H: Le traitement des hemangiomes vertebraux. L'actualite rhumatologique (expansion scientifique) 30:332–346, 1993.

177. Persson BM, Ekelund L, Lovdahl A, et al: Favorable results of acrylic cementation for giant cell tumors. Acta Orthop Scand 55:209–214, 1984.

178. Barr JD, Barr MS, Lemley TJ, McCann RM: Percutaneous vertebroplasty for pain relief and spinal stabilization. Spine 25:923–928, 2000.

179. Cotten A, Deramond H, Cortet B, et al: Preoperative percutaneous injection of methyl methacrylate and N-butyl cyanoacrylate in vertebral hemangiomas. AJNR 17:137–142, 1996.

180. Deramond H, Darrasson R, Galibert P: Percutaneous vertebroplasty with acrylic cement in the treatment of aggressive spinal angiomas. Rachis 1:143–153, 1989.

181. Deramond H, Debussche-Depriester C, Pruvo JP, Galibert P: La vertebroplastie. Feuillets de Radiol 30:262–268, 1990.

182. Galibert P, Deramond H: La vertebroplastie percutanee comme traitement des angiomes vertebraux et des affections dolorigenes et fragilisantes du rachis. Chirurgie 116:326–335, 1990.

183. Bascoulergue Y, Duquesne J, et al: Percutaneous injection of methyl methacrylate in the vertebral body for treatment of various diseases: percutaneous vertebroplasty [abstract]. Radiology 169(P):372, 1988.

184. Corwin J, Lindberg RD: Solitary plasmacytoma of bone vs. extramedullary plasmacytoma and their relationship to multiple myeloma. Cancer 43:1007–1013, 1979.

185. Sundaresen N, Krol G, Hughes JEO: Primary malignant tumors of the spine. In Youmans J (ed): Neurological Surgery. WB Saunders, Philadelphia, 1990, pp 3548–3573.

186. Weinstein JN: Differential diagnosis and surgical treatment of primary benign and malignant neoplasms. In Frymoyer JW (ed): The Adult Spine: Principles and Practices. Raven Press, New York, 1991, pp 829–860.

187. Sheperd S: Radiotherapy and the management of metastatic bone pain. Clin Radiol 39:547–550, 1988.

188. Gilbert HA, Kagam AR, Nussbaum H, et al: Evaluation of radiation therapy for bone metastases: Pain relief and quality of life. AJR 129:1095–1096, 1977.

189. Murray JA, Bruels MC, Lindberg RD: Irradiation of polymethylmethacrylate: In vitro gamma radiation effect. J Bone Joint Surg 56:311–312, 1974.

190. Fox M, Onofrio B: The natural history and management of symptomatic and asymptomatic vertebral hemangiomas. J Neurosurg 78:36–45, 1993.

191. Schwartz D, Nair S, Hershey B, et al: Vertebral arch hemangioma producing spinal cord compression during pregnancy. Diagnosis by magnetic resonance imaging. Spine 14:888–890, 1989.

192. Foley K: The treatment of cancer pain. N Engl J Med 313:84–95, 1985.

193. Melton LJ: Epidemiology of spinal osteoporosis. Spine 22:2S–11S, 1997.

194. Lane JM, Riley EH, Wirganowicz PZ: Osteoporosis: Diagnosis and treatment. J Bone Joint Surg 78A:618–632, 1996.

195. Barr JD, Barr MS, Lemley TJ: Combined CT and fluoroscopic guidance for percutaneous vertebroplasty. Presented at the 34th Annual Meeting of the American Society of Neuroradiology, Seattle, WA, 21–27 June 1996.

196. Gangi A, Kastler BA, Dietemann JL: Percutaneous vertebroplasty guided by a combination of ct and fluoroscopy. AJNR 15:83–86, 1994.

197. Deramond H, Depriester C, Galibert P, Le Gars D: Percutaneous vertebroplasty with polymethylmethacrylate. Radiol Clin North Am 36:533–546, 1998.

198. Stringham D, Hadjipavlou A, Dzioba RB, et al: Percutaneous transpedicular biopsy of the spine. Spine 19:1985–1991, 1994.

199. Jensen ME, Evans AJ, Mathis JM, et al: Percutaneous polymethylmethacrylate vertebroplasty in the treatment of osteoporotic vertebral body compression fractures: Technical aspects. Am J Neuroradiol 18:1897–1904, 1997.

200. Kaemmerlen P, Thiesse P, Bouvard H, et al: Vertebroplastie percutanee dans le traitement des metastases: Technique et resultats. J Radiol 70:557–562, 1989.

201. Cortet B, Cotten A, Boutry N, et al: Percutaneous vertebroplasty in the treatment of osteoporotic vertebral compression fractures: an open prospective study. J Rheumatol 26:2222–2228, 1999.

202. Grados F, Depriester C, Cayrolle G, et al: Long-term observations of vertebral osteoporotic fractures treated by percutaneous vertebroplasty. Rheumatology (Oxford) 39(12):1410–1414, 2000.

203. Wang GW, Wilson CS, Hubbard SL, et al: Safety of anterior cement fixation in the cervical spine: in vivo study of dog spine. South Med J 77:178–179, 1984.

204. Debussche-Depriester C, Deramond H, Fardellone P, et al: Percutaneous vertebroplasty with acrylic cement in the treatment of osteoporotic vertebral crush fracture syndrome. Neuroradiology 33:149–152, 1991.

205. Amar AP, Larsen DW, Teitelbaum GP: Use of a screw-syringe injector for cement delivery during kyphoplasty: technical report. Neurosurgery 53:380–383, 2003.

206. Belkoff SM, Mathis JM, Fenton DC, et al: An ex vivo biomechanical evaluation of an inflatable bone tamp used in the treatment of compression fracture. Spine 26:151–156, 2001.

207. Belkoff SM, Mathis JM, Deramond H, Jasper LE: An ex vivo biomechanical evaluation of a hydroxyapatite cement for use with kyphoplasty. Am J Neuroradiol 22:1212–1216, 2001.

208. Peh WCG, Gelbart MS, Gilula LA, Peck DD: Percutaneous vertebroplasty: Treatment of painful vertebral compression fractures with intraosseous vacuum phenomena. Am J Radiol 180: 1411–1417, 2003.

209. Belkoff SM, Jasper LE, Stevens SS: An ex vivo evaluation of an inflatable bone tamp used to reduce fractures within vertebral bodies under load. Spine 27:1640–1643, 2002.

210. Phillips FM, Wetzel FT, Lieberman I, Campbell-Hup PM: An in vivo comparison of the potential for extravertebral cement leak after vertebroplasty and kyphoplasty. Spine 27:2173–2179, 2002.

211. Lane JM, Johnson CE, Khan SN, et al: Minimally invasive options for the treatment of osteoporotic vertebral compression fractures. Orthop Clin N Am 33:431–438, 2002.

212. Phillips FM: Minimally invasive treatments of osteoporotic vertebral compression fractures. Spine 28:S45–S53, 2003.

213. Hardouin P, Fayada P, Leclet H, Chopin D: Kyphoplasty. Joint Bone Spine 69:256–261, 2002.

214. Kang JD, An H, Boden S, et al: Cement augmentation of osteoporotic compression fractures and intraoperative navigation. Spine 28:S62–S63, 2003.

215. Garfin SR, Yuan HA, Reiley MA: Kyphoplasty and vertebroplasty for the treatment of painful osteoporotic compression fractures. Spine 26:1511–1515, 2001.

216. Fourney DR, Schomer DF, Nader R, et al: Percutaneous vertebroplasty and kyphoplasty for painful vertebral body fractures in cancer patients. J Neurosurgery (Spine I) 98:21–30, 2003.

217. Theodorou DJ, Theodorou SJ, Duncan TD, et al: Percutaneous balloon kyphoplasty for the correction of spinal deformity in painful vertebral body compression fractures. J Clin Imaging 26:1–5, 2002.

218. Coumans JVCE, Reinhardt MK, Lieberman IH: Kyphoplasty for vertebral compression fractures: 1-year clinical outcomes from a prospective study. J Neurosurg (Spine 1) 99:44–50, 2003.

219. Ahmad Z, Abbasi F, Mitsunaga M, Portner B: Pain reduction and functional improvement after kyphoplasty: A retrospective study of 50 patients [abstract]. Arch Phys Med Rehabil 84:A21, 2003.

220. Lieberman IH, Dudeney S, Reinhardt MK, Bell G: Initial outcome and efficacy of kyphoplasty in the treatment of painful osteoporotic vertebral compression fractures. Spine 26:1631–1638, 2001.

221. Ledlie JT, Fenfro M: Balloon kyphoplasty: One-year outcomes in vertebral body height restoration, chronic pain, and activity levels. J Neurosurg (Spine 1) 98:36–42, 2003.

Fluoroscopy and Radiation Safety

Honorio T. Benzon, M.D.

The use of fluoroscopy has revolutionized interventional pain management. Fluoroscopy is required in the more difficult procedures where precise needle placement is required. These procedures include interventions for back pain such as epidural steroid injection, facet joint injection, facet nerve block and rhizotomy, sacroiliac joint injection, discography, placement of spinal cord stimulator, and the newer interventional procedures such as intradiscal electrothermal coagulation (IDET) procedure, nucleoplasty, and vertebroplasty. Fluoroscopy is also used in lumbar paravertebral sympathetic block, visceral sympathetic blocks such as celiac plexus block, superior hypogastric plexus block, and ganglion impar block.

Several studies on epidural steroid injections showed the usefulness of fluoroscopy. Anatomical landmarks can be difficult to recognize especially in obese, elderly, or arthritic patients.[1] Epidural steroid injections are not straightforward especially in the sacral region where the surface landmarks are not clearly delineated. Occasionally, the patient may not be able to give a complete history. For example, one patient who was treated by the author who had a laminectomy did not realize that she had a bone stimulator placed (Fig. 62-1). The patient had a right L1 radiculopathy and a right paramedian epidural steroid injection was performed with the needle insertion at a distance from the bone stimulator (Fig. 62-2).

In a nationwide survey in the USA the investigators found that there was a wide variability in the use of fluoroscopy. Private practitioners used fluoroscopy more than those in academic centers. In the cervical region 73% of private practitioners used fluoroscopy compared to only 39% in academic institutions.[2] The transforaminal approach to epidural injections are employed in patients who had previous laminectomy by 61% of private practitioners compared to 15% of those in academic institutions.[2] For transforaminal epidural steroid injections, confirmation of correct needle placement and spread of the dye in the anterior epidural space can only be demonstrated by fluoroscopy.

One of the earlier studies on epidural steroid injections showed that blind placements were accurate in 83 of 100 patients.[1] In this study where 85% of the injections were performed in the lumbar area, experienced anesthesiologists performed the interlaminar epidural placements yet the incidence of inaccurate placement was 17%. Another study where the epidurals were placed by experienced anesthesiologists and an orthopedic surgeon showed a 75% success rate with blind epidural placements.[3]

In cervical epidural placements a study noted that there was a 47% success rate on the first attempt of needle placement.[4] In 63% of the placements (24 of 38 epidurals) a second attempt was required. The lack of reliability of the loss of resistance technique may be partially due to the lack of continuity of the

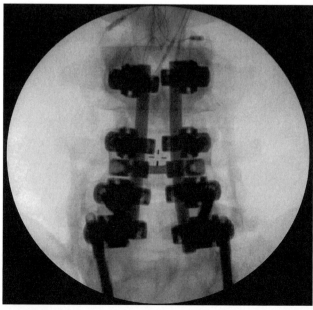

FIGURE 62-1. Fluoroscopic image of a patient who had a lumbar laminectomy and fusion. In addition, a bone stimulator was placed.

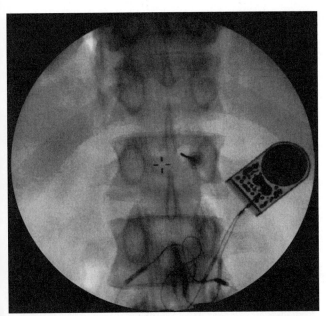

FIGURE 62-2. Fluoroscopic image of the patient wherein a right T12–L1 paramedian epidural steroid injection was performed; the needle was inserted close to the bone stimulator. A lead wire is seen obscuring the L1–L2 interspace.

ligamentum flavum in the cervical area.[5] Another finding in the study[4] was a 51% incidence (19 of 38) of unilateral spread of the contrast, although the authors inserted their needle slightly lateral to the midline. In addition to the slight lateral insertion of the needle, the unilateral spread may also be caused by the plica mediana dorsalis, a thin septum dividing the posterior epidural space. The presence of the plica mediana dorsalis has not been demonstrated in the cervical region, but in the lumbar and thoracic levels the plica mediana dorsalis has been shown to divide the posterior epidural space into compartments hindering the free flow of the injected solution.[6–8] One of the more interesting findings in the study by Stojanovic et al.[4] is the spread of the contrast in the ventral epidural space in only in 28% of the patients (11 out of 38 epidurograms). The spread of the injectate in the anterior epidural space is important since this is the location of the herniated intervertebral disc and the interface between the herniated disc and the nerve root. The placement of the drug in the anterior epidural space is the rationale for transforaminal epidural steroid injections (see Chapter 41 on transforaminal epidural steroid injections).

Caudal epidural steroid injections are ideally performed under fluoroscopic control. Experienced radiologists incorrectly place the caudal needle 38% of the time.[9] Renfrew et al.[9] showed that the experience of the physician improved the success rate of blind epidural placements. Physicians who performed less than 10 epidurals had a success rate of 48% compared to 62% by experienced physicians.[9] Another study showed that senior physiatrists successfully placed the caudal needle in 74% of their first attempts.[10] Their success rate improved to 88% when landmarks were identified easily. It appears that the most common site of incorrect needle placement is in the subfascial plane posterior to the sacrum.[10] Correct placement of the caudal needle is obviously improved when fluoroscopy is utilized. In a study of 116 caudal steroid injections done under fluoroscopy, radiologists found that the success rate was 97%.[11] In this study[11] it was found that the injection of 9 to 15 mL volume reached the mid to upper lumbar spine unless the patient has a severely stenotic spinal canal.

In patients who had previous laminectomy it was noted that the mean number of attempts to place successfully the needle in the epidural space is 2 ± 1.[12] The difficulty in placing the epidural needle may be due to fibrosis and adhesions within the epidural space making the loss of resistance sign equivocal. In 25 of 48 patients the Touhy needle and epidural catheter were placed one or two intervertebral spaces above or below the desired level. The unreliability of the landmarks may be due to removal of the posterior spinous process during the surgery making the count of the vertebral levels difficult. When 5 mL contrast medium was injected, the contrast reached the level of pathology in 26% (12 of 47) of the patients probably because the postoperative adhesions prevented the spread of the dye.[12] The success rates of needle placements in the different studies[1,3,4,9–12] is shown in Table 62-1.

Machikanti et al.[13] emphasized the necessity of using fluoroscopy in epidural steroid injections. The low incidence of the dye reaching the level of pathology requires the use of fluoroscopy to eliminate the question of incorrect needle placement with blind injections. Documentation of the spread of the dye can be correlated with the response of the patient. It should be noted, however, that there are differences in the flow characteristics between the contrast media and the steroid solution and that the flow of the dye may not completely predict the flow of the steroid medication. The steroid solution may be more limited in its distribution because it tends to precipitate in the diluent drug, either a local anesthetic or saline. In addition to confirmation of correct needle placement, one additional advantage in using fluoroscopy is the determination of intravascular injections. Unintentional intravascular injection may occur in spite of negative aspiration through the needle. The vascular uptake of the dye can be documented when live fluoroscopy is used during the injections or can be suspected when there is immediate disappearance of the dye after injection.

There are several reasons for not utilizing fluoroscopy in epidural steroid injections. These include the avoidance of radiation, cost of the use of fluoroscopy, inconvenient scheduling, location of the X-ray facility, and allergy to contrast agents. However, the potential for false loss of resistance and inaccurate vertebral level of entry makes fluoroscopy desirable in epidural steroid injections. The added benefits of fluoroscopy include the documentation of spread of the contrast whether it is unilateral, located in the ventral epidural space, or whether it reached the desired level of pathology. The documentation of correct needle placement and ideal spread of the injectate eliminates technical factors as a cause of lack of response of the patient. For these reasons, the use of fluoroscopy is becoming the standard of care in epidural steroid injections.

FLUOROSCOPY MACHINE

X-rays are generated by a current, which is measured in milliamperes (mA), passing through an electrically heated negatively charged filament (the cathode).[14] This process produces electrons. A high voltage (kilovolt peak, kVp) passes through the X-ray tube towards the positive electrode (anode). The electrode–anode interaction produces energy that is converted

TABLE 62-1. **SUCCESS RATES IN EPIDURAL PLACEMENTS**

Route	Blind/Fluoroscopy	Physician	Experience/Faculty	Success Rate	Reference
Cervical	Fluoroscopy	Anesthesiologists	Faculty/house staff	100%*	4
Lumbar†	Blind	Anesthesiologists	Experienced	83%	1
Lumbar	Blind	Anesthesiologists and an orthopedic surgeon	Experienced	75%	3
Lumbar, s/p surgery	Blind	Anesthesiologists	Attending	92%	12
Caudal	Blind	Radiologists	Attending	48–62%‡	9
Caudal	Blind/fluoroscopy	Radiologists	Attending	74–88%	10
Caudal	Fluoroscopy	Radiologists	Attending	97%	11

* Up to four attempts were made in successfully placing the needle in the epidural space.
† 85% of the injections were in the lumbar area.
‡ Experienced radiologists had a success rate of 62% compared to 48% for the inexperienced anesthesiologists (see text).

to X-radiation. The X-radiation that passes through the body enters an image intensifier where it is converted to a visible image that is displayed on a monitor screen.

The important parts of the fluoroscopy machine include the X-ray tube, image intensifier, C-arm, and the control panel (Fig. 62-3).[15] The X-ray tube fires the beam of electrons through a high-voltage vacuum tube, forming X-rays that are emitted through a small opening. The image intensifier collects the electromagnetic particles and translates them into a usable image that can be viewed on a television monitor. The C-arm facilitates positioning of the fluoroscope for the physician to get posteroanterior, oblique, and lateral views of the patient. The control panel (Fig. 62-4) contains the controls for the technician to adjust manually the quality of the image or leave it to the "automatic brightness control," or ABC, system. Also located in the control panels are the controls for magnification and collimation of the image.

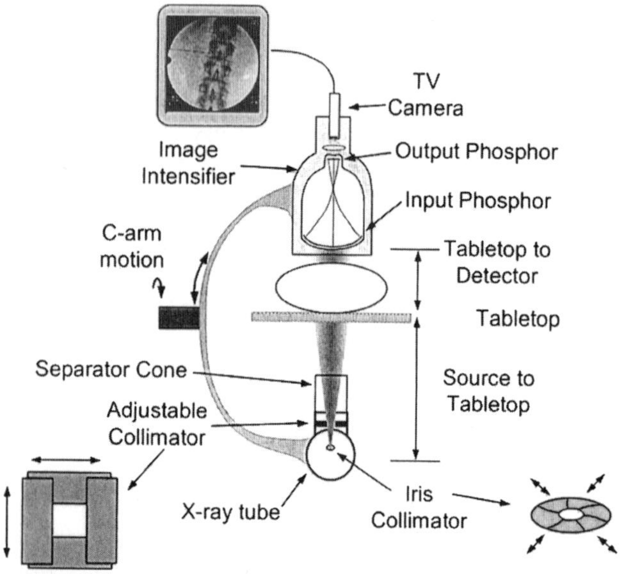

The quality of image contrast depends on the balance between the tube voltage or kVp and the tube current.[15] The kVp is the high voltage through which the electron beam passes in the X-ray vacuum tube. Increased kVp increases the penetrability of the X-ray beam, decreases the contrast, and produces brighter pictures. The fluoroscopic examination of the back of a normal sized adult starts with the kVp set at 75; bigger patients require a higher kVp. The typical settings are 80 to 100 kVp for the back, 50 kVp for the hands, and 70 kVp for the abdomen. Broadman[14] recommends the highest kVp setting that produces the adequate contrast or gray scale ordering to minimize X-ray exposure for the patient and personnel. The tube current reflects the number of electrons fired through the high-voltage vacuum tube. Higher tube currents mean more X-rays are produced and emitted. The tube current is set between 1 and 5 mA; lower settings are adequate for most interventional fluoroscopy procedures.

The image contrast is obtained by balancing the tube voltage or kVp against the tube current.[14] Higher kVp settings reduce the number of emitted X-rays but reduce the image contrast. A nice component of fluoroscopy machines is the ABC system where the computer automatically analyzes the image contrast and makes the appropriate tube current adjustments balancing image contrast and patient safety. It is

FIGURE 62-3. Reprinted from Reg Anesth Pain Med, Vol 27: Fishman SM, et al: Radiation safety in pain medicine, pp 296–305. Copyright (2002), with permission from the American Society of Regional Anesthesia and Pain Medicine.

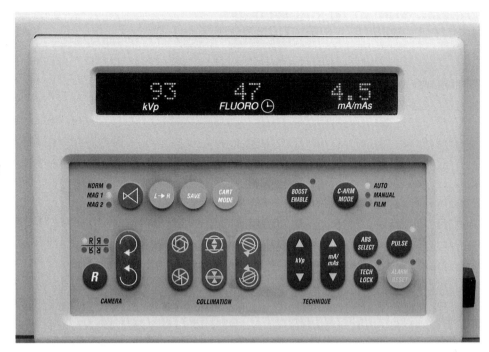

FIGURE 62–4. Control panel of the fluoroscopy machine.

recommended that the interventional pain physician leave the machine on the ABC system during the performance of interventional procedures to limit the number of images taken.

RADIATION SAFETY

The increasing use of fluoroscopy implies that the pain physician is aware of radiation safety to limit the number of radiations to the patient and the personnel.[16] A review article, book chapters, monographs, and government publications are available to help the interventional pain physician better understand the concept of radiation safety.[14,15,17–21]

Radiation is the process by which energy, in the forms of waves or particles, is emitted from a source.[15] Radiation includes X-rays, gamma rays, ultraviolet, infrared, radar, microwaves, and radio waves. Radiation absorbed dose (rad) is the unit of measure that expresses the amount of energy deposited in tissue from ionizing radiation sources. Units of gray (Gy) are preferred, instead of rad, in the International System (SI) of units. A gray is defined as the quantity of radiation that results in an energy deposition of 1 joule per kilogram (1 J/kg) within the irradiated material; 1 Gy is equivalent to 100 rad and to 1,000 mGy.

Different types of radiation may have similar absorbed doses but produce different biologic effects.[15] To predict occupational exposure from radiation, the term radiation absorbed dose (rad) is converted to radiation equivalent man (rem). The unit of dose equivalent to rem in the SI system is the sievert (Sv); 1 rem is equivalent to 1 rad and 100 rem is equivalent to 1 Sv.

Radiobiology: The biologic effects of radiation are caused by the ionization of water molecules within cells, producing highly reactive free radicals that damage macromolecules such as DNA. Acute effects (nonstochastic or deterministic) occur at relatively high dose levels such as those given during radiotherapy treatments or in accidents. Chronic effects are the results of long-term low-dose effects. The severity of these effects is unrelated to the dose; hence they are called stochastic or nondeterministic effects. Doses lower than 1 Gy generally do not cause noticeable acute effects other than slight cellular changes. However, there is increased probability of induced cancer or leukemia in the exposed individual. A radiation dose equivalent of 25 rem (0.25 Sv) may lead to a measurable hematologic depression.[15,19] A whole body total radiation dose exceeding 100 rem (1 Sv) may lead to nausea, fatigue, radiation dermatitis, alopecia, intestinal disturbances, and hematologic disorders. The average annual radiation dose from medical X-rays is approximately 40 mrem (0.4 mSv).[15,19]

Maximum Permissible Dose (MPD): The MPD is the upper limit of allowed radiation dose one may receive without the risk of significant side effects. The annual whole body dose limit for physicians is 50 mSv. Table 62-2 shows the annual maximum permissible dose per target area.[15] For the fetus, the annual maximum permissible dose is 0.5 rem or 5 mSv. Assuming proper techniques, the scattered radiation dose to the patient and the medical personnel should be less than the above radiation doses. Reduction of the amount of radiation implies selection of the type of examination and imaging modality to minimize the dose to the patient and personnel. These include knowledge of the value of the radiologic examinations and the views that are necessary, selection of the equipment to be as dose-efficient as possible, and proper installation and regular and correct maintenance of the equipment. The principle involved in reducing the amount of radiation dose is ALARA (as low as reasonably achievable) or ALARP (as low as reasonably practicable) implying the use of the lowest amount of tube current, compatible with a good image, to reduce radiation.

Radiation Protection of the Patient: Several precautions can be observed to minimize the exposure of the patient to radiation. The beam-on time should be reduced since radiation

TABLE 62-2. ANNUAL MAXIMUM TARGET ORGAN PERMISSIBLE RADIATION DOSE

Organ/Area	Annual Maximum Permissible Dose	
	rem	mSv
Whole body	5	50
Lens of eye	15	150
Thyroid	50	500
Gonads	50	500
Extremities	50	500

Reproduced with permission from Fishman SM, Smith H, Meleger A, Sievert JA: Radiation safety in pain medicine. Reg Anesth Pain Med 27:296–305, 2002.

exposure increases linearly with time and total exposure is equal to the exposure rate times the time. It is recommended that the fluoroscopy machine be equipped with a laser pointer; this is attached to the image intensifier. The laser pointer allows the technician to mark the area of interest reducing the number of scout fluoroscopy views before the area of interest is viewed. The X-ray tube should be kept as far away from the patient as possible. Increasing the distance between the X-ray tube and the patient reduces radiation to the patient and improves the quality of the image. It has been recommended that the X-ray tube be at least 30 cm away from the patient. The image intensifier should be positioned as close to the patient as possible. Collimation should be used to reduce the area being irradiated thereby reducing the amount of X-rays received by the patient. The use of live fluoroscopy should be minimized; freeze frames should be relied on as frequently as possible. Finally, magnification should be limited since magnifying the image ×1 increases the amount of radiation 2.25 times while magnifying the image ×2 increases the amount of radiation 4 times.[15]

As stated, the MPD to the fetus is 5 mSv per year. An old theory is the "10-day rule" wherein it was thought that X-ray examination of the abdomen of a woman of child-bearing age should be carried out within 10 days of the onset of menstruation since this time represents the least likelihood of conception taking place. If conception took place, the embryo would be most sensitive to the effect of radiation. The "10-day rule" is probably erroneous. The fetus is relatively insensitive to the effects of radiation in the early stages of pregnancy. The period when the fetus is most sensitive to radiation is at 8 to 15 weeks' gestation when the rate of proliferation of DNA within the brain is at a maximum.[17] Any significant deleterious effect of radiation during conception is likely to lead to spontaneous abortion.

Radiation Protection of Personnel: The factors affecting radiation exposure to personnel include the time or duration of X-ray exposure, distance from the source of the X-rays, and protection from the radiation. It should be noted that the major source of radiation is the patient who serves as conduit for scattered radiation. The radiation dose to the patient and subsequent scatter can be reduced by using the lowest tube current (mA) compatible with a good X-ray image. The beam-on time should be kept to a minimum; there is a 5-minute alarm in most fluoroscopy machines. Only necessary personnel should be present in the fluoroscopy room. The personnel should be notified each time before fluoroscopy is on. The personnel should step back from field whenever possible when the fluoroscopy machine is turned on. The intensity of ionizing radiation decreases exponentially as the distance from the source is increased. The inverse square law states that the radiation is inversely proportional to the square of the distance (the space between the individual and the X-ray source). Therefore, as the distance is doubled, the exposure rate is reduced by one fourth.[15] Finally, barriers or screens can be employed; these are utilized mostly in the orthopedic, urology, and radiology suites.

Undercouch and Overcouch Fluoroscopy: The conventional undercouch fluoroscopy arrangement occurs when the X-ray tube is located beneath the fluoroscopy table and the image intensifier is above the table (Fig. 62-5). In this arrangement and with the table horizontal, most of the scattered

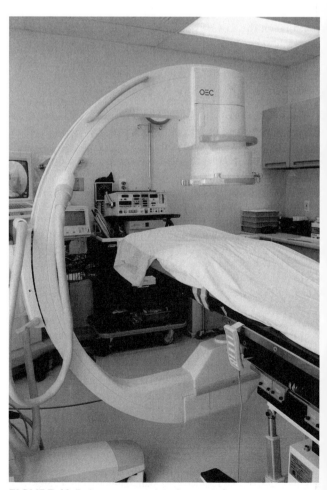

FIGURE 62-5. A conventional undercouch fluoroscopy arrangement wherein the X-ray tube is located beneath the fluoroscopy table and the image intensifier is above the table.

radiation is in the downward direction and absorbed in the floor or the side panels of the table. In the overcouch fluoroscopy arrangement the position of the X-ray tube and image intensifier is reversed or the oblique and lateral views are employed. In this arrangement it is difficult to get adequate shielding to the medical personnel. The maximum amount of scattered radiation is normally backwards from the entrance surface of the radiation and the side of the patient receiving most of the primary beam (i.e., the side of the X-ray tube). Scattered radiation is 2 to 3 times higher at the side of the X-ray tube. The physician should preferably stand on the side of the image intensifier when lateral views are taken. Also, the image intensifier has a lead–plastic apron attached to its edge which serves to absorb much of the scattered radiation that emerges from the patient shielding the physician from some of the scattered radiation.

Barriers and Shielding: Shielding refers to radiation protection afforded by equipments that absorb X-rays. The categories of shielding include fixed, mobile, and personal shielding.[17] Fixed shielding includes the thickness of walls, which should have a lead equivalence of 1 to 3 mm, the doors, and protective cubicles. Mobile shielding is appropriate during fluoroscopy procedures where a member of staff needs to remain near the patient. Personal shielding includes lead aprons, gloves, thyroid shields, and glass spectacles.

LEAD APRONS: For reasons of weight, lead aprons generally have shielding equivalence equal to 0.25 to 0.5 mm lead barrier and will only attenuate the radiation. Lead aprons absorb 90% to 95% of scattered radiation that reaches them (Table 62-3). "Wrap-around" lead aprons are useful when the medical personnel spend a lot of time with their backs turned away from the patient. When wrap-around aprons are not used, the personnel wearing them should not turn unshielded backs toward the X-ray beam. Lead aprons should be worn properly and stored properly. They should not be folded or thrown on the floor since it may produce creases that develop into breaks in the protective barrier.

LEAD RUBBER GLOVES AND LEADED GLASSES: Lead rubber gloves usually have a minimum lead equivalence of 0.25 mm since thicker leaded gloves make manipulations that require dexterity more difficult. The protection offered by "radiation-resistant" gloves may not be significant and the gloves may only give a false sense of security. The use of leaded gloves may actually increase the X-ray exposure when the fluoroscopy machine is in the ABC mode. In this scenario the machine senses the poor contrast between the bones of the gloved hand and the surrounding soft tissue and the ABC system automatically adjusts the tube current setting to produce a better contrast but a higher radiation dose.

The use of leaded glasses with side shields may reduce the risk of cataract formation. However, the effectiveness of glass spectacles may be overrated and ordinary eyeglasses may give adequate reduction in the eye doses. A single dose of 200 rem (2 Sv) or a total exposure of 800 rem (8 Sv) has been related to cataract formation and the latent period between the radiation exposure and the appearance of cataracts is approximately 8 years.[15,19]

Minimizing and Monitoring Radiation: Wagner and Archer recommended 10 measures to reduce risks from fluoroscopic X-rays (Table 62-4). Federal and state regulations in the USA require that anyone who works in a station where he or she may receive over 25% of the allowable quarterly limit (1.25 rem or 1,250 mrem) must be supplied with monitoring equipment or a radiation badge or film badge. A radiation badge is a pack of photographic film that measures radiation exposure for personnel monitoring. It measures the quantity and the quality of radiation (beta or gamma radiation). It is read with a densitometer, the amount of darkening of the film is proportional to the amount of radiation absorbed by the film. The film inside the badge is easily damaged by pen or moisture and the badge cannot be used for periods exceeding 8 weeks because the image fades.

There are usually two badges worn by the physician during the fluoroscopy procedure. The "collar badge" is worn outside the apron on the upper portion of body, usually on the upper

TABLE 62-3. PERCENTAGE PRIMARY X-RAY BEAM TRANSMISSION FOR KILOVOLTAGES AND LEAD APRONS

Lead Thickness (mm)	Single-Phase Generator (1 or 2 pulse)		
	75 kVp	100 kVp	125 kVp
0.22	4.5	12.1	12.8
0.44	0.7	3.7	5.1
0.5	<0.1	3.1	4.4
0.72	<0.1	1.4	2
1	<0.1	0.3	0.6

From Robinson A: Diagnostic protection and patient doses in diagnostic radiology. *In* Grainger RG, Allison D (eds): Grainger & Allison's Diagnostic Radiology: A Textbook of Medical Imaging. Churchill-Livingstone, New York, 1997, pp 169–189.

TABLE 62-4. TEN MEASURES FOR MINIMIZING RISKS FROM FLUOROSCOPIC X-RAYS

1. Dose rates are greater and dose accumulates faster in larger patients.
2. Keep the tube current as low as possible.
3. Keep the kVp as high as possible (and mA as low as possible) to achieve the appropriate compromise between image quality and low patient dose.
4. Keep the patient at maximum distance from the X-ray tube.
5. Keep the image intensifier as close to the patient as possible.
6. Do not overuse geometric or electronic magnification.
7. If the image quality is not compromised, remove the grid during procedures on small patients or when the image intensifier cannot be placed close to the patients.
8. Always collimate down to the area of interest.
9. Personnel must wear protective aprons, use shielding, monitor their doses, and know how to position themselves and the machines for minimum dose.
10. Keep beam-on time to an absolute minimum.

From Wagner LK, Archer BR: Minimizing Risks from Fluoroscopic X-rays, ed 3. RM Partnership, Woodlands, TX, 2000.

edge of the thyroid shield. This badge approximates radiation exposure to the lens of eye. The "behind the apron" badge is worn behind the apron, usually on the waist of the physician. The X-ray reading in this badge represents the actual dose to the gonads and the major blood-forming organs. The film badges should be placed correctly. It is not uncommon for the physician to interchange the placement of the badge resulting in a gross error in the interpretation of the X-ray risk to the physician.

The badges should be returned on time: old badges give inaccurate results. It should be realized that all the radiation badges from all departments in the hospital (e.g., radiology, cardiology, operating rooms, etc.) are sent for readings at the same time and that a delay in returning the badges from one department unnecessarily delays the reading of all the badges. The reports are issued in the form of monthly computer print-outs (Fig. 62-6).

Organization of Radiation Protection: Each hospital has a radiation safety office. The office usually has a clinical director, a radiation adviser, and a radiation protection supervisor.[17] The clinical director is usually a radiologist or clinician in charge responsible for establishing protocols and procedures for the examination of patients and is involved in the selection of equipment as well as day-to-day decisions. The radiation protection adviser (RPA) is usually an experienced physicist who gives advice on the design of X-ray rooms, monitoring of doses to patients and staff, and performs calibration and safety checks on radiology equipment. The radiation protection supervisor (RPS) is usually an experienced full-time member of the radiology staff who will, in collaboration with the RPA, write local rules and ensure their compliance by the staff, ensure that the staff wear radiation monitoring devices, and report to the department chair, administration, or RPA any incident in the hospital that is related to radiation safety.

RADIOLOGICAL CONTRAST MEDIA (RCM)

Iodine is the only element that has proved satisfactory for general use as an intravascular radiological contrast medium. The maximum recommended concentration of iodine is 300 mg iodine per mL and the maximum recommended dose is 3 g of iodine. The absorption of iodine is variable. Its mean half-life is 12 hours and 80% to 90% is excreted via the kidneys within 24 hours. There are two kinds of contrast media with respect to their osmolality: the high-osmolality contrast media (HOCM) and the low-osmolality contrast media (LOCM) (Table 62-5).[22,23] The HOCM are ionic monomers and include various concentrations of sodium, meglumine, or sodium-meglumine salts of diatrizoic and iothalamic salts. These media provide 3 iodine atoms for 2 ions, giving an iodine:particle ratio of 3:2; their osmolalities range between 433 mOsm/kg and 2,400 mOsm/kg.[22] The LOCM are non-ionic monomers, i.e., a molecule that does not dissociate in solution, and are ideal for myelography. The LOCM provide an iodine:particle ratio of 3:1 and their osmolalities range between 411 mOsm/kg and 796 mOsm/kg.[22] The LOCM cause less nausea and vomiting, produce less pain on peripheral arterial injection, and are associated with a lower incidence of mild, moderate, and severe adverse reactions compared to the HOCM (the incidence of adverse reaction rate with LOCM is 0.03% compared to 0.36% with HOCM).

Adverse Reactions to Contrast Media: The concerns regarding the use of contrast media include an adverse reaction to the contrast media and unintentional intrathecal injection. The patients considered at greater risk of an adverse reaction to the contrast media are listed in Table 62-6.[22] Patients who have a history of allergic reaction to the radiologic contrast media should be premedicated. Greenberger and Patterson[24] recommended that the patient be given three doses of oral prednisone 50 mg at 13, 7, and 1 hour before the procedure. They also recommended that diphenhydramine (Benadryl) 50 mg be given 1 hour before injection of the contrast.[24] Lasser et al.[25] recommended two oral doses of methylprednisolone 32 mg given at 12 and 2 hours before the procedure.

Unintentional Intrathecal Injection: The contrast media are actually not licensed for intrathecal use. It is recommended that water-soluble contrast media such as iohexol (Omnipaque) or iopamidol (Isovue) be used since adhesive arachnoiditis has not been observed with the nonionic water-soluble contrast media. The risk of seizure is virtually eliminated with the new agents and neurotoxicity is low but not negligible.

NORTHWESTERN MEM HOSP
251 E HURON
RADIATION SAFETY OFC
GALTER RM 8-138
CHICAGO IL 60611

LANDAUER ®

Landauer, Inc. 2 Science Road Glenwood, Illinois 60425-1586
Telephone: (708)755-7000 Facsimile: (708)755-7016
www.landauerinc.com

RADIATION DOSIMETRY REPORT

luxel®

ACCOUNT NO.	SERIES CODE	ANALYTICAL WORK ORDER	REPORT DATE	DOSIMETER RECEIVED	REPORT TIME IN WORK DAYS	PAGE NO.
79397	ATH	0126800010	10/04/01	09/25/01	7	1

** DUPLICATE **

PARTICIPANT NUMBER	NAME			DOSIMETER	USE	RADIATION QUALITY	DOSE EQUIVALENT (MREM) FOR PERIODS SHOWN BELOW			QUARTERLY ACCUMULATED DOSE EQUIVALENT (MREM)			YEAR TO DATE DOSE EQUIVALENT (MREM)			LIFETIME DOSE EQUIVALENT (MREM)			RECORDS FOR YEAR	INCEPTION DATE (MM/YY)
	ID NUMBER	BIRTH DATE	SEX				DEEP DDE	EYE LDE	SHALLOW SDE	DEEP DDE	EYE LDE	SHALLOW SDE	DEEP DDE	EYE LDE	SHALLOW SDE	DEEP DDE	EYE LDE	SHALLOW SDE		
FOR MONITORING PERIOD:							08/10/01 - 09/09/01			QTR 3			2001							
07377				P	COLLAR		M	M	M										8	07/99
			M	P	WAIST		M	M	M				18	11	13	18	14	18		07/99
					ASSIGN		M	M	M	M	M	M								
					NOTE		ASSIGNED DOSE BASED ON EDE 1 CALCULATION													
07379				P	COLLAR		M	M	M										8	07/99
					NOTE		ESTIMATED													
			M	P	WAIST		M	M	M											07/99
					NOTE		ESTIMATED													
					ASSIGN		M	M	M	M	M	M	13	10	11	13	10	13		
					NOTE		ESTIMATED													
					NOTE		ASSIGNED DOSE BASED ON EDE 1 CALCULATION													
07380				P	COLLAR		M	M	M										9	07/99
					NOTE		ESTIMATED													
			M	P	WAIST		M	M	M											07/99
					NOTE		ESTIMATED													
					ASSIGN		M	M	M	M	M	M	14	34	34	14	198	208		
					NOTE		ESTIMATED													
					NOTE		ASSIGNED DOSE BASED ON EDE 1 CALCULATION													
07507				P	COLLAR		M	M	M										8	02/00
			M	P	WAIST		M	M	M				15	9	10	16	10	11		02/00
					ASSIGN		M	M	M	M	M	M								
					NOTE		ASSIGNED DOSE BASED ON EDE 1 CALCULATION													

M: MINIMAL REPORTING SERVICE OF 1 MREM   QUALITY CONTROL RELEASE: VG   2S - PR 7326 - RPT130 - N1 C   - 09552

Accredited by the National Institute of Standards and Technology through NVLAP *

FIGURE 62-6. A sample of a printout of radiation exposure of medical personnel.

TABLE 62-5. **CONTRAST MEDIA, THEIR IODINE CONCENTRATIONS, AND OSMOLALITIES**

Contrast Medium	Iodine (mg/mL)	Osmolality
HOCM		
Diatriazoate Na (Hypaque)	300	1522–1550
Diatriazoate Na (8%)-meglumine (52%) (Renografin)	292	1422–1539
Iothalamate meglumine (60%) (Conray)	282	1400
LOCM		
Iohexol (Omnipaque)	300	709
Iopamidol (Isovue)	300	616
Ioversol (Optiray)	320	702
Ioxaglate sodium (19.6%)-meglumine (39.3%) (Hetabrix)	320	600

From Drug Reviews from the Formulary. Intravascular contrast media. Hospital Pharmacy 26:275–278, 1991.

TABLE 62-6. **PATIENTS AT GREATER RISK OF A SEVERE ADVERSE REACTION TO RADIOLOGIC CONTRAST MEDIA (RCM)**

Patients with history of a previous adverse reaction to RCM (excluding mild flushing, nausea)
Asthmatic patients
Allergic and atopic patients
Cardiac patients with decompensation, unstable arrhythmia, recent MI
Renal failure, diabetic nephropathy
Feeble infants and the elderly
Patients with severe general debility or dehydration
Patients with metabolic hematologic disorders

From Grainger RG: Intravenous contrast media. In Grainger RG, Allison D (eds): Grainger & Allison's Diagnostic Radiology: A Textbook of Medical Imaging. Churchill-Livingstone, New York, 1997, pp 35–45.

REFERENCES

1. Mehta M, Salmon N: Extradural block: Confirmation of injection site by X-ray monitoring. Anaesthesia 40:1009–1012, 1985.
2. Cluff R, Mehio AK, Cohen SP, et al: The technical aspects of epidural steroid injections: A national survey. Anesth Analg 95:403–408, 2002.
3. White AH, Derby R, Wynne G: Epidural injections for the treatment of low back pain. Spine 5:78–86, 1980.
4. Stojanovic MP, Vu TN, Caneris O, et al: The role of fluoroscopy in cervical epidural steroid injections. Spine 27:509–514, 2002.
5. Hogan QH: Epidural anatomy examined by cryomicrotome section. Influence of age, vertebral level, and disease. Reg Anesth 21:395–406, 1996.
6. Bloomberg R: The dorsomedian connective tissue band in the lumbar epidural space of humans: An anatomical study using epiduroscopy in autopsy cases. Anesth Analg 65:747–752, 1986.
7. Gallart L, Blanco D, Samso ER, et al: Clinical and radiologic evidence of the epidural plica mediana dorsalis. Anesth Analg 71;698–701, 1990.
8. Savolane ER, Pandya JB, Greenblatt SH, et al: Anatomy of the human lumbar epidural space: New insights using CT-epidurography. Anesthesiology 68:217–220, 1988.
9. Renfrew DL, Moore TE, Kathol MH, et al: Correct placement of epidural steroid injections: Fluoroscopic guidance and contrast administration. Am J Neuroradiol 12:1003–1007, 1991.
10. Stitz MY, Sommer HM: Accuracy of blind versus fluoroscopically guided caudal epidural injection. Spine 24:1371–1376, 1999.
11. El-Khoury GY, Ehara S, Weinstein JN, et al: Epidural steroid injection: A procedure ideally performed with fluoroscopy control. Radiology 168:554–557, 1988.
12. Fredman B, Ben Nun M, Zohar E, et al: Epidural steroids for treating failed back surgery syndrome: Is fluoroscopy necessary? Anesth Analg 88:367–372, 1999.
13. Machikanti L, Bakhit CE, Fellows B: Fluoroscopy is medically necessary for the performance of epidural steroid injections. Anesth Analg 89:1330–1331, 1999.
14. Broadman L: Radiation safety. *In* Raj PP, Abram BM, Benzon HT, et al (eds): Practical Management of Pain, ed 2. Mosby, St Louis, 2000, pp 834–837.
15. Fishman SM, Smith H, Meleger A, Seibert JA: Radiation safety in pain medicine. Reg Anesth Pain Med 27:296–305, 2002.
16. Rathmell JP: Imaging in regional anesthesia and pain medicine: We have much to learn. Reg Anesth Pain Med 27:240–241, 2002.
17. Robinson A: Diagnostic protection and patient doses in diagnostic radiology. *In* Grainger RG, Allison D (eds): Grainger & Allison's Diagnostic Radiology: A Textbook of Medical Imaging. Churchill-Livingstone, New York, 1997, pp 169–189.
18. Goetz BB, Murphy CH: Radiation safety. *In* Murphy CH, Murphy MR (eds): Radiology for Anesthesia and Critical Care. Churchill-Livingstone, New York, 1987, pp 257–262.
19. National Council on Radiation Protection and Measurements (NCRP): Report no. 116. Limitation of exposure to ionizing radiation. NCRP Publications, Bethesda, MD, 1993.
20. International Commission on Radiological Protection: Recommendations of the International Commission on Radiological Protection, ICRP Publication No. 60. Ann ICRP 21:1–3, 1991.
21. Wagner LK, Archer BR: Minimizing Risks from Fluoroscopic X-rays, ed 3. RM Partnership, Woodlands, TX, 2000.
22. Grainger RG: Intravenous contrast media. *In* Grainger RG, Allison D (eds): Grainger & Allison's Diagnostic Radiology: A Textbook of Medical Imaging. Churchill-Livingstone, New York, 1997, pp 35–45.
23. Drug Reviews from the Formulary. Intravascular contrast media. Hospital Pharmacy 26:275–278, 1991.
24. Greenberger PA, Patterson R: The prevention of immediate generalized reactions to radiocontrast media in high-risk patients. Clin Immunol 87:867–872, 1991.
25. Lasser EC, Berry CC, Talner LB, et al: Pretreatment with corticosteroids to alleviate reactions to intravenous contrast media. N Engl J Med 317:845–849, 1987.

Approach to the Management of Cancer Pain

Jay R. Thomas, M.D., Ph.D.,
Frank D. Ferris, M.D., and
Charles F. von Gunten, M.D., Ph.D., F.A.C.P.

While this chapter reviews the pharmacological management of cancer pain, medications are not the only important component of comprehensive cancer pain management. In an attempt to simplify the subject of cancer pain management, pathophysiological processes have been separated from psychological, social, and spiritual factors. While this separation may be useful for heuristic and conceptual purposes, it has led to the unfortunate labeling of the former as "real" pain and the latter as "not real" pain. It has also led to the inappropriate extrapolation of research on acute pain, particularly in laboratory animals, to the management of chronic pain, and to the general avoidance of emotional, psychological, social, and spiritual issues by physicians trained in the scientific method. Optimal pain control may not be possible unless suffering in these other dimensions is addressed. Appropriate referral to allied health providers, such as counselors, social workers, chaplains, or hospices may be required.

ASSESSMENT OF CANCER PAIN

Since pain perception is inherently subjective, the gold standard for assessing pain is the patient's self report.[1] Whereas acute pain is accompanied by signs of adrenergic stimulation such as tachycardia and hypertension, chronic cancer pain may fail to display any of these changes even though the patient reports severe pain.

To guide decision-making regarding the appropriate strategies to manage pain, during each evaluation the location, type, temporal profile, and severity of each significant pain should be assessed.

Type: Cancer pain can be classified as nociceptive, neuropathic, or a combination of the two.[2] Each type typically presents with a number of relatively distinct qualities.

Nociceptive pain results when pain-sensing neuronal pathways are stimulated and function normally. Specialized receptors at the distal end of neuronal axons, termed nociceptors, detect noxious mechanical, chemical, and thermal stimuli and generate neuronal electrical activity. These signals are transmitted normally along neuronal pathways to the brain. Within the brain they are integrated with other cortical activity and lead to the patient's perception of pain.

Nociceptive pain can originate from somatic or visceral sources, or both. Somatic pain originates from skin, muscle, bone, and fascia. It is mediated by the somatic nervous system. As innervation is highly specific, localization of the pain is precise. Somatic pain is often described as sharp, aching, or throbbing. Visceral pain originates from internal structures such as the organs of the gastrointestinal tract. It is mediated by the autonomic nervous system. As there is a lack of specificity of innervation, and considerable neuronal crossover, visceral pain is typically difficult to localize or describe, and may encompass an area that is much larger than might be expected for a single organ. Visceral pain involving hollow visci is often characterized as crampy.

Neuropathic pain has been defined as a primary lesion or dysfunction of the pain-sensing nervous system.[3] The lesion can be either peripheral in the somatic or visceral nervous system, or central. The nerves themselves may be subject to damage from compression, infiltration, ischemia, metabolic injury, or transection.[4] The myelin sheath that insulates one nerve from another may also be damaged. As an example, in a post-thoracotomy pain syndrome the pain may be due to the formation of a neuroma in the somatic nerves caused by aberrant healing postoperatively. This can lead to erratic electrical activity, cross transmission from one neuron to another (ephaptic transmission), and an experience of pain by the patient.

Alternatively, neuropathic pain may also be caused by dysfunction of the nervous system. As an example, chronic nociceptive pain can lead to increased sensitivity of spinal cord neurons in a process called central facilitation or "wind-up."[5] Although the nerves are not damaged, an abnormal signaling system is set up such that a given noxious stimulus produces a greater pain experience than normal, and/or normally non-noxious stimuli lead to pain. This exaggerated neuronal state at least partially explains the phenomenon of allodynia, where an event that is normally not painful, such as the pressure from a bed sheet or clothing on the chest of patient with recurrent breast cancer, causes pain.[6] The enzyme cyclooxygenase (COX) and the neurotransmitter glutamate, the N-methyl-D-aspartate (NMDA) receptor, and the recruitment of previously silent neurons are thought to be involved in perpetuating this abnormal experience of pain. Neuropathic pain is often described as burning, shooting, stabbing, or electric-like and may be associated with numbness, tingling, and/or sensory deficits.

Temporal Profile: The temporal profile of a pain will provide further clues to its etiology.[1] As an example, spontaneous pain of short duration could be the paroxysmal firing of a neuroma. Back pain that occurs only with weight bearing could indicate a spinal bony metastasis. These insights may help conceptualize the pathophysiology that underlies the pain, and influence the medications prescribed and the route by which they are administered.

Most cancer pain is continuous over time with some variation in intensity, particularly at night. Without intervention, it rarely disappears completely. Cancer pain is also frequently associated with intermittent paroxysms of pain that occur with activity (e.g., movement, chewing, swallowing, breathing, defecating, urinating, dressing, touch, etc.), or during a procedure.

If this is the first assessment, the patient should be asked about the duration of the pain. When did it first start? How long has it been present? Did it come on slowly, or suddenly? During each assessment, the temporal profile of the pain should be established. One can ask what the baseline or background pain is like. Does it vary over time, e.g., worse at night? Is the patient ever pain-free? Are there times when the pain gets much worse? What factors exacerbate or relieve the pain, e.g., activity, touch, clothing, cold/heat, procedures, etc.

Severity: Sequential measurement of severity using one of a number of different validated severity assessment scales will provide an indication of the changing intensity of the pain experienced by a given patient over time. It will also guide analgesic management. In a given patient, the same tool should be used for each assessment.

A numerical analogue scale is the simplest. The patient is asked to indicate the severity of the pain on a 10-point scale where 0 represents "no pain" and 10 represents the "worst possible pain."

Alternatively, a visual analogue scale can provide more visual cues, and be more reliable. The patient is asked to indicate the severity of the pain by marking a 100 mm line at a point that indicates the intensity of her/his pain (delimited by the descriptors "no pain" at one end (usually the left) and "worst possible pain" at the other end). A few patients will find it easier to understand a vertical line where "no pain" is at the bottom and "worst possible pain" is at the top.

For children, and adults who do not understand numerical or visual analogue scales, the Wong–Baker or other faces scales are similarly reliable assessment tools.

To understand how the pain varies over time, one can ask about the intensity of the continuous pain now, the worst it has been in the last 24 hours, the best it has been in the last 24 hours, and the intensity of intermittent pain at its peak.

Total Pain: Together with a careful physical examination and select laboratory and imaging studies, it is usually possible to identify the relevant pathophysiology leading to a pain state. However, a particular pain syndrome is part of a whole person's experience. The concept of "total pain" emphasizes that multiple nonphysical factors can also contribute to pain, i.e., psychologic factors (e.g., anxiety, depression), social factors (e.g., familial estrangement), and spiritual or existential factors (e.g., loss of meaning in life, fear of death). It may not be possible to control pain successfully without also addressing each of these other sources of suffering.[7]

TREATMENT OF CANCER PAIN

World Health Organization Three-Step Ladder: In 1988 the World Health Organization (WHO) first promoted the Canadian three-step ladder for cancer pain management (see Fig. 63-1).[8] Recent pain guidelines from the Royal College of Physicians and the European Association for Palliative Care both use the WHO guidelines as a basis.[9,10] Today, it is the

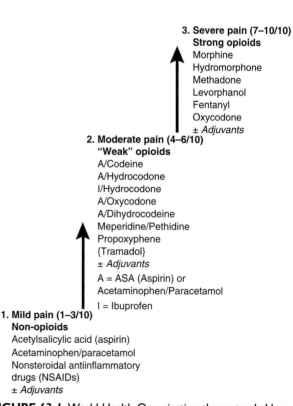

3. **Severe pain (7–10/10)**
Strong opioids
Morphine
Hydromorphone
Methadone
Levorphanol
Fentanyl
Oxycodone
± *Adjuvants*

2. **Moderate pain (4–6/10)**
"Weak" opioids
A/Codeine
A/Hydrocodone
I/Hydrocodone
A/Oxycodone
A/Dihydrocodeine
Meperidine/Pethidine
Propoxyphene
{Tramadol}
± *Adjuvants*

A = ASA (Aspirin) or
Acetaminophen/Paracetamol
I = Ibuprofen

1. **Mild pain (1–3/10)**
Non-opioids
Acetylsalicylic acid (aspirin)
Acetaminophen/paracetamol
Nonsteroidal antiinflammatory
drugs (NSAIDs)
± *Adjuvants*

FIGURE 63-1. World Health Organization three-step ladder.

cornerstone for the WHO's public health initiative to treat cancer pain worldwide.

The ladder provides a clinically useful strategy for classifying the available analgesics, and guiding initial analgesic selection based on the severity of the patient's pain. If the pain is mild (1/10 to 3/10) an analgesic can be chosen from step one. If it is moderate (4/10 to 6/10), one can start with an analgesic from step two. If it is severe (7/10 to 10/10), one can start with an opioid from step three. At any step, adjuvant analgesics can be added to optimize pain control.[11]

STEP ONE: Acetaminophen and the nonsteroidal anti-inflammatory drugs (NSAIDs) including acetylsalicylic acid (ASA) are the mainstay of step one of the WHO analgesic ladder for the management of mild pain. They obey first-order kinetics and may be dosed up to recommended maximums (see Table 63-1). Many are available without prescription. Sustained-release preparations or NSAIDs with longer half-lives, e.g., Piroxicam, that require less frequent dosing may encourage adherence. When pain is more than mild, step-one analgesics can be combined with opioids at steps two and three.

STEP TWO: Several opioid analgesics are conventionally available in combination with acetaminophen, ibuprofen, or ASA and are commonly used to manage moderate pain. They are listed in Fig. 63-1 under step two of the WHO analgesic ladder. With the exceptions of propoxyphene (that truly has weak analgesic activity), tramadol (that has a unique combination of very weak opioid activity with other analgesic properties), meperidine, and codeine (methyl morphine, which has one-tenth the potency of morphine), the opioids in this class are close in potency to morphine (mg for mg).[12] However, they have been called "weak" opioids because, in combination, they have a ceiling to their analgesic potential due to the maximum amounts of acetaminophen or ASA that can be administered per 24 hours (e.g., 4 g acetaminophen per 24 hours).[13]

The combination medications of step two all obey first-order kinetics and may be dosed up to recommended maximums (see Table 63-2). The potential adverse effects are those of the component drugs.[14,15]

Frequently, patients are simultaneously given prescriptions for several step-two drugs even though pain is poorly controlled. This usually occurs when physicians are reluctant to prescribe a step-three opioid. Aside from propoxyphene, there is no evidence that maximal dosing of any "step-two" medication is better than another and trials of several step-two medications are likely to prolong the patient's pain. In addition, when a step-two drug inadequately relieves pain, patients may combine two or more medications, or take more than the prescribed amount in an attempt to obtain pain relief. In doing so they may unknowingly put themselves at increased risk for significant toxicity from either the acetaminophen or ASA component of the medication.

If pain persists, or increases, despite a maximum dose of a step-two drug, a step-three drug should be prescribed instead.

STEP THREE: The pure agonist opioid analgesics comprise step three of the WHO analgesic ladder. Morphine is the prototypical drug because of its ease of administration and wide availability. Other widely prescribed opioids are listed in step three of Fig. 63-1. Many patients with chronic pain are best managed with an appropriately titrated strong opioid that is combined with one or more coanalgesics. In contrast with the

step-one and step-two analgesics, there is no ceiling effect or upper limit to the dose of opioids when titrating to relieve pain.

"STEP FOUR": Several studies of the WHO three-step ladder have demonstrated that its application results in the adequate control of up to 90% of patients with cancer pain.[1] Several authors have informally invoked "step four" to indicate approaches that should be reserved for patients whose pain is not controlled by competent use of the analgesic approaches outlined in the first three steps. In general, "step four" involves invasive approaches for pain relief that can be summarized as follows.

TABLE 63-1. SELECTED STEP-ONE ANALGESICS

Drug	Suggested Maximum Dose
Acetaminophen (APAP, Tylenol)	650 mg PO q4h
Acetylsalicylic acid (ASA, aspirin)	650 mg PO q4h
Ibuprofen (Motrin)	800 mg PO qid
Choline magnesium trisalicylate (Trilisate)	1500 mg PO tid
Celecoxib (Celebrex)	100 mg PO qd
Diclofenac (Cataflam) Diclofenac: extended release (Voltaren)	50 mg PO qid 75 mg PO tid
Diflunisal (Dolobid)	500 mg PO tid
Etodolac (Lodine)	400 mg PO tid
Indomethacin (Indocin)	50 mg PO qid
Ketoprofen (Orudis)	75 mg PO qid
Nabumetone (Relafen)	1 g PO bid
Naproxen (Naprosyn)	500 mg PO tid
Oxaprozin (Daypro)	1800 mg PO qd
Rofecoxib (Vioxx)	25 mg PO qd
Sulindac (Clinoril)	200 mg PO bid
Salsalate (Disalcid)	1500 mg PO tid
Ketorolac (Toradol)	60 mg IM/IV then 30 mg IV/IM q6h; 10 mg PO qid; not to exceed 5 days

TABLE 63-2. **SELECTED STEP-TWO ANALGESICS**

Drug	Suggested Maximum Dose
Codeine	60 mg PO q4h
Codeine 30 mg/325 mg APAP (Tylenol #3); codeine 30 mg/325 mg ASA (Empirin #3)	2 PO q4h
Hydrocodone 5 mg/500 mg APAP (Vicodin) Hydrocodone 10 mg/650 mg APAP (Lortab)	2 PO q6h 1 PO q6h
Hydrocodone 7.5 mg/200 mg ibuprofen (Vicoprofen)	1 PO q4h
Oxycodone 5 mg/325 mg APAP (Percocet); oxycodone 5 mg/325 mg ASA (Percodan)	2 PO q4h
Tramadol 50 mg (Ultram)	2 PO q6h

Subcutaneous (SC) or intravenous (IV) administration of opioid analgesics and coanalgesics may be required for patients where oral (PO), buccal mucosal, rectal (PR), or transcutaneous approaches are not possible or practical, or where doses of oral opioids lead to undesirable adverse effects. Adverse effects may be minimized as a result of the uniform delivery of the drug parenterally, the change in route of administration, or the reduction in first-pass metabolite production.

Subcutaneous delivery is the preferred parenteral route of administration. It can be accomplished with a small-gauge needle that causes little pain at insertion, requires minimal skill to place, and can be left in situ for up to a week with minimal risk of local or systemic infection.

Intraspinal administration of opioid analgesics either epidurally or intrathecally may be required in selected patients.

Intraventricular application of opioid analgesics and other drugs has been investigated for selected central pain syndromes.

Neuroablative techniques such as peripheral neurolytic blockade, ganglionic blockade, cordotomy, and cingulotomy may be appropriate in highly selected patients.

Common Analgesics

ACETAMINOPHEN: Despite its wide use, the precise mechanism of action remains unclear. Although it is analgesic and antipyretic, it is not anti-inflammatory, at least systemically. Its analgesic activity is additive to other analgesic agents, including the NSAIDs and opioids.

Acetaminophen is associated with significant liver toxicity. It is generally recommended that the total dose not exceed 4 g per 24 hours.

NSAIDs INCLUDING ASA: Normally, the enzyme COX catalyzes the conversion of arachidonic acid to prostaglandins and thromboxanes. These inflammatory mediators sensitize nerve endings to painful stimuli and stimulate a group of silent nociceptors that only fire in an inflammatory milieu. In the spinal cord, COX plays a role in setting up the dysfunctional signaling pattern involved in neuropathic pain.

NSAIDs are potent anti-inflammatory medications that inhibit the activity of COX and decrease the levels of these inflammatory mediators. As a result, there is less sensitization of nerve endings, less recruitment of silent nociceptors, and less risk of central "wind-up." While primary analgesia may be achieved at low doses, for their anti-inflammatory effects maximum doses should be used. As they act through an alternate mechanism to opioids and other adjuvant analgesics, NSAIDs may be combined with other analgesics to achieve better pain relief than is possible with a single medication.

The morbidity and mortality associated with NSAIDs, including ASA, are significantly higher than for any of the other analgesics. The adverse effects of NSAIDs are related to their mechanism of action. Inhibition of COX leads to inhibition of platelet aggregation and micro-arteriolar constriction/decreased perfusion, particularly in the stomach and kidneys. In the stomach the relative ischemia compromises the production of gastric mucus by the chief cells, and significantly increases the risk of gastric erosions and bleeding. In the kidneys the relative ischemia increases the risk of renal papillary necrosis and renal failure.

COX exists in two forms: a constitutive form, COX-1, and a form that is inducible under conditions of inflammation, COX-2. There are both COX-2-selective and nonselective NSAIDs that target both forms of COX. Whereas renal insufficiency is a risk of both nonselective and COX-2-selective NSAIDs, the risk of gastropathy and platelet inhibition is significantly decreased with COX-2-selective NSAIDs.

Patients (particularly the elderly) who are dehydrated, malnourished, cachectic, or have a history of nausea, gastritis, or gastric ulceration with NSAIDs are at increased risk for adverse effects from NSAIDs. However, the dyspepsia and abdominal pain that limit use of the NSAIDs in some patients do not correlate with significant gastric erosions and gastrointestinal bleeding.

To minimize the risk of ischemia, the patient should be well hydrated. The use of an H_2 blocking antacid (e.g. cimetidine or ranitidine) to treat NSAID dyspepsia and abdominal pain does not prevent gastric erosions and gastrointestinal bleeding. Only misoprostol, a prostaglandin-E analogue that reverses the effect of NSAIDs on the micro-arteriolar circulation of the stomach, and the proton-pump inhibitors (such as omeprazole, pantoprazole) have been shown to heal gastric erosions and reduce the risk of significant gastric bleeding.

The nonacetylated salicylates (choline magnesium trisalicylate and salsalate), nabumetone, and the COX-2 inhibitors do not significantly affect platelet aggregation. They may be useful in patients who are thrombocytopenic and for whom other NSAIDs are contraindicated. Sulindac is thought to be least likely to induce renal failure because of its minimal effect on prostaglandin synthesis at the level of the proximal renal tubule.

In contrast to the opioids, the NSAIDs and acetaminophen have a ceiling effect to their analgesic potential, do not produce pharmacological tolerance, and are not associated with physical or psychological dependence.

OPIOIDS: Opioid analgesics act by binding to opioid receptors of three subtypes (mu, kappa, and delta) both peripherally and centrally. The central receptors in the spinal cord and brain are most important for mediating analgesia. The opioid analgesics in common usage may be divided into those that are full agonists, partial agonists, and mixed agonist–antagonists. The pure agonist drugs are the most useful in chronic intractable pain.

OPIOIDS TO AVOID: The mixed agonist–antagonist opioids (such as pentazocine, butorphanol, and nalbuphine) and the partial agonist opioids (such as buprenorphine) are poor choices for patients with severe pain. They have no advantages over the pure agonist opioids. Besides having a ceiling effect to the analgesia they produce, they have the significant disadvantage that, if combined with a pure opioid agonist, they may precipitate acute pain and opioid withdrawal symptoms.

Meperidine (Demerol) is a synthetic pure agonist opioid that is widely used in the postoperative management of acute pain. However, its continued use has been questioned for three reasons. First, because of its short duration of action in comparison with morphine or other pure agonist opioids it must be dosed too frequently to provide convenient, adequate analgesia. Second, because its oral absorption is unpredictable, a reliable oral dose cannot be prescribed that corresponds to parenteral doses. Third, and most significant, the major liver metabolite normeperidine, which has a longer half-life (approximately 6 hours) than meperidine (approximately 3 hours), accumulates with repeat dosing q3h for analgesia and frequently causes significant subclinical or clinical toxicity, including impaired concentration, restlessness, agitation, excessive dreams, hallucination, myoclonic jerks, or even seizures. This accumulation is particularly accentuated in patients with compromised renal function. The assertions that meperidine is associated with less constipation or spasm of the sphincter of Oddi are not supported by evidence. Its use is best limited to small doses (25 to 50 mg) parenterally to treat rigors associated with fever, drugs, or blood product transfusions.

Analgesic Pharmacology: Pharmacological principles guide the dosing of systemic analgesics to treat and prevent cancer pain.

ROUTES OF ADMINISTRATION: The oral route of administration is preferred for the management of cancer pain. It provides the simplest, least expensive way to manage up to 90% of all cancer pain. When it is not available, analgesics can be administered buccally and rectally before resorting to more invasive and expensive routes of delivery. In a small number of patients (<5%) subcutaneous, intravenous, or intraspinal administration may be required.

ROUTINE DOSING FOR CONSTANT PAIN: One should distinguish between constant and intermittent pain. For chronic

cancer pain analgesics should be prescribed on a regular schedule at doses sufficient to keep the pain controlled. Dosing solely on an "as needed" or "prn" basis is inappropriate as it subjects the patient to unnecessary pain and may increase both the patient's anxiety and the total dose required to control the pain.

Most of the short-acting drugs used for analgesia, particularly acetaminophen, the NSAIDs including ASA, and the opioids, follow first-order kinetics. When prescribing them on a routine schedule, they should be administered once every half-life in order to achieve steady state and maintain constant serum levels, i.e., q4h for PO opioid dosing. Methadone, with its longer half-life is administered every 8 to 12 hours.[16–18]

TITRATION: When initiating, titrating, or changing analgesic therapy, drugs that follow first-order kinetics take 5 half-lives to reach pharmacological steady state. Changes in dosages should only be made once the serum level has reached steady state, e.g., once every 20 to 24 hours when morphine is given PO, or even SC. Waiting longer will not improve pain control. Increasing dosages before steady state is reached may lead to unnecessarily high serum levels and undesired adverse effects.

SUSTAINED-RELEASE PRODUCTS: Sustained-release medications should not be used alone to adjust or titrate a patient's uncontrolled pain. Using them for titration unduly prolongs the process to bring the pain under control. However, once the pain is controlled, changing to a sustained-release product may enhance the patient's quality of life and improve compliance and adherence due to the decreased frequency of dosing (e.g., q8h, q12h, q24h, etc.).

Sustained-release preparations of codeine, hydromorphone, morphine, and oxycodone are (or soon will be) available for PO administration and should be administered in accordance with the instructions of the manufacturer.

Transdermal fentanyl patches are convenient when patients are receiving stable opioid dosing, but should not be used to titrate unrelieved pain. Approximately 12 to 18 hours are needed for significant serum levels of fentanyl to accumulate, so appropriate doses of opioids need to be maintained during this window of time. Fentanyl patches may be changed every 72 hours, although a small number of patients may need to have their patch(es) changed every 48 hours.

BREAKTHROUGH OR RESCUE DOSING FOR INTERMITTENT PAIN: Changes in pain severity may occur spontaneously because of activity (e.g., movement) or a procedure (e.g., venipuncture, wound dressing change). If the duration and severity of the change is sufficient, extra short-acting doses of the same or similar medication (breakthrough or rescue doses) on an "as needed" or "prn" basis may be appropriate. If a patient regularly requires more than 2 to 4 breakthrough doses per 24 hours, then the routine dose should be adjusted upwards. For intermittent pain of short duration (seconds to a few minutes) breakthrough dosing, particularly of the opioids, may lead to undesired adverse effects without increased analgesia.

For most analgesics the time to reach maximum serum concentration (C_{max}) after a given dose of medication correlates closely with the maximum analgesic effect. Breakthrough doses of an analgesic can be given safely with a frequency equivalent to the time required to reach C_{max}. For example, a bolus of IV morphine achieves its maximum serum concentration (C_{max}) in 5 to 10 minutes, SC doses take 20 to 30 minutes, and PO morphine achieves its maximum in 45 to 65 minutes. Therefore, breakthrough doses can be given q5–10min IV (e.g., the usual settings for patient-controlled analgesia pumps in the postoperative setting), q30min SC, or q60min PO. Making the patient wait any longer when the pain is not controlled simply prolongs the time required to establish optimal pain control.

The size of the breakthrough dose should be related to the routine dose. For the strong opioids such as morphine, hydromorphone, and oxycodone, a simple rule-of-thumb is: for the oral route administer 10% of the total 24-hour dose per breakthrough dose every 1 hour as needed. For the intravenous route, administer 50% to 100% of the hourly infusion rate every 5 to 10 minutes as needed. The dose is then adjusted as the routine dose changes or as the intensity of the intermittent pain requires.

Oral transmucosal fentanyl has kinetics similar to intravenous delivery. It is supplied in a candy matrix lozenge on an applicator stick that is twirled against the buccal mucosa. Although expensive, its quick onset and offset make it useful to treat short-lived breakthrough pain. Dosing must be individualized: it cannot be calculated as an equianalgesic dose.[19,20]

EQUIANALGESIC DOSING: The relative abilities of opioid analgesics to relieve pain have been correlated (Table 63-3). These relationships are not scientifically precise, as there is significant interpatient variability. Further, the data from which these equivalencies are derived are often not directly applicable to chronic cancer pain. Nevertheless, the equianalgesic tables are useful to approximate the dose of a new analgesic when changes are contemplated. The dose should then be adjusted based on patient response.[21]

When changing between opioids, there is incomplete cross-tolerance. To correct for this when pain is controlled, some advocate reducing the dose of the new medication by 25% to 50% after calculating the equianalgesic dose.[22]

Methadone, an opioid with a half-life that ranges from 15 to 40 hours or more, is an important exception.[23] Its apparent

TABLE 63-3. EQUIANALGESIC DOSING

Oral Dose (mg)	Analgesic	Parenteral Dose (mg) IV/SC/IM
150	Meperidine	50
100	Codeine	60
15	Hydrocodone	–
15	Morphine	5
10	Oxycodone	–
4	Hydromorphone	1.5
2	Levorphanol	1
–	Fentanyl	0.050

equianalgesic efficacy varies with the dose of opioid. In acute dosing, or at low doses, it appears to be a 1:1 ratio of methadone to morphine. For doses of morphine less than 500 mg/day, the relative potency of methadone to morphine is about 5:1. For patients taking between 500 and 1,000 mg of morphine per day, the relative potency of methadone becomes 10:1. For patients taking greater than 1,000 mg of morphine per day, the relative potency could be from 15:1 to 20:1. Because of its long and variable half-life, care must be taken when switching from one opioid to methadone and while titrating to an effective dose. Because of its long half-life, adverse effects may appear several days after doses are adjusted. Without continuous review these may be serious: methadone is the opioid most associated with respiratory depression when dosed on a regular basis.[24,25]

Attempts have been made to correlate the relative analgesia provided by acetaminophen, the NSAIDs, and the opioids. Ketorolac 10 mg orally seems to be roughly equivalent to the combination tablet 60 mg codeine/650 mg acetaminophen PO or 6 to 9 mg morphine PO in cancer pain. Transdermal fentanyl 25 µg/h is approximately 50 mg morphine PO q24h.

When changing routes of administration, differences in opioid metabolism (e.g., less first-pass catabolism IV/IM/SC compared to PO) necessitate adjustments to the opioid dose as indicated in Table 63-3. For example, an equivalent dose of morphine IV/IM/SC will be one-half to one-third that given PO.

CLEARANCE/BUILDUP: Acetaminophen is metabolized in the liver and becomes toxic if catabolic pathways become saturated (usually at doses > 4 g per 24 hours). Therefore its use is contraindicated in liver failure or in the setting of significant liver injury.

ASA and many of the commonly used NSAIDs (such as naproxen and ibuprofen) are also primarily metabolized and/or eliminated by the liver (exceptions include piroxicam).

The opioids are conjugated in the liver and >90% of the metabolites excreted renally. While most of the opioid metabolites are inactive, some (such as morphine 6-glucuronide) have analgesic activity and several (such as morphine 3-glucuronide) may be responsible for observed adverse effects (e.g., central nervous system excitation).[26] Mild elevation in transaminases should not have a significant impact on opioid dosing. Patients with severe liver failure should have their opioid doses decreased and/or dosing intervals increased.

Impaired renal excretion will reduce opioid clearance.[27] This may lead to buildup of metabolites and undesired adverse effects. Analgesia will be sustained and risk of adverse effects increased. To reduce the risk of buildup, patients receiving morphine should be well hydrated and maintain adequate urine output. If renal function is impaired, morphine doses should be decreased and dosing intervals increased. The patient with anuria may require very little or no extra morphine to maintain analgesia. Routine dosing should be discontinued.

Methadone is not renally excreted and fentanyl does not have active metabolites.

OPIOID ADVERSE EFFECTS: The common and uncommon adverse effects of opioid analgesics are listed in Table 63-4.

Common adverse effects of the opioid analgesics are easily managed.[28] In the majority of patients, pharmacological tolerance develops to all of the common adverse effects except constipation, within one to two weeks. Consequently, nausea and

TABLE 63-4. ADVERSE EFFECTS OF OPIOID ANALGESICS

Common	Uncommon
Constipation	Dysphoria/delirium
Nausea/vomiting	Bad dreams/hallucinations
Drowsiness	Pruritus/urticaria
Dry mouth	Urinary retention
Sweats	Myoclonic jerks/seizures
	Respiratory depression

vomiting may be treated expectantly with antiemetics for the short period that these symptoms are problematic. If nausea and/or vomiting persist, changing the opioid or the route of administration may resolve the problem.

Similarly, patients should be counseled that the drowsiness they experience when initiating an opioid will usually dissipate after the first week or so. Patients can often tolerate a little drowsiness if they are assured that it will not persist for the entire time they are taking opioid analgesics. In fact, once a stable dose of an opioid has been reached drowsiness will likely settle completely, and function will normalize. Most patients on a stable dose of opioid who have no adverse effects may safely drive a car. Persistent somnolence may be managed by ensuring adequate hydration and renal clearance, changing to a sustained-release product to minimize peak effects, changing the opioid, changing the route of administration, or by adding a psychostimulant (such as methylphenidate or pemoline).

As patients given opioid analgesics will not develop tolerance to constipation, they should be treated with stimulant laxatives (e.g., Senna or Bisacodyl), osmotic laxatives (e.g., magnesium salts or lactulose), or prokinetic agents (e.g., metoclopramide) on a routine basis. Simple stool softeners (e.g., sodium docusate) are usually ineffective.

Persistent adverse effects from opioids seem to be somewhat idiosyncratic to the drug and individual. Simply changing to an alternative opioid at an equianalgesic dose will often resolve the problem.

The uncommon adverse effects of the opioids are also manageable. The dysphoria and confusion that occasionally occur may be managed by ensuring adequate hydration and renal clearance (thereby minimizing metabolite buildup), lowering the opioid dose, changing the opioid analgesic, or by adding low doses of a neuroleptic drug such as haloperidol, chlorpromazine, or risperidone.

The pruritus and urticaria that occur with opioids are not immune mediated, but a nonspecific release of histamine from mast cells in the skin. This may be managed with long-acting antihistamines, doxepin 10 to 30 mg PO qhs, or by changing to an alternative opioid analgesic. True allergy presenting as bronchospasm leading to anaphylaxis is extremely rare. Most patients who report allergy have had poorly managed adverse effects (usually nausea/vomiting and/or constipation) or too much medication too fast (leading to drowsiness and/or confusion).

The risk of respiratory depression from opioid analgesics in patients with pain is frequently misunderstood. Pain is a potent stimulus to breathe and a significant stressor. While we cannot be certain of the effects of the first dose in an opioid-naive patient, patients develop pharmacological tolerance to the respiratory depressant effects of opioids over the same time course as other adverse effects. Consequently, in the patient taking opioid analgesics for any significant length of time it is difficult to demonstrate significant respiratory depression when opioids are administered to manage pain.

Too frequently opioids have been withheld or underdosed because of unsubstantiated fear of respiratory depression or the mismanagement of adverse effects. In the patient with uncontrolled pain, opioid analgesics can be judiciously but expeditiously and safely titrated until adequate relief is obtained or intolerable adverse effects encountered.

OPIOID EXCESS/OVERDOSE: In the setting of pain management, opioid excess presents first as mild drowsiness, proceeds to persistent somnolence, then to a poorly arousable state, and finally to respiratory depression. These changes may be associated with increasing restlessness, agitation, confusion, dreams, hallucinations, myoclonic jerks, or even sudden onset of seizures.

When assessing a patient for respiratory depression, it should be remembered that a respiratory rate of 8 to 12 per minute is frequently normal, particularly at night time. One should first check for arousability: the patient may be sleeping. If early, or even moderate excess is present without major compromise, the opioid can be held and normal metabolism will clear the excess opioid, particularly if the patient is adequately rehydrated. Naloxone reversal is not normally necessary.

If the patient is not arousable, has a respiratory rate less than 6 to 8 per minute or there is significant hypoxemia or hypotension present, opioid reversal with naloxone may be warranted. A 0.4 or 1.0 mg ampule of naloxone can be diluted with 10 ml of saline and 0.1 to 0.2 mg IV boluses administered every 1 to 2 minutes. SC or PO administration is not appropriate. As naloxone has a high affinity for opioid receptors, titration any faster, or with larger boluses, may precipitate opioid withdrawal that presents as an acute pain crisis, psychosis, or severe abdominal pain and precipitates pulmonary edema or even myocardial infarction. Only if several 0.1 to 0.2 mg boluses are ineffective should the bolus size be increased.

Naloxone has a high affinity for lipids and will redistribute itself into adipose tissue within 10 to 15 minutes of administration. Any improvement frequently disappears within this time frame and signs of toxicity return. Repeated naloxone dosing may be necessary to sustain the reversal until the patient has cleared sufficient of the opioid to be out of danger. If the overdose is severe and considerable naloxone is required, a continuous infusion of naloxone may be required until the crisis is over.

If a patient who has been well managed on a stable dose of opioid for some time suddenly develops signs of overdose, the opioid should be stopped and sepsis or other causes should be ruled out. It is unlikely that the opioid alone will be the cause of the "effective overdose."

ADDICTION VS. TOLERANCE: Addiction, the psychological dependence on the drug, is a vastly overrated and misunderstood consequence of using opioid analgesics.[1] In patients with chronic cancer pain, the incidence of addiction is less than 1:1,000 and is usually related to preexisting dependency. Because of its rarity, it is not listed in Table 63-1 with the other adverse effects of the opioids.

Physical dependence, meaning the development of a withdrawal syndrome upon abrupt discontinuation of the drug, is not evidence of addiction. Physical dependence occurs over the same time course as tolerance develops to the adverse effects of the opioid analgesics and is the result of changes in the numbers and function of opioid neuroreceptors in the presence of exogenous opioid.

If opioid analgesics are tapered instead of abruptly withdrawn, withdrawal symptoms do not occur. Usually the opioid dose can be reduced by 50 to 75% q2–3days without ill effect. Occasionally a small dose of a benzodiazepine (e.g., 0.5 to 1.0 mg of lorazepam) or of methadone (with its longer half-life) may be necessary to settle the feeling of slight uneasiness or restlessness that accompanies a rapid tapering process. If restlessness or agitation is anything more than very mild, the rate of tapering should be slowed.

ADJUVANT PAIN MEDICINES: Adjuvant analgesics are used to enhance the analgesic efficacy of opioids, treat concurrent symptoms that exacerbate pain, and/or provide independent analgesia for specific types of pain. They may be used at all stages of the analgesic ladder. Some of the adjuvants, such as acetaminophen, the NSAIDs, the tricyclic antidepressants, and perhaps the antiepileptics, have primary analgesic activity themselves and may be used alone or as coanalgesics.

Two cancer pain syndromes bear particular mention in this regard. Bone pain from bone metastases is thought to be, in part, prostaglandin mediated. Consequently, the NSAIDs and/or steroids may be particularly helpful in combination with opioids. Cord compression should always be considered if the pain is severe, increasing quickly, or associated with motor, bowel, or bladder dysfunction.

Neuropathic pain is rarely controlled with opioids alone. The tricyclic antidepressants, antiepileptics, and steroids are often required in combination with the opioids to achieve adequate relief. Commonly used agents are listed below with a few comments about their use.

- *NSAIDs* and/or *acetaminophen* may be added to the opioids for adjuvant analgesia, particularly when inflammatory or peripheral mechanisms are thought to be responsible for the painful stimulus.
- *Corticosteroids* provide a range of effects including anti-inflammatory activity, mood elevation, antiemetic activity, and appetite stimulation. They reduce pain both by their anti-inflammatory effect of reducing arachidonic acid release to form prostaglandins as well as decreasing swelling and pressure on nerve endings. Undesirable effects such as hyperglycemia, weight gain, myopathy, and dysphoria or psychosis may complicate prolonged therapy.[29–31]
- *Anticonvulsants* (such as gabapentin, carbamazepine, valproate, lamotrigine, clonazepam, and phenytoin) are used either alone, or in addition to opioids or other coanalgesics to manage neuropathic pain. They have been particularly advocated for neuropathic pain with a shooting or lancinating quality (such as trigeminal neuralgia or nerve root compression).[32–36]
- *Tricyclic antidepressants* (such as amitriptyline, desipramine, imipramine, and nortriptyline) are useful in pain management in general, and neuropathic pain in particular. They have innate analgesic properties and are effective through mechanisms that include enhanced inhibitory modulation of nociceptive impulses at the level of the dorsal horn. If the anticholinergic adverse effects of tertiary amine tricyclics (amitriptyline, imipramine) are undesirable or troublesome, the secondary amine tricyclics (nortriptyline, desipramine) may be effective analgesics and produce fewer adverse effects. The selective serotonin reuptake inhibitor class of antidepressants has not been shown to be useful in similar ways to the tricyclic antidepressants. Newer atypical antidepressants (such as venlafaxine) may have a role, but have not been well studied.[37,38]
- *Bisphosphonates* (such as pamidronate) and *calcitonin* have been used as adjuvant analgesics in the management of bone pain from bone metastases.[39] In cancer, bone pain is caused in large part by osteoclast-induced bone resorption rather than the direct effects of the tumor on periosteal or medullary nerve endings. Both the bisphosphonates and calcitonin inhibit osteoclast activity on bone and have been reported to reduce pain significantly in at least some patients.

Neuroleptic medications (such as haloperidol, chlorpromazine, or risperidone) and anxiolytics (such as lorazepam) are used for the management of specific psychiatric disorders that complicate pain management such as delirium, psychosis, or anxiety disorders. With the exception of methotrimeprazine and clonazepam, none have been shown to have intrinsic analgesic activity.

NMDA receptor antagonists, such as dextromethorphan, ketamine, and methadone, may affect the spinal neural circuitry that leads to a neuropathic pain state resistant to high-dose opioids.[40] Clinical studies with dextromethorphan and ketamine have shown some mild pain effects but have been significantly limited by dose-related adverse effects, particularly drowsiness. Methadone, however, is inexpensive and well tolerated. It exists as a racemic mix of levo and dextro isomers. The levo form binds at opioid receptors, while both forms can block the NMDA receptor. It is hypothesized that its NMDA receptor antagonist activity explains the variable potency observed when changing from other opioids to methadone.

Local anesthetics, such as systemic lidocaine, that are non-selective inhibitors of Na-channels have also been utilized to treat neuropathic pain.[41,42] Oral anesthetics such as mexiletine have also been used in neuropathic pain, but clinical trials to date have not been definitive. Topical lidocaine patches have been approved for use in postherpetic neuralgia. Research has identified many subtypes of Na-channels. In the future it may be possible to block a specific subset involved in mediating pain transmission.

Alpha-2-adrenergic agonists such as clonidine can also be effective adjuvant analgesics for both nociceptive and neuropathic pain.[43] They act at the level of the spinal cord in two ways. First, they act in a mechanistically similar way to the opioids. They act on the same neurons in the cord and lead to the same intracellular events but act through a different receptor. Thus, it is likely that they can enhance the nociceptive effects of opioids. Second, researchers believe alpha-2-adrenergic agonists also decrease sympathetic outflow which is involved with neuropathic pain. Clonidine can be given systemically or delivered intraspinally. Systemic delivery may be limited by the adverse effects of lethargy, dry mouth, and hypotension.

CONCLUSIONS

Although cancer pain is a prevalent and severe problem there are a multitude of effective tools to treat nociceptive, neuropathic, and mixed pain syndromes. The opioids remain the first-line therapy for moderate to severe pain. However, when unsuccessful or limited by adverse effects multiple classes of adjuvant analgesics are available to help optimize pain control. If one class alone is insufficient to control pain or is limited by adverse effects, it is rational to try combining classes. This combination may result in synergistic treatment of pain and may allow individual doses to be decreased thus lowering the risk of adverse effects. Using these guidelines and keeping in mind the concept of total pain, most cancer pain can be controlled with oral drugs.

KEY POINTS

- Successful treatment of cancer pain is possible most of the time.
- The cancer pain syndrome should be determined: nociceptive, neuropathic, or mixed.
- Cancer pain should be assessed and managed within the dimensions of suffering that a patient and his or her family experience: physical, psychological, social, and spiritual.
- Daily evaluation includes an assessment of the location, type, temporal profile, and severity of each significant pain.
- The World Health Organization's three-step approach to cancer pain management using systemic analgesics has been demonstrated to be effective at managing 90% of the pain experienced by patients worldwide.
- Opioids are essential for the management of moderate to severe cancer pain. Familiarity with each opioid's pharmacokinetics, equianalgesic dosing, adverse effects, and cost are necessary for their safe, effective, and cost-efficient use.
- Adjuvant analgesics combined with opioids will improve cancer pain control, especially in neuropathic and mixed pain syndromes.

REFERENCES

1. Jacox A, Carr DB, Payne R, et al: Management of Cancer Pain. Clinical Practice Guideline No. 9. AHCPR Publication No. 94-0592. Agency for Health Care Policy and Research, US Department of Health and Human Services, Public Health Service, Rockville, MD, March 1994.
2. Yaksh TL, Wallace MS: Advances in pain research. In Wallace MS, Dunn JS, Yaksh TL (eds): Anesthesiology Clinics of North America (Pain: Nociceptive and Neuropathic Mechanisms with Clinical Correlates). WB Saunders, Philadelphia, 1997, pp 229–234.
3. Merskey H, Bogduk N (eds): Classification of Chronic Pain, ed 2. IASP Task Force on Taxonomy. IASP Press, Seattle, 1994.
4. Yaksh TL, Chaplan SR: Physiology and pharmacology of neuropathic pain. In Wallace MS, Dunn JS, Yaksh TL (eds): Anesthesiology Clinics of North America (Pain: Nociceptive and Neuropathic Mechanisms with Clinical Correlates). WB Saunders, Philadelphia, 1997, pp 335–352.
5. Michaelis M, Habler HJ, Jaenig W: Silent afferents: A separate class of primary afferents? Clin Exp Pharmacol Physiol 23:99–105, 1996.
6. Yaksh TL: The spinal pharmacology of facilitation of afferent processing evoked by high-threshold afferent input of the postinjury pain state. Curr Opin Neurol Neurosurg 6:250–256, 1993.
7. Saunders C: Care of patients suffering from terminal illness at St. Joseph's Hospice. Nursing Mirror 14:7–10, 1964.
8. WHO: Cancer Pain Relief. ed 2. WHO, Geneva, 1996.
9. Principles of pain control in palliative care for adults. Guidance prepared by a working group of the Ethical Issues in Medicine Committee of the Royal College of Physicians. J R Coll Physicians Lond 34:350–352, 2000.
10. Hanks GW, Conno F, Cherny N, et al: Morphine and alternative opioids in cancer pain: The EAPC recommendations. Br J Cancer 84:587–593, 2001.
11. Emmanuel LL, von Gunten CF, Ferris FF (eds): Module 4: Pain management. In EPEC (Education for Physicians on End-of-Life Care). EPEC Project, Robert Wood Johnson Foundation, 1999, M4-1-35. Available at www.epec.net.
12. Raffa RB, Friderichs E, Reimann W, et al: Opioid and nonopioid components independently contribute to the mechanism of action of tramadol, an 'atypical' opioid analgesic. J Pharmacol Exp Ther 260:275–285, 1992.
13. Mitchell JR, Potter WZ: Drug metabolism in the production of liver injury. Med Clin North Am 59:877–885, 1975.
14. Carson JL, Willett LR: Toxicity of nonsteroidal anti-inflammatory drugs. An overview of the epidemiological evidence. Drugs 46(Suppl 1):243–248, 1993.
15. Peura DA: Gastrointestinal safety and tolerability of nonselective nonsteroidal anti-inflammatory agents and cyclooxygenase-2-selective inhibitors. Cleve Clin J Med 69(Suppl 1):SI31–SI39, 2002.
16. Collins SL, Faura CC, Moore RA, McQuay HJ: Peak plasma concentrations after oral morphine: A systematic review. J Pain Symptom Manage 16:388–402, 1998.
17. Stuart-Harris R, Joel SP, McDonald P, et al: The pharmacokinetics of morphine and morphine glucuronide metabolites after subcutaneous bolus injection and subcutaneous infusion of morphine. Br J Clin Pharmacol 49:207–214, 2000.
18. Du X, Skopp G, Aderjan R: The influence of the route of administration: A comparative study at steady state of oral sustained release morphine and morphine sulfate suppositories. Ther Drug Monit 21:208–214, 1999.
19. Streisand JB, Varvel JR, Stanski DR, et al: Absorption and bioavailability of oral transmucosal fentanyl citrate. Anesthesiology 75:223–229, 1991.
20. Gourlay GK, Kowalski SR, Plummer JL, et al: The transdermal administration of fentanyl in the treatment of postoperative pain: Pharmacokinetics and pharmacodynamic effects. Pain 37:193–202, 1989.
21. Levy MH: Pharmacologic treatment of cancer pain. N Engl J Med 35:1124–1132, 1996.
22. Pasternak GW: Incomplete cross tolerance and multiple mu opioid peptide receptors. Trends Pharmacol Sci 22:67–70, 2001.
23. Verebely K, Volavka J, Mule S, Resnick R: Methadone in man: Pharmacokinetic and excretion studies in acute and chronic treatment. Clin Pharmacol Ther 18:180–190, 1975.
24. Davis MP, Walsh D: Methadone for relief of cancer pain: A review of pharmacokinetics, pharmacodynamics, drug interactions and protocols of administration. Support Care Cancer 9:73–83, 2001.
25. Vigano A, Fan D, Bruera E: Individualized use of methadone and opioid rotation in the comprehensive management of cancer pain associated with poor prognostic indicators. Pain 67:115–119, 1996.
26. Pereira J, Bruera E: Emerging neuropsychiatric toxicities of opioids. J Pharm Care Pain Symptom Control 5:3–29, 1997.
27. Osborne RJ, Joel SP, Slevin ML: Morphine intoxication in renal failure: The role of morphine-6-glucuronide. BMJ 292:1548–1549, 1986.
28. O'Mahony S, Coyle N, Payne R: Current management of opioid-related side effects. Oncology (Huntingt) 15:61–73, 2001.
29. Demoly P, Chung KF: Pharmacology of corticosteroids. Respir Med 92:385–394, 1998.
30. Patten SB, Neutel CI: Corticosteroid-induced adverse psychiatric effects: Incidence, diagnosis and management. Drug Safety 22:111–122, 2000.
31. Sorensen PS, Helweg-Larsen S, Mouridsen H, et al: Effect of high-dose dexamethasone in carcinomatous metastatic spinal cord compression treated with radiotherapy: A randomised trial. Eur J Cancer 30A:22, 1994.

32. Backonja M, Beydoun A, Edwards K, et al: Gabapentin for the symptomatic treatment of painful neuropathy in patients with diabetes mellitus: A randomized controlled trial. JAMA 280:1831–1836, 1998.

33. Rowbathm M, Harden N, Stacey B, et al: Gabapentin for the treatment of postherpetic neuralgia. JAMA 280:1837–1842, 1998.

34. Caccia MR: Clonazepam in facial neuralgia and cluster headache. Clinical and electrophysiological study. Eur Neurol 13:560–563, 1975.

35. McQuay H, Carroll D, Jadad AR, et al: Anticonvulsant drugs for management of pain: A systematic review. BMJ 311:1047–1052, 1995.

36. Eisenberg E, Lurie Y, Braker C, et al: Lamotrigine reduces painful diabetic neuropathy: A randomized, controlled study. Neurology 57:505–509, 2001.

37. Max MB, Lynch SA, Muir J, et al: Effects of desipramine, amitriptyline, and fluoxetine on pain in diabetic neuropathy. N Engl J Med 326:1250–1256, 1992.

38. Tasmuth T, Hartel B, Kalso E: Venlafaxine in neuropathic pain following treatment of breast cancer. Eur J Pain 6:17–24, 2002.

39. Coleman RE: Management of bone metastases. Oncologist 5:463–470, 2000.

40. Nelson KA, Park KM, Robinovitz E, et al: High-dose oral dextromethorphan versus placebo in painful diabetic neuropathy and postherpetic neuralgia. Neurology 48:1212–1218, 1997.

41. Galer BS, Harle J, Rowbotham MC: Response to intravenous lidocaine infusion predicts subsequent response to oral mexiletine: a prospective study. J Pain Symptom Manage 12:161–167, 1996.

42. Rowbotham MC, Davies PS, Verkempinck C, Galer BS: Lidocaine patch: Double-blind controlled study of a new treatment method for post-herpetic neuralgia. Pain 65:39–44, 1996.

43. Eisenach JC, Rauck RL, Buzzanell C, Lysak SZ: Epidural clonidine analgesia for intractable cancer pain: Phase I. Anesthesiology 71:647–652, 1989.

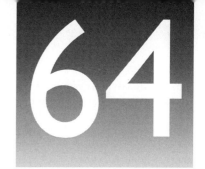

Management of Pain at End of Life

Judith A. Paice, Ph.D., R.N.

Pain is a serious problem for people with life-threatening illnesses. In studies exploring symptoms experienced near the end of life, pain, dyspnea, anxiety, and depression are common.[1–3] Cancer pain has been well characterized, representing a wide array of syndromes. These range from acute episodes related to procedures, such as bone marrow aspiration, to chronic syndromes emanating from direct tumor involvement or cancer therapies. Although it may be common during advanced disease, cancer pain can be relieved in 80% to 90% of patients.[4] Less is known about pain occurring in persons with other life threatening illnesses ordinarily seen in palliative care or hospice, such as congestive heart failure, end-stage renal disease, or neuromuscular disorders. An awareness of the most common syndromes in these populations, specific assessment techniques, as well as therapies used to treat these conditions is essential to providing relief.

Until recently experimental models that analyzed the neurobiology of pain due to cancer or other life-threatening illnesses did not exist, limiting our understanding of the unique mechanisms of these phenomena. The development of rodent models of bone pain[5] and chemotherapy-induced neuropathies[6] will provide insights into the neurobiology of cancer pain, eventually leading to the development of targeted, mechanism-based therapies. Furthermore, greater understanding of cancer pain biology may enhance knowledge related to other symptoms common in end of life care. For example, initial evidence surrounding the role of inflammatory cytokines suggests a common biological mechanism between pain, fatigue, depression, and other symptoms.[7] These investigations will be critical to complete our understanding of symptom management for those in palliative care or hospice.

PALLIATIVE CARE AND HOSPICE

All health care professionals, regardless of their specialty area, are responsible for care of the dying, and, therefore, must gain necessary knowledge and skills to care appropriately for those patients. Pain and symptom management, along with

advance care planning, are key elements of this care. Resources, such as palliative care services and hospices, are available to assist clinicians as they provide care to these patients and their families.

Palliative care is the "active total care of patients whose disease is not responsive to curative treatment. Control of pain, of other symptoms, and of psychological, social, and spiritual problems is paramount. Palliative care affirms life and regards dying as a normal process."[8] Palliative care is best integrated into the patient's care early in the course of the disease, rather than being segregated to the last days or weeks of a person's life. Palliative care is often provided through consultation services, inpatient units, outpatient clinics, day programs, and other creative models.[9]

Hospice care in the USA is a philosophy of care with similar tenets to palliative care. Goals include attention to alleviation of physical and emotional suffering, along with focus on the patient and family as the unit of care. Most hospice care in the USA is provided within the home, although a few free-standing units exist for patients unable to be cared for in the home. Hospice is reimbursed through the Medicare hospice benefit. Qualified patients must be certified as having a life expectancy of six months if the disease takes its natural course.[10]

PAINFUL SYNDROMES IN CANCER AND OTHER LIFE-THREATENING ILLNESSES

Awareness of the painful syndromes seen in those with cancer and other life-threatening illnesses promotes accurate diagnosis and management. Other chapters in this book describe a variety of pain syndromes that, although primarily seen in the general population, also may occur in people with life-threatening illnesses. However, several syndromes occur uniquely in those with cancer or other advanced diseases.

Cancer: Cancer pain syndromes can be grouped in a variety of categories: acute vs. chronic, somatic vs. neuropathic, and disease vs. treatment related[11] (see Chapter 63). Acute pain is generally due to invasive procedures, such as diagnostic or surgical interventions, and is not unlike the experience of patients with nonmalignant disease. Examples of treatment-related acute pain unique to individuals with cancer are noted in Table 64-1. Chronic pain syndromes often include involvement of bone, soft tissue, the viscera, and the nervous system. Bone metastases are common sources of pain, particularly in patients with breast, lung, or prostate cancers. Lymphedema, occurring in approximately 20% of women who undergo axillary node dissection, is an example of soft tissue pain associated with significant physical and psychological morbidity.[12] Visceral pain may arise from involvement of tumor within the liver, intestine, kidney, peritoneum, bladder, or other organs. Neuropathic pains can evolve from numerous causes, may be difficult for patients to describe, and are often complex to treat (see Table 64-2).[13–15] Finally, many people with cancer experience syndromes unrelated to the cancer or its treatment, such as osteoarthritis.

Other Life-Threatening Illnesses: The prevalence and types of pain experienced by patients with specific nonmalignant diseases at the end of life have not been fully characterized. Examples include neuropathic pain associated with multiple sclerosis, chest pain due to end-stage cardiac disease, and pain due to pressure ulcers or immobility in those who are debilitated (Table 64-3).

TABLE 64-1. ACUTE CANCER PAIN SYNDROMES

Chemotherapy
  Arthralgia and myalgia induced by paclitaxel
  Cold allodynia induced by oxaliplatin
  Headache due to methotrexate or L-aspariginase
  Mucositis commonly due to pre transplant chemotherapy regimen
  Pain due to infusion of chemotherapy into peritoneum or bladder

Growth factors
  Myalgia, bone pain, fever, headache

Hormonal therapy
  Flare syndrome (myalgia, arthralgia, and headache) in prostate or breast cancer

Immunotherapy
  Myalgia, arthralgia, and headache due to interferon

Radiation
  Bone pain flare (due to radionuclides)
  Enteritis and proctitis
  Mucositis
  Myelitis when spinal cord is irradiated

Adapted from Portenoy RK, Conn M: Cancer pain syndromes. In Bruera E, Portenoy RK (eds): Cancer Pain: Assessment and Management. Cambridge University Press, Cambridge, 2003, pp 89–108. Reprinted with the permission of Cambridge University Press.

TABLE 64-2. CHRONIC NEUROPATHIC PAIN SYNDROMES SEEN AT END OF LIFE[14,47,48]

Cancer-related
  Brachial, cervical, or sacral plexopathies
  Chemotherapy-induced neuropathy
    Cisplatin
    Oxaliplatin
    Paclitaxel
    Vincristine
    Vinblastine
  Cranial neuropathies
  Postherpetic neuropathy
  Postradiation plexopathies
  Surgical neuropathies
    Phantom pain
    Postmastectomy syndrome
    Post-thoracotomy syndrome

Noncancer causes of neuropathies
  Alcohol-induced neuropathy
  Brachial plexus avulsion (trauma)
  Carpal tunnel syndrome
  Complex regional pain syndrome
  Diabetic neuropathy
  Fabry's disease
  Failed back syndrome
  Guillain Barré
  HIV-associated neuropathy
    Viral involvement
    Antiretrovirals
  Poststroke pain
  Trigeminal neuralgia
  Vitamin deficiencies

ASSESSMENT OF PAIN AT THE END OF LIFE

The assessment techniques described in other chapters should be applied to patients with cancer or other life-threatening illnesses. Intensity, location (or often, multiple locations), quality, temporal nature of the pain, and factors that alter the pain are critical to ascertain.[11] As with all other pain syndromes, a thorough history is followed by a comprehensive physical examination, with particular emphasis on the neurological evaluation.[16] Radiographic, laboratory, and other diagnostic techniques may be indicated, although in caring for those at the end of life, treatment decisions may be made empirically to avoid uncomfortable scans or invasive procedures.

When patients are unable to verbalize or describe their pain, clinicians can use the furrowed brow as a proxy measure of pain.[17] If there is no response to adequate doses of opioids or other analgesics, additional sources of distress (e.g., distended bladder or fecal impaction) should be explored.

While the general assessment of pain is universal, several additional dimensions are critical at end of life. A psychosocial assessment is indicated, directed towards the meaning of the pain as well as the effect of pain on the patient and their caregiver

TABLE 64-3. **PAIN SYNDROMES SEEN IN PEOPLE WITH NONCANCER DIAGNOSES AT END OF LIFE**

Disorder	Pain Syndromes
Cardiovascular disease • Cardiomyopathy • Congestive heart disease • Peripheral vascular disease	• Chest pain • Ischemia
Cirrhosis	• Abdominal pain due to portal hypertension, esophageal varices
Debility	• Myalgias due to immobility • Painful pressure ulcers • Abdominal pain due to constipation, impaction • Suprapubic pain due to distended bladder
End-stage renal disease	• Painful pruritus
HIV	• Abdominal pain due to infectious gastrointestinal disorders • Chest pain from pneumocystis pneumonia • Headaches • Herpetic neuropathy • Myalgia • Neuropathies due to antiretrovirals and the virus
Neuromuscular disorders • ALS • Multiple sclerosis • Spinal cord injury	• Painful spasticity • Lower extremity dysesthesias • Periorbital pain and trigeminal neuralgia (MS)
Pulmonary disease • Emoblism • Infection • Pneumothorax	• Chest pain • Dyspnea

The findings of this assessment may suggest the need for education, to mediate fears of addiction, for example. The results of this questioning may also prompt referral to social workers, chaplains, or others who are trained to address the existential distress or suffering experienced by the patient or their family.[18,19]

Pain does not exist in isolation and symptom clusters are common, particularly at end of life. Several instruments have been designed to measure clinically multiple symptoms, including the Edmonton Symptom Assessment Scale (ESAS),[20,21] the M.D. Anderson Symptom Inventory (MDASI),[22] the Memorial Symptom Assessment Scale (MSAS),[23] and others. A recently developed tool, the Distress "Thermometer," is a vertical visual analogue scale designed to look like a thermometer, with 0 meaning "no distress" and 10 (at the top of the thermometer) indicating "extreme distress."[24] Accompanying the distress scale is a checklist of various physical, psychological, practical, family support, and spiritual/religious concerns. These are brief, clinically useful tools that quantify the intensity of a variety of symptoms common at end of life (see Table 64-4). The specific needs of people enrolled in hospice are addressed in the Brief Hospice Inventory (BHI). The BHI assesses outcomes of hospice patients, including physical and psychological symptoms, patient's perceptions of hospice care, as well as ratings of their quality of life.[25] Each statement is measured using an 11-point scale.

Benefits of these instruments include the systematic assessment of pain and other symptoms. These data inform the clinician as a treatment plan is developed, particularly when managing complex pain syndromes that occur at the end of life.

COMPLEX PAIN SYNDROMES AT END OF LIFE

The management of pain in palliative care and hospice incorporates the same analgesics, routes, and principles described in Chapter 63.[26] The majority of patients will obtain relief from these therapies or with the addition of interventional techniques. Unfortunately, a small percentage of patients will experience complex syndromes that do not respond to traditional approaches, such as bone pain, intractable neuropathic pain, or malignant bowel obstruction, or will develop severe opioid-induced toxicity.

TABLE 64-4. **PAIN AND OTHER SYMPTOM ASSESSMENT TOOLS USED IN PALLIATIVE CARE**

Assessment Tool	Description
Edmonton Symptom Assessment Scale (ESAS)	• Consists of 9 symptoms; can add 1 to individualize • Measures severity using a 0 to 10 visual analogue or numeric scales • Sum of 9 symptoms = distress • Valid and reliable[21,49] • www.palliative.org for instructions
M. D. Anderson Symptom Inventory (MDASI)	• Consists of 13 items; ranked from 0 "not present" to 10 "as bad as you can imagine" • Includes 6 interference items; ranked from 0 "did not interfere" to 10 "interfered completely" • Valid and reliable[22] • www.mdanderson.org/departments/prg
Memorial Symptom Assessment Scale (MSAS)	• Measures 32 physical and psychological symptoms using Likert scales • Evaluates prevalence, severity, and distress • Total score is average of all 32 symptoms • Valid and reliable[23,50,51] • Pediatric versions available[52,53] • www.promotingexcellence.org
Distress thermometer	• Measures distress using a vertical visual analogue designed to look like a thermometer • 0 indicates "no distress" and 10 (at the top of the thermometer) indicates "extreme distress" • Includes a checklist of physical, psychological, practical, family support, and spiritual/religious concerns • www.nccn.org

Bone Pain: Bone pain is often difficult to treat, in that patients may obtain good relief of movement associated pain from higher-dose opioid therapy, yet will be extremely sedated when they stop moving or placing pressure on the bone. Patients at risk include those with cancers that frequently metastasize to bone, including breast, lung, prostate, or multiple myeloma.[5] Table 64-5 lists treatment options.

Intractable Neuropathic Pain: Neuropathies can be difficult to treat. Standard therapies include opioids and adjuvant analgesics, including corticosteroids (see Table 64-5).[16,27] Additionally, nerve blocks and other interventional techniques can be useful.[28] In more refractory cases intravenous lidocaine infusions are used to treat intractable pain.[29] Using techniques and protocols originating from pain clinics, intravenous lidocaine 1 to 2 mg/kg is given over 15 to 30 minutes. If effective, a continuous infusion of 1 to 2 mg/kg/hour is started. The analgesic effects can be as prolonged as weeks of relief. Perioral numbness is an early warning sign of potential toxicity. Hepatic dysfunction and significant cardiac conduction abnormalities are relative contraindications to the treatment, viewed in balance with the patient's goals of care and prognosis.

Malignant Bowel Obstruction: Bowel obstruction is common in progressive gynecologic and colorectal malignancies.

The majority of patients with bowel obstruction will die within 6 months. Palliation can include surgery in selected cases, or, more commonly, intravenous or subcutaneous octreotide, nasogastric tube suction, and venting gastrostomy, in addition to analgesics and antiemetics.[30] Table 64-5 lists specific treatment options.

Opioid Neurotoxicity: The neuroexcitatory effects of opioids include myoclonus, hyperalgesia, delirium, and grand mal seizures. These toxicities have been reported in association with morphine, hydromorphone, hydrocodone, fentanyl, and methadone.[31,32] The 3-glucuronide metabolites are implicated as contributing to these neuroexcitatory effects.[33] Both morphine-3-glucuronide (M3G) and hydromorphone-3-glucuronide (H3G) are believed to produce myoclonus and seizures.[34] Renal failure appears to be a significant risk factor, as patients are unable to clear the metabolite.[35] Case reports suggest that H3G plasma levels are greatly increased in the presence of renal failure, with the ratio of H3G to parent compound four times higher than the ratio seen in patients with normal renal function.[35]

The treatment of mild myoclonus generally includes switching to another opioid, lowering the dose of the opioid, and adding a benzodiazepine. Clonazepam 0.5 mg orally twice daily with upward titration may be effective. If the patient is

TABLE 64-5. **MANAGEMENT OF COMPLEX PAIN SYNDROMES AT END OF LIFE**

Malignant bone pain[5,54,55]
Dexamethasone 8–20 mg PO, IV, SQ every morning (not to be used in conjunction with NSAIDs)
Opioids
Bisphosphonates such as pamidronate or zoledronic acid
Radiation therapy (may be given as single fraction in some cases)
Radionuclides such as strontium-89
Orthotics for braces or slings
Physical or occupational therapy for assistive devices

Intractable neuropathic pain[16,27,29,47,56,57]
Dexamethasone 8–20 mg PO, IV, SQ every morning (not to be used in conjunction with NSAIDs)
Opioids can be effective but higher doses are indicated (methadone may provide additional benefit over other opioids)
Anticonvulsants
Tricyclic antidepressants, including novel or atypical agents such as venlafaxine
Local anesthetics (e.g., LidoDerm patch, intraspinal infusions in combinations with opioids, or parenteral infusions)

Malignant intestinal obstruction[30]
Dexamethasone 8–20 mg PO, IV, SQ every morning to reduce inflammation and nausea (not to be used in conjunction with NSAIDs)
Opioids
Octreotide 20 µg/hour IV or SQ to decrease intestinal secretions; increase dose as needed
Scopolamine transdermal patches (1.5 mg, up to 2 patches) may reduce secretions
Nasogastric tube or venting gastrostomy if consistent with patient goals

NSAIDs, nonsteroidal anti-inflammatory drugs.

unable to swallow, midazolam or lorazepam may be used. Hyperalgesia frequently is misdiagnosed and the first response by well-meaning clinicians often is to increase the opioid dose. This generally results in greater pain, with potential progression to delirium and possibly seizures.

When these more severe neurotoxicities occur, the opioid dose should be reduced by at least 50%. Some advocate stopping the opioid altogether, since the half-life of these metabolites is long and the patient is unlikely to experience the abstinence syndrome.[36] Naloxone appears to be ineffective in reversing this toxicity. Should seizures occur, first- and second-line therapies include phenytoin and benzodiazepines, such as diazepam or lorazepam.[37] In some cases the seizures will progress in frequency and intensity, advancing to status epilepticus.[38] Refractory status epilepticus treatment may require midazolam, barbiturates, and propofol.[39]

- Midazolam is particularly useful in palliative care due to its rapid onset and short duration, as well as its ability to be given subcutaneously, intravenously, orally, bucally, sublingually, or rectally. Furthermore, its only known drug incompatibility is with corticosteroids, particularly betamethasone, dexamethasone, and methylprednisolone.[39]
- The standard dose of phenobarbital in the management of seizures is 20 mg/kg intravenous infusion, with a maximum rate of 50 to 100 mg/minute.
- The recommended dose of propofol to treat refractory status epilepticus is 1 to 2 mg/kg via intravenous injection over 5 minutes and repeated if necessary. A maintenance intravenous infusion of 2 to 10 mg/kg per hour is then

started, using the lowest dose needed to suppress seizure activity.[39]

OTHER SYMPTOMS COMMON AT END OF LIFE

Dyspnea, anxiety, depression, and other symptoms are common in the face of advanced illness. Palliation of these symptoms, which are frequently linked with pain, can result in improved pain control and enhanced quality of life.

Dyspnea: Dyspnea, or air hunger, can occur as a result of a variety of illnesses, including cancer, congestive heart failure, or pulmonary diseases.[2] Opioids are the first drug of choice, often in small doses that do not cause sedation.[40] Short-acting anxiolytics are indicated in the face of severe anxiety. Simple measures such as bedside fans can provide additional comfort.

Anxiety: Anxiety is highly correlated with unrelieved pain.[41] Additionally, many medications commonly used in palliative care, such as corticosteroids, neuroleptics (including metoclopramide), bronchodilators, antihistamines, digitalis, and occasionally benzodiazepines (which can cause a paradoxical reaction in elderly patients), can result in motor restlessness and agitation. Abrupt withdrawal from alcohol, opioids, benzodiazepines, and nicotine also produce agitation. Hypoxia, pulmonary embolus, sepsis, hypoglycemia, thyroid abnormalities, and heart failure are associated with anxiety, as are certain tumors, including pheochromocytomas, and some pancreatic cancers. Primary or metastatic lung cancers and chronic cardiopulmonary conditions can lead to dyspnea, which can also produce anxiety.

Pharmacologic treatment of anxiety usually consists of benzodiazepines, particularly lorazepam as it has a short duration of action and produces fewer adverse effects. A typical initial dosage is 0.5 to 2 mg orally 3 or 4 times daily. Lorazepam can be placed sublingually, which is useful when patients have difficulty swallowing, or given parenterally as a bolus or infusion. Haloperidol is frequently used for short-term management of severe anxiety and as an antipsychotic, with initial dosage starting at 0.5 to 1 mg orally twice daily.[41] Frank discussion of patients' fears in a supportive environment, along with the use of relaxation strategies, such as audiotapes, breathing exercises, and guided imagery, may alleviate anxiety.[42]

Depression: Depression is often poorly recognized in people at end of life.[43] Diagnosis may be difficult in advanced disease, as the usual physical symptoms of depression (fatigue, anorexia, and sleep disturbance) can result from the disease itself or its treatment. Psychological symptoms suggestive of depression in the patient with life-threatening illness include loss of self-worth, unremitting sadness and hopelessness, and suicidal ideation. There is evidence that a simple screening question "Are you depressed?" or "Are you sad?" is the most valid measure of a patient's depression.[44] Supportive psychotherapy may be of benefit, although limited life span may be a barrier. Antidepressant medications, such as serotonin specific reuptake inhibitors (SSRIs), e.g., citalopram, fluoxetine, paroxetine, and sertraline, are usually well tolerated. However, the two to four weeks required for the drug to take effect is often too long for patients with advanced disease and a very short life span. Newer, "atypical antidepressants" (bupropion, mirtazepine, and venlafaxine) have a relatively rapid onset of action and few reported side effects. However, for patients with a very limited lifespan, stimulants such as methylphenidate and pemoline provide rapid relief, usually within hours to days.[45,46]

CONCLUSION

Pain, dyspnea, anxiety, and depression are serious symptoms experienced by people with life-threatening illnesses. All health care professionals are responsible for care of the dying, and, therefore, must be aware of the most common syndromes occurring in this population, able to conduct specific assessment techniques, and knowledgeable about the therapies used to treat these symptoms. Resources, such as palliative care services and hospices, can assist physicians as they provide care to these patients and their families.

KEY POINTS

- All physicians, regardless of specialty, are responsible for care of patients with life-threatening illnesses.
- Assessment of pain and other symptoms at end of life requires knowledge of common syndromes, as well as skill to conduct a thorough history and physical examination, with particular attention to the neurological evaluation.
- Complex pain syndromes require novel drug therapies, in addition to standard nonopioid, opioid, and adjuvant analgesics.
- Adequate pain control in those with life-threatening illness requires attention to related symptoms such as dyspnea, anxiety, and depression.

REFERENCES

1. Desbiens NA, Wu AW: Pain and suffering in seriously ill hospitalized patients. J Am Geriatrics Soc 48(Suppl 5):S183–S186, 2000.
2. Potter J, Hami F, Bryan T, et al: Symptoms in 400 patients referred to palliative care services: Prevalence and patterns. Palliat Med 17:310–314, 2003.
3. Ng K, von Gunten CF: Symptoms and attitudes of 100 consecutive patients admitted to an acute hospice/palliative care unit. J Pain Symptom Manage 16:307–316, 1998.
4. WHO expert committee: Cancer Pain Relief and Palliative Care, ed 2. World Health Organization, Geneva, 1996.
5. Clohisy DR, Mantyh PW: Bone cancer pain. Cancer 97 (Suppl 3):866–873, 2003.
6. Polomano RC, Mannes AJ, Clark US, et al: A painful peripheral neuropathy in the rat produced by the chemotherapeutic drug, paclitaxel. Pain 94:293–304, 2001.
7. Cleeland CS, Bennett GJ, Dantzer R, et al: Are the symptoms of cancer and cancer treatment due to a shared biologic mechanism? A cytokine-immunologic model of cancer symptoms. Cancer 97:2919–2925, 2003.
8. WHO: Cancer Pain Relief and Palliative Care. World Health Organization, Geneva, 1990.
9. Bosanquest N, Salisbury S: Providing a Palliative Care Service: Towards an Evidence Base. Oxford University Press, Oxford, 1999.
10. Field MJ, Cassel CK, Institute of Medicine Committee on Care at End of Life: Approaching Death: Improving Care at the End of Life. National Academy Press, Washington, DC, 1997.
11. Cherny N, Portenoy R: Cancer pain: Principles of assessment and syndromes. In Wall P, Melzack R (eds): Textbook of Pain, ed 4. Churchill Livingstone, Edinburgh, 1999, pp 1017–1064.
12. Ververs JM, Roumen RM, Vingerhoets AJ, et al: Risk, severity and predictors of physical and psychological morbidity after axillary lymph node dissection for breast cancer. Eur J Cancer 37: 991–999, 2001.
13. Backonja M-M: Painful neuropathies. In Loeser J, Butler S, Chapman C, Turk D (eds): Bonica's Management of Pain, ed 3. Lippincott Williams & Wilkins, Philadelphia, 2001, pp 371–387.
14. Portenoy RK, Conn M: Cancer pain syndromes. In Bruera E, Portenoy RK (eds): Cancer Pain: Assessment and Management. Cambridge University Press, Cambridge, 2003, pp 89–108.
15. Bruera E, Kim HN: Cancer pain. JAMA 290:2476–2479, 2003.
16. Dworkin RH, Backonja M, Rowbotham MC, et al: Advances in neuropathic pain: Diagnosis, mechanisms, and treatment recommendations [see comment]. Arch Neurol 60:1524–1534, 2003.
17. Education for Physicians on End-of-life care: Available at www.epec.net.
18. Chang VT, Hwang SS, Feuerman M, et al: Symptom and quality of life survey of medical oncology patients at a veterans affairs medical center: A role for symptom assessment. Cancer 88:1175–1183, 2000.
19. Cherny NI, Coyle N, Foley KM: Suffering in the advanced cancer patient: A definition and taxonomy. J Palliat Care 10:57–70, 1994.
20. Bruera E, Schoeller T, Wenk R, et al: A prospective multicenter assessment of the Edmonton staging system for cancer pain. J Pain Symptom Manage 10:348–355, 1995.
21. Chang VT, Hwang SS, Feuerman M: Validation of the Edmonton Symptom Assessment Scale. Cancer 88:2164–2171, 2000.
22. Cleeland CS, Mendoza TR, Wang XS, et al: Assessing symptom distress in cancer patients: The M.D. Anderson Symptom Inventory. Cancer 89:1634–1646, 2000.
23. Portenoy RK, Thaler HT, Kornblith AB, et al: The Memorial Symptom Assessment Scale: An instrument for the evaluation of symptom prevalence, characteristics and distress. Eur J Cancer 30A:1326–1336, 1994.

24. Holland JC, Jacobsen PB, Riba MB, et al: NCCN: Distress management. Cancer Control 8(6 Suppl 2):88–93, 2001.

25. Guo H, Fine PG, Mendoza TR, et al: A preliminary study of the utility of the brief hospice inventory. J Pain Symptom Manage 22:637–648, 2001.

26. American Pain Society: Principles of Analgesic Use in the Treatment of Acute Pain and Cancer Pain, ed 5. American Pain Society, Glenview, IL, 2003.

27. Farrar JT, Portenoy RK: Neuropathic cancer pain: The role of adjuvant analgesics. Oncology (Huntington) 15:1435–1442, 2001.

28. Furlan AD, Lui PW, Mailis A: Chemical sympathectomy for neuropathic pain: Does it work? Case report and systematic literature review. Clin J Pain 17:327–336, 2001.

29. Ferrini R, Paice JA: Infusional lidocaine for severe and/or neuropathic pain. J Support Oncol 2:90–94, 2004.

30. Randall TC, Rubin SC: Management of intestinal obstruction in the patient with ovarian cancer. Oncology (Huntington) 14:1159–1163, 2000.

31. Han PK, Arnold R, Bond G, et al: Myoclonus secondary to withdrawal from transdermal fentanyl: Case report and literature review. J Pain Symptom Manage 23:66–72, 2002.

32. Sarhill N, Davis MP, Walsh D, et al: Methadone-induced myoclonus in advanced cancer. Am J Hospice Palliat Care 18:51–53, 2001.

33. Wright AW, Mather LE, Smith MT: Hydromorphone-3-glucuronide: A more potent neuro-excitant than its structural analogue, morphine-3-glucuronide. Life Sci 69:409–420, 2001.

34. Smith MT: Neuroexcitatory effects of morphine and hydromorphone: Evidence implicating the 3-glucuronide metabolites. Clin Exper Pharmacol Physiol 27:524–528, 2000.

35. Lee MA, Leng ME, Tiernan EJ: Retrospective study of the use of hydromorphone in palliative care patients with normal and abnormal urea and creatinine. Palliat Med 15:26–34, 2001.

36. EPERC: Fast Fact and Concept #58: Neuroexcitatory effects of opioids: Treatment. www.eperc.mcw.edu, 2003.

37. Chang BS, Lowenstein DH: Epilepsy. N Engl J Med 349:1257–1266, 2003.

38. Lowenstein DH, Alldredge BK: Status epilepticus. N Engl J Med 338:970–976, 1998.

39. Golf M, Paice JA, Feulner E, et al: Refractory status epilepticus. J Palliat Med 7:85–88, 2004.

40. Thomas JR, von Gunten CF: Clinical management of dyspnoea. Lancet Oncol 3:223–228, 2002.

41. Payne DK, Massie MJ: Anxiety in palliative care. In Chochinov HM, Breitbart W (eds): Handbook of Psychiatry in Palliative Medicine. Oxford University Press, New York, 2000, pp 63–74.

42. Buckman R: Communication in palliative care: A practical guide. In Doyle D, Hanks GWC, MacDonald N (eds): Oxford Textbook of Palliative Medicine, ed 2. Oxford University Press, New York, 1998.

43. Pirl WF, Roth AJ: Diagnosis and treatment of depression in cancer patients. Oncology (Huntington) 13:1293–1301, 1999.

44. Chochinov HM, Wilson KG, Enns M, Lander S: "Are you depressed?" Screening for depression in the terminally ill. Am J Psychiatry 154:674–676, 1997.

45. Bruera E, Driver L, Barnes EA, et al: Patient-controlled methylphenidate for the management of fatigue in patients with advanced cancer: A preliminary report. J Clin Oncol 21:4439–4443, 2003.

46. Breitbart W, Rosenfeld B, Kaim M, et al: A randomized, double-blind, placebo-controlled trial of psychostimulants for the treatment of fatigue in ambulatory patients with human immunodeficiency virus disease. Arch Intern Med 161:411–420, 2001.

47. Paice J: Mechanisms and management of neuropathic pain in cancer. J Support Oncol 1:107–120, 2003.

48. Mendell JR, Sahenk Z: Clinical practice. Painful sensory neuropathy [see comment]. N Engl J Med 348:1243–1255, 2003.

49. Rees E, Hardy J, Ling J, et al: The use of the Edmonton Symptom Assessment Scale (ESAS) within a palliative care unit in the UK. Palliat Med 12:75–82, 1998.

50. Hwang SS, Chang VT, Fairclough DL, et al: Longitudinal quality of life in advanced cancer patients: Pilot study results from a VA medical cancer center [see comment]. J Pain Symptom Manage 25:225–235, 2003.

51. Chang VT, Hwang SS, Feuerman M, et al: The Memorial Symptom Assessment Scale short form (MSAS-SF). Cancer 89:1162–1171, 2000.

52. Collins JJ, Byrnes ME, Dunkel IJ, et al: The measurement of symptoms in children with cancer. J Pain Symptom Manage 19:363–377, 2000.

53. Collins JJ, Devine TD, Dick GS, et al: The measurement of symptoms in young children with cancer: The validation of the Memorial Symptom Assessment Scale in children aged 7–12. J Pain Symptom Manage 23:10–16, 2002.

54. Berenson JR: Zoledronic acid in cancer patients with bone metastases: Results of phase I and II trials. Semin Oncol 28 (2 Suppl 6):25–34, 2001.

55. Jeremic B: Single fraction external beam radiation therapy in the treatment of localized metastatic bone pain. A review. J Pain Symptom Manage 22:1048–1058, 2001.

56. Rowbotham MC, Twilling L, Davies PS, et al: Oral opioid therapy for chronic peripheral and central neuropathic pain. N Engl J Med 348:1223–1232, 2003.

57. Tasmuth T, Hartel B, Kalso E: Venlafaxine in neuropathic pain following treatment of breast cancer. Eur J Pain 6:17–24, 2002.

Neurolytic Visceral Sympathetic Blocks

Celiac Plexus Block, Superior Hypogastric Block, Ganglion Impar Block

Oscar de Leon-Casasola, M.D.,
Robert E. Molloy, M.D., and
Mark Lema, M.D., Ph.D.

Pain associated with cancer may be somatic, visceral, and neuropathic in origin and about 50% of all cancer patients have a combination of pain types at the time of diagnosis. When visceral structures are stretched, compressed, invaded, or distended, a poorly localized noxious pain is reported. Patients experiencing visceral pain often describe the pain as vague, deep, squeezing, crampy, or colicky in nature. Other signs and symptoms include referred pain, such as shoulder pain that appears when the diaphragm is invaded with tumor, and nausea/vomiting.

Visceral pain associated with cancer may be relieved with oral pharmacologic therapy that includes combinations of nonsteroidal anti-inflammatory agents, opioids, and coadjuvant therapy. Neurolytic blocks of the sympathetic axis are also extremely effective in controlling visceral cancer pain. Thus, neurolysis of the sympathetic axis should be judged as an important adjunct to pharmacologic therapy for the relief of severe pain experienced by cancer patients. As such, these blocks can rarely eliminate cancer pain, because patients also frequently experience coexisting somatic and neuropathic pain. Thus, oral pharmacologic therapy must be continued albeit at lower doses. The goal of performing a neurolytic block of the sympathetic axis is to (1) maximize the analgesic effect of opioid and nonopioid analgesics and (2) reduce the dosage of these agents to alleviate untoward side effects.

Neurolytic techniques have a narrow risk–benefit ratio. Thus, sound clinical judgment and complete patient understanding are essential to minimize undesirable effects. The detailed description of the techniques for these blocks is beyond the scope of this review. Thus, the reader is directed to other publications for this purpose.[1]

INTERPLEURAL PHENOL BLOCK

The role of interpleural analgesia (IPA) in both acute and chronic pain management is still undergoing clinical scrutiny. Original work with this technique showed that IPA could provide analgesia in patients with subcostal incisions and fractured ribs.[2,3]

The technique for insertion of an interpleural catheter is relatively easy, and an epidural tray can be utilized. Local anesthetics (0.5% bupivacaine or 2% lidocaine) have been traditionally utilized via intermittent bolus or a continuous infusion. Recently, interpleural phenol[4] has been described as an alternative for the treatment of visceral pain associated with esophageal cancer. Unpublished data suggest that this is an effective technique to treat visceral pain associated with cancer of the esophagus, liver, biliary tree, stomach, and pancreas. A multicenter study is under way to determine the efficacy of this block in the treatment of pain associated with the above-mentioned malignancies.[5]

Drugs and Dosing: For neurolytic blocks the utilization of increasing concentrations of phenol is recommended. Since patients with cancer of the esophagus or the chest wall frequently exhibit pleural effusions, several injections through a catheter are indicated. Initially, 10 mL of 6% phenol is recommended; and progressive increase up to 10% according to the results is encouraged, because the pleural effusion acts as a diluting agent. However, further experience with patients with pleural effusions suggests that administration of 5 to 10 mL of 6% phenol will render adequate results.[5]

For analgesia associated with cancer, a continuous infusion of 0.25% to 0.375% bupivacaine (8 to 10 mL/hour) or intermittent bolus doses of 0.5% bupivacaine (10 to 15 mL every 8 hours) also provide adequate analgesia. However, if the 0.5% concentration of bupivacaine is chosen, the risk of toxicity is higher. Thus, the use of 0.375% to 0.5% ropivacaine for a continuous infusion, and 0.5% ropivacaine for intermittent bolus dosing, 10 to 15 mL every 8 hours, may be a better choice in these patients.

Technique: The key to a successful analgesic response is proper patient positioning. For all blocks except multiple intercostal rib blocks sparing the thoracic sympathetic chain, the patient should be positioned with the affected side up. Since the block sets up by mass action, delivery of the agent is by gravity to thoracic spinal nerves emanating from the paravertebral area. The patient is turned to an oblique position, with the side to be blocked uppermost. The operator stands to face the patient's back. The head may be placed up or down 20° depending on the area to be blocked, to facilitate the spread of the injectate by gravity. For upper abdominal visceral pain, and for sympathetic block of pain originating from the upper abdominal viscera, the patient can be placed in a sitting position. The block is then performed on the left side for pancreatic, gastric, or splenic pain and on the right side for hepatic pain.

Once the patient is positioned properly and supported by a pillow, a skin wheal is raised immediately superior to the eighth rib in the seventh intercostal space, approximately 8 to 10 cm lateral to the midline. If a continuous technique is selected, a needle allowing passage of a catheter (often epidural) is selected. If a single injection technique is used, then a short beveled needle of sufficient length is used. The epidural needle is inserted perpendicular to the skin over the eighth rib and walked cephalad until contact with the superior edge of the rib is lost. Before slowly advancing the needle further, a syringe containing approximately 2 mL of saline is attached, and then entry into the pleural space is identified using a passive loss of resistance technique. When the needle tip is in the pleural space, the syringe plunger and contained saline are pulled down by the negative interpleural pressure, and injection will be easy. If a catheter is used, it should be threaded approximately 10 cm into the pleural space, taking care to reduce air entrained through the needle.

Complications: Complications from this procedure can be divided into two categories, those produced by traumatic injuries of either the needle or the catheter and those produced by the neurolytic agent injected in the interpleural space. Thus, pneumothorax may occur in 2% of patients,[6] and lung injury has been reported when a rigid catheter is utilized.[7] Phrenic nerve palsy resulting in respiratory failure may also occur following this block. Thus, bilateral blocks should be avoided.

Systemic effects from drug absorption may also occur since the pleural membranes are highly vascularized. Thus, we limit the doses of phenol to 10 mL of a 10% solution.

Efficacy: There is no outcome information to determine the efficacy of this block for the treatment of visceral pain. The published experienced with this block is limited to a case report, and the effects in a large population have not been reported.

CELIAC PLEXUS BLOCK

The celiac plexus is situated retroperitoneally in the upper abdomen. It is at the level of the T12 and L1 vertebrae, anterior to the crura of the diaphragm. It surrounds the abdominal aorta and the celiac and superior mesenteric arteries. The plexus continues inferiorly to form the superior and the inferior mesenteric plexus.

The celiac plexus is composed of a network of nerve fibers, both from the sympathetic and parasympathetic systems. It contains one to five large ganglia, which receive sympathetic fibers from the three splanchnic nerves (greater, lesser, and least). The thoracic splanchnic nerves lie above and posterior to the diaphragm, anterior to the T12 vertebra. The celiac plexus also receives parasympathetic fibers from the vagus nerve.

Autonomic supply to the liver, pancreas, gallbladder, stomach, spleen, kidneys, intestines, and adrenal glands, as well as to the blood vessels, arises in the celiac plexus.

Indications: Neurolytic blocks of the celiac plexus have been used for malignant and chronic nonmalignant pain. In patients with acute or chronic pancreatitis it has been used with significant success.[8] Likewise, patients with cancer in the upper abdomen who have a significant visceral pain component have responded well to this block.[9]

Technique: There are multiple posterior percutaneous approaches to block nociceptive impulses from the viscera of the upper abdomen. These include the classic retrocrural approach, block of the splanchnic nerves, the anterocrural (or transcrural) approach, and the transaortic approach. With the common posterior approaches, the two needles are inserted at the level of the first lumbar vertebra, 5 to 7 cm from the midline. The tip of the needle is then directed towards the body of L1 for the retrocrural and anterocrural approaches and to the body of T12 for neurolysis of the splanchnic nerves. The left needle is positioned just posterior to the aorta and the right needle is advanced 1 cm deeper with a retrocrural or splanchnic nerve approach. Fluoroscopy reveals spread of contrast above the diaphragm and anterior to the vertebral body. The needles must be advanced through the diaphragm using the anterocrural approach. This is relatively easy on the right side, but more difficult on the left side, because of the position of the aorta. Two solutions have been described, confirmation with computed tomography (CT) scan[10] and use of a single-needle, transaortic injection on the left side.[11] The left needle is inserted closer to the midline and placed anterolateral to the aorta with CT scan, or into and through the aorta with the transaortic approach. Figures 65-1 to 65-4 illustrate the final position of the needles and the expected spread of contrast medium after successful placement. More recently, CT[12] and ultrasound[13] techniques have allowed pain specialists to perform neurolysis of the celiac plexus via a transabdominal approach. This approach is frequently used when patients are not able to tolerate either the prone or lateral decubitus position, or when the liver is so enlarged that a posterior approach is not feasible.

Drug and Dosing: For neurolytic blocks, 50% to 100% alcohol, 20 mL per side, is utilized. When injected by itself, alcohol can produce severe pain. Thus, it is recommended to first inject 5 to 10 mL of 0.25% bupivacaine 5 minutes

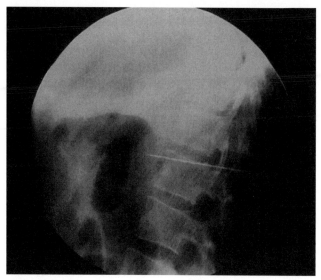

FIGURE 65-1. Lateral radiograph showing placement of the needle tip 1.0 to 1.5 cm anterior to the body of the L1 vertebra.

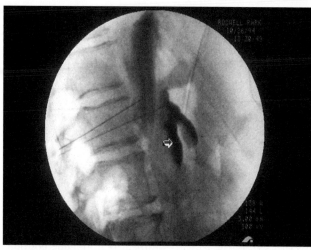

FIGURE 65-3. Lateral radiograph showing that spread of contrast through the right-sided needle is anterior to the aorta, while spread from the left needle travels cephalad, above and posterior to the diaphragm. (Same patient as in Fig. 65-2.)

prior to the injection of alcohol, or to dilute 100% alcohol by 50% with local anesthetic (0.25% bupivacaine). Phenol in a 10% final concentration may also be used, and it has the advantage of being painless on injection. Both agents appear to have the same efficacy.

Complications: Complications associated with celiac plexus blocks appear to be related to the technique used: retrocrural, transcrural,[10,14] or transaortic.[11] In a prospective, randomized study of 61 patients with cancer of the pancreas, Ischia et al.[9] compared the efficacy and the incidence of complications associated with three different approaches to celiac plexus neurolysis. Orthostatic hypotension was more frequent in patients who had a retrocrural (50%) or splanchnic nerve block technique (52%) than those who underwent an anterocrural approach

(10%). In contrast, transient diarrhea was more frequent in patients who had an anterocrural approach (65%) than those having a splanchnic nerve block technique (5%), but not the retrocrural approach (25%). The incidence of dysesthesia, interscapular back pain, reactive pleurisy, hiccoughing, or hematuria was not statistically different among the three groups.

The incidence of complications from neurolytic celiac plexus blocks was recently determined by Davis[15] in 2,730 patients having blocks performed from 1986 to 1990. The overall incidence of major complications, such as paraplegia and bladder and bowel dysfunction, was 1 in 683 procedures. However, the report does not describe which approach or approaches were utilized for the performance of the blocks.

Important aspects in the diagnosis and management of specific complications include:

1. Malposition of the needle should always be ruled out with radiologic imaging prior to the injection of a neurolytic

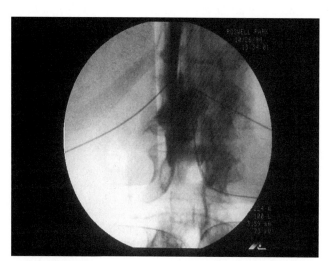

FIGURE 65-2. Posteroanterior radiograph showing bilateral caudad spread of contrast medium through the right-sided needle, which is anterocrural, and unilateral cephalad spread through the needle on the left side, which is retrocrural. (See also Fig. 65-3.)

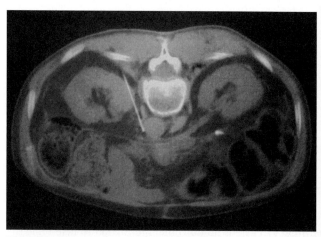

FIGURE 65-4. Computed tomographic (CT) scan showing the needle adjacent to the lateral wall of the aorta, anterior to the crura of the diaphragm.

agent, as the needle's tip may be intravascular, in the peritoneal cavity, or in a viscus. Imaging techniques currently used include biplanar fluoroscopy, CT, or ultrasound guidance. However, no study has evaluated the superiority of one technique over the others. Wong and Brown[16] suggested that the use of radiologic imaging does not alter the quality of the block or the incidence of complications based on a retrospective study of 136 patients with pancreatic cancer pain treated with a celiac plexus block with or without radiologic control of the position of the needle's tip. However, it is not clear how many of those patients had radiologic imaging. Assuming that half of the patients did not, the upper 95% confidence limit for complications is 5%.[17]

2. Orthostatic hypotension may occur in 1% to 3% of patients after the block for up to 5 days. Treatment includes bed rest, avoidance of sudden changes in position, and fluid replacement. Once compensatory vascular reflexes are fully activated, this side effect disappears. Wrapping of the lower extremities from the toe to the upper thighs with elastic bandages has been used with success in patients who developed orthostatic hypotension and needed to ambulate during the first week after the block.

3. Backache may result from: (a) local trauma during the needle placement resulting in a retroperitoneal hematoma, (b) alcohol irritation of the retroperitoneal structures, or (c) injury to the lumbar plexus. Patients with a backache should have at least two hematocrit measurements at a one-hour interval. If there is a decrease in the hematocrit, radiologic imaging is indicated to rule out a retroperitoneal hematoma. A urine analysis positive for red cells suggests renal injury.

4. Retroperitoneal hemorrhage is rare but has also been reported. Thus, in patients who present with orthostatic hypotension, one must rule out hemorrhage before assuming that it is a physiologic response to the block. Patients who present with backache and orthostatic hypotension after a celiac plexus block should be admitted to the hospital for serial hematocrit monitoring. If a low or a decreasing hematocrit is demonstrated, patients should undergo radiologic evaluation to rule out injury to the kidneys, the aorta, or other vascular structures. A surgical consult should be obtained as soon as feasible.

5. Diarrhea may occur due to sympathetic block of the bowel. Treatment includes hydration and antidiarrheal agents. Oral loperamide is a good choice, although any anticholinergic may be used. Matson et al.[18] have reported near-fatal dehydration from diarrhea after this block. Thus, in debilitated patients, diarrhea must be treated aggressively.

6. Abdominal aortic dissection has also been reported.[19,20] The mechanism of aortic injury is direct damage with the needle during the performance of the block. As expected, the anterocrural approach is more frequently associated with this complication. Thus, if there were evidence of atherosclerotic disease of the abdominal aorta, it would seem appropriate to avoid this approach.

7. Paraplegia and transient motor paralysis have occurred after celiac plexus block.[21–27] Current thinking is that these neurologic complications may occur due to spasm of the lumbar segmental arteries that perfuse the spinal cord.[27] In fact, canine lumbar arteries undergo sustained contraction when exposed to both alcohol and phenol.[28] The magnitude of the response to phenol was directly related to concentration, while the alcohol-induced response was inversely related to concentration. Low concentrations of ethanol produce significant contractile effects in human aortic smooth muscle cells by increasing the intracellular concentration of ionized calcium.[29] Thus, it may be empirically suggested that alcohol should not be used if there is evidence of significant atherosclerotic disease of the aorta, suggesting that the circulation to the spinal cord may also be impaired. However, there is also a report of paraplegia after phenol use,[21] suggesting that other factors, such as direct vascular or neurologic injury or retrograde spread to the spinal cord, may come into play. These complications further support the use of radiologic imaging during the performance of the block.

Efficacy: There are only three randomized controlled trials[9,30,31] and one prospective study[32] evaluating the efficacy of celiac plexus neurolysis in pain due to cancer of the upper abdomen. One of the studies evaluated the efficacy of three different approaches to celiac plexus neurolysis in pancreatic cancer in a prospective, randomized fashion.[9] In this study 48% (29 of 61 patients) experienced *complete* pain relief after the neurolytic block, while 52% (32 of 61 patients) required further therapy for residual visceral pain. This was attributed to technical failure in 15 patients (20%) and to neuropathic/somatic pains in 17 patients (28%). The second study[30] compared the procedure with oral pharmacologic therapy in 20 patients. The author concluded that celiac plexus neurolysis resulted in an equal reduction in visual analogue pain scores as therapy with a nonsteroidal anti-inflammatory drug (NSAID)–opioid combination. However, opioid consumption was significantly lower in the group of patients who underwent neurolysis, when compared to the group receiving oral pharmacologic therapy, during the 7 weeks of the study. Moreover, the incidence of side effects was greater in the group of patients receiving oral pharmacologic therapy when compared to those in the block group. The third randomized controlled trial[31] also compared the procedure with drug therapy in 24 patients. Celiac plexus block was associated with better short-term pain relief, and transient diarrhea and hypotension. There were no persistent analgesia benefits when compared to the patients using drug therapy alone, but the block patients had lower analgesic consumption and fewer side effects such as nausea, vomiting, and constipation.

In the other prospective, nonrandomized study[32] 41 patients treated according to the World Health Organization (WHO) guidelines for cancer pain relief were compared with 21 patients treated with a neurolytic celiac plexus block. The authors concluded that this technique could play an important role in the management of pancreatic cancer pain.

Since one of the three studies that used a randomized controlled design compared different approaches to the celiac plexus and had no control group,[9] and the other two compared the procedure with an analgesic drug,[30,31] it is not possible to estimate the success rate of this technique. In contrast, the results of a meta-analysis that evaluated the results of 21 *retrospective* studies in 1,145 patients concluded that adequate to excellent pain relief can be achieved in 89% of the patients during the first 2 weeks after the block.[33] Partial to complete pain relief continued in approximately 90% of the patients who were alive at the 3-month interval and in 70% to 90% until death, even if beyond 3 months after celiac plexus block. Moreover, the efficacy was similar in patients with pancreatic cancer and in those with other intra-abdominal malignancies of the upper abdomen. However, it is important to recognize that these results are based on *retrospective* evaluations, which may not yield reliable information or may be subject to publication bias. In addition, statistical techniques used for the analysis must account for the heterogeneity produced by the patient selection criteria, technical differences in the performance of the blocks, choice of neurolytic agents and doses, diversity in the tools for the evaluation of pain, goals of therapy, etc. Thus, the meta-analysis must be interpreted with caution, as the results may be overly encouraging.

The efficacy of celiac plexus neurolysis appears to be related to the site and extent of pancreatic tumor involvement. Rykowski and Hilgier[34] demonstrated that sustained, effective pain relief occurred in 92% (33 of 36) of patients with cancer of the head of the pancreas but in only 29% (4 of 14) of patients with cancer of the body and tail of the pancreas. Block failure in 13 patients appears to be explained by the extent of tumor growth around the celiac axis, which was confirmed by CT scan.

New Perspectives: As previously discussed, oral pharmacological therapy with oral opioids, NSAIDs, and coadjuvants is frequently used for the treatment of cancer pain. However, there is evidence to suggest that chronic use of high doses of opioids may have a negative effect on immunity.[35] Thus, analgesic techniques that lower opioid consumption should have positive effects on patient outcomes. Lillimoe et al.[36] showed in a prospective, randomized trial that patients with nonresectable cancer of the pancreas receiving splanchnic neurolysis had a longer survival than patients that did not. These findings may be the result of lower opioid use in the group of patients randomized to neurolysis, resulting in (1) better preserved immune function and (2) lower incidence of side effects, such as nausea and vomiting, that allows patients to eat better. This hypothesis is currently being tested in a prospective, randomized trial.

SUPERIOR HYPOGASTRIC PLEXUS BLOCK

Cancer patients with tumor extension into the pelvis may experience severe pain unresponsive to oral or parenteral opioids. Moreover, some patients may complain of excessive sedation or other side effects that limit the acceptability and usefulness of oral opioid therapy. Thus, a more invasive approach may be needed to control pain and improve quality of life.

Both pelvic pain associated with cancer and that seen with chronic nonmalignant conditions may be alleviated by blocking the superior hypogastric plexus.[37–40] Analgesia to the organs in the pelvis is possible because the afferent fibers innervating these structures travel with the sympathetic nerves, trunks, ganglia, and rami and are accessible for neurolytic block. Thus, a sympathectomy for visceral pain is analogous to a peripheral neurectomy or dorsal rhizotomy for somatic pain. A recent study has suggested that, even in advanced stages, visceral pain is an important component of the cancer pain syndrome experienced by patients with cancer of the pelvis.[38] Thus, it appears that percutaneous neurolytic blocks of the superior hypogastric plexus should be offered more frequently to patients with advanced stages of pelvic cancer.

The superior hypogastric plexus is situated in the retroperitoneum, bilaterally, extending from the lower third of the fifth lumbar vertebral body to the upper third of the first sacral vertebral body. The technique for the blockade has been described elsewhere.[37–39]

Technique: Patients are placed in the prone position with a pillow under the pelvis to flatten the lumbar lordosis. Plancarte et al. preceded some of their blocks with a "single-shot" L4–L5 epidural injection of 8 to 10 mL of 1% lidocaine to enhance patient cooperation, reduce reflex muscle spasm, and ameliorate discomfort. Alternatively, local infiltration of the intervening muscle planes can be performed. Needle insertion sites are 5 to 7 cm lateral to the midline, depending on patient's height and girth, at the level of the L4–L5 interspace. Two 7 to 9 inch, 22-gauge short beveled needles (Chiba type) are inserted with the bevel directed medially, 45° mesiad and 30° caudad, so that the needle tips lie anterolateral to the L5–S1 intervertebral space. Aspiration is important to avoid injection into the iliac vessels. If blood is aspirated, a transvascular approach can be used.

Biplanar fluoroscopy is used to verify accurate needle placement. Anteroposterior (AP) views should reveal the tip of the needle at the level of the junction of the L5 and S1 vertebral bodies. Lateral views will confirm placement of the needle tip just beyond the vertebral body's anterolateral margin. The injection of 2 to 3 mL of water-soluble contrast medium is used to verify accurate needle placement and to rule out intravascular injection. In the AP view the spread of contrast should be confined to the midline region. In the lateral view a smooth posterior contour corresponding to the anterior psoas fascia indicates that the needle is at the appropriate depth. Figures 65-5 and 65-6 show adequate needle placement and contrast medium spread prior to neurolysis of the superior hypogastric plexus.

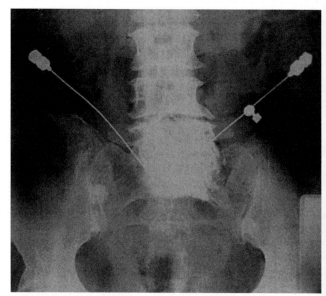

FIGURE 65-5. Posteroanterior radiograph demonstrating bilateral correct needle placement and adequate spread of the contrast medium.

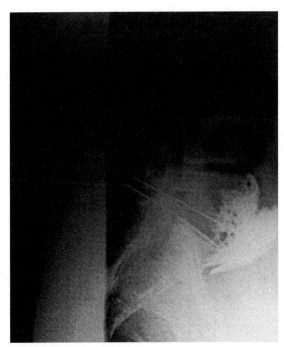

FIGURE 65-6. Cross-lateral radiograph demonstrating correct needle placement and adequate spread of the contrast medium.

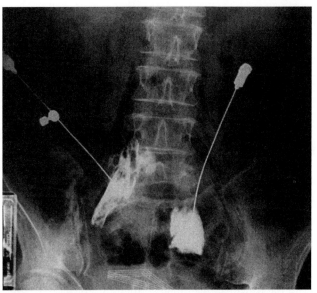

FIGURE 65-7. Anteroposterior radiograph showing correct needle placement but inadequate spread of the contrast medium due to tumor spread.

For a prognostic hypogastric plexus blockade a volume of 6 to 8 mL of 0.25% bupivacaine through each needle is recommended. For therapeutic purposes a total of 6 to 8 mL of 10% aqueous phenol can be injected through each needle.

Complications: Potential complications include retroperitoneal hematoma formation and acute ischemia of the foot, due to the dislodgement of an atherosclerotic plaque from the iliac vessels. A combined experience of more than 200 cases from the Mexican Institute of Cancer, Roswell Park Cancer Institute, and M.D. Anderson Cancer Center has failed to detect neurologic complications associated with this block.[39]

Efficacy: The effectiveness of the block was originally demonstrated by documenting a significant decrease in pain scores via a visual analogue pain scale (VAS).[37] In this study Plancarte et al. showed that this block was effective in reducing VAS scores in 70% of the patients with pelvic pain associated with cancer.[37] The great majority of the patients enrolled had a diagnosis of cervical cancer. In a subsequent study 69% of the patients experienced a decrease in VAS scores. Moreover, a mean daily morphine dose reduction of 67% was seen in the success group (736 ± 633 to 251 ± 191 mg/day), and 45% in the failure group (1443 ± 703 to 800 ± 345 mg/day).[38] In a more recent multicentric study 159 patients with pelvic pain associated with cancer were evaluated. Overall, 115 patients (72%) had satisfactory pain relief after one or two neurolytic procedures. Mean opioid use decreased by 40% from 58 ± 43 to 35 ± 18 equianalgesic mg/day of morphine, 3 weeks after treatment in all the studied patients. The decrease in opioid consumption was significant for both the success group (56 ± 32 to 32 ± 16 mg/day) and the failure group (65 ± 28 to 48 ± 21 mg/day).[39] Success was defined in these two studies as the ability to reduce opioid consumption by at least 50% in the 3 weeks following the block and a decrease in the pain scores below 4/10 in the VAS.[38,39]

Three important conclusions may be drawn from the results of these studies. First, reductions in pain scores and in opioid consumption are significant even in advanced stages of pelvic cancer. This suggests that visceral pain may be an important component of cancer pain even in the late stages of the disease, when differentiation of somatic pain from visceral pain is very difficult. Second, neurolysis is not as effective in the presence of significant retroperitoneal lymph node involvement (20% vs. 70% response rate). This lack of success may reflect involvement of nerve tissue or tumor spread to somatic structures within the pelvis (see Fig. 65-7). However, patients with extensive retroperitoneal pelvic involvement who showed a confluence of contrast material in the midline, on PA fluoroscopic views, experienced good results in one of the studies.[38] Third, use of this neurolytic block early in the management of pelvic visceral pain associated with cancer may be economically sound, based on the opioid reduction experienced by patients in both the failure and the success groups.[38,39]

In a recent case report Rosenberg et al.[40] reported on the efficacy of this block in a patient with severe chronic nonmalignant penile pain after transurethral resection of the prostate. Although the patient did not receive a neurolytic agent, a diagnostic block performed with 0.25% bupivacaine and 20 mg of methylprednisolone acetate was effective in relieving the pain for more than 6 months. The usefulness of this block in chronic benign pain conditions has not been adequately documented.

GANGLION IMPAR BLOCK

The ganglion impar is a solitary retroperitoneal structure located at the level of the sacrococcygeal junction. This ganglion marks the end of the two sympathetic chains.

Visceral pain in the perineal area associated with malignancies may be effectively treated with neurolysis of the ganglion impar (the ganglion of Walther).[41,42] Patients who will benefit from this blockade will frequently present with vague and poorly localized pain, which is burning in character and frequently accompanied by sensations of urgency. However, the clinical value of this block is not clear as the published experienced is limited (3 case series).

Technique: This block may be performed with the patient in the left lateral decubitus position with the knees flexed, in the litothomy position, or in the prone position. The initial technique employs a 22-gauge, 3.5-inch spinal needle that is manually bent to facilitate placement of the needle tip anterior to the concavity of the sacrum and coccyx. The needle is introduced through the anococcygeal ligament with its concavity oriented posteriorly and, under fluoroscopic guidance, is directed along the midline to contact bone at or near the sacrococcygeal junction (Fig. 65-8). Contrast dye confirms retroperitoneal spread; on the lateral view, it is shaped like a comma. An easier, transcoccygeal approach is performed with the patient in the prone position. A 20-gauge, 1.5-inch needle is inserted through the sacrococcygeal ligament in the midline. The needle is then advanced until the tip is placed posterior to the rectum. For diagnostic blocks, 4 to 8 mL of 1% lidocaine or 0.25% bupivacaine is selected, and for neurolytic block 4 (to 8) mL of 10% phenol is used. Although the technique is relatively straightforward, care is needed to prevent perforation of the rectum and injection into the periosteum.

Complications: No complications or side effects have been reported with this block.

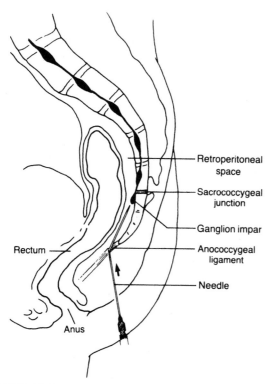

FIGURE 65-8. Lateral schematic view of correct needle placement for blockade of the ganglion impar.

Labels in figure:
- Retroperitoneal space
- Sacrococcygeal junction
- Ganglion impar
- Anococcygeal ligament
- Needle
- Rectum
- Anus

CONCLUSIONS

Neurolysis of the sympathetic axis is a safe and cost-effective way to treat visceral pain associated with cancer. The benefits are not limited to improved analgesia but also include a decrease in opioid consumption. These results may have both economic implications and additional important clinical effects due to the actions of high-dose chronic opioid therapy in the immune and gastrointestinal systems. The knowledge and refined techniques, currently used to perform these blocks, allow patients to undergo these procedures in a safe and expeditious manner. Thus, pain practitioners should consider them as adjuvant therapy for the successful treatment of cancer pain.

KEY POINTS

- Neurolytic blocks of the sympathetic axis are an important adjunct to pharmacologic therapy for the relief of severe visceral pain experienced by cancer patients. The goal of performing these blocks is to maximize the analgesic effect of opioid and nonopioid analgesics while reducing their dosage to alleviate untoward side effects.
- Neurolytic celiac plexus block for patients with pancreatic cancer pain results in excellent analgesia, reduced opioid utilization, and decreased side effects such as nausea, vomiting, and constipation when compared to systemic analgesic therapy.
- Patients with nonresectable cancer of the pancreas receiving splanchnic neurolysis had longer survival than patients not blocked. This may result from their lower opioid use, resulting in better-preserved immune function as well as improved nutrition due to fewer opioid side effects.
- Complications of neurolytic celiac plexus block include diarrhea, postural hypotension, back pain, aortic injury, hemorrhage, and paraplegia.
- Neurolytic superior hypogastric plexus block has proven effective, with minimal complications, in reduction of pain and opioid consumption in patients with advanced pelvic cancer, suggesting that a significant component of visceral pain is present even with advanced disease.

REFERENCES

1. de Leon Casasola OA: Regional anesthetic techniques for the management of cancer pain. Techniques Reg Anesth Pain Manage 1:27–31, 1997.
2. Reiestad F, Stromskag KE: Interpleural catheter in the management of postoperative pain. A preliminary report. Reg Anesth 11:89–91, 1986.
3. Rocco A, Reiestad F, Gudman J, et al: Intrapleural administration of local anesthetics for pain relief in patients with multiple rib fractures. Preliminary report. Reg Anesth 12:10–14, 1987.
4. Lema MJ, Myers DP, de Leon-Casasola OA: Interpleural phenol therapy for the treatment of chronic esophageal cancer pain. Reg Anesth 17:166–170, 1992.
5. Silva H, Plancarte R, de Leon-Casasola OA: Personal communication.
6. Stromskag KE, Minor B, Steen PA: Side effects and complications related to interpleural analgesia: An update. Acta Anaesthesiol Scand 34:473–477, 1990.
7. Stromskag KE, Reiestad F, Holmquist EVO, et al: Intrapleural administration of 0.25%, 0.375%, and 0.5% bupivacaine with epinephrine after cholecystectomy. Anesth Analg 67:430–444, 1988.
8. Rykowski JJ, Hilgier M: Continuous celiac plexus block in acute pancreatitis. Reg Anesth 20:528–532, 1995.

9. Ischia S, Ischia A, Polati E, et al: Three posterior percutaneous celiac plexus block techniques: A prospective randomized study in 61 patients with pancreatic cancer pain. Anesthesiology 76:534–540, 1992.

10. Singer RC: An improved technique for alcohol neurolysis of the celiac plexus block. Anesthesiology 56:137–141, 1982.

11. Ischia S, Luzzani A, Ischia A, et al: A new approach to the neurolytic block for coeliac plexus: The transaortic technique. Pain 16:333–341, 1983.

12. Romanelli DF, Beckmann CF, Heiss FW: Celiac plexus block: Efficacy and safety of the anterior approach. Am J Roentgenol 160:497–500, 1993.

13. Gimenez A, Martina-Noguera A, Donoso L, et al: Percutaneous neurolysis of the celiac plexus via the anterior approach with sonographic guidance. Am J Roentgenol 161:1061–1063, 1993.

14. Hilgier M, Rykowski JJ: One needle transcrural celiac plexus block: Single shot, or continuous technique, or both. Reg Anesth 19:277–283, 1994.

15. Davis DD: Incidence of major complications of neurolytic coeliac plexus block. J R Soc Med 86:264–266, 1993.

16. Wong GY, Brown DL: Celiac plexus block for cancer pain. Techniques Reg Anesth Pain Manage 1:18–26, 1997.

17. Hanley JA, Lippman-Hand A: If nothing goes wrong, is everything all right. JAMA 249:1743–1745, 1983.

18. Matson JA, Ghia JN, Levy JH: A case report of potentially fatal complications associated with Ischia's transaortic method of celiac plexus block. Reg Anesth 10:193–196, 1985.

19. Sett SS, Taylor DC: Aortic pseudoaneurysm secondary to celiac plexus block. Ann Vasc Surg 5:88–91, 1991.

20. Kaplan R, Schiff-Keren B, Alt E: Aortic dissection as a complication of celiac plexus block. Anesthesiology 83:632–635, 1995.

21. Galizia EJ, Lahiri SK: Paraplegia following coeliac plexus block with phenol. Br J Anaesth46:539–540, 1974.

22. Lo JN, Buckley JJ: Spinal cord ischemia a complication of celiac plexus block. Reg Anesth 7:66–68, 1982.

23. Cherry DA, Lamberty J: Paraplegia following coeliac plexus block. Anaesth Intens Care 12:59–72, 1984.

24. Woodham MJ, Hanna MH: Paraplegia after coeliac plexus block. Anaesthesia 44:487–489, 1989.

25. Van Dongen RTM, Crul BJP: Paraplegia following coeliac plexus block. Anaesthesia 46:862–863, 1991.

26. Jabbal SS, Hunton J: Reversible paraplegia following coeliac plexus block. Anaesthesia 47:857–858, 1992.

27. Wong GY, Brown DL: Transient paraplegia following alcohol celiac plexus block. Reg Anesth 20:352–355, 1995.

28. Brown DL, Rorie DK: Altered reactivity of isolated segmental lumbar arteries of dogs following exposure to ethanol and phenol. Pain 56:139–143, 1994.

29. Johnson ME, Sill JC, Brown DL, et al: The effect of the neurolytic agent ethanol on cytoplasmic calcium in arterial smooth muscle and endothelium. Reg Anesth 21:6–13, 1996.

30. Mercadante S: Celiac plexus block versus analgesics in pancreatic cancer pain. Pain 52:187–192, 1993.

31. Polati E, Finco G, Gottin L, et al: Prospective randomized double-blind trial of neurolytic coeliac plexus block in patients with pancreatic cancer. Br J Surg 85:199–201, 1998.

32. Ventafridda GV, Caraceni AT, Sbanotto AM, et al: Pain treatment in cancer of the pancreas. Eur J Surg Oncol 16:1–6, 1990.

33. Eisenberg E, Carr DB, Chalmers TC: Neurolytic celiac plexus block for the treatment of cancer pain: A meta-analysis. Anesth Analg 80:290–295, 1995.

34. Rykowski JJ, Hilger M: Efficacy of neurolytic celiac plexus block in varying locations of pancreatic cancer: Influence on pain relief. Anesthesiology 92:347–354, 2000.

35. Yeager MP: Morphine inhibits spontaneous and cytokine-enhanced natural killer cell cytotoxicity in volunteers. Anesthesiology 83:500–508, 1995.

36. Lillimoe KD, Cameron JL, Kaufman HS, et al: Chemical splanchnicectomy in patients with unresectable pancreatic cancer. Ann Surg 217:447–457, 1993.

37. Plancarte R, Amescua C, Patt RB, et al: Superior hypogastric plexus block for pelvic cancer pain. Anesthesiology 73:236–239, 1990.

38. de Leon-Casasola OA, Kent E, Lema MJ: Neurolytic superior hypogastric plexus block for chronic pelvic pain associated with cancer. Pain 54:145–151, 1993.

39. Plancarte R, de Leon-Casasola OA, El-Helealy M, et al: Neurolytic superior hypogastric plexus block for chronic pelvic pain associated with cancer. Reg Anesth 22:562–568, 1997.

40. Rosenberg SK, Tewari R, Boswell MV, et al: Superior hypogastric plexus block successfully treats severe penile pain after transurethral resection of the prostate. Reg Anesth Pain Med 23:618–620, 1998.

41. Plancarte R, Amescua C, Patt RB: Presacral blockade of the ganglion of Walther (ganglion impar). Anesthesiology 73:A751, 1990.

42. Swofford JB, Ratzman DM: A transarticular approach to blockade of the ganglion impar (ganglion of Walther). Reg Anesth 23(Suppl 3):203, 1998.

Intrathecal and Epidural Neurolysis

Agents Used for Neurolytic Block

Robert E. Molloy, M.D.

Neurolytic blockade is a valuable tool, useful in managing intractable cancer pain. Its use presupposes a thorough assessment of the patient's overall medical condition and application of a multimodal approach to address the patient's many needs. The use of appropriate anticancer therapy, opioid analgesics, and adjuvant drugs is all presumed, as is consideration of other potential invasive therapies and the potential benefits and risks of each intervention. This must be followed by a thorough discussion of reasonable expectations for a neurolytic block; the limitations to any expected pain relief; the probable need for use of analgesic and other drugs in reduced doses; and an honest description of potential complications. Diagnostic or prognostic local anesthetic blocks are also desirable before neurolytic blockade. These procedures should be performed by well-trained, experienced physicians. The patient's response should be monitored by assessing pain levels, pain relief, activity levels, appetite, sleep, mood, and drug intake before and after blockade. The potential for respiratory depression and narcotic withdrawal syndrome after sudden cessation of pain requires carefully titrated opioid withdrawal.[1] The agents available for neurolytic block, and their intrathecal and epidural administration, are considered in this chapter.[2–4]

ALCOHOL

Ethyl alcohol is commercially available in undiluted (absolute or 100% alcohol) vials. When exposed to the atmosphere, it absorbs water. The effective concentration is 50% to 100%. Alcohol is the classic neurolytic agent, reported by Dogliotti for subarachnoid injection in 1931. It produces destruction of nerve fibers and subsequent wallerian degeneration of axonal fibers. A series of events occurs, including neural swelling and dissolution of cellular elements, followed by collapse and digestion of the myelin sheath. However, the basal lamina of the Schwann cell sheath remains intact, allowing for new Schwann cell proliferation and providing a framework for subsequent nerve fiber growth. Therefore, regeneration of axons

can occur unless the cell bodies of these nerves have been completely destroyed.[1] Schlosser studied alcohol block of the trigeminal nerve and reported in 1907 that the entire nerve, except for the neurolemma, degenerates and is absorbed.[5] More dilute solutions produce less complete neural destruction of somatic neurons. The concentration of alcohol needed to provide adequate relief of pain with somatic block seems to be 50% to 70%, although Labat and Greene found a 33% concentration to be effective on peripheral nerves without producing significant muscle paralysis.[6] Attempts to find a relatively low concentration of alcohol capable of producing complete sensory loss without any motor deficits have not been ultimately successful.

Alcohol extracts neural cholesterol, phospholipids, and cerebrosides, and it causes precipitation of lipoproteins and neuropeptides.[7] This results in sclerosis of the nerve fibers and myelin sheath. Merrick described the effects of alcohol injection on sympathetic nerves.[8] Injection of the sympathetic ganglion cells produced permanent nerve destruction, whereas injection of preganglionic and postganglionic fibers produced axonal degeneration with limited destruction of ganglionic cell bodies and recovery of many neurons. Sympathetic neurons regenerated over the course of 3 to 5 months or longer.

Alcohol, in contrast to phenol, is readily soluble in body fluids, and it spreads from the injection site quite rapidly. This may limit the ability to restrict the injectate and alters the volume required to produce adequate neurolysis. An alcohol block requires larger volumes than phenol.[4] Large volumes may favor spread of agent to adjacent sites. Alcohol is readily absorbed into the bloodstream after celiac plexus block. Thompson measured alcohol blood levels after celiac plexus block using 50 mL of 50% ethyl alcohol. He found that blood alcohol levels rose acutely over the first 20 minutes to a peak level of 0.021 g/dL.[9] This is only one-fifth of the common legal limit for alcohol intoxication.

Intrathecal alcohol injection results in rapid uptake of alcohol, resultant destruction of the dorsal roots, and variable injury to the surface of the spinal cord and the posterior columns. Alcohol is rapidly absorbed from cerebrospinal fluid (CSF) such that only 10% of the injected dose remains in the CSF after 10 minutes, and 4% after 30 minutes.[10] Alcohol is hypobaric with respect to CSF and quickly floats to the top when injected in CSF. The effective concentration is almost 100% for intrathecal use and 50% for celiac plexus block.

Clinically, alcohol neurolysis is employed more often for lumbar sympathetic and celiac plexus blocks, although epidural and cranial nerve applications have been reported to be successful. Alcohol produces significant pain on injection, requiring the prior injection of a local anesthetic into tissues. Alcohol injection may be followed by burning or shooting neuropathic pain which can last for weeks or months. This may occur after peripheral nerve block or with spread to somatic nerve roots after lumbar sympathetic block. Unintended spread of alcohol to adjacent tissues can produce cellular injury or necrosis. Alcohol may also produce arterial vasospasm. This may be related to a potential ischemic cause of paraplegia after celiac plexus block.[4]

Alcohol neurolytic injection may induce a disulfiram-like toxic reaction in patients being treated with drugs that inhibit alcohol dehydrogenase. Umeda and Arai reported a reaction with temporary flushing, sweating, dizziness, vomiting, and hypotension following an alcohol celiac plexus block with 15 mL 67% alcohol. The patient had received the antibiotic moxalactam, an inhibitor of this enzyme.[11] Other agents that have this property include: disulfiram, metronidazole, chloramphenicol, tolbutamide, chlorpropamide, and β-lactam-type antibiotics.[4]

PHENOL

Mandl reported the use of phenol for sympathetic ganglion block in animals in 1947,[12] and Maher described the results of intrathecal phenol in humans in 1955.[13] Mandl observed complete necrosis within 24 hours, progressive degeneration over 45 days, and regeneration in less than 3 months. This suggested that recovery from sympathetic block with phenol occurs more rapidly than with alcohol. It was initially supposed that phenol selectively blocked small nerve fibers while sparing large fibers. Subsequent reports documented transient local anesthetic blockade by dilute intrathecal phenol, but widespread neural damage with clinically relevant concentrations. In essence, phenol appears to be just as neurotoxic as alcohol, producing nonselective damage to neural tissues. Phenol coagulates proteins as its primary mechanism of injury.

Stewart and Lourie observed nonselective degeneration of spinal nerve roots after phenol, suggesting that nerve damage was proportional to the concentration used.[14] Nathan et al. confirmed the nonselective effects of phenol by histological studies and electrophysiological evidence of damage to A-alpha and A-beta fibers.[15] In studies of intrathecal injection in both cats and humans Smith demonstrated that hyperbaric phenol primarily destroyed axons in posterior sensory rootlets, in the posterior columns of the cord, and to a lesser extent in the anterior root axons. It produces nonselective destruction by denaturing proteins of axons and adjacent blood vessels. Degeneration occurred over 2 weeks, and regeneration progressed over 14 weeks.[16] Maher and Mehta observed mostly sensory block after intrathecal injection of 5% phenol, but motor block also at higher concentrations.[17]

Injected phenol in glycerin appears to fix rapidly within the subarachnoid space. Ichiyanagi and colleagues found that phenol concentrations decreased to 30% of the initial concentration within 1 minute and to 0.1% by 15 minutes.[18] Phenol injection near peripheral nerves produces protein coagulation, axonal degeneration, and subsequent wallerian degeneration. Axonal regeneration occurs more rapidly than after alcohol. Gregg and co-workers performed in vivo electrophysiological studies of the effects of alcohol and phenol peripheral nerve injections in cats. Alcohol produced significant depression of compound action potentials at 2 months.[19] The effects of phenol seen at 2 weeks had returned to normal by 8 weeks.[20] It has been suggested but not confirmed that phenol affects vascular tissue more than nerves. Heavner and Racz found that phenol caused much greater nerve tissue destruction after intrathecal versus epidural injection, without evidence of primary vascular injury as the mechanism of tissue damage.[21]

Phenol is usually prepared by the hospital pharmacy for clinical use. Various concentrations are prepared with saline, distilled sterile water, glycerin, and contrast dyes. Phenol is relatively insoluble in water. At room temperature the maximum aqueous concentration achieved is 6.7%, unless glycerin is added. Supersaturated solutions of 10% phenol prepared in distilled water or in bupivacaine are also used.[4] The aqueous solution of phenol has a greater ability to penetrate the rat sciatic nerve perineurium and produce endoneurial damage than the glycerin preparation, but results are identical with intraneural injections.[22] Phenol in glycerin is hyperbaric relative to CSF. A biphasic action is observed clinically. An initial local anesthetic effect produces warmth and numbness that diminishes over 24 hours, leaving a less intense neurolytic effect. This is an advantage for intrathecal neurolysis, because the painless warmth and numbness provide feedback on the area to be affected by the block. Concentrations between 4% and 10% phenol are typically used for neurolytic block. Phenol is used clinically for lumbar sympathetic, celiac plexus, hypogastric plexus, somatic nerve, epidural, and intrathecal neurolytic blocks. The relative potencies of these two neurolytic agents are such that 3% phenol is equivalent to 40% alcohol.[23] Toxicity from phenol may be seen at systemic doses of at least 8.5 g, causing convulsions, central nervous system depression, and cardiovascular collapse. Chronic poisoning can cause skin, gastrointestinal, and renal toxicity. Normal clinical doses are unlikely to cause toxicity, if accidental intravenous injection is avoided.

Vascular effects of neurolytic agents are also of concern. An added risk is incurred when a neurolytic agent is injected near a prosthetic vascular graft. Dacron woven grafts exhibited diminished tensile strength after 72-hour exposure to 50% alcohol or 6% phenol, whereas Gor-Tex grafts were unchanged. Electron microscopy had demonstrated significant fiber degeneration of Dacron and much less degradation of Gore-Tex by higher concentrations of these agents.[24] Occasional paraplegia after neurolytic celiac plexus block has been postulated to occur because of spinal cord ischemia. Vasospasm of segmental lumbar arteries has been induced in dogs after exposure to ethanol and phenol.[25] This appears to be unrelated to synaptic neurotransmitters or to sodium channels. Johnson and colleagues demonstrated that low concentrations of ethanol induce significant contractile effects in human aortic smooth muscle cells along with increased intracellular concentration of cytoplasmic ionized calcium.[26] The fact remains that phenol and alcohol will destroy all types of tissue and may cause a contractile response in blood vessels which may lead to loss of function. Therefore, extreme care is required when they are used.

INDICATIONS FOR NEURAXIAL NEUROLYTIC BLOCK

The goal of these blocks is interruption of nociceptive input from injured tissues at the spinal or epidural level. The desired result is selective destruction of dorsal roots and rootlets between the spinal cord and the dorsal root ganglion. The combined selection of patient position, level of injection, and baricity of the neurolytic agent is designed to produce predictable, segmental sensory loss. The resultant analgesia should be prolonged but not permanent; axonal regeneration does occur over a period of weeks to months. Only a very small minority of cancer patients are candidates for neurolytic blockade.[1] Neurolytic subarachnoid blockade should be reserved for intractable cancer pain, particularly when it is well localized in a patient with a short life expectancy.[27] Appropriate anticancer therapy measures should be employed, along with basic analgesic drug therapy. The World Health Organization analgesic ladder should be employed with appropriate adjuvant drug therapy. Neurolytic spinal blockade is ideal for patients with advanced or terminal malignancy; for patients with pain resistant to usual analgesic measures or intolerable side effects of analgesic therapy; for patients with visceral and somatic rather than neuropathic pain; and for patients with unilateral pain localized to a few adjacent dermatomes, ideally situated in the trunk, away from the innervation of the extremities and sphincters[27] (Table 66-1). Additional favorable factors are a primary somatic pain mechanism; absence of midline, axial pain; and demonstrated relief with prognostic local anesthetic blocks. The presence of intraspinal tumor is associated with failure of neurolytic spinal blockade. Informed consent from the patient and relatives is essential. Patients must be aware of the expected benefits and potential risks of intrathecal neurolysis.

TABLE 66-1. INTRATHECAL NEUROLYSIS: INDICATIONS FOR NEUROLYTIC SPINAL BLOCK

Intractable cancer pain
Failure of analgesic therapy
Intolerable side effects of analgesic therapy
Advanced or terminal malignancy
Unilateral pain
Pain limited to a few dermatomes
Pain located in the trunk, thorax, abdomen
Primary somatic pain mechanism
Absence of intraspinal tumor spread
Effective analgesia with prognostic block
Fully informed consent of patient
Realistic expectations of patient and family

Data from Bonica JJ, Buckley FP, Moricca G, et al: Neurolytic blockade and hypophysectomy. In Bonica JJ, Chapman CR, et al (eds): The Management of Pain, ed 2. Lea & Febiger, Philadelphia, 1990, p 1980.

Reasonable expectations of localized analgesia, decreased analgesic requirements, and diminished side effects should be tempered by understanding that the malignancy may continue to progress and produce pain at other sites and that the block will gradually lose effectiveness over time and may have to be repeated. Potential problems include inadequate initial pain relief, inadequate duration of relief, and weakness of the limb muscles or the rectal and bladder sphincters. Any available alternative analgesic strategies should also be discussed with the patient in a similar fashion.[1]

Techniques: An accurate pain diagnosis after comprehensive evaluation of the patient is necessary to select a technique of neurolytic spinal blockade. Documentation of preblock neurological function is essential along with the location of all malignant lesions. Prognostic spinal anesthetic blockade with a small amount of local anesthetic should be performed in a fashion that mimics the planned neurolytic block as much as possible.[28]

Anesthetic baricity and volume, injection site, and patient position should be considered to achieve this goal. In general, neurolytic blockade produces less dramatic effects than the initial prognostic local anesthetic injection. The choice of hypobaric alcohol or hyperbaric phenol is based on the location of the pain and practical patient positioning considerations. There is no clear difference in efficacy (Table 66.2).

Intrathecal Alcohol: The specific gravity of absolute alcohol is less than 0.8, and that of spinal fluid is almost 1.007. Therefore, alcohol is hypobaric to and tends to move upward in CSF, in a direction opposite to that of gravity. Dermatome and sclerotome charts (for bone metastases) aid in the selection of nerve roots to be blocked.[29] Neurolytic spinal block is carried out at the level where the target dorsal root leaves the spinal cord, not where the spinal nerve passes through the intervertebral foramen (Table 66-3). This distinction is important only for lower thoracic and lumbosacral nerve root destruction. The patient must be positioned to place the target rootlets uppermost in the subarachnoid space. The patient is placed in the lateral position with the side to be blocked uppermost. A combination of pillows, kidney rests, and table extension is used below the injection site to raise it above adjacent spinal levels. The patient is also turned 45° toward the prone position to raise the dorsal nerve rootlets into a horizontal position, superior to their adjacent ventral rootlets. This position is maintained by restraining the patient with adequate tape to prevent movement at an inappropriate time.

Once the patient is in position, a short-bevel 22-gauge needle is inserted at the selected interspace. The epidural space is identified, and then cautious entry into the subarachnoid space is detected by continuous aspiration of the syringe's plunger. The needle is adjusted to ensure the bevel's location just anterior to the arachnoid membrane. Alcohol is then injected in 0.1 mL aliquots using a tuberculin syringe and at least 60 to 90 seconds between injections. Alcohol elicits temporary dermatomal burning, which can be used to confirm needle placement at the painful area. If burning is reported at a level distant from the patient's complaint, a new needle may be placed at involved sites, and 0.1 mL aliquots of alcohol may be injected through each properly placed needle. The total dose of alcohol injected for pain localized to one or two dermatomes should not exceed 0.5 to 0.7 mL. The patient remains

TABLE 66-2. **AGENTS FOR NEUROLYTIC SPINAL BLOCK**

	Alcohol	Phenol
Physical properties	Low water solubility	Absorbs water on air exposure
Stability at room temperature	Unstable	Stable
Concentration	100%	4–7%
Diluent	None	Glycerin
Relative to CSF	Hypobaric	Hyperbaric
Patient position	Lateral	Lateral
Added tilt	Semiprone	Semisupine
Painful side	Uppermost	Most dependent
Injection sensations	Immediate burning pain	Painless, warm feeling
Onset of neurolysis	Immediate	Delayed 15 minutes
CSF uptake ends	30 minutes	15 minutes
Full effect	3 to 5 days	1 day

CSF, cerebrospinal fluid.

immobilized for 30 minutes after injection to allow complete fixation of alcohol to the selected nerve roots, preventing subsequent spread to other levels. The efficacy of alcohol blockade should be assessed after 3 to 5 days. Repeat injection may be necessary in some patients after this time interval.

Intrathecal Phenol: Phenol in glycerin is hyperbaric relative to CSF, and its spread after injection is determined by gravity (specific gravity of glycerin is 1.25). The patient must be positioned with the painful side dependent and the affected rootlets most dependent. Invariably the head of the table is elevated, and often the table is flexed under the injection site. The patient is also turned 45° toward the supine position to place the target dorsal rootlets in the most dependent position. Hyperbaric phenol seems well suited to treat pelvic and perineal pain with unilateral blocks on each side or, alternatively, with a saddle block performed in one sitting.[30] This procedure may be ideal for any patient at end of life having intractable pelvic cancer pain, especially when prior or planned performance of a bladder diversion procedure obviates concerns about development of incontinence.[31] The solution is extremely viscous and hard to inject, even when a 20-gauge, short-bevel needle is used. Phenol is injected in 0.1 mL increments up to a total dose similar to that used with alcohol.[30] With both agents, the needle should be cleared with 0.2 mL of air before it is withdrawn. Phenol fixes within 15 minutes, but the patient should remain in position for 30 minutes after injection. Phenol produces an initial local anesthetic effect, but no

injection pain occurs. The resultant analgesia can be assessed after 1 day, allowing for earlier decisions about repeat injection than after alcohol spinal blockade.

Intrathecal phenol injection may be modified to treat severe lower extremity spasticity, due to a neurological disease such as multiple sclerosis. This might be considered in a severe case if maximum doses of oral medications have been tried; other treatment options such as intrathecal baclofen pump are not suitable; effective management of bladder and bowel dysfunction is in place; and the patient is aware of the risks for loss of sensation and sexual function. The procedure is modified to target the ventral motor rootlets, and the patient is turned 30° to 40° toward the prone position to accomplish this goal.[32] Jarrett et al. reported easier positioning and relief of spasms in 84% of patients, but 24% also developed recurrence of skin breakdown. Repeated injection may be employed to achieve bilateral effect or after regression of initial benefit.[32]

Results: Neurolytic spinal blockade can produce profound unilateral segmental analgesia. Frequently incomplete analgesia occurs, but this may be remedied by repeating the injection. The most likely causes of treatment failure are unreasonable expectations and poor patient selection. The results of published series are difficult to interpret because of differences in tumor type and site; neurolytic agent, dose, and site of injection; and definitions of pain relief. Specific data on drug intake, pain scores, nausea and sleep scales, activity levels, and severity and duration of side effects are not uniformly reported.

TABLE 66-3. RELATIONSHIPS OF SPINAL VERTEBRAE TO SPINAL CORD LEVELS

Interspace Used for Injection	Nerve Rootlets Arising from Cord
C5–C6	C6, C7
C6–C7	C8
C7–T1	T1, T2
T1–T2	T2, T3
T2–T3	T3, T4
T3–T4	T5
T4–T5	T6
T5–T6	T7
T6–T7	T8, T9
T7–T8	T9, T10
T8–T9	T10, T11
T9–T10	T11, T12
T10–T11	T12 to L2
T11–T12	L2 to L5
T12–L1	L5 to S5

Adapted from Bonica JJ, Buckley FP, Moricca G, et al: Neurolytic blockade and hypophysectomy. In Bonica JJ, Chapman CR, et al (eds): The Management of Pain, ed 2. Lea & Febiger, Philadelphia, 1990, p 1980; Patt RB, Cousins MJ: Techniques for neurolytic neural blockade. In Cousins MJ, Bridenbaugh PO (eds): Neural Blockade in Clinical Anesthesia and Management of Pain, ed 3. Lippincott-Raven, Philadelphia, 1998, pp 1007–1061; Winnie AP, Candido KD: Subarachnoid neurolytic blocks. In Waldman SD (ed): Interventional Pain Management. WB Saunders, Philadelphia, 2001, pp 554–559.

Bonica and colleagues attempted to compare the best studies reporting the results of subarachnoid alcohol and phenol in three broad categories: good, fair, and poor pain relief.[1] Their conclusions are summarized in Table 66-4. The outcomes with alcohol and phenol seem to be similar, with good to excellent results reported in one-half to two-thirds of patients. The duration of pain relief is highly variable. Overall, the average duration of relief is 4 months; but it may be much shorter, particularly with phenol. The superiority of one neurolytic agent over the other has not been established. Many authors believe that pain relief may be better and last longer with alcohol, but that phenol may be safer, more versatile, and their agent of choice.

Complications: The most common complication of neurolytic block is persistent pain, due either to the underlying disease or to tissue damage at the site of injection. Side effects of neurolytic spinal blockade include postdural puncture headache, rare meningitis, loss of touch and position sense, persistent numbness and paresthesias, and loss of motor function due to unintended neurolysis of ventral rootlets. The most serious complications are muscle weakness of the extremities, and paresis of the urinary and rectal sphincters. These latter complications occur relatively frequently. Fortunately, they are usually transient occurrences, resolving within 1 week in many patients. Persistent complications are present at 1 month in about 2% of patients. There seems to be little to choose between phenol and alcohol as the agent employed and the risk of these potentially serious complications.[33] Gerbershagen reviewed reports that provided data on the duration of 303 complications after intrathecal neurolysis and observed when they disappeared: 28% did so within 3 days, 23% within 1 week, 21% within 1 month, 9% within 4 months, and 18% after more than 4 months.[34] Bonica and associates summarized the incidence of serious neurological complications after intrathecal neurolysis based on 11 studies;[1] these data are adapted and summarized in Table 66-5. The overall incidence of each condition is recorded along with the figure for prolonged or permanent conditions when available. Thoracic intrathecal neurolysis is associated with a low incidence of complications. There is a moderate risk of limb paresis when the procedure is performed at the cervical and especially at the lumbar level. Acute paraplegia may occur immediately after intrathecal neurolysis when undiagnosed metastatic spinal tumor is present before blockade.[35,36] The acute neurological deterioration may be related to traumatic needling of tumor but may also occur even when spinal injection is performed many segments away from the spinal metastatic disease.

TABLE 66-4. SUBARACHNOID BLOCKS FOR CANCER PAIN RELIEF

Agent	No. of Studies	No. of Patients	Good Results (%)	Fair Results (%)	Poor Results (%)
Alcohol	13	1634	61	24	15
Phenol	12	1982	58	16	28

Adapted from Bonica JJ, Buckley FP, Moricca G, et al: Neurolytic blockade and hypophysectomy. In Bonica JJ, Chapman CR, et al (eds): The Management of Pain, ed 2. Lea & Febiger, Philadelphia, 1990, Table 96-3, p 2007 and Table 96-4, p 2008.

TABLE 66-5. SUBARACHNOID BLOCKADE FOR CANCER PAIN RELIEF

Agent	No. of Studies	No. of Patients	Bladder Paresis*	Bowel Paresis*	Motor Weakness*
Alcohol	7	3123	5.7/0.7	1.1/0.3	4.9/0.8
Phenol	4	874	9.7/0.8	1.6/0.3	4.7/1.5

* Complications given as total %/prolonged %.
Adapted from Bonica JJ, Buckley FP, Moricca G, et al: Neurolytic blockade and hypophysectomy. In Bonica JJ, Chapman CR, et al (eds): The Management of Pain, ed 2. Lea & Febiger, Philadelphia, 1990, Table 96-25, p 2009.

EPIDURAL NEUROLYTIC BLOCK

Epidural neurolysis has been used as an alternative approach to subarachnoid blockade. It provides relief of pain that is bilateral, but analgesia may be less profound than after intrathecal neurolysis. It may be effective for abdominal cancer pain of visceral or mixed somatic and visceral origin.[37] Some of the proposed advantages of this technique are better efficacy for thoracic and cervicothoracic junction pain, increased safety, and ease of repeated injections. Some of these advantages remain theoretical. Placement of a thoracic epidural catheter may be less demanding to some practitioners than positioning of multiple needles just barely into the subarachnoid space but not within the substance of the spinal cord.

Technique: Injection may be made through an epidural needle or catheter. The needle should be placed near the vertebral levels corresponding to the dermatomal levels that supply the patient's painful lesion. A large needle is required to inject phenol in glycerin, but a smaller needle or catheter is adequate for ethyl alcohol, aqueous phenol, or phenol in saline. Confirmation of correct needle placement can be made with contrast-enhanced radiologic imaging and a test dose of local anesthetic. Use of an epidural catheter allows careful confirmation of epidural position and pain relief with a small volume (3 to 4 mL) of local anesthetic. Epidural neurolysis can then be performed through the same catheter at a later time. Racz and colleagues developed a soft, nonkinking, wire-embedded epidural catheter for this purpose; it is designed to help prevent false-negative aspiration tests before injection.[38] Aspiration without repeat local anesthetic test dosing can then be used before each injection of 5.5% phenol in saline. The volume injected should correspond to the effective dose of local anesthetic used previously. From 2 to 5 mL may be adequate depending on the injection level.[39] Racz and colleagues recommended daily repeat injection until increasingly positive responses cease to occur or the patient is free of pain after 24 hours. Korevaar used a similar technique but injected ethyl alcohol on a daily basis for up to 3 days through a thoracic epidural catheter inserted 3 to 5 cm into the epidural space. Local anesthetic test doses were used before each daily dose of 3 to 5 mL of alcohol given over 20 to 30 minutes in 0.2 mL increments.[37] Success was defined as at least 70% pain relief and decease in narcotic dose of ≥25%. Initial relief occurred in all cancer patients, and mean duration of relief in survivors was 4.4 months. Results were less impressive in patients with chronic nonmalignant pain.[37]

Results: In four studies the results of thoracic epidural phenol or alcohol neurolysis were positive for management of cancer pain. Initial pain relief was obtained in about 80% of patients (range 65% to 100%).[1] The duration of benefit varied with severity of patient disease and in many cases lasted until the time of death. Among survivors, the average duration of analgesia varied from less than 1 month to longer than 3 months in different patient groups. Although some authors noted no serious complications, a greater margin of safety for epidural versus intrathecal neurolysis has not been established. Katz and associates questioned the safety of epidural phenol in a study of the effects of lumbar epidural phenol on primate spinal cord 2 weeks after injection. They demonstrated lower extremity motor weakness clinically. Predominant[40] posterior nerve root damage was observed, but anterior root and spinal cord damage also was seen. Hayashi and colleagues reported necropsy results in a patient who died 24 days after a series of three transcatheter thoracic epidural alcohol injections. There was no abnormality of the spinal nerve roots and spinal cord; but the laminar structure of the dura was destroyed at the outer third of the dura.[41] Adequate information to support the superiority of epidural versus intrathecal neurolysis is lacking.

PATIENT CARE AFTER INTRASPINAL NEUROLYTIC BLOCK

The patient may experience profound pain relief after the neurolytic block procedure. Failure to decrease long-acting analgesic therapy may result in relative overdose and predictable side effects. However sudden cessation of all opioid drugs is likely to lead to a withdrawal syndrome. Careful attention to gradual drug withdrawal and individual titration of opioids to manage any residual pain at the target area or at distant sites is required. Assessment of the procedure's success should include the extent of change in the patient's verbal pain score, 24-hour opioid consumption, side-effect profile, sleep, activity tolerance, and the objective assessment of relatives and caregivers. Careful neurological examination to document the extent and duration of any sensory or motor deficits is also required. Should such complications occur, the neurological deficits can be expected to resolve over time. Many do so quickly, and most will resolve after nerve regeneration has occurred. Patient reassurance, analgesia, and protective physical therapy should be provided in such cases. If analgesia is incomplete after appropriate evaluation, repeat injection may be offered.

Because of the anatomic separation of sensory and motor roots in the subarachnoid space, particularly at thoracic levels, intrathecal neurolytic blocks offer the unique potential to provide relatively selective unilateral sensory blockade without concomitant motor blockade. Phenol saddle block for intractable cancer pain at the end of life may be effective for selected patients. Epidural neurolytic blocks allow for repeat injections at thoracic levels and for treatment of bilateral pain. Transcatheter epidural neurolysis may be an option for cancer patients with mixed somatic and visceral pain who are resistant to neurolytic visceral sympathetic blockade.[37,38] Both procedures have potential neurological complications. It is essential that these be discussed with the patient and family before the procedure, and informed consent should be documented. There has been a trend to avoid these procedures and to maximize the use of opioids by the oral, subcutaneous, intravenous, transdermal, and intraspinal routes of administration. Recognizing the risks of inadequate analgesia, early recurrence of pain, and serious neurological complications, the indications, if any, for neurolytic spinal or epidural blockade in patients *with nonmalignant pain* are extremely limited. However, neurolytic blocks are simple, low-technology procedures with a high success rate and potential great efficacy.[33] There are selected patients who remain good candidates for neurolytic blockade for intractable cancer pain. Ventafridda and colleagues used neurolytic blockade in 29% of patients entered into a 2-year validating study of the World Health Organization cancer pain treatment guidelines.[42]

KEY POINTS

- The neurolytic agents alcohol and phenol produce nonselective damage to neural tissues. Alcohol extracts lipids and precipitates proteins, while phenol primarily coagulates proteins. Alcohol is hypobaric relative to CSF, while phenol in glycerin is hyperbaric to CSF.
- Both alcohol and phenol may produce a contractile response in blood vessels which may lead to serious ischemic neural tissue damage.
- The goal of neurolytic spinal block is selective destruction of dorsal roots and rootlets between the spinal cord and the dorsal root ganglion. Neurolytic spinal blockade is ideal for patients with advanced malignancy and intractable visceral or somatic pain which is localized to a few adjacent, unilateral dermatomes ideally situated in the trunk.
- Hyperbaric subarachnoid phenol may be well suited to treat a patient at end of life having intractable pelvic cancer pain, especially when performance of a bladder diversion procedure obviates concerns about development of incontinence.
- The most common complication of neurolytic spinal block is persistent pain. The most serious complications are lower extremity muscle weakness and paresis of the urinary and rectal sphincters. These latter complications occur relatively frequently but are usually only transient occurrences.

REFERENCES

1. Bonica JJ, Buckley FP, Moricca G, et al: Neurolytic blockade and hypophysectomy. *In* Bonica JJ, Chapman CR, et al (eds): The Management of Pain, ed 2. Lea & Febiger, Philadelphia, 1990, p 1980.
2. Jain S, Gupta R: Neurolytic agents in clinical practice. *In* Waldman SD (ed): Interventional Pain Management. WB Saunders, Philadelphia, 2001, pp 220–225.
3. Myers RR: Neuropathology of neurolytic agents. *In* Cousins MJ, Bridenbaugh PO (eds): Neural Blockade in Clinical Anesthesia and Management of Pain, ed 3. Lippincott-Raven, Philadelphia, 1998, pp 985–1006.
4. De Leon-Casasola OA, Ditonio E: Drugs commonly used for nerve blocking: Neurolytic agents. *In* Raj PP (ed): Practical Management of Pain, ed 3. Mosby, St Louis, 2000, pp 575–578.
5. Schlosser H: Erfahrungen in der neuralgiebehandlung mit alkoholeinspritzungen. Verh Cong Innere Med 24:49, 1907.
6. Labat G, Greene MB: Contribution to modern method of diagnosis and treatment of so-called sciatic neuralgias. Am J Surg 11:435, 1931.
7. Rumsby MG, Finean JB: The action of organic solvents on the myelin sheaths of peripheral nerve tissue: Short chain aliphatic alcohols. J Neurochem 13:1509, 1966.
8. Merrick RL: Degeneration and recovery of autonomic neurons following alcoholic block. Ann Surg 113:298, 1941.
9. Thompson GE, Moore DC, Bridenbaugh DL, et al: Abdominal pain and alcohol celiac plexus nerve block. Anesth Analg 56:1, 1985.
10. Matsuki M, Kato Y, Ichiyanagi K: Progressive changes in the concentration of ethyl alcohol in the human and canine subarachnoid spaces. Anesthesiology 36:617, 1972.
11. Umedi S, Arai T: Disulfiram-like reaction to moxalactam after celiac plexus alcohol block. Anesth Analg 64:377, 1985.
12. Mandl F: Aqueous solution of phenol as a substitute for alcohol in sympathetic block. J Int Coll Surg 13:566, 1950.
13. Maher RE: Relief of pain in incurable cancer. Lancet 1:18, 1955.
14. Stewart WA, Lourie H: An experimental evaluation of the effects of subarachnoid injections of phenol-Pantopaque in cats. J Neurosurg 20:64–72, 1963.
15. Nathan PW, Sears TA, Smith MC: Effects of phenol solutions on the nerve roots of the cat: An electrophysiological and histological study. J Neurol Sci 2:7–29, 1965.
16. Smith MC: Histological findings following intrathecal injections of phenol solutions for the relief of pain. Anaesthesia 36:387, 1964.
17. Maher RM, Mehta M: Spinal (intrathecal) and extradural analgesia. *In* Lipton S (ed): Persistent Pain: Modern Methods of Treatment. Grune & Stratton, New York, 1977, p 61.
18. Ichiyanagi K, Matsuki M, Kinefuchi J, et al: Progressive changes in the concentration of phenol and glycerin in the human subarachnoid space. Anesthesiology 42:622–624, 1975.
19. Gregg RV, Constantini CH, Ford DJ, et al: Electrophysiologic and histopathologic investigation of alcohol as a neurolytic agent. Anesthesiology 63:A250, 1985.
20. Gregg RV, Constantini CH, Ford DJ, et al: Electrophysiologic and histopathologic investigation of phenol in renograffin as a neurolytic agent. Anesthesiology 63:A239, 1985.
21. Heavner JE, Racz GB: Gross and microscopic lesions produced by phenol neurolytic procedures. *In* Racz GB (ed): Techniques of Neurolysis. Kluwer Academic, Boston, 1989, p 27.
22. Westerlund T, Vuorinen V, Kirvela O, et al: The endoneurial response to neurolytic agents is highly dependent on the mode of application. Reg Anesth Pain Med 24:294–302, 1999.
23. Moller JE, Helweg-Larson J, Jacobsen G: Histopathological lesions in the sciatic nerve of the rat following perineural application of phenol and alcohol solutions. Dan Med Bull 16:116–119, 1969.
24. Gale DW, Valley MA, Rogers JN, et al: Effects of neurolytic concentrations of alcohol and phenol on Dacron and Gore-Tex vascular prosthetic grafts. Reg Anesth 19:395–401, 1994.
25. Brown DL, Rorie DK: Altered reactivity of isolated segmental lumbar arteries of dogs following exposure to ethanol and phenol. Pain 56:139–143, 1994.
26. Johnson ME, Sill JC, Brown DL, et al: The effect of the neurolytic agent ethanol on cytoplasmic calcium in arterial smooth muscle and endothelium. Reg Anesth 21:6–13, 1996.

27. Patt RB, Cousins MJ: Techniques for neurolytic neural blockade. *In* Cousins MJ, Bridenbaugh PO (eds): Neural Blockade in Clinical Anesthesia and Management of Pain, ed 3. Lippincott-Raven, Philadelphia, 1998, pp 1007–1061.

28. Swerdlow M: Complications of neurolytic neural blockade. *In* Cousins MJ, Bridenbaugh PO (eds): Neural Blockade in Clinical Anesthesia and Management of Pain, ed 2. JB Lippincott, Philadelphia, 1988, p 719.

29. Winnie AP, Candido KD: Subarachnoid neurolytic blocks. *In* Waldman SD (ed): Interventional Pain Management. WB Saunders, Philadelphia, 2001, pp 554–559.

30. Swerdlow M: Intrathecal and extradural block and pain relief. *In* Swerdlow M (ed): Relief of Intractable Pain. Elsevier, Amsterdam, 1983, p 175.

31. Slatkin NE, Rhiner M: Phenol saddle blocks for intractable pain at end of life: Report of four cases and literature review. Am J Hosp Pall Care 20:62–66, 2003.

32. Jarrett L, Nandi P, Thompson AJ: Managing severe lower limb spasticity in multiple sclerosis: Does intrathecal phenol have a role? J Neurol Neurosurg Psychiatry 73:705–707, 2002.

33. Charlton JE, Macrae WA: Complications of neurolytic neural blockade. *In* Cousins MJ, Bridenbaugh PO (eds): Neural Blockade in Clinical Anesthesia and Management of Pain, ed 3. Lippincott-Raven, Philadelphia, 1998, pp 663–672.

34. Gerbershagen HY: Neurolysis: subarachnoid neurolytic blockade. Acta Anesthesiol Belg 1:45, 1981.

35. Hay RC: Subarachnoid alcohol block in the control of intractable pain: Report of results in 252 patients. Anesth Analg 41:12, 1962.

36. Kuzucu EY, Derrik WS, Wilber SA: Control of intractable pain with subarachnoid alcohol block. JAMA 195:541–544, 1966.

37. Korevaar WC: Transcatheter thoracic epidural neurolysis using ethyl alcohol. Anesthesiology 69:989–993, 1988.

38. Racz GB, Sabongy M, Gintautas J, et al: Intractable pain therapy using a new epidural catheter. JAMA 248:579–581, 1982.

39. Racz GB, Heavner J, Haynsworth R: Repeat epidural phenol injections in chronic pain and spasticity. *In* Lipton S (ed): Persistent Pain: Modern Methods of Treatment, vol 5. Grune & Stratton, New York, 1985, p 157.

40. Katz JA, Selhorst S, Blisard KS: Histopathological changes in primate spinal cord after single and repeated epidural phenol administration. Reg Anesth 20:283–290, 1995.

41. Hayashi I, Odashiro M, Sasaki Y: Two cases of epidural neurolysis using ethyl alcohol and histopathologic changes in the spinal cord. Masui 49:877–880, 2000.

42. Ventafridda V, Tamburini M, Caraceni A, et al: A validation study of the WHO method for cancer pain relief. Cancer 59:850–856, 1987.

67

Local Anesthetics: Clinical Aspects

Spencer S. Liu, M.D.

Local anesthetics are commonly used in the clinical practice of pain medicine. This chapter discusses clinical pharmacology, pharmacokinetics, and toxicity of local anesthetics.

MECHANISMS OF ACTION OF LOCAL ANESTHETICS

Anatomy of Nerves: Local anesthetics are often used to block nerves either peripherally or centrally at the spinal and epidural space. Knowledge of the anatomy of nerves will aid in understanding the mechanism of action of local anesthetics. Peripheral nerves are mixed nerves containing afferent and efferent fibers that may be myelinated or unmyelinated. Each individual axon within the nerve fiber is surrounded by endoneurium composed of non-neural glial cells. Individual nerve fibers are gathered into fascicles and surrounded by perineurium composed of connective tissue. Finally, the entire peripheral nerve is encased by epineurium composed of dense connective tissue. In addition to the enveloping connective tissue, all mammalian nerves with a diameter greater than 1 μm are myelinated. Myelinated nerve fibers are segmentally enclosed by Schwann cells forming a bilayer lipid membrane that is wrapped several hundred times around each axon. Thus, myelin accounts for over half the thickness of nerve fibers greater than 1 μm. Separating the myelinated regions are the nodes of Ranvier where structural elements for neuronal excitation are concentrated. Unmyelinated nerve fibers (diameter smaller than 1 μm) are encased by a Schwann cell that covers several (5 to 10) fibers at once. These fibers are continuously encased by Schwann cells and do not possess interruptions (nodes of Ranvier). The existence of multiple protective layers around both myelinated and unmyelinated nerve fibers presents a substantial barrier to the entry of clinically used local anesthetics. For example, animal models suggest that performance of peripheral nerve blocks result in only 1.6% of the injected dose of local anesthetic penetrating into the nerve.[1] In general, increasing myelination and nerve diameter leads to increased conduction velocity. The presence of myelin accelerates conduction velocity due to increased electrical insulation of nerve fibers and saltatory conduction. Increased nerve diameter accelerates conduction velocity both by increased myelination and by improved electrical cable conduction properties of the nerve. Both afferent and efferent functions are carried out by both myelinated and unmyelinated nerves.

Electrophysiology of Neural Conduction: Ionic disequilibria across semipermeable membranes form the basis for neuronal resting potentials and for the potential energy needed to initiate and maintain electrical impulses. The resting potential of neural membranes averages −60 to −70 mV with the interior being negative to the exterior. This resting potential is predominantly maintained by a potassium gradient with 10 times greater concentration of potassium within the cell. This gradient is maintained by an active protein pump that transports potassium into the cell and sodium out of the cell through voltage-gated potassium channels that are open at resting potentials.[2] In contrast to the dependence of resting membrane potential to potassium disequilibria, generation of action potentials is primarily due to voltage-gated sodium channels. Sodium channels exist in several conformations depending on membrane potential and time. At resting membrane potential, sodium channels predominantly exist in a resting (closed) conformation. Following activation (opening) of the sodium channel and depolarization, the channel will spontaneously close into an inactivated state in a time-dependent fashion to allow repolarization and then revert to a resting conformation.

An action potential will be generated by depolarization when the impulse firing threshold of the axon is reached. Once an action potential is generated, propagation of the potential along the nerve fiber is required for information to be transmitted. Both impulse generation and propagation are an "all or nothing" phenomenon. In the case of impulse propagation, either the locally generated action potential reaches the threshold potential of adjacent segments and causes propagation along the nerve, or the local depolarization ends. Nonmyelinated fibers require achievement of threshold potential at the immediately adjacent membrane, whereas myelinated fibers require generation of threshold potential at a subsequent node of Ranvier.

Repolarization after action potential generation and propagation rapidly follows due to increasing equilibria of internal and external sodium ions, time-controlled decrease in sodium conductance, and a voltage-controlled increase in potassium conductance. In addition, active internal concentration of potassium occurs via the membrane bound enzyme Na^+/K^+ ATPase which extrudes three sodium ions for every two potassium ions that are absorbed.

Molecular Mechanisms of Action of Local Anesthetics:

Most evidence indicates that the sodium channel is the key target of local anesthetic activity. The wide variety of compounds that exhibit local anesthetic activity combined with the different effects of neutral and charged local anesthetics suggest that local anesthetics may act on the sodium channel either by modification of the lipid membrane surrounding it or by direct interaction with its protein structure.[2]

Previous studies have demonstrated that anesthetics can reduce sodium conductance through sodium channels by interacting with the surrounding lipid membrane. Alterations in neuronal membranes by local anesthetics can occur by altering the fluidity of the membrane which causes membrane expansion and subsequent closure of the sodium channel. Such observations can account for local anesthetic actions of neutral and lipophilic local anesthetics, but do not explain the different activity of clinically used, tertiary amine local anesthetics (e.g., lidocaine). Instead, the mechanisms of action of these local anesthetics are best explained by direct interaction with the sodium channel (modulated receptor theory). The commonly used tertiary local anesthetics exist in free equilibrium as both a lipid-soluble neutral form and a hydrophilic, charged form depending on pKa and environmental pH. Although the neutral form may exert anesthetic actions as described above, the cationic species is clearly the more potent form. These tertiary local anesthetics also all demonstrate greater sodium channel blockade when the neural membrane is repetitively depolarized (1 to 100 Hz), whereas neutral local anesthetics exhibit little change in activity with increased frequency of stimulation (use-dependent block). Increasing frequency of stimulation increases the probability that sodium channels will exist in the open and inactive forms as compared to the unstimulated state. Thus, differences in activity of tertiary local anesthetics between use-dependent (repetitive stimulation) and tonic (unstimulated) block are well explained by the existence of a single local anesthetic receptor within the sodium channel that possesses different affinities during different channel conformations (resting–medium, open–high, inactive–low).

Mechanism of Blockade of Peripheral Nerves:

Local anesthetics may block function of peripheral nerves through several mechanisms. As discussed above, sodium channel blockade leads to attenuation of neural action potential formation and propagation. Although it remains unknown in humans by what percentage the neural action potential must be decreased before functional block occurs, recent animal studies suggest that the action potential must be decreased by at least 50% before measurable loss of function is observed. During clinical applications, it is likely that greater than 1 cm of the peripheral nerve is exposed to local anesthetic. For example, sciatic nerve blocks in humans probably result in 5 to 10 cm of affected nerve length. In such a situation the exposure length of the nerve fiber becomes an important determinant of blocking susceptibility.[1] Smaller nerve fibers require a shorter length of fiber exposed to local anesthetic for block to occur than do large fibers. This observation is theorized to occur due to decremental conduction. This phenomenon describes the decreased ability of successive nodes of Ranvier to propagate an impulse in the presence of local anesthetic. As internodal distances become greater with increasing nerve fiber size, larger nerve fibers will demonstrate increasing resistance to local anesthetic block. Thus, this theory well explains the clinical occurrence of differential sensory block.

A final mechanism whereby local anesthetics may block peripheral nerve function is via degradation of transmitted electrical patterns. It is theorized that a large part of the sensory information transmitted via peripheral nerves is carried via coding of electrical signals in after-potentials and after-oscillations. Evidence for this theory is found in studies demonstrating loss of sensory nerve function after incomplete local anesthetic blockade. For example, sensation of temperature of the skin can be lost despite unimpeded conduction of small fibers.[3]

Mechanism of Blockade of Central Neuraxis:

Central neuraxial block via spinal or epidural administration of local anesthetics involves the same mechanisms as discussed above at the level of spinal nerve roots either intra- or extradural. In addition, central neuraxial administration of local anesthetics allows multiple potential actions of local anesthetics within the spinal cord at different sites. For example, within the dorsal horn, local anesthetics can exert familiar ion channel block of sodium and potassium channels in dorsal horn neurons and inhibit generation and propagation of nociceptive electrical activity. Similar actions in the ventral horn may contribute to block of motor activity from central neuraxial administration of local anesthetics. Other spinal cord neuronal ion channels such as calcium channels are also important for afferent and efferent electrical activity. Administration of calcium channel blockers to spinal cord N (neuronal) calcium channels results in hyperpolarization of cell membranes, resistance to electrical stimulation from nociceptive afferents, and intense analgesia. Local anesthetics appear to have similar actions on calcium channels which may contribute to analgesic actions of central neuraxially administered local anesthetics.

In addition to ion channels, multiple neurotransmitters are involved in nociceptive transmission in the dorsal horn of the spinal cord. For example, substance P, the archetypal tachykinin, is an important neurotransmitter that modulates nociception from C fibers and is released from presynaptic terminals of dorsal root ganglion cells. Administration of local anesthetics in concentrations that occur after spinal and epidural anesthesia inhibits release of substance P and may exert analgesic actions by presynaptic actions. Other neurotransmitters that are important for nociceptive processing in the spinal cord such as acetylcholine and gamma-aminobutyric acid (GABA) are also affected by local anesthetics in the presynaptic area. Local anesthetics can affect these analgesic pathways by either directly binding to receptors or by altering local pharmacokinetics of endogenous agonists. Finally, local anesthetics can also affect the postsynaptic effects of nociceptive neurotransmitters. Administration of clinically relevant concentrations of local anesthetics inhibits binding of substance P to its receptor in the central neuraxis in a noncompetitive fashion. These studies suggest that antinociceptive effects of central neuraxial local anesthetic block may be mediated via complex interactions at neural synapses in addition to ion channel blockade.[2]

PHARMACOLOGY

Clinical Potencies of Local Anesthetics: Clinical effects of local anesthetics depend on numerous factors other than in vitro potency.[1] Local factors affecting diffusion and spread of local anesthetic will have a great impact on clinical potencies of local anesthetics and will vary with different applications (e.g., peripheral nerve block vs. spinal injection).[2] Furthermore, clinical use may not require absolute suppression of the compound action potential, but rather a disruption of information coding in the pattern of discharges.[3] Thus, clinical potencies may not exactly concur with potencies determined in experimental models, but will more acurately reflect clinical effects (Table 67-1).

Tachyphylaxis: Tachyphylaxis to local anesthetics is a clinical phenomenon, whereby repeated injection of the same dose of local anesthetic leads to decreasing efficacy. Tachyphylaxis has been described after central neuraxial blocks, peripheral nerve blocks, and for many different local anesthetic agents (amides, esters, short acting, long acting). Recent evidence suggests a potential phamacokinetic mechanism for tachyphylaxis.[4] Radiolabelled lidocaine was used in rat models for repeated peripheral nerve block and infiltration anesthesia. As expected, repeated injections of a constant dose of lidocaine resulted in marked decrease in the durations of anesthesia. This marked decrease in duration of anesthesia was coupled with an accelerated decline in lidocaine content in the nerves and skin after repeated injections. In addition to pharmokinetic mechanisms, pharmacodynamic mechanisms may also be involved in tachyphylaxis. An interesting clinical feature of tachyphylaxis to local anesthetics is its dependence on dosing interval. If dosing intervals are short enough such that pain does not occur then tachyphylaxis does not develop. Conversely, longer periods of patient discomfort before redosing hastens development of tachyphylaxis. The clinical observation of the importance of pain for the development of tachyphylaxis suggests a central mechanism of tachyphylaxis via spinal cord sensitization (windup), and recent studies lend support to this theory.[5] Further work is needed to elucidate fully the mechanisms of tachyphylaxis to local anesthetics.

Additives to Increase Local Anesthetic Activity

EPINEPHRINE: Addition of epinephrine to local anesthetics can prolong the duration of local anesthetic block, increase the intensity of block, and decrease the systemic absorption of local anesthetic.[6] The mechanism whereby epinephrine exerts its effects on local anesthetics remains uncertain. Vasoconstrictive effects of epinephrine probably play an important role, as most local anesthetics (except ropivacaine) produce local vasodilation.[7] Local vasoconstriction would theoretically inhibit systemic absorption of local anesthetic, thus allowing a greater amount available for blocking activity. Further analgesic effects from epinephrine may also occur via interaction with α-2-adrenergic receptors in the brain and spinal cord, especially since local anesthetics increase the vascular uptake of epinephrine.[8] Although most reports support the practice of adding epinephrine, reported effectiveness depends on amount of epinephrine added, local anesthetic used, and type of regional block (Table 67-2).

ALKALINIZATION: The initial rationale for alkalinization was to increase the percentage of local anesthetic existing as the lipid-soluble, neutral form able to access neural sodium channels. The pH of commercial preparations of local anesthetics ranges from 3.9 to 6.47 and is especially acidic if prepackaged with epinephrine.[9] As the pKa of commonly used local anesthetics ranges from 7.6 to 8.9, less than 3% of the commercially prepared local anesthetic exists as the lipid-soluble, neutral form. However, local anesthetics cannot be alkalinized beyond a pH of 6.05 to 8 before precipitation occurs; thus such pH values will increase the neutral form to around 10%.[9]

Other effects of alkalinization can also increase the clinical effects of local anesthetics.[10] In general, clinical studies demonstrate increased activity of alkalinized local anesthetic primarily when epinephrine is present, either prepackaged or freshly added. Although prepackaged epinephrine-containing solutions are quite acidic, fresh addition of epinephrine does not alter

TABLE 67-1. RELATIVE POTENCY OF LOCAL ANESTHETICS FOR DIFFERENT CLINICAL APPLICATIONS

| | Short Duration 2-Chloroprocaine | Medium Duration | | Long Duration | | |
		Lidocaine	Mepivacaine	Bupivacaine, levobupivacaine	Ropivacaine	Tetracaine
Peripheral nerve	N/A	1	2.6	3.6	3.6	N/A
Spinal	1	1	1	9.6	5	6.3
Epidural	2	1	1	4	4	N/A

N/A, not available.
Data from Liu SS, Hodgson PS: Local anesthetics. *In* Barash PG, Cullen BF, Stoelting RF (eds): Clinical Anesthesia. Lippincott-Raven, Philadelphia, 2001, pp 449–472.

TABLE 67-2. **EFFECTS OF ADDITION OF EPINEPHRINE TO LOCAL ANESTHETICS**

	Increase Duration	Decrease Blood Levels (%)	Dose/Concentration of Epinephrine
Peripheral nerve block			
Bupivacaine	+/−	10–20	1:200,000
Lidocaine	++	20–30	1:200,000
Mepivacaine	++	20–30	1:200,000
Ropivacaine	−	0	1:200,000
Epidural			
Bupivacaine	+/−	10–20	1:300,000 – 1:200,000
Levobupivacaine	+/−	10–20	1:200,000 – 1:400,000
Chloroprocaine	++		1:200,000
Lidocaine	++	20–30	1,600,000 – 1:200,000
Mepivacaine	++	20–30	1:200,000
Ropivacaine	−	0	1:200,000
Spinal			
Bupivacaine	+/−		0.2 mg
Lidocaine	++		0.2 mg
Tetracaine	++		0.2 mg

++, overall supported; −, overall not supported; +/−, unclear.
Data from Liu SS, Hodgson PS: Local anesthetics. *In* Barash PG, Cullen BF, Stoelting RF (eds): Clinical Anesthesia. Lippincott-Raven, Philadelphia, 2001, pp 449–472.

the pH of the more alkaline plain local anesthetic solutions. Thus, the association between increased local anesthetic activity with alkalinization and epinephrine does not appear to be solely due to increased acidity with epinephrine-containing solutions. On the other hand, the vasoconstrictive effects of epinephrine are also pH dependent. At a pH less than 5.6, little vasoconstriction is seen, and maximum vasoconstriction occurs around a pH of 7.8. Therefore, alkalinization may affect the activity of local anesthetic by activation of vasoconstrictive effects of epinephrine.

Clinical effects of alkalinizing plain solutions of local anesthetics will depend on the type of local anesthetic and type of regional block.[11] Variability between local anesthetics and type of block can be expected due to the pKa and commercial pH of each local anesthetic, type of nerves to be blocked, length and diameter of nerves to be blocked, and surrounding vascular and depot structures around the anatomic area of block. Clinical trials suggest that alkalinization most affects lidocaine for axillary block, lidocaine and bupivacaine for epidural block, and mepivacaine for sciatic and femoral blocks.

OPIOIDS: Addition of opioids to local anesthetics has recently gained popularity. Opioids have multiple central neuraxial and peripheral mechanisms of analgesic action. Supraspinal administration of opioids results in analgesia via opiate receptors in multiple sites, via activation of descending spinal pathways, and via activation of nonopioid analgesic pathways. Spinal administration of opioids provides analgesia primarily by attenuating C fiber nociception, and is independent of supraspinal mechanisms.[12] Coadministration of opioids with local anesthetics epidurally and intrathecally results in synergistic analgesia.[13]

The recent discovery of peripheral opioid receptors offers yet another avenue where the coadministration of local anesthetics and opioids may be useful.[14] The most promising clinical results have been from intra-articular administration of local anesthetic/opioid for postoperative analgesia, whereas combining local anesthetics and opioids for nerve blocks appears to be ineffective. There are several reasons for a predicted lack of effect of coadministration of local anesthetic and opioid for peripheral nerve blocks. Anatomically, peripheral opioid receptors are found primarily at the end terminals of afferent fibers. However, peripheral nerves are commonly blocked by deposition of anesthetic proximal to the end terminals of nerve fibers. In addition, common sites for peripheral nerve blocks are encased in multiple layers of connective tissue which the anesthetics must traverse before accessing peripheral opioid receptors. Finally, previous studies have demonstrated the importance of concomitant local tissue inflammation for analgesic effectiveness of peripheral opioid receptors.[15] The mechanism for the underlying dependence on local inflammation is speculative and may involve upregulation or activation of peripheral opioid receptors or "loosening" of intercellular junctions to allow passage of opioids to receptors. Nonetheless, lack of inflammation at the site of a peripheral nerve block may also reduce the effects of coadministration of local anesthetic and opioid. All of these factors combine to decrease the theoretical effectiveness of combinations of local anesthetics and opioids for peripheral nerve blocks.

α-2 AGONISTS: α-2 agonists may also be useful adjuvants to local anesthetics. α-2 agonists, such as clonidine, produce analgesia via supraspinal and spinal adrenergic receptors.[16] Clonidine also has direct inhibitory effects on peripheral nerve conduction (A and C nerve fibers). Thus, addition of clonidine may have multiple routes of action depending on type of application. Preliminary evidence suggests that coadministration of α-2 agonist and local anesthetic results in central neuraxial and peripheral nerve analgesic synergy, whereas systemic (supraspinal) effects are additive.[17] Central neuraxial synergy may be partially due to reductions in spinal cord metabolism and vasoconstriction of spinal cord blood flow by clonidine. Overall, clinical trials indicate that addition of clonidine to intrathecal, epidural, and peripheral applications of local anesthetics enhances local anesthetic activity.

Systemic Analgesia from Local Anesthetics: Intravenous administration of lidocaine (1 to 5 mg/kg) has been used to treat postoperative, cancer, and chronic neuropathic pain. The mechanism of analgesia remains unclear, but does not involve blockade of impulse conduction in peripheral nerves.[18] In fact, multiple mechanisms of systemic analgesia have been proposed. A peripheral mechanism has been demonstrated, as systemic local anesthetics at sub-blocking concentrations (1 to 20 μg/mL) reversibly depress generation of spontaneous electrical activity in injured C and A-delta nerve fibers and dorsal root ganglia. The ability of sub-blocking concentrations of local anesthetic to inhibit electrical coding of sensory information represents another peripheral mechanism for systemic analgesia.[3] Central mechanisms have also been demonstrated by inhibition of tonic electrical activity of hippocampal pyramidal cells, and inhibition of nociceptive reflexes and central sensitization in the spinal cord.[19] In addition, orally administered tocainide and mexiletine (class I anti-arrhythmic agents that are structurally and electrophysiologically similar to lidocaine) have been successfully used to treat chronic pain conditions.

CLINICAL PHARMOCOKINETICS

Systemic absorption of local anesthetics after clinical use can produce blood levels resulting in central nervous system and cardiovascular toxicity. In general, local anesthetics with decreased systemic absorption will have a greater margin of safety. The rate and extent of absorption will depend on numerous factors, the most important of which are: (1) site of injection, (2) dose of local anesthetic, (3) physicochemical properties of local anesthetic, and (4) addition of epinephrine.

The relative amounts of fat and vascularity surrounding the site of injection will interact with the physicochemical properties of the local anesthetic to affect the rate of systemic uptake. In general, areas with greater vascularity will have more rapid and complete uptake, as compared to those with more fat, regardless of type of local anesthetic. Thus, rates of absorption generally decrease in the following order: intercostal > caudal > epidural > brachial plexus > sciatic/femoral (Table 67-3).

TABLE 67-3. TYPICAL PEAK BLOOD LEVELS (C$_{MAX}$) AFTER CLINICAL USE OF LOCAL ANESTHETICS

Local Anesthetic	Technique	Dose (mg)	Cmax (μg/mL)	Tmax (min)	Approximate Threshold Toxic Plasma Concentration (μg/mL)
Bupivacaine	Brachial plexus	150	1.0	20	3
	Celiac plexus	100	1.50	17	
	Epidural	150	1.26	20	
	Intercostal	140	0.90	30	
	Lumbar sympathetic	52.5	0.49	24	
	Sciatic/femoral	400	1.89	15	
Levobupivacaine	Brachial plexus	250	1.2	55	3
	Epidural	75	0.36	50	
Lidocaine	Brachial plexus	400	4.00	25	5
	Epidural	400	4.27	20	
	Intercostal	400	6.8	15	
Mepivacaine	Brachial plexus	500	3.68	24	5
	Epidural	500	4.95	16	
	Intercostal	500	8.06	9	
	Sciatic/femoral	500	3.59	31	
Ropivacaine	Brachial plexus	190	1.3	53	3
	Epidural	150	1.07	40	
	Intercostal	140	1.10	21	

Data from Liu SS, Hodgson PS: Local anesthetics. *In* Barash PG, Cullen BF, Stoelting RF (eds): Clinical Anesthesia. Lippincott-Raven, Philadelphia, 2001, pp 449–472.

The greater the total dose of local anesthetic injected, the greater the systemic absorption and peak blood levels (C_{max}). This relationship is nearly linear, and is relatively unaffected by anesthetic concentration and speed of injection.

Physicochemical properties of local anesthetics will affect systemic absorption. In general, the more potent agents with greater lipid solubility and protein binding will result in lower systemic absorption and C_{max}. Increased binding to neural and non-neural tissue probably explains this observation.

Epinephrine can counteract the inherent vasodilating characteristics of most local anesthetics. The reduction in C_{max} with epinephrine is most effective for the less potent, shorter-acting agents (Table 67-2), as increased tissue binding rather than local blood flow may be a greater determinant of absorption for the long-acting agents.

TOXICITY OF LOCAL ANESTHETICS

Central Nervous System (CNS) Toxicity of Local Anesthetics

SYSTEMIC CNS TOXICITY: Systemic CNS toxicity due to local anesthetics is dose dependent (Table 67-4). Local anesthetic potency for systemic CNS toxicity approximately parallels action potential blocking potency (Table 67-5). External factors can increase potency for CNS toxicity, such as acidosis and increased pCO_2, perhaps via increased cerebral perfusion or decreased protein binding of local anesthetic. There are also external factors that can decrease local anesthetic potency for generalized CNS toxicity. For example, seizure thresholds of local anesthetics are increased by administration of barbiturates and benzodiazepines in animal models.[20]

LOCAL CNS TOXICITY: Recent interest has focused on potential local CNS toxicity from administration of local anesthetics. Previous studies have demonstrated that local anesthetics in clinically used concentrations are safe for peripheral nerves. However, all clinically used local anesthetics can cause concentration-dependent nerve fiber damage in peripheral nerves when used in high enough concentrations.[21]

TABLE 67-4. SYSTEMIC EFFECTS OF LIDOCAINE

Plasma Concentration (μg/mL)	Effect
1–5	Analgesia
5–10	Lightheadedness; tinnitus; numbness of tongue
10–15	Seizures; unconsciousness
15–25	Coma; respiratory arrest
>25	Cardiovascular depression

Data from Liu SS, Hodgson PS: Local anesthetics. In Barash PG, Cullen BF, Stoelting RF (eds): Clinical Anesthesia. Lippincott-Raven, Philadelphia, 2001, pp 449–472.

TABLE 67-5. RELATIVE POTENCY FOR SYSTEMIC CENTRAL NERVOUS SYSTEM TOXICITY BY LOCAL ANESTHETICS AND RATIO OF DOSAGE NEEDED FOR CARDIOVASCULAR SYSTEM:CENTRAL NERVOUS SYSTEM (CVS:CNS) TOXICITY

Agent	Relative Potency for CNS Toxicity	CVS:CNS
Bupivacaine	4	2.0
Levobupivacaine	2.9	2.0
Chloroprocaine	0.3	3.7
Etidocaine	2.0	4.4
Lidocaine	1.0	7.1
Mepivacaine	1.4	7.1
Prilocaine	1.2	3.1
Procaine	0.3	3.7
Ropivacaine	2.9	2.2
Tetracaine	2.0	

Data from Liu SS, Hodgson PS: Local anesthetics. In Barash PG, Cullen BF, Stoelting RF (eds): Clinical Anesthesia. Lippincott-Raven, Philadelphia, 2001, pp 449–472.

Mechanisms for local anesthetic neurotoxicity remain speculative, but previous studies have demonstrated local anesthetic-induced injury to Schwann cells, inhibition of fast axonal transport, and disruption of the blood–nerve barrier. Local anesthetics may also indirectly damage nerves by decreasing neural bloodflow and thus causing ischemia possibly through effects on prostaglandin metabolism.

Intrathecal use of lidocaine (5% in 7.5% dextrose) has received special interest due to reports of persistent sensory deficits after administration via small-bore intrathecal catheter and single injection. In particular, the potentially high incidence (20% to 40%) of transient neurologic symptoms (TNS) after single-shot spinal anesthesia with 5% lidocaine has raised concerns for potential neurotoxicity.[22] Multiple factors increase the risk of TNS such as ambulatory anesthesia status, use of lidocaine, and patient positioning (e.g., lithotomy). Although animal studies demonstrate concentration-dependent electrophysiologic toxicity with lidocaine beginning at approximately 1%, TNS do not appear to be concentration dependent. This contradictory feature coupled with the lack of development of neurologic deficits, lack of electrophysiologic neural changes during TNS, and successful treatment with nonsteroidal anti-inflammatory drugs (NSAIDs) and trigger point injections have led many to question the presumed neurologic etiology of TNS.[22]

Cardiovascular System (CVS) Toxicity of Local Anesthetics: In general, much greater doses of local anesthetics are required to produce CVS toxicity then CNS toxicity. Similar to CNS toxicity, potency for CVS toxicity reflects the anesthetic potency of the agent (Table 67-5). The more potent, more lipid-soluble agents (bupivacaine, etidocaine, levobupivacaine, ropivacaine) appear to have a different sequence of CVS toxicity than less potent agents. For example, increasing doses of lidocaine lead to hypotension, bradycardia, and hypoxia, whereas bupivacaine often results in sudden cardiovascular collapse due to ventricular dysrhythmias that are resistant to resuscitation.[23] Recently, ropivacaine and levobupivacaine have been released as alternatives to bupivacaine. Both of these agents are single-isomer preparations (levo), are approximately equipotent to bupivacaine for regional blocks requiring large doses of local anesthetic (epidural anesthesia and peripheral nerve blocks),[24,25] and are approximately 30% to 50% less cardiotoxic but are still capable of causing sudden cardiovascular collapse.[26] There are several possible systemic and local mechanisms for increased cardiotoxicity from potent local anesthetics.

SYSTEMIC CVS TOXICITY: Recent studies have demonstrated that the central and peripheral nervous systems may be involved in the increased cardiotoxicity with bupivacaine and to a lesser degree levobupivacaine and ropivacaine. The nucleus tractus solitarii in the medulla is an important region for autonomic control of the CVS. Neural activity in the nucleus tractus solitarii of rats is markedly diminished by intravenous doses of bupivacaine immediately prior to development of hypotension. Furthermore, direct intracerebral injection of bupivacaine can elicit sudden dysthymias and cardiovascular collapse.[27,28] Peripheral effects of bupivacaine on the autonomic and vasomotor systems may also augment its CVS toxicity. Bupivacaine possesses a potent peripheral inhibitory effect on sympathetic reflexes that have been observed even at blood concentrations similar to those measured after uncomplicated regional anesthesia.[29] Finally, bupivacaine also has potent direct vasodilating properties which may exacerbate cardiovascular collapse.

LOCAL CVS TOXICITY: The more potent local anesthetics appear to possess greater potential for electrophysiologic toxicity. A previous study examining lidocaine, bupivacaine, and ropivacaine in rats has demonstrated equivalent peak effects on myocardial contractility but much greater effects on electrophysiology (prolongation of QRS) from bupivacaine and ropivacaine than lidocaine.[30] Although all local anesthetics block the cardiac conduction system via a dose-dependent block of sodium channels, two features of bupivacaine's sodium channel blocking abilities may enhance its cardiotoxicity. First, bupivacaine exhibits a much stronger binding affinity to resting and inactivated sodium channels than lidocaine. Second, bupivacaine dissociates slowly from sodium channels during cardiac diastole, and bupivacaine conduction block accumulates at physiologic heart rates (60 to 180 beats per minute). In contrast, lidocaine fully dissociates from sodium channels during diastole and little accumulation of conduction block occurs at physiologic heart rates.

Increased potency for direct myocardial depression from bupivacaine and to a lesser degree levobupivacaine and ropivacaine is another contributing factor to increased cardiotoxicity.[31] Bupivacaine is the most completely studied potent local anesthetic, and possesses a high affinity for sodium and potassium channels in the cardiac myocyte.[32] Furthermore, bupivacaine inhibits calcium channels, release of calcium from sarcoplasmic reticulum, and mitochondrial energy metabolism.[33] Thus, multiple direct effects of bupivacaine on activity of the cardiac myocyte may enhance the cardiotoxicity of bupivacaine.

Treatment of Bupivacaine Toxicity: The multiple mechanisms for cardiovascular toxicity for bupivacaine and to a lesser degree levobupivacaine and ropivacaine have led to no optimal method of treatment. Obviously, oxygenation and ventilation must be immediately instituted with cardiopulmonary resuscitation if needed. Ventricular dysrhythmias may be difficult to treat and may need large and multiple doses of electrical cardioversion, epinephrine, bretyllium, and magnesium. A new and potentially promising therapy is administration of 20% intravenous lipid. Mechanisms are unclear but animal models have been highly successful at rescue after intentional bupivacaine cardiotoxicity.[34]

KEY POINTS

- Local anesthetics have differing potencies with regional anesthesia and pain medicine procedures than their in vitro potencies.
- Depending on application, local anesthetics can be potentiated by epinephrine, alkalinization, opioids, and α-2 agonists.
- TNS from spinal lidocaine are unlikely due to concentration-dependent electrophysiologic neural toxicity.
- Newer, long-acting agents such as ropivacaine and levobupivacaine are approximately equipotent to bupivacaine for peripheral nerve blocks and epidural anesthesia and have less cardiotoxicity.

REFERENCES

1. Gokin AP, Philip B, Strichartz GR: Preferential block of small myelinated sensory and motor fibers by lidocaine: In vivo electrophysiology in the rat sciatic nerve. Anesthesiology 95:1441–54, 2001.
2. Liu SS, Hodgson PS: Local anesthetics. *In* Barash PG, Cullen BF, Stoelting RF (eds): Clinical Anesthesia. Lippincott-Raven, Philadelphia, 2001, pp 449–472.
3. Raymond SA: Subblocking concentrations of local anesthetics: Effects on impulse generation and conduction in single myelinated sciatic nerve axons in frog. Anesth Analg 75:906, 1992.
4. Choi RH, Birknes JK, Popitz-Bergez FA, et al: Pharmacokinetic nature of tachyphylaxis to lidocaine: Peripheral nerve blocks and infiltration anesthesia in rats. Life Sci 61:PL 177–184, 1997.
5. Lee K-C, Wilder RT, Smith RL, Berde CB: Thermal hyperalgesia accelerates and MK-801 prevents the development of tachyphylaxis to rat sciatic nerve blockade. Anesthesiology 81:1284, 1994.
6. Tucker GT: Safety in numbers. The role of pharmacokinetics in local anesthetic toxicity: The 1993 ASRA Lecture. Reg Anesth 19:155, 1994.
7. Sinnott CJ, Cogswell III LP, Johnson A, Strichartz GR: On the mechanism by which epinephrine potentiates lidocaine's peripheral nerve block. Anesthesiology 98:181–188, 2003.
8. Ueda W, Hirakawa M, Mori K: Acceleration of epinephrine absorption by lidocaine. Anesthesiology 63:717, 1985.
9. Ikuta PT, Raza SM, Durrani Z, et al: pH adjustment schedule for the amide local anesthetics. Reg Anesth 14:229, 1989.
10. Wong K, Strichartz GR, Raymond SA: On the mechanisms of potentiation of local anesthetics by bicarbonate buffer: Drug structure–activity studies on isolated peripheral nerve. Anesth Analg 76:131, 1993.

11. Capogna G, Celleno D, Laudano D: Alkalinization of local anesthetics: Which block, which local anesthetic? Reg Anesth 20:369–377, 1995.

12. Niv D, Nemirovsky A, Rudick V, et al: Antinociception induced by simulataneous intrathecal and intraperironeal administration of low doses of morphine. Anesth Analg 80:886, 1995.

13. Walker SM, Goudas LC, Cousins MJ, Carr DB: Combination spinal analgesic chemotherapy: A systematic review [review; 158 refs]. Anesth Analg 95:674–715, 2002.

14. Stein C, Machelska H, Binder W, Schafer M: Peripheral opioid analgesia [review; 42 refs]. Curr Opin Pharmacol 1:62–65, 2001.

15. Machelska H, Stein C: Immune mechanisms in pain control [review; 70 refs]. Anesth Analg 95:1002–1008, table of contents, 2002.

16. Eisenach JC, De Kock M, Klimscha W: Alpha-2-adrenergic agonists for regional anesthesia. A clinical review of clonidine (1984–1995). Anesthesiology 85:655, 1996.

17. Pertovaara A, Hamalainen MM: Spinal potentiation and supraspinal additivity in the antinociceptive interaction between systemically administered α2-adrenoreceptor agonist and cocaine in the rat. Anesth Analg 79:261, 1994.

18. Wallace MS, Laitin S, Licht D, Yaksh TL: Concentration–effect relations for intravenous lidocaine infusions in human volunteers: Effects on acute sensory thresholds and capsaicin-evoked hyperpathia. Anesthesiology 86:1262–1272, 1997.

19. Abram SE, Yaksh TL: Systemic lidocaine blocks nerve injury-induced hyperalgesia and nociceptor driven spinal sensitization in rats. Anesthesiology 80:383, 1994.

20. Bernards CM, Artruu AA: Hexamethonium and midazolam terminate dysrhythmias and hypertension caused by intracerebroventricular bupivacaine in rabbits. Anesthesiology 74:89, 1991.

21. Kalichman MW: Physiologic mehanisms by which local anesthetics may cause injury to nerve and spinal cord. Reg Anesth 18:448, 1993.

22. Liu SS, McDonald SB. Current issues in spinal anesthesia. Anesthesiology 94:888–906, 2001.

23. Groban L, Deal DD, Vernon JC, et al: Cardiac resuscitation after incremental overdosage with lidocaine, bupivacaine, levobupivacaine, and ropivacaine in anesthetized dogs. Anesth Analg 92:37–43, 2001.

24. McClellan KJ, Faulds D: Ropivacaine: An update of its use in regional anaesthesia [review; 161 refs]. Drugs 60:1065–1093, 2000.

25. Foster RH, Markham A: Levobupivacaine: A review of its pharmacology and use as a local anaesthetic [review; 71 refs]. Drugs 59:551–579, 2000.

26. Ohmura S, Kawada M, Ohta T, et al: Systemic toxicity and resuscitation in bupivacaine-, levobupivacaine-, or ropivacaine-infused rats [comment]. Anesth Analg 93:743–748, 2001.

27. Pickering AE, Waki H, Headley PM, Paton JF: Investigation of systemic bupivacaine toxicity using the in situ perfused working heart–brainstem preparation of the rat. Anesthesiology 97:1550–1556, 2002.

28. Ladd LA, Chang DH, Wilson KA, et al: Effects of CNS site-directed carotid arterial infusions of bupivacaine, levobupivacaine, and ropivacaine in sheep. Anesthesiology 97:418–428, 2002.

29. Chang KSK, Yang M, Andresen MC: Clinically relevant concentrations of bupivacaine inhibit rat aortic baroreceptors. Anesth Analg 78:501, 1994.

30. Reiz S: Cardiotoxicity of ropivacaine – A new amide local anaesthetic agent. Acta Anaesthesiol Scand 33:93, 1989.

31. Graf BM, Abraham I, Eberbach N, et al: Differences in cardiotoxicity of bupivacaine and ropivacaine are the result of physicochemical and stereoselective properties. Anesthesiology 96:1427–1434, 2002.

32. Berman MF, Lipka LJ: Relative sodium current block by bupivacaine and lidocaine in neonatal rat myocytes. Anesth Analg 79:350, 1994.

33. Sztark F, Tueux O, Emy P, et al: Effects of bupivacaine on cellular oxygen consumption and adenine nucleotide metabolism. Anesth Analg 78:335, 1994.

34. Groban L, Butterworth J: Lipid reversal of bupivacaine toxicity: Has the silver bullet been identified? Reg Anesth Pain Med 28:167–169, 2003.

Spinal Anesthesia

Francis Salinas, M.D.

This chapter reviews the relevant clinical anatomy, technical aspects, pharmacology, and physiology of spinal anesthesia. Special aspects of spinal anesthesia are covered in detail in other chapters: intrathecal opioid injections for postoperative pain (Chapter 29), postdural puncture (Chapter 40), combined spinal–epidural technique (Chapter 70), complications after neuraxial blockade, including transient neurological symptoms (TNS) and cauda equina syndrome (Chapter 82), and neuraxial blocks in the setting of pharmacologic anticoagulation (Chapter 83).

ANATOMY

Vertebral Column and Ligaments: The spinal column is bound together and stabilized by several ligaments (Fig. 68-1).[1] Beneath the skin and subcutaneous tissue, the supraspinous ligament runs between the tips of the spinous processes. The interspinous ligament connects adjacent spinous processes, blending posteriorly with the supraspinous ligament and anteriorly with the ligamentum flavum. The ligamentum flavum connects adjacent lamina firmly together and it forms, together with the lamina, the posterior wall of the spinal canal. The anterior and posterior longitudinal ligaments run along the anterior and posterior surfaces of the vertebral bodies.

Meninges and Spinal Cord: Within the bony spinal canal, the spinal meninges form three connective tissue membranes that cover and protect the spinal cord. The dura mater is the outermost meningeal layer and consists of fibroelastic fibers arranged in both a longitudinal and circumferential arrangement. The inner layer of the dura mater is closely attached to the middle meningeal layer, the arachnoid mater. There is a potential space between the dura mater and the arachnoid mater called the subdural space, which normally contains minute amounts of serous fluid that moistens the surfaces of the opposing layers. The structure of the arachnoid mater allows for easy separation of the arachnoid mater from the inner surface of the dura. This has important clinical implications as this can potentially allow subdural injection of spinal

agents despite free return of cerebrospinal fluid (CSF) during intended spinal injection, leading to unanticipated effects of spinal anesthesia.[2] The arachnoid mater is the middle meningeal layer and is composed of overlapping layers of epithelial cells connected by tight junctions, which allows the arachnoid mater to function as the principal physiologic barrier to substances traversing in and out of the CSF.[3] The pia mater is the innermost meningeal layer and is composed of a thin layer of highly vascular connective tissue adherent to the

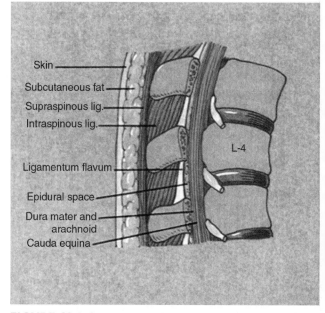

FIGURE 68-1. Sagittal view of the structures the spinal needle passes through before reaching the subarachnoid space. (Reproduced with permission from Brown DL: Spinal block. In Brown DL (ed): Atlas of Regional Anesthesia, ed 1. WB Saunders, Philadelphia, 1992, pp 267–281.)

Skin
Subcutaneous fat
Supraspinous lig.
Intraspinous lig.
L-4
Ligamentum flavum
Epidural space
Dura mater and arachnoid
Cauda equina

spinal cord. In contrast to the arachnoid mater, the pia mater is fenestrated, which allows the spinal cord to communicate freely with the CSF.

In the majority of adults the caudal tip of the spinal cord (conus medullaris) ends between L1 and L2. However, both cadaver studies and magnetic resonance imaging (MRI) studies have shown that in 2% to 5% of adults the conus medullaris extends below the L2 vertebral body.[4–6] Given the inability of even experienced anesthesiologists to identify accurately the correct intervertebral space (one space higher than presumed in 51% of cases) and the frequency with which the conus medullaris terminates below L2, it is not surprising that there are now published reports of significant damage to the distal spinal cord after administration of spinal anesthesia.[4,7–9] Thus, to avoid possible trauma to the distal spinal cord, spinal anesthesia should not be routinely performed above L2. However, spinal anesthesia performed at the L2–L3 intervertebral space is not completely devoid of risk of trauma to the spinal cord as a small percentage of adults will have a conus medullaris that terminates below L2.

PHYSIOLOGY OF CEREBROSPINAL FLUID

Cerebrospinal Fluid Volume: Local anesthetic solutions injected at the lumbar level will become diluted in the volume of the lumbosacral CSF before reaching their site of action within the central nervous system. Thus, individual variations in lumbosacral CSF volumes can have a significant effect on the extent and duration of spinal anesthesia. Recent studies utilizing fast spin-echo MRI demonstrate a wide variability between individuals in the volume of lumbosacral CSF, with a mean volume of 50 ± 20 mL, but a range of 28 to 81 mL. Individuals considered obese, with an average body mass index of 33.1, had a significantly lower CSF volume (42.9 ± 9.5 mL

vs. 53.5 ± 12.9 mL) compared to nonobese individuals.[10] Further MRI studies have demonstrated that the physiologic maneuver of external abdominal compression leading to inferior vena cava obstruction (as would be seen in the term parturient) has been shown to decrease dynamically the lumbosacral CSF volume by as much as 28%.[11] The mechanism for the decreased lumbosacral CSF volume was shown to be the result of direct compression of the thecal sac by engorged epidural venous plexus. The venous engorgement and compression of the thecal sac were reversible, as demonstrated by the return to baseline CSF volumes immediately after removal of external abdominal compression.[11] In a small volunteer study lumbosacral CSF volume and the extent and duration of spinal anesthesia showed excellent clinical correlation, with CSF volume accounting for 80% of the variability for peak block height and regression of sensory and motor block. Unfortunately, lumbosacral CSF volume did not correlate well with external physical measurements, except possibly for body mass index.[12] As a consequence, lumbosacral CSF volume cannot be easily estimated from individual patient's body habitus.

Cerebrospinal Fluid Density, Specific Gravity, and Baricity: Solutions that have the same density as CSF have a baricity of 1.0000 and are classified isobaric. Solutions that are denser than CSF are classified as hyperbaric, whereas solutions that are less dense than CSF are termed hypobaric. Recent studies have reported normal values for human CSF densities, which show clinically significant variations between specific patient population subgroups (Table 68-1).[13–15] The mean CSF density for males (1.00063 ± 0.00013) is very similar to postmenopausal females (1.00062 ± 0.00016). The mean CSF density for premenopausal females (1.00048 ± 0.00006) is slightly lower than for postmenopausal females. Women at term pregnancy and immediately postpartum have been shown to

TABLE 68-1. DENSITIES AND BARICITIES OF COMMONLY USED LOCAL ANESTHETICS FOR SPINAL ANESTHESIA

Solution	Density	Baricity
CSF	1.0003*/1.0006†	1.0000
Hyperbaric		
Lidocaine 5% in 7.5% dextrose	1.0265	1.0262/1.0260
Bupivacaine 0.75% in 8.25% dextrose	1.0247	1.0244/1.0241
Isobaric‡		
Lidocaine 2%	0.9999	0.9996/0.9993
Bupivacaine 0.5%	0.9994	0.9991/0.9988
Hypobaric		
Lidocaine 0.5% in water	0.9985	0.9985/0.9980
Bupivacaine 0.35% in water	0.9973	0.9970/0.9967
Tetracaine 0.2% in water	0.9925	0.9922/0.9920

* Average density for pregnant females.
† Average density for males and nonpregnant females.
‡ The plain solutions are hypobaric relative to CSF, but are used clinically as "isobaric solutions."
Data from references 13–16, 22–26.

have significantly lower mean CSF densities (1.00033 ± 0.00007) than either men or nonpregnant women. A recent study using plain hypobaric bupivacaine in supine patients demonstrated excellent clinical correlation between CSF density and peak block height. This study indicated that the higher the CSF density, the higher the level of peak block height observed.[16] However, despite the level of clinical correlation, CSF density was poorly predictive of peak block height, suggesting that CSF density is only one of a number of factors influencing the extent of spinal anesthesia.

TECHNICAL ASPECTS OF SPINAL ANESTHESIA

Needle Design: Spinal needles utilized for lumbar puncture are classified into two main categories based on those that are designed to cut though dural fibers ("cutting needles") or to spread dural fibers ("pencil-point needles"). Typical cutting-type spinal needles, such as the Quincke spinal needle, have a sharp point with a medium-length cutting bevel. Commonly used pencil-point needles (Whitacre, Sprotte, and Gertie-Marx) have a rounded noncutting solid tip, with an opening on the side of the needle, 2 to 4 mm proximal to the needle tip. The type and size of spinal needle chosen by the majority of anesthesiologists is based on the desire to minimize leakage of CSF after dural puncture, so as to minimize the incidence of postdural puncture headache (PDPH). In an in vitro investigation pencil-point needles demonstrated 2 to 3 times less CSF leakage compared to Quincke cutting needles of corresponding size.[17] Furthermore, a meta-analysis and a large prospective randomized study have shown both a lower risk and lower severity of PDPH with pencil-point needles compared to cutting needles of comparable size.[18,19] However, attention to technique also plays an important role in reducing the risk of PDPH, as a large prospective analysis of 8,034 spinal anesthetics demonstrated that repeated attempts at dural puncture conferred a 2.6-fold increased risk of PDPH (4.2% vs. 1.6%) compared to a single dural puncture.[20]

Approaches to the Subarachnoid Space: The midline approach is the most widely used one as it is technically the easiest to learn and perform for most anesthesiologists. With the patient in the lateral, sitting, or prone position, the anesthesiologist must advance the spinal needle toward the subarachnoid space by judging the needle direction in both the sagittal plane (parallel to the spinous process) and horizontal plane (relative to the course and angle of spinal needle direction in the cephalad and caudad orientation of the interspinous space). With the spinal needle inserted in the truly midline sagittal plane and in the middle of the interspinous space, the spinal needle should advance, in order, through the skin, subcutaneous tissue, supraspinous ligament, interspinous ligament, ligamentum flavum, and then the dura and arachnoid matter before entering the subarachnoid space (Fig. 68-1).[1]

Although less commonly performed, the paramedian approach is more useful in clinical circumstances where advancing a spinal needle through the midline interspinous space is difficult, such as degenerative calcification of interspinous ligament in elderly patients. The paramedian approach is also ideally suited when optimal patient positioning cannot be achieved due to either pain (fractures and dislocations of the hip and lower extremities) or patient characteristics (obesity, term pregnancy, or scoliosis). Anatomically, the paramedian approach takes advantage of a much larger target area to allow access to the subarachnoid space (see Fig. 69-4).[21] For the paramedian approach, the spinous process forming the lower border of the desired interspace is identified, with the spinal needle insertion site 1 cm lateral to this point. The spinal needle is directed slightly cephalad and 10° to 15° toward the midline to compensate for the lateral insertion point. There should be minimal resistance to advancement until the ligamentum flavum is encountered. The lumbosacral (Taylor) approach is a variation of the paramedian approach designed to enter the subarachnoid space via the L5–S1 interlaminar space (the largest in the vertebral column). The spinal needle is inserted 1 cm medial and 1 cm caudal to the most caudad aspect of the posterior superior iliac spine. The spinal needle is then angled 45° to 55° cephalad and medial enough to access the L5–S1 interspace.

PHARMACOLOGY OF LOCAL ANESTHETICS AND ADJUNCTS

Factors Influencing Block Height: Successful spinal anesthesia requires a block that not only provides sensory anesthesia and/or motor blockade appropriate for the surgical procedure and site, but also of sufficient duration for the expected time course of the procedure. In addition, the block must predictably recede, so as to allow for timely discharge from the recovery room. Thus, knowledge of the factors that determine block height and duration is essential in choosing the proper local anesthetic solution for an individual patient.

Baricity: Many factors have been postulated to influence peak block height.[22] However, only a few factors are of clinical importance and the baricity of the local anesthetic solution relative to the patient position is the most important. Baricity is important because gravity causes hyperbaric solutions to gravitate to the most dependent areas of the subarachnoid space, whereas hypobaric solutions float upward to nondependent areas of the subarachnoid space. Therefore, it is possible, by choosing the appropriate baricity and patient position, to "direct" the local anesthetic solution to the dermatomal segments that require anesthesia. Clinically, hypobaric solutions have been defined as those with densities less than three standard deviations below mean patient CSF density and hyperbaric solutions as those with densities greater than three standard deviations above mean patient CSF density.[13,14] Because of the variability in mean CSF density, a local anesthetic solution must have a density of less than 0.9990 to function reliably as a hypobaric spinal anesthetic. In contrast, solutions with a density of greater than 1.0015 can be expected to function reliably as hyperbaric spinal anesthetics.[22]

HYPERBARIC SOLUTIONS: Hyperbaric solutions are formulated by mixing the local anesthetic solution in 5% to 8% dextrose (Table 68-1).[22–26] The distribution of hyperbaric solutions is determined by the position of the patient after injection of the local anesthetic solution into the subarachnoid space. In the level supine position, the typical curvature of the spinal column influences the distribution so that hyperbaric solutions injected at the apex of the lumbar lordosis will flow caudad toward the sacral kyphosis, and, more importantly, cephalad toward the lowest point of the thoracic kyphosis (Fig. 68-2).[21]

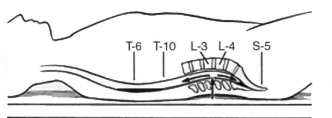

FIGURE 68-2. In the level horizontal supine position the typical curvature of the spinal column influences the distribution so that hyperbaric solutions injected at the apex of the lumbar lordosis will flow caudad toward the sacral kyphosis and cephalad toward the thoracic kyphosis. Pooling of hyperbaric solutions in the thoracic kyphosis is thought to explain the clinical observation that hyperbaric spinal anesthesia will typically result in an average block height of T4–T6. (Reproduced with permission from Stevens RA: Neuraxial blocks. *In* Brown DL (ed): Regional Anesthesia and Analgesia, ed 1. WB Saunders, Philadelphia, 1996, pp 319–322.)

Thus, pooling of hyperbaric solutions in the thoracic kyphosis is thought to explain the clinical observation that hyperbaric spinal anesthesia will typically result in an average block height of T4–T6. Injection at or above the apex of the lumbar lordosis, or placing the patient in the supine head down position after injection will facilitate movement toward the thoracic kyphosis. Injection of hyperbaric solutions with the patient in the sitting position will result in pooling of hyperbaric solutions in the lumbosacral segments to produce a "saddle block," which is appropriate for perineal and perianal surgery performed in the lithotomy position.

HYPOBARIC SOLUTIONS: Hypobaric solutions are typically formulated by diluting the local anesthetic solution in distilled water. They are ideally suited for surgical procedures in either the head down (prone jackknife) position or with the patient in the lateral position where the operative side is nondependent (total hip arthoplasty).[23,24] Hypobaric solutions can be injected with the patient in the same position as that required for surgery, thus minimizing the need to change the position after induction of spinal anesthesia. Hypobaric spinal anesthesia for total hip arthoplasty has been shown to provide longer sensory block than isobaric spinal anesthesia, despite no difference in peak block height or the degree of motor block.[23] Use of hypobaric spinal anesthesia for the prone jackknife position also provides a "saddle block" for the operative procedure. When the procedure is completed, the patient must be allowed to recover with the head down in the supine position as the block has the potential to rise if the patient's upper body is placed upright.[24]

ISOBARIC SOLUTIONS: The major clinical advantage of isobaric solutions is that the position of the patient during and after the injection has no effect on the distribution of the anesthetic and therefore has no effect on the final level of block height. Isobaric spinal anesthesia is particularly well suited when levels of sensory anesthesia to T10 or below are required. Tetracaine, in niphanoid crystalline form (20 mg), can be diluted with patient CSF and the desired dose can be injected in an isobaric fashion. More commonly, the plain commercial formulations of bupivacaine (0.5%) and lidocaine (2%) are clinically used as "isobaric" solutions. However, recent work

determining the reference values for human CSF densities and densities of commonly used local anesthetic indicates that they are actually hypobaric relative to human CSF.[14,25,26]

Minor Factors Influencing Block Height: Patient characteristics such as age, height, weight, and anatomic configuration of the spine have all been postulated to have an effect on block height, but none of these have been shown to be either clinically important or a reliable predictor of block height. The effect of the interdependent variables of local anesthetic dose, volume, and concentration on the distribution within the subarachnoid space has been extensively studied, and it appears that the dose (mass) is the most important factor of the three in influencing the peak block height of isobaric solutions within the subarachnoid space.[27,28] The dose of local anesthetic is relatively less important in influencing the peak block height of hyperbaric solutions, as baricity relative to patient position predominates over the dose in determining peak block height.

Factors Influencing Duration of Spinal Anesthesia

LOCAL ANESTHETIC: The primary factor in determining block duration is the choice of local anesthetic agent. Lidocaine, procaine, and chloroprocaine are short- to intermediate-acting local anesthetics depending on the dose used. Lidocaine has traditionally been the most widely used local anesthetic for short- to intermediate-duration surgery, but its associated risk of TNS has limited it recent use (see Chapter 82 on the complications of neuraxial blockade). Although currently approved by the US Food and Drug Administration (FDA), 2-chloroprocaine is not yet specifically indicated for use in spinal anesthesia. However, recent volunteer data indicate that preservative-free spinal 2-chloroprocaine in the dose range 30 to 60 mg is effective and has an anesthetic profile appropriate for use in the ambulatory setting, with minimal risk of TNS.[29,30] Mepivacaine is an intermediate-acting local anesthetic with a similar profile to lidocaine, but is not commonly used for spinal anesthesia. Bupivacaine and tetracaine are long-acting local anesthetics that are commonly used for spinal anesthesia. Ropivacaine is an L-isomer of racemic bupivacaine and appears to be 50% less potent than bupivacaine for spinal anesthesia, but in equipotent doses has a similar duration of sensory anesthesia and recovery profile. Levobupivacaine is the S-enantiomer of racemic bupivacaine and appears to be similar to bupivacaine in potency and duration of spinal anesthesia.

DOSE AND BLOCK HEIGHT: Increasing the dose clearly increases duration of the spinal anesthesia for all the commonly used spinal local anesthetics (Table 68-2).[31–36] For a given dose of local anesthetic, higher peak blocks tend to regress faster than blocks. Thus, isobaric local anesthetic solutions usually produce blocks of longer duration than hyperbaric blocks using the same dose. In addition, hyperbaric spinal anesthesia can be manipulated by patient position to decrease peak block height and also result in a block of longer duration.[37] It is thought that the lower cephalad spread results in a relatively higher local anesthetic concentration in the CSF and spinal nerve roots, which requires more time for the local anesthetic to decrease below the minimally effective concentration.

SPINAL ANALGESIC ADJUNCTS: The addition of local anesthetic adjuncts for spinal anesthesia was originally used to prolong the duration of sensory anesthesia. However, the use

TABLE 68-2. DOSE AND DURATION OF LOCAL ANESTHETICS COMMONLY USED FOR SPINAL ANESTHESIA IN THE USA

Local Anesthetic Solution	Dose (mg)	Peak Block Height	Duration of Sensory Anesthesia*		
			Onset of Two-Dermatome Regression (minutes)	Regression to L1–L2 (minutes)	Regression to S2–S3 (minutes)
Hyperbaric 2-chloroprocaine	30	T7	47 ± 8	53 ± 30	98 ± 20
	45	T5	45 ± 3	75 ± 14	116 ± 15
	60	T2	43 ± 5	92 ± 13	132 ± 23
Plain lidocaine	40	T12	44 ± 17	60 ± 24	142 ± 27
	60	T8	40 ± 16	67 ± 14	157 ± 28
	80	T4	33 ± 16	104 ± 23	188 ± 27
Hyperbaric lidocaine	50	T4	50 ± 16	80 ± 30	123 ± 21
	75	T4	75 ± 4	†	136 ± 6
	100	T2	59 ± 11	134 ± 38	198 ± 60
Plain mepivacaine	60	T4	95 ± 21	150 ± 32	210 ± 18
	80	T4	100 ± 20	160 ± 20	225 ± 23
Plain bupivacaine	10	T7	33 ± 16	100 ± 20	180 ± 10
Hyperbaric bupivacaine	4	T8	21 ± 4	45 ± 12	120 ± 25
	5	T7	53 ± 14	†	120 ± 25
	8	T5	59 ± 13	135 ± 51	198 ± 33
	12	T5	65 ± 32	123 ± 44	164 ± 30
	15	T3	110 ± 30	216 ± 46	300 ± 55
Hyperbaric ropivacaine	4	T12	25 ± 13	30 ± 12	38 ± 32
	8	T9	37 ± 12	60 ± 20	80 ± 33
	12	T4	47 ± 12	115 ± 30	143 ± 23

* Duration of anesthesia is dependent on dose, peak block height, and location of surgery.
† Data unavailable.
Data from references 29–36.

of spinal anesthetic adjuncts is now used primarily to decrease the dose of local anesthetics used for ambulatory anesthesia in order to provide a faster recovery while maintaining or improving anesthetic success.[38,39] In addition, spinal analgesic adjuncts can also prolong and improve postoperative analgesia. The useful spinal analgesic adjuncts include vasoconstrictors (epinephrine and phenylephrine), opioids (fentanyl and morphine), and the alpha-2-adrenergic agonist clonidine. Spinal administration of neostigmine improves postoperative analgesia (by inhibiting the breakdown of the spinal neurotransmitter acetylcholine). However, the high incidence of refractory nausea and vomiting associated with spinal administration of neostigmine precludes its use as a clinically useful analgesic adjunct for spinal anesthesia.[40,41]

The addition of 0.2 mg of epinephrine has been shown to prolong the duration of lumbosacral anesthesia for both lidocaine and low-dose bupivacaine by 20% to 35%.[38]

Unfortunately, the usefulness of epinephrine at traditional doses (0.2 mg) is hampered by the prolongation of recovery from both motor block and the ability to void to a disproportionate degree as compared with the anesthetic benefit.[38,42] However, recent data demonstrate that very low doses of intrathecal epinephrine (15 μg) may improve the anesthetic success of low-dose lidocaine/fentanyl spinal anesthesia without prolonging the time to void and achieve discharge criteria.[43] Phenylephrine has significantly decreased in popularity as an intrathecal adjunct due to the fact that its use has been associated with a 10-fold increase in the risk of TNS.[44]

Intrathecally administered opioids selectively bind to mu-opioid receptors in the spinal cord and produce spinal analgesia by decreasing nociceptive afferent input from A-delta and C fibers without affecting dorsal nerve roots or somatosensory evoked potentials.[45] Hydrophilic opioids, such as morphine, produce good spinal analgesia, and are characterized by slow onset of action (greater than 30 minutes), long duration of action (up to 24 hours), and a small risk of delayed respiratory depression caused by cephalad spread within CSF.[45] There is evidence that 0.1 mg of intrathecal morphine produces a clinically relevant reduction in postoperative pain and analgesic consumption, while minimizing the associated effects of pruritis, nausea, vomiting, urinary retention, and respiratory depression.[46,47] Fentanyl is a lipophilic opioid that produces rapid onset of dose-dependent analgesia with a minimally effective dose of 10 μg, and with the risk of respiratory depression minimal up to 25 μg. Addition of 10 to 25 μg of fentanyl to local anesthetic solutions allows the use of very small doses of local anesthetics, improves the quality and success of surgical anesthesia, and does not lengthen duration until discharge in ambulatory surgery.[38,39]

Intrathecal-administered clonidine acts synergistically with local anesthetics and provides dose-dependent sensory analgesia and side effects of hypotension, bradycardia, and sedation.[48] Clonidine is well absorbed, with almost 100% bioavailability, and, interestingly, a similar spinal anesthetic augmentation can be achieved by administering 150 to 200 μg clonidine orally 1 to 3 hours before induction of spinal anesthesia.[49] Dose–response studies for intrathecal clonidine indicate that 15 μg is an optimal dose for low-dose ambulatory spinal anesthesia, and is not associated with delays in either recovery of motor block or spontaneous voiding.[50,51]

PHYSIOLOGIC EFFECTS OF SPINAL ANESTHESIA

An understanding of the physiologic effects of spinal anesthesia is essential in order to differentiate them from true complications that can potentially lead to adverse patient outcomes.[52] The degree to which these physiologic effects determine the risk–benefit ratio of choosing spinal anesthesia is dependent on the patient's comorbidity, surgical procedure, clinical setting (inpatient vs. ambulatory), and dose and choice of local anesthetic solutions.

Cardiovascular Physiology: Hypotension and bradycardia are both well-recognized physiologic effects of the sympathetic blockade from spinal anesthesia, although their clinical presentations are usually mild and respond rapidly to intervention. The incidence of hypotension (defined as a systolic blood pressure below 85 to 90 mmHg or a decrease from baseline levels of more than 30%) in large prospective studies ranges from 8.2% to 33%, with 81% of the episodes occurring when the peak sensory block height is above T5.[53–55] Hypotension is due to a decrease in both cardiac output (CO) and systemic vascular resistance (SVR). The marked decrease in the vasomotor tone within the venous capacitance vessels results in a redistribution of the central blood volume to the splanchnic and lower extremity vasculature.[56,57] The resulting decrease in venous return to the heart leads to a decrease in CO. In young healthy subjects SVR decreases only moderately (15% to 18%), even with significant sympathetic blockade. In contrast, SVR has been shown to decrease by as much as 23% to 26% in older patients (average age 68 to 72 years) with T4–T6 sensory levels of spinal anesthesia.[58,59] The higher degree of resting sympathetic tone exhibited by older patients may explain the exaggerated decrease in SVR to sympathetic blockade compared with younger patients.

Heart rate is physiologically controlled within the vasomotor center of the medulla oblongata. Spinal anesthesia that blocks efferent connections from the medulla to the sympathetic cardioaccelerator fibers at the T1 to T5 levels results in unopposed parasympathetic tone and will normally result in only mild to moderate decreases in heart rate. The overall incidence of moderate bradycardia (defined as a heart rate below 50 beats/minute) in large prospective studies is 9% to 13%, with almost 75% of these episodes occurring when peak sensory block height is above T5.[53,54] More importantly, the sympathectomy induced by spinal anesthesia can lead to a marked decrease in venous return to the heart that paradoxically further enhances parasympathetic tone, potentially leading to episodes of unexpected marked bradycardia/asystole and cardiovascular collapse.[60] The mechanisms leading to an unexpected abrupt onset of bradycardia/asystole are believed to be due to a complex interaction of cardiovascular reflexes mediated by baroreceptors within the sinoatrial node, right atrium, and left ventricle.[60, 61]

Despite the frequency of mild to moderate decreases in both blood pressure and heart rate, severe episodes of hypotension and sudden onset of marked bradycardia/asystole are uncommon, but not rare. In two large prospective surveys designed to evaluate the incidence of serious complications during spinal anesthesia only 28 cardiac arrests occurred in 42,521 patients for an overall incidence of 0.07%, but with a mortality rate of 21% of those suffering a cardiac arrest.[62,63]

Given the mortality rate associated with cardiac arrest occurring during spinal anesthesia, awareness of, and attention to, the factors that lead to hypotension and bradycardia are essential for proper patient selection and patient management. Large prospective studies have identified a peak sensory block height above T5 as the most predictive risk factor for developing hypotension during spinal anesthesia.[53,54,62] Other risk factors identified, in order of predictive strength, include emergency surgery, alcohol consumption, age greater than 40 years, baseline systolic blood pressure of less than 120 mmHg, history of hypertension, combined spinal/general anesthesia, dural puncture at or above the L2–L3 intervertebral space, and addition of phenylephrine to the local anesthetic.[53,54,62] The risk factors for developing moderate bradycardia in order of predictive strength include a baseline heart rate less than 60 beats/minute, ASA physical status I vs. III/IV, prolonged PR interval, use of beta-blockers, and block height greater than T5.[53,54,62] In contrast to a sensory block level above T5 being the most significant risk factor for hypotension, a sensory block level above T5 is a weak predictor of moderate bradycardia and does not correlate with the severity of bradycardia.[54] When two or more risk factors for bradycardia are present, the risk for severe bradycardia/asystole may significantly increase.

The use of prophylactic volume loading with crystalloid solutions prior to induction of spinal anesthesia in order to prevent hypotension is largely ineffective due to the known pharmacokinetic properties of infused crystalloid solutions.[64] Even large volumes of infused crystalloids rapidly redistribute from the intravascular compartment to the extravascular compartment.[65] Thus, a more rational approach to crystalloid administration based on pharmacokinetics may be to administer crystalloids rapidly either at the time of or just after induction of spinal anesthesia.[52] In contrast to crystalloid solutions, prophylactic volume loading with 500 to 1,000 mL colloid solutions prior to induction of spinal anesthesia has been consistently shown to maintain blood pressure and volume expansion in both surgical and obstetric patients.[66,67] Colloid administration results in a sustained increase of intravascular volume due to the slower redistribution from the intravascular to the extravascular compartment.[52,64] However, the increased efficacy of colloid therapy must be weighed against its increased cost and the small but significant risk of anaphylaxis.

The treatment of hypotension includes measures for correcting the underlying mechanisms of decreased venous return, SVR, and CO.[52] Studies have shown that optimal pharmacologic correction of these mechanisms is best achieved by the use of the combined alpha-adrenergic and beta-adrenergic agonist effects of ephedrine.[68] Ephedrine may be administered intravenously in 5 to 10 mg boluses or as a continuous infusion (50 mg/250 to 1,000 mg crystalloid). Phenylephrine is a direct-acting alpha-adrenergic agonist, and intravenous administration results in dose-dependent increases in systolic, diastolic, and mean arterial pressure that are accompanied by decreases in CO and heart rate. Thus, phenylephrine may be best suited for the hypotensive, tachycardic patient in whom the potential chronotropic effects of ephedrine are not desired. Moderate bradycardia may be treated with either intravenous ephedrine (5 to 20 mg boluses) or intravenous atropine (0.4 to 1.0 mg). In the case of severe bradycardia, particularly if unresponsive to the previously mentioned treatments or in the setting of a precipitous decrease in heart rate, intravenous epinephrine (5 to 20 μg) should be administered promptly and may require even higher doses (0.2 to 0.3 mg) to achieve a desired response.

Thermoregulatory Physiology: Perioperative hypothermia associated with spinal anesthesia can approach the same magnitude as with general anesthesia.[69] Despite the associated increased incidence of myocardial ischemia, cardiac morbidity, wound infection, blood loss, transfusion requirements, and patient discomfort associated with perioperative hypothermia, an observational study revealed that only 27% of patients were monitored for temperature during a central neuraxial block.[70] In this study 77% of the patients were hypothermic (core temperature less than 36°C) upon arrival to the recovery room and 22% had a core temperature below 35°C. The three principal mechanisms that contribute to heat loss during spinal anesthesia are redistribution of core heat to the periphery caused by vasodilatation from the sympathetic blockade, loss of thermoregulation due to decreased thresholds for vasoconstriction and shivering below the level of blockade, and increased heat loss from vasodilatation below the level of sympathetic blockade. It has been demonstrated that incremental increases in block height leads to proportional decreases in core temperature.[69,71] Strategies to minimize heat loss include accurate (core) temperature monitoring, active warming with forced air warmers, warming of intravenous fluids, covering exposed skin, and limiting block height when possible.[52] Active measures should be instituted routinely as they are not only effective in minimizing heat loss, but have also been shown to decrease recovery room stays by 50% to 60%.[72]

Pulmonary Physiology: Spinal blockade to even midthoracic levels has been shown to have minimal effect on inspiratory muscle function, with little change in respiratory rate, tidal volume, resting minute ventilation, and mean inspiratory flow.[52] In contrast, active expiratory muscle function as measured by peak expiratory flow has been shown to decrease in proportion to the height of spinal blockade. Midthoracic blocks associated with anterior abdominal and intercostal muscle relaxation limit active expiratory muscle function and can potentially impair the ability to cough and clear tracheal or bronchial secretions. In the absence of sedation, spinal anesthesia has a minimal clinical effect on gas exchange.[73] In clinical settings the use of intrathecal morphine is not associated with an increased risk of hypoxemia or depression of respiratory rate as compared to intravenous morphine.[74] In a volunteer study the use of intrathecal morphine has been shown to depress the ventilatory response to hypoxia in similar magnitude to, but longer lasting than, that after equianalgesic doses of intravenous morphine.[75]

Central Nervous System Effects: Spinal anesthesia has been shown to have sedative effects in the absence of intravenous sedation.[76] In addition, central neuraxial anesthesia has been show to decrease the hypnotic requirements of midazolam, thiopental, and potent inhaled anesthetics.[77–79] The proposed mechanism for this independent sedative effect of spinal anesthesia is a decrease in reticular activating system activity due to interruption of ascending afferent sensory input to the brain. Animal studies support the mechanism of deafferentation as hypnotic requirements and EEG measurements of electrical activity in the reticular formation are decreased during spinal anesthesia without detection of local anesthetics in the brain.[79,80] Clinically, the degree of sedation correlates with the level of peak block height, with greater sedation observed with greater block heights.[77] The clinical relevance of these observations is the decreased requirements for pharmacological sedation during spinal anesthesia.

REFERENCES

1. Brown DL: Spinal block. *In* Brown DL (ed): Atlas of Regional Anesthesia, ed 1. WB Saunders, Philadelphia, 1992, pp 267–281.
2. Hogan QH: Anatomy of the spinal anesthesia: some old and new findings. Reg Anesth Pain Med 23:340–343, 1998.
3. Bernards CM, Hill HF: Morphine and alfentanil permeability through the spinal dura, arachnoid, and pia mater of dogs and monkeys. Anesthesiology 73:1214–1219, 1990.
4. Broadbent CR, Maxwell WB, Ferrie R, et al: Ability of anaesthetists to identify a marked lumbar interspace. Anaesthesia 55: 1122–1126, 2000.
5. Saifuddin A, Burnett SJ, White J: The variation of the position of the conus medullaris in an adult population: A magnetic resonance imaging study. Spine 23:1452–1456, 1998.
6. Reimann AF, Anson BJ: Vertebral level of termination of the spinal cord with report of a case of a sacral cord. Anat Rec 88:127–138, 1944.
7. Render CA: The reproducibility of the iliac crest as a marker of lumbar spine level. Anaesthesia 51:1070–1071, 1996.
8. Reynolds F: Damage to the conus medullaris following spinal anaesthesia. Anaesthesia 56:235–247, 2001.
9. Hamandi K, Mottershead J, Lewis T, et al: Irreversible damage to the spinal cord following spinal anesthesia. Neurology 59: 624–626, 2002.
10. Hogan QH, Prost RP, Kulier A, et al: Magnetic resonance imaging of the cerebrospinal fluid volume and the influence of body habitus and abdominal pressure. Anesthesiology 84:1341–1349, 1996.
11. Lee RR, Abraham RA, Quinn CB: Dynamic physiologic changes in lumbar CSF volume quantitatively measured by three-dimensional fast spin-echo MRI. Spine 10:1172–1178, 2001.

12. Carpenter RL, Hogan QH, Liu SS, et al: Lumbosacral cerebrospinal fluid volume is the primary determinant of sensory block extent and duration during spinal anesthesia. Anesthesiology 89:24–29, 1998.

13. Richardson MG, Wissler RN: Density of lumbar cerebrospinal fluid in pregnant and nonpregnant humans. Anesthesiology 85:326–330, 1996.

14. Lui ACP, Polis TZ, Cicutti NJ: Densities of cerebrospinal fluid and spinal anaesthetic solutions in surgical populations at body temperature. Can J Anaesth 45:297–303, 1998.

15. Schiffer E, Van Gessel E, Gamulin Z: Influence of sex on cerebrospinal fluid density in adults. Br J Anaesth 83:943–944, 1999.

16. Schiffer E, Van Gessel E, Fournier R, et al: Cerebrospinal fluid density influences extent of plain bupivacaine spinal anesthesia. Anesthesiology 96:1325–1330, 2002.

17. Holst D, Mollman M, Ebel C: In vitro investigation of cerebrospinal fluid leakage after dural puncture with various spinal needles. Anesth Analg 87:1331–1335, 1998.

18. Halpern S, Preston R: Postdural puncture headache and spinal needle design. Meta-analyses. Anesthesiology 81:1376–1383, 1994.

19. Vallejo MC, Mandell GL, Sabo DP, et al: Postdural puncture headache: A randomized comparison of five spinal needles in obstetric patients. Anesth Analg 91:916–920, 2000.

20. Seeberger MD, Kaufmann M, Staender S, et al: Repeated dural puncture increases the incidence of postdural puncture headache. Anesth Analg 82:302–305, 1996.

21. Stevens RA: Neuraxial blocks. *In* Brown DL (ed): Regional Anesthesia and Analgesia, ed 1. WB Saunders, Philadelphia, 1996, pp 319–322.

22. Greene NM: Distribution of local anesthetic solutions within the subarachnoid space. Anesth Analg 64:715–730, 1985.

23. Faust A, Fournier R, Van Gessel E, et al: Isobaric versus hypobaric spinal bupivacaine for total hip arthoplasty in the lateral position. Anesth Analg 97:589–594, 2003.

24. Bodily M, Carpenter RL, Owens BD: Lidocaine 0.5% spinal anaesthesia: A hypobaric solution for short-stay perirectal surgery. Can J Anaesth 39:770–773, 1992.

25. Horlocker TT, Wedel DJ: Density, specific gravity, and baricity of spinal anesthetic solutions at body temperature. Anesth Analg 76:1015–1018, 1993.

26. Richardson MG, Wissler RN: Densities of dextrose-free intrathecal local anesthetics, opioids, and combinations measured at 37°C. Anesth Analg 84:95–99, 1997.

27. Van Sunder AA, Grouls RJ, Korsten HH, et al: Spinal anesthesia: Volume or concentration – What matters? Reg Anesth 21:112–118, 1996.

28. Malinovsky JM, Renaud G, Le Corre P, et al: Intrathecal bupivacaine in humans: Influence of volume and baricity. Anesthesiology 91:1260–1266, 1999.

29. Smith KN, Kopacz DJ, McDonald SB: Spinal 2-chloroprocaine: A dose ranging study and the effect of epinephrine. Anesth Analg 98:81–88, 2004.

30. Na KB, Kopacz DJ: Spinal 2-chloroprocaine solutions: Density at 37°C and pH titration. Anesth Analg 98:70–74, 2004.

31. Liam BL, Yim CF, Chong JL: Dose response study of 1% lidocaine for spinal anaesthesia for lower limb and perineal surgery. Can J Anaesth 45:645–650, 1998.

32. Markey JR, Montiague R, Winnie AP: A comparative efficacy of hyperbaric 5% lidocaine and 1.5% lidocaine for spinal anesthesia. Anesth Analg 85:1105–1107, 1997.

33. Pawloski J, Sukhani R, Pappas A, et al: The anesthetic and recovery profile of two doses (60 and 80 mg) of plain mepivacaine for ambulatory anesthesia. Anesth Analg 91:580–584, 2000.

34. McDonald SB, Liu SS, Kopacz DJ, et al: Hyperbaric spinal ropivacaine: A comparison to bupivacaine in volunteers. Anesthesiology 90:971–977, 1999.

35. Alley EA, Kopacz DJ, McDonald SB, et al: Hyperbaric spinal levobupivacaine: A comparison to racemic bupivacaine in volunteers. Anesth Analg 94:188–193, 2002.

36. Frey K, Holman S, Mikat-Stevens M, et al: The recovery profile of hyperbaric spinal anesthesia with lidocaine, tetracaine, and bupivacaine. Reg Anesth Pain Med 23:159–163, 1998.

37. Kooger Infante NE, Van Gessel E, Forster A, et al: Extent of hyperbaric spinal anesthesia influences the duration of spinal block. Anesthesiology 92:1319–1323, 2000.

38. Salinas FV, Liu SS: Spinal anaesthesia: Local anaesthetics and adjuncts in the ambulatory setting. Best Pract Res Clin Anaesthesiol 16:195–2002, 2002.

39. Pitkanen M, Rosenberg PH: Local anaesthetics and additives for spinal anaesthesia – Characteristics and factors influencing the spread and duration of the block. Best Pract Res Clin Anaesthesiol 17:305–322, 2003.

40. Liu SS, Hodgson PH, Moore JW, et al: Dose–response effects of spinal neostigmine added to bupivacaine spinal anesthesia in volunteers. Anesthesiology 90:710–717, 1999.

41. Lauretti GR, Hood DD, Eisenach JC, et al: A multi-center study of intrathecal neostigmine for analgesia following vaginal hysterectomy. Anesthesiology 89:913–918, 1998.

42. Moore JM, Liu SS, Pollock JE, et al: The effect of epinephrine on small-dose hyperbaric bupivacaine spinal anesthesia: Clinical implications for ambulatory surgery. Anesth Analg 86:973–977, 1998.

43. Turker G, Unkunkaya N, Yilmazlar A, et al: Effects of adding epinephrine plus fentanyl to low-dose lidocaine for spinal anesthesia in outpatient knee arthroscopy. Acta Anaesthesiol Scand 47:986–992, 2003.

44. Sakura S, Sumi M, Sakaguchi Y, et al: The addition of phenylephrine contributes to the development of transient neurological symptoms after spinal anesthesia with 0.5% tetracaine. Anesthesiology 87:771–778, 1997.

45. Hamber EA, Vsicomi CM: Intrathecal lipophilic opioids as adjuncts to surgical spinal anesthesia. Reg Anesth Pain Med 24:255–263, 1999.

46. Dahl JB, Jeppesen IS, Jorgensen H, Wetterslev J, et al: Intraoperative and postoperative analgesic efficacy and adverse effects of intrathecal opioids in patients undergoing cesarean section with spinal anesthesia: A qualitative and quantitative systematic review of randomized controlled trials. Anesthesiology 91:1919–1927, 1999.

47. Slappendel R, Weber EWG, Dirksen R, et al: Optimization of the dose of intrathecal morphine in total hip surgery: A dose-finding study. Anesth Analg 88:822–826, 1999.

48. Chiari A, Eisenach JC: Spinal anesthesia: Mechanisms, agents, methods, and safety. Reg Anesth Pain Med 23:1353–1359, 1998.

49. Liu SS, Chiu AA, Neal JM, et al: Oral clonidine prolongs lidocaine spinal anesthesia in human volunteers. Anesthesiology 82:1353–1359, 1995.

50. DeKocK M, Gautier P, Fanard L, et al: Intrathecal ropivacaine and clonidine for ambulatory knee arthroscopy: A dose response study. Anesthesiology 94:574–578, 2001.

51. Dobrydnjov I, Axelsson K, Thorn SE, et al: Clonidine combined with small-dose bupivacaine during spinal anesthesia for inguinal herniorrhaphy: A randomized double-blinded study. Anesth Analg 96:1496–1503, 2003.

52. Salinas FV, Sueda LA, Liu SS: Physiology of spinal anaesthesia and practical suggestions for successful spinal anaesthesia. Best Pract Res Clin Anaesthesiol 17:289–303, 2003.

53. Tarkkila PJ, Isola J: A regression model for identifying patients at high risk of hypotension, bradycardia, and nausea during spinal anaesthesia. Acta Anaesthesiol Scand 36:554–558, 1992.

54. Carpenter RL, Caplan RA, Brown DL, et al: Incidence and risk factors for side effects of spinal anesthesia. Anesthesiology 76:916–922, 1992.

55. Hartmann B, Junger A, Klasen J, et al: The incidence and risk factors for hypotension after spinal anesthesia: An analysis with automated data collection. Anesth Analg 94:1521–1529, 2002.

56. Hogan QA: Venous capacitance changes in the lower extremities during spinal anesthesia. Reg Anesth 21:376, 1996.

57. Arndt JO, Hock A, Stanton-Hocks M, et al: Peridural anesthesia and the distribution of blood in supine humans. Anesthesiology 63:616–623, 1985.

58. Critchley LAH, Stuart JC, Short TG, et al: Haemodynamic effects of subarachnoid block in elderly patients. Br J Anaesth 73:464–470, 1994.

59. Rooke GA, Freun PR, Jacobson AF: Hemodynamic response and change in organ blood volume during spinal anesthesia in elderly men with cardiac disease. Anesth Analg 85:99–105, 1997.

60. Evans RG, Ventura S, Dampney RAL, et al: Neural mechanisms in the cardiovascular responses to acute central hypovolaemia. Clin Exp Pharmacol Physiol 28:479–487, 2001.

61. Stienstra R: Mechanisms behind and treatment of sudden, unexpected circulatory collapse during central neuraxis blockade. Acta Anaesthesiol Scand 44:965–971, 2000.

62. Tarkkila PJ, Kaukinen S: Complications during spinal anesthesia. Reg Anesth 16:101–106, 1991.

63. Auroy Y, Narchi P Messiah A, et al: Serious complications related to regional anesthesia; results of a prospective survey in France. Anesthesiology 87:479–486, 1997.

64. Griffel MI, Kaufman BS: Pharmacology and physiology of colloids and crystalloids. Crit Care Clin 8:235–253, 1992.

65. Svensen C, Hahn RG: Volume kinetics of ringer solution, dextran 70, and hypertonic saline in male volunteers. Anesthesiology 87:204–212, 1997.

66. Sharma SK, Gajraj NM, Sidawi ES: Prevention of hypotension during spinal anesthesia: A comparison of hetastarch and lactated Ringer's solution. Anesth Analg 84:111–114, 1997.

67. Marhofer P, Faryniak B, Oismuller C, et al: Cardiovascular effects of 6% hetastarch and lactated Ringer's solution during spinal anesthesia. Reg Anesth Pain Med 24:399–404, 1999.

68. Butterworth JF, Piccione W, Berrizbeitia LD, et al: Augmentation of venous return by adrenergic agonists during spinal anesthesia. Anesth Analg 85:126–133, 1986.

69. Sessler DI: Perioperative heat balance. Anesthesiology 92:578–596, 2000.

70. Arkilic CF, Akca O, Taguchi A, et al: Temperature monitoring and management during neuraxial anesthesia: An observational study. Anesth Analg 91:662–666, 2000.

71. Frank SM, El-Rahmany HK, Cattanea CG, et al: Predictors of hypothermia during spinal anesthesia. Anesthesiology 92:1330–1334, 2000.

72. Casati A, Fanelli G, Ricci A, et al: Shortening the discharging time after total hip replacement under combined spinal/epidural anesthesia by actively warming the patient during surgery. Minerva Anestesiol 65:507–514, 1999.

73. Steinbrook RA, Concepcion MA: Respiratory effects of spinal anesthesia. Anesth Analg 72:182–186, 1991.

74. Cole PJ, Craske DA, Wheatley RG: Efficacy and respiratory effects of low-dose spinal morphine for postoperative analgesia following knee arthoplasty. Br J Anaesth 85:233–237, 2000.

75. Bailey PL, Lu JK, Pace NL, et al: Effects of intrathecal morphine on the ventilatory response to hypoxia. N Eng J Med 343:1228–1234, 2000.

76. Pollock JE, Neal JM, Liu SS, et al: Sedation during spinal anesthesia. Anesthesiology 93:728–734, 2000.

77. Gentili M, Huu PC, Enel D, et al: Sedation depends on the level of sensory block induced by spinal anesthesia. Br J Anaesth 81:970–971, 1998.

78. Hodgson PH, Liu SS, Gras TW: Does epidural anesthesia have general anesthetic effects? Anesthesiology 91:1687–1692, 1999.

79. Eappen S, Kissin I: Effect of subarachnoid bupivacaine block on anesthetic requirements for thiopental in rats. Anesthesiology 88:1036–1042, 1998.

80. Antognini JF, Jinks SL, Atherley R, et al: Spinal anaesthesia indirectly depresses cortical activity associated with electrical stimulation of the reticular formation. Br J Anaesth 91:233–238, 2003.

Epidural Anesthesia

Rom A. Stevens, M.D., and
Nigel E. Sharrock, M.B. Ch.B.

Epidural anesthesia has been used in one form or another since shortly after the start of the 20th century.[1] The advent of the Tuohy needle and epidural catheter in the 1940s led to an interest in caudal and lumbar epidural anesthesia for the provision of labor analgesia. During the past 20 years a great deal of new information about the physiology and anatomy relevant to the practice of epidural anesthesia has led to greater clinical success with this technique. Currently, in North America and Europe epidural anesthesia with or without "light general anesthesia" is a very popular technique for operative anesthesia with the ability to extend epidural analgesia into the postoperative period for several days or weeks.

ANATOMY

The epidural space is a potential space that exists within the bony confines of spinal canal outside the dura mater. For this reason, the term "extradural anesthesia" is used in the UK and Ireland and "peridural anesthesia" is used in the German-speaking countries. The epidural space extends from the sacrococcygeal ligament to the foramen magnum. This space contains fat and blood vessels at some levels, but is only a potential space at other levels (Fig. 69-1). Work by Hogan has demonstrated the discontinuous nature of the epidural space.[2] Fortunately for anesthesiologists and patients, this discontinuous space can be made continuous by injection of local anesthetic (or contrast dye), and small-gauge catheters can be passed for some distance cephalad to the insertion point, provided radiologic guidance is used.

Starting from the plane of the back, there are three ligaments through which an epidural needle must pass to reach the epidural space: (1) the supraspinous ligament, a thin ligament of little consequence that joins the tips of the spinous processes, (2) the interspinous ligament, which connects adjacent spinous process and can degenerate to form cavities, sometimes resulting in a false loss-of-resistance test, and (3) the ligamentum flavum, which is an embryologically bilateral structure fused in the midline, sometimes incompletely.[3] As the epidural needle is advanced from the interspinous ligament into the denser ligamentum flavum, an increase in the resistance to injection is felt, and sometimes a "gritty" sensation is noted. Loss of resistance should occur within approximately 5 mm of needle entry into the ligamentum flavum.

The depth from skin to the epidural space in adults is dependent upon the amount of adipose tissue present. Gutierrez measured the distance from skin to loss of resistance

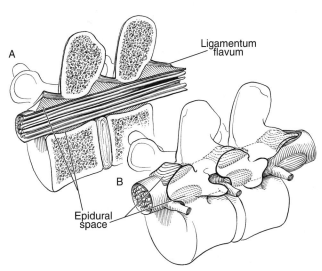

FIGURE 69-1. *A*, Sagittal section of the epidural space demonstrates that the contents of the epidural space depend upon the level of section. *B*, Three-dimensional representation of the epidural space shows the discontinuity of the epidural contents. However, this potential space can be dilated by injection of fluid into the epidural space and made continuous. (Reproduced from Stevens RA: Neuraxial blocks. *In* Brown DL (ed): Regional Anesthesia and Analgesia. WB Saunders, Philadelphia, 1996, pp 319–357 by permission of Mayo Foundation for Medical Education and Research.)

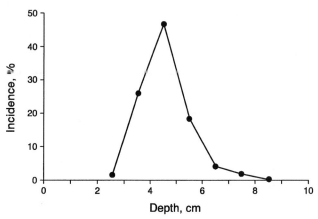

FIGURE 69-2. Depth of epidural space from skin. Data from Gutierrez.[4] (Reproduced from Stevens RA: Neuraxial blocks. *In* Brown DL (ed): Regional Anesthesia and Analgesia. WB Saunders, Philadelphia, 1996, pp 319–357 by permission of Mayo Foundation for Medical Education and Research.)

in adults[4] (Fig. 69-2). The most frequently encountered distance was 5 cm, but the distance ranged from 2.5 to 9 cm in his study population.

SELECTION OF INTERSPACE AND APPROACH

The epidural space can in theory be entered at any vertebral interspace between C2 and the sacral hiatus (L5/S1). In usual clinical practice the most cephalad interspace used is C7/T1 and the most caudad is the sacral hiatus. The guiding principle behind the choice of the interspace is to place the epidural catheter closest to the dermatome in the middle of the surgical incision (Fig. 69-3). For example, if the patient is to undergo a gastrectomy (incision: T6–T11), the epidural catheter should ideally be placed between T8 and T10. Following this principle will result in the maximum concentration of local anesthetic or opioid delivered at the dermatomes where anesthesia, analgesia, and motor block are required.

There are two standard approaches to the epidural space: midline and paramedian. They differ in the angle of the needle with respect to the plane of the back and in the exact location of needle puncture of the skin. The actual point of needle entry into the epidural space does not differ substantially between these two approaches. For the beginner, the midline

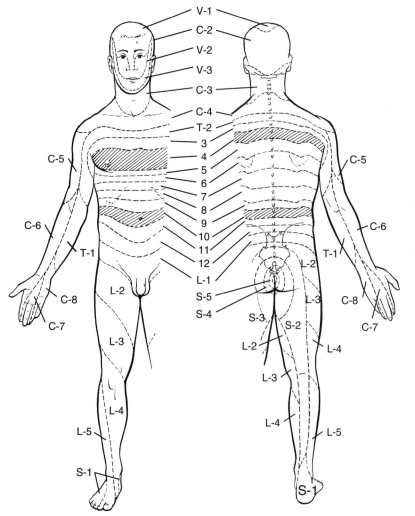

FIGURE 69-3. Dermatome chart. When testing the upper limit of block on the chest, note that the T2 dermatome borders on the C4 dermatome. Dermatomes C5 through T1 comprise the brachial plexus. (Reproduced from Stevens RA: Neuraxial blocks. *In* Brown DL (ed): Regional Anesthesia and Analgesia. WB Saunders, Philadelphia, 1996, pp 319–357 by permission of Mayo Foundation for Medical Education and Research.)

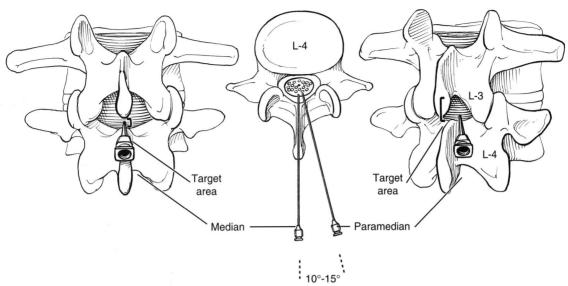

FIGURE 69-4. Paramedian approach for lumbar neuraxial block. The target area when the needle is angled 10° to 15° from midline is larger than the target area for the midline approach. This approach is particularly useful in elderly patients who may have osteoarthritic changes narrowing the interspace or degenerative interspinous ligaments, which could produce a false-positive loss of resistance to injection. This approach is also very useful for thoracic epidural anesthesia. (Reproduced from Stevens RA: Neuraxial blocks. In Brown DL (ed): Regional Anesthesia and Analgesia. WB Saunders, Philadelphia, 1996, pp 319–357 by permission of Mayo Foundation for Medical Education and Research.)

approach is the easiest, because the needle is inserted perpendicular to the skin and parallel to the spinous processes at that spinal level (Fig. 69-3, bony anatomy of the spinous processes). For epidural punctures in the midthoracic region (T5–T10) angulation of spinous processes and in some cases overlapping spinous processes require a very acute angle of insertion when the midline approach is attempted. A paramedian approach is often easier in this region. In the elderly population degeneration of the interspinous ligaments may result in cavitation and a false loss of resistance to injection.[5] Additionally, osteophytic growth of the laminae may result in narrowing of the "target area" available with the midline approach. The paramedian approach will provide a larger "target area" (Fig. 69-4).

The largest interspace in the body is the L5/S1 interspace. The paramedian approach to this interspace is called the "Taylor approach." The needle is inserted at a point 1 cm medial and 1 cm caudal to the posterior superior iliac spine, and inserted at a 45° angle cephalad and medial toward the interspace. In patients with advanced stages of calcification of the spine the Taylor approach may provide the best opportunity to gain access to the lumbar epidural space.

IDENTIFICATION OF THE EPIDURAL SPACE

A variety of different techniques for identifying needle entry into the epidural space have been described.[6] The most commonly used techniques are the "hanging drop" technique of Gutierrez[7] and the "loss of resistance" technique. Studies have shown that the thoracic epidural space has a subatmospheric pressure, probably related to the negative intrapleural pressure, and will "suck" a drop of fluid placed at the hub of the Tuohy needle as the needle is advanced from the ligamentum flavum into the epidural space. Presence of a negative pressure in the lumbar epidural space is not as reliable; therefore Bromage does not recommend the use of the hanging drop technique in the lumbar region, particularly in laboring females, where the pressure may be increased during contractions of the uterus.[6]

Loss of resistance to air or saline is probably the most widely used technique to identify needle entry into the epidural space. The sensation felt on the syringe when using air or saline is quite different. Air is compressible and the feeling is "bouncy" and the epidural needle is advanced through the interspinous and yellow ligaments. Saline is not compressible and provides a rapid change from resistance to no resistance to injection when the needle enters the epidural space. Loss of resistance to air has the advantage that no fluid is injected into the epidural space; thus if fluid is aspirated from the Tuohy needle, it will be clear that this fluid is cerebrospinal fluid (CSF). In addition, any saline that is injected into the epidural space will dilute local anesthetic subsequently injected. Disadvantages of using air include rare cases of venous air embolus, pneumocephalus, nerve root compression, persistence of epidural air bubbles for greater than 24 hours, expansion of these air bubbles if nitrous oxide is inhaled, and possibly resultant inadequate anesthesia.[8] The authors believe that in the hands of an expert there is no clear advantage of one technique over the other, as long as large volumes (>3 mL) of air are not injected. Whether air or saline is used is the personal preference of the anesthesiologist (Fig. 69-5).

FACTORS AFFECTING SPREAD OF LOCAL ANESTHETICS WITHIN THE EPIDURAL SPACE

Major factors that have been generally accepted to affect spread of block after epidural injection of local anesthetic *in the adult patient* are:[9] (1) dose of local anesthetic (volume × concentration), (2) age of patient, and (3) site of injection (thoracic vs. lumbar). Minor factors are: (1) morbid obesity,

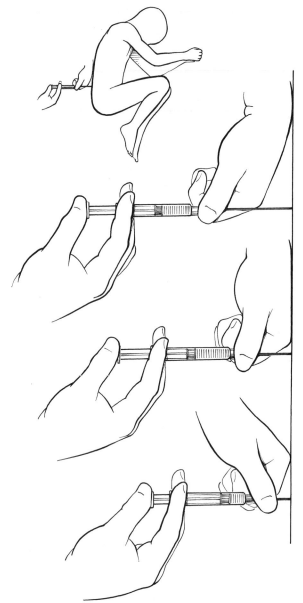

FIGURE 69-5. "Bromage grip" for advancing the epidural needle. The needle is firmly gripped between the thumb and index finger of the nondominant hand. The dorsum of the wrist is placed against the patient's back, and the needle is advanced by extension of the wrist. The dominant hand provides intermittent (for loss of resistance to air) or constant (for loss of resistance to saline) pressure on the plunger of the needle. Needle advancement is halted as soon as resistance to injection is lost. (Reproduced from Stevens RA: Neuraxial blocks. *In* Brown DL (ed): Regional Anesthesia and Analgesia. WB Saunders, Philadelphia, 1996, pp 319–357 by permission of Mayo Foundation for Medical Education and Research.)

(2) pregnancy, and (3) position of patient. Factors that have been shown to have no effect upon spread are: (1) gender, (2) height, (3) weight (except for morbid obesity), (4) direction of Tuohy needle orientation, (5) speed of injection, (6) arteriosclerosis, and (7) mode of injection (fractionated vs. bolus injection). Doses of local anesthetics should be reduced with

thoracic vs. lumbar injection in patients older than 70 years, and to a lesser extent in morbidly obese and in pregnant patients. To calculate roughly anesthetic spread after lumbar injection of 2% lidocaine in a young adult, the figures of 1.25 mL/segment for lumbar injection and 0.75 mL/segment for thoracic injection can be used.[10]

CHOICE OF DRUG, DOSE, AND DURATION OF ACTION

For epidural anesthesia, the choice of drug is essentially a question of how long is the desired duration of anesthesia. Generally, for outpatient surgery, 2-chloroprocaine 3% and lidocaine 2%, with or without epinephrine, are the drugs of choice, because the patient will generally meet discharge criteria within 3 to 4 hours after a 20 mL dose.[11] Mepivacaine 2% produces a longer duration of sensory anesthesia than lidocaine 2%, and a significantly longer time to discharge from the ambulatory surgery center. Bupivacaine or levobupivacaine 0.5 to 0.75% and ropivacaine 0.75 to 1.0% are the drugs of choice for inpatient surgery, because of their longer duration of action. The 1% solution of ropivacaine and the 0.75% solution of bupivacaine are roughly equivalent in terms of duration and quality of sensory and motor block.[12] The time to obtaining surgical anesthesia and motor block is somewhat longer with the less concentrated solutions. The concentrated solutions produce more complete motor block and more complete block of the S1 nerve root, which sometimes remains unblocked after lumbar epidural anesthesia.[13] Anesthesia of this dermatome is important for ankle surgery, and must be confirmed by sensory testing before the patient is draped for surgery.

Epinephrine (1:200,000) is added by the authors to all epidural solutions because it serves as a marker for intravascular injection should either the epidural needle or catheter be placed into a blood vessel at any time. By monitoring the heart rate during and for 2 minutes after epidural local anesthetic injection, and by injecting no more than a 5 mL aliquot at once, an intravascular injection of local anesthetic can be detected, and catastrophic local anesthetic toxicity can be avoided.

A convenient way to compare the duration of action among different local anesthetics is "time to two-segment regression" (Fig. 69-6). Table 69-1 lists the times to two-segment regression for commonly used local anesthetics.[14]

COMPLICATIONS

Amongst beginners, the most common complication of epidural anesthesia is a failed block. In experienced hands the failure rate of epidural anesthesia should be less than 3%. The most common explanation for failure, in the opinion of the authors, is encountering a false loss of resistance, insertion of the epidural catheter and subsequent local anesthetic injection into a space other than the epidural space. A false loss of resistance can be encountered with the Tuohy needle tip in a variety of places, including in a cavitated interspinous ligament,[5] in the paravertebral space, and in the prevertebral space. To avoid a failed epidural block in the practice of surgical anesthesia, the following procedures are recommended by the authors:

1. A thorough knowledge of spinal anatomy is necessary.
2. The level of needle puncture should be guided by the dermatomal site of surgery (see above).

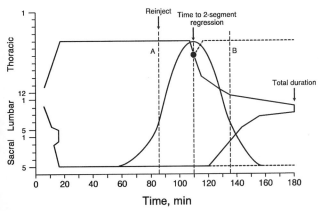

FIGURE 69-6. Analgesia–time plot of lumbar epidural analgesia. Note time to initial onset (latency), time to maximum spread, time to two-segment regression, and time to complete resolution of analgesia. The optimum time to reinjection, to avoid regression of anesthesia, is calculated as mean time to two-segment regression minus 1.5 times standard deviation. (Reproduced from Stevens RA: Neuraxial blocks. In Brown DL (ed): Regional Anesthesia and Analgesia. WB Saunders, Philadelphia, 1996, pp 319–357 by permission of Mayo Foundation for Medical Education and Research.)

3. An adequate dose of concentrated local anesthetic (0.75% bupivacaine or levobupivacaine, 1.0% ropivacaine, 3% 2-chloroprocaine, or 2% lidocaine) should be injected via the needle to set up the block with minimal delay and to facilitate passage of the epidural catheter.
4. The epidural catheter must be tested for intravascular and intrathecal placement by injection, after a negative aspiration test of 3 mL of a local anesthetic solution containing epinephrine 15 μg, while monitoring the heart rate.
5. Within 10 minutes, obvious evidence of a bilateral motor and sensory block should be evident, appropriate to the dermatomal level and dose of local anesthetic injection.

The level of analgesia should be symmetrical. If the foregoing is found not to be present, the block should be repeated, if appropriate to the clinical situation. Waiting longer than 10 minutes for evidence of a block has no value.

Dural puncture should occur with less than 1% frequency in experienced hands. In training programs an incidence of unintentional dural puncture as high as 3% might be acceptable. Unfortunately, in patients under the age of 40 years the rate of postdural puncture headache after puncture of the dura with a 17-gauge epidural needle may be as high as 75%.[15] If a dural puncture occurs, an epidural catheter can be inserted one interspace higher, and carefully tested to rule out intrathecal placement. If properly placed, this new epidural catheter can be used to provide surgical or obstetrical anesthesia/analgesia. At the end of surgery or labor, a prophylactic autologous blood patch using 10 to 15 mL sterile autologous blood can be injected via the epidural catheter. This approach is greater than 50% successful in preventing a postdural puncture headache.[16] The epidural catheter is then removed. If a positional headache presents, a conventional epidural blood patch, injecting 10 to 15 mL sterile autologous blood via a Tuohy needle inserted at or near the interspace of dural puncture can be performed. The success rate of a conventional blood patch in treating a postdural puncture headache is greater than 95%.[17] The authors believe that early treatment of a postdural puncture headache is important because it will decrease time to discharge from hospital, and may prevent a postdural puncture headache from becoming a chronic problem.[18]

OTHER COMPLICATIONS

Hypothermia can occur in patients with epidural and spinal anesthesia due to vasodilation of blood vessels to the skin of the lower extremities and abdomen, and increased heat loss.[19] In addition, patients with extensive central neuraxis blocks will have a lowered shivering threshold. During epidural and spinal

TABLE 69-1. REGRESSION TIMES FOR LUMBAR EPIDURAL ANESTHESIA

Local Anesthetic	Time to Two-segment Regression (Plain)	Time to Two-segment Regression with Epi	Duration – 1.5 × SD With Epi
3% 2-chloroprocaine	45	57 ± 7	47
2% lidocaine	46 ± 5	97 ± 19	70
2% mepivacaine	–	117	–
0.5% bupivacaine and levobupivacaine	165	196 ± 31	150
0.75% bupivacaine and levobupivacaine	165 ± 46	201 ± 40	141
1% ropivacaine (plain)	178	–	–

All times are in minutes. Data expressed as means or means ± standard deviation (SD).

anesthesia, patients are at similar risk for hypothermia as patients under general anesthesia.[20] Therefore, monitoring of body temperature and proactive warming of intravenous fluids and of the patient using a warming blanket is important in patients with prolonged epidural and spinal anesthetics.

Hypotension can be a serious problem if the patient is or becomes hypovolemic during the course of epidural anesthesia. Hypotension during epidural or spinal fluid is usually treated with intravenous ephedrine 5 to 10 mg boluses and volume replacement using a balanced salt solution. Blood volume should be monitored by assessing urine output via a Foley catheter or by measuring central venous pressures if large blood losses are expected or if bleeding or third space losses are expected to continue into the postoperative period. Sudden bradycardia can occur during epidural or spinal anesthesia in the presence of hypovolemia (Bezold–Jarrisch reflex).[21] To prevent bradycardia, which can lead to cardiac arrest, avoidance of hypovolemia and prophylactic treatment with an intravenous infusion of epinephrine 1 to 4 μg/minute can be helpful.[22]

SPINAL EPIDURAL HEMATOMA

Epidural hematoma is a serious but fortunately very rare complication of epidural and spinal anesthesia. In the absence of antiplatelet medications or anticoagulants, Tryba has estimated the incidence of spinal hematoma associated with regional anesthesia to be 1:190,000 epidural anesthetics.[23] Almost all of the reported cases of this complication in patients with central neuraxis anesthesia have received heparin, coumadin, or a potent antiplatelet drug, such as ticlodipine, prior to the initiation of the block. Studies performed at the Mayo Clinic convincingly suggest that preoperative use of nonsteroidal anti-inflammatory drugs (NSAIDs) do not place the patient at risk for this complication.[24] Intraoperative anticoagulation with heparin is probably safe, so long as the epidural catheter is neither inserted nor removed while the patient has an abnormal coagulation profile.[25]

Definitive diagnosis of epidural hematoma is made by computerized tomography (CT) or magnetic resonance imaging (MRI) scan. Clinical signs are: (1) new development of a motor and sensory block of the lower extremities, or persistence of a motor or sensory block after the anesthesia should have dissipated, (2) loss of deep tendon reflexes in the lower extremities, and (3) possibly severe back pain localized to the level of the hematoma. Should this complication be suspected, a CT or MRI scan should be done immediately. If the diagnosis is confirmed a neurosurgeon or orthopedic spine surgeon should be consulted to decompress the spinal canal. There are cases of full neurological recovery if decompression is carried out within 4 to 6 hours of the onset of the symptoms.[26] Late decompression usually does not result in functional recovery, and poor neurological outcome is a poor prognostic indicator for longevity.

Use of anticoagulants may be a risk factor for development of epidural hematoma. A consensus statement and recommendations are available on the American Society of Regional Anesthesia and Pain Medicine website (www.asra.com).

EPIDURAL ABSCESS AND SKIN INFECTION

Catheter site infection and epidural abscess are also thankfully very rare complications of epidural and spinal anesthesia. DuPen et al. studied the incidence and etiologic organisms of epidural catheter tract infections in cancer patients with indwelling epidural catheters.[27] They found that the responsible organism is almost always a skin contaminant. The risk of catheter tract infection increases the longer an epidural catheter is in place. Therefore, in the practices of the authors, epidural catheters left in place for postoperative pain control are inspected daily by the Acute Pain Service. If signs of infection are detected, the catheter is discontinued, the catheter insertion site is cleaned with an iodine solution, and consideration is given to treating the patient using a first-generation cephalosporin. In general, unless an epidural catheter is tunneled, the authors do not recommend leaving an epidural catheter in place for postoperative analgesia longer than 4 days.

Very rarely, an epidural catheter tract infection may progress to an epidural abscess. CT or MRI scan again makes the definitive diagnosis. Clinical signs and symptoms are: (1) severe pain at the vertebral level of the abscess, (2) fever and leukocytosis, and (3) new onset of sensory and/or motor block of the lower extremities. Treatment of an epidural abscess is usually by decompression and intravenous antibiotics. However, DuPen's group reported several cases in cancer patients treated with antibiotics via the indwelling epidural catheter.

INTRAOPERATIVE MANAGEMENT

If the surgery continues beyond the expected time to two-segment regression for the local anesthetic being used, a re-dose ("top-up") will be necessary. Bromage has recommended that the "top-up" dose be given prior to the time to two-segment regression to avoid intraoperative dissipation of the block. Thus for 2-chloroprocaine with epinephrine the time to reinjection is 45 minutes, for lidocaine with epinephrine it is 60 minutes, and for bupivacaine it is 120 minutes. One-half to two-thirds of the initial volume is given as a "top-up" dose. For surgical procedures lasting more than 3 hours, a continuous infusion of 0.5% bupivacaine, levobupivacaine, or 0.75% ropivacaine can be given at a rate of 3 to 4 mL/hour depending upon the extent of block desired, the location of the epidural catheter, and the dermatome location of surgery. Use of a continuous infusion vs. "top-up" dosing has the advantage that it avoids hypotension normally observed 10 to 15 minutes after the "top-up" dose.

COMBINED EPIDURAL/GENERAL ANESTHESIA

For surgical procedures lasting 2.5 hours or more, addition of "light" general anesthesia to the epidural or spinal anesthetic is often indicated and preferable to intravenous sedation. For surgical procedures of the thorax and upper abdomen, endotracheal intubation and mechanical ventilation is indicated. For procedures involving the lower abdomen and lower extremities, a laryngeal mask airway and spontaneous ventilation is often perfectly adequate. Whichever option of airway management is selected, it is important that the epidural catheter provides anesthesia and motor block, while the general anesthetic agent provides amnesia and ability to tolerate the artificial airway. Thus, only low concentrations of anesthetic gases are needed to maintain general anesthesia, usually less than one-half the Minimal Alveolar Concentration (MAC) required to prevent movement in response to a surgical stimulus. Neuromuscular blocking agents are used only for insertion of the endotracheal tube, and then allowed to dissipate. In this way, should the patient have too little general anesthetic, movement of the head, neck, or upper extremities will alert the anesthesiologist that a higher inspired anesthetic concentration is necessary to prevent potential recall of intraoperative events. The major advantages of this technique of epidural plus "light" general anesthesia are: (1) an awake and cooperative patient who can cough, deep breathe, and participate in his or her care in the immediate postoperative period, even after prolonged surgery, (2) excellent peri- and postoperative analgesia, (3) ability to provide intraoperative controlled hypotension to reduce blood loss, (4) decreased risk of deep venous thrombosis and pulmonary embolism for patients undergoing total joint replacement,[28] and (5) decreased time to return of bowel function after colon surgery,[29] and functional exercise capacity as well as quality of life after colonic surgery.[30]

KEY POINTS

- For segmental anesthesia/analgesia, the vertebral level of the epidural catheter should be matched to the dermatomal level of the surgical incision.
- Major factors that affect spread of epidural block are dose of local anesthetic, age of patient, and site of injection.
- Epidural hematoma and abscess are severe but rare complications that classically present with pain and neurologic changes.

REFERENCES

1. Bromage PR: Epidural Analgesia. WB Saunders, Philadelphia, 1978, pp 1–4.
2. Hogan Q, Toth J: Anatomy of soft tissues of the spinal canal. Reg Anesth Pain Med 24:303–310, 1999.
3. Hogan Q: Epidural anatomy examined by cryomicrotome section: Influence of age, vertebral level, and disease. Reg Anesth 21:395–406, 1996.
4. Gutierrez A: Anesthesia Extradural. Rev Cir Buenos Aires 1939, p 52.
5. Sharrock NE: Recording of, and an anatomical explanation for false positive loss of resistance during lumbar extradural anesthesia. Br J Anaesth 51:253–258, 1979.
6. Bromage PR: Identification of the epidural space. *In* Epidural Analgesia. WB Saunders, Philadelphia, 1978, pp 176–214.
7. Gutierrez A: Valor de la aspiracion liquida en el espacio peridural en la anestesia peridural. Rev Cir Buenos Aires 12:225, 1933.
8. Saberski LR, Kondamuri S, Osinubi OYO: Identification of the epidural space: Is loss of resistance to air a safe technique? A review of the complications related to use of air. Reg Anesth 22:3–15, 1997.
9. Park WY: Factors influencing distribution of local anesthetics in the epidural space. Reg Anesth 13:49–57, 1988.
10. Bromage PR: Mechanism of action. *In* Epidural Analgesia. WB Saunders, Philadelphia, 1978, pp 131–135.
11. Kopacz DJ, Mulroy MF: Chloroprocaine and lidocaine decrease hospital stay and admission rate after outpatient epidural anesthesia. Reg Anesth 15:19–25, 1990.
12. Wood MB, Rubin AP: A comparison of epidural 1% ropivacaine and 0.75% bupivacaine for lower abdominal gynecologic surgery. Anesth Analg 76:1274–1278, 1993.
13. Galindo A, Benavides O, Ortega de Munoz S, et al: Comparison of anesthetic solutions used in lumbar and caudal peridural anesthesia. Anesth Analg 57:175–179, 1978.
14. Stevens RA: Neuraxial blocks. *In* Brown DL (ed): Regional Anesthesia and Analgesia., WB Saunders, Philadelphia, 1996, p 342.
15. Lambert DH, Hurley RJ, Hertwig L, Datta S: Role of needle gauge and tip configuration in the production of lumbar puncture headache. Reg Anesth 22:66–72, 1997.
16. Cheek T, Banner R, Sauter J, et al: Prophylactic extradural blood patch is effective. A preliminary communication. Br J Anaesth 61:340–342, 1988.
17. Ostheimer GW, Palahnuik RJ, Snider SM: Epidural blood patch for post lumbar puncture headache. Anesthesiology 41:307, 1974.
18. Stevens RA, Jorgensen N: Successful treatment of dural puncture headache with epidural saline infusion after failure of epidural blood patch. Acta Anaesthiol Scand 32:429–431, 1988.
19. Glosten B, Sessler DI, Faure EAM, et al: Central temperature changes are not perceived during epidural anesthesia. Anesthesiology 77:10–16, 1992.
20. Sessler DI: Perioperative heat balance [review; 39 refs]. Anesthesiology 92:578–596, 2000.
21. Campagna JA, Carter C: Clinical relevance of the Bezold–Jarisch reflex. Anesthesiology 98:1250–1260, 2003.
22. Sharrock NE, Mineo R, Urquhart B: Hemodynamic response to low-dose epinephrine infusion during hypotensive epidural anesthesia for total hip replacement. Reg Anesth 15:295–299, 1990.
23. Horlocker TT, Wedel DJ, Benzon HT, et al: Proceedings of the 2nd ASRA consensus conference on neuraxial anesthesia and anticoagulation. RAPM 28:172–198, 2003.
24. Horlocker TT: Thromboprophylaxis and neuraxial anesthesia [review; 36 refs]. Orthopedics 26(Suppl 2):s243–s249, 2003.
25. Rao TKL, El-Etr AA: Anticoagulation following placement of epidural and subarachnoid catheters: An evaluation of neurologic sequelae. Anesthesiology 55:618–620, 1981.
26. Horlocker TT, Wedel DJ: Neurologic complications of spinal and epidural anesthesia [review; 80 refs]. Reg Anesth Pain Med 25:83–98, 2000.
27. DuPen SL, Peterson DG, Williams A, et al: Infection during chronic epidural catheterization: Diagnosis and treatment. Anesthesiology 70:905–909, 1990.
28. Sharrock NE, Ranawat CS, Urquhart B: Factors influencing deep vein thrombosis following total hip arthroplasty. Anesth Analg 76:765–771, 1993.
29. Liu SS, Carpenter R, Mackey D, et al: Effects of perioperative analgesic technique on rate of recovery after colon surgery. Anesthesiology 83:757–765, 1995.
30. Carli F, Mayo N, Klubien K, et al: Epidural analgesia enhances functional exercise capacity and health-related quality of life after colonic surgery. Anesthesiology 97:540–549, 2002.

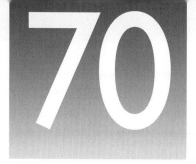

Combined Spinal–Epidural Techniques

Susan McDonald, M.D.

Combined spinal–epidural anesthesia (CSEA) has become an increasingly popular regional anesthetic technique over the past decade.[1] It can successfully combine the rapid and profound onset of neuraxial anesthesia with the ability to titrate or prolong the blockade. Low intrathecal doses can be used which may offer more hemodynamic stability or a more rapid recovery in ambulatory surgery. Its use in obstetrical anesthesia as a "walking epidural" has gained wide acceptance. CSEA has some unique disadvantages including increased failure rate of the spinal anesthetic, intrathecal migration of epidural drug and/or catheter, and decreased reliability of epidural test dosing. However, it is relatively simple to perform and various techniques and needle configurations have been described for its numerous clinical applications.

TECHNIQUES

CSEA can be performed either with the needle-through-needle or the double-segment technique. The needle-through-needle approach is more extensively described in the literature. A number of commercial kits are available, and although they vary in design, they all are performed through one puncture in a single interspace (Fig. 70-1). With the double-segment technique, the epidural and spinal portions are performed separately.

The double-segment technique allows the epidural catheter to be placed first at one interspace with the spinal anesthetic following at another, usually more caudad, interspace. An epidural test dose may be more reliable if done first, and confirmation of a well-placed epidural catheter is certainly an advantage of this approach. This approach, however, has its disadvantages when compared to the needle-through-needle approach. Introducing the spinal needle after catheter placement carries the risk of damaging the catheter with the spinal needle, as studies have shown the direction in which the epidural catheter lies cannot be predicted.[1,2] Cook describes a double-segment technique using a single interspace that avoids this potential needle damage: the spinal needle is first introduced and once cerebrospinal fluid (CSF) is identified, the stylet is replaced and then the epidural needle is placed more cephalad in the same interspace; the epidural catheter is threaded before the spinal needle stylet is removed and intrathecal injection performed.[1] Theoretically, by creating two separate punctures there may be an increased incidence of adverse events such as backache, headache, infection, and hematoma.[3] There is controversy as to whether or not the double-segment technique decreases the failure rate of spinal anesthesia.[4–6]

The needle-through-needle technique is quicker and simpler to perform and may have greater acceptance by surgical patients than the double-segment approach.[4] Different needle configurations have been designed. The simplest version is a Tuohy needle (or equivalent) through which a long, small-gauge spinal needle (24 to 30 gauge) is passed. Once the epidural space is identified, the spinal needle, which is a few millimeters longer than conventional spinal needles, is introduced through the needle for the intrathecal injection. Then, the spinal needle is withdrawn and the epidural catheter is threaded through the epidural needle. Locking adapters are available that fix the spinal needle in place prior to injection, with the assumption that accidental movement of the needle during injection is a reason for block failure.[7,8] Another type of epidural needle has a "back-eye." The design was meant to provide a better "feel" for dural puncture and reduce the risk of threading the epidural catheter through the dural hole.[9] It should be noted that successful exit through the back-eye varies between 50% and 100%.[1] The double-barrel needle has a separate 20-gauge conduit for the spinal needle laser welded to an 18-gauge epidural needle.[10] Having observed that the spinal needle created notches in epidural needle tips as it passed through, Eldor designed this needle to reduce the perceived risk of toxicity from metal fragments caused by needle friction.[11,12] One advantage to this double-barrel needle is the ability to perform the spinal anesthetic after the epidural catheter has been placed and tested without needing the separate puncture of the double-segment technique.

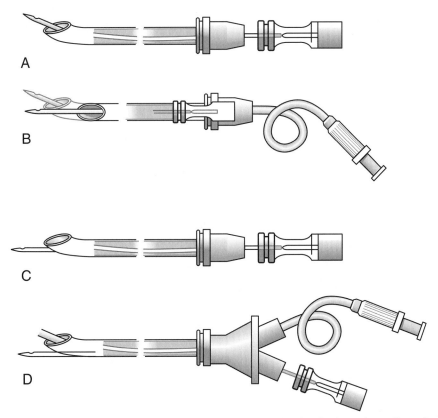

A

B

C

D

FIGURE 70–1. Various configurations for combined spinal–epidural needles. *A,* Needle-through-needle technique; *B,* double-barrel needle by Eldor; *C,* epidural needle with "back-eye" for spinal needle; *D,* Coomb's combined needle. (Reproduced from Eldor J: The evolution of combined spinal-epidural anesthesia needles. Reg Anesth Pain Med 22:294–296, 1997 with permission from the American Society of Regional Anesthesia and Pain Medicine.)

POTENTIAL COMPLICATIONS

Metal Toxicity: Eldor designed the double-barrel needle because of his belief that the friction from passing the spinal needle through the Tuohy needle causes metal fragments to be deposited in the epidural and intrathecal spaces.[10,11] He also surmised this metal toxicity may cause aseptic meningitis.[12] However, recent evaluations using atomic absorption spectrography and photomicrography did not demonstrate metal fragments even after five spinal needle passes and suggested the notches were due to malleability of the metal.[13,14]

Catheter Migration: It has been believed that the intentional dural puncture with the spinal needle would increase the risk of intrathecal placement of the epidural catheter. The risk is essentially no greater than any continuous epidural technique. It is virtually impossible to fit an 18-gauge catheter through a single dural hole made by a 25- or 27-gauge needle, and this has been confirmed by electron microscopy imaging and epiduroscopy.[13,15] The catheter, however, can pass through the accidental dural puncture made by the epidural needle up to 45% of the time in a cadaveric model.[16] Migration of the catheter later in the anesthetic course is no more likely than with conventional epidural techniques.

Failure of the Spinal Block: Recent data suggest the failure rate of spinal anesthesia with the combined technique to be about 5%.[1] While certainly higher than with conventional spinal anesthesia, this failure rate is improved from previous reports of 10% to 25%, and may be due to greater familiarity with the technique and with the development of better equipment. For example, the Luer lock apparatus that was previously available to help secure the needle in place did so only at a fixed needle length that may not have been long enough to reach the dura. Now variable extension adapters are available to allow the needle to be fixed at the needed length.[7,17]

The needle-through-needle technique creates some unique reasons for failure (Fig. 70-2). The spinal needles used are typically 25 to 27 gauge and longer than conventional needles which results in a slower rate of CSF and in greater resistance to injection. Instability of the spinal needle has been blamed for increasing the failure rate since in placing the delicate spinal needle through the epidural needle there is no tissue to anchor it in place.[7,8] Using saline for a loss-of-resistance method to identify the epidural space can lead to a false return of saline in the needle hub rather than CSF. While using air for the loss of resistance can reduce this risk, Kopacz et al. have described a modification of the hanging-drop technique to aid in identification of dural puncture when saline is used: a drop of fluid in the epidural needle hub will move inwardly as a result of the negative pressure generated when the spinal needle tents the dura, until the needle passes through the dura and CSF returns.[18] Since the epidural needle is the conduit for the spinal needle, any deviation from midline can make it

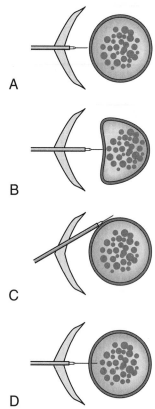

FIGURE 70–2. Reasons for failure of the combined spinal–epidural technique. *A,* The spinal needle does not reach the dura (spinal needle length too short or epidural needle not far enough into epidural space); *B,* spinal needle dents but does not penetrate the dura (may be an increased incidence when pencil-point needles are used); *C,* epidural needle not oriented midline; *D,* successful technique. (Reproduced from Rawal N, Van Zundert A, Holmstrom B, et al: Combined spinal-epidural technique. Reg Anesth Pain Med 22:406–423, 1997 with permission from the American Society of Regional Anesthesia and Pain Medicine.)

difficult to reach the dura.[3] Some propose using an even longer spinal needle for better success,[19] while others believe longer needles only result in higher incidence of parasthesia.[8]

The baricity of the spinal anesthetic and the patient position during block placement must be taken into consideration when carrying out a needle-through-needle technique. When the spinal block is placed before the epidural catheter is threaded, the length of time between spinal drug injection and final step of securing the epidural catheter in place may be crucial to the block's spread. This time period may be increased significantly if there is difficulty threading the catheter due to paresthesia, resistance, or even return of blood within the catheter.[1] For example, if the patient is sitting and a hyperbaric spinal agent is chosen, the final block height may not reach the desired level if it takes too long to place the catheter and reposition the patient. Elevated sensory block with increased hypotension has been seen in patients who had isobaric bupivacaine administered while in the sitting position, presumably because of the extra time it took to complete the CSEA block.[20,21]

Failure of the Epidural Block: When the spinal block is performed first, as in the needle-through-needle approach, the reliability of the epidural catheter test dose is reduced. First, it will not help identify an intrathecal catheter if a spinal block is already in place. In fact, it may result in a dangerously high block.[1] Second, the magnitude of hemodynamic response may be reduced if the catheter is intravascular, although the heart rate and systolic blood pressure response remains intact in healthy individuals.[22] No controlled randomized prospective studies have addressed the failure of epidural anesthesia or analgesia with the combined technique;[23] however, the incidence of failure is not likely to be higher with the combined technique. Retrospective data suggest that the incidence of failure may even be lower in the obstetric population, presumably because the midline approach is more carefully used and because CSF in the spinal needle is evidence that the epidural space has been reached.[24–26]

Aspiration of the epidural catheter may yield CSF even when the catheter is not intrathecally placed.[27] The unreliability of the test dose and aspiration tests plus the potential for leakage of epidural drugs into the intrathecal space (see below) make it essential that all epidural drugs be carefully administered with the unintentional subarachnoid injection always in mind and that all patients be closely monitored.

Dural Spread of Epidural Drugs: Enhancement of the spinal block has been seen with injection of epidural agents. This can be a result of either intrathecal spread of these drugs or from a pressure effect. It is unlikely that there would be significant clinical effects from leakage of drugs through a small-gauge dural puncture.[28,29] The greater pressure of the subarachnoid space makes it more likely that fluid will leak into the epidural space, as presumed with postdural puncture headaches, than the reverse.[16] If the epidural needle creates a dural rent, however, then significant leakage of epidural agents can occur.[30,31]

The pressure effect comes from the observation that injecting volume into the epidural space increases the pressure around the dural sac and therefore "squeezes" the CSF compartment. A recent myelographic evaluation demonstrated that the subarachnoid space's diameter decreased to 40% after 5 mL and to 25% after 10 mL normal saline was injected through an epidural catheter.[32] This "squeeze" essentially promotes the cephalad spread of the spinal anesthetic, but the effect appears to be time dependent. Sensory block extension can be significant (three to four dermatomes) if epidural saline is injected within 20 minutes of bupivacaine spinal anesthesia.[28,33,34] However, once a block has settled at its maximum height, adding saline as volume results in no increase in block height,[28,35] and if delayed until two-segment regression has begun, it can even result in shorter duration of anesthesia.[36]

Risk of Postdural Puncture Headache: The risk of postdural puncture headache (PDPH) in parturients is higher than in the surgical population. However, there is some evidence that the risk of PDPH after CSE may be less than with single-shot spinal techniques. While the use of smaller-gauge needles may contribute to this reduced incidence, it may be that the volume administered then increases the pressure in the epidural space.[16,24] Others believe the oblique angle that the spinal needle traverses the dura may also help.[1,16] There are also reports that epidural or intrathecal opioids may be protective against PDPH.[16,37]

CLINICAL APPLICATIONS

The Surgical Patient: There are practical advantages to employing CSEA in surgical anesthesia. The intrathecal component can provide profound sensory and motor blockade necessary for surgery and the epidural component can be used to prolong the anesthetic duration. The epidural catheter can then be used for postoperative epidural analgesia on the ward.

While more often the "full dose" of the spinal drug is chosen, another way to manage the CSEA technique is through "sequential" dosing. This "sequential" method uses low intrathecal doses followed by incremental epidural doses to create a slow, deliberate rise of the block height until the desired level is reached. Thus, the sympathetic blockade may be limited and a lower incidence of hypotension may be seen, which may be useful in high-risk patients, such as those with cardiac disease. However, the onset of anesthesia takes longer to establish.[1,16]

This concept of sequential dosing can be taken one step further for ambulatory surgery patients. Since dose of local anesthetic determines both anesthetic success and duration of recovery, the availability of the epidural catheter for a rescue anesthetic allows use of low, marginal doses of spinal local anesthetic. This dosing strategy may result in more rapid recovery and discharge. If the CSEA technique takes more time than conventional spinal anesthesia, however, the relative cost benefit from decreased recovery time may not overcome this increased induction time.[38]

The Obstetrical Patient: Over the past decade CSEA has gained the most acceptance in obstetrical anesthesia. Known as the "walking epidural," CSEA is used most often for labor and delivery, as it offers more rapid pain relief than conventional epidural analgesia with lower incidence of motor blockade. CSEA has also been recommended for anesthesia for caesarean section.

When used for labor and delivery, CSEA often combines intrathecal opioids with an epidural local anesthetic infusion. Typically a lipid-soluble opioid, such as fentanyl (up to 25 μg) or sufentanil (up to 10 μg), is chosen because it provides rapid onset of analgesia, often before the next contraction.[39,40] Such pain relief usually lasts about 90 minutes, but can be prolonged an additional 30 minutes or more with a variety of adjuncts such as 2.5 mg bupivacaine, 2 mg ropivacaine, 200 μg of epinephrine, or 50 μg of clonidine.[39,41] Most patients maintain their ability to sit, stand, or walk with assistance, and micturate. Studies have shown patients have intact proprioception and balance with low intrathecal doses such as 2.5 mg bupivacaine plus 5 μg fentanyl.[42,43] However, if a traditional lidocaine/epinephrine test dose is given through the epidural catheter at the time of placement, there may be significant impairment in mobility.[44]

Recent studies have shown that CSEA does not have any increased risk of instrumental delivery or side effects, including PDPH, when compared with conventional epidural analgesia.[40,45] Others have shown actual advantages to the use of CSEA, such as reducing incidence of instrumental vaginal delivery,[46] faster progression of labor,[47] lower anxiety with CSEA block placement,[48] and decrease incidence of PDPH

rate possibly due to the volume effect of epidural administration.[24] Incidence of pruritus is significantly higher (>80%), however, in those receiving intrathecal opioids.[24,39] Other side effects of intrathecal opioids need to be considered, including hypotension, fetal bradycardia, and respiratory depression.[16,39]

As an anesthetic for caesarean section, CSEA offers a rapid, titratable block with good muscle relaxation.[16] With its potentially denser block, the technique may reduce the conversion rate of regional to general anesthesia.[1] Recently, Davies et al. found that when compared to conventional epidural anesthesia, CSEA provided more rapid onset, better motor block, decreased anxiety levels, decreased shivering, and greater patient satisfaction.[48] The sequential dosing regimen may be useful in some high-risk parturients.[1]

CONCLUSION

Over the past decade CSEA has gained wide acceptance as a regional anesthetic technique, especially in the obstetric population. It combines the benefits of a subarachnoid block with those of an epidural technique. While it may have its unique disadvantages, familiarity with the technique and its equipment may reduce the failure risk.

KEY POINTS

- CSEA combines the rapid onset and profound anesthesia of a spinal block with the epidural catheter's ability to titrate and prolong the block.
- CSEA can be done as a needle-through-needle technique or as a double-segment method.
- Unique disadvantages may include failure of spinal or epidural components, potential intrathecal catheter placement, and leakage of epidural drugs through a dural hole.
- Clinical applications for CSEA include labor and delivery (as "walking epidurals") and ambulatory surgery.

REFERENCES

1. Cook TM: Combined spinal-epidural techniques. Anaesthesia 55:42–64, 2000.
2. Hogan Q: Epidural catheter tip position and distribution of injectate evaluated by computed tomography. Anesthesiology 90:964–970, 1999.
3. Rawal N, Van Zundert A, Holmstrom B, et al: Combined spinal-epidural technique. Reg Anesth Pain Med 22:406–423, 1997.
4. Casati A, D'Ambrosio A, De Negri P, et al: A clinical comparison between needle-through-needle and double-segment techniques for combined spinal and epidural anesthesia. Reg Anesth Pain Med 23:390–394, 1998.
5. Lyons G, Macdonald R, Mikl B: Combined epidural/spinal anaesthesia for caesarean section. Through the needle or in separate spaces? Anaesthesia 47:199–201, 1992.
6. Puolakka R, Pitkanen MT, Rosenberg PH: Comparison of technical and block characteristics of different combined spinal and epidural anesthesia techniques. Reg Anesth Pain Med 26:17–23, 2001.
7. Stocks GM, Hallworth SP, Fernando R: Evaluation of a spinal needle locking device for use with the combined spinal epidural technique. Anaesthesia 55:1185–1188, 2000.
8. Levy N, Fernando R: Reducing the incidence of technical failures and paraesthesia in combined spinal-epidural techniques. Anaesthesia 55:1230–1231, 2000.

9. Joshi GP, McCarroll SM: Evaluation of combined spinal-epidural anesthesia using two different techniques. Reg Anesth 19: 169–174, 1994.

10. Eldor J: The evolution of combined spinal-epidural anesthesia needles. Reg Anesth Pain Med 22:294–296, 1997.

11. Eldor J: Eldor combined spinal/epidural needle. Anaesthesia 48:173, 1993.

12. Eldor J, Guedj P: Aseptic meningitis due to metallic particles in the needle-through-needle technique. Reg Anesth 20:360, 1995.

13. Holst D, Molmann M, Schymroszcyk B, et al: No risk of metal toxicity in combined spinal-epidural anesthesia. Anesth Analg 88:393–397, 1999.

14. Herman N, Molin J, Knape KG: No additional metal particle formation using the needle-through-needle combined epidural/spinal technique. Acta Anaesth Scand 40:227–231, 1996.

15. Holmstrom B, Rawal N, Axelsson K, et al: Risk of catheter migration during combined spinal epidural block: Percutaneous epiduroscopy study. Anesth Analg 80:747–753, 1995.

16. Rawal N, Holmstrom B, Crowhurst JA, et al: The combined spinal-epidural technique. Anesthesiology Clin N Am 18:267–295, 2000.

17. Hoffman VLH, Vercauteran MP, Buczkowski PW, et al: A new combined spinal epidural apparatus: Measurement of the distance to the epidural and subarachnoid spaces. Anaesthesia 52:350–355, 1997.

18. Kopacz DJ, Bainton BG: Combined spinal epidural anesthesia: A new "hanging drop." Anesth Analg 82:433–434, 1996.

19. Riley ET, Hamilton CL, Ratner EF, et al: A comparison of the 24-gauge Sprotte and Gertie Marx spinal needles for combined spinal-epidural analgesia during labor. Anesthesiology 97:574–577, 2002.

20. Klasen J, Junger A, Hartmann B, et al: Differing incidences of relevant hypotension with combined spinal-epidural anesthesia and spinal anesthesia. Anesth Analg 96:1491–1495, 2003.

21. Holmstrom B, Laugaland K, Rawal N, et al: Combined spinal epidural block versus spinal and epidural block for orthopaedic surgery. Can J Anaesth 40:601–606, 1993.

22. Liu SS, Stevens RA, Vasquez J, et al: The efficacy of epinephrine test doses during spinal anesthesia in volunteers: Implications for combined spinal-epidural anesthesia. Anesth Analg 4:780–783, 1997.

23. Correll DJ, Viscusi ER, Witkowski TA: Success of epidural catheters placed for postoperative analgesia: Comparison of a combined spinal-epidural vs. standard epidural technique. Anesthesiology 89:A1095, 1998.

24. Norris MC, Grieco WM, Borkowski M: Complications of labor analgesia: Epidural versus combined spinal epidural techniques. Anesth Analg 79:529–537, 1994.

25. van de Velde M, Teunkens A, Hanssens M, et al: Post dural puncture headache following combined spinal epidural or epidural anaesthesia in obstetric patients. Anaesth Int Care 29:595–599, 2001.

26. Eappen S, Blinn A, Segal S: Incidence of epidural catheter replacement in parturients: A retrospective chart review. Int J Ob Anesth 7:220–225, 1998.

27. Isaac R, Coe AJ, Hornsby VP: False-positive epidural catheter aspiration tests in needle through needle combined spinal-epidural anaesthesia. Anaesthesia 56:772–776, 2001.

28. Stienstra R, Dilrosun-Alhadi BZR, Dahan A, et al: The epidural "top-up" in combined spinal-epidural anesthesia: The effect of volume versus dose. Anesth Analg 88:810–814, 1999.

29. Suzuki N, Koganemaru M, Onizuka S, et al: Dural puncture with a 26-gauge spinal needle affects spread of epidural anesthesia. Anesth Analg 82:1040–1042, 1996.

30. Swenson JD, Wisniewski M, McJames S, et al: The effect of prior dural puncture on cisternal cerebrospinal fluid morphine concentrations in sheep after administration of lumbar epidural morphine. Anesth Analg 83:523–525, 1996.

31. Bernards CM, Kopacz DJ, Michel MZ: Effect of needle puncture on morphine and lidocaine flux through the spinal meninges of the monkey in vitro. Implications for combined spinal-epidural anesthesia. Anesthesiology 80:853–858, 1994.

32. Takiguchi T, Okano T, Egawa H, et al: The effect of epidural saline injection on analgesic level during combined spinal and epidural anesthesia assessed clinically and myelographically. Anesth Analg 85:1097–1100, 1997.

33. Choi DH, Park NK, Cho HS, et al: Effects of epidural injection on spinal block during combined spinal and epidural anesthesia for cesarean delivery. Reg Anesth Pain Med 25:591–595, 2000.

34. Mardirosoff C, Dumont L, Lemedioni P, et al: Sensory block extension during combined spinal and epidural. Reg Anesth Pain Med 23:92–95, 1998.

35. Leeda M, Stienstra R, Arbous MS, et al: The epidural "top-up": Predictors of increase of sensory blockade. Anesthesiology 96:1310–1314, 2002.

36. Trautman WJ, Liu SS, Kopacz DJ: Comparison of lidocaine and saline for epidural top-up during combined spinal-epidural anesthesia in volunteers. Anesth Analg 84:574–577, 1997.

37. Eldor J, Guedj P, Cotev S: Epidural morphine injections for the treatment of postspinal headache. Can J Anaesth 37:710–711, 1990.

38. Liu SS, McDonald SB: Current issues in spinal anesthesia. Anesthesiology 94:888–906, 2001.

39. Paech M: Newer techniques of labor analgesia. Anesthesiology Clin N Am 21:1–17, 2003.

40. Comparative Obstetric Mobile Epidural Trial (COMET) Study Group UK: Randomized controlled trial comparing traditional with two "mobile" epidural techniques: anesthetic and analgesic efficacy. Anesthesiology 97:1567–1575, 2002.

41. Eisenach JC: Combined spinal-epidural analgesia in obstetrics. Anesthesiology 91:299–302, 1999.

42. Pickering AE, Parry MG, Ousta B, et al: Effect of combined spinal-epidural ambulatory labor analgesia on balance. Anesthesiology 91:436–441, 1999.

43. Davies J, Fernando R, McLeod A, et al: Postural stability following ambulatory regional analgesia for labor. Anesthesiology 97:1576–1581, 2002.

44. Calimaran AL, Strauss-Hoder TP, Wang WY, et al: The effect of epidural test dose on motor function after a combined spinal-epidural technique for labor analgesia. Anesth Analg 96:1167–1172, 2003.

45. Norris MC, Fogel ST, Conway-Long C: Combined spinal-epidural versus epidural labor analgesia. Anesthesiology 95:913–920, 2001.

46. Nageotte MP, Larson D, Rumney PJ, et al: Epidural analgesia compared with combined spinal-epidural analgesia during labor in nulliparous women. N Engl J Med 337:1715–1719, 1997.

47. Tsen LC, Thue B, Datta S, et al: Is combined spinal-epidural analgesia associated with more rapid cervical dilation in nulliparous patients when compared with conventional epidural analgesia? Anesthesiology 91:920–925, 1999.

48. Davies SJ, Paech MJ, Welch H, et al: Maternal experience during epidural or combined spinal-epidural anesthesia for caesarean section: A prospective, randomized trial. Anesth Analg 85:607–613, 1997.

Caudal Anesthesia

**Kenneth D. Candido, M.D.,
and Antoun Nader, M.D.**

Caudal anesthesia was described at the turn of the last century by two French physicians, Fernand Cathelin and Jean-Anthanase Sicard, and predated the lumbar approach to epidural block by several years.[1] However, it did not gain popularity immediately after its inception. The difficulties arose from the confusion associated with the wide variety of arrangement of sacral bones encountered in the general population, and the subsequent high failure rate associated with attempts to locate the sacral hiatus. The unpredictability of the technique along with a failure rate of 5% to 10% made caudal epidural anesthesia unpopular until a resurgence of interest occurred in the 1940s led by Hingson and colleagues, primarily for use in obstetrical anesthesia. The approach has many applications, including surgical anesthesia in children and adults, as well as the management of acute and chronic pain conditions. Infants and young children before the age of puberty, as well as lean adults, are usually easy subjects for caudal anesthesia, and an acceptable success rate of 98% to 100% can be expected in this selected patient population.[1] The technique of caudal epidural block in pain management has been greatly enhanced by the use of fluoroscopic guidance and epidurography. Unfortunately, clinical indications, and especially therapeutic interventions for the relief of chronic pain in individuals with failed back surgery syndrome, are often most prevalent in patients with difficult caudal landmarks. It has been suggested that traditional lumbar peridural block should not be attempted employing an approach requiring needle placement through a spinal surgery scar, either for the placement of corticosteroids and adjuvants, or for the performance of surgical anesthesia (due to the likelihood of tearing the dura, and the possibility of inducing hematoma formation over the cauda equina when blood from the procedure gets trapped between the layers of tough scar and connective tissues).[2] Under these circumstances it is recommended that fluoroscopically guided caudal epidural block be performed. The second resurgence in popularity of caudal anesthesia parallels the increasing need to find safe alternatives to conventional lumbar epidural block in selected patient populations.

ANATOMICAL CONSIDERATIONS

The sacrum is a large triangular-shaped bone formed by the fusion of the five sacral vertebrae. It has a blunted, caudal apex that articulates with the coccyx. Its superior, wide base articulates with the fifth lumbar vertebra at the lumbosacral angle (Fig. 71-1). Its dorsal surface is convex and has a raised interrupted median crest with four (sometimes three) spinous tubercles representing fused sacral spines. Flanking the median crest, the posterior surface is formed by fused laminae. Lateral to

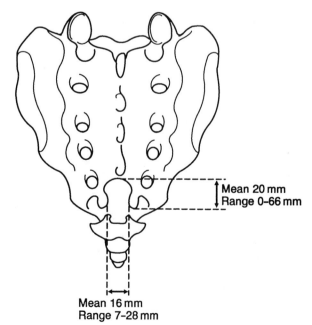

FIGURE 71-1. Dorsal surface of the sacrum. (From Martín LVH: Sacral epidural (caudal) block. In Wildsmith JAW, Armitage EN (eds): Principles and Practice of Regional Anesthesia. Churchill-Livingstone, New York, 1987, pp 127–134.)

the median crest, four pairs of dorsal foramina lead into the sacral canal through intervertebral foraminae; each transmits the dorsal ramus of a sacral spinal nerve. Below the fourth (or third) spinous tubercle an arched sacral hiatus is identified in the posterior wall of the sacral canal, due to the failure of the fifth pair of laminae to meet, exposing the dorsal surface of the fifth sacral vertebral body. The caudal opening of the canal is the sacral hiatus, roofed by the firm elastic membrane, the sacrococcygeal ligament, which is an extension of the ligamentum flavum. The fifth inferior articular processes project caudally and flank the sacral hiatus as sacral cornuae, connected to the coccygeal cornua by intercornual ligaments.

The sacral canal is formed by the sacral vertebral foramina and is triangular in shape. It is a continuation of the lumbar spinal canal. Each lateral wall presents four intervertebral foramina, through which the canal is in continuity with pelvic and dorsal sacral foramina. The posterior sacral foramina are smaller than their anterior counterparts. The sacral canal contains the cauda equina (including the filum terminale) and the spinal meninges (Fig. 71-2). Near its midlevel (typically the middle one-third of S2, but varying from S1 to S3)[3,4] the subarachnoid and subdural spaces cease to exist and the lower sacral spinal roots and filum terminale pierce the arachnoid and dura maters. The lowest margin of the filum terminale emerges at the sacral hiatus and traverses the dorsal surface of the fifth sacral vertebra and sacrococcygeal joint to reach the coccyx. The fifth spinal nerves also emerge through the hiatus medial to the sacral cornua. The sacral canal contains the epidural venous plexus, which generally terminates at S4 but which may continue more caudad (Fig. 71-2). Most of these vessels are concentrated in the anterolateral portion of the canal. The remainder of the sacral canal is filled with adipose tissue, which is subject to an age-related decrease in its density. This change may be responsible for the transition from the predictable spread of local anesthetics administered for caudal anesthesia in children, to the limited and unpredictable segmental spread seen in adults.[5]

There is significant variability in sacral hiatus anatomy among individuals of seemingly similar backgrounds, race, and stature.[1] As individuals age there is significant thickening of the overlying ligaments and the cornua. The hiatal margins often defy recognition by even skilled fingertips. The practical problems related to caudal anesthesia are mainly referable to the wide anatomical variations in size, shape, and orientation of the sacrum. Trotter[3] summarized the major anatomical variations of the sacrum. The sacral hiatus may be almost closed, asymmetrically open, or widely open secondary to anomalies in the pattern of fusion of the laminae of the sacral arches. Sacral spina bifida was noted in about 2% of males, and in 0.3% of females. The anteroposterior depth of the sacral canal may vary from less than 2 mm to greater than 1 cm. Individuals with sacral canals having anteroposterior diameters less than 3 mm may not be able to accommodate anything larger than a 21-gauge needle (5% of the population).[1] Additionally, the lateral width of the sacral canal varies significantly. Since the depth and width may vary, the volume of the canal itself may also vary. Trotter found that sacral volumes varied between 12 and 65 mL, with a mean volume of 33 mL.[3] A magnetic resonance imaging (MRI) study in 37 adult patients found the volume (excluding the foramina and dural sac) to be 14.4 mL with a range of 9.5 to 26.6 mL.[6] Patients with smaller capacities may not be able to accommodate the typical volumes of local anesthetics administered for epidural anesthesia via the caudal route. In a cadaver study of 53 specimens the mean distance between the tip of the dural sac and the upper edge of the sacral hiatus as denoted by the sacrococcygeal membrane was 45 mm with a range of 16 to 75 mm.[3] In the MRI study mentioned above, the mean distance was found to be 60.5 mm, with a range of 34 to 80 mm.[6] The sacrococcygeal membrane could not be identified in 10.8% of subjects using MRI.[6]

The sacral foramina afford anatomical passages permitting the egress of injected solutions such as local anesthetics and adjuvants. The posterior sacral foramina are essentially sealed by the multifidus and sacrospinalis muscles, but the anterior foramina are unobstructed by muscles and ligaments, permitting ready egress of solutions through them.[7] The sacral curvature varies substantially.[8] This variability tends to be more severe in males than in females. The clinical significance of this finding is that a noncurving epidural needle will more likely

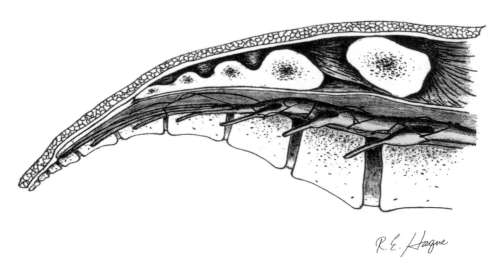

FIGURE 71-2. Lateral view of the sacrum demonstrating the filum terminale and the sacral venous plexus enveloping the nerve roots and extending to the sacral hiatus.

pass easily into the canal of females than males. The angle between the axis of the lumbar canal and the sacral canal varies between 7° and 70° in subjects with marked lordosis. The clinical implication of this finding is that the cephalad flow of caudally injected solutions may be more limited in lordotic patients with exaggerated lumbosacral angles than in those with flatter lumbosacral angles, where the axes of the lumbar and sacral canals are more closely aligned.

INDICATIONS FOR CAUDAL EPIDURAL BLOCK

The indications for caudal epidural block are essentially the same as for lumbar epidural block, but its use may be preferred when sacral nerve spread of anesthetics and adjuvants is sought preferentially over lumbar nerve spread. The unpredictability of ascertaining consistent cephalad spread of anesthetics administered through the caudal canal limits the use of this technique in situations where it is essential to provide lower thoracic and upper abdominal neuraxial blockade. Though this modality is described for perioperative use (diminishing role) and for managing chronic pain scenarios in adults (increasing role), it is essential to recognize that caudal block has an extremely wide range of applicability[9–12] (Table 71-1).

Other newer indications in adults bear special mention and will be described later, including the performance of percutaneous epidural neuroplasty;[13,14] the use of caudal analgesia following lumbar spinal surgery;[15] caudal analgesia after emergency orthopedic lower extremity surgery;[16] administration of local anesthetic adjuvants for postoperative analgesia;[17] and caudal block for performing neurolysis for intractable cancer pain.[18]

TECHNIQUE OF CAUDAL EPIDURAL BLOCK

The technique of caudal epidural block involves palpation, identification, and puncture.[1] Candidates are evaluated as for any epidural block and the indications and relative and absolute contraindications to its performance are identical. A full complement of noninvasive monitors is applied, and baseline vital signs are assessed. In pediatric patients blocks may be performed with the patient fully anesthetized; the same is not recommended for older children and adults. One must decide whether a continuous or single-shot technique will be employed. For continuous techniques, a Tuohy-type needle with a lateral facing orifice is appropriate. Patient positioning is undertaken next, realizing that several positions are available

TABLE 71-1. **CLINICAL APPLICATIONS OF CAUDAL EPIDURAL NERVE BLOCK**

General uses
1. Administration of anesthesia in infants, children, and adults, especially for surgery of the perineum, anus, and rectum; inguinal and femoral herniorrhaphy; cystoscopy and urethral surgery; hemorrhoidectomy; vaginal hysterectomy
2. Prognostic neural blockade to evaluate pelvic, bladder, perineal, genital, rectal, anal, and lower extremity pain
3. Provide sympathetic block for individuals suffering from acute vascular insufficiency of lower extremities secondary to vasospastic or vasocclusive disease, including frostbite and ergotamine toxicity
4. Relief of labor pain (mostly historical)
5. Conditions requiring epidural block where extensive segmental block is not important

Acute pain management
1. Management of pelvic and lower extremity pain secondary to trauma (without evidence of pelvic fracture)
2. Postoperative pain management
3. Temporizing measure for pain secondary to acute lumbar vertebral compression fractures

Chronic pain management
1. Injection of local anesthetics and/or medications for lumbar radiculopathy secondary to herniated discs and spinal stenosis
2. Approach to the epidural space in failed back surgery syndrome
3. Postherpetic neuralgia
4. Complex regional pain syndromes
5. Orchalgia; pelvic pain syndromes
6. Percutaneous epidural neuroplasty

Cancer pain management
1. Chemotherapy-related peripheral neuropathy
2. Bony metastases to the pelvis
3. Injection therapy for pain secondary to pelvic, perineal, genital, rectal malignancy
4. Prognostic indicator prior to performing neurodestructive sacral nerve ablation(s)
5. Injection of hyperbaric phenol solutions for management of sacral pain

Adapted from Waldman S: Caudal epidural nerve block. *In* Waldman S (ed): Interventional Pain Management, ed 2. WB Saunders, Philadelphia, 2001, p 520.

for adults, compared to the lateral decubitus position in neonates and children. The lateral position is efficacious in pediatrics because it permits easy access to the airway in cases where general anesthesia or heavy sedation has been administered prior to performing the block. In adults, the prone position is the most frequently utilized, but the lateral decubitus position or the knee-chest (also known as "knee-elbow") position may be employed. In the prone position the procedure or operating room table should be flexed or a pillow may be placed beneath the symphysis pubis and iliac crests to produce slight flexion of the hips. This maneuver makes palpation of the caudal canal easier. The legs are separated with the heels rotated outwards, to smooth out the upper part of the anal cleft, while simultaneously relaxing the gluteal muscles. For placement of caudal epidural block in the parturient, the woman is in the lateral (Sim's position) or in the knee-elbow position. A dry gauze swab is placed in the anal cleft to protect the anal area and genitalia from betadine or other disinfectants (especially alcohol) used to sterilize the skin. The anatomical landmarks are assessed next. The skin folds of the buttocks are useful guides in locating the underlying sacral hiatus. Alternatively, a triangle may be marked on the skin over the sacrum, using the posterior superior iliac spines (PSIS) as the base, with the apex pointing inferiorly (caudally). Normally, this apex sits over or immediately adjacent to the sacral hiatus. The hiatus is marked and the tip of the index finger is placed on the tip of the coccyx in the natal cleft while the thumb of the same hand palpates the two sacral cornua located 3 to 4 cm more rostrally at the upper end of the natal cleft. The sacral cornua may be identified by gently moving the palpating index finger from side to side. The palpating thumb should sink into the hollow between the two cornua, as if between two knuckles of a fist.[1] A sterile skin preparation and draping of the entire region is performed in the usual fashion. A fine-gauge 1.5-inch needle is then utilized to infiltrate the skin over the sacral hiatus using 3 to 5 mL of 1% to 1.5% plain lidocaine HCl. If fluoroscopy is utilized, a lateral view is obtained to demonstrate the anatomical boundaries of the sacral canal. The authors routinely leave the local anesthetic infiltration needle in situ for this view, since it offers a guide as to whether the approach is at the appropriate level for subsequent advancement of the epidural needle. With fluoroscopy, the caudal canal appears as a translucent layer posterior to the sacral segments. The median sacral crest is visualized as an opaque line posterior to the caudal canal. The sacral hiatus is usually visualized as a translucent opening at the base of the caudal canal. The coccyx may be seen articulating with the inferior surface of the sacrum. The authors utilize the anteroposterior view once the epidural needle is safely situated within the confines of the canal, and the epidural catheter is advanced cephalad (Fig. 71-3). In this projection the intermediate sacral crests appear as opaque vertical lines on either side of the midline. The sacral foramina are visualized as translucent and nearly circular areas lateral to the intermediate sacral crests. The presence of intestinal gas may obfuscate the recognition of these structures.

Once the tissues overlying the hiatus have been anesthetized, a 17- or 18-gauge Tuohy-type needle is inserted either in the midline, or, using a lateral approach, into the caudal canal. A feeling of a slight "snap" may be appreciated when the advancing needle pierces the sacrococcygeal ligament. Once the needle reaches the ventral wall of the sacral canal, it is slowly withdrawn and redirected, directing it more cranially

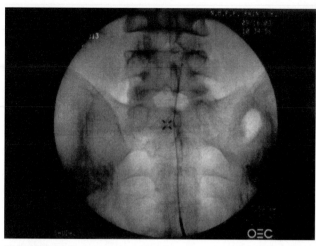

FIGURE 71-3. Anteroposterior fluoroscopic view of the sacrum demonstrating an epidural catheter advanced to the superior surface of the L5 vertebral body. Note the sacral foramina, seen as translucent and nearly circular areas on either side of the advancing catheter.

(by depressing hub and advancing) for further insertion into the canal (Fig. 71-4). The cranioventral direction of the needle is a 45° angle to the sacrococcygeal ligament (120° angle to the back). A syringe loaded with either air or saline containing a small air bubble is then attached to the needle, and the loss-of-resistance technique is used to establish entry into the epidural space. The needle tip should stay below the S2 level to avoid tearing the dura and the needle should never be advanced in the space to the full length of the shaft. The skin corresponding to about 1 cm inferior to the PSIS indicates the S2 level (caudal-most extension of the dura mater). The dural sac extends lower in children than in adults and epidural needles should be very carefully advanced no deeper than the S3 or S4 level in this patient population.

A "whoosh" test has been described for identifying correct needle placement in the caudal canal. This characteristic sound has been noted during auscultation of the thoracolumbar region during the injection of 2 to 3 mL of air into the caudal epidural space.[19] In pediatric patients electrical stimulation has been used to ascertain correct needle placement in the caudal canal. Anal sphincter contraction (corresponding to stimulation of S2–S4) is sought with 1 to 10 mA currents.[20] If the needle has been inserted correctly, it will swing easily from side to side at the hub while the shaft is held like a fulcrum at the sacrococcygeal membrane and the tip moves freely in the sacral canal. If cerebrospinal fluid (CSF) is aspirated through the needle, it should be withdrawn and injection should not be undertaken. If blood is aspirated, the needle should be withdrawn and reinserted until no blood is apparent at the hub. If injection of air (or saline) for the loss-of-resistance technique results in a bulging over the sacrum, the needle tip most probably lies dorsal to the sacrum in the subcutaneous tissues (Fig. 71-5). If the needle tip is subperiosteal, the injection will meet with significant resistance, and the patient will experience pain. The cortical layer of the sacral bone is often quite thin, particularly in infants and older subjects, and puncture of cancellous bone is relatively easy, especially if force is exerted while advancing the needle. The sensation of entering cancellous

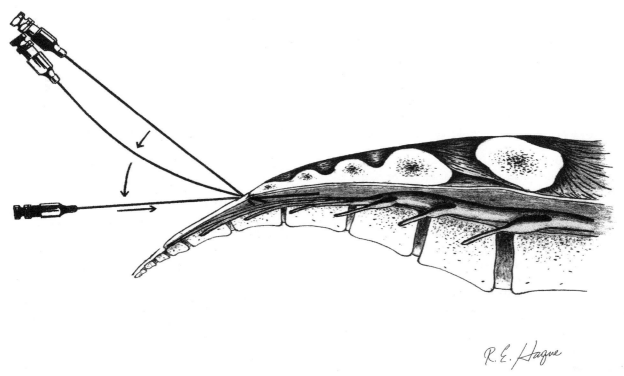

FIGURE 71-4. Caudal epidural needle placement seen in lateral projection. Note that the needle is directed cranioventrally at a 45° angle to the sacrococcygeal ligament. Upon reaching the ventral wall of the sacral canal, it is withdrawn and redirected.

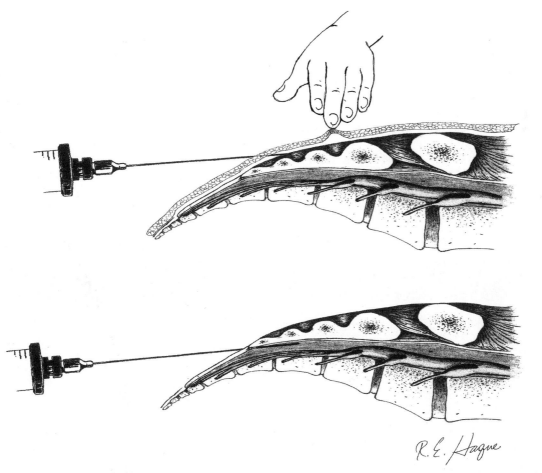

FIGURE 71-5. Caudal epidural needle placed dorsal to the sacrum in subcutaneous tissue. Injection of air or saline for the loss-of-resistance test results in bulging over the sacrum.

bone is not unlike penetrating the sacrococcygeal membrane; there is a feeling of resistance that is suddenly overcome and the needle advances more freely and subsequent injection is unhampered. Injected solutions may be absorbed very rapidly from bone marrow and toxic drug reactions result. In this situation, pain is typically noted over the caudal part of the sacrum during the injection. If this occurs, the needle should be withdrawn slightly and rotated on its axis until it can be reinserted in a slightly different direction.[21-23] If injection is made anterior to the sacrum (between the sacrum and coccyx), it is possible to perforate the rectum, or, in parturients, the baby's head may be injured. This limits the use of caudal block in laboring women once the presenting part has descended into the perineum. Inadvertent venous puncture also may occur, and the incidence of this has been reported to be about 0.6%.[24]

Caudal block may be a single-shot or continuous catheter technique. For continuous block, the catheter may be advanced anterograde (conventionally) or retrograde. Continuous caudal block may be performed in retrograde fashion using needle insertion into the lumbar epidural space, but directed inferiorly instead of superiorly. One study of 10 patients had epidural catheters advanced through 18-gauge Tuohy-type epidural needles in retrograde fashion from the L4–L5 interspace. This technique was associated with a 20% failure rate with the catheter going into the paravertebral or retrorectal spaces, despite easy epidural space entry.[25] Using the conventional approach a Huber-tipped Tuohy needle is used as a conduit to pass the epidural catheter into the canal. This needle has a ski-like tip that limits its being caught or snagged on the sacral periosteum. The needle is inserted with its shoulder anteriorly and its orifice facing dorsally. Alternatively, a standard 16- or 17-gauge catheter-over-needle (angiocatheter) may serve as the introducing needle for subsequent catheter placement. The catheter is advanced with fluoroscopic guidance especially when it is performed for chronic pain management in failed back surgery syndrome. The catheters should be advanced gently, since there have been reports of dural puncture with rapid or aggressive advancement. The lateral and anteroposterior views should be obtained to demonstrate placement of the catheter is in the epidural space (lateral view) and to follow its path in a cephalad or cephalolateral direction (anteroposterior view). When the desired level is attained, iodinated contrast media may be injected, followed by the injection of local anesthetics, corticosteroids, or adjuncts. We usually do not advance the catheter higher than the level of the L4 vertebral body, although we have occasionally advanced it to the L1 or L2 level. Some authorities suggest avoiding advancement more than 8 to 12 cm cephalad.

CAUDAL EPIDURAL BLOCK IN ADULTS

Caudal epidural local anesthetic block in adults may be chosen for surgeries of the lower abdomen, perineum, or lower extremities. The local anesthetics used are as for lumbar epidural block (Table 71-2). Spread of local anesthetics may be influenced by volume, speed of injection, or patient posture.[1] Caudal epidural block results in sensory and motor block of the sacral roots and limited autonomic block. The sacral contribution of the parasympathetic nervous system will be blocked. This causes loss of visceromotor function of the bladder and intestines distal to the colonic splenic flexure. Sympathetic block, though limited compared to lumbar or thoracic epidural block, does occur. The sympathetic outflow from the spinal cord ends at the L2 level, and therefore caudal block should not routinely cause peripheral vasodilatation of the lower extremities to the degree seen with lumbar epidural. Caudal block is indicated whenever the area of surgery involves the sacral and lower lumbar nerve roots. The technique is suitable for anal surgery (hemorrhoidectomy and anal dilatation), gynecological procedures, surgery on the penis or scrotum, and lower limb surgeries. Using a catheter technique, it is possible to use caudal epidural block for vaginal hysterectomy and inguinal herniorrhaphy.

Caudal epidural block is used less frequently than lumbar or even thoracic epidural block for providing perioperative analgesia in adults. The pelvis enlarges markedly in puberty while the epidural fat in the lumbosacral region undergoes compaction and increased fibrous content. This hinders cephalad spread of solutions particularly when compared with the spread in children.

The large capacity of the sacral canal accommodates correspondingly large volumes of solution; significant volumes may

TABLE 71-2. LOCAL ANESTHETICS COMMONLY USED FOR CAUDAL ANESTHESIA IN ADULTS

Agent	Concentration (%)	Dose (mg)	Sensory Onset (Four-Segment Spread) (minutes)	Duration (Two-Segment Regression) (minutes)
Lidocaine	1.5–2	300–600	10–20	90–150
Chloroprocaine	2–3	400–900	8–15	45–80
Mepivacaine	2	400–600	10–20	90–240
Ropivacaine	0.75–1	150–300	15–25	120–210
Bupivacaine/ levobupivacaine	0.5–0.75	100–225	10–25	180–270

All solutions with epinephrine 1:200,000, except ropivacaine. All doses and times approximate.

be lost through the wide anterior sacral foramina. Therefore, the caudal dose requirements of local anesthetics are significantly larger to effect the same segmental spread than are the corresponding lumbar doses. Roughly, twice the lumbar epidural local anesthetic dose is needed for caudal block to attain similar levels of analgesia and anesthesia, and solutions injected in the caudal space take longer to spread (Table 71-2). Bromage noted that age is not correlated with caudal segmental spread in adults and the upper level of analgesia resulting from 20 mL doses of local anesthetic solution varies widely between S2 and T8.[1] This unpredictability limits the usefulness of applying caudal anesthesia for surgical procedures that require cephalad analgesia levels above the pelvic level or the umbilicus.

CAUDAL BLOCK IN PREGNANCY

The sacral canal shares in the general engorgement of extradural veins that occurs in late pregnancy, or in any clinical condition in which the inferior vena cava (IVC) is partially obstructed. Since the effective volume of the caudal canal is markedly diminished during the latter part of pregnancy, the caudal dosage should be reduced proportionately in women at term. There may be a substantial increase in the segmental spread of local anesthetics in pregnant women at term, necessitating a 28% to 33% decrease of dose requirement in this patient population.[1] The choice of a continuous catheter or a single-shot technique during active labor is limited by the relative lack of sterility at the sacral hiatus which may be contaminated by feces and meconium.

Rare cases of Horner's syndrome have been noted when large doses of local anesthetics are injected caudally during labor.[1] This is most likely to occur if injection is made with the patient on her back (engorgement of epidural venous plexus and IVC compression are maximum). The so-called "dual technique" (lumbar and caudal) of epidural block for labor is no longer used. Since the pain of uterine contractions is mediated by sympathetic nervous system fibers originating from T10 to L2, a lumbar epidural catheter suffices for both stage I and stage II of parturition, with dosage adjustments being made depending upon the exact circumstances and requirements.

CAUDAL EPIDURAL BLOCK IN CHILDREN

The sacral hiatus is usually very easy to palpate in infants and children, and caudal epidural block is an integral part of the intra- and postoperative management of children undergoing a wide range of surgical procedures below the diaphragm. The technique is easily learned; one study demonstrated an 80% success rate in resident trainees after completing 32 procedures performed without fluoroscopic guidance.[26] In infants and small children a 21-gauge short-beveled 1-inch needle may be used for single-injection techniques. For continuous blocks, a standard epidural catheter may be advanced through an 18-gauge angiocatheter, or a thin-walled 18-gauge epidural needle. It has been noted that by the age of 4 or 5 years the sacral canal is usually large enough to accept such a needle for passage of a catheter.[1] There are three groups of individuals for whom this technique is used: those requiring sacral block (circumcision, anal surgery), those requiring lower thoracic block (inguinal herniorrhaphy), and, rarely, those requiring analgesia

of the upper thoracic dermatomes (reserved for special situations). Caudal block is usually combined with light general anesthesia with spontaneous ventilation. Unlike in adults, the segmental spread of analgesia following caudal administration is more predictable in children up to about 12 years of age. Studies suggest that the cephalad spread of caudal solutions in children is not hampered by the same anatomical constraints that develop from puberty onwards. Before puberty, anatomical impedance at the lumbosacral junction has not yet developed to a marked degree and caudal solutions can flow freely upward into the higher recesses of the spinal canal. As a consequence, the rostral spread of caudal anesthesia is more extensive and more predictable in children than in adults.

Anesthetic dose requirements are about 0.1 mL/segment per year for 1% lidocaine or 0.25% bupivacaine.[1] The dose may also be calculated based upon body weight. The relationship between age and dose requirements is strictly linear with a high degree of correlation up to 12 years old.[1] Plasma bupivacaine concentrations in children receiving caudal block with 0.2% of the local anesthetic, 2 mg/kg, were less than equivalent doses administered via ilioinguinal–iliohypogastric block for pain control following herniotomy or orchidopexy. Additionally, the times to peak plasma concentrations were faster in the peripheral nerve block group indicating that caudal block is a safe alternative to local infiltration techniques in inguinal surgery.[27] In a study of children aged 1 to 6 years of age who underwent orchidopexy a caudal block using larger volumes of dilute bupivacaine (0.2%) was shown to be more effective than a smaller volume of the standard (0.25%) concentration in blocking the peritoneal response to spermatic cord traction, with no change in the quality of postoperative analgesia. In that study the total bupivacaine dose was identical in both groups (20 mg).[28] Ropivacaine 0.5% was shown to provide a significantly longer duration of analgesia following inguinal herniorrhaphy in children aged 1.5 to 7 years when compared to 0.25% ropivacaine or 0.25% bupivacaine.[29] All the children received 0.75 mL/kg of the local anesthetic. Unfortunately, however, the times to first voiding and to standing were significantly delayed in the group receiving 0.5% ropivacaine and there was one case of motor block of the lower extremities. This demonstrates the trade-off when one attempts to maximize analgesia by altering local anesthetic concentration or total dose.[29]

The success of a caudal block in pediatrics may be predicted from the laxity of the anal sphincter secondary to the reduction in sphincter tone from the local anesthetic block. This is a good sign since most caudal blocks in children are performed while the child is anesthetized, and it is not possible to assess the effectiveness of the block by testing for sensory analgesia levels. One study demonstrated that the presence of a lax anal sphincter at the termination of surgery correlated with the reduced need to administer opioids perioperatively.[30]

Even though caudal block is a mainstay of pain management in pediatric surgery and represents probably 60% of all regional anesthetic techniques in this patient population, not all studies demonstrated a marked benefit of caudal block for postoperative analgesia when compared to other modalities. Following unilateral inguinal herniorrhaphy, caudal block was shown to provide effective, but not superior, pain management when compared to local wound infiltration in 54 children. The side effects and rescue analgesia requirements did not differ between the two groups.[31]

TABLE 71-3. **TYPICAL LOCAL ANESTHETICS FOR CAUDAL BLOCK IN PEDIATRICS (SINGLE SHOT)**

Agent (and reference)	Concentration (%)	Dose	Onset (minutes)	Duration of Action (minutes)
Ropivacaine[33]	0.2	2 mg/kg	9	520
Bupivacaine[33]	0.25	2 mg/kg	12	253
Ropivacaine[34]	0.2	0.7 mg/kg	11.7	491
Bupivacaine[34]	0.25	0.7 mg/kg	13.1	457
Ropivacaine[35]	0.2	1 mL/kg	8.4	NR
Levobupivacaine[35]	0.25	1 mL/kg	8.8	NR
Bupivacaine[35]	0.25	1 mL/kg	8.8	NR

NR, not recorded.

Caudal epidural block in children may induce significant changes in descending aortic blood flow while maintaining heart rate and mean arterial blood pressure. In a study of 10 children aged 2 months to 5 years a transesophageal Doppler probe was used to calculate hemodynamic variables after the injection of 1 mL/kg of 0.25% bupivacaine with epinephrine 5 μg/mL. The aortic ejection volume increased, while aortic vascular resistance decreased by about 40%.[32] These data suggest that caudal block results in vasodilatation secondary to sympathetic nervous system blockade.

The local anesthetics typically administered for single-shot caudals in pediatrics are listed in Table 71-3.[33–35]

UNIQUE APPLICATIONS OF CAUDAL EPIDURAL BLOCK: CHRONIC AND ACUTE PAIN MANAGEMENT

Percutaneous epidural neuroplasty uses a caudal catheter left in place for up to three days to inject hypertonic solutions into the epidural space to treat radiculopathy with low back pain and epidural scarring, typically from previous lumbar spinal surgery. In addition to local anesthetics and corticosteroids, hypertonic saline and hyaluronidase are added to the injectate. This treatment was associated with a reduction of pain in subjects with radiculopathy who were refractory to conventional therapies. The technique relies upon fluoroscopic guidance and caudal epidurography, since this was noted to be effective in correlating a filling defect of injected iodinated contrast media with the patient's reported level of pain.[14] Injection of solutions into the epidural space of a patient with adhesions is usually quite painful because of distention of affected nerve roots.[13] Triamcinolone acetate has been recommended instead of methylprednisolone since particulate steroids can occlude an epidural catheter or possibly cause infarction of spinal tissue via vascular injection.[13] Hypertonic saline is used to prolong pain relief due to its local anesthetic effect and its ability to reduce edema in previously scarred or inflamed nerve roots.[13]

The authors recommend a lateral needle placement into the caudal canal, directing the needle and catheter towards the affected side. Lateral placement tends to minimize the likelihood of penetrating the dural sac or subdural area. When 5 to 10 mL of contrast media are injected into the caudal canal through an epidural catheter, a "Christmas-tree" appearance (Fig. 71-6) develops as dye spreads into the perineural structures inside the bony canal and along the nerves as they exit the vertebral column.[13] Epidural adhesions prevent dye spread so there is no outline of the involved nerve roots (Fig. 71-7). If the needle is in the subarachnoid space, the dye spreads centrally and cephalad to a level higher than that attained with epidural spread. Once correct catheter placement in the epidural space is ensured, 1,500 units of hyaluronidase in 10 mL

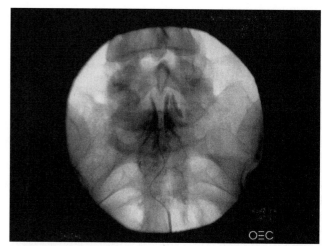

FIGURE 71-6. Anteroposterior view of a caudal catheter epidural injection of 2 mL of contrast. Note the characteristic "Christmas tree" appearance of the spreading dye.

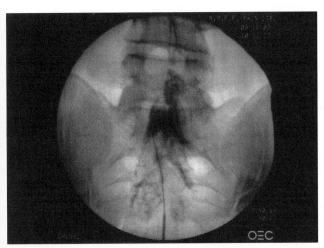

FIGURE 71-7. Anteroposterior fluoroscopic view of a patient with failed back surgery syndrome who underwent L5–S1 laminectomy and is now selected for percutaneous epidural neuroplasty. There is a significant filling defect from epidural adhesions at that level preventing left-sided dye spread so that there is no outline of the left S1 nerve root.

of preservative saline are injected followed by 10 mL of 0.2% ropivacaine and 40 mg of triamcinolone. Following these two injections, an additional injection of 9 mL of 10% hypertonic saline is infused over 20 to 30 minutes. On the second and third days, the local anesthetic (ropivacaine) injection is followed up by the hypertonic saline solution. Antibiotic coverage is provided to reduce the possibility of epidural abscess formation.

Another unique application of caudal block is to provide postoperative analgesia in patients undergoing lumbar spine surgeries. In one series patients received 20 mL of 0.25% bupivacaine with 0.1 mg buprenorphine via the caudal epidural approach, performed prior to surgical incision.[15] The patients underwent posterior interbody fusion and laminotomy for spinal stenosis, and postoperative pain control was compared in the caudal group with a group treated with conventional parenteral opioids. The caudal group required less rescue analgesic medication doses for the first 12 hours following surgery.[15] A reduction in blood pressure in the caudal group patients undergoing laminotomy, but not fusion, was noted in the patients with prolonged-duration (24 hours) postoperative analgesia.

Caudal epidural block has also been compared with intramuscular opioids in the treatment of pain after emergency lower extremity orthopedic surgery. The caudal group who received 20 mL of 0.5% bupivacaine had 8 hours of superior analgesia and also had a significant reduction in the need for rescue opioid medications.[16]

Caudal injection of clonidine 75 µg with 7 mL bupivacaine 0.5% and 7 mL lidocaine 2% with epinephrine 5 µg/mL has been used for postoperative analgesia after elective hemorrhoidectomy. Thirty-two adults received the clonidine/local combination while a control group received local anesthetic alone. Analgesia averaged 12 hours in the clonidine group, compared to <5 hours in the local anesthetic-only group. Bradycardia occurred in about 22% of patients in the clonidine group.[17]

Caudal injections of alcohol or phenol have been used to treat intractable pain due to cancer. In a study of 67 blocks it was found that the lower sacral roots were easily reached with the caudal, and that the S1 and S2 roots (contribution from the lumbosacral plexus) were spared.[18]

COMPLICATIONS ASSOCIATED WITH CAUDAL EPIDURAL BLOCK

The complications of caudal block are the same as those occurring following lumbar epidural block and may include those related to the technique itself and those related to the local anesthetic or other injected substance. Fortunately, most serious complications occur infrequently. Possibilities include epidural abscess, meningitis, epidural hematoma, dural puncture and postdural puncture headache, subdural injection, pneumocephalus and air embolism, back pain, and broken or knotted epidural catheters. The incidence of local anesthetic-induced seizures occurs more frequently following caudal block than it does following lumbar or thoracic approaches. In a retrospective study of 25,697 patients who received brachial plexus blocks or caudal or lumbar epidural blocks from 1985 to 1992 Brown et al. noted 26 seizures.[36] The frequency of seizures in adults was caudal > brachial plexus block > lumbar or thoracic epidural block. There were 9 overall seizures attributed to local anesthetic injection in the caudal space, 8 occurring with chloroprocaine, and 1 occurring with lidocaine. There was a 70-fold incidence (0.69%) of local anesthetic toxic reactions with caudal epidural anesthesia than with lumbar or thoracic epidural anesthesia in adults. In children, however, one retrospective review identified only 2 toxic reactions (i.e., local anesthetic-induced seizures) in 15,000 caudal blocks.[37] Dalens' group found that inadvertent intravascular injection occurs in up to 0.4% of pediatric caudals,[38] demonstrating the importance of performing epinephrine-containing test dosing in this age group. It has been suggested that an elevation of heart rate greater than 10 beats per minute, or an increase in systolic blood pressure greater than 15 mmHg should be taken as indicative of systemic injection. T-wave changes on the ECG occur earliest following intravascular injection, followed by HR changes, and, lastly, by blood pressure changes. These changes may be delayed for up to 90 seconds following the injection.[38]

Total spinal anesthesia occasionally occurs, as in the case report of an 18-month-old, 10 kg child who received a caudal block postoperatively after undergoing emergency repair of a recurrent diaphragmatic hernia. The child had a history of craniofacial dystosis. An amount of 4 mL of 0.5% bupivacaine and 2.5 µg/kg of buprenorphine was injected in a total volume of 10 mL. Eye opening and hand movement were delayed for 3 hours following this complication.[39]

SUMMARY

Caudal epidural block is a technique of providing analgesia and anesthesia of the lumbosacral nerve roots that predates conventional lumbar approaches. The block has gone through several periods of acceptability and although it is infrequently applied to routine surgical cases in adults, it is the most commonly performed regional anesthetic technique in infants and children. Caudal block has enjoyed a resurgence lately, due to its role in gaining access to the lumbar epidural space below the scar tissue from spinal surgeries and for performing epiduroscopy. The technique is here to stay, and pain medicine clinicians who routinely utilize fluoroscopy will find that it has many applications, both for routine and complicated cases.

KEY POINTS

- The sacral canal contains the cauda equina (including the filum terminale), the spinal meninges, adipose tissue, and the sacral venous plexus.
- The volume of the sacral canal averages 14.4 mL, but varies from 9.5 to 26.6 mL.
- The indications for performing caudal epidural block are essentially the same as for lumbar epidural block.
- Percutaneous epidural neuroplasty is a technique of administering local anesthetics, corticosteroids, hyaluronidase, and hypertonic saline through a caudal catheter for the purpose of lysing epidural adhesions.
- Adult patients are typically placed prone for the block, while the lateral decubitus position is preferred for pediatrics.
- The use of caudal block in pediatrics is primarily for perioperative pain control, whereas in adults it is primarily used for chronic pain management.
- In adults roughly twice the local anesthetic dose is required compared to lumbar epidural block to attain the same segmental spread.

ACKNOWLEDGMENT

Artwork for this chapter was provided by Robert Haque.

REFERENCES

1. Bromage PR: Epidural Analgesia. WB Saunders, Philadelphia, 1978, pp 258–282.
2. Racz G: Personal communication. American Society of Anesthesiologists Annual Meeting, San Francisco, CA, 12 October 2003.
3. Trotter M: Variations of the sacral canal: Their significance in the administration of caudal analgesia. Anesth Analg 26:192–202, 1947.
4. MacDonald A, Chatrath P, Spector T, Ellis H: Level of termination of the spinal cord and the dural sac: A magnetic resonance study. Clin Anat 12:149–152, 1999.
5. Igarashi T, Hirabayashi Y, Shimizu R, et al: The lumbar extradural structure changes with increasing age. Br J Anaesth 78:149–152, 1997.
6. Crighton I, Barry B, Hobbs G: A study of the anatomy of the caudal space using magnetic resonance imaging. Br J Anaesth 78:391–395, 1997.
7. Bryce-Smith R: The spread of solutions in the extradural space. Anaesthesia 9:201–205, 1954.
8. Brenner E: Sacral anesthesia. Ann Surg 79:118–123, 1924.
9. Waldman S: Caudal epidural nerve block. In Waldman S (ed): Interventional Pain Management, ed 2. WB Saunders, Philadelphia, 2001, p 520.
10. Winnie A, Candido KD: Differential neural blockade for the diagnosis of pain. In Waldman S (ed): Interventional Pain Management, ed 2. WB Saunders, Philadelphia, 2001, pp 162–173.
11. Candido KD, Stevens RA: Intrathecal neurolytic blocks for the relief of cancer pain. Best Practice Res Clin Anaesthesiol 17:407–428, 2003.
12. Lou L, Racz G, Heavner J: Percutaneous epidural neuroplasty. In Waldman S (ed): Interventional Pain Management, ed 2. WB Saunders, Philadelphia, 2001, pp 434–445.
13. Heavner J, Racz G, Raj P: Percutaneous epidural neuroplasty: Prospective evaluation of 0.9% NaCl versus 10% NaCl with or without hyaluronidase. Reg Anesth Pain Med 24:202–207, 1999.
14. Manchikanti L, Bakhit C, Pampati V: Role of epidurography in caudal neuroplasty. Pain Digest 8:277–281, 1998.
15. Kakiuchi M, Abe K: Pre-incisional caudal epidural blockade and the relief of pain after lumbar spine operations. Int Orthop 21:62–66, 1997.
16. McCrirrick A, Ramage D: Caudal blockade for postoperative analgesia: A useful adjunct to intramuscular opiates following emergency lower leg orthopaedic surgery. Anaesth Intensive Care 19:551–554, 1991.
17. Van Elstraete A, Pastureau F, Lebrun T, Mehdaoui H: Caudal clonidine for postoperative analgesia in adults. Br J Anaesth 84:401–402, 2000.
18. Porges P, Zdrahal F: Intrathecal alcohol neurolysis of the lower sacral roots in inoperable rectal cancer (German). Anaesthetist 34:627–629, 1985.
19. Chan S, Tay H, Thomas E: "Whoosh" test as a teaching aid in caudal block. Anaesth Intensive Care 21:414–415, 1993.
20. Tsui B, Tarkkila P, Gupta S, Kearney R: Confirmation of caudal needle placement using nerve stimulation. Anesthesiology 91:374–378, 1999.
21. Digiovanni A: Inadvertent interosseous injection – A hazard of caudal anesthesia. Anesthesiology 34:92–94, 1971.
22. Lofstrom B: Caudal anaesthesia. In Ejnar Eriksson (ed): Illustrated Handbook of Local Anaesthesia. AB Astra, Copenhagen, 1969, pp 129–134.
23. Caudal block. In Covino BG, Scott DB (eds): Handbook of Epidural Anaesthesia and Analgesia. Grune & Stratton, 1985, pp 104–108.
24. Dawkins C: An analysis of the complications of extradural and caudal block. Anaesthesia 24:554–563, 1969.
25. Chung Y, Lin C, Pang W, et al: An alternative continuous caudal block with caudad catheterization via lower lumbar interspace in adult patients. Acta Anaesthesiol Scand 36:221–227, 1998.
26. Schuepfer G, Konrad C, Schmeck J, et al: Generating a learning curve for pediatric caudal epidural blocks: An empirical evaluation of technical skills in novice and experienced anesthesiologists. Reg Anesth Pain Med 25:385–388, 2000.
27. Stow P, Scott A, Phillips A, White J: Plasma bupivacaine concentrations during caudal analgesia and ilioinguinal-iliohypogastric nerve block in children. Anaesthesia 43:650–653, 1988.
28. Verghese S, Hannallah R, Rice LJ, et al: Caudal anesthesia in children: Effect of volume versus concentration of bupivacaine on blocking spermatic cord traction response during orchidopexy. Anesth Analg 95:1219–1223, 2002.
29. Koinig H, Krenn C, Glaser C, et al: The dose–response of caudal ropivacaine in children. Anesthesiology 90:1339–1344, 1999.
30. Verghese S, Mostello L, Patel R: Testing anal sphincter tone predicts the effectiveness of caudal analgesia in children. Anesth Analg 94:1161–1164, 2002.
31. Schindler M, Swann M, Crawford M: A comparison of postoperative analgesia provided by wound infiltration or caudal analgesia. Anaesth Intensive Care 19:46–49, 1991.
32. Larousse E, Asehnoune K, Dartayet B, et al: The hemodynamic effects of pediatric caudal anesthesia assessed by esophageal Doppler. Anesth Analg 94:1165–1168, 2002.
33. Ivani G, Mereto N, Lampugnani E, et al: Ropivacaine in paediatric surgery: Preliminary results [abstract]. Paediatr Anaesth 8:127–129, 1998.

34. Ivani G, Lampugnani E, De Negri P, et al: Ropivacaine vs. bupivacaine in major surgery in infants [abstract]. Can J Anaesth 46:467–469, 1999.

35. Ivani G, DeNegri P, Conio A, et al: Comparison of racemic bupivacaine, ropivacaine and levobupivacaine for pediatric caudal anesthesia. Effects on postoperative analgesia and motor blockade. Reg Anesth Pain Med 27:157–161, 2002.

36. Brown D, Ransom D, Hall J, et al: Regional anesthesia and local anesthetic-induced systemic toxicity: Seizure frequency and accompanying cardiovascular changes. Anesth Analg 81:321–328, 1995.

37. Giaufre E, Dalens B, Gombert A: Epidemiology and morbidity of regional anesthesia in children: A one-year prospective survey of the French-language Society of Pediatric Anesthesiologists. Anesth Analg 83:904–912, 1996.

38. Dalens B, Hansanoui A: Caudal anesthesia in pediatric surgery: Success rate and adverse effects in 750 consecutive patients. Anesth Analg 8:83–89, 1989.

39. Afshan G, Khan F: Total spinal anaesthesia following caudal block with bupivacaine and buprenorphine. Paediatr Anaesth 6:239–242, 1996.

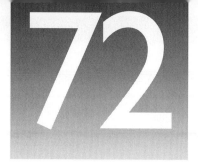

Head and Neck Blocks

Umeshraya T. Pai, M.D.,
Rajeshri Nayak, M.D., and
Robert E. Molloy, M.D.

TRIGEMINAL NERVE

The trigeminal nerve is the fifth cranial nerve and has three divisions: ophthalmic, maxillary, and mandibular. It is predominantly a sensory nerve, with a small motor component that is contained in the mandibular division. Proximally, the sensory component of the trigeminal nerve is connected to the ventral aspect of the pons. Distally, the sensory component leaves from the medial concave border of the trigeminal (semilunar) ganglion. The trigeminal ganglion is located at the apex of the petrous temporal bone in the posterior medial part of the middle cranial fossa. The ganglion is also related to the inferior lateral aspect of the cavernous sinus. The minor motor component of the trigeminal nerve is at the medial side of the nerve at the attachment to the pons and runs inferior to the ganglion to exit through the foramen ovale, with the mandibular division as its motor branches.[1]

MAXILLARY NERVE BLOCK

Anatomy: The maxillary nerve is the second division of the trigeminal nerve and is also known as the V2 division. This nerve is the middle division of the trigeminal nerve and is attached to the distal convex border of the trigeminal ganglion. The maxillary nerve exits from the cranial cavity through the foramen rotundum. From this point, the nerve traverses the superior part of the pterygopalatine fossa and swings laterally to traverse the inferior orbital fissure toward the maxillary sinus. As the nerve runs along the roof of the maxillary sinus, it supplies the maxillary sinus itself and the anterior teeth of the upper jaw via the anterior and middle superior alveolar nerves. The nerve then exits through the infraorbital foramen to innervate the skin of the face and the underlying mucosa extending from the lower eyelid to the upper lip. While the nerve is at the pterygopalatine fossa, it is connected to the pterygopalatine ganglion, through which it gives off branches to the nasal cavity, pharynx, and palate. In addition, the nerve gives off the zygomatic nerve and the posterior superior alveolar nerve. The zygomatic nerve supplies the lateral portion of the face and the posterior superior alveolar nerve, which supplies the upper molar region.[2]

Indications
- Maxillofacial procedures.
- Surgical procedures on the teeth of the upper jaw.
- Chronic pain conditions involving tumors of the maxillary sinus.
- Assessment and diagnosis of pain syndromes in the distribution of the nerve; i.e., trigeminal neuralgia, acute herpes zoster.

Contraindications
- Infection at the site of entry.
- Coagulopathy.
- Preexisting neurologic deficits.

Landmarks
- Midpoint of the zygomatic arch of the temporal bone.
- Condyle of the mandibular head.
- Coronoid process of the mandible.
- Mandibular notch between the condyle and the coronoid process.

Technique: There are two approaches in performing a maxillary nerve block, both of which are discussed here (Fig. 72-1).

LATERAL APPROACH: The patient is supine with the head turned away from the side of the intended block. The side of the face is prepared and draped in a sterile manner. The landmarks are palpated, and the midpoint of the zygomatic arch is marked. The skin is infiltrated with local anesthetic in the area of the mandibular notch between the condyle and the coronoid process of the mandible below the midpoint of the zygomatic arch.

After infiltration, a 22-gauge, 3-inch needle is introduced perpendicular below the midpoint of the zygomatic arch and walked onto the lateral pterygoid plate. A depth marker can be placed on the needle to the anticipated depth (approximately

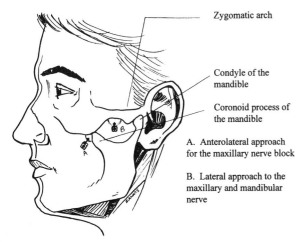

FIGURE 72-1. Two approaches to performing a maxillary nerve block.

0.5 to 1 cm from the initial depth to the lateral pterygoid plate). The needle is then withdrawn and redirected and advanced anteromedially into the pterygopalatine fossa (Fig. 72-2). A nerve stimulator may be helpful, because paresthesias may or may not be elicited. After aspiration to rule out intravascular placement of the needle, 2 to 3 mL of local anesthetic is deposited for the desired effect.

ANTEROLATERAL APPROACH: The patient is positioned and prepared in the manner described above. The angle between the inferior border of the zygomatic bone and the coronoid process of the mandible is located and marked. After a skin wheal is raised at this angle, a 3-inch, 22-gauge needle is directed medially, superiorly, and posteriorly to lie along the posterior surface of the maxilla and further advanced approximately 4 to 5 cm, depending on the extent of subcutaneous tissue.

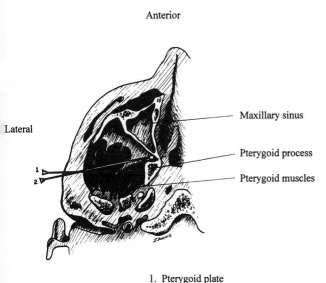

Maxillary Nerve Block

1. Pterygoid plate
2. Maxillary nerve

FIGURE 72-2. Maxillary nerve block, transverse section.

Once the needle tip walks off the maxilla, a paresthesia may be elicited when the needle tip reaches the pterygopalatine fossa. As before, a nerve stimulator may be helpful to verify the position of the needle. Once the position is determined, local anesthetic is deposited after negative aspiration.

Complications
- If the needle is placed too deep and anterior, direct injection into the optic nerve is possible resulting in transient blindness with local anesthetic use or permanent blindness with the use of neurolytic agent.
- Because of vascularity of the region secondary to the rich venous plexus and the third part of the maxillary artery and its five to six branches, intravascular injection is a possibility.
- Hematoma can develop, the extent of which depends on the size of the needle.

MANDIBULAR NERVE BLOCK

Anatomy: The mandibular nerve is the third division of the trigeminal nerve and is also referred to as the V3 division. It arises from the lower part of the distal convexity of the trigeminal ganglion and then joins the motor component. From this point, the nerve exits through the foramen ovale to enter the infratemporal fossa. It then divides into a smaller anterior division and a larger posterior division. The anterior division is predominantly motor, except for the buccal branch, which provides sensation to the cheek. The motor branches innervate the muscles of mastication. The posterior division is predominantly sensory, except for the myelohyoid branch, which provides motor innervation to the myelohyoid muscle and the anterior belly of the digastric muscle. The sensory portion of the mandibular nerve innervates the meninges (via the recurrent meningeal branch), the temporomandibular joint, the ear, and the outer surface of the tympanic membrane, anterior two-thirds of the mouth, and adjoining part of the floor of the mouth, and the mandible with its associated teeth. The sensory portion terminates as the mental nerve, which supplies the chin. All of these areas are innervated through the following branches: auriculotemporal, lingual, and inferior alveolar.

Indications
- Surgical procedures in the cutaneous distribution of the nerve.
- Surgery of the mandible (i.e., open reduction and internal fixation of the mandible), associated teeth and gums, and anterior two-thirds of the tongue.
- Postoperative pain control in the area of distribution of the nerve.
- Treatment of chronic pain syndromes; i.e., carcinoma of the tongue, lower jaw, and floor of the mouth; trigeminal neuralgia; or acute herpes zoster.

Contraindications: Contraindications are similar to those described for the maxillary nerve block.

Landmarks: Landmarks are similar to those described for the maxillary nerve block.

Technique: The patient is positioned and prepared in a manner similar to that described for the maxillary nerve block. The landmarks are palpated, and a point below the midpoint of

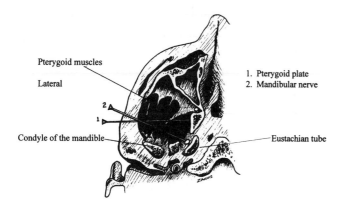

Pterygoid muscles

Lateral

1. Pterygoid plate
2. Mandibular nerve

Condyle of the mandible

Eustachian tube

Mandibular Nerve Block

FIGURE 72-3. Mandibular nerve block, transverse section.

the zygomatic arch in the mandibular notch is marked. After infiltration of the overlying skin with local anesthetic, a 22-gauge, 3-inch needle is inserted perpendicular to the skin and advanced posteromedially to a depth of approximately 4 to 5 cm, at which point paresthesias in the distribution of the nerve may be elicited. Local anesthetic is deposited after negative aspiration to achieve the desired effect. On the other hand, if bone (lateral pterygoid plate) is contacted, the needle is withdrawn and redirected more posteriorly in an attempt to elicit paresthesia (Fig. 72-3). Once again, a nerve stimulator may be useful if there is difficulty in eliciting paresthesias. The landmarks for this block are similar to those for the lateral approach to the maxillary block, the difference between the two being the direction of advancement of the needle. The lateral approach to the maxillary block involves advancing the needle anteromedially, whereas the mandibular block involves advancing the needle posteromedially.

Complications

- Intravascular injection is a potential complication because of the proximity of the pterygoid plexus of veins, maxillary artery, and its branch, the middle meningeal artery.
- If the needle is inserted too deep, the superior constrictor muscle can be pierced, resulting in entry into the pharynx.

GLOSSOPHARYNGEAL NERVE BLOCK

Anatomy: The glossopharyngeal nerve is the ninth cranial nerve. It arises from the cranial part of the medulla and exits from the cranial cavity through the intermediate compartment of the jugular foramen. The nerve then runs between the internal carotid artery and internal jugular vein, after which it swings around the stylopharyngeus muscle toward the pharynx and the tongue. During its course, it lies deep to the styloid process. The nerve supplies motor fibers to the pharyngeal muscles and sensory fibers to the middle ear, posterior third of the tongue, and the pharynx. It also innervates the carotid sinus and the carotid body. The nerve is in close proximity to the vagus nerve, accessory nerve, and sympathetic trunk.[3]

Indications

- Diagnosis and treatment of glossopharyngeal neuralgia.
- Control of pain arising from cancer of the tongue and pharynx.
- Control of pain during awake endoscopy.

Contraindications: Contraindications are similar to those mentioned for the blocks described above.

Landmarks

- Mastoid process, posteriorly.
- Angle of the mandible, anteriorly.
- Styloid process of the temporal bone, in the middle.

Technique

EXTRAORAL APPROACH: Appropriate monitoring and intravenous access are required before proceeding with the block. The patient is supine, with the head turned to the side opposite of the block. The lateral face and portion of the neck below the ear are prepared in sterile manner.

The angle of the mandible and the mastoid process are marked. The point midway between these two landmarks inferior to the ear corresponds to the position of the styloid process of the temporal bone. The skin overlying the styloid process is infiltrated with local anesthetic. A 22-gauge, 3-inch needle is then inserted perpendicular to the skin and advanced toward the styloid process. Once the styloid process is contacted, a depth marker is placed 0.5 cm from the skin. The needle is then withdrawn and reinserted anterior to the styloid process to the depth marker. This corresponds to the location of the glossopharyngeal nerve as it curves around the stylopharyngeus muscle (Fig. 72-4). An amount of 2 to 3 mL of local anesthetic is injected after negative aspiration.[4]

INTRAORAL APPROACH: This approach uses a tongue depressor or laryngoscope for exposure after topical local anesthetic application to the tongue. A tonsil needle or a 22-gauge, 3.5-inch spinal needle with a distal 25° bend is used for injection at a depth of 0.5 cm under the mucosa. The landmark for injection is the lower lateral portion of the posterior tonsillar pillar. An amount of 2 to 3 mL of local anesthetic is injected after negative aspiration.

Complications

- Intravascular injection into the internal carotid artery or internal jugular vein is a potential risk. Injection into the carotid artery can result in seizures and possible cardiovascular collapse.
- Hematoma from trauma to the above-mentioned vessels can occur.
- Inadvertent nerve block can occur due to proximity to the vagus, hypoglossal, and accessory nerves. This may result, respectively, in dysphonia and tachycardia, weakness of the tongue, and weakness of the trapezius muscle.
- Bilateral block of the glossopharyngeal nerves can result in total pharyngeal paralysis with associated risk of aspiration; severe upper airway obstruction after extubation has been reported in children following tonsillectomy.[5]

PHRENIC NERVE BLOCK

Anatomy: The phrenic nerve is formed from the ventral roots of C3–C5; its primary component arises from the C4 anterior primary ramus. The three roots join at the lateral border of the anterior scalene muscle, and the phrenic nerve passes inferiorly along the anterior surface of this muscle, posterior to the sternomastoid and omohyoid muscles, and into the chest. It travels close to the internal mammary artery, the

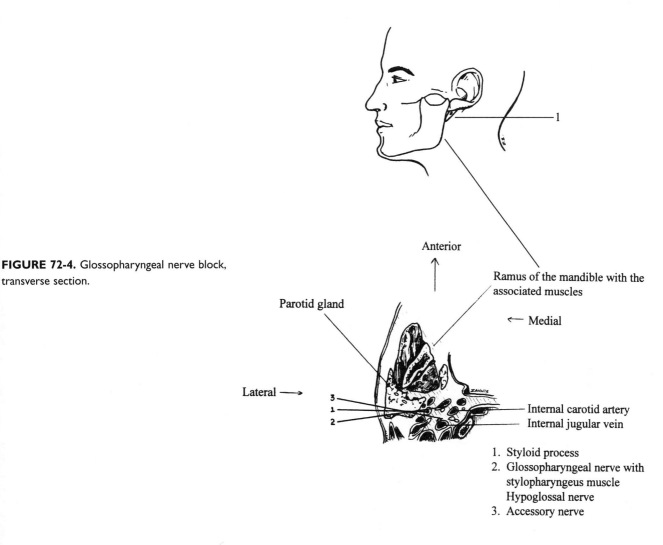

FIGURE 72-4. Glossopharyngeal nerve block, transverse section.

Anterior

Ramus of the mandible with the associated muscles

Parotid gland

← Medial

Lateral →

Internal carotid artery
Internal jugular vein

1. Styloid process
2. Glossopharyngeal nerve with stylopharyngeus muscle
   Hypoglossal nerve
3. Accessory nerve

---

root of the lung, and the pericardium. It communicates with the sympathetic chain, the accessory nerve, and the hypoglossal nerve.[6]

Indications
- Treatment of intractable hiccups by interruption of both afferent and efferent limbs of the hiccup reflex.
- Diagnosis and treatment of cancer pain due to diaphragmatic invasion.

Landmarks
- Posterior border of the sternomastoid muscle.
- Anterior border of the anterior scalene muscle.
- Groove between these muscles, one inch above the clavicle.

Technique: Patient monitoring, intravenous access, and skin preparation are as above. The approach is very similar to that for interscalene block. The patient is supine and asked to lift his/her head off the bed and to turn to the opposite side. The groove between the sternomastoid and anterior scalene muscles is identified, about 2.5 cm above the clavicle. A 22-gauge, 1.5-inch block needle is inserted medially and slightly inferiorly, parallel to the anterior surface of the anterior scalene muscle. An infiltration block may be performed at a depth of 2.5 cm, in a fan-like manner along this surface. A peripheral nerve

stimulator with an insulated block needle may be used to accurately locate the nerve. The endpoint is production of unilateral diaphragmatic contraction.[7]

Complications
- Accidental intravascular injection.
- Hematoma formation, particularly after trauma to the inaccessible subclavian vessels.
- Unilateral paralysis of the diaphragm, with reduction of vital capacity by 20%.
- Recurrent laryngeal nerve block and hoarseness.
- Unintentional spinal or epidural block resulting from needle insertion too deeply.
- Horner's syndrome.
- Pneumothorax, or chylothorax on the left side.

CERVICAL PLEXUS BLOCK

Anatomy: Kappis reported the original cervical plexus block technique in 1912, using a posterior approach. Heidenbeim described a lateral technique for this block in 1914, and this general approach has gained widespread acceptance.[8] The cervical plexus is formed from the upper four cervical nerves. Their dorsal and ventral roots join to form a spinal nerve as they exit through an intervertebral foramen. The cervical spinal

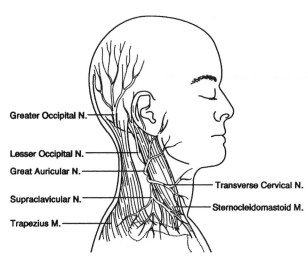
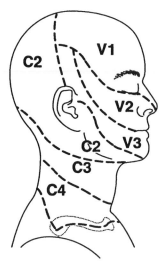

FIGURE 72-5. Peripheral cutaneous (left) and dermatomal (right) innervation of the head and neck, including the branches of the superficial cervical plexus and the greater occipital nerve.

nerves then split into anterior and posterior divisions. The C1 spinal nerve is formed almost entirely from a ventral root, and it is primarily a motor nerve. It actually emerges between the occiput and the arch of the atlas as the suboccipital nerve, and it is not directly blocked during cervical plexus block. The anterior primary rami of C2–C4 travel laterally along the sulcus in their respective transverse processes, passing posterior to the vertebral artery. Lateral to the transverse process, these cervical nerves are enclosed in a fascial space derived from the fascia of the muscles attached to the tubercles of the transverse processes. This space is continuous with the interscalene fascial plane inferior to it, allowing for single-injection techniques of cervical plexus block.

The anterior primary rami of C2–C4 form three loops, which are referred to as the cervical plexus. This plexus lies behind the sternomastoid muscle, giving off both superficial and deep branches (Fig. 72-5). The superficial branches pierce the deep cervical fascia posterior to the sternomastoid muscle and supply skin and superficial tissues in the head, neck, and shoulder. The four distinct branches of the superficial cervical plexus are the lesser occipital, the great auricular, the transverse cervical, and the supraclavicular nerves. The first two branches pass superiorly to the area of the ear, the mastoid, and the angle of the mandible. The transverse cervical nerve passes anteriorly to supply most of the anterolateral neck between the chin and the sternal notch and clavicles. The supraclavicular nerves descend to supply the anterolateral shoulder and the upper pectoral region. The deep branches of the cervical plexus innervate the deeper structures, including the muscles of the anterior and lateral neck as well as the diaphragm via the phrenic nerve.

Indications: Cervical plexus blockade is indicated for many surgical procedures of the anterior and lateral neck and the supraclavicular fossa (Table 72-1). Unilateral block is adequate for procedures that do not extend to the midline. For surgery of the thyroid gland,[9] larynx, and trachea, bilateral block and intravenous sedation are required. Bilateral deep cervical plexus block is usually avoided because of the added risks involved, particularly respiratory compromise. Superficial cervical plexus block facilitates awake placement of pulmonary artery catheters[10] and central venous catheters.[11] Combined with

midazolam, superficial cervical plexus block has been found to be a safe, reliable, and well-tolerated alternative to general anesthesia in pediatric patients with mediastinal masses.[12]

Various types of carotid artery surgery have been performed under combined superficial and deep cervical plexus block.[13–18] The major advantages of performing carotid endarterectomy with this approach include the ability to assess neurologic function (and therefore the need for vascular shunting) in the awake patient. Davies and colleagues reported high patient acceptance of this technique, a low incidence of neurologic complications, and an acceptable rate of cardiovascular complications. Corson and colleagues observed an apparent decrease in the incidence of neurologic complications after carotid endarterectomy performed with cervical plexus block when compared with general anesthesia. Benjamin and associates reported that awake neurologic monitoring during carotid endarterectomy allowed for prompt, accurate identification of patients with cerebral ischemia who would clearly benefit from intraoperative shunting. Preoperative clinical status and vascular

TABLE 72-1. POTENTIAL INDICATIONS FOR CERVICAL PLEXUS BLOCK

Superficial neck procedures
Neck dissection procedures
Thyroglossal and branchial cysts
Thyroidectomy
Lymph node excision
Cervical node biopsy in a child with a mediastinal mass
Insertion of a pulmonary artery catheter
Internal jugular and subclavian venous cannulation
Percutaneous carotid balloon angioplasty
Carotid endarterectomy with awake neurological monitoring
Relief of metastatic pharyngeal cancer pain
Relief of occipital and other neuralgias
Relief of postoperative pain after neurosurgical operations[44]
Transvenous cardiac pacemaker insertion[14]

anatomy were not reliable predictors of the need for shunting. Adequate anesthesia for transvenous pacemaker insertion has been observed after cervical plexus block combined with block of the second through the fourth intercostal nerves.[19] Complete anesthesia of the dermatomes from C3 to T4 was obtained, without anesthesia of the brachial plexus.

Technique

SUPERFICIAL CERVICAL PLEXUS BLOCK: For superficial cervical plexus block,[20,21] the patient is placed in the supine position with the arms resting at the sides and the head turned slightly away from the side to be blocked. The head is lifted off the table to bring the sternomastoid muscle and its posterior border into prominence. The midpoint of the muscle's posterior border is identified, and a 22-gauge, 4 to 5 cm needle is inserted subcutaneously, posterior and immediately deep to the sternomastoid muscle, injecting 5 mL of local anesthetic. Two additional 5 mL injections are made along the posterior border of the muscle as the needle is redirected both superiorly and inferiorly. A lower concentration of local anesthetic is effective, such as 0.5% to 0.75% lidocaine with epinephrine 5 µg/mL.

DEEP CERVICAL PLEXUS BLOCK: The patient is positioned just as for superficial cervical plexus block. This procedure is essentially a cervical paravertebral somatic block of the C2, C3, and C4 spinal nerves at the lateral edge of their transverse processes (Fig. 72-6). A lateral approach has been proven to be simple and more reliable than the posterior approach for deep cervical plexus block. Traditionally three needles are inserted at the C2–C4 levels. The insertion sites are located along a reference line drawn on the patient's neck. This line connects the tip of the mastoid process to the anterior tubercle of the C6 transverse process, which is easily palpated at the level of the cricoid cartilage. Some authors recommend drawing a second reference line parallel to and 1 cm posterior to the original line to better approximate the location of the underlying transverse processes, which are then located by palpation. The C2 transverse process is located 1 to 2 cm below the mastoid along the reference line, while C3 and C4 are sought 1.5 cm and 3 cm inferior to C2. The C3 transverse process is located at the level of the hyoid bone. The C4 transverse process may be found at the level of the upper border of the thyroid cartilage or, alternatively, at the lower level of the mandibular ramus.

The deep cervical plexus block is performed with a 22-gauge needle directed medially and caudally to avoid an excessive depth of insertion and unintentional spinal, epidural, or subdural blockade or vertebral artery injection. The first end point for needle placement is contact with the bony transverse processes at a depth of 1.5 to 3 cm; the more inferior processes tend to become more superficial. The second end point is production of a paresthesia, which may require redirecting the needle in anterior and posterior directions along the tip of the transverse process. At each level, 3 to 5 mL of local anesthetic is injected, using a relatively higher concentration such as 1.5% lidocaine with epinephrine 5 µg/mL. The superficial and deep cervical plexus block techniques appear to be equally effective for carotid endarterectomy with no difference in supplemental local anesthetic requirements.[22]

Deep cervical plexus block can also be produced with a single injection at one level using a larger volume of local anesthetic. A single-needle interscalene cervical plexus block has been described with injection at the C4 level.[23] The interscalene cervical plexus block is performed in a fashion similar to

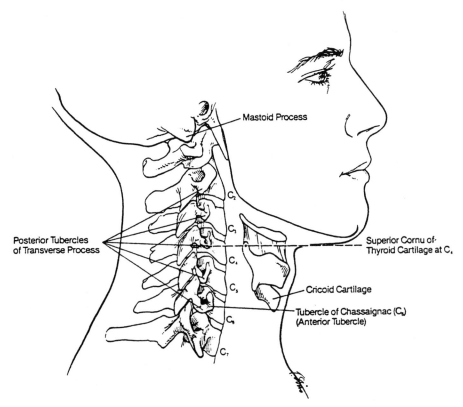

FIGURE 72-6. Bony landmarks for deep cervical plexus block. (From Raj PP, Pai D, Rawal N: Techniques of regional anesthesia in adults. *In* Raj PP (ed): Clinical Practice of Regional Anesthesia. Churchill Livingstone, New York, 1991, p 271.)

that for brachial plexus block but at a more cephalad level. If a nerve stimulator is used, a deltoid muscle motor response is sought, and 10 to 15 mL of local anesthetic is injected. The interscalene approach is simple, less painful, associated with less systemic absorption of local anesthetic, and equally effective when compared to the classic multiple-injection technique.[24] Incomplete analgesia may occur during procedures such as carotid endarterectomy. This is occasionally noted at the upper extent of a cervical incision, where glossopharyngeal nerve innervation is encountered. Incision of the carotid sheath may also produce pain during an otherwise satisfactory block. This sheath is traversed by branches of the upper and lower roots of the ansa cervicalis.[25] Local infiltration by the surgeon is often effective in these situations.

LOCAL ANESTHETICS: Shorter-duration block may be produced with lidocaine or mepivacaine, longer block with bupivacaine or ropivacaine. More dilute solutions can be used for superficial cervical plexus block. Several studies have measured blood levels of local anesthetic after cervical plexus block without detecting clinical or laboratory evidence of toxicity.[26–29] Dawson and colleagues observed mean peak lidocaine blood levels of about 5 μg/mL after injection of 6 mg/kg of 1.5% lidocaine with epinephrine 5 μg/mL. These levels are similar to those found after multiple, bilateral intercostal nerve blockade, the regional anesthetic technique widely considered to produce the highest systemic levels of local anesthetic. Molnar and colleagues demonstrated the effect of epinephrine 5 μg/mL on lidocaine blood levels. After 7 mg/kg of 1.5% lidocaine, mean peak blood levels were about 7.5 μg/mL with clonidine added and 4.5 μg/mL with epinephrine.

Complications: Because of the proximity of the vertebral artery, accidental intra-arterial injection may result in almost instantaneous central nervous system toxicity consisting of convulsions, loss of consciousness, and blindness.[30] Intraneural or transforaminal needle placement may result in unintentional spinal anesthesia. Local anesthetic may spread to the epidural or subdural space, resulting in bilateral cervicothoracic anesthesia.[31,32] Phrenic nerve block can be anticipated, with a resultant decrement in inspiratory capacity.[33] Bilateral cervical plexus block is generally avoided to prevent serious respiratory compromise, particularly in the presence of pulmonary disease. Bradycardia from bilateral sympathetic block and airway obstruction may also occur.[34] Local anesthetic deposition or spread superficial to the deep cervical fascia can block the sympathetic chain and the recurrent laryngeal nerve, resulting in Horner's syndrome and hoarseness. Systemic toxicity may occur after accidental injection of the vertebral, external jugular, or internal jugular veins with either deep or superficial cervical plexus blocks. Careful aspiration tests and the initial injection of 1 mL of anesthetic with deep cervical plexus block are used to detect intrathecal, intravascular, or vertebral artery injection. Limiting needle insertion to the depth of the lateral edge of the transverse process may also decrease the chance of complications.

OCCIPITAL NERVE BLOCK

Blockade of the greater occipital nerve provides anesthesia of the medial part of the posterior scalp. It is most often employed in the diagnosis and therapy of chronic pain conditions.

Most headaches are either muscular or vascular in nature. Occipital pain may rarely occur with cranial malignancy, infection, or congenital abnormalities, and a careful history and physical examination are always indicated to rule out serious underlying causes of headache.[35] Myofascial trigger points in the posterior cervical muscles (e.g., the upper semispinalis cervicis) produce dull, aching occipital pain, whereas trigger points in the splenius capitis produce referred headache near the vertex. They may be managed with better posture, massage, stretching exercises, and trigger point injections. Arthritis of the cervical spine may also be associated with occipital headaches. Exaggerated muscle tension or contraction of the semispinalis capitis muscle may be theorized to produce occipital neuralgia by direct compression of the greater occipital nerve. However, the role of greater occipital nerve compression may be relatively minor.[36] Occipital neuralgia produces continuous throbbing pain in the suboccipital area, perhaps aggravated by pressure over the greater occipital nerve.[37] By definition, occipital neuralgia is relieved by diagnostic blockade of the greater occipital nerve.[38] This may include referred pain to the head and neck outside the typical distribution of the greater occipital nerve. A series of occipital nerve blocks with local anesthetic and depot steroid may be therapeutic for occipital neuralgia.[39]

Bovim and Sand[40] evaluated the response to diagnostic greater occipital nerve block in patients with cervicogenic headache, migraine without aura, and tension-type headache. They defined cervicogenic headache according to the criteria proposed by Sjaastad and associates, the most important of which are as follows:

- Unilateral headache; always on the same side.
- Symptoms and signs of neck involvement—Pain due to neck pressure or head position; ipsilateral neck, shoulder, or arm pain; reduced cervical flexibility.
- Pain characteristics—Episodic or continuous pain; moderate, nonthrobbing neck pain with radiation; history of neck trauma; female sex.

Occipital nerve block reduced pain in 19 of 22 patients with cervicogenic headache. At least 40% pain relief (visual analogue scale) was noted in 80% of cervicogenic headache patients, but in none of those with migraine or tension-type headache. Forehead pain was also relieved in 17 of 22 patients with cervicogenic headache, suggesting the presence of referred pain to the trigeminal nerve distribution. Pain relief outside the area blocked was rare with the other two headache types.

Anthony evaluated 796 patients with idiopathic headache and no history of whiplash or head injury. Cervicogenic headache was diagnosed in 128 patients (16.1%). Depot methylprednisolone injections of the greater and lesser occipital nerves produced complete relief of headache in 169 of 180 patients with cervicogenic headache for an average of 23.5 (10 to 77) days.[41] Inan et al. reported long-lasting relief of cervicogenic headache after repeated blocks, with equal efficacy for greater occipital nerve block and C2/C3 nerve blocks.[42]

Anatomy: The sensory innervation of the posterior head and neck arises from the second and third cervical nerves.[1] The lateral section of the posterior scalp is supplied by the lesser occipital and great auricular nerves, branches of the cervical

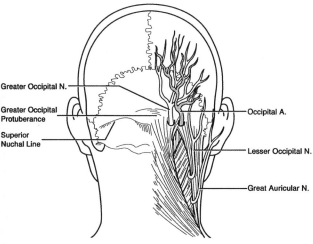

FIGURE 72-7. Technique of greater occipital nerve block, demonstrating the position of the greater occipital nerve and the occipital artery above the superior nuchal line. (Modified from Tucker JH, Flynn JF: Head and neck regional anesthesia. *In* Brown DL (ed): Regional Anesthesia and Analgesia. WB Saunders, Philadelphia, 1996, p 240.)

plexus (see Fig. 72-5). They are accessible for blockade laterally near the superior nuchal line or, alternatively, at the posterior edge of the sternomastoid muscle, in its middle third. The medial section of the posterior scalp is supplied by the greater occipital nerve, the termination of the medial branch of the dorsal ramus of C2. This nerve arises between the atlas and axis laterally and travels posteriorly and medially before turning cephalad, deep to the semispinalis capitis muscle.[43] Near the base of the skull, the greater occipital nerve passes posteriorly through the semispinalis capitis muscle and then continues under the trapezius muscle to travel cephalad and laterally, passing between the insertions of the trapezius and sternomastoid muscles to reach a subcutaneous position. In its subcutaneous course over the posterior scalp, the nerve lies adjacent and medial to the occipital artery, which serves as the prime landmark for blockade of the greater occipital nerve (Fig. 72-7).

Technique: The greater occipital nerve is blocked with the seated patient's head and neck flexed forward, chin to chest. Three landmarks are identified: the mastoid process, the greater occipital protuberance, and the superior nuchal line. The occipital arterial pulse is identified along this line, approximately one-third of the distance from the greater occipital protuberance toward the mastoid. Injection of 3 to 5 mL of local anesthetic just medial to the artery, with or without prior elicitation of paresthesia, produces occipital anesthesia. An initial diagnostic block is best performed with only 1 to 2 mL of drug after a paresthesia has been obtained. When the arterial pulse is not palpable, a wider area of subcutaneous infiltration may be required. Anesthesia of the scalp should develop in 5 to 10 minutes.

There are no common complications to this block that do not apply to any superficial, perivascular injections. This presumes that the skull is intact and that an accidental suboccipital injection is avoided.

KEY POINTS

- Bilateral block of the glossopharyngeal nerves can result in total pharyngeal paralysis with associated risk of aspiration and severe upper airway obstruction.
- Carotid artery surgery may be performed under combined superficial and deep cervical plexus block, allowing for assessment of neurological function in a conscious patient. This technique has achieved a high rate of patient acceptance, a low incidence of neurological complications, and an acceptable rate of cardiovascular morbidity.
- Occipital nerve block is utilized for both diagnosis and therapy of occipital neuralgia.

REFERENCES

1. Tucker JT, Flynn JF: Head and neck regional blocks. *In* Brown DL (ed): Regional Anesthesia and Analgesia. JB Saunders, Philadelphia, 1996, pp 240–253.
2. Waldman SD: Blockade of the trigeminal nerve and its branches. *In* Waldman SD (ed): Interventional Pain Management, ed 2. WB Saunders, Philadelphia, 2001, pp 321–329.
3. Waldman SD: Glossopharyngeal nerve block. *In* Waldman SD (ed): Interventional Pain Management. WB Saunders, Philadelphia, 2001, pp 331–334.
4. Romanoff M: Somatic nerve blocks of the head and neck. *In* Raj PP (ed): Practical Management of Pain, ed 3. Mosby, St Louis, 2000, pp 579–596.
5. Bean-Lijewski JD: Glossopharyngeal nerve block for pain relief after pediatric tonsillectomy: Retrospective analysis and two cases of life-threatening upper airway obstruction from an interrupted trial. Anesth Analg 84:1232–1238, 1997.
6. Greenfield MA: Phrenic nerve block. *In* Waldman SD (ed): Interventional Pain Management, ed 2. WB Saunders, Philadelphia, 2001, pp 337–339.
7. Okuda Y, Kitajima T, Asai T: Use of a nerve stimulator for phrenic nerve block in treatment of hiccups. Anesthesiology 88:525–527, 1998.
8. Pappas JL, Warfield CA: Cervical plexus blockade. *In* Waldman SD (ed): Interventional Pain Management, ed 2. WB Saunders, Philadelphia, 2001, pp 342–361.
9. LoGerfo P, Ditkoff BA, Chabot J, et al: Thyroid surgery using monitored care: An alternative to general anesthesia. Thyroid 4:437–439, 1994.
10. Brull SJ: Superficial cervical plexus block for pulmonary artery catheter insertion. Crit Care Med 20:1362–1363, 1992.
11. Chauhan S, Baronia AK, Maheshwari A, et al: Superficial cervical plexus block for internal jugular and subclavian venous cannulation in awake patients. Reg Anesth 20:459, 1995.
12. Brownlow RC, Berman J, Brown RE: Superficial cervical plexus block for cervical node biopsy in a child with a large mediastinal mass. J Ark Med Soc 90:378–380, 1994.
13. Alessandri C, Bergeron P: Local anesthesia in carotid angioplasty. J Endovasc Surg 3:31–34, 1996.
14. Benjamin ME, Silva ME, Watt C, et al: Awake patient monitoring to determine the need for shunting during carotid endarterectomy. Surgery 114:673–679, 1993.
15. Davies MJ, Mooney PH, Scott DA, et al: Neurologic changes during carotid endarterectomy under cervical plexus block predict a high risk of postoperative stroke. Anesthesiology 78:829–833, 1993.
16. Davies MJ, Murrell GC, Cronin KD, et al: Carotid endarterectomy under cervical plexus block: A prospective clinical audit. Anaesth Intensive Care 18:219–223, 1990.
17. Corson JD, Chang BB, Karmody AM: The influence of anesthetic choice on carotid endarterectomy outcome. Arch Surg 122:807–812, 1987.

18. Castresana MR, Balser JS, Newman WH, et al: Cervical block for carotid endarterectomy followed immediately by general anesthesia for coronary artery bypass and aortic valve replacement. Anesth Analg 77:186–187, 1993.

19. Raza SM, Vasireddy AR, Candido KD, et al: A complete regional anesthesia technique for cardiac pacemaker insertion. J Cardiothorac Vasc Anesth 5:54–56, 1991.

20. Murphy TM: Somatic blockade of head and neck. In Cousins MJ, Bridenbaugh PO (eds): Neural Blockade in Clinical Anesthesia and Management of Pain, ed 2. JB Lippincott, Philadelphia, 1988, p 533.

21. Raj PP, Pai D, Rawal N: Techniques of regional anesthesia in adults. In Raj PP (ed): Clinical Practice of Regional Anesthesia. Churchill Livingstone, New York, 1991, p 271.

22. Stoneham MD, Doyle AR, Knighton JD: Prospective, randomized comparison of deep or superficial cervical plexus block for carotid endarterectomy surgery. Anesthesiology 89:907–912, 1999.

23. Winnie AP, Ramamurthy S, Durrani Z, et al: Interscalene cervical plexus block: A single injection technique. Anesth Analg 54:370–375, 1975.

24. Merle JC, Mazoit JX, Desgranges P, et al: A comparison of two techniques for cervical plexus blockade: Evaluation of efficacy and systemic toxicity. Anesth Analg 89:1366–1370, 1999.

25. Einav S, Landesberg G, Prus D, et al: A case of nerves. Reg Anesth 21:168–170, 1996.

26. Dawson AR, Dysart RH, Amerena JV, et al: Arterial lignocaine concentrations following cervical plexus blockade for carotid endarterectomy. Anaesth Intensive Care 19:197–200, 1991.

27. Molnar RR, Davies M, Scott DA, et al: Comparison of clonidine and epinephrine in lidocaine for cervical plexus block. Reg Anesth 22:137–142, 1997.

28. Tissot S, Frering B, Gagnieu MC, et al: Plasma concentrations of lidocaine and bupivacaine after cervical plexus block for carotid surgery. Anesth Analg 84:1377–1379, 1997.

29. Neill RS, Watson R: Plasma bupivacaine concentration during combined. Regional and general anesthesia for resection and reconstruction of head and neck carcinomata. Br J Anaesth 56:485–492, 1984.

30. Szeinfeld M, Laurencio M, Pallares VS: Total reversible blindness following stellate ganglion block. Anesth Analg 60:689–690, 1981.

31. Kumar A, Battit GE, Froese AB, et al: Bilateral cervical and thoracic epidural blockade complicating interscalene brachial plexus block: Report of two cases. Anesthesiology 35:650–652, 1971.

32. Huang KC, Fitzgerald MR, Tsueda K: Bilateral block of cervical and brachial plexuses following interscalene block. Anaesth Intensive Care 14:87–88, 1986.

33. Castresana MR, Masters RD, Castresana E, et al: Incidence and clinical significance of hemidiaphragmatic paresis in patients undergoing carotid endarterectomy during cervical plexus block anesthesia. J Neurosurg Anesthesiol 6:21–23, 1994.

34. Levelle P, Martinez OA: Airway obstruction after bilateral carotid endarterectomy. Anesthesiology 63:220–222, 1985.

35. Brown DL, Wong GY: Occipital nerve block. In Waldman SD, Winnie AP (eds): Interventional Pain Management. WB Saunders, Philadelphia, 1996, pp 226–229.

36. Bovim G, Bonamico L, Fredriksen TA, et al: Topographic variations in the peripheral course of the greater occipital nerve. Spine 16:475–478, 1991.

37. Sjaastad O, Fredriksen TA, Pfaffenrath V: Cervicogenic headache: Diagnostic criteria. Headache 30:725–726, 1990.

38. Headache Classification Committee of the International Headache Society: Classification and diagnostic criteria for headache disorders, cranial neuralgias, and facial pain. Cephalalgia 8(Suppl 7):1–96, 1988.

39. Anthony M: Headache and the greater occipital nerve. Clin Neurol Neurosurg 4:297–301, 1992.

40. Bovim G, Sand T: Cervicogenic headache, migraine without aura and tension-type headache: Diagnostic blockade of greater occipital and supra-orbital nerves. Pain 51:43–48, 1992.

41. Anthony M: Cervicogenic headache: Prevalence and response to local steroid therapy. Clin Exp Rheumatol 18(Suppl 19):S59–S64, 2000.

42. Inan N, Ceyhan A, Inan L, et al: C2/C3 nerve blocks and greater occipital nerve block in cervicogenic headache treatment. Funct Neurol 16:239–243, 2001.

43. Vital JM, Grenier F, Dantheribes M, et al: An anatomic and dynamic study of the greater occipital nerve (n. of Arnold): Applications to the treatment of Arnold's neuralgia. Surg Radiol Anat 11:205–210, 1989.

44. Niijima K, Malis U: Preventive superficial cervical plexus block for postoperative cervicocephalic pain in neurosurgery. Neurol Med Chir (Tokyo) 33:365–367, 1993.

Brachial Plexus Blocks: Techniques Above the Clavicle

Kenneth D. Candido, M.D.

ANATOMICAL CONSIDERATIONS

The brachial plexus is formed by the anterior primary rami of cervical nerve roots C5–C8 and thoracic nerve root T1. The fourth cervical nerve (C4) contributes to about 67% of plexuses, and, if significant, may shift the plexus in a craniad direction ("prefixed plexus"). The second thoracic nerve (T2) contributes to about 33% of plexuses, and may shift the plexus in a caudad direction ("postfixed plexus"). Through a complex series of dividing and reuniting, the principal elements of the plexus interact in a manner analogous to the components of a tree; roots, trunks, divisions, cords, and terminal branches (Fig. 73-1). The roots of C5–C8 and T1 travel along the groove between the anterior and posterior tubercles of the transverse processes of the cervical vertebrae, pass posterior to the vertebral artery (Fig. 73-2), and descend towards the first rib. Along the way, they are enveloped by the posterior fascia of the anterior scalene muscle and the anterior fascia of the middle scalene muscle: the so-called "interscalene space"[1,2] (Fig. 73-3). The anterior scalene muscle arises from the anterior tubercles of the transverse processes of C3–C6 and inserts on the scalene tubercle of the first rib. It separates the subclavian vein and artery (Fig. 73-4). The middle scalene muscle arises from the posterior tubercles of the transverse processes of C2–C7 and inserts on the first rib just posterior to the subclavian groove on the rib. After arriving at the distal end of their respective transverse processes, the five roots converge to form the three trunks (superior, middle, inferior), which together with the subclavian artery invaginate the scalene fascia to form a "subclavian space."[2] The superior trunk of the plexus is formed by the union of the C5 and C6 nerve roots, the middle trunk is the distal continuation of C7, and the inferior trunk is formed by the union of the C8 and T1 nerve roots. As these three trunks pass over the first rib and under the clavicle, each divides into an anterior and posterior division (there are

a total of six divisions) (Fig. 73-1). It is at this level that separation of fibers destined for the anterior arm (flexor or volar surface of the upper extremity) and the posterior arm (extensor or dorsal surface) occurs. As the plexus emerges from beneath the clavicle, the fibers recombine to form the three cords of the brachial plexus. The lateral cord is formed by the union of the anterior divisions of the superior and middle trunks; the medial cord is simply the continuation of the anterior division of the inferior trunk; and the posterior cord is composed of the posterior divisions of all three trunks (Figs. 73-1 and 73-5). The medial and lateral cords then give rise to nerves that supply the flexor surface of the upper extremity while those nerves arising from the posterior cord supply the extensor surface of the arm. Each of the three cords of the plexus gives off a branch that contributes to or becomes one of the major nerves to the upper extremity, and then terminates as another major nerve. The lateral and medial cords give off branches that become the lateral and medial heads of the median nerve (C5–C8) (major terminal branch). The lateral cord continues as the musculocutaneous nerve (C5–C7) (major terminal branch), while the medial cord continues on as the ulnar nerve (C7–T1) (major terminal branch). The posterior cord gives off the axillary nerve (C5–C6) (major terminal branch) and then continues on as the radial nerve (C5–T1) (major terminal branch) (Fig. 73-1).

When performing brachial plexus blocks above the clavicle using peripheral nerve stimulator techniques, it is important to appreciate several of the anatomical branches from the roots that, while not essential to successful brachial plexus anesthesia, have considerable significance since they may be stimulated when one is seeking an evoked motor response prior to injecting local anesthetic solutions. The long thoracic nerve, arising from C5, C6, and C7 innervates the serratus anterior muscle. Its stimulation may result in contraction of the muscular wall enveloping the ribs, and may be mistaken for

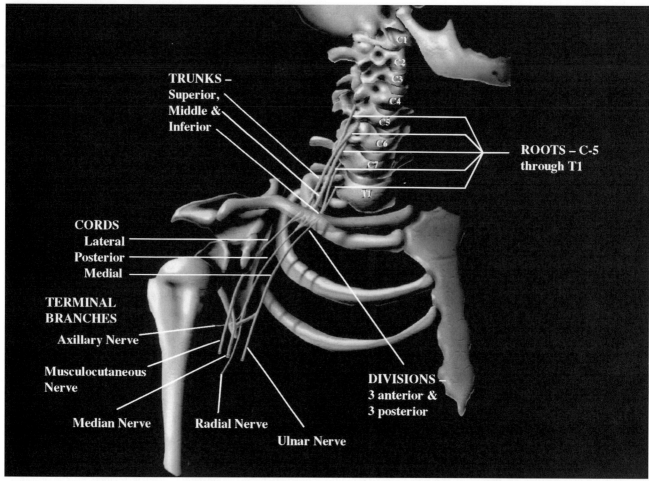

FIGURE 73-1. Anatomy of the brachial plexus: roots (5); trunks (3); divisions (6); cords (3); major peripheral nerves (5).

diaphragmatic contraction resulting from stimulation of the phrenic nerve (C3, C4, C5). The dorsal scapular nerve, arising from C5 and innervating the major and minor rhomboids and the levator scapulae, may be stimulated, resulting in a contraction of the musculature of the back and shoulder blade. The trunks also supply two branches, the nerve to the subclavius (C5–C6) and the suprascapular nerve (C5–C6). The suprascapular nerve has significance in the performance of brachial plexus blocks above the clavicle, since in addition to motor branches to the supraspinatus and infraspinatus muscles, it also supplies the only sensory fibers (to the shoulder joint) that arise above the clavicle. Since the nerve may leave the brachial plexus shortly after arising from the superior trunk, a paresthesia resulting from its stimulation is an unreliable indicator that a stimulating needle is correctly placed within the confines of the sheath.[3] As a general rule of thumb when using a nerve stimulator technique, diaphragmatic contraction requires a more posterior reinsertion of the needle (the phrenic nerve sits outside the sheath on the anterior scalene muscle) while trapezius or posterior deltoid contraction requires reinsertion of the needle more anteriorly in the interscalene space.

Brachial plexus block in addition to providing sensory analgesia and anesthesia and motor block also blocks the sympathetic outflow to the upper extremity. Postganglionic sympathetic nerve fibers reach the nerve roots as gray rami communicantes from the middle and inferior cervical sympathetic ganglia and stellate ganglion (Fig. 73-6), and are subsequently distributed to the upper extremity. Additional contributions may arise from the vertebral artery (fibers given off to C4, C5, C6), and from the nerve of Kuntz (branch from T2).[2] Ultimately, postganglionic fibers to the upper extremity are derived from two potential sources. The first is a distal innervation that is carried to the peripheral vessels by the somatic nerves of the plexus. The second mode is a proximal innervation (not extending beyond the proximal part of the brachial artery) arising from the cervical sympathetic chain, particularly via the stellate ganglion. This supplies the proximal one-third of the extremity. The distal innervation (distal two-thirds of the arm) mediates vasoconstriction of resistance vessels, implying that brachial plexus block produces vasodilatation of veins of the upper extremity, increases the amount of blood pooling in the distal arm, and increases skin temperature.

Supraclavicular techniques of brachial plexus block rely upon anatomical considerations at the root and trunk levels, as opposed to infraclavicular techniques (cords) or axillary approaches (major peripheral branches). Single-injection techniques above the clavicle rely upon the concept of a continuous fascial compartment from the prevertebral fascia of the cervical vertebrae passing distally to (and beneath) the clavicle (Fig. 73-7).

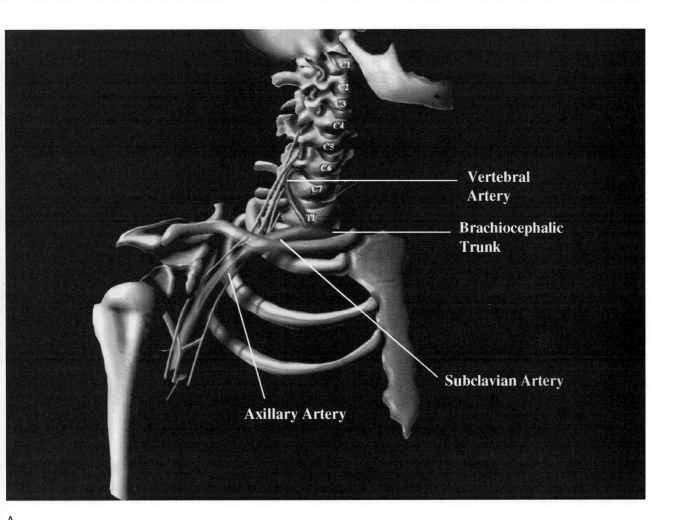

Vertebral
Artery

Brachiocephalic
Trunk

Subclavian Artery

Axillary Artery

A

FIGURE 73-2. *A,* Relationship of relevant arterial structures to the brachial plexus above the clavicle. Note that the brachial plexus is posterior to both the subclavian artery as well as to the vertebral artery.

TECHNIQUES OF BRACHIAL PLEXUS BLOCK ABOVE THE CLAVICLE

Interscalene Techniques: Dating back to at least 1912 (Kappis), interscalene techniques were described that blocked the plexus at the root level. While Kappis was attempting to block spinal nerves at the level where they emerged from the vertebral column, Mulley may have described the first true lateral paravertebral interscalene block in 1919.[2] Probably the true forerunner of the contemporary interscalene approach was Etienne who described a single-injection technique involving the omotrapezoid triangle formed by the lateral edge of the sternocleidomastoid muscle and the anterior edge of the trapezius.[2]

Due to the proximity of the central neuraxis, interscalene block requires the least volume of local anesthetic and has the shortest latency of onset of any brachial block approach. There have been many modifications over the years, all attempting to improve the success rate and reduce the incidence of complications. The approach is above both the cupola of the lung and subclavian artery and is least likely to result in pneumothorax or vascular complications.

The author's technique is as described by Winnie[1,2] and is as follows. The patient lies supine with the head turned *slightly* towards the opposite side, is told to relax the shoulder, and to reach towards the ipsilateral knee with the hand. A full complement of noninvasive hemodynamic monitors is applied and an intravenous cannula is secured in a distal vein on the contralateral (i.e., nonsurgical) extremity. Intravenous administration of modest doses of a rapidly acting, short-duration benzodiazepine (midazolam) is acceptable prior to commencing the block. The patient should be alert enough to report verbally any paresthesias, dysesthesias, or other abnormal sensations, both during the needle insertion(s) as well as during the subsequent injection of local anesthetic solution. The interscalene groove is palpated and the C6 level is estimated by dropping a line laterally from the cricoid cartilage (Fig. 73-8). The external jugular vein typically crosses the interscalene groove at C6, but this occurs with some variability. An "anesthetic line" has been described to locate the plexus along its proximal to distal length, but this appears to nullify the inherent simplicity in locating the scalene muscles as the primary landmark in supraclavicular techniques.[4] With the palpating index and middle fingers straddling and indenting the

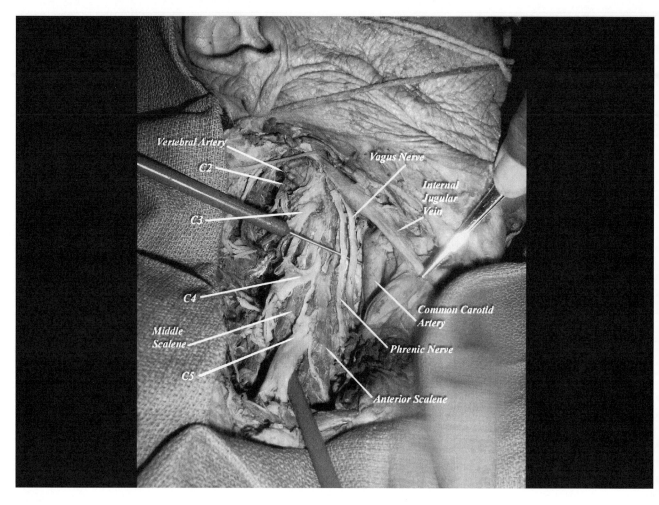

B

FIGURE 73-2. *B,* Anatomical dissection of the right side of the neck depicting the relationships seen in *A.* Note the proximity of the vertebral artery to the C2 nerve root, and the location of the phrenic nerve sitting on the anterior surface of the anterior scalene muscle. Also note the significant girth of the cervical nerves 4 and 5.

interscalene groove (to minimize the distance from the skin to the cervical transverse processes), the opposite hand advances a 22-gauge, 2-inch Stimuplex (B. Braun, Bethlehem, PA) needle into the groove, using nerve stimulator assistance (Fig. 73-9). Although the fingers compress the skin towards the nerve roots and central neuraxis, it should be appreciated that cadaver dissections have demonstrated that the minimum distances from the skin to the C6 foramen and vertebral column are 23 mm and 35 mm, respectively.[5] The direction of the needle should be perpendicular to the skin with a slightly posterior (dorsad), medial (mesiad), and inferior (caudad) direction until a motor response is observed at 0.5 mA or less (Fig. 73-10). Whereas an evoked motor response of the shoulder, elbow, or hand is acceptable prior to injecting local anesthetic, a shoulder *paresthesia* should not be used as a sole endpoint since it may indicate that the stimulating needle is stimulating the supra-scapular nerve, either within or outside the brachial plexus sheath.[3,6] The roots lie slightly closer to the middle than to the anterior scalene muscle, and the needle should therefore be in closer proximity to the middle scalene. Blockade of C8 and T1 may be delayed unless significant volumes of local anesthetic

are utilized (40 mL for individuals 68 to 74 inches tall). The resultant anesthesia and analgesia will be in the distribution of the nerve roots C5–C8 and T1. Therefore, assessing the patient requires knowledge of peripheral dermatomes of the upper extremity. The block is ideal for shoulder surgery, and, if the surgeon is performing arthroscopy, where a posterior port is frequently utilized (Fig. 73-11), one simply makes the injection at C4 instead of C6. The C4 level can be estimated by moving our lateral line to the interscalene space from the most prominent aspect of the thyroid cartilage, instead of the cricoid (Fig. 73-12). Although palpation of the interscalene groove is more difficult as one progresses more cephalad, it has been found that the groove is easily *followed* from an inferior (caudad) point upwards on the neck.[7] Alternatively, C4 may be blocked separately by an additional injection of 5 mL of local anesthetic. A recent study at the author's institution confirmed Kerr's anatomical data indicating that 7% of brachial plexuses have no C4, and only partial C5 contributions to the trunks.[8] Thus, a supplemental C4 block may be needed if the clinician does not wish to perform cervical plexus block. Hemidiaphragmatic paresis and concomitant 25% to 30%

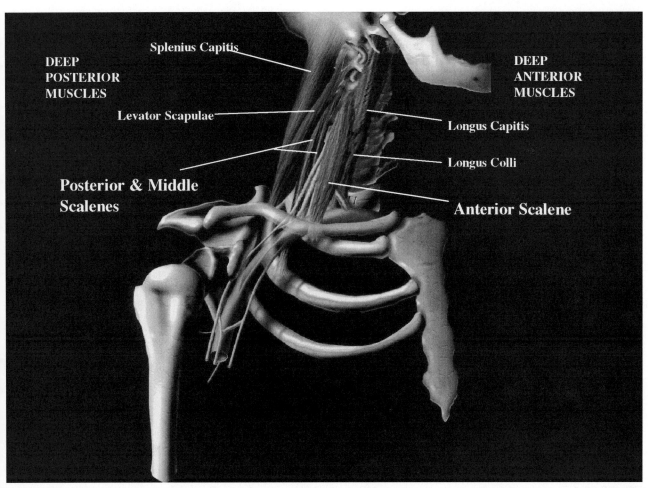

DEEP
POSTERIOR
MUSCLES

Splenius Capitis

DEEP
ANTERIOR
MUSCLES

Levator Scapulae

Longus Capitis

Longus Colli

Posterior & Middle
Scalenes

Anterior Scalene

FIGURE 73-3. The brachial plexus above the clavicle is "sandwiched" between the anterior and middle scalene muscles and is enclosed in their respective fascial envelope.

reduction in pulmonary function occurs routinely following this technique,[9] which limits its usefulness in patients who cannot tolerate unilateral, impaired diaphragmatic function. For prolonged postoperative analgesia, clonidine 150 µg or buprenorphine 300 µg may be added to the local anesthetic solution, or continuous catheter techniques may be used.[10–12] First described by Winnie in 1970, extracath or intracath continuous techniques may be used, with the former having greater inherent safety. As with single-injection techniques, side effects like hemidiaphragmatic paresis, Horner's syndrome, and recurrent laryngeal nerve block are all possible using continuous catheter techniques, as are complications like hematoma, infection, nerve injury, hemopneumothorax, subcutaneous and mediastinal emphysema, and spinal subarachnoid and epidural block.[2] The incidence of side effects like Horner's syndrome, hoarseness, and subjective breathing difficulties related to the spread of local anesthetic to neural structures may be slightly higher following right-sided blocks than it is for left-sided interscalene brachial blocks, but the mechanism for this is unclear at present. The recurrent laryngeal nerve, on the right side, leaves the vagus nerve and loops around the subclavian artery several centimeters higher than the nerve on the left side, which is not given off until the carotid has joined the aorta lower in the chest[2] (Fig. 73-13).

This might explain the higher incidence of hoarseness on the right side versus the left. The cupola of the lung is normally higher on the right than on the left side, but the effect, if any, of this phenomenon on neural side effects is unknown. Serious complications such as death, cardiac arrest, and respiratory arrest are rare following interscalene and supraclavicular techniques. In a study from France the authors identified two complications that occurred after 5,358 total interscalene (ISB) or supraclavicular (SCB) brachial blocks.[13] There was 1 neurologic injury out of 3,459 ISBs and 1 seizure out of 1,899 SCBs for an overall incidence of 3.7 complications per 10,000 blocks. The single-injection technique can be used to minimize these complications associated with multiple injection techniques (stated to be 1.7%).[14] The syndrome of sudden hypotension and bradycardia (vasovagal syncope) during shoulder surgery with the patients in the beach-chair position is of continuing concern, and has been attributed to activation of the Bezold–Jarisch reflex, although this remains controversial.[15] The incidence of this complication has been reported to range from 13% to 24% of awake patients in the sitting position who are undergoing shoulder arthroscopy with interscalene brachial plexus anesthesia.[16,17]

For most cases the local anesthetic chosen for single-injection brachial block is levobupivacaine (the S (–) enantiomer of

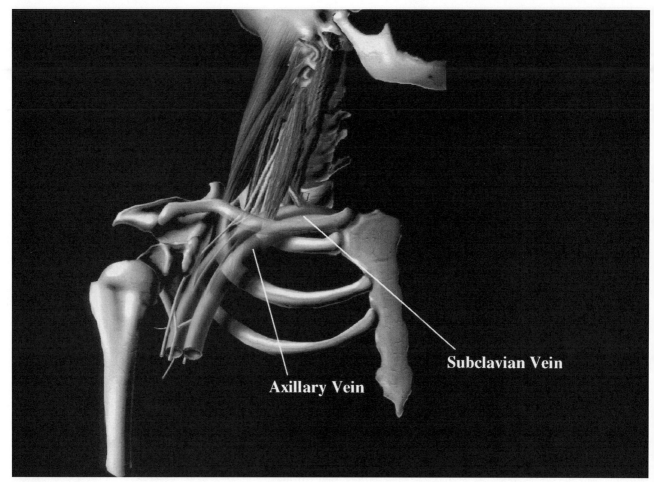

FIGURE 73-4. The subclavian vein and artery separated by the anterior scalene muscle. The artery, then, is within the confines of the perivascular space; the vein is not.

bupivacaine) 0.625% with epinephrine 1:200,000 to 1:300,000 (5 μg/mL or 3.75 μg/mL),[18,19] although some patients prefer to avoid the 18 to 30 hours of postblock paresis routinely seen with this agent. In these cases one can use 1.5% mepivacaine with epinephrine, but buprenorphine 0.3 mg/40 mL is usually added for prolonging postoperative analgesia.[20,21] Ropivacaine, an aminoamide local anesthetic that is highly protein bound and lipid soluble, may be an alternative anesthetic in institutions without access to levobupivacaine, as it is purported to have less propensity for cardiotoxicity than racemic bupivacaine while having a similar anesthetic profile (in equipotent concentrations) for brachial plexus anesthesia.[22]

Subclavian (Supraclavicular) Techniques: Kulenkampff described the first percutaneous supraclavicular block in 1911, a single-injection technique using an approach above the clavicle in the scalene triangle.[2] Labat, in 1922, advocated multiple injections (three) while avoiding the paresthesia technique of Kulenkampff.[2] Over the ensuing years it was noted that approaches near the clavicle were associated with an incidence of pneumothorax as high as 6%.[23] Anatomically, the traditional approach, whereby the needle is inserted 1 cm above the midpoint of the clavicle, is flawed since this point frequently does not lie over the first rib (as suggested) thereby negating the protection afforded to the cupola of the lung by

the rib. The anatomy of the scalene muscles, and the orientation of the three trunks of the brachial plexus vertically (stacked, one above the other) in the scalene space, lend themselves ideally to approaches whereby the needle is advanced dorsally tangential to the subclavian artery (i.e., directly caudad). Since the direction of the needle insertion is parallel to the borders of the scalene muscles and since these muscles always insert on the first rib, the locations of the plexus, subclavian artery, and rib are located more precisely using this approach than with any of the other supraclavicular techniques. The author's approach is as described by Winnie,[2,24] and is as follows. The patient lies supine with the shoulder completely relaxed and the head turned slightly towards the opposite side, as noted for interscalene block discussed above. The interscalene groove is palpated after the patient elevates the head off the bed to demonstrate the prominence of the clavicular head of the sternocleidomastoid muscle (Fig. 73-14). The palpating finger(s) now sit on the anterior belly of the anterior scalene muscle, and must be rolled laterally towards the middle scalene muscle until the finger(s) "slip into the groove" between the two muscles. The groove is traced inferiorly until the subclavian arterial pulse is felt, or until the omohyoid muscle (running obliquely and inferiorly across the groove) obscures further palpation (Figs. 73-15 and 73-16). At the approximate level of C6, a 22-gauge, 2-inch Stimuplex needle is advanced inferiorly

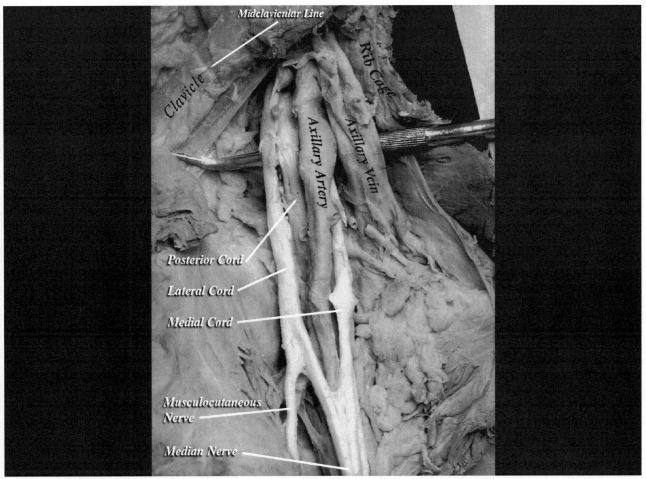

FIGURE 73-5. The three cords (lateral, posterior, medial) of the brachial plexus immediately beneath the clavicle, entwined around the axillary artery.

(caudad, but not mesiad or dorsad). The needle is now in the longest dimension of the interscalene space (parallel to the scalene muscles), while observing the arm for an appropriate motor response at 0.5 mA or less. Aspiration of bright red blood through the needle signifies that the needle is situated too far anteriorly (subclavian artery), and needs to be withdrawn and reinserted closer to the middle scalene muscle. An amount of 40 mL of local anesthetic is now injected in divided doses. Levobupivacaine, or mepivacaine, is used as detailed above. Since the plexus exists in its fewest component parts (three trunks) at this level, theoretically a lesser volume of local anesthetic should be necessary compared to the interscalene block (where five nerve roots are attempted to be blocked), although clinically most practitioners continue to inject at least 40 mL as above for interscalene block. The resultant anesthesia and analgesia will be in the distribution of the trunks (superior, middle, inferior). This block is appropriate for surgeries below the shoulder, specifically for procedures at the elbow or distally. Even though pneumothorax remains the most dreaded potential complication associated with this approach, Franco and Vieira, in a recent article, found *no clinically apparent* pneumothoraces in 1,001 consecutive supraclavicular blocks.[25] This supported earlier work performed at two other institutions where no pneumothoraces were encountered in a

combined total of 237 subclavian perivascular brachial blocks.[2] Anatomically, it would also appear that phrenic nerve block (with resultant hemidiaphragmatic paresis) is less likely with this approach than with interscalene block. Neal et al. demonstrated, in fact, that the incidence of phrenic nerve block following supraclavicular brachial block is about 50%.[26] For prolonged analgesia/anesthesia following supraclavicular block, clonidine or buprenorphine may be added to the local anesthetic, or, alternatively, continuous catheter techniques may be used.[10] Subclavian perivascular brachial block is ideal for continuous catheter insertion and maintenance, since the catheter may be sutured or secured flat against the neck and does not protrude from it at right angles, as it does with interscalene catheters. The author uses an extracath technique, and, since the plexus is compartmentalized at this level, has found that continuous catheter techniques require a smaller volume of local to be effective than do other approaches.[10] Other side effects and complications are similar to those listed above for interscalene block.

Alternative Techniques Above the Clavicle: Using the techniques of brachial plexus block discussed above (and simply modifying the volume, concentration, and type of local anesthetic), one is able to provide anesthesia for any surgical

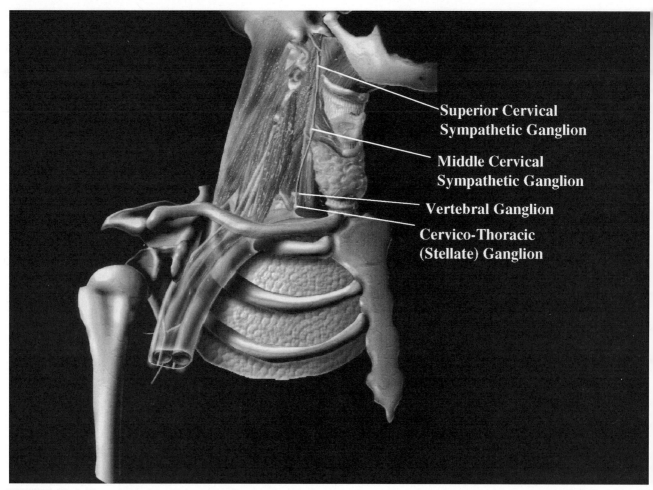

FIGURE 73-6. The relationship of the cervical sympathetic nerves to the roots and trunks of the brachial plexus on the right side of the neck.

procedure from carotid endarterectomy (cervical plexus block), to total shoulder arthroplasty, to arthroscopy and open shoulder work (interscalene block at C6), to surgical procedures on the humerus, elbow, or forearm/hand (subclavian perivascular block). Nevertheless, new techniques continue to be sought and developed in the quest to improve on success rates and minimize complications inherent to regional block anesthesia. The parascalene technique of Vongvises and Panijayanond[27] was the first of several of these modifications. They advocated an approach at a site similar to the subclavian perivascular block, but chose to advance the needle in a direction *vertically*, i.e., perpendicular to the long-axis of the body. The technique employs a similar patient positioning to that of subclavian perivascular block, including palpation of the sternocleidomastoid muscle to identify the anterior scalene muscle, and hence the groove between it and the middle scalene muscle. At a point 1.5 to 2 cm above the clavicle, a 22-gauge needle is advanced in an anteroposterior direction until a paresthesia is elicited. The local anesthetic is injected at this point after careful aspiration. The authors state that the first rib acts as a barrier if the plexus is missed by the advancing needle. If, after multiple unsuccessful attempts, no paresthesia can be elicited, the local anesthetic is simply injected along the lateral edge of the anterior scalene muscle above the first rib in a "fanlike manner." The authors reported a 97%

success rate, but needed a second injection to attain this high percentage.

In 1987 Dalens et al.[28] modified the parascalene technique for use in children. They determined from pediatric cadavers that the technique of Vongvises and Panijayanond resulted in injury to the cupola of the lung in greater than 50% of pediatric cases. A rolled towel is placed under the child's shoulders with the child in the supine position. The head is turned somewhat to the opposite side, and a line is drawn from the midpoint of the clavicle to Chassaignac's tubercle, which is located either by palpation or by dropping a line drawn laterally from the cricoid cartilage to the lateral border of the sternocleidomastoid muscle. This line is trisected and the needle is inserted at the junction of the lower and middle thirds of the line. A 22-gauge, short, insulated needle is advanced directly posterior, and using a nerve stimulator an appropriate motor response is sought. Dalens et al. reported a 98% success rate using this approach, with no major complications.

Brown, in 1993,[29] described his plumb-bob technique, which is another parascalene technique. This approach uses an injection site even lower than the two techniques mentioned above. Although the blocks of both Vongvises and Dalens are discussed in the Brown paper, those techniques are stated to require more complex measurements or equipment than the plumb-bob block. The patient is placed supine with the head

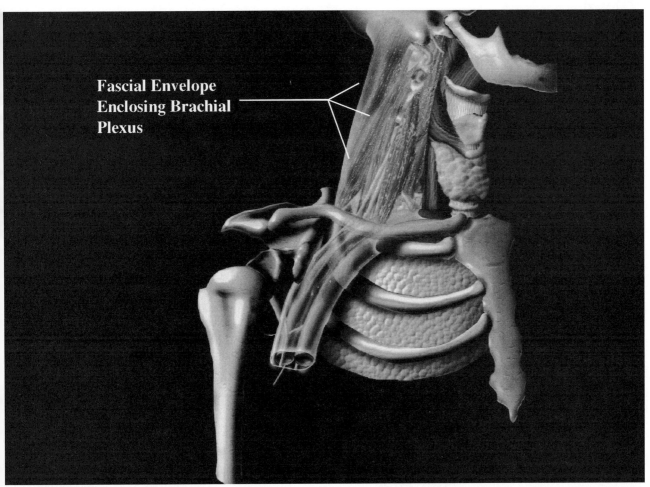

Fascial Envelope Enclosing Brachial Plexus

FIGURE 73-7. A continuous fascial compartment from the cervical prevertebral fascia to the distal axilla, enclosing and enveloping all the major elements of the brachial plexus. The "brachial plexus sheath" may be entered at any level (analogous to peridural anesthesia) and forms the foundation for single-injection techniques.

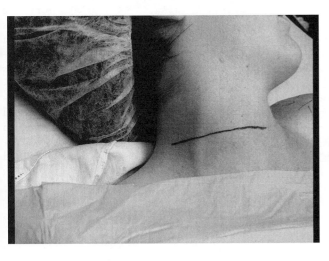

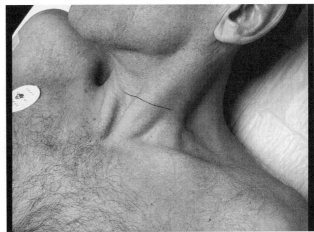

A   B

FIGURE 73-8. A, Anatomical landmarks for interscalene brachial plexus block on the right side of the neck including the external jugular vein, crossing the interscalene groove at about the level of the cricoid cartilage (C6). B, The head has been elevated from the gurney, tensing the sternocleidomastoid muscle. The lateral line at approximately C6 indicates the level of needle insertion for interscalene brachial plexus block (left-side view).

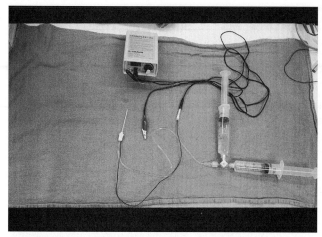

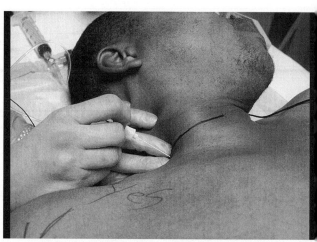

FIGURE 73-9. A peripheral nerve stimulator and insulated 22-gauge block needle. Notice the "immobile needle" (extension tubing) that serves to free the operator's hand and isolate the needle from the rest of the syringe system containing the local anesthetic.

FIGURE 73-10. Insertion of the insulated regional block needle for right-sided interscalene brachial plexus block. The direction of needle insertion is slightly mesiad, slightly dorsad, and slightly caudad.

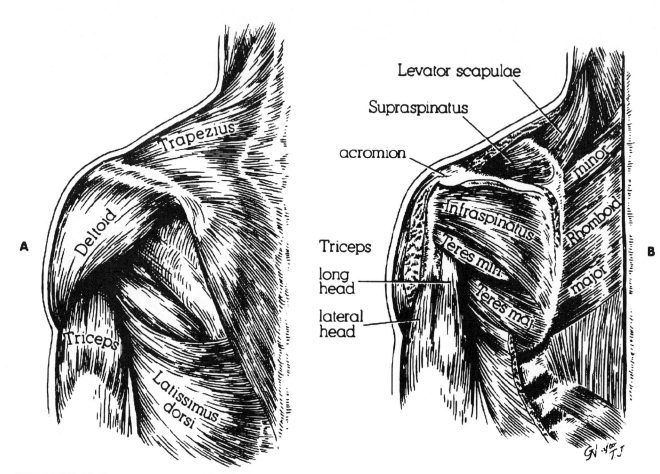

FIGURE 73-11. Posterior view of the left shoulder demonstrating the muscles beneath dermatomes C4–C7, particularly the posterior deltoid and the superior segment of the trapezius.

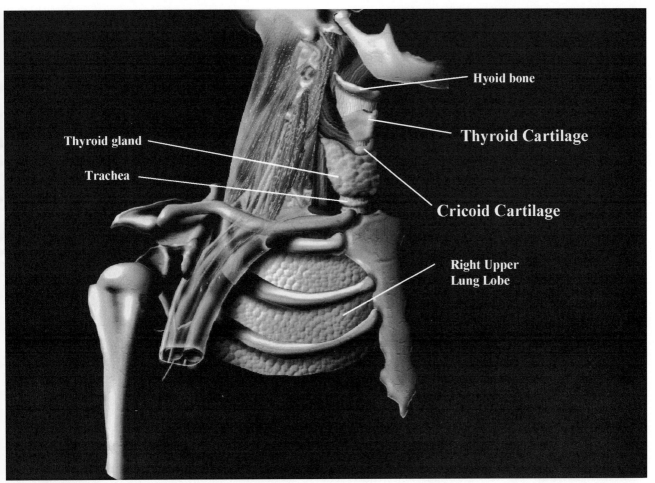

Hyoid bone

Thyroid gland

Trachea

Thyroid Cartilage

Cricoid Cartilage

**Right Upper
Lung Lobe**

FIGURE 73-12. Distinction between the cricoid cartilage (C6) landmark for interscalene block and the thyroid cartilage (C4) landmark for cervical plexus block.

turned to the opposite side. The point at which the lateral border of the sternocleidomastoid muscle joins the superior aspect of the clavicle is marked, and a 22-gauge, 5 to 6 cm blunt needle is inserted at this point (Fig. 73-17). The direction is directly posterior (perpendicular to the bed). The needle is advanced until a paresthesia is elicited, after which the local anesthetic is injected, or until the needle is angled about 30° cephalad. If the plexus is not contacted then the needle is redirected caudad in small steps until a paresthesia is obtained or until the 30° angle is reached. The success rate of this technique was not stated in the original report. Recently, a reevaluation of this technique using magnetic resonance imaging (MRI) scanning and needle direction simulation suggested that the direction of the needle in the original description of the technique would have resulted in *pleural contact in 60% of volunteers*, without prior contact with the subclavian artery or the brachial plexus, but always with subclavian vein contact.[30] Importantly, these investigators found that the plumb-bob trajectory very rarely contacted the brachial plexus, usually passing it by 12 mm. They recommended changing the needle direction to one aimed much more cephalad (45°) than originally described.

The intersternocleidomastoid approach[31] attempts to minimize the risk of pneumothorax by directing the needle anterior and superior to the dome of the lung towards the distal trunks. Subclavian arterial puncture may occur. Direct pressure over

the artery may be difficult because of its position behind the clavicle. The insertion site is at the medial border of the clavicular head of the sternocleidomastoid muscle, 3 cm above the sternal notch. The insulated needle is attached to a nerve stimulator and is directed caudally, dorsally, and laterally toward the midpoint of the clavicle, passing posterior to the clavicular head of the muscle and forming a 45° angle with the plane of the operating room table. The goal is to pass the needle deep to the clavicular head of the sternocleidomastoid muscle, pass through the posterior and caudal portion of the anterior scalene muscle, and to approximate the plexus just superior to the first rib. Usually, a 90 mm (3.5 inch) needle is employed versus the 50 mm (2 inch) needle used in the interscalene and subclavian perivascular techniques. The needle is advanced until an appropriate motor response is obtained. The possibility of permanently injuring or impaling the phrenic nerve as it crosses the anterior scalene muscle may occur with this technique.[31]

COMPLICATIONS

Complications of brachial plexus techniques above the clavicle have been discussed. Perioperative nerve injury remains a significant concern following brachial plexus block. In Auroy's retrospective analysis all neurologic complications of regional

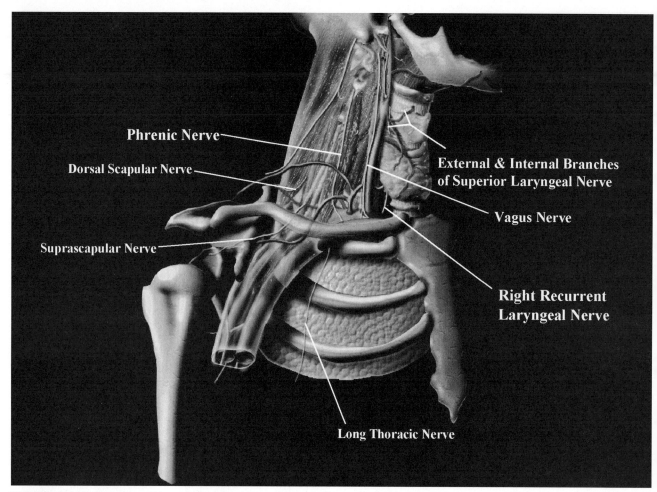

FIGURE 73-13. Relative position of the right recurrent laryngeal nerve and its relationship to the vagus nerve and to the roots and trunks of the brachial plexus.

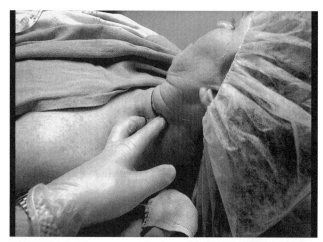

FIGURE 73-14. Initial patient position for left-sided subclavian perivascular brachial plexus block. As for interscalene block, the interscalene groove is the major cutaneous landmark, and is identified by indenting the skin lateral to the clavicular head of the sternocleidomastoid muscle. The fingers are then rolled laterally from the belly of the anterior scalene muscle into the groove between the anterior and middle scalene muscles.

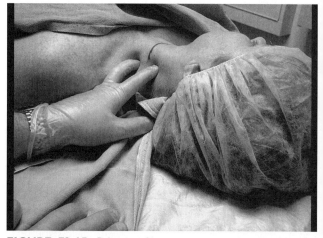

FIGURE 73-15. Palpating fingers appropriately seated in the interscalene groove on the left side.

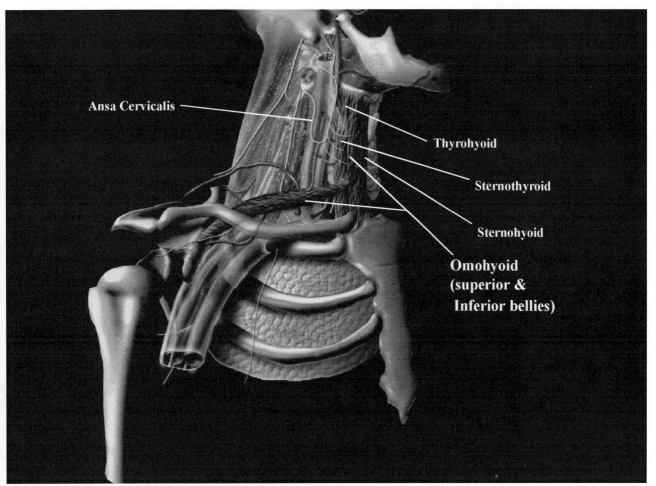

FIGURE 73-16. Demonstration of the obliquely situated omohyoid muscle, an impediment to tracing the interscalene groove inferiorly to the clavicle in some individuals.

anesthesia occurred within 48 hours of surgery, and 85% resolved within 3 months.[13] In Cheney's report 31% of brachial plexus injuries associated with regional anesthesia followed a paresthesia either during the needle insertion or during the injection of local anesthetic.[32] It has been suggested that perineural hematoma, intraneural edema, tissue reaction, or scar formation may be causative factors in neural injury. Importantly, positioning and surgical trespass, including the use of tourniquets or retractors intraoperatively and the application of casts postoperatively, may be etiological factors in many nerve dysfunction cases that are erroneously attributed to regional anesthesia. Certainly, injection of local anesthetic onto an elicited paresthesia should be undertaken very gently. The roles of epinephrine-induced neural ischemia, intrafascicular (intraneuronal) injections, and chemical injury due to local anesthetics themselves have been exhaustively reviewed.[33]

SUMMARY AND CONCLUSIONS

Consistent and reliable anesthesia of the entire upper extremity with either the interscalene or subclavian perivascular techniques of brachial plexus block can be performed with few complications. These techniques are easy to learn and subsequently teach to resident trainees in a busy clinical setting, and have a very high patient acceptance. Anatomically, these

techniques make sense since the needle is advanced towards and enters the very narrow interscalene space in its long axis. Alternatively, the parascalene techniques advocate placing the needle *across* the interscalene space in its *narrowest* dimension. The slightest movement of the needle, therefore, will result in the needle exiting this space, and hence the bulk of the volume of local anesthetic could theoretically be deposited outside the intended fascial compartment. Recall that the interscalene block is carried out at the level of the roots, while the subclavian perivascular block is carried out at the level of the nerve trunks. Therefore, assessing the dermatomal spread of the block is appropriate following an interscalene block, while anesthesia along the distribution of the superior, middle, or inferior trunks should be undertaken following a subclavian block. The C8 and T1 nerve roots are not infrequently missed following interscalene block, although increasing the volume of local anesthetic occasionally overcomes this problem, which is inconsequential if surgery is planned on the shoulder area.

From a safety standpoint, all the newer parascalene techniques were originally developed to minimize the incidence of pneumothorax (stated to be 0.5% to 6%). Interestingly, this high incidence was the one quoted prior to the introduction of the subclavian perivascular technique of brachial plexus block. There appears to be no report of pneumothorax after interscalene or subclavian perivascular brachial plexus block if the

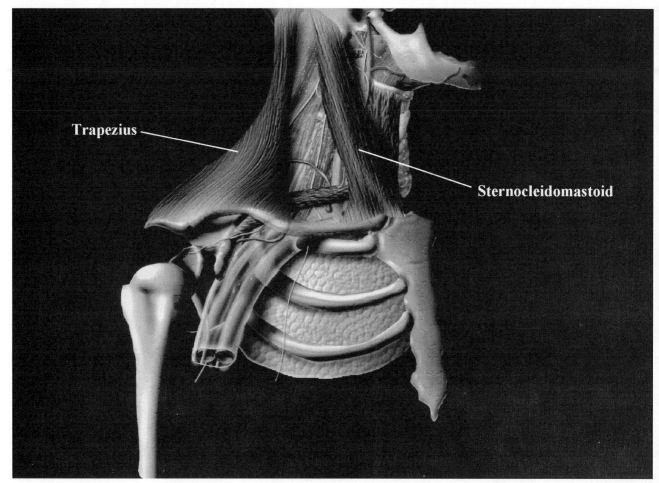

FIGURE 73-17. Major anatomical landmarks for the parascalene techniques of brachial plexus block, including the sternocleidomastoid muscle and midpoint of the clavicle, two important landmarks for the "plumb-bob" technique of Brown.[29]

technique, as originally described, is followed. As far as safety is concerned, the interscalene approaches have an unrivaled track record and we are yet to find an alternative technique that has proven to have a superior success rate with less likelihood of complications.

KEY POINTS

- The C4 nerve root contributes to about two-thirds of brachial plexuses and shifts the plexus cephalad (prefixed plexus). The T2 nerve root contributes to about one-third of plexuses and shifts the plexus caudad (postfixed plexus).
- The minimum distances from the skin to the C6 vertebral foramen and to the spinal cord are 23 mm and 35 mm, respectively, implying that inserting a needle for interscalene brachial block to a depth of less than 25 mm may result in nerve root contact.
- The incidence of neural side effects such as Horner's syndrome and hoarseness appears to be greater with right- as compared to left-sided interscalene brachial block.
- Continuous catheter techniques are better accomplished using the subclavian perivascular block technique than the interscalene technique since in the former approach the catheter may be sutured directly to the skin of the neck, minimizing the likelihood of dislodgement.

- The incidence of phrenic nerve block (and hence hemidiaphragmatic paralysis) occurs about one-half as frequently following supraclavicular block as it does following interscalene block.
- The needle trajectory in the original description of the "plumb-bob" technique of brachial plexus block was recently demonstrated by an MRI study to contact infrequently the brachial plexus elements.
- Needle insertion in the intersternocleidomastoid technique of brachial plexus block through the anterior scalene muscle places the phrenic nerve in jeopardy of being directly contacted.

ACKNOWLEDGMENT

The author thanks Dr. Naveen Nathan for his contribution to the medical illustrations appearing in this chapter.

REFERENCES

1. Winnie AP: Interscalene brachial plexus block. Anesth Analg 49:455–466, 1970.
2. Winnie AP: Plexus anesthesia. *In* Perivascular Techniques of Brachial Plexus Block, vol 1. WB Saunders, Philadelphia, 1983, p 49.

3. Sukhani R, Candido KD: Interscalene brachial plexus block: Shoulder paresthesia versus deltoid motor response – Revisiting the anatomy to settle the controversy. Anesth Analg 95:1818–1819, 2002.

4. Grossi P: The anesthetic line: A guide for new approaches to block the brachial plexus. Tech Reg Anesth Pain Manage 7:56–60, 2003.

5. Lombard T, Couper J: Bilateral spread of analgesia following interscalene brachial plexus block. Anesthesiology 58:472–473, 1983.

6. Choquet O, Jochum D, Estebe JP, et al: Motor response following paresthesia during interscalene block: Methodological problems may lead to inappropriate conclusions. Anesthesiology 98:587–588, 2003.

7. Candido KD, Sultana S, Sreekumar S: Regional versus general anesthesia for carotid endarterectomy surgery. Prog Anesthesiol XV:199–228, 2001.

8. Kerr AT: The brachial plexus of nerves in man, the variations in its formation and branches. Am J Anat 23:285–395, 1918.

9. Urmey W, Talts K, Sharrock N: One hundred percent incidence of hemidiaphragmatic paresis associated with interscalene brachial plexus anesthesia diagnosed by ultrasonography. Anesth Analg 72:498–503, 1991.

10. Winnie AP, Candido KD, Torres M: Continuous peripheral nerve blocks for the management of trauma to the extremities. *In* Grande CM, Rosenberg AD, Bernstein RL (eds): Perioperative Pain Management and Regional Anesthesia for the Trauma Patient. WB Saunders, New York, 1999, pp 209–238.

11. Borgeat A, Tewes E, Biasca N, Gerber C: Patient-controlled interscalene analgesia with ropivacaine after major shoulder surgery: PCIA vs PCA. Br J Anaesth 81:603–605, 1998.

12. Haasio J, Rosenberg P: Continuous supraclavicular brachial plexus anesthesia. Tech Reg Anesth Pain Manage 1:157–162, 1997.

13. Auroy Y, Benhamou D, Bargues L, et al: Major complications of regional anesthesia in France. Anesthesiology 97:1274–1280, 2002.

14. Fanelli G, Casati A, Garancini P, et al: Nerve stimulator and multiple injection technique for upper and lower limb blockade: Failure rate, patient acceptance, and neurologic complications. Anesth Analg 88:847–852, 1999.

15. D'Alessio J, Weller R, Rosenblum M: Activation of the Bezold–Jarisch reflex in the sitting position for shoulder arthroscopy using interscalene block. Anesth Analg 80:1158–1162, 1995.

16. Kahn R, Hargett M: Beta-adrenergic blockers and vasovagal episodes during shoulder surgery in the sitting position under interscalene block. Anesth Analg 88:378–381, 1999.

17. Ligouri G, Kahn R, Gordon J, et al: The use of metoprolol and glycopyrrolate to prevent hypotension/bradycardic events during shoulder arthroscopy in the sitting position under interscalene block. Anesth Analg 87:1320–1325, 1998.

18. Foster RH, Markham A. Levobupivacaine: A review of its pharmacology and use as a local anesthetic. Drugs 59:551–579, 2000.

19. Casati A, Borghi B, Fanelli G, et al: Interscalene brachial plexus anesthesia and analgesia for open shoulder surgery: A randomized, double-blinded comparison between levobupivacaine and ropivacaine. Anesth Analg 96:253–259, 2003.

20. Candido KD, Franco C, Khan M, et al: Brachial plexus block with buprenorphine for postoperative pain relief. Reg Anesth Pain Med 26:352–356, 2001.

21. Candido KD, Winnie AP, Ghaleb A, et al: Buprenorphine added to the local anesthetic for axillary brachial plexus block prolongs postoperative analgesia. Reg Anesth Pain Med 27:162–167, 2002.

22. Hickey R, Candido KD, Ramamurthy S, et al: Brachial plexus block with a new local anesthetic: 0.5% ropivacaine. Can J Anaesth 37:732–738, 1990.

23. Moore DC: *In* Complications of Regional Anesthesia. Clinical Anesthesia: Regional Anesthesia. FA Davis, Philadelphia, 1969, Chapter 12, p 233.

24. Winnie AP, Collins VJ: The subclavian perivascular technic of brachial plexus anesthesia. Anesthesiology 25:353–363, 1964.

25. Franco C, Vieira Z: 1,001 subclavian perivascular brachial plexus blocks: Success with a nerve stimulator. Reg Anesth Pain Med 25:41–46, 2000.

26. Neal J, Kopacz D, Liu S, et al: Quantitative analysis of respiratory, motor and sensory function after supraclavicular block. Anesth Analg 86:1239–1244, 1998.

27. Vongvises P, Panijayanond T: A parascalene technique of brachial plexus anesthesia. Anesth Analg 58:267–273, 1979.

28. Dalens B, Vanneuville G, Tanguy A: A new parascalene approach to the brachial plexus in children: Comparison with the supraclavicular approach. Anesth Analg 66:1264–1271, 1987.

29. Brown DL, Cahill DR, Bridenbaugh LD: Supraclavicular nerve block: Anatomic analysis of a method to prevent pneumothorax. Anesth Analg 76:530–534, 1993.

30. Klaastad Ø, VadeBoncouer T, Tillung T, Smedby Ö: An evaluation of the supraclavicular plumb-bob technique for brachial plexus block by magnetic resonance imaging. Anesth Analg 96:862–867, 2003.

31. Pham-Dang C, Gunst JP, Gouin F, et al: A novel supraclavicular approach to brachial plexus block. Anesth Analg 85:111–116, 1997.

32. Cheney F, Domino K, Caplan R, Posner K: Nerve injury associated with anesthesia. Anesthesiology 90:1062–1069, 1999.

33. Neal J, Hebl J, Gerancher J, Hogan Q: Brachial plexus anesthesia: Essentials of our current understanding. Reg Anesth Pain Med 27:402–428, 2002.

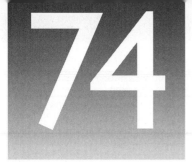

Brachial Plexus Blocks: Techniques Below the Clavicle

**Kenneth D. Candido, M.D., and
Edward Yaghmour, M.D.**

ANATOMICAL CONSIDERATIONS

Brachial plexus blocks below the clavicle involve blockade of the cords or peripheral nerves and include the techniques of axillary block and infraclavicular block. There are no currently described techniques of brachial block wherein the divisions of the plexus are intentionally or primarily blocked, principally because of their relatively isolated anatomical location beneath the clavicle and above the first rib (Fig. 74-1). As the plexus emerges from beneath the clavicle the fibers from the divisions recombine to form the three cords of the plexus (Fig. 74-2). The lateral cord is formed by the union of the anterior divisions of the superior and middle trunks; the medial cord is merely the continuation of the anterior division of the inferior trunk; and the posterior cord is composed of the posterior division of all three trunks. Thus, because of their derivation, the medial and lateral cords give rise to nerves that supply the flexor (volar or anterior) surface of the upper extremity whereas nerves arising from the posterior cord supply the extensor (dorsal) surface of the arm.[1] Next, each of the three cords of the plexus gives rise to a branch that becomes one of the major nerves to the upper extremity, and then terminates as another major terminal nerve. The lateral and medial cords are the origins of the lateral and medial heads of the median nerve (C5–C8) (major terminal branch). The lateral cord continues on as the musculocutaneous nerve (C5–C7) (major terminal branch), whereas the medial cord continues on as the ulnar nerve (C7–T1) (major terminal branch). The posterior cord gives off the axillary nerve as its branch (C5–C6) (major terminal branch) and then continues on as the radial nerve (C5–T1) (major terminal branch).

The musculocutaneous nerve (C5–C7) is the major terminal branch of the lateral cord (Fig. 74-3). After the lateral cord gives off its contribution to the median nerve, the musculocutaneous nerve leaves the plexus and dives into the substance of the coracobrachialis muscle. Then, it courses down the arm between the biceps and brachialis muscles, sending motor fibers to the powerful flexors of the forearm (Table 74-1). It terminates as the lateral antebrachial cutaneous nerve. Injury to the musculocutaneous nerve typically results in paralysis of the coracobrachialis, biceps, and brachialis muscles with resultant inability to flex the forearm. The musculocutaneous nerve has particular significance in axillary techniques of brachial plexus block that employ a peripheral nerve stimulator, where stimulation of this nerve and resultant flexion of the arm at the elbow often confuse the novice trainee into believing they are safely situated within the confines of the axillary perivascular sheath of the brachial plexus. In reality, the stimulating needle is in the coracobrachialis muscle, and injection of local anesthetic using this response as an endpoint inevitably results in a partial, or failed, block. The nerve must be routinely blocked separately by an injection into the substance of the coracobrachialis muscle since the usual takeoff of the nerve is proximal enough that its fibers are not bathed by local anesthetic solutions administered at more distal levels in the perivascular sheath.

The median nerve consists of motor fibers originating primarily from C6–C8, with occasional contributions from C5 and T1 (Fig. 74-3). Sensory fibers originate from C6–C8.[1] The lateral cord contributes to the lateral head of the median nerve, which joins the medial head contributed by the medial cord. Thus this nerve may be considered as a branch of both the cords derived from the anterior divisions. The two contributing divisions of the nerve, at their most cephalad point of origin, straddle the third part of the axillary artery before uniting on its ventral surface. The nerve then continues its course along the brachial artery into the forearm, where it ultimately divides into muscular and cutaneous branches in the hand.

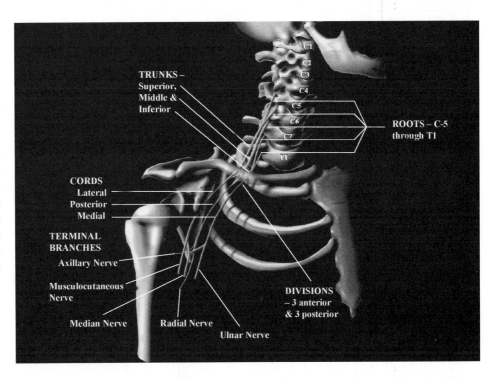

FIGURE 74-1. Relationship of the various elements of the brachial plexus to the bony skeleton. From roots, trunks, divisions, and cords to terminal nerves. Note the relatively isolated location of the divisions of the brachial plexus beneath the clavicle and above the first rib. No currently described techniques of brachial plexus block are performed at the level of the divisions.

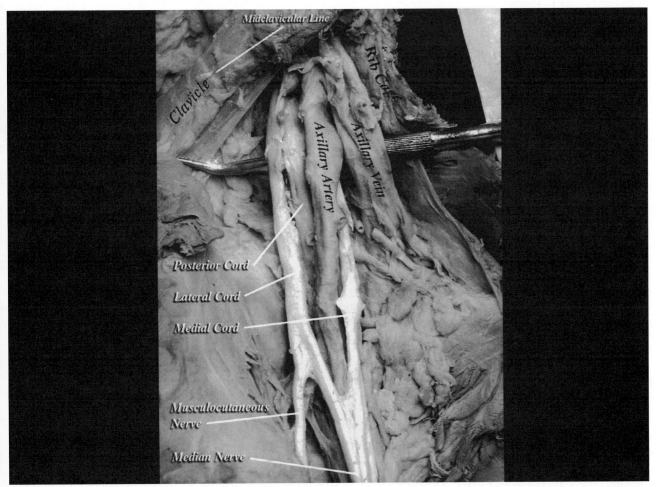

FIGURE 74-2. Anatomical dissection of the right side of the infraclavicular region demonstrating the derivation of the three cords of the brachial plexus.

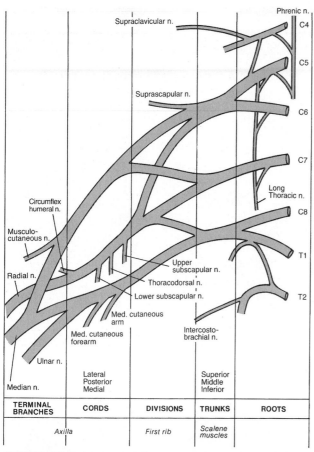

FIGURE 74-3. Anatomy of the brachial plexus. (From Hughes JJ, Desgrand DA: Upper limb blocks. *In* Wildsmith JAW, Armitage EN (eds): Principles and Practice of Regional Anesthesia, ed 2. Churchill Livingstone, Edinburgh, 1993, p 169.)

The median nerve provides motor branches to most of the flexor and pronator muscles of the forearm (Table 74-1). It also supplies all the superficial volar muscles except the flexor carpi ulnaris, and all of the deep volar muscles except the ulnar half of the flexor digitorum profundus. The motor branches in the hand supply the first two lumbricales and the thenar muscles that lie superficial to the tendon of the flexor pollicis longus. Sensory branches supply the skin of the palmar aspect of the thumb, the lateral two and a half fingers and the distal end of the dorsal aspect of the same fingers. Occasionally, the median nerve may encroach upon the sensory area normally innervated by the ulnar nerve, or that innervated by the radial nerve. Injury to the median nerve results in the so-called "ape hand deformity."

The medial brachial cutaneous nerve is derived from C8–T1. It is the second collateral derivation of the medial cord. It supplies the medial portion of the upper arm as far distally as the medial epicondyle. High in the axilla, part of this nerve forms a loop with the intercostobrachial nerve, with which it shares a reciprocal size and innervation area relationship. The medial antebrachial cutaneous nerve is also derived from C8–T1. It is another branch from the medial cord and arises just medial to the axillary artery. It passes down through the arm medial to the brachial artery to supply the skin over the entire medial aspect of the forearm to the wrist. A segment

of this nerve may also innervate the skin over the biceps muscle to the elbow.

The ulnar nerve is the major terminal branch of the medial cord (Fig. 74-3). It arises from the medial cord after the medial head of the median nerve has branched off the cord at the lower border of the pectoralis minor muscle. It descends the arm medial to the artery, running parallel to and between the median and medial antebrachial cutaneous nerves. It passes distally through a groove on the medial head of the triceps and passes behind the medial epicondyle. It then passes down the medial aspect of the lower forearm into the hand. Motor branches in the forearm supply the flexor carpi ulnaris and the ulnar head of the flexor digitorum profundus (Table 74-1). In the hand motor branches supply all of the small muscles deep and medial to the long flexor tendon of the thumb except the first two lumbricales. There are no sensory branches in the forearm, but in the hand the skin of the fourth and fifth fingers and the medial half of the hand are usually supplied by the ulnar nerve. Ulnar nerve injury typically results in the deformity known as "clawhand."

The posterior cord gives off one major terminal branch, the axillary nerve, before continuing on as the radial nerve. The axillary nerve (C5–C6) leaves the plexus high in the axilla in the quadrilateral space bounded by the surgical head of the humerus, the teres major and minor muscles, and the long head of the triceps. Its sensory fibers supply the skin overlying the lower two-thirds of the posterior deltoid, and its motor fibers supply the teres major and minor (Table 74-1). An articular branch supplies the shoulder joint in most cases. Injury to the axillary nerve results in an inability to abduct the arm. The radial nerve is the largest branch of the entire plexus and is the terminal continuation of the posterior cord. It accompanies the profunda artery behind and around the humerus in the musculospiral groove. Motor branches supply the triceps (the powerful extensor of the forearm), the anconeus, and the upper portion of the extensor–supinator group of muscles. The major sensory branches include the dorsal antebrachial cutaneous nerve that innervates the posterior aspect of the forearm as far as the wrist, as well as the posterolateral aspect of the upper arm. Branches to the hand innervate the dorsal aspect of the lateral hand, including the first two and a half fingers as far as the distal interphalangeal joint. Injury of the radial nerve results in "wrist drop."

As axillary and infraclavicular blocks of the brachial plexus block the sympathetic nerves to the arm and hand, recall that a dual system of innervation exists for the upper arm. Postganglionic sympathetic fibers are distributed distally via the somatic nerves of the plexus to the peripheral vessels. About 23% of fibers in a peripheral nerve are sympathetic postganglionic axons, where they are bundled together by Schwann cells.[2] Efferent sympathetic fibers supplying a cutaneous region do not necessarily arrive via the same pathway as the sensory afferents supplying that same area. The proximal sympathetics arise directly from the cervical sympathetic chain, particularly from the middle and inferior cervical sympathetic ganglia. The postganglionic sympathetic fibers pass directly to the subclavian artery and are conveyed in a plexiform manner along the outer coat of the vessel and subsequently into the axillary artery. Whereas the proximal innervation is the mechanism of sympathetic supply to the proximal third of the arm, distal innervation through the sympathetic fibers traveling with the somatic nerves of the brachial plexus

TABLE 74-1. **MOTOR INNERVATION OF THE UPPER EXTREMITY**

Nerve	Muscle Group(s)	Function/Action
Axillary nerve (C5–C6)	Deltoid	Abducts arm; flexes and medially rotates arm (anterior fibers); extends and laterally rotates arm (posterior fibers)
	Teres minor	Rotates arm laterally, adduction
Musculocutaneous nerve (C5–C6)	Coracobrachialis	Flexes, adducts arm
	Biceps (long head)	Flexes arm and forearm
	Biceps (short head)	Supinates hand
	Brachialis	Flexes forearm
Radial nerve (C5–C8)	Triceps (long head)	Extends, adducts arm
	Triceps (lateral head)	Extends forearm
	Triceps (medial head)	Extends forearm
	Brachioradialis	Flexes forearm
	Extensor carpi radialis	Extends, abducts hand
	Extensor digiti	Extends fingers
	Extensor carpi ulnaris	Extends, adducts hand
	Supinator	Supinates forearm
	Abductor pollicis longus	Abducts, extends thumb
Median nerve (C6–T1)	Pronator teres	Pronates, flexes forearm
	Flexor carpi radialis	Flexes, abducts hand
	Palmaris longus	Flexes hand at wrist
	Flexor digitorum superficialis	Flexes hand, first, second phalanges
	Flexor policis longus	Flexes hand, phalanges
	Pronator quadratus	Pronates forearm
Ulnar nerve (C8–T1)	Flexor carpi ulnaris	Flexes, adducts hand
	Flexor digitorum profundus	Flexes phalanges, hand at wrist
	Intrinsic hand muscles	Flex, extend, abduct, adduct phalanges

Adapted from Neal J, Hebl J, Gerancher J, Hogan Q: Brachial plexus anesthesia: Essentials of our current understanding. Reg Anesth Pain Med 27:402–428, 2002.

control the constrictor impulses to the resistance vessels in the extremity. Blockade of the brachial plexus, then, results in complete blockade of the vasoconstrictor fibers to the capacitance vessels (i.e., the veins), which allows blood to pool peripherally in the arm. A study showed that there is an increase in skin temperature of the hand by 1.5°C after axillary block, accompanied by an increase in skin blood flow of 73% as determined by laser Doppler flowmetry.[3] Thomas et al.[4] demonstrated that axillary block increased upper limb blood flow by 23% and increased transcutaneous PO_2 from 41 to 54 mmHg in room air. This suggested that the blood flow increase was not all through shunts. Sympathetic block, however, dramatically increased the transcutaneous PO_2 in hyperbaric oxygen, presumably by prevention of vasoconstriction during hyperoxia. A study using strain gauge plethysmography demonstrated that axillary block increased blood flow to the hand by 296% compared with 132% produced by stellate ganglion block.[5] Smaller flow changes were noted in the forearm and no changes were noted in the venous capacitance vessels.

The subclavian artery becomes the axillary artery beneath the clavicle at the lateral border of the first rib (Fig. 74-4). The axillary artery lies central to the three major peripheral nerves of the plexus (ulnar, median, and radial nerves). The cords are not truly medial, lateral, and posterior with respect to their positions around the artery until they pass behind the pectoralis minor muscle. Also, above the first rib, the subclavian vein lies outside of the neurovascular sheath; however, as it passes over the first rib and beneath the clavicle the subclavian vein joins the neurovascular bundle. This has significance for axillary and infraclavicular techniques of brachial plexus block since the vein forms the anterior wall of the compartment within the perivascular sheath, anterior to the ulnar nerve and anterior to the axillary artery. At the lateral edge of the pectoralis minor muscle, the cords give rise to the terminal nerves as described above. Importantly, two of the major terminal nerves, the musculocutaneous and the axillary, are excluded from the axillary perivascular space. These two nerves leave the sheath high in the axilla under the pectoralis minor muscle at

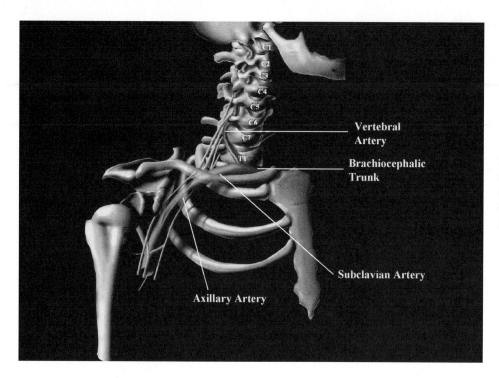

FIGURE 74-4. Evolution of the axillary artery from the subclavian artery. Note the relationship of the arteries to the clavicle and the lateral border of the first rib.

the level of the coracoid process and therefore must be blocked separately. The intercostobrachial and medial brachial cutaneous nerves likewise travel parallel to the axillary perivascular compartment, but are separated from it and must therefore be blocked separately if necessary. In summary, the contents of the axillary perivascular space are enclosed by three muscles (the biceps, triceps, and coracobrachialis), and by the shaft of the humerus. These structures surround and envelop two vessels (the axillary vein and artery) and three nerves (median,

radial, ulnar). The axillary sheath, a collection of connective tissue surrounding the neurovascular structures, is a continuation of the prevertebral fascia that separates the anterior and middle scalene muscles (Fig. 74-5). DeJong demonstrated that the axillary perivascular sheath of cadavers accommodated a volume of 42 mL to extend circumferentially to the three major nerves of the plexus as well as to spread proximally high enough to reach the musculocutaneous nerve.[6] This concept has implications for determining the appropriate volume of

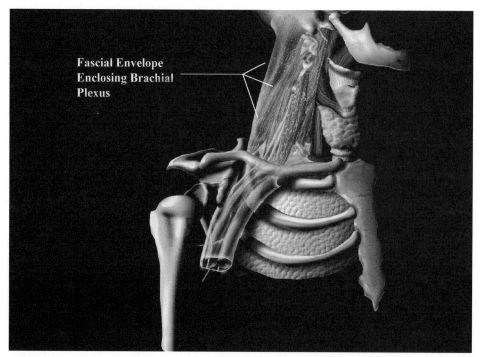

FIGURE 74-5. Derivation of the axillary perivascular sheath. The sheath is derived from the prevertebral fascia of the cervical vertebrae, and extends from the interscalene space to the level of the distal axilla. It may be entered at any level to provide brachial plexus anesthesia using single-injection techniques.

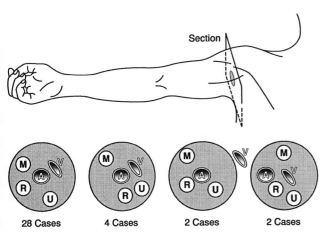

FIGURE 74-6. Variable anatomy of the axillary sheath seen in 36 axillary dissections in cadavers. Cross-sections taken at labeled site in proximal arm demonstrate the relative positions of the axillary artery (A) and vein (V), and the median (M), ulnar (N), and radial (R) nerves. (Modified from Partridge B, Katz J, Benirschke K: Functional anatomy of the brachial plexus: Implications for anesthesia. Anesthesiology 66:743, 1987.)

local anesthetic to inject for both axillary, as well as for infraclavicular blocks of the brachial plexus. Within the neurovascular space, the usual relationship of the structures has the axillary vein medial, the median nerve superior, the ulnar nerve anterior and inferior, and the radial nerve inferior and posterior to the axillary artery.

There are multiple variations in the distribution of the three nerves in the inferior segment of the axillary artery. Partridge et al.[7] were among the first to depict the "classic" orientation of the three major nerves surrounding the axillary artery in quadrants (median nerve superior; ulnar nerve inferomedial; radial nerve inferoposterior), and found that this arrangement was only apparent in about 78% of cadaver dissections (Fig. 74-6). If one conceptualizes the axilla to be divided into eight sectors with the axillary artery at its epicenter, the nerve distribution around it may be somewhat variable.[8] Typically, the median nerve occupies sector 1; the axillary vein occupies sector 2; the ulnar nerve is in sector 3; and the radial nerve is in sector 4. The remaining sectors are occupied, with significant overlap, by the muscles named above. As one progresses distally, from the level of the pectoralis major, through the biceps towards the elbow, the orientation of the major nerves dramatically changes, further emphasizing the utility of attempting the block at the most cephalad level to maintain the spatial relationships described above. Klaastad et al.[9] describe four quadrants surrounding the brachial artery. In their schema the median nerve occupies quadrant 2; the ulnar nerve occupies 3; the radial nerve occupies 4; and the musculocutaneous nerve occupies quadrant 1. Their description relies upon an insertion site 4 cm distal to the lateral border of the pectoralis major muscle, a site far removed (i.e., more distal) from that advocated by the present authors.

AXILLARY TECHNIQUE OF BRACHIAL PLEXUS BLOCK

The authors perform axillary brachial plexus block for surgery of the arm below the elbow, including the wrist and hand. We use the transarterial or nerve stimulator techniques as follows:

The patient lies supine with the arm abducted to approximately 90° and externally rotated to permit the dorsum of the hand to lie flat on the gurney while supported on one or two pillows. The forearm should be parallel to the long axis of the patient's body. Noninvasive monitors are applied, and baseline vital signs are recorded. An intravenous cannula is inserted, and modest doses of a rapid-acting, short-duration benzodiazepine (e.g., midazolam) may be administered for amnesia and sedation. It is important that the patient maintain verbal communication during the performance of the procedure to relay information such as the presence of paresthesias during needle insertion or the subjective sensation(s) of light-headedness or circumoral numbness if rapid systemic levels of local anesthetics are attained. Hyperabduction of the hand and arm is avoided since it tends to obliterate the axillary arterial pulse, a critical landmark in the successful performance of the technique. It has been shown that hyperabduction obliterated the pulse in 83% of individuals.[1] Hyperabduction causes stretching, torsion, and pinching of the subclavian–axillary vessels and the brachial plexus at three distinct locations: where the subclavian vessels and plexus trunks pass between the clavicle and first rib; at the point where the cords and vessels pass around the tendinous insertion of the pectoralis minor muscle to the coracoid process; and at the level where both vessels and plexus pass around the head of the hyperabducted humerus.[1] After the axillary arterial pulse has been identified, it is traced proximally as far beneath the pectoralis major muscle as possible, using the index finger of the left hand (for right-sided axillary block), or of the right hand (for left-sided axillary block). A Doppler probe may be used to appreciate adequately the pulse in those who are obese or who have poorly palpable peripheral pulses. Reducing the degree of abduction sometimes makes palpation of the pulse easier as one proceeds more proximally. It is important to attempt to trace the pulse as high proximally as possible, since injection of local anesthetic above the level of the head of the humerus tends to favor cephalad spread of the local anesthetic and tends to promote blockade of the nerves (i.e., musculocutaneous and axillary) that leave the plexus high in the axilla. While maintaining continual palpation of the pulse, the opposite hand guides a short-beveled 22-gauge, 1.5- to 2-inch needle towards the maximally appreciated pulse, superior and tangential to it. The needle should be directed along the long axis of the humerus, and should not be directed perpendicularly, since it will then be crossing the axillary perivascular space in its shortest dimension (i.e., will "bisect" it). The chances for successfully blocking all three major nerves at this level (median, ulnar, radial) are increased by guiding the needle into the perivascular space in the same orientation as the direction of the artery itself. The plexus may be approached until one of several endpoints is attained. Cockings et al.[10] noted that the transarterial technique was associated with the highest degree of success, but other authorities report lower success rates (60% to 90% successful block for each individual nerve).[11] In two retrospective studies the transarterial technique was associated with 88% and 94% success rates, respectively.[12,13] In this technique the axillary artery is transfixed between the index and middle fingers of the palpating hand, and the artery is intentionally entered using the short-beveled needle. Aspiration of bright red blood indicates that the anterior (medial) wall of the artery has been entered, and the needle should then be advanced through the posterior arterial wall. Digital pressure applied over the artery should then be released, and the artery is re-entered by withdrawing the needle to verify its placement. It is then passed once again through the posterior wall of the artery while maintaining continual aspiration. When continual aspiration ceases to reveal bright red blood, but only a "wisp" of blood, it is acceptable to incrementally inject the contents of the syringe into the perivascular space. Alternatively, half the contents of the syringe may be injected posteriorly, and the other half anterior to the artery after withdrawing the needle tip back towards the skin.

Multiple Injection Techniques in the Transarterial Approach: Some authorities suggest that the dual injection technique offers the highest degree of success of blocking all three nerves, without increasing the likelihood of complications. Hickey et al. found no overall difference in success rates between single and multiple transarterial injection techniques; however, there was a lower incidence of blockade and a longer latency of median nerve anesthesia in the group receiving a single injection of local anesthetic behind the artery.[14] Some have found lower overall success rates, however, when criteria are standardized to include blockade of three or four peripheral nerves of the forearm or hand. When compared to the so-called "fascial click" technique of identifying correct needle placement in the axillary perivascular space, the transarterial approach provided a similar (and low) rate of successful blockade of all four peripheral nerves of the forearm using a single injection.[15] In that study there was only a 48% successful blocking of all four nerves with the transarterial approach, vs. 59% with the single injection fascial click or paresthesia technique. Goldberg et al.[16] compared the two-injection transarterial technique to a single-injection paresthesia or single-injection nerve stimulator-guided technique. These techniques resulted in 79%, 80%, and 70% success rates, respectively. There was no statistically significant difference in the number of unblocked nerves between the three approaches. These results were subsequently confirmed by Pere et al.[17] who compared two-injection transarterial techniques to a single-injection nerve stimulator approach. There was greater spread of contrast media using the transarterial method, as well as better circumferential spread and greater distal and proximal spread within the sheath. However, the spread of contrast did not correlate with block success. In two studies by Koscielniak-Nielsen et al.[18,19] a two-injection transarterial technique was compared with four-nerve peripheral nerve stimulation technique. In both their studies the four-nerve method resulted in a higher success rate of complete surgical anesthesia of the forearm (88%, 94%) vs. the transarterial, two-injection method (62%, 64%). They also found a shorter latency of onset with the four-nerve stimulator technique but a shorter time to perform the block using the transarterial technique. Since the latency to onset was shorter with the four-nerve stimulating technique, the longer time to perform the block was deemed inconsequential.

Paresthesia Technique: The techniques of fascial click, field block with nerve and injection "fanning," and the paresthesia-seeking approach, while of historical interest, will not be discussed in detail. Paresthesia elicitation may be associated with neural injury, but there is some controversy regarding this issue. Axonal degeneration and a damaged blood–nerve barrier are inconsistent or absent after needle tip penetration without injection,[20] or even with the intrafascicular injection of saline.[21,22]

The elicitation of paresthesias during axillary plexus block is probably of minimal consequence as long as local anesthetic is not injected intrafascicularly, although the clinical data are contradictory.[22,23] Although the intentional elicitation of a paresthesia may represent direct needle trauma and theoretically may increase the risk of neurologic injury, there are no prospective, randomized clinical studies that are able to definitely support or refute these claims.[13,22–26] Selander and colleagues[24] performed one of the early prospective investigations examining the role of paresthesias and nerve injury. They reported a higher incidence of postoperative neurologic complications in patients where a paresthesia was intentionally sought during axillary blockade (2.8%) compared to those undergoing a perivascular technique (0.8%). While the difference was not found to be statistically significant, it bears mentioning that unintentional paresthesias were elicited and injected upon in patients within the perivascular group who experienced postoperative nerve injury. Overall, 40% of patients within the perivascular group reported unintentional paresthesias during performance of the procedure, demonstrating the difficulty standardizing the technique and analysis of nerve injury.

Use of Peripheral Nerve Stimulation: In our technique we seek an evoked motor response via peripheral nerve stimulation. The advantages cited with using a nerve stimulator include a high success rate, the ability to perform the block on sedated or uncooperative patients, the avoidance of paresthesias and the potential for neurologic injury, and the avoidance of arterial puncture and subsequent vascular insufficiency or hematoma formation.[16,27–30] It has been suggested that the use of the nerve stimulator avoids altogether the possibility of neuropathy from nerve trauma.[31,32] This may not be true, as demonstrated by Choyce et al.[33] They used noninsulated needles and intentionally sought paresthesias. Once obtained, they turned on a peripheral nerve stimulator to obtain an evoked motor response. In 25% of patients a current of >0.5 mA was required to manifest a motor response while 42% required currents of 0.75 to 3.3 mA. The site of the original paresthesia was concordant to the evoked motor response in 81% of patients. This implies that a nerve stimulator response may not exclude neural injury from the unintentional contact of the needle to the nerve. Their use of noninsulated needles, however, may be questioned since Ford et al.[34] demonstrated that the use of insulated needles resulted in more precise localization of the needle tip than does use of noninsulated ones. In one randomized, prospective analysis comparing the efficacy and safety of various techniques of axillary block including transarterial, single paresthesia, or nerve stimulator technique Goldberg et al.[16] failed to encounter a single case of postoperative neural injury between the three groups. The total number of patients was small (59), so the validity of the results needs to be interpreted cautiously. Fortunately, axillary block may not be associated with as high an incidence of neural injury as other approaches to the brachial plexus. Indeed, Fanelli et al.[35] reported a higher incidence of neural complications (4% vs. 1%) in the interscalene technique vs. the axillary approach when both techniques are performed using the nerve stimulator. In that report complete recovery of neurologic function occurred in all patients within 3 months (range 4 to 12 weeks).

In our technique the 22-gauge, insulated stimulating needle is connected by a sterile extension tubing set ("immobile needle") to a 20 or 30 mL syringe loaded with local anesthetic. Although it has been suggested that a properly placed needle will pulsate, this sign cannot be taken as definitive evidence that the needle is correctly seated. A nerve stimulator response is sought with a current of <0.4 mA in the distributions of the median, radial, or ulnar nerves. Riegler,[36] in a retrospective review, suggested that the predominant response elicited by the nerve stimulator during axillary block is finger motion (61% of cases) and wrist movement (flexion, extension, or deviation) (35% of cases). Stimulation of the median nerve, typically located at the superior border of the artery, results in an evoked motor response characterized by pronation of the arm, wrist flexion, finger adduction, flexion of the lateral two fingers, and thumb opposition. Stimulation of the radial nerve, typically located inferior and posterior to the artery, results in wrist extension, supination of the arm, metacarpophalangeal extension, and thumb abduction. In our experience stimulation of the ulnar nerve is rarely encountered using the nerve stimulator technique. The ulnar nerve is typically situated inferior and anterior to the artery, and its stimulation results in deviation of the wrist in an ulnar or medial direction, metacarpophalangeal flexion, and thumb adduction.

Local Anesthetics Used: Following aspiration in several quadrants, 40 to 50 mL of local anesthetic are injected incrementally with frequent intermittent aspiration tests being performed at least after every 3 mL. Speed of injection seems to be important, with rapid injection (15 mL in 10 seconds vs. over 20 to 30 seconds) resulting in reduced anesthetic spread and increased axillary block failure rates.[37] Other physical modalities attempting to speed block onset, such as warming the local anesthetic prior to performing axillary block, have not been shown to decrease latency of onset.[38] Our local anesthetic of choice is levobupivacaine 0.5% with epinephrine, 1:300,000. We found that this provides an acceptable latency of onset. We add buprenorphine 300 μg/40 mL, or alternatively clonidine 150 μg/40 mL, if we use shorter-acting agents and still desire prolonged postoperative analgesia.[39,40] Alternatives to levobupivacaine are racemic bupivacaine or ropivacaine. Plain bupivacaine 0.5% has been demonstrated to provide prolonged anesthesia and analgesia vs. plain ropivacaine 0.5% for axillary block.[41] Raeder et al.[42] showed that 0.5% bupivacaine is approximately equivalent to 0.75% ropivacaine for axillary block. We tend to avoid using mixtures of local anesthetics, agreeing with the opinion of Covino and Wildsmith[43] that these combinations provide few clinically significant advantages. Axillary block with bupivacaine 0.25% was shown by Martin et al.[44] to have a significantly longer duration of action than when it was combined with 1% lidocaine. The uncertainties and complexities of adding chemicals with distinct pKa values, lipid solubilities, and protein binding qualities to produce an intermediate-onset and intermediate-duration local anesthetic are intuitive. We make our injection as proximal as possible over the axillary arterial pulse, with our palpating fingers deeply situated beneath the pectoralis major muscle. A single-injection technique using this approach has resulted in a high degree of successful anesthesia of all the major peripheral nerve components of the brachial plexus.

Multiple Injection Techniques with Peripheral Nerve Stimulation: Some authorities continue to advocate for multiple injection techniques of axillary block. Inberg et al.[45]

stated that the success rate of single-injection techniques is much lower than two injection techniques. Gaertner et al.[46] concurred that a three-nerve injection technique of axillary block was more efficacious than single-injection techniques. Coventry et al.[47] showed a 97% rate of complete anesthesia of all peripheral nerves of the forearm and hand when a three-nerve electrical stimulation technique was used. They stimulated the musculocutaneous, median, and radial nerves. However, there was only a 53% block success rate when only the musculocutaneous and median nerves were electrically stimulated in the same study. Kosceilniak-Nielsen et al. similarly demonstrated improved success, reduced latency, and shortened time to readiness for surgery when comparing three-nerve stimulation vs. one-nerve stimulation axillary blocks, even though the three-nerve technique took longer to perform.[48] Other investigators suggest that it is the specific nerve(s) sought, and not particularly the number of nerves stimulated that influences latency and success. Lavoie et al.[49] found that four- or two-nerve stimulation techniques were equally successful, as long as one of the two nerves being sought in the latter technique was the musculocutanoues nerve. Sia et al.[50] noted that four- and three-nerve stimulation techniques (without searching for ulnar nerve stimulation) were virtually identical in overall success rates (92% vs. 90%). Additionally, since the four-nerve stimulation technique required significantly longer time to perform, their work suggests it is unnecessary to seek deliberately stimulation of the ulnar nerve. These same investigators[51] noted that their four-nerve axillary technique resulted in significantly shorter time to perform the block, as well as shorter latency to onset and time to readiness for surgery, than did a multiple paresthesia technique. Complete surgical anesthesia was also more likely (91%) with the nerve stimulator technique than for the multiple paresthesia technique (76%).

Determinants of Success: Axillary block success is volume dependent up to 40 to 60 mL; most authorities agree that low-volume block frequently fails to block one or more nerves. Vester-Andersen et al. demonstrated that musculocutaneous nerve block was improved following axillary block by increasing the volume of injectate from 20 mL to 40 mL (52% vs. 75%), as was block of the axillary nerve, but there was no additional improvement by increasing the volume (while maintaining the same total dose of local anesthetic) to 80 mL.[52] The same group, in a different study, found that increasing the volume and total dose of 1% mepivacaine from 40 mL (400 mg) to 50 mL (500 mg) to 60 mL (600 mg) had minimal effect on the incidence of sensory or motor block latency or success rates, and, further, that the incidence of musculocutaneous nerve block was similar in all three groups.[53] The same group noted a progressive increase in successful motor block using 40 mL volumes while increasing the concentration (hence, total dose) of local anesthetic (mepivacaine with epinephrine).[54] The results of these studies imply that drug mass (i.e., volume × concentration) is the most important determinant of block efficacy. The actual volume of injectate should depend upon the patient's size, sex, and age. An amount of 20 mL of local anesthetic is probably not a large enough volume to reach consistently the cords of the plexus in most adults, a level indicated by the coracoid process.[1] Some 40 mL more consistently spreads cephalad towards the level of the first rib.[1] Some advocate placing firm digital pressure directly behind the needle during and immediately following injection to minimize the likelihood of retrograde flow of local anesthetic distally in the axillary perivascular space, but this is of questionable efficacy. Controversy exists regarding the efficacy of using a distally placed tourniquet or applying digital pressure distal to the regional block needle. Whereas Eriksson advocated using a tourniquet, Winnie demonstrated that this was an ineffective means of minimizing distal spread of local and enhancing cephalad spread.[1] He suggested applying firm digital pressure immediately distal to the inserted block needle, and, further, showed via a series of X-rays of the axilla following dye instillation that this modality effectively prevented retrograde flow and promoted centrad flow.[1] Lang et al. verified that digital pressure, and not the use of a distally placed tourniquet, prevented distal spread of local anesthetic.[55] Yang et al.[56] suggested that this maneuver did not improve sensory block following axillary block. Successful blockade of the musculocutaneous nerve was not improved using digital pressure distal to the needle.[57]

With either the transarterial or nerve stimulator techniques, once the injection of the appropriate volume of local anesthetic has been accomplished, the needle is withdrawn until it lies in the subcutaneous tissue directly over the artery, and its orientation is changed so that it runs from the biceps to the triceps. At this point, 3 to 5 mL of local anesthetic are deposited. This is to block the intercostobrachial nerve and the medial brachial cutaneous nerve, if it lies outside the sheath. This supplemental block is suited for those individuals who require a tourniquet placed on the upper arm. The intercostobrachial nerve supplies cutaneous analgesia to the superior portion of the axilla, and often extends distally to the anterior border of the axilla and to the anterior shoulder. As soon as the subcutaneous injection has been made, the needle should be withdrawn while maintaining the digital pressure, and the arm is brought down alongside the body to reduce the obstruction imposed by the humeral head to central spread of the local anesthetic.[1] It was suggested that the arm should be brought down alongside the patient's body immediately upon completing injecting the volume of local anesthetic to enhance central flow by minimizing the barrier provided by the head of the abducted humerus.[1] Yamamoto et al.[58] showed that adduction of the arm to 0° increased centrad flow of local anesthetic after axillary block, but there was no effect on sensory block when using this maneuver. They did note, however, that there was improved motor block of the radial nerve using arm adduction. Once the block begins to "set-up" an inability to extend the forearm from the flexed position will be noted, representing motor blockade of the muscles subserved by the radial nerve.

Other approaches to block peripheral branches of the brachial plexus below the clavicle have been developed. The midhumeral approach of Bouaziz et al.[59] was recently compared to conventional axillary block (Fig. 74-7). The midhumeral approach had a higher success rate of blocking four nerves of the hand and forearm compared to the axillary approach (88% success vs. 54%). The conventional axillary block, however, was characterized by a shorter time to attain complete anesthesia, possibly due to ulnar nerve sparing using the midhumeral approach.

INFRACLAVICULAR TECHNIQUE OF BRACHIAL PLEXUS BLOCK

The indications for infraclavicular block of the brachial plexus are essentially the same as for axillary block, i.e., surgery of the forearm or hand. The major benefit of this approach, when compared to traditional blocks above the clavicle, is the unlikely risk of encroaching upon the pleural space or lung parenchyma and causing a pneumothorax, while maintaining the high success rate of blocking the axillary and musculocutaneous nerves prior to their departure from the sheath of the brachial plexus.[60,61] The ulnar segment of the medial cord is also blocked. The technique is ideally suited for continuous catheter insertion and maintenance, since the patient may move the head and arm without dislodging the catheter.[62] The major disadvantages with the technique are increased pain, since the pectoralis major and minor muscles are traversed by the needle, and the necessity of using a nerve stimulator. The recently described coracoid approach[63] uses ultrasonic needle guidance instead of peripheral nerve stimulation and may obviate these disadvantages. In its final position, the block needle should be situated at the level of the distal cords (i.e., in the middle of the brachial plexus) using Raj's technique (Fig. 74-8). Using the coracoid approach, studies have demonstrated a 75% to 85% blockade of the axillary nerve and an 80% to 100% blockade of the musculocutaneous nerve[64,65] (Fig. 74-9). Additionally, the incidence of phrenic nerve block and resultant hemidiaphragmatic paralysis has been stated to be minimal.[66]

In our technique, the patient lies supine with the head in a neutral position or turned slightly towards the contralateral (nonblocked) side. The arm may be adducted, abducted, or extended out away from the body, but it is typically abducted at 90° as for axillary block. This helps localize the axillary arterial pulse, a useful landmark for completing this block. The clavicle

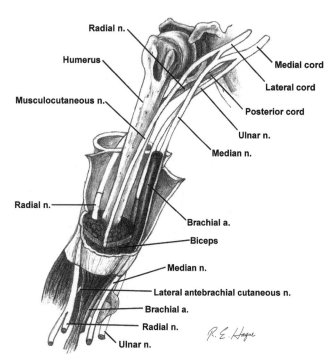

FIGURE 74-7. Anatomical separation of the peripheral nerves for blockade using the midhumeral approach. At this level, the major peripheral nerves of the upper extremity do not share a common fascial sheath as they do at more cephalad levels, and therefore they must each be blocked individually.

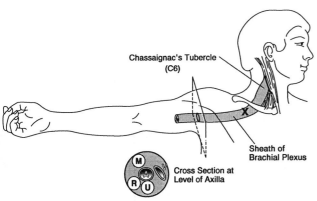

FIGURE 74-8. Landmarks and technique involved in the classic approach to infraclavicular brachial plexus blockade. The needle is inserted at X. The cross-section at the level of the axilla shows the orientation of the artery (A), vein (V), and medial (M), radial (R), and ulnar (U) nerves within the axillary sheath.

is measured and divided into thirds using a sterile marking pen. The lung typically lies beneath the medial one-third of the clavicle, hence the benefit of dividing that structure into thirds. The physician stands on the opposite side from the arm to be blocked. A line is drawn from the C6 tubercle to the brachial artery in the arm. After the skin is infiltrated, the intended needle tract is anesthetized. A 100 mm (4 inch) insulated stimulator needle is inserted on the chest wall 2 cm medial and 2 cm caudad from the most lateral aspect of the coracoid process (where the pectoralis major and minor muscles are thin), aiming for the axillary arterial pulse.[62] The plane of needle insertion lies laterally to the rib cage and lung, and intersects the plexus at the level of the distal cords rather than at the level of the nerve trunks or divisions. The needle is passed directly posteriorly through the substance of the pectoralis major muscle and is a potentially painful procedure. When the nerve stimulator is activated, there is direct motor

stimulation of this large muscle mass at a depth of about 1 to 3 cm. Advancing an additional 3 to 7 cm, the brachial plexus cords are usually encountered by the stimulating needle. Often the suprascapular, axillary, or musculocutaneous nerves are first encountered, since they exit the brachial plexus sheath at a site close to the coracoid process. Accepting their stimulation as an endpoint results in a higher failure rate than accepting an evoked motor response of the hand, which indicates a more central location of the needle tip.[64,65] If no neural elements are stimulated on the initial pass of the needle, the needle should be redirected progressively more caudad until hand movement is noted. Since the needle is advanced lateral to the ribcage, pneumothorax remains an unlikely consequence of caudad advancement.[63] Continued lateral redirection may result in blockade of only one or two nerves in a manner analogous to partial axillary block. We use the same volume, concentration, and local anesthetic(s) as described for axillary block. There have been recent attempts to "fine-tune" the technique of infraclavicular block, but it remains to be seen whether these modifications, particularly the vertically directed needle technique, gain widespread acceptability.[67,68]

INFRACLAVICULAR VS. AXILLARY BRACHIAL PLEXUS BLOCK

When the infraclavicular block is compared to axillary block for surgery of the arm and hand, approaches relying upon a single nerve-evoked motor response failed to demonstrate a difference in success, latency, or duration of blockade.[64] Further, at least two nerves were blocked in 100% of the infraclavicular blocks vs. in 85% of the axillary blocks. Musculocutaneous nerve block, as expected, was more successful following infraclavicular block, as compared to axillary block. In another study, however, the success rate of infraclavicular block was decidedly lower than it was for axillary block, with 57% of patients in the former group having anesthesia in the distributions of four nerves of the forearm and hand vs. 87% in the latter group.[65] Latency of onset was shorter in the axillary group, while times to perform the block, and duration of action, did not differ significantly. The authors used a two-nerve injection technique for the infraclavicular block, and a four-nerve technique for the axillary block.

CONTINUOUS TECHNIQUES

Prolonging the duration of perioperative anesthesia and postoperative analgesia is the function of continuous catheter techniques. Originally designed in response to the need to provide antinociception for patients with chronic pain or with vascular insufficiency,[69–71] their use has been expanded to include routine catheter placement and management in otherwise healthy outpatients.

Most reports of the use of continuous devices are simple observational analyses based upon the aggregate clinical experience of practitioners who employ these techniques.[72–4]

There are a wide variety of manufacturers currently developing and producing kits for this purpose. In addition to the stimulating insulated needle and various needle tip designs, as well as the catheter device itself, there are a variety of pumps that permit the administration of local anesthetic and/or adjuvants for prolonged periods of time. Detailed studies have looked at serum concentrations of local anesthetics to gauge

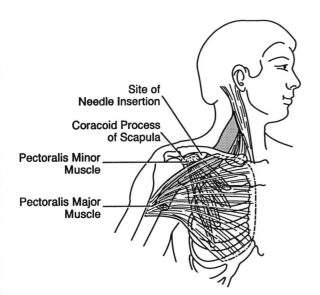

FIGURE 74-9. Landmarks and needle position involved in the modified technique of infraclavicular brachial plexus blockade.

the effect of alterations in delivery rates and local anesthetic concentrations on outcome and side effects. Other investigators have performed comparisons of local anesthetic infusions vs. saline controls to gauge the efficacy of relieving postoperative pain following upper extremity surgery. Salonen et al.[75] prospectively evaluated 60 elective hand surgery patients receiving continuous catheter axillary blocks with ropivacaine. Postoperatively, three continuous infusion study groups were evaluated, including two distinct ropivacaine concentrations (0.1% and 0.2%) and a normal saline control. They found no apparent advantage to the two ropivacaine concentrations vs. control as regards analgesia occurring after the initial 12 hours postoperatively. This demonstrates the need for additional studies on continuous catheter techniques for postoperative analgesia before advocating for their routine use.

COMPLICATIONS

Axillary block is the technique of brachial plexus block most likely to be associated with intravascular injection. This is because it is the only site where the major, large vein lies within the sheath.[1] However, the axillary vein lies anterior and slightly inferior to the artery (Fig. 74-2) and therefore is easily compressible beneath appropriately situated palpating fingers. Techniques advocating multiple injections or injections above and below the axillary artery enhance the likelihood of encountering the vein, and hence injecting into it. With the transarterial techniques the possibility is real that the volume of local anesthetic might be injected directly intra-arterially, but due to the fractionation of injectate volumes that typically occurs with this approach, this should rarely occur. Stan et al. reported[13] that the total incidence of vascular complications following axillary block is 1.4%, including 0.2% incidence of intravascular injection, even with test dosing and aspiration. Brown et al.[76] suggested that the incidence of local anesthetic-induced seizures is 1/10,000 axillary blocks, which is less than that reported for supraclavicular or interscalene blocks, and which approximates the incidence during epidural block. Carles et al.[77] stated that the incidence of seizure was 1.2/1,000 to 1.3/1,000 following axillary block vs. 7.6/1,000 after interscalene and 7.9/1,000 for supraclavicular block. The axillary data was similar regardless of technique chosen (transarterial, peripheral nerve stimulator, humeral). There is no evidence that the site of injection of local anesthetic (axillary vs. supraclavicular vs. interscalene) affects the actual blood level of local anesthetic,[78] although the peak blood level may occur more rapidly following injection with interscalene vs. axillary block.[79] Hematoma is certainly a possibility with axillary block, but, fortunately, the area of injection (unlike for subclavian perivascular plexus block) is readily compressible. Ben-David and Stahl[80] reported on a case of radial nerve dysfunction associated with a large axillary hematoma following axillary block and the transarterial technique. Neurologic function was impaired for up to 6 months following this procedure. Hematoma formation needs to be considered in any patient with neurologic impairment following axillary or infraclavicular brachial blocks. Pseudoaneurysm formation may also complicate axillary block,[81,82] and may occur in the artery as well as in the axillary vien.[83] The consequences of pseudoaneurysm formation include pressure-induced neural ischemia. In the case report of Groh et al.[81] the patient continued to experience severe median nerve dysfunction persisting 4 months postoperatively.

A case of axillary artery dissection and subsequent thrombotic obliteration following axillary block without arterial puncture has been reported.[84] Vascular insufficiency is not an infrequent accompaniment of the transarterial technique, and results in severe blanching of the skin of the hand and wrist. We have seen several cases where the patient's hand takes on a "cadaveric" appearance. Additionally, the peripheral pulses (radial and ulnar arterial) are distant or absent. Stan et al. noted that the incidence of transient arterial vasospasm may approach 1% in selected patient populations.[13] We have observed this phenomenon in at least 50% of individuals receiving transarterial axillary blocks as described above. Merrill et al. reported on a case of arterial vasospasm lasting 15 minutes after axillary block with 20 mL of 1% lidocaine and 0.05% tetracaine with epinephrine 1:200,000.[85] Fortunately, this phenomenon is reversible, in that we have not yet encountered a patient in whom this does not spontaneously reverse itself within about 15 minutes. This likely results from the intra-arterial injection of epinephrine-containing solutions, producing profound vasoconstriction of the axillary artery. The phenomenon reverses itself when the increase in blood flow from the sympathetic nervous system block produced by the axillary block results in effective dilution and washout of the locally injected epinephrine.

Pulmonary complications following axillary or infraclavicular block are virtually unheard of, yet must always be considered if the needle is directed away from the axilla and towards the chest wall, a decidedly unwise maneuver. Rodriguez et al. found that respiratory function is not affected by axillary or infraclavicular block.[66]

Neural injury following axillary block is gratefully a rare occurrence. Auroy's group performed a large, retrospective analysis of complications related to regional anesthesia in France.[86] In 11,024 axillary brachial blocks there were only 2 instances of neurologic injury noted, for an incidence of 1.9/10,000. All neurologic complications, in their review, occurred within 48 hours of surgery, and in 85% of cases the complications resolved within 3 months. They concluded that needle trauma and local anesthetic neurotoxicity were the etiologies of most neurologic complications. In that same study there was only one reported seizure, for an incidence of 0.9/10,000.[86]

The design of needles may have a bearing on nerve injury. It is clearly easier to enter a nerve fascicle with a sharply pointed needle,[24] but greater injury may be done when a blunt needle succeeds in penetrating the perineurium, even without injection.[87]

Paresthesia techniques and injecting upon elicited paresthesias may contribute to perioperative neural injury. Selander et al. found that unintentional paresthesias were elicited and injected upon in patients who ultimately experienced postoperative nerve injury.[23] Yet, even without eliciting notable paresthesias, 19% of patients receiving axillary blocks had paresthesias persisting into the first postoperative day.[25] These were not associated with the type of local anesthetic, number of needle advances, anesthetic technique (paresthesia vs. transarterial), or duration of tourniquet inflation. However, there was a significant increase in the incidence of acute paresthesias in patients who had preoperative neurologic symptoms within an extremity. At 2 weeks, only 5% of patients continued to experience new postoperative paresthesias. Symptoms consisted solely of numbness and tingling in the fingers as well as forearm hyperesthesia.

By 4 weeks, all patients except for 1 (0.4%) had resolution of their symptoms. Stan et al.[13] reported an incidence of 0.2% neurologic complications in almost 1,000 patients undergoing axillary block using the transarterial approach. If a paresthesia was elicited, the local anesthetic was not injected, and the needle was redirected. In the 12% of patients who did have a periprocedural paresthesia there were no instances of postoperative neurologic complications, leading them to speculate that those individuals who did develop this complication experienced unintentional/unobserved mechanical trauma or intraneuronal injection during block supplementation.

Ischemia may be a mechanism contributing to damage that follows intrafascicular injection of local anesthetics. Selander and Sjostrand[88] demonstrated that intrafascicular injections might lead to compressive nerve sheath pressures greater than 600 mmHg. This transient elevation in endoneural fluid pressure may exceed capillary perfusion pressure for up to 15 minutes, interfering with the nerve's endoneural microcirculation. Elevated pressures may also alter the permeability of the blood–nerve barrier within the endoneurium, possibly contributing to axonal degeneration, Schwann cell injury, and fibroblast proliferation.

In any case of suspected neural injury following axillary or infraclavicular block the following steps ("mini-neurologic examination") should be undertaken immediately: the median nerve may be tested by using a pinprick over the palmar surface of the distal phalanx of the index finger; the ulnar nerve may be tested in similar fashion by pinprick testing of the palmar surface of the distal phalanx of the fifth finger; the radial nerve may be tested by asking the patient to extend the distal phalanx of the thumb; the musculocutaneous nerve function can be assessed by asking the patient to flex the forearm; and the axillary nerve may be assessed by abduction of the arm.[1] It is important to obtain electromyographic studies as quickly as possible following a suspected nerve injury, for the purposes of establishing a time frame of when the injury might have occurred. Electrodiagnostic studies should be obtained as expeditiously as possible to rule out the likelihood of preexisting lesions playing an integral part in the etiology of these processes.

SUMMARY

Techniques of brachial plexus block below the clavicle offer many unique advantages vs. the supraclavicular approaches. They spare diaphragmatic function and are not associated with pneumothorax, recurrent laryngeal nerve block, Horner's syndrome, or shoulder weakness. Some studies suggest that the incidence of neuropathy following their implementation is less than that of the supraclavicular blocks. Infraclavicular techniques are ideally suited for continuous catheter insertion and maintenance, since patient movement does not easily dislodge the devices. Future developments will focus on improving our understanding of how to maximize success rates and improve blockade of all four of the major nerves of the forearm and hand.

KEY POINTS

- There are no currently described techniques of brachial plexus block that rely upon blockade at the level of the divisions of the plexus.
- It has been demonstrated that the capacity of the axillary perivascular sheath is 42 mL.

- Axillary and infraclavicular blocks of the brachial plexus are appropriate for surgeries of the upper extremity from the elbow to the fingers.
- The transarterial technique of axillary block has consistently been associated with the highest success rate of complete block.
- Paresthesias occur in up to 40% of cases of axillary perivascular block, even when not intentionally sought.
- Axillary block is volume dependent up to 40 to 60 mL; local anesthetic drug mass (volume × concentration) is the main determinant of efficacy of the block.
- The infraclavicular technique blocks the brachial plexus at the level of the cords.
- The infraclavicular technique is anatomically the most suitable of all brachial block techniques, including those performed above the clavicle, for the insertion and maintenance of continuous catheters.
- Of all the techniques of brachial block, axillary block is associated with the highest incidence of intravascular injection of local anesthetics.

ACKNOWLEDGMENT

The authors wish to thank Dr. Naveen Nathan for his outstanding contribution to the anatomical diagrams presented in this chapter. Additional artwork was provided by Robert Haque.

REFERENCES

1. Winnie AP: Plexus anesthesia. Perivascular Techniques of Brachial Plexus Block, vol 1. WB Saunders, Philadelphia, 1983.
2. Schmalbruch H: Fiber composition of the rate sciatic nerve. Anat Record 215:71–81, 1986.
3. Katz J: Skin blood flow after axillary brachial plexus block: The use of laser Doppler flowmetry. Reg Anesth 9:68–69, 1984.
4. Thomas PS, Hakim TS, Trang LQ, et al: The synergistic effect of sympathectomy and hyperbaric oxygen exposure on transcutaneous PO_2 in healthy volunteers. Anesth Analg 88:67–71, 1999.
5. Zenz M, Tryba M, Horch C: Sympathicusblockade nach plexus-anaesthesie. Reg Anaesth 9:84–87, 1986.
6. DeJong R: Axillary block of the brachial plexus. Anesthesiology 22:215–225, 1961.
7. Partridge B, Katz J, Benirschke K: Functional anatomy of the brachial plexus sheath: Implications for anesthesia. Anesthesiology 66:743–747, 1987.
8. Ritz G, Kapral S, Greher M, Mauritz W: Ultrasonographic findings of the axillary part of the brachial plexus. Anesth Analg 92:1271–1275, 2001.
9. Klaastad O, Smedby O, Thompson G, et al: Distribution of local anesthetics in axillary brachial plexus block: A clinical and magnetic resonance imaging study. Anesthesiology 96:1315–1324, 2002.
10. Cockings E, Moore P, Lewis R: Transarterial brachial plexus blockade using high doses of 1.5% mepivacaine. Reg Anesth 12:159–164, 1987.
11. Urmey W: Upper extremity blocks. *In* Brown D (ed): Regional Anesthesia and Analgesia. WB Saunders, Philadelphia, 1996, pp 254–278.
12. Aantaa R, Kirvela O, Lahdenpera A, Nieminen S: Transarterial brachial plexus anesthesia for hand surgery: A retrospective analysis of 346 cases. J Clin Anesth 6:189–192, 1994.
13. Stan T, Krantz M, Solomon D, et al: The incidence of neurovascular complications following axillary brachial plexus block using a transarterial approach. A prospective study of 1,000 consecutive patients. Reg Anesth 20:486–492, 1995.

14. Hickey R, Hoffman J, Tingle L, et al: Comparison of the clinical efficacy of three perivascular techniques for axillary brachial plexus block. Reg Anesth 18:355–358, 1993.

15. Youssef M, Desgrand D: Comparison of two methods of axillary brachial plexus anaesthesia. Br J Anaesth 60:841–844, 1988.

16. Goldberg M, Gregg C, Larijani G, et al: A comparison of three methods of axillary approach to brachial plexus blockade for upper extremity surgery. Anesthesiology 66:814–816, 1987.

17. Pere P, Pitkanen M, Tuominen M, et al: Clinical and radiological comparison of perivascular and transarterial techniques of axillary brachial plexus block. Br J Anaesth 70:276–279, 1993.

18. Koscielniak-Nielsen Z, Hesselbjerg L, Fejlberg V: Comparison of transarterial and multiple nerve stimulation techniques for an initial axillary block by 45 mL of mepivacaine 1% with adrenaline. Acta Anaesthesiol Scand 42:570–575, 1998.

19. Koscielniak-Nielsen Z, Nielsen P, Nielsen S, et al: Comparison of transarterial and multiple nerve stimulation techniques for axillary block using a high dose of mepivacaine with adrenaline. Acta Anaesthesiol Scand 43:398–404, 1999.

20. Lofstrom B, Wennberg A, Wien L: Late disturbances in nerve function after block with local anaesthetic agents. Acta Anaesthesiol Scand 10:111–122, 1966.

21. Gentili F, Hudson A, Hunter D, Kline: Nerve injection injury with local anesthetic agents: A light and electron microscopic, fluorescent microscopic, and horseradish peroxidase study. Neurosurg 6:263–272, 1980.

22. Selander D, Brattsand R, Lundborg G, et al: Local anesthetics: Importance of mode of application, concentration, and adrenaline for the appearance of nerve lesions. Acta Anaesthesiol Scand 23:127–136, 1979.

23. Winchell S, Wolfe R: The incidence of neuropathy following upper extremity nerve blocks. Reg Anesth 10:12–15, 1985.

24. Selander D, Dhuner K-G, Lundborg G: Peripheral nerve injury due to injection needles used for regional anesthesia: an experimental study of the acute effects of needle point trauma. Acta Anaesthesiol Scand 21:182–188, 1977.

25. Urban M, Urquhart B: Evaluation of brachial plexus anesthesia for upper extremity surgery. Reg Anesth 19:175–182, 1994.

26. Pearce H, Lindsay D, Leslie K: Axillary brachial plexus block in two hundred consecutive patients. Anaesth Intens Care 24:453–458, 1996.

27. Baranowski A, Pither C: A comparison of three methods of axillary brachial plexus anaesthesia. Anaesthesia 45:362–365, 1990.

28. Davis W, Lennon R, Wedel D: Brachial plexus anesthesia for outpatient surgical procedures on an upper extremity. Mayo Clin Proc 66:470–473, 1991.

29. Eeckelaert J, Filliers E, Alleman J, Hanegreefs G: Supraclavicular brachial plexus block with the aid of nerve stimulator. Acta Anaesth Belgica 35:5–17, 1984.

30. McClain D, Finucane B: Interscalene approach to the brachial plexus: Paresthesia versus nerve stimulator. Reg Anesth 12:80–83, 1987.

31. Winnie AP: Does the transarterial technique of axillary block provide a higher success rate and lower complication rate than a paresthesia technique? Reg Anesth 20:482–485, 1995.

32. Gentili M, Wargnier J: Peripheral nerve damage and regional anaesthesia. Letter to the editor. Br J Anaesth 70:594, 1993.

33. Choyce A, Chan V, Middleton W, et al: What is the relationship between paresthesia and nerve stimulation for axillary brachial plexus block? Reg Anesth Pain Med 26:100–104, 2001.

34. Ford D, Pither C, Raj P: Comparison of insulated and uninsulated needles for locating peripheral nerves with a peripheral nerve stimulator. Anesth Analg 63:925–928, 1984.

35. Fanelli G, Casati A, Garancini P, Torri G: Nerve stimulator and multiple injection technique for upper and lower limb blockade: Failure rate, patient acceptance, and neurologic complications. Study Group on Regional Anesthesia. Anesth Analg 88:847–852, 1999.

36. Riegler F: Brachial plexus block with the nerve stimulator: Motor response characteristics at three sites. Reg Anesth 17:295–299, 1992.

37. Rucci F, Pippa P, Baccaccini A, Barbagli R: Effect of injection speed on anaesthetic spread during axillary block using the orthogonal two-needle technique. Eur J Anaesth 12:505–511, 1995.

38. Chilvers C: Warm local anaesthetic – Effect on latency of onset of axillary brachial plexus block. Anaesth Intensive Care 21:795–798, 1993.

39. Candido KD, Franco C, Khan M, et al: Brachial plexus block with buprenorphine for postoperative pain relief. Reg Anes Pain Med 26:352–356, 2001.

40. Candido KD, Winnie AP, Ghaleb A, et al: Buprenorphine added to the local anesthetic for axillary brachial plexus block prolongs postoperative analgesia. Reg Anesth Pain Med 27:162–167, 2002.

41. McGlade D, Kalpokas M, Mooney P, et al: A comparison of 0.5% ropivacaine and 0.5% bupivacaine for axillary brachial plexus anaesthesia. Anaesth Intensive Care 26:515–520, 1998.

42. Raeder J, Drosdahl S, Klaastad O, et al: Axillary brachial plexus block with ropivacaine 7.5 mg/ml. A comparative study with bupivacaine 5 mg/ml. Acta Anaesth Scand 43:794–798, 1999.

43. Covino B, Wildsmith JAW: Clinical pharmacology of local anesthetic agents. In Cousins MJ, Bridenbaugh PO (eds): Neural Blockade in Clinical Anesthesia and Management of Pain. Lippincott-Raven, Philadelphia, 1998, pp 97–128.

44. Martin R, Dumais R, Cinq-Mars S, Tetrault J: Bloc axillaire par blocage simultane de plusieurs neris II. Evaluation du mélange lidocaine-bupivacaine. Ann Fr Anesth Reanim 12:233–236, 1993.

45. Inberg P, Annila I, Annila P: Double-injection method using peripheral nerve stimulator is superior to single injection in axillary plexus block. Reg Anesth Pain Med 24:509–513, 1999.

46. Gaertner E, Estebe J, Cuby C, Launoy A: Triple-injection method using peripheral nerve stimulator is superior to single injection in infraclavicular plexus block: A preliminary study [abstract]. Reg Anesth Pain Med 26S:30A, 2001.

47. Coventry D, Barker K, Thomson M: Comparison of two neuro-stimulation techniques for axillary brachial plexus blockade. Br J Anaesth 86:80–83, 2001.

48. Koscielniak-Nielsen Z, Stens-Pedersen H, Lippert F: Readiness for surgery after axillary block: Single or multiple injection techniques. Eur J Anaesth 14:164–171, 1997.

49. Lavoie J, Martin R, Tetrault J: Axillary plexus block using a peripheral nerve stimulator: Single or multiple injections. Can J Anaesth 39:583–586, 1992.

50. Sia S, Bartoli M: Selective ulnar nerve localization is not essential for axillary brachial plexus block using a multiple nerve stimulation technique. Reg Anes Pain Med 26:12–16, 2001.

51. Sia S, Bartoli M, Lepri A, et al: Multiple-injection axillary brachial plexus block: A comparison of two methods of nerve localization-nerve stimulation versus paresthesia. Anesth Analg 91:647–651, 2000.

52. Vester-Andersen T, Christiansen C, Sorensen M, et al: Perivascular axillary block: II. Influence of injected volume of local anaesthetic on neural blockade. Acta Anaesthesiol Scand 27:95–98, 1983.

53. Vester-Andersen T, Husum B, Lindeburg T, et al: Perivascular axillary block: IV. Blockade following 40, 50 or 60 ml of mepivacaine 1% with adrenaline. Acta Anaesthesiol Scand 28:99–105, 1984.

54. Vester-Andersen T, Eriksen C, Christiansen C: Perivascular axillary block: III. Blockade following 40 ml of 0.5%, 1% or 1.5% mepivacaine with adrenaline. Acta Anaesthesiol Scand 28:95–98, 1984.

55. Lang E, Theiss D, Jankovic D: The extent of blockade following various techniques of brachial plexus block. Anesth Analg 62:55–58, 1983.

56. Yang W, Chui P, Metreweli C: Anatomy of the normal brachial plexus revealed by sonography and the role of sonographic guidance in anesthesia of the brachial plexus. Am J Roentgenol 171: 1631–1636, 1998.

57. Koscielniak-Nielsen Z, Christensen L, Pedersen H, Brusho J: Effect of digital pressure on the neurovascular sheath during perivascular axillary block. Br J Anaesth 75:702–706, 1995.

58. Yamamoto K, Tsubokawa T, Ohmura S, Kobayashi T: The effects of arm position on central spread of local anesthetics and on quality of the block with axillary brachial plexus block. Reg Anes Pain Med 24:36–42, 1999.

59. Bouaziz H, Narchi P, Mercier F, et al: Comparison between conventional axillary block and a new approach at the midhumeral level. Anesth Analg 84:1058–1062, 1997.

60. Whiffler K: Coracoid block – A safe and easy technique. Br J Anaesth 53:845–848, 1981.

61. Sims J: A modification of landmarks for infraclavicular approach to brachial plexus block. Anesth Analg 56:554–555, 1997.

62. Raj P: Infraclavicular approaches to brachial plexus anesthesia. Tech Reg Anesth Pain Manage 1:169–177, 1997.

63. Wilson J, Brown D, Wong G: Infraclavicular brachial plexus block: Parasagittal anatomy important to the coracoid technique. Anesth Analg 87:870–873, 1998.

64. Kapral S, Jandrasits O, Schabernig C, et al: Lateral infraclavicular plexus block vs. axillary block for hand and forearm surgery. Acta Anaesthesiol Scand 43:1047–1052, 1999.

65. Koscielniak-Nielsen Z, Totboll Nielsen P, Risby Mortensen C: A comparison of coracoid and axillary approaches to the brachial plexus. Acta Anaesthesiol Scand 44:274–279, 2000.

66. Rodriguez J, Barcena M, Rodriguez V, et al: Infraclavicular brachial plexus block effects on respiratory function and extent of the block. Reg Anesth Pain Med 23:564–568, 1998.

67. Geiger P, Mehrkens HH: Vertical infraclavicular brachial plexus blockade. Tech Reg Anesth Pain Manag. 7:67–71, 2003.

68. Haro F, Rodriguez J, De Andres J: Alternatives to the vertical approach for intraclavicular brachial plexus block. Tech Reg Anesth Pain Manage 7:72–80, 2003.

69. Selander D: Catheter technique in axillary plexus block. Acta Anaesthesiol Scand 21:324–329, 1977.

70. Sarma J: Long-term continuous axillary plexus blockade using 0.25% bupivacaine. Acta Anaesthesiol Scand 34:511–513, 1990.

71. Aguilar J, Mendiola M, Valdivia J, De Paz J: Long-term continuous axillary brachial plexus blockade using an implanted port. Tech Reg Anesth Pain Manage 2:74–78, 1998.

72. Winnie AP, Candido KD, Torres M: Continuous peripheral nerve blocks for the management of trauma to the extremities. *In* Grande C, Rosenberg A, Bernstein R (eds): Perioperative Pain Management and Regional Anesthesia for the Trauma Patient. WB Saunders, New York, 1999, pp 209–238.

73. Rosenquist R, Finucane B: Axillary brachial plexus anesthesia using a bullet-tipped needle/catheter device. Tech Reg Anesth Pain Manage 1:182–184, 1997.

74. Macaire P: Axillary block: Single shot or continuous technique. Tech Reg Anesth Pain Manage 7:81–86, 2003.

75. Salonen M, Haasio J, Bachmann M, et al: Evaluation of efficacy and plasma concentrations of ropivacaine in continuous axillary brachial plexus block: High dose for surgical anesthesia and low dose for postoperative analgesia. Reg Anesth Pain Med 25:47–51, 2000.

76. Brown D, Ransom D, Hall J, et al: Regional anesthesia and local anesthetic-induced systemic toxicity: Seizure frequency and accompanying cardiovascular changes. Anesth Analg 81:321–328, 1995.

77. Carles M, Pulcini A, Macchi P, et al: An evaluation of the brachial plexus block at the humeral canal using a neurostimulator (1417 patients): The efficacy, safety, and predictive criteria of failure. Anesth Analg 92:194–198, 2001.

78. Maclean D, Chambers W, Tucker G, Wildsmith JAW: Plasma prilocaine concentrations after three techniques of brachial plexus blockade. Br J Anaesth 60:136–139, 1988.

79. Vester-Andersen T, Christiannsen C, Hansen A, et al: Interscalene brachial plexus block: Area of analgesia, complications and blood concentrations of local anesthetics. Acta Anaesthesiol Scand 25:81–84, 1981.

80. Ben-David B, Stahl S: Axillary block complicated by hematoma and radial nerve injury. Reg Anesth Pain Med 24:264–266, 1999.

81. Groh G, Gainor B, Jeffries J, et al: Pseudoaneurysm of the axillary artery with median nerve deficit after axillary block anesthesia. JBJS (Am) 72:1407–1408, 1990.

82. Zipkin M, Backus W, Scott B, Poppers P: False aneurysm of the axillary artery following brachial plexus block. J Clin Anesth 3:143–145, 1991.

83. Restelli L, Pinciroli D, Conoscente F, Cammelli F: Insufficient venous drainage following axillary approach to brachial plexus blockade. Br J Anaesth 56:1051–1053, 1984.

84. Ott B, Neuberger L, Frey H: Obliteration of the axillary artery after axillary block. Anaesthesia 44:773–774, 1989.

85. Merrill D, Brodsky J, Hentz R: Vascular insufficiency following axillary block of the brachial plexus. Anesth Analg 60:162–164, 1981.

86. Auroy Y, Benhamou D, Bargues L, et al: Major complications of regional anesthesia in France. Anesthesiology 97:1274–1280, 2002.

87. Rice A, McMahon S: Peripheral nerve injury caused by injection needles used in regional anaesthesia: Influence of bevel configuration, studied in a rat model. Br J Anaesth 9:433–438, 1992.

88. Selander D, Sjostrand J: Longitudinal spread of intraneurally injected local anesthetics. Acta Anaesthesiol Scand 22:622–634, 1978.

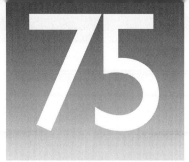

Truncal Blocks: Intercostal, Paravertebral, Interpleural, Suprascapular, Ilioinguinal, and Iliohypogastric Nerve Blocks

Robert E. Molloy, M.D.

INTERCOSTAL NERVE BLOCK

Regional anesthesia of the trunk may be applied using multiple varying block techniques. This chapter considers a selection of the available approaches. Intercostal nerve blocks provide analgesia of the chest wall for patients with surgical incisions, rib fractures, chest tubes, thoracic herpes zoster, and rib lesions.[1–4] Intercostal block has been combined with light general anesthesia and celiac plexus block to provide analgesia for abdominal surgical procedures. Repeated blocks may be required for acute traumatic pain states. The utility of this block would be markedly enhanced by the introduction of a safe, ultra-long-acting local anesthetic agent or slow-release preparation. This advance in local anesthetic pharmacology should allow for prolonged postoperative chest wall analgesia after intercostal blocks, while minimizing the side effects (nausea, urinary retention, hypotension, pruritis) frequently seen with epidural opioid and local anesthetic techniques. Intercostal nerve block may be helpful as one diagnostic tool in the evaluation of patients with abdominal or thoracic pain, particularly in detection of somatic rather than visceral mechanisms of pain.

Intercostal blocks produce minimal effects on pulmonary function studies in healthy volunteers.[5] They do reduce the decline in 1-second forced expiratory volume (FEV_1) seen in the initial postoperative period after truncal incisions when compared to systemic opioids,[6,7] and they may decrease the incidence of postoperative pulmonary complications.[8] The analgesia from T3–T9 intercostal blocks with 20 mL 0.5%

bupivacaine was equal or superior to that from epidural fentanyl 2 µg/mL, with 0.125% bupivacaine infused at 6 to 10 mL per hour during the first 24 hours after thoracotomy.[9] Pain relief was superior with epidural infusion during the second 24 hours after surgery, which can be explained by the fact that intercostal nerve blocks were not repeated. Bilateral intercostal nerve blocks are infrequently performed because of the possibility of bilateral pneumothorax and local anesthetic toxic effects.

Anatomy: Thoracic nerve roots emerge from the intervertebral foramina into the paravertebral space. Here they send white rami communicantes to the sympathetic chain, receive gray rami communicantes in return, and send a posterior cutaneous branch to supply the paravertebral skin and muscles and the posterior ligaments and articulations of the vertebral column. As the nerves leave the paravertebral space, they enter the intercostal space below the respective rib of each, lying between the innermost intercostal muscle and the pleura. Lateral to the paravertebral muscles, the prominent angles of the ribs are palpable as the primary landmark for intercostal nerve block. At the angle of the rib, the nerve lies between the innermost intercostal muscle and the inner intercostal muscle. At this distance, the thickness of the rib is about 8 mm, and the costal groove is widest.[10] Here the nerve is positioned below the intercostal vein and artery, under or below the rib (Fig. 75-1). A cadaver study found that the intercostal nerve remained in a classic subcostal position only 17% of the time.[11] It was shown

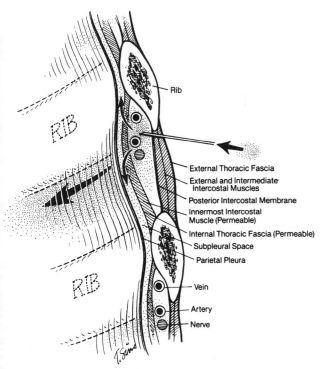

FIGURE 75-1. Anatomy of the intercostal nerve at the angle of the rib, the site of needle placement for classic intercostal nerve block. (From Raj PP, Pai U, Rawal N: Techniques of regional anesthesia in adults. *In* Raj PP (ed): Clinical Practice of Regional Anesthesia. Churchill Livingstone, New York, 1991, p 271.)

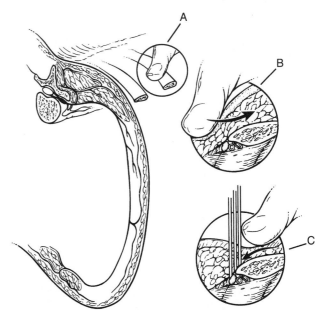

FIGURE 75-2. Anatomy of the intercostal nerve and technique of classic intercostal nerve block near the angle of the rib. (From Thompson GE: Intercostal nerve block. *In* Waldman SD, Winnie AP (eds): Interventional Pain Management. WB Saunders, Philadelphia, 1996, p 311.)

to be in a midcostal location most frequently (73%), and it was supracostal in some cadavers (10%). Just beyond the midaxillary line, the lateral cutaneous branch of the nerve arises, providing sensory innervation anteriorly and posteriorly to much of the thorax and abdomen[12] (Fig. 75-2).

The ideal location for intercostal nerve block is at the posterior angle of the rib, just lateral to the paravertebral muscle mass, except for the uppermost nerves, because of the interposition of the scapulae. Block may also be performed just posterior to the midaxillary line without missing the lateral cutaneous nerve.[13] However, the intercostal space is narrower here, and the lower edge of the rib becomes sharper and more narrow.[14]

The intercostal nerves are the primary rami of thoracic nerves T1–T11. Most of the T1 nerve fibers combine with C8 to form the lower trunk of the brachial plexus. Fibers from T2 and T3 form the intercostobrachial nerve; they also supply the upper chest wall above the nipple line, along with the supraclavicular nerves from the cervical plexus. Intercostal nerves T4–T11 supply the thoracoabdominal wall from the nipple line to below the umbilicus. The T12 nerve is actually a subcostal nerve that contributes branches to the iliohypogastric and ilioinguinal nerves.[15]

Technique: The ideal patient position is prone, with a pillow under the abdomen and both upper extremities hanging over the sides of the table, which maximizes retraction of the scapulae away from the upper ribs. This allows for bilateral blockade and posterior access to the angles of the ribs to enhance safety

and success of the procedure. The lateral decubitus position is also quite satisfactory for unilateral blockade after rib fractures and lateral thoracotomy and for chest tube placement. The supine position has been utilized for bilateral block under general anesthesia, which avoids the need to turn the patient. The anatomy of the intercostal space is less ideal near the midaxillary line (Table 75-1).

After intravenous access has been established, with the patient positioned and monitored, the landmarks for block are drawn with a marking pen. The midline spinous processes are marked, and bilateral lines are drawn through the angles of the ribs where they are first easily palpated lateral to the paraspinal muscles. This may be 8 cm lateral to the midline inferiorly and less than 6 cm superiorly, to avoid the scapula. An intersecting line is drawn at the inferior border of each rib to be blocked, beginning with the 12th rib. Appropriate intravenous sedation is required, and skin wheals are raised at each intersecting line. A 22- to 25-gauge short-bevel needle attached to a control syringe is used, beginning at the most caudal nerve to be blocked. The index finger of the left (nondominant) hand pulls the skin up over the rib, and the right (dominant) hand inserts the needle with syringe, angled slightly cephalad, close to the tip of the left index finger and onto the rib. The left hand now grasps the needle hub, anchored to the chest wall, and both controls the needle and "walks" it off the lower rib margin. It is advanced about 3 mm beyond the lower rib margin. The right hand injects 3 to 5 mL of local anesthetic while the left hand either remains motionless or moves the needle in and out about 1 mm. The needle is then replaced on the same rib or removed altogether, before the left hand begins to palpate the next rib margin in a cephalad direction (see Fig. 75-2). This process is repeated for each nerve to be blocked. It is important to retain control of the syringes and needle at all times, so that

TABLE 75-1. **POSITIONING THE PATIENT FOR INTERCOSTAL NERVE BLOCK**

Patient Position	Site of Block	Advantages and Disadvantages
Prone	Angle of ribs	Best access for bilateral block; simplest technique
Lateral	Angle of ribs	Ideal for patient comfort and unilateral block; position change for bilateral blocks
Supine	Midaxillary line	Bilateral blocks under general anesthesia, avoids position change, more difficult
Intrathoracic	Intrapleural; direct injection of nerve	Technically difficult to inject; total spinal anesthesia may occur

the physician's advancement of the syringes and the patient's unexpected movements will not allow the needle to penetrate the pleura.

Side Effects and Complications and Dosing: Intercostal block is avoided by many physicians to avoid the risk of pneumothorax, which has been thought to occur relatively frequently, in 1% to 2% of patients. The rate of pneumothorax detected by X-ray has been reported to be 0.42% by Moore and Bridenbaugh,[16] and clinically obvious pneumothorax occurs at a much lower rate. Chest tube insertion is rarely needed, even when a small pneumothorax occurs. Systemic local anesthetic toxic effects are a concern with multiple intercostal nerve blocks because of multiple injections and relatively rapid absorption from this site. The local anesthetic agent selected and the total dose employed are important contributing factors. Epinephrine, 5 µg/mL, decreases absorption of the local anesthetic agent.

The effective concentration of bupivacaine is between 0.25% and 0.5%. Drug concentration must be reduced when large volumes are used to avoid exceeding maximum recommended doses for the drug selected (2 to 3 mg/kg for bupivacaine). Postblock patient monitoring should continue for at least 20 minutes. Accidental widespread neuraxial block has been reported after intraoperative intrathoracic block by the surgeon.[17] Injection under direct vision by the surgeon at a medial location may result in local anesthetic placement into a dural cuff or into the nerve itself, with resultant occurrence of spinal anesthesia (Table 75-2). The duration of bupivacaine may be extended from hours to days by its incorporation into liposomes and polymer microspheres. This has been demonstrated for intercostal block using the sheep model.[18] Chronic intercostal neuralgia after surgery or herpes zoster has been treated effectively with intercostal nerve block using 5% tetracaine.[19]

TABLE 75-2. **COMPLICATIONS OF INTERCOSTAL BLOCK**

Pneumothorax
Local anesthetic toxicity
Total spinal anesthesia

PARAVERTEBRAL NERVE BLOCK

Blockade of the paravertebral space offers an alternative regional anesthetic to intercostal and epidural nerve blockade.[20] Patients with chronic pain who require diagnostic or therapeutic nerve blocks[21] and patients who undergo operative procedures of the chest and upper abdomen[22–24] may benefit. The utility of this procedure is controversial, largely due to concern for pneumothorax and the wide variation of the anatomy of the paravertebral space.

Anatomy: The thoracic paravertebral space is a narrow, triangular space lateral to the vertebral column. It is bounded posteriorly by the superior costotransverse ligament, anteriorly by the parietal pleura, and superiorly and inferiorly by the heads and necks of adjoining ribs. The base is formed by the posterolateral aspect of the body of the vertebra and the intervertebral foramen, which communicates with the epidural space. The paravertebral space contains the sympathetic chain, rami communicantes, and dorsal and ventral roots of the spinal nerve. Local anesthetic injection provides sensory, motor, and sympathetic blockade.[25]

Because the paravertebral space is continuous with the surrounding spaces, injection of local anesthetic can provide anesthesia to several dermatomes through the following means (Fig. 75-3):

- Lateral diffusion into the intercostal space.
- Superior or inferior spread into adjacent paravertebral space.
- Medial diffusion into the epidural space.
- A combination of these.

If unilateral blockade is maintained, anesthesia and sympathetic blockade are unilateral, and the risk of hypotension is significantly reduced. After injection of 5 mL of contrast into the paravertebral space, the contrast medium will be confined to the paravertebral space about 20% of the time. Epidural and intercostal spread will occur in about 70% and 10% of cases, respectively. A wide range of sensory losses may be seen. This inconsistency in the spread of the solution makes the use of diagnostic blocks without fluoroscopic confirmation a controversial endeavor. Depth from the skin to the transverse process varies significantly, depending on the thickness of the subcutaneous fat layer. The distance from the spinous process laterally to the tip of the transverse process ranges from 2 to 4 cm.

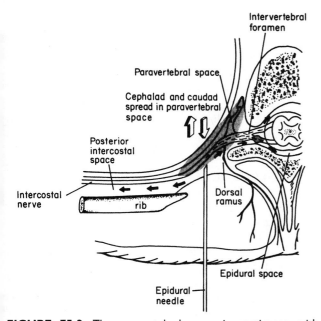

FIGURE 75-3. The paravertebral space is contiguous with surrounding spaces. *Arrows* depict spread of local anesthetic to the intercostal, epidural, and inferior and superior paravertebral spaces. (From Chan VW, Ferrante FM: Continuous thoracic paravertebral block. *In* Ferrante FM, VadeBoncoeur TR (eds): Postoperative Pain Management. Churchill Livingstone, New York, 1993, p 408.)

A negative pressure gradient exists from the paravertebral space to the epidural space.

Technique: With the patient in the decubitus or prone position, the back is prepared as for an epidural block placement. Two landmarks are used to enter the paravertebral space at the thoracic level. The inferior portion of the spinous process of the vertebral body corresponding to the desired somatic nerve block is identified. A line is drawn 3 cm laterally and a point is marked as the needle entry site. This point overlies the transverse process of the vertebral body inferior to the desired paravertebral space.

Local anesthetic infiltration is performed, in all planes perpendicular to the skin, and the same needle is used to seek the transverse process. It is usually 1.5 to 2 cm below the skin, but it may be deeper, depending on the size of the patient. The needle of choice is placed in the same location, and the transverse process is again contacted. The needle is "walked" superiorly until it slips off of the transverse process. A loss-of-resistance technique, using saline or air, is used to identify the paravertebral space as the epidural needle passes through the superior costotransverse ligament. "Walking" off the transverse process superiorly, as opposed to inferiorly, allows entry into the paravertebral space at an angle perpendicular to the superior costotransverse ligament, which allows the best loss-of-resistance technique (Fig 75-4). The needle will also enter the portion of the paravertebral space that is the deepest, which minimizes the risk of pneumothorax. A needle placed superior to the identified transverse process is immediately inferior to the transverse process of the vertebra whose spinous process was used as the original landmark.

If a continuous infusion of local anesthetic is planned for postoperative pain, a standard epidural needle is used. After negative aspiration to check for blood, cerebrospinal fluid, and

FIGURE 75-4. Direction of the epidural needle. The needle strikes the transverse process and then angles superiorly to pass through the superior costotransverse ligament. (From Chan VW, Ferrante FM: Continuous thoracic paravertebral block. *In* Ferrante FM, VadeBoncoeur TR (eds): Postoperative Pain Management. Churchill Livingstone, New York, 1993, p 410.)

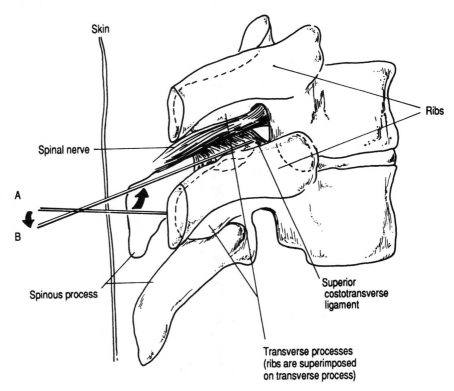

air, a standard epidural catheter is placed 2 to 3 cm into the space. A double-catheter technique (bilateral) has been described for abdominal procedures. Paravertebral blocks, as single injections, have been described for patients having breast surgery. These patients have a higher incidence of nausea and vomiting, which may be significantly less with regional anesthesia.

Dosing: Absorption of local anesthetic from the paravertebral space is difficult to predict. Analgesia has varied from 1 to 10 hours after a single injection. Usually, 15 mL of 0.5% bupivacaine provides analgesia of four dermatomes at the thoracic level.[26] Infusions of 0.25% to 0.5% bupivacaine at 4 to 8 mL/hour have been reported, at an average rate of 0.1 mL/kg/hour. On average, bupivacaine blood levels are similar to those after epidural bolus injections and continuous infusions, although on an individual basis, larger variations in plasma concentrations may be observed from paravertebral local anesthetics.[27]

Complications: The overall failure rate is estimated to be 10%, similar to that for epidural catheter placement.[28] Dural puncture and subarachnoid injection are potential complications. The incidence would likely increase if the needle were directed more medially. This is the widest portion of paravertebral space, which may minimize the risk of pneumothorax. Pneumothorax is estimated to occur in 0.5% of cases. Vascular injection is thought to occur in about 3% to 7% of cases. Hypotension occurs in about 5% of cases, which is much less common than with epidural local anesthetic injection. Urinary retention is infrequent; it was cited to be 10% in one study, as opposed to 60% in patients with epidural analgesia. This is due to the near unilateral block of the paravertebral space. In general, the rate of complications is similar to, if not less than, that seen with placement of epidural catheters. The incidence of vascular puncture and pneumothorax is significantly increased when bilateral paravertebral techniques are used.[29]

Continuous paravertebral infusion should remain an option for patients who cannot tolerate the potential respiratory depression of epidural or intravenous opioids, and would have difficulty managing the potential hypotension from epidural local anesthetics. With proper technique, and confirmation by fluoroscopy if necessary, complications can be minimized. As a single-injection technique, paravertebral somatic nerve block remains an alternative to epidural injection and intercostal nerve block for the treatment of chronic pain syndromes.

Continuous Extrapleural Intercostal Nerve Block:
Another possible variation of both paravertebral and intercostal nerve block is continuous extrapleural intercostal nerve block. This technique requires placement of a catheter during surgery, when the patient's chest is open. Before closing the thoracotomy incision, an epidural needle can be placed percutaneously into the thorax via an intercostal space, near the incision, in the midclavicular line. At the level of the thoracotomy incision, the parietal pleura is opened with a 1 cm incision over the sympathetic nerve trunk. An extrapleural pocket is constructed two spaces above and below the incision. A standard epidural catheter is placed in this pocket and sutured with absorbable suture, and the parietal pleura is closed. Efficacy of this procedure appears to be related to absence of local pleural disease or surgical disruption and to effective localization of

injected local anesthetic in the extrapleural pocket. Confirmation of correct catheter placement may be done with contrast medium and fluoroscopy. This technique reduced post-thoracotomy pain and systemic analgesic intake, and it significantly improved pulmonary function when compared to placebo in two randomized, controlled studies.[30,31] Recommended doses are similar to those for paravertebral block discussed above. Bupivacaine is employed in 0.25% to 0.5% concentration. An initial bolus dose of 0.2 to 0.3 mL/kg may be followed with a continuous infusion of 0.1 mL/kg/hour.[32]

INTERPLEURAL BLOCK

Interpleural block may be used to provide unilateral perioperative analgesia during and after cholecystectomy, renal, or breast surgery. After cholecystectomy, interpleural analgesia reduces opioid consumption and visual analogue scale (VAS) pain scores while improving measures of pulmonary function.[33,34] The duration of interpleural analgesia is significantly reduced after thoracotomy with chest tube placement.[35] Interpleural analgesia after unilateral rib fractures is accompanied by dramatic improvement in pulmonary function.[36] Interpleural analgesia has been effective in case reports for upper extremity ischemic and neuropathic pain, thoracic herpes zoster, pancreatitis, and thoracic cancer pain. Neurolytic phenol interpleural block was effective for a patient with resistant pain from esophageal cancer.[37] When compared to intercostal blockade, interpleural block produces analgesia which is less intense and of shorter duration.[38]

Anatomy: The visceral layer of pleura surrounds the lung and reflects back on the chest wall and diaphragm to form the parietal pleura. The interpleural space is a potential site for local anesthetic administration. Local anesthetics may block free nerve endings in the pleura and diffuse across the pleura to act on adjacent nerves. The intercostal nerves are present posteriorly and laterally, while the splanchnic nerves, sympathetic chain, phrenic and vagus nerves are medial to the pleura. The lowest roots of the brachial plexus pass superiorly, over the cupula.

Technique: Interpleural catheters are ideally placed in the lateral or semiprone position with the affected side uppermost. The ipsilateral arm should hang across the body or off the table to retract the scapula anteriorly. The endpoint for entry into the interpleural space is detection of negative interpleural pressure, which is present during spontaneous ventilation. Placement should be avoided during controlled ventilation to prevent catheter misplacement, lung injury, and pneumothorax.[39]

Once the patient is positioned properly and supported by a pillow, the skin is prepared and draped. The site for catheter insertion is selected from the fifth through eighth intercostal spaces, and a skin wheal is raised immediately superior to the selected rib, approximately 8 to 10 cm lateral to the midline. Deeper infiltration is performed with a 22-gauge needle to anesthetize the superior surface of the rib. A 17- or 18-gauge epidural needle is then inserted at the same site, with its bevel aimed in the direction of intended catheter insertion. The epidural needle is placed perpendicular to the skin, over the rib, and walked cephalad until contact with the superior edge of the rib is lost. Before slowly advancing the needle further, the needle stylet is removed, and a glass syringe containing approximately 2 mL of saline (or air) is attached. Then entry into the pleural space is identified using a passive loss-of-resistance technique. It is important to detect a plugged needle or a sticky syringe barrel, to prevent accidental placement of the needle through the visceral pleura into the lung parenchyma. When the needle tip is in the pleural space, the negative interpleural pressure pulls down the syringe plunger and contained saline, and injection will be easy. The interpleural catheter should be threaded approximately 5 to 10 cm into the pleural space, taking care to reduce air entrained through the needle. An alternative technique utilizes a saline-filled syringe with its plunger removed. Entry into the pleural space is detected by a fall in the saline column, and the catheter may be introduced without having to remove the syringe.[40]

Dosing: The key to a successful analgesic response is proper patient positioning before local anesthetic injection. Injection with the operative side uppermost favors medial spread of solution and unilateral sympathetic block. Since the block sets up by mass action, delivery of the agent is influenced by gravity to thoracic spinal nerves emanating from the paravertebral area. Injection in the supine position favors block of the intercostal nerves with less sympathetic block. The head may be placed up or down 20° depending on the area to be blocked, to facilitate the spread of the injectate by gravity. A head-down position favors upper thoracic and cervical spread. For upper abdominal visceral pain, the patient can be placed in head-up or in a sitting position. The block is then performed on the left side for pancreatic, gastric, or splenic pain and on the right side for hepatic or gallbladder pain. An initial test dose is used to detect accidental intravascular catheter placement. A therapeutic dose of 20 to 30 mL of 0.25% to 0.5% bupivacaine is delivered over 2 to 3 minutes, and patient position is subsequently maintained for 20 to 30 minutes. Epinephrine does not decrease blood levels or prolong analgesia. Duration of analgesia is proportional to the mass of injected drug, and 100 mg bupivacaine produces analgesia for 8 hours.[41] Repeated bolus doses may be given every 6 to 8 hours, or as needed. A continuous infusion of 0.25% bupivacaine at 0.125 mL/kg/hour produced better analgesia after cholecystectomy, with lower blood levels, than intermittent bolus dosing.[42]

Complications: Complications from this procedure can be divided into two categories, those produced by traumatic injuries of either the needle or the catheter and those produced by systemic absorption of local anesthetic injected in the interpleural space. Thus, pneumothorax may occur in up to 2% of patients.[43] Pneumothorax or catheter malposition appear to be more likely with use of sharper needles, stiffer epidural catheters, and positive-pressure ventilation during needle and catheter placement. The following steps may minimize catheter-related risks: slow introduction of a soft, flexible tip catheter; use of a blunt epidural needle; and use of a heavy glass syringe barrel to better detect entry into the interpleural space.[44] Systemic effects from drug absorption may occur, particularly with inflammation of pleural membranes. Local anesthetic toxicity was reported in 1.3% by Stromskag et al. Peak local anesthetic levels occur after 20 to 30 minutes, and they exceed those seen after multiple intercostal blocks using equal doses. Pleural effusion has been reported infrequently, with a 0.4% incidence. Horner's syndrome occurs often after successful interpleural block. Phrenic nerve palsy, bronchopleural fistula formation,

empyema, and injury to the neurovascular bundle may also occur following this block. For these reasons, many physicians prefer to avoid bilateral blocks.

SUPRASCAPULAR NERVE BLOCK

Suprascapular nerve block (SSNB) is indicated for relief of pain in the shoulder, which may be due to bursitis, capsular tear, or other causes.[45] Thirty-four patients with frozen shoulder, trained in a home shoulder exercise program, received a series of three weekly suprascapular nerve blocks using 10 mL 0.5% bupivacaine or saline. A 64% reduction in the McGill Pain Questionnaire multidimensional pain descriptors score was observed in the treatment group, versus 13% in the placebo group, after 1 month.[46] There was also a nonsignificant 15.8% improvement in shoulder function in the treatment group versus 4% in the placebo group. In another randomized, controlled trial 83 patients with chronic shoulder pain due to rheumatoid arthritis or degenerative arthritis received a single SSNB, for a total of 108 affected shoulders, using either 10 mL of 0.5% bupivacaine with 40 mg of methylprednisolone acetate or saline. Clinically significant improvements in all VAS pain scores, the shoulder pain disability index, the Short Form-36, and some range of movement scores were seen at weeks 1, 4, and 12 in the treatment group shoulders compared to placebo.[47] The author has found this block useful in patients who have had stroke and developed adhesive capsulitis of the shoulder. The block is performed before physical therapy, which is used to increase the range of motion of the involved shoulder.

Anatomy: The suprascapular nerve originates from the upper trunk of the brachial plexus (C4–C6), crosses the posterior triangle of the neck, and passes deep to the trapezius muscle. The nerve traverses the suprascapular notch and descends deep to the supraspinatus and the infraspinatus muscles,[48] supplying the two muscles and about 70% of the shoulder joint. Sensory innervation includes the posterior and posterosuperior regions of the shoulder joint and capsule, and the acromioclavicular joint (Fig. 75-5).

Technique: The patient sits on the table or cart, preferably with the arms folded across the abdomen. A line is drawn along the spine of the scapula from the tip of the acromion to the scapular border. The midpoint of this line is noted, and a vertical line, parallel to the vertebral spines, is drawn through it. The angle of the upper outer quadrant is bisected with a line; the site of insertion of the needle is 2.5 cm from the apex of the angle. The area is prepared and draped, and a skin wheal is made. A 3-inch (7.5 cm), 22-guage needle is inserted perpendicular to the skin in all planes, (i.e., downward, inward, and forward) (Fig. 75-5). After contacting bone (i.e., the area surrounding the suprascapular notch) at approximately 5 to 6.5 cm, the needle is slightly withdrawn and redirected medially, laterally, or superiorly until it is felt to slide into the notch. Local anesthetic (10 mL) is injected. The position of the needle tip is checked by withdrawing the needle and reinserting it laterally or medially to contact the walls of the suprascapular notch. Pneumothorax, which occurs in less than 1% of cases, is caused by deeper-than-recommended advancement of the needle.

The subjective relief of the patient's symptoms and the ability of the patient to tolerate manipulation of the shoulder indicate

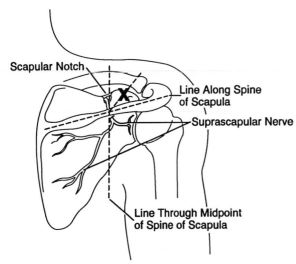

FIGURE 75-5. Anatomy and landmarks involved in suprascapular nerve block. *X* is the site of needle insertion. (Adapted from Moore DC: Regional Block: A Handbook for Use in the Clinical Practice of Medicine and Surgery, ed 4. Charles C Thomas, Springfield, IL, 1979, pp 300–303.)

a successful block. No skin analgesia results from the block. Weakness of external shoulder rotation also confirms successful block.[49]

ILIOINGUINAL AND ILIOHYPOGASTRIC NERVE BLOCKS

Ilioinguinal and iliohypogastric nerve blocks may be used in diagnosis and treatment of chronic suprapubic and inguinal pain after lower abdominal surgery or hernia repair. They may be combined with genitofemoral nerve block in the similar evaluation and treatment of chronic inguinal and testicular pain after hernia repair.[50] These blocks may be applied in the management of patients with neuralgias and nerve entrapment syndromes. Iliohypogastric and ilioinguinal nerve blocks are also important components of regional anesthesia of the inguinal region, most typically performed for inguinal herniorrhaphy. Preoperative wound infiltration decreased analgesic requirements and pain scores at 1, 2, and 10 days after inguinal hernia repair when compared with general anesthesia alone.[51] Preincisional local anesthetic infiltration, compared to similar block at the end of hernia repair, delayed the first demand for postoperative analgesia and increased the number of patients not requiring supplemental analgesics in a single study.[52] This apparent demonstration of preemptive analgesia was not confirmed in a second study.[53] Intraoperative bilateral ilioinguinal nerve block with 0.5% bupivacaine also decreased analgesic requirements and pain scores for 24 hours after cesarean section performed under general anesthesia.[54]

Anatomy: The iliohypogastric (T12–L1) and ilioinguinal (L1) nerves emerge from the lateral border of the psoas major muscle, travel around the abdominal wall, and penetrate the transverse abdominal and the internal oblique muscles to innervate the hypogastric and inguinal areas. The anterior cutaneous branch of the iliohypogastric nerve passes through the internal oblique muscle just medial to the anterior superior iliac spine (ASIS), to lie between it and the external oblique muscle. It then passes through the external oblique above the superficial inguinal ring, and it supplies the suprapubic area. The ilioinguinal nerve remains between the deeper two muscle layers until it is much closer to the inguinal canal. It travels through the inguinal canal below the spermatic cord, and it supplies the upper medial thigh and superior inguinal region. An effective block of both nerves performed medial to the ASIS must be made at multiple depths, in various fascial planes. The genitofemoral (L1–L2) nerve passes through and along the anterior surface of the psoas major muscle, and it divides into genital and femoral branches above the inguinal ligament. Its genital branch travels with the spermatic cord and innervates the genitalia inferior to the area supplied by the ilioinguinal nerve.

Technique: The primary landmark for both approaches to hernia block is the ASIS, palpated with the patient reclining in the supine position. The first technique uses an injection site 2 to 3 cm along a line from the ASIS to the umbilicus, which should also be about 2 cm medial and 2 cm cephalad to the ASIS. A 22-gauge, 2-inch needle is inserted perpendicular to the skin, noting the feel when each layer of muscle fascia is penetrated. Infiltration, using 10 mL of local anesthetic, is performed at each depth and, subsequently, in both directions along this line. A second technique uses a 22-gauge, 3-inch needle, inserted at a site 3 cm medial and 3 cm inferior to the ASIS. The needle is initially directed slightly cephalad and laterally, aiming to contact the medial edge of the iliac crest. It is inserted along the medial edge of the iliac crest, injecting local anesthetic as it is withdrawn. Subsequent injection is made in a more medial direction through the various muscle layers. Supplemental infiltration of the incision and/or field block may be needed for surgery of the inguinal region.

The genital branch of the genitofemoral nerve block can be blocked by infiltration of 5 to 10 mL local anesthetic, using a 22-gauge, 5 cm needle inserted through the skin just lateral to the pubic tubercle and below the inguinal ligament. Infiltration around the spermatic cord at its exit from the inguinal canal is also an effective technique.[55]

Complications: Systemic toxicity may occur due to the large volumes of local anesthetic that are often employed. A lower concentration of local anesthetic may be used to decrease this risk. Local infection may occur. Accidental block of the lateral femoral cutaneous nerve and partial block of the femoral nerve may also occur.

KEY POINTS

- The introduction of a safe, ultra-long-acting local anesthetic preparation would allow for prolonged postoperative chest wall analgesia after intercostal blocks, while minimizing the side effects (nausea, urinary retention, hypotension, pruritus) frequently seen with epidural opioid and local anesthetic techniques.

- Intercostal blocks produce minimal effects on pulmonary function studies in healthy volunteers; reduce the decline in FEV_1 seen in the initial postoperative period after truncal incisions when compared to systemic opioids; and they may decrease the incidence of postoperative pulmonary complications.

- After injection of 5 mL into the paravertebral space, contrast medium will be confined to the paravertebral space about 20% of the time; epidural and intercostal spread will occur in about 70% and 10% of cases, respectively.
- Suprascapular nerve block has proven efficacy for significant pain relief and some functional improvement in patients with shoulder arthritis or frozen shoulder.

REFERENCES

1. Moore DC, Bridenbaugh LD: Intercostal nerve block in 4,333 patients: Indications, techniques, and complications. Anesth Analg 41:1–11, 1962.
2. Moore DC: Intercostal nerve block for postoperative somatic pain following surgery of the thorax and upper abdomen. Br J Anaesth 47:S284–S286, 1975.
3. Nunn JF, Slavin C: Posterior intercostal nerve block for pain relief after cholecystectomy. Br J Anaesth 52:253–260, 1980.
4. Bunting P, McGeachie JF: Intercostal nerve blockade producing analgesia after appendectomy. Br J Anaesth 61:169–172, 1988.
5. Jakobson S, Fridriksson H, Hedenstrom H, et al: Effects of intercostal nerve blocks on pulmonary mechanics in healthy men. Acta Anaesthesiol Scand 24:482–486, 1980.
6. Faust RJ, Nauss LA: Post-thoracotomy intercostal nerve block: Comparison of its effects on pulmonary function with those of intramuscular meperidine. Anesth Analg 55:542–546, 1976.
7. Engberg G: Respiratory performance after upper abdominal surgery: A comparison of pain relief with intercostal block and centrally acting analgesics. Acta Anaesthesiol Scand 29:427–433, 1985.
8. Engeberg G, Wiklund L: Pulmonary complications after upper abdominal surgery: Their prevention with intercostal blocks. Acta Anaesthesiol Scand 32:1–9, 1988.
9. Wurnig PN, Lackner H, Teiner C, et al: Is intercostal nerve block for pain management in thoracic surgery more successful than epidural anaesthesia? Eur J Cardiothorac Surg 21:1115–1119, 2002.
10. Kopacz DJ, Thompson GE: Intercostal nerve block. In Waldman SD (ed): Interventional Pain Management, ed 2. WB Saunders, Philadelphia, 2001, pp 401–408.
11. Hardy PA: Anatomical variation in the position of the proximal intercostal nerve. Br J Anaesth 61:338–339, 1988.
12. Thompson GE: Intercostal nerve block. In Waldman SD, Winnie AP (eds): Interventional Pain Management. WB Saunders, Philadelphia, 1996, p 311.
13. Moore DC: Intercostal nerve block: Spread of India ink injected into the subcostal groove. Br J Anaesth 53:325–329, 1981.
14. Kopacz DJ: Regional anesthesia of the trunk. In Brown DL (ed): Regional Anesthesia and Analgesia. WB Saunders, Philadelphia, 1996, pp 292–318.
15. Thompson GE, Moore DC: Celiac plexus, intercostal, and minor peripheral blockade. In Cousins MJ, Bridenbaugh PO (eds): Neural Blockade in Anesthesia and Management of Pain, ed 2. JB Lippincott, Philadelphia, 1988, p 503.
16. Moore DC, Bridenbaugh LD: Pneumothorax: Its incidence following intercostal nerve block. JAMA 182:1005–1008, 1962.
17. Benumof JL, Semenza J: Total spinal anesthesia following intrathoracic intercostal nerve blocks. Anesthesiology 43:124–125, 1975.
18. Drager C, Benzinger D, Gao F, et al: Prolonged intercostal nerve blockade in sheep using controlled-release of bupivacaine and dexamethasone from polymer microspheres. Anesthesiology 89:969–979, 1998.
19. Doi K, Nikai T, Sakura S, et al: Intercostal nerve block with 5% tetracaine for chronic pain syndromes. J Clin Anesth 14:39–41, 2002.
20. Perttunen K, Nilsson E, Heinonen J, et al: Extradural, paravertebral and intercostal nerve blocks for post-thoracotomy pain. Br J Anaesth 75:541–547, 1995.
21. Purcell-Jones G, Pither CE, Justins DM: Paravertebral somatic nerve block: A clinical, radiologic, and computed tomographic study in chronic pain patients. Anesth Analg 68:32–39, 1989.
22. Weltz CR, Greengrass RAA, Lyerly HK: Ambulatory surgical management of breast carcinoma using paravertebral block. Ann Surg 222:19–26, 1995.
23. Richardson J, Vowden P, Sadanathan S: Bilateral paravertebral analgesia for major abdominal vascular surgery: A preliminary report. Anaesthesia 50:995–998, 1995.
24. Matthews PJ, Govenden V: Comparison of continuous paravertebral and extradural infusions of bupivacaine for pain relief after thoracotomy. Br J Anaesth 62:204–205, 1989.
25. Chan VW, Ferrante FM: Continuous thoracic paravertebral block. In Ferrante FM, VadeBoncoeur TR (eds): Postoperative Pain Management. Churchill Livingstone, New York, 1993, p 408.
26. Eason MJ, Wyatt R: Paravertebral thoracic block – A reappraisal. Anaesthesia 34:638–642, 1979.
27. Berrisford RG, Sabanathan S, Mearns, et al: Plasma concentrations of bupivacaine and its enantiomers during continuous extrapleural and intercostal nerve block. Br J Anaesth 70:201–204, 1993.
28. Longquist PA, MacKenzie J, Soni AK: Paravertebral blockade: Failure rate and complications. Anaesthesia 50:813–815, 1995.
29. Naja Z, Lonnqvist PA: Somatic paravertebral nerve block: Incidence of failed block and complications. Anaesthesia 56:1184–1188, 2001.
30. Sabanathan S, Mearns AJ, Bickford Smith PJ, et al: Efficacy of continuous intercostal nerve block on post-thoracotomy pain and pulmonary mechanics. Br J Surg 77:221–225, 1990.
31. Barron DJ, Tolan MJ, Lea RE: A randomized controlled trial of continuous extra-pleural analgesia post-thoracotomy: Efficacy and choice of local anesthetic. Eur J Anaesthesiol 16:236–245, 1999.
32. Dauphin A, Lubanska-Hubert E, Young JE, et al: Comparative study of continuous extrapleural intercostal nerve block and lumbar epidural morphine in post-thoracotomy pain. Can J Surg 40:431–436, 1997.
33. Rademaker BM, Sih IL, Kalkman CJ, et al: Effects of interpleurally administered bupivacaine 0.5% on opioid analgesic requirements and endocrine response during and after cholecystectomy: A randomized double-blind controlled study. Acta Anaesthesiol Scand 35:108–112, 1991.
34. Frenette L, Boureault D, Guay J: Interpleural analgesia improves pulmonary function after cholecystectomy. Can J Anaesth 38:71–74, 1991.
35. Symreng T, Gomez MN, Rossi N: Intrapleural bupivacaine v saline after thoracotomy – Effects on pain and lung function – a double blind study. J Cardiothorac Anesth 3:144–149, 1989.
36. Rocco A, Reiestad F, Gudman J, et al: Intrapleural administration of local anesthetics for pain relief in patients with multiple rib fractures. Reg Anesth 12:10–14, 1987.
37. Lema MJ, Meyers DP, De Leon-Casasola OA, et al: Pleural phenol therapy for the treatment of chronic esophageal cancer pain. Reg Anesth 17:166–170, 1992.
38. Van Kleef JW, Burm AG, Vletter AA: Single-dose interpleural versus intercostal blockade: Nerve block characteristics and plasma concentration profiles after administration of 0.5% bupivacaine with epinephrine. Anesth Analg 70:484–448, 1990.
39. Symreng T, Gomez MN, Johnson B, et al: Intrapleural bupivacaine – Technical considerations and intraoperative use. J Cardiothorac Anesth 3:139–143, 1989.
40. Ben-David B, Lee E: The falling column: a new technique for interpleural catheter placement. Anesth Analg 71:212, 1990.
41. Stromskag KE, Reistad F, Holmquist EL, et al: Intrapleural administration of 0.25%, 0.375%, and 0.5% bupivacaine with epinephrine after cholecystectomy. Anesth Analg 67:430–434, 1988.

42. Laurito CE, Kirz LI, Vadeboncouer RE, et al: Continuous infusion of interpleural bupivacaine maintains effective analgesia after cholecystectomy. Anesth Analg 72:516–521, 1991.

43. Stromskag KE, Minor B, Steen PA: Side effect and complications related to interpleural analgesia: An update. Acta Anaesthesiol Scand 34:473–477, 1990.

44. O'Leary KA, Yarussi AT, Myers DP: Interpleural catheters: Indications and techniques. *In* Waldman SA (ed): Interventional Pain Management, ed 2. WB Saunders, Philadelphia, 2001, pp 409–414.

45. Moore DC: Regional Block: A Handbook for Use in the Clinical Practice of Medicine and Surgery, ed 4. Charles C Thomas, Springfield, IL, 1979, pp 300–303.

46. Dahan TH, Pelletier M, Petit M, et al: Double blind randomized clinical trial examining the efficacy of bupivacaine suprascapular nerve blocks in frozen shoulder. J Rheumatol 27:1464–1469, 2000.

47. Shanahan EM, Ahern M, Smith M, et al: Suprascapular nerve block (using bupivacaine and methylprednisolone acetate) in chronic shoulder pain. Ann Rheum Dis 62:400–406, 2003.

48. Ellis H, Feldman S: Anatomy for Anaesthetists, ed 3. Blackwell Scientific, London, 1977, p 186.

49. Neal JM, McDonald SB, Larkin SL: Suprascapular nerve block prolongs analgesia after nonarthroscopic shoulder surgery but does not improve outcome. Anesth Analg 96:982–986, 2003.

50. Reynolds L, Kedlaya D: Ilioinguinal-iliohypogastric and genitofemoral nerve blocks. *In* Waldman SA (ed): Interventional Pain Management, ed 2. WB Saunders, Philadelphia, 2001, pp 508–511.

51. Tverskoy M, Cozacov C, Ayache M, et al: Postoperative pain after inguinal herniorrhaphy with different types of anesthesia. Anesth Analg 70:29–35, 1990.

52. Ejlersen E, Andersen HB, Elaisen K, et al: A comparison between preincisional and postincisional lidocaine infiltration and postoperative pain. Anesth Analg 74:495–498, 1992.

53. Dierking GW, Dahl JB, Kanstrup J, et al: Effect of pre- vs. postoperative inguinal field block on postoperative pain after herniorrhaphy. Br J Anaesth 68:344–348, 1992.

54. Bunting P, McConachie I: Ilioinguinal nerve blockade for analgesia after cesarean section. Br J Anaesth 61:773–775, 1988.

55. Kuzma PJ, Kline MD: Upper and lower extremity neural blockade. *In* Raj PP (ed): Practical Management of Pain, ed 3. Mosby, St Louis, 2000, p 608.

Lumbar Plexus, Femoral, Lateral Femoral Cutaneous, Obturator, Saphenous, and Fascia Iliaca Blocks

Kenneth D. Candido, M.D., and
Honorio T. Benzon, M.D.

LUMBAR PLEXUS BLOCK

Anatomic Considerations: Unlike the situation for the upper extremity where the roots of the brachial plexus are consistently sandwiched between the fasciae of the anterior and middle scalene muscles and hence are readily accessible to single-injection techniques of neural blockade, the roots of the lumbar plexus course through the substance of one large muscle, the psoas major, in their journey from the lumbar paravertebral space to the lower extremity (Fig. 76-1).[1,2] The fasciae of the large psoas major muscle (anteriorly) and quadratus lumborum muscle (posteriorly) invest the lumbar plexus from its origin at the anterior primary rami of the L1, L2, L3, and L4 nerve roots. However, this relationship is inconsistent and somewhat unreliable for routine utilization in single-injection posterior approaches to the plexus. In one study successful lumbar plexus catheters were found within the substance of the psoas major muscle in 74% of patients (59/80) and in the space between the psoas major and quadratus lumborum muscles in 22% (18/80) of patients when evaluated radiographically.[3] Occasionally, the lumbar plexus receives contributions from T12 or from L5, analogous to the so-called "prefixed" or "postfixed" brachial plexus scenarios described in Chapter 73. The upper part of the lumbar plexus supplies the iliohypogastric and ilioinguinal nerves, which are in series with the thoracic nerves and innervate the trunk above the level of the leg. The iliohypogastric nerve supplies the skin of the buttock and the muscles of the abdominal wall. The ilioinguinal nerve supplies the skin of the perineum and adjoining inner thigh.

The genitofemoral nerve (from L1 and L2) supplies the genital area and adjacent thigh.

Unlike the situation for the upper extremity where the nerves remain in close proximity to each other between the scalene muscles, the three major components of the lumbar plexus (femoral, lateral femoral cutaneous, obturator nerves) take widely divergent courses down through the pelvis towards their ultimate destinations in the leg. Computed tomographic data indicate that the depths of the femoral nerve (situated medially between the lateral femoral cutaneous nerve and the obturator nerve) from the skin of the back and psoas major landmarks are as follows: femoral nerve, 9.01 ± 2.43 cm; psoas major medial border, 2.73 ± 0.64 cm from the medial sagittal plane; lateral psoas border, 6.41 ± 1.61 cm from the medial sagittal plane.[2] Of the three nerves, only the largest branch of the lumbar plexus, the femoral nerve remains in close proximity to the psoas muscle as it descends into the leg. The lateral femoral cutaneous nerve leaves the lateral border of the psoas major muscle at about its midpoint and enters the lateral thigh at a very superficial level. The obturator nerve leaves the medial border of the psoas major and enters the medial thigh at a very deep level.

The femoral nerve is derived from the dorsal portions of L2, L3, and L4, and descends from its origins to appear at the lateral margin of the psoas major at approximately the junction of the middle and lower thirds of that muscle. As the nerve continues on its descent towards the leg, it remains between the psoas major and the iliacus muscles so that, above the inguinal ligament, the femoral nerve is surrounded laterally by

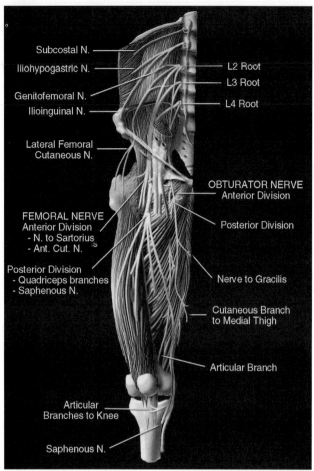

FIGURE 76-1. The lumbar plexus. Anterior view of the right leg. The three main roots (L2, L3, L4) are shown passing from their origins towards the psoas major muscle (transected in the figure) which they run through on their way towards the inguinal ligament. Demonstrated are the primary derivations of the plexus, the obturator, femoral, and lateral femoral cutaneous nerves, as well as the terminal branch of the femoral nerve, the saphenous nerve.

the iliacus fascia, medially by the fascia of the psoas major, and anteriorly by the transversalis fascia. Beneath the inguinal ligament, the fused iliopsoas fascia continues to provide a posterior and lateral wall of this compartment; the inguinal ligament and, below it, the fascia lata continue to provide an anterior wall; and the thick iliopectineal fascia provides a continuation of the medial wall. The lumbar plexus may therefore be blocked utilizing an anterior approach beneath the inguinal ligament (the inguinal paravascular technique) that attempts to block the three major nerves using a modification of the standard femoral nerve block technique (see below). It may also be blocked posteriorly using a psoas compartment approach or a paravertebral approach. Unlike the situation for axillary brachial plexus block, where there is a close neurovascular relationship of the terminal plexus in the axilla and where the axillary sheath envelops the entire neurovascular bundle, in the inguinal region the neural and vascular elements are separated and this separation is reinforced by the femoral sheath. This anatomical consideration makes single-injection anterior lumbar plexus block more challenging than single-injection brachial

plexus block. It is possible that when three nerves are successfully blocked with this approach, the local anesthetic actually spreads laterally along fascial planes rather than ascending to the roots of the lumbar plexus.

Theoretically, the fascial envelope around the femoral nerve is used as a conduit for the injected local anesthetic to spread upwards towards the forming elements of the lumbar plexus when the anterior approach is used (3-in-1 block). In clinical practice, however, routine block of the femoral, lateral femoral cutaneous, and obturator nerves using a single injection of local anesthetic does not occur. In actual practice, the lateral femoral cutaneous nerve is blocked only 96% and the obturator nerve 4% to 47% of the time despite the use of a large volume of local anesthetic.[4] Other studies have demonstrated poorer results of attaining obturator nerve block with the single-injection technique, ranging from 0% obturator nerve block to 4%.[5,6] A cadaver study of 6 specimens asserts that no single sheath encompasses all three nerves in the inguinal region,[7] and a clinical study in patients undergoing muscle biopsy showed no evidence of obturator nerve block.[8] However, a recent magnetic resonance imaging (MRI) study in 7 volunteers did demonstrate that the anterior branch of the obturator nerve is blocked using this technique, in addition to the femoral and lateral femoral cutaneous nerves, even though the spread of 30 mL of local anesthetic did not reach the lumbar plexus.[9] If all three nerves are blocked, the resultant analgesia will encompass the entire anterior, medial, and lateral surfaces of the leg, i.e., all but the area innervated by the sciatic and posterior femoral cutaneous nerves. Motor block will include the quadriceps muscles and the adductors of the thigh.

Indications for Lumbar Plexus Block: Lumbar plexus block is appropriate for surgeries of the thigh or knee, including above-the-knee amputation,[10] as a diagnostic and therapeutic tool for chronic pain disorders, or to provide analgesia for painful conditions of the proximal leg including herpes zoster.[11] Since the resultant sympathetic nerve block is unilateral and postganglionic, the degree of blood pressure fluctuations should not approximate those seen following neuraxial block in a given individual. Lumbar plexus block, therefore, is indicated for any unilateral proximal lower extremity procedure where a subarachnoid or epidural block might be undesirable or contraindicated. It has also been utilized to provide bilateral analgesia following bilateral femoral shaft surgery.[12] Postoperative analgesia after total knee and hip replacement surgery or open-reduction and internal fixation of acetabular fractures is significant when this technique is employed.[13-17] It may be one component of multimodal analgesia following total knee arthroplasty to avoid opioid use postoperatively.[18] Surgery of the hip and lower extremity has been successfully performed in patients using either lumbar plexus anesthesia (variety of approaches) or a combination of lumbar plexus and sciatic nerve block.[5,19-22] However, this combination of techniques may not be sufficient for total knee arthroplasty, as demonstrated in one study where 22% of patients required general anesthesia due to inadequate analgesia intraoperatively.[23] Blood loss following total hip arthroplasty is reduced using this block as compared to general anesthesia.[24]

Techniques of Lumbar Plexus Block: Psoas compartment block of the lumbar plexus is carried out as follows. The patient is placed in the lateral decubitus position with the

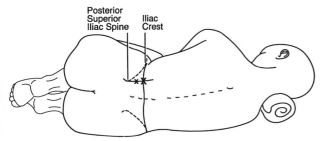

FIGURE 76-2. Psoas compartment block of Chayen and co-workers *(x)* and lumbar plexus block of Winnie and co-workers *(X)*. See text for details of the technique.

intended surgical site uppermost. The upper thigh is flexed at the hip and the knee is flexed, i.e., Sim's position. A line is drawn between the iliac crests (intercristal line) and another one is drawn through the lumbar spinous processes. The posterior superior iliac spine (PSIS) is identified and marked. A line is drawn, parallel to that connecting the lumbar spinous processes from about L3 inferiorly, bisecting the PSIS. The site of needle insertion is where the parallel spinous line (or "paraspinous line") bisects the intercristal line. An alternative technique, that of Chayen et al., moves the point of insertion about 3 cm distal to the intercristal line at the transverse process of L5[25] (Fig. 76-2). In this technique it is necessary to contact the L5 transverse process and then slide the needle superiorly and anteriorly above it. Several investigators have found that this technique reliably produces blockade of the femoral, lateral femoral cutaneous, and obturator nerves in almost 100% of patients.[26,27] In either approach, after the usual skin disinfectant is applied, a 4-inch, 22-gauge insulated regional block needle is advanced using nerve stimulator guidance through the marked site in a direction that is perpendicular to the back and all planes. While it may be tempting to consider ultrasonography to identify the lumbar plexus using a posterior approach, a study showed that this was not feasible.[28] A quadriceps femoris contraction, indicated by a "patellar snap," is the sought after endpoint when using a stimulating current of ≤0.4 mA. The femoral nerve is usually contacted at a depth of 4–9 cm from the skin, and, since it forms the medial component of the lumbar triplex, is the basis for injecting the

local anesthetic solution. If the initial needle insertion fails to elicit the desired response, then the needle is withdrawn and redirected slightly more medially in 1 cm increments until the patellar snap is found. The usual volume of local anesthetic is 30 mL, and the agents typically utilized are listed in Table 76-1. Successful blockade of the femoral nerve, obturator nerve, and lateral femoral cutaneous nerve was found in 95%, 90%, and 85% of patients, respectively, when using 0.4 mL/kg of 0.2% ropivacaine.[3] Using variable volumes of 0.35% bupivacaine, psoas compartment block produced 100%, 77%, and 97% successful blockade of the same three nerves.[29] In that same study the 3-in-1 block resulted in successful sensory analgesia in 93%, 47%, and 63% of the three nerves.[29] Continuous catheter techniques for major hip, thigh, or knee surgery were evaluated radiographically to determine catheter tip location.[30] Of the catheters inserted, 1.8% ended up in the epidural space while the other 98.2% produced successful lumbar plexus block.[30] Complications of this technique include cases of systemic local anesthetic toxicity from levobupivacaine[31] and retroperitoneal hematoma in a patient who was anticoagulated following the block.[32]

The inguinal paravascular technique of lumbar plexus block was described by Winnie[33] and is carried out as follows. The patient lies supine and the physician stands on the contralateral side of the anticipated surgery. After applying hemodynamic monitors and recording baseline vital signs, a modest dose of a short-acting sedative may be administered intravenously. The skin over the femoral triangle is disinfected in standard fashion, after which the lateral edge of the femoral arterial pulse is palpated about 1 to 2 cm beneath the inguinal ligament. A small skin wheal may be raised over the intended injection site using a 25-gauge needle and 1 to 2 mL of lidocaine. A 22-gauge, 2-inch insulated regional block needle is advanced using nerve stimulator guidance in a cephalad direction at about a 30° angle to the skin. Alternatively, a standard short-beveled needle may be used if one is undertaking the paresthesia approach. The needle is advanced lateral to the palpating index finger beneath the inguinal ligament until either a paresthesia of the femoral nerve is obtained, or a brisk motor response of the quadriceps muscle at ≤0.4 mA occurs ("patellar snap"—see section on femoral nerve block) indicating proximity of the needle tip to the femoral nerve. Ultrasonic guidance has been used successfully to reduce the time to perform the block, improve

TABLE 76-1. TYPICAL LOCAL ANESTHETICS USED FOR LUMBAR PLEXUS BLOCK

Local Anesthetic Agent	Surgical Anesthesia (Time to Onset) (minutes)	Surgical Anesthesia (Duration) (hours)	Duration of POA* (hours)
Mepivacaine 1.5%	10–15	2.5–3	5–6
Mepivacaine 1.5% + tetracaine 0.2%	10–15	3–4	8–12
Levobupivacaine 0.5%	20–30	4–5	12–16
Levobupivacaine 0.625%	10–15	5–7	16–24

* POA, postoperative analgesia.
All local anesthetics include epinephrine 1:200,000 (5 μg/mL).

complete sensory block, and reduce the amount of local anesthetic necessary for 3-in-1 block when compared to a nerve stimulator technique.[34,35] Following appropriate verification that the needle tip is situated in proximity to the femoral nerve (and is advanced sufficiently cephalad to assure that the tip is under the inguinal ligament), the needle is immobilized[36] and the desired volume of local anesthetic is injected while maintaining firm digital pressure distal to the needle to prevent retrograde flow and encourage cephalad spread of the local anesthetic.[37] The agent routinely chosen by the present authors is levobupivacaine, 0.625% with epinephrine 1:200,000 for a total volume of 20 to 30 mL.[38] Alternatively, the volume may be estimated by dividing the height of the patient in inches by three (i.e., for a 72-inch tall person, the dose would be about 72 divided by 3 = 24 mL). Increasing the volume of local anesthetic injected from 20 to 40 mL (mepivacaine 1%) produced a small but statistically insignificant increase in successful blockade of all three nerves. The obturator nerve was blocked in 62% of the low-volume group, and in 78% of the higher-volume group.[39] In one study the use of 0.25% ropivacaine was equivalent to 0.5% ropivacaine and 0.25% bupivacaine in providing 48-hour analgesia following total knee replacement using a single-injection technique.[40] Following total knee arthroplasty, the addition of epinephrine, 1:200,000 to variable ropivacaine concentrations (0.2% and 0.5%) for 3-in-1 block did not prolong postoperative analgesia.[41] For hip fracture repair in 10 patients over the age of 80 years, bupivacaine 2 mg/kg provided excellent analgesia without signs or symptoms of systemic toxicity or plasma levels exceeding 1.83 μg/mL.[42] Following arthroscopic knee surgery, ropivacaine 0.2% for 3-in-1 block was found not to be superior to intra-articular ropivacaine for postoperative analgesia.[43]

The major difference between 3-in-1 block and femoral nerve block is that a larger volume of local anesthetic and distal digital pressure are used for the former, in the hope that in addition to the femoral nerve, the obturator and lateral femoral cutaneous nerves are blocked. When compared to femoral nerve block for knee surgery, the 3-in-1 block provided a greater degree of muscle relaxation and a longer duration of postoperative analgesia.[44] The benefit of a single-injection technique of lumbar plexus block versus separate blocks of the femoral, lateral femoral cutaneous, and obturator nerves is that it avoids the multiple needle sticks to which the patient is exposed, with their inherent risk of neuropathy, as well as the larger volume of local anesthetic needed for individual blocks as compared to one single stick. The possibility of intravascular injection may also be less with single-injection techniques versus multiple individual nerve injections.

Continuous Techniques: If desired, continuous catheter techniques can be employed to prolong perioperative analgesia indefinitely.[45] First described by Rosenblatt in 1980,[46] the technique may utilize an intracath or an extracath or one of the currently available customized regional anesthesia catheter systems. For use of the continuous technique in patients with femoral fracture, care should be taken to minimize the strength of the current applied for evoked motor stimulation, since vigorous quadriceps muscle contraction occurring with larger currents may be quite painful. The limitation of the extracath technique is the inability to advance the catheter much beyond the level of the inguinal ligament. Because of the greater distance between the needle entry site and the lumbar plexus than

for example for axillary brachial plexus block, the intracath technique has become more popular when continuous techniques are desired.[47,48] The local anesthetic of choice for continuous lumbar plexus techniques following knee surgery may be bupivacaine 0.125%, since this is the concentration found to be as effective as 0.25% bupivacaine, but which is associated with lower plasma bupivacaine levels.[49] In early studies most intracaths were advanced 15 to 20 cm into the femoral sheath, and the results were uniformly good. Singelyn et al. compared catheter advancement 13 ± 2 cm versus 26 ± 3 cm from the skin.[50] They found that complete "3-in-1" block was more likely following less cephalad catheter placements. Twenty-three percent (23/100) continuous catheters advanced using the inguinal paravascular approach and advanced from between 16 to 20 cm actually reached the lumbar plexus when evaluated using contrast media and pelvic radiography.[51] Whether or not 3-in-1 blocks do in fact block three nerves, at least two studies have documented lower pain scores with less opioid use postoperatively in patients who received continuous 3-in-1 blocks added to a general anesthetic compared to those individuals who received general anesthesia alone.[52,53] When compared to parenteral opioids or intraarticular analgesia for postoperative pain relief following knee surgery, continuous 3-in-1 blocks provides better analgesia with less side effects.[54–56] The technique has been shown comparable to epidural analgesia for providing postoperative analgesia.[57]

Complications of continuous techniques are similar to those occurring after single-shot blocks and include femoral neuropathy and femoral nerve compression from a subfascial hematoma.[58,59] Systemic toxic reactions to local anesthetic may also occur from intravascular injection or from exceeding the recommended local dosing limits.[60] Arterial puncture and intravascular catheter placement, although rare, do occur, as does epidural block from advancing the catheter too far cephalad.[60]

FEMORAL NERVE BLOCK

Anatomic Considerations: The femoral nerve (L2–L4) courses from the lumbar plexus in the groove between the psoas major and iliacus muscles, where it enters the thigh by passing deep to the inguinal ligament. At the level of the groin crease, the femoral nerve lies anterior to the iliopsoas muscle and slightly lateral to the femoral artery (Figs. 76-3 and 76-4). At or above the inguinal ligament the femoral nerve divides into anterior and posterior divisions; the anterior (superficial) division innervates the skin over the anterior thigh and supplies the sartorius muscle, and the posterior (deep) division innervates the quadriceps femoris muscle, the knee joint and its medial ligament, and also is the division from which the saphenous nerve is derived. Therefore, posterior division block is essential for successful femoral nerve block for procedures of the anterior thigh and knee. The two divisions may lay one behind the other (Fig. 76-3) (as their names suggest, respectively), or side-by-side at the level of the groin crease (Fig. 76-4). Both divisions lie deep to the fascia iliaca. Stimulation of the anterior division results in muscle contraction of the medial thigh ("sartorius twitch"). The branches from the anterior division are primarily sensory and the branches from the posterior division, primarily motor. The technique of femoral nerve block is similar to the inguinal paravascular block of the lumbar plexus as described above. Recently, an algorithm has been developed to maximize the likelihood of attaining success

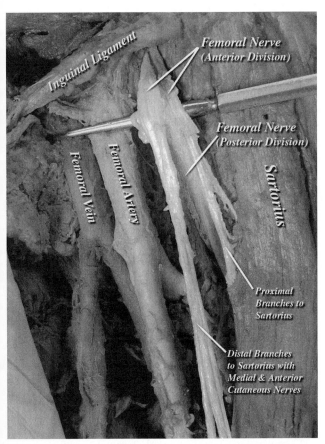

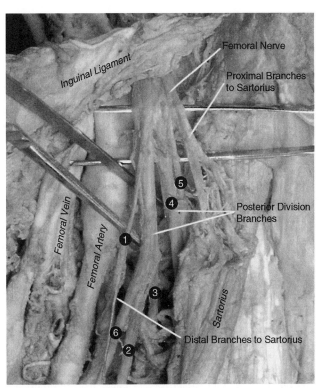

FIGURE 76-3. Cadaver dissection of the left femoral nerve, associated vascular structures, and the inguinal ligament. The posterior division of the femoral nerve is truly posterior to the anterior division, and is seated somewhat medially.

FIGURE 76-4. Cadaver dissection of a left femoral nerve, demonstrating a femoral nerve where the anterior and posterior divisions are seated side by side. 1, Distal branches to the sartorius; 2, saphenous nerve; 3, nerve to the vastus lateralis; 4, 5, intermediate and medial femoral cutaneous nerves; 6, nerve to the vastus medialis.

when the nerve stimulator guided approach is used[61] (Fig. 76-5). The algorithm was derived following cadaver dissections that determined that the nerve supply to the quadratus femoris (posterior division of the femoral nerve) is truly posterior (50%), posterolateral (29%), or posteromedial (21%) to that supplying the sartorius muscle (anterior division of the femoral nerve).

Indications for Femoral Nerve Block: Femoral nerve block is appropriate for managing pain due to a fractured shaft of the femur, for perioperative pain management following knee surgeries including total knee arthroplasty[62-64] or anterior cruciate ligament reconstruction,[65-67] or for skin graft donor sites of the anterior thigh. It may also suffice for analgesia following quadriceps tendon repair and in hemiplegic patients for the reduction of quadriceps spasticity.[68] It has been used in a patient-controlled analgesia (PCA) mode for analgesia following total hip arthroplasty.[69] Combined with a sciatic nerve block, femoral nerve block typically provides outstanding perioperative analgesia for a variety of procedures both above and below the knee joint. One study demonstrated reduced opioid use in patients who received femoral nerve injections versus systemic opioid infusions following total knee arthroplasty.[70] Compared to spinal block for saphenous vein stripping surgery, femoral and genitofemoral nerve blocks provided superior analgesia and faster recovery times.[71] Although one study

suggested that femoral nerve block is minimally effective in reducing analgesic requirements following anterior cruciate ligament reconstruction,[67] a large review of 1,200 cases seems to indicate that this is a valuable modality for reducing pain following complex knee surgeries.[72]

Technique of Femoral Nerve Block: The technique of femoral nerve block is carried out as follows. The patient lies supine with the leg on the operative side extended and resting upon the gurney. After uncovering the intended injection side (continuing to cover the genitalia and perineum), the anesthesiologist standing on the contralateral side palpates the femoral arterial pulsation. The skin is marked using a felt-tipped marking pen, and is disinfected in standard fashion. After administering a small dose of a sedative-hypnotic and ascertaining that baseline vital signs are stable, a small skin wheal is raised 2 to 3 cm beneath the inguinal ligament at the level of the groin crease,[73] 1 cm lateral to the arterial pulsation, using a 25-gauge needle and 1 to 3 mL of lidocaine. The advantages of performing the block at the inguinal crease level versus the level of the inguinal ligament (as for the inguinal paravascular lumbar plexus block described above) include the superficial and easy access of the femoral nerve and artery at the inguinal crease; the width of the nerve at this level is greatest; and, the more consistent relationship of the femoral nerve to the artery.[74] A 22-gauge, short-beveled, 2-inch insulated regional block needle is advanced from the injection site in a cephalad direction at a 60° angle to the skin surface. A peripheral nerve stimulator

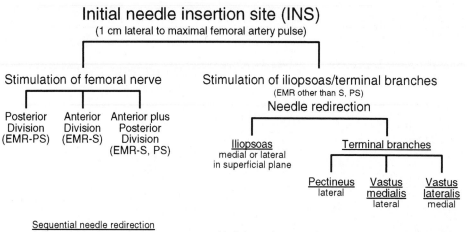

FIGURE 76-5. Algorithm for maximizing success using neuro-stimulation-assisted femoral nerve block (FNB).

is used to isolate the "patellar snap" (quadriceps femoris muscle contraction) at a stimulating current of ≤0.4 mA. If the sartorius twitch is observed on the lower medial thigh, the stimulating needle should be advanced an additional 5 to 10 mm to stimulate the posterior division of the nerve, since that branch is deep to the fascia iliaca, and it is possible that the stimulating needle is stimulating the anterior division through the fascia. If simple advancement of the needle fails to still elicit a patellar snap, the needle should be withdrawn and advanced in a posterolateral direction in 2 to 3 mm increments. If the patellar snap is still not attained, or if direct stimulation of the sartorius muscle occurs indicated by local muscle contraction, the needle is too far laterally situated, and must be withdrawn and reinserted in a posteromedial direction. This situation corresponds to a posterior division that is most likely behind and medial to the anterior division (Fig. 76-3). Once a brisk patellar snap is observed, a volume of 20 to 25 mL of local anesthetic is incrementally injected with continual intermittent aspiration every 2 mL. The agent most frequently utilized by the present authors is levobupivacaine, 0.5% with epinephrine, 1:200,000. Alternatively, for shorter-duration block, 1% to 1.5% lidocaine or mepivacaine with epinephrine may be employed (Table 76-1). Casati et al. found that the minimal local anesthetic volume resulting in successful femoral nerve block in 50% of patients was 14 ± 2 mL of 0.5% ropivacaine and 15 ± 2 mL of bupivacaine 0.5%.[75] Mulroy et al. noted that 25 mL of 0.25% bupivacaine provided equivalent duration analgesia to 0.5% of the same agent when anterior cruciate ligament surgery was performed using epidural anesthesia.[76] Patient-controlled femoral nerve analgesia using 0.2% ropivacaine following major knee surgery was equivalent to continuous infusion techniques, but was associated with lower total ropivacaine doses.[77] Successful block is indicated by saphenous nerve sensory analgesia, since the saphenous nerve is the terminal branch of the posterior division of the femoral nerve and provides sensory innervation to the medial malleolus and medial side of the leg, and quadriceps muscle weakness which ensures motor block of the posterior division. Patients, when asked to "kick out their leg like a dancing Rockette" will be

unable to extend the flexed leg below the knee joint. If the femoral nerve block is inadequate for surgery or analgesia (i.e., the saphenous nerve sensory block is absent or spotty, and/or the muscles innervated by the quadriceps are not paretic), the nerve block may be supplemented using the fascia iliaca block (see below).

Complications associated with femoral nerve block are identical to inguinal paravascular block described above and include vascular perforation with hematoma formation, intravascular injection, femoral nerve palsy, and even epidural block if a continuous catheter is advanced from the injection site more than 20 cm cephalad. Some 57% of 208 continuous catheters removed at 48 hours tested positive for bacterial colonization, although no cellulitis or abscesses occurred.[78] It is important to recall that femoral nerve block is not appropriate for patients who have previously undergone ilioinguinal surgery including vascular grafting and resection of tumors or large inguinal lymph nodes, nor is it appropriate in cases of preexisting femoral neuropathy or if local skin infection or peritoneal infection is noted.

LATERAL FEMORAL CUTANEOUS NERVE BLOCK

Anatomic Considerations: The lateral femoral cutaneous nerve (LFCN) is a purely sensory nerve that is derived from L2–L3 caudad to the ilioinguinal nerve. After emerging from the lateral border of the psoas major muscle, the LFCN lies deep to the fascia lata, medial and inferior to the anterior superior iliac spine (ASIS). The LFCN enters the thigh below the inguinal ligament, medial or lateral to the ASIS. This inconsistent location of the nerve implies that a relatively large volume of local anesthetic may need to be deposited beneath the shelving iliac crest when blocking the nerve using the ASIS as the landmark and proceeding blindly. However, the relationship of the LFCN to the tendinous origin of the sartorius muscle is consistent (Fig. 76-6), and beneath the inguinal ligament the infiltration of local anesthetic between the skin and the sartorius typically results in LFCN block. The LFCN divides

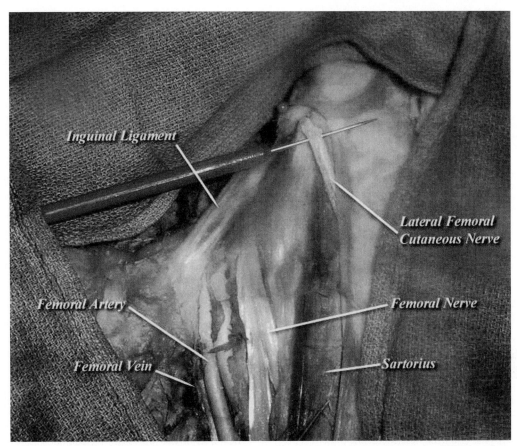

FIGURE 76-6. Cadaver dissection of the left thigh demonstrating the lateral femoral cutaneous nerve (LFCN) and its relationship to the sartorius muscle beneath the inguinal ligament.

into anterior and posterior branches about 7 to 10 cm below the ASIS. The anterior branch supplies the skin over the anterolateral aspect of the thigh as low as the knee, and the posterior branch passes through the fascia lata before passing rearwards to supply the skin on the lateral aspect of the thigh from just below the greater trochanter to about the middle of the thigh. Although both branches are sensory, a peripheral nerve stimulator may be used to identify the posterior branch of the LFCN. In this regard, LFCN stimulator-guided block is highly successful (100%) using a smaller volume of local anesthetic than for the blind infiltration technique.

Indications for LFCN Block: Indications for block of the LFCN include analgesia of a skin graft donor site on the lateral thigh, for performing muscle biopsies during work-up of malignant hyperthermia, or as a supplement to femoral and sciatic nerve blocks for lower extremity surgery where a thigh tourniquet will be required. LFCN block is an important aid in diagnosing the syndrome of meralgia paresthetica. Lack of significant pain relief in the presence of demonstrable analgesia in the lateral thigh area following the block may indicate a more proximal source of lateral thigh pain, including lumbar radiculopathy or intrapelvic pathology. Treatment of meralgia paresthetica may include repeated LFCN blocks using combinations of local anesthetics and corticosteroids. Since the anterior branch of the LFCN forms part of the patellar plexus, LFCN block is indicated along with other blocks

for successful analgesia following surgery on the knee including anterior cruciate ligament reconstruction and total knee arthroplasty. Following femoral neck surgery, LFCN block reduced opioid requirements postoperatively in a group of elderly patients.[79]

Technique of LFCN Block: The sensory stimulation LFCN technique is undertaken as follows.[80] The patient lies in the supine position, and the ASIS is marked using a felt-tipped marking pen. A point 2 cm medial and inferior to the ASIS is identified and also marked.[81] The negative lead of a neuromuscular blockade monitor is placed on the marked site, and the monitor is set to deliver a 2 to 3 mA current using a single-twitch cycle. The lead is moved from medial to lateral until a paresthesia is elicited corresponding to the innervation of the lateral thigh in the distribution of the posterior branch of the LFCN. This should represent an area variably described as an oblong spheroid shape on the lateral thigh from the greater trochanter inferiorly to the knee. The paresthesia should coincide with the nerve stimulation, i.e., the "beep" of the blockade monitor. An uninsulated 22-gauge, 2-inch regional block needle connected to the nerve stimulator is then introduced and the same paresthesia should be elicited at 0.5 to 0.6 mA at 1 Hz. A total volume of 5 to 8 mL of local anesthetic should be incrementally injected in divided doses. Success rates have been reported to be higher (100% versus 40%) with this approach as compared to the classic technique.[80]

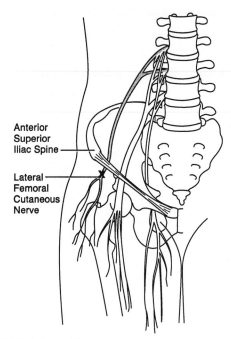

Anterior Superior Iliac Spine

Lateral Femoral Cutaneous Nerve

FIGURE 76-7. Lateral femoral cutaneous nerve block. The needle is inserted 2 cm medial and 2 cm inferior to the anterior superior iliac spine.

The blind infiltration technique of LFCN block (so-called "classic approach") has also been described. The patient is positioned as above, and the ASIS is again marked. A second point, 2 cm medial and 2 cm caudad to the ASIS is also marked. A 22-gauge, 2-inch short beveled needle is advanced through a local anesthetic skin wheal at this second point in a direction towards the ASIS (point one). As the needle traverses the fascia lata, a distinct "pop" will be felt. The local anesthetic may be deposited in a fanwise manner, both above and below the fascia lata, specifically between the fascia lata and the sartorius (Fig. 76-7). An acceptable volume of local anesthetic for complete LFCN block is about 15 to 20 mL. Alternatively, the needle may be introduced as described above and may be directed laterally and cephalad to place its tip beneath the iliac bone, inferior and medial to the ASIS. At this point, the local anesthetic is deposited in a fanwise manner beneath the shelving iliac crest. Spillover of local anesthetic is always a possibility when performing LFCN block, and one study suggested that 35% of patients blocked using the traditional "fanwise injection" technique and 5% of those blocked with a nerve stimulator demonstrated quadriceps muscle weakness following the block.[80]

OBTURATOR NERVE BLOCK

Anatomic Considerations: The obturator nerve is derived from L2–L4, although the contribution from L2 is frequently small or even nonexistent.[81] The nerve emerges at the upper level of the medial border of the psoas major muscle at the approximate level of the sacroiliac joint and passes behind the iliac vessels from which it is separated by the fascia iliaca (Fig. 76-1). It continues its downward course with the iliac vessels and obturator artery and vein along the obturator groove and passes through the obturator foramen into the thigh.

At the level of the obturator foramen or canal, the nerve divides into two terminal branches (anterior and posterior) that supply the medial thigh. The anterior branch supplies an articular branch to the hip joint, and anterior adductor muscles (pectineus, adductor longus, adductor brevis) and a small cutaneous contribution to the medial and inferior thigh. The posterior branch innervates the deep adductor muscles (adductor brevis and magnus, obturator externus) and frequently sends a contribution to the knee joint. This small contribution may be important for determining analgesia following knee surgeries. Up to 30% of individuals may have a small, accessory obturator nerve derived from the ventral rami of L3 and L4. This accessory branch may give off rami to the pectineus and hip joint.[82]

Indications for Obturator Nerve Block: The obturator nerve is a mixed nerve with a significant motor function. Indications for blocking the nerve include diagnosis and management of painful conditions of the hip and for the relief of adductor spasm of the hip. Radiofrequency lesioning of sensory branches of the nerve was successfully used to treat hip joint pain in 14 patients.[83] The block is also a valuable adjunct to femoral and lateral femoral cutaneous nerve blocks for surgeries of the knee as detailed above, or for analgesia for surgical tourniquets placed on the thigh. In a group of 60 patients, obturator block provided superior analgesia when combined with femoral and sciatic nerve blocks for total knee replacement, versus those cases unaccompanied by obturator block.[84] The block is used as a diagnostic aid for painful syndromes of the hip joint, inguinal area or lumbar spine, or for relief of pain due to severe osteoarthritis of the hip. The nerve may also be blocked as an adjunct for transurethral surgeries for bladder tumors, since subarachnoid block or general anesthesia without the aid of muscle relaxants does not routinely prevent adductor muscle contractions that could contribute to bladder perforation, bleeding, or incomplete resection.[85,86] A study showed that isolated obturator nerve block proved superior to 3-in-1 block for preventing thigh adduction during operative electrocautery for transurethral surgery.[87] In a subsequent study by the same investigators, however, the two were roughly equivalent with regards preventing adduction, and, furthermore, the 3-in-1 block produced lower mean and peak plasma lidocaine levels even though the dose administered was 133% higher than that used for bilateral obturator blocks.[88]

Technique of Obturator Nerve Block: The nerve is blocked with the patient in the supine position and the leg to be blocked slightly abducted. The pubic tubercle is palpated and a local anesthetic skin wheal is raised 1 to 2 cm below and 1 to 2 cm lateral to it. A short-beveled, 22-gauge, 3.5-inch needle is advanced through the skin wheal in a slightly mesiad direction until the ramus of the pubis is contacted. Once the horizontal ramus is identified, typically at a depth of about 1.5 to 4 cm, the needle is withdrawn and re-advanced cephalad to attempt to enter the obturator canal. This should occur at a depth about 2 to 3 cm deeper than that at which the ramus was contacted. Once the canal has been contacted, the needle must again be withdrawn and redirected slightly laterally and inferiorly until it enters the obturator canal (Fig. 76-8). Once within the canal, the needle is advanced 2 to 3 cm, and, after ascertaining via negative aspiration that the obturator vessels

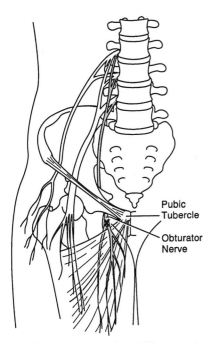

FIGURE 76-8. Obturator nerve block. The site of needle insertion is 1 to 2 cm inferior and 1 to 2 cm lateral to the pubic tubercle. The needle is redirected in a lateral and superior direction after the horizontal ramus of the pubic bone is contacted.

have not been punctured, 10 to 15 mL of local anesthetic are incrementally injected. It is essential to identify the bony wall of the obturator canal to verify that the needle has not entered contiguous structures such as the rectum or vagina, which lie medially and superiorly.[81] As an alternative technique, a peripheral nerve stimulator may be used to find the nerve. In this approach, the 22-gauge insulated regional block needle is advanced until adduction of the thigh is noted at stimulating currents of ≤0.4 mA. Successful block is heralded by the onset of weakness of thigh adduction. Reliance upon testing the medial inferior thigh for sensory analgesia is faulty, since the obturator nerve makes a variable and inconsistent contribution to sensory innervation in that area.[81] Bouaziz et al. injected 7 mL of 0.75% bupivacaine directly over the obturator nerve and found that there was no sensory branch from the nerve in 57% of patients (17/30).[89] Their conclusion was that the only way to assess obturator nerve block is to check adductor strength. Using this approach with lidocaine, it was determined that up to 300 mg (15 mL of 2% solution) provided plasma lidocaine concentrations that were safe and effective following bilateral block.[90] A modification of the above-mentioned techniques is the use of the upper end of the adductor longus muscle as a landmark for needle insertion.[91] The needle was directed laterally and cephalad using nerve stimulator guidance, and resulted in a higher success rate (80% versus 60%) than the traditional block.

Potential side effects and complications of obturator block include intravascular injection, nerve injury with resultant neuropraxia or neurotmesis, and the aforementioned injection into contiguous, unintentional sites such as the rectum or vagina. Obturator arterial injury has also been reported in a patient undergoing resection of a bladder tumor.[92]

SAPHENOUS NERVE BLOCK

Anatomic Considerations: The saphenous nerve is the only cutaneous branch of the posterior division of the femoral nerve. It arises in the femoral triangle, descends lateral to the femoral artery, then enters the adductor canal of Hunter where it crosses in front of the artery.[93] The nerve exits the lower part of the canal by emerging between the sartorius and gracilis muscles. Immediately upon leaving the adductor canal, the saphenous nerve gives off its infrapatellar branch which pierces the sartorius muscle and is distributed to the skin immediately below the knee. The saphenous nerve then runs down the medial border of the tibia immediately behind the saphenous vein, crosses with the vein in front of the medial malleolus and reaches the base of the great toe. The saphenous nerve supplies an extensive cutaneous area over the medial side of the knee, leg, ankle, and foot.[93]

Indications for Saphenous Nerve Blockade: The saphenous nerve is usually blocked below the knee as part of the ankle block. In the pain clinic the nerve is blocked individually in patients with saphenous neuralgia or saphenous nerve entrapment at the adductor canal.[94]

Techniques of Saphenous Nerve Blockade: There are several approaches to blockade of the saphenous nerve. The saphenous nerve can be blocked above the knee, at the level of the knee, below the knee, and just above the medial malleolus. Blockade above the knee includes the perifemoral, subsartorial, and transsartorial approaches,[95–98] while blockade at the level of the knee includes the paracondylar saphenous field block (PSFB)[99,100] and the nerve stimulator technique[101] where the nerve is blocked at the level of the medial femoral condyle. The saphenous nerve has also been blocked by subcutaneous infiltration below the knee distal to the medial condyle of the tibia (below the knee field block (BKFB))[102,103] and the paravenous approach.[104] Finally, the saphenous nerve can be blocked just above the medial malleolus of the foot.[102,103]

PERIFEMORAL APPROACH: The site of needle insertion is 5 to 6 cm below the inguinal crease, 0.5 cm lateral to the femoral artery.[105] At 2 to 4 cm depth, the nerve to the vastus medialis muscle is stimulated with a nerve stimulator, at ≤0.4 mA, resulting in the contraction of the medial aspect of the thigh. The vastus medialis muscle contracts secondary to stimulation of the nerve to the vastus medialis muscle which runs alongside the saphenous nerve. The nerve to the vastus medialis muscle is used as a landmark to locate the saphenous nerve since the saphenous nerve is purely a sensory nerve.[95] Other investigators insert their needle on the line of the inguinal fold.[97] The higher needle insertion may block the other muscular branches of the femoral nerve resulting in thigh muscle weakness.

SUBSARTORIAL APPROACH: The needle is inserted in the middle third of the thigh, in the groove between the vastus medialis muscle and the sartorius muscle.[95] The groove is felt by rolling the finger from the lateral to the medial side of the middle of the thigh. Identification of the site of needle insertion is difficult although the sartorius muscle can be made more prominent by flexing the knee and laterally rotating the hip in semiflexion and abduction, i.e., squatting position.[95,96]

Weakness of the thigh muscles is less with this approach because of the more distal site of local anesthetic injection. However, it is more difficult to perform because of the difficulty in locating the groove between the sartorius and the vastus medialis muscles.

TRANSSARTORIAL APPROACH: The sartorius muscle is identified; this is facilitated in the supine patient who elevates the extended leg. The site of needle insertion is 3 to 4 cm superior and 6 to 8 cm posterior to the superomedial border of the patella.[105] The insulated needle is inserted at an angle of 45° caudally and directed slightly posteriorly. Paresthesia is elicited with a nerve stimulator at ≤0.6 mA at 3 to 5 cm depth.

In the original description of the transsartorial technique, a 17-gauge Touhy needle is inserted at one fingerwidth above the patella.[98] The needle is inserted at an angle of 45° from the coronal plane and advanced in a caudad direction, through the belly of the sartorius muscle, until a loss of resistance is felt at a depth of 1.5 to 3 cm. This implies that the needle tip is at the adductor hiatus and the local anesthetic is injected. In our study[105] we found that paresthesia to the medial leg and foot with the nerve stimulator was a very reliable indicator of saphenous nerve stimulation and consequent blockade.

PARACONDYLAR APPROACH: The medial condyle of the femur is palpated. The needle is inserted perpendicular to the skin and advanced slowly until paresthesia along the saphenous nerve is elicited or until bone is contacted.[99] Local anesthetic is injected while the needle is inserted until it reaches the patella and when paresthesia is elicited. Several fanwise insertions are apparently sufficient to locate the nerve. Local anesthetic is also injected posterior to the medial femoral condyle.[100] The success rate of this approach in anesthetizing the medial aspect of the leg is 25% to 40%.

BELOW THE KNEE FIELD BLOCK: A linear subcutaneous injection of local anesthetic is made immediately below the insertion of the sartorius tendon at the tibial tubercle.[102,103] The infiltration is made in an anterior and posterior direction up to the anteromedial aspect of the gastrocnemius muscle.

Another approach in this area is the paravenous approach[104] wherein the saphenous vein is identified in the medial head of the gastrocnemius muscle at the level of the tibial tubercle. Subcutaneous infiltration is made lateral and medial to the saphenous vein. In this technique the patient's leg hangs down and a tourniquet is used to make the saphenous vein prominent. A success rate of 100% has been reported with this technique. The disadvantages of the technique include the difficulty of identifying the vein in obese patients and the absence of the vein in patients who had varicose vein stripping.

BLOCKADE AT THE MEDIAL MALLEOLUS: Local anesthetic is injected subcutaneously above the medial malleolus of the foot.[102,106] The injection extended anteriorly and posteriorly above the medial malleolus. Other authors recommended a subcutaneous infiltration around the great saphenous vein, immediately above the medial malleolus.[107]

A 10 mL volume of local anesthetic is injected with each of the above approaches. The reported success rates of the different approaches ranged from 80% with the perifemoral approach, 90% with the transsartorial approach, 40% with the paracondylar approach, and 40% to 65% with the below the knee

field block. We compared the different approaches of saphenous nerve blockade using a nerve stimulator technique and confirmed the effectiveness of the transsartorial approach.[105] In some instances, supplementary blockade of the medial cutaneous nerve of the superficial peroneal nerve may have to be performed to ensure complete numbness of the medial side of the foot.[105]

FASCIA ILIACA BLOCK

Anatomical Considerations: The femoral nerve, LFCN, and obturator nerve run a considerable part of their course close to the inner aspect of the fascia iliaca. The fascia iliaca is attached medially to the vertebral column and upper part of the sacrum. It covers the psoas muscle and iliacus muscle and is attached to the inner lip of the iliac crest and pelvic brim. At the groin the fascia iliaca is continuous with the posterior margin of the inguinal ligament. Laterally it attaches to the ASIS. Medially, it blends with the pectineal fascia. The fascia iliaca reflection thus forms a triangular potential space, the "fascia iliaca compartment." Through this compartment the three major terminal nerves of the lumbar plexus pass. Distally at the level of the femoral triangle, the fascia iliaca becomes narrow. It is covered by the fascia lata and forms the roof of an adipose-filled space known as the lacuna musculorum, which lies adjacent to the femoral vessels. It is postulated that the injection of a sufficient volume of local anesthetic solution into the lacuna musculorum favors cephalad migration towards the iliacus muscle, facilitating spread of local anesthetic within the entire fascia iliaca compartment and resulting in blockade of all three component nerves (femoral, obturator, LFCN) that lie within it.[108]

Indications for Fascia Iliaca Block: The indications for fascia iliaca block are identical to those of inguinal paravascular lumbar plexus block. The technique has been successfully used in the prehospital treatment of femoral fractures in 27 patients and was found to provide excellent analgesia.[109] A case report detailed the use of this block in an elderly patient with a history of epidural abscess undergoing bilateral total knee arthroplasty.[110] In a study of 62 patients undergoing total knee arthroplasty catheters advanced 15 to 20 cm using this approach and infused with 0.2% bupivacaine resulted in excellent analgesia and opioid-sparing effects.[111] Forty percent of the catheter tips were situated superior to the upper third of the sacroiliac joint as determined by computed tomography.[111]

Technique of Fascia Iliaca Block: The technique of fascia iliaca block is as follows. The patient lies supine as for inguinal paravascular lumbar plexus block or for femoral nerve block. Anatomical landmarks are assessed including the projection of the inguinal ligament (the line between the pubic tubercle and the ASIS). This line is drawn using a felt-tipped marking pen, and it is then trisected. The needle entry site is 1 cm distal to the point where the middle and lateral thirds of the inguinal line meet. To simplify the block concept, the injection point can be considered to be midway between traditional femoral nerve block and traditional lateral femoral cutaneous nerve block. After raising a local anesthetic skin wheal as for the techniques previously described, the 22-gauge short-beveled regional block needle is inserted at the marked site and advanced in a cephalad direction at a 75° angle to the skin.

Alternatively, a 20-gauge Tuohy-type needle may be substituted. The "loss of resistance" (tissue "pop") will be appreciated as the needle tip traverses the fascia lata.[112] The needle continues to be advanced, however, until a second loss of resistance is experienced. This second loss of resistance corresponds to the needle entering and passing through the fascia iliaca. The 75° angle of the needle to the skin is then reduced to about 30° and the needle is advanced an additional 1 cm cephalad. After negative aspiration tests, a volume of local anesthetic (25 to 30 mL) is incrementally injected in divided doses. In 20 children receiving the fascia iliac block for thigh surgery plasma bupivacaine levels were significantly lower when epinephrine 1:200,000 was added to the local anesthetic.[113]

Fascia iliaca block has compared favorably to 3-in-1 block for a variety of scenarios in children and adults.[112] In Dalens' early report, the fascia iliaca block was effective in >90% of children undergoing lower limb surgery, versus a much lower 20% rate of successful analgesia using the 3-in-1 block.[112] In adults the fascia iliaca block using lidocaine was more effective than 3-in-1 blocks for simultaneously blocking the LFCN and the femoral nerve. Dye spread beneath the fascia iliaca was observed in 10% of the 3-in-1 blocks and in 36% of the fascia iliaca group.[108] Some 44 patients undergoing upper leg surgery had continuous catheters placed either using the 3-in-1 approach to the lumbar plexus, or the fascia iliaca block. No significant difference was observed in the location of the catheter tips beneath the fascia iliaca, and analgesia was also similar in the two groups, further blurring the distinction in evaluating the efficacy of similar techniques such as these two.[114]

KEY POINTS

- The lumbar plexus originates from the anterior primary rami of L1 through L4 and courses between the psoas major muscle and quadratus lumborum muscle, with the proximal plexus lying in the substance of the former.
- The obturator nerve is unreliably blocked when using the inguinal paravascular approach (3-in-1 block) to lumbar plexus block.
- The femoral nerve is derived from L2 through L4 and at the groin crease lies anterior to the iliopsoas muscle and slightly lateral to the femoral artery. The anterior division of the nerve innervates the sartorius muscle, and the posterior division innervates the quadriceps femoris muscle.
- The LFCN is a pure sensory nerve and is derived from L2 to L3 anterior primary rami. It divides into anterior and posterior branches 7 to 10 cm below the ASIS. LFCN block is a useful diagnostic and therapeutic modality for the syndrome known as meralgia paresthetica.
- The major contributing branches to the obturator nerve are the anterior primary rami of L3 and L4. The anterior branch of the obturator nerve supplies an articular branch to the hip joint and anterior adductor muscles; the posterior branch innervates the deep adductor muscles. Obturator nerve block is useful for relieving spastic conditions of the thigh.
- The saphenous nerve is the only cutaneous branch of the posterior division of the femoral nerve. Of the different approaches to saphenous nerve blockade, the transsartorial approach seems to be the most effective without causing weakness of the thigh muscles. The use of a nerve stimulator aids in identifying the saphenous nerve. There may be a

cross-innervation of the medial aspect of the foot. In some patients the superficial peroneal nerve also innervates the area.
- Fascia iliaca block is a technique of blocking the femoral, lateral femoral cutaneous, and obturator nerves using a single-injection technique. A double loss-of-resistance technique is utilized through the fascia lata and the fascia iliaca to access the nerves. The technique is useful for treating painful femoral fractures and for providing postoperative analgesia following total knee arthroplasty.

REFERENCES

1. Farny J, Drolet P, Girard M: Anatomy of the posterior approach to the lumbar plexus block. Can J Anaesth 41:480–485, 1994.
2. Dietemann J, Sick H, Wolfram-Gabel R, et al: Anatomy and computed tomography of the normal lumbosacral plexus. Neuroradiology 29:58–68, 1987.
3. Capdevila X, Macaire P, Dadure C, et al: Continuous psoas compartment block for postoperative analgesia after total hip arthroplasty: New landmarks, technical guidelines, and clinical evaluation. Anesth Analg 94:1606–1613, 2002.
4. Lang S, Yip R, Chang P: The femoral 3-in-1 block revisited. J Clin Anesth 5:292–296, 1993.
5. Parkinson S, Mueller J, Little W, et al: Extent of blockade with various approaches to the lumbar plexus. Anesth Analg 68:243–248, 1989.
6. Spillane W: 3-in-1 blocks and continuous 3-in-1 blocks. Reg Anesth 17:175–176, 1992.
7. Ritter J: Femoral nerve "sheath" for inguinal paravascular lumbar plexus block is not found in human cadavers. J Clin Anesth 7:470–473, 1995.
8. Madej T, Ellis F, Halsall P: Evaluation of the "3-in-1" lumbar plexus block in patients having muscle biopsy. Br J Anaesth 62:515–517, 1989.
9. Marhofer P, Nasel C, Sitzwohl C, Kapral S: Magnetic resonance imaging of the distribution of local anesthetic during the three-in-one block. Anesth Analg 90:119–124, 2000.
10. Marhofer P, Schrogendorfer K, Andel H, et al: Combined sciatic nerve–3 in 1 block in high risk patient (German). Anasthesiol Intensivmed Notfallmed Schmerzther 33:399–401, 1998.
11. Hadzic A, Vloka J, Saff G, et al: The "three-in-one block" for treatment of pain in a patient with acute herpes zoster infection. Reg Anesth 22:575–578, 1997.
12. Capdevila X, Biboulet P, Bouregba M, et al: Bilateral continuous 3-in-1 nerve blockade for postoperative pain relief after bilateral femoral shaft surgery. J Clin Anesth 10:606–609, 1998.
13. Edwards N, Wright E: Continuous low-dose 3-in-1 nerve blockade for postoperative pain relief after total knee replacement. Anesth Analg 75:265–267, 1992.
14. Fournier R, Van Gessel E, Gaggero G, et al: Postoperative analgesia with "3-in-1" femoral nerve block with prosthetic hip surgery. Can J Anaesth 45:34–38, 1998.
15. Singelyn F, Deyaert M, Joris D, et al: Effects of intravenous patient-controlled analgesia with morphine, continuous epidural analgesia, and continuous three-in-one block on postoperative pain and knee rehabilitation after unilateral total knee arthroplasty. Anesth Analg 87:88–92, 1998.
16. Chelly J, Casati A, Al-Samsam T, et al: Continuous lumbar plexus block for acute postoperative pain management after open reduction and internal fixation of acetabular fractures. J Orthop Trauma 17:362–367, 2003.
17. Ho A, Karmakar M: Combined paravertebral lumbar plexus and parasacral sciatic nerve block for reduction of hip fracture in a patient with severe aortic stenosis. Can J Anaesth 49:946–950, 2002.

18. Horlocker T, Hebl J, Kinney M, Cabanela M: Opioid-free analgesia following total knee arthroplasty – A multimodal approach using continuous lumbar plexus (psoas compartment) block, acetaminophen, and ketorolac. Reg Anesth Pain Med 27:105–108, 2002.

19. Vaghadia H, Kapnoudhis P, Jenkins L, et al: Continuous lumbosacral block using a Tuohy needle and catheter technique. Can J Anaesth 39:75–78, 1992.

20. Ben-David B, Lee E, Critoru M: Psoas block for surgical repair of hip fracture: A case report and description of a catheter technique. Anesth Analg 71:298–301, 1990.

21. Elmas C, Atanassoff P: Combined inguinal paravascular (3-in-1) and sciatic nerve blocks for lower limb surgery. Reg Anesth 18:88–92, 1993.

22. Buckenmaier CC 3rd, Xenos J, Nilsen S: Lumbar plexus block with perineural catheter and sciatic nerve block for total hip arthroplasty. J Arthroplasty 17:499–502, 2002.

23. Luber M, Greengrass R, Vail T: Patient satisfaction and effectiveness of lumbar plexus and sciatic nerve block for total knee arthroplasty. J Arthroplasty 16:17–21, 2001.

24. Stevens R, Van Gessel E, Flory N, et al: Lumbar plexus block reduces pain and blood loss associated with total hip arthroplasty. Anesthesiology 93:115–121, 2000.

25. Chayen D, Nathan H, Chayen M: The psoas compartment block. Anesthesiology 45:95–99, 1976.

26. Farny J, Girard M, Drolet P: Posterior approach to the lumbar plexus combined with a sciatic nerve block using lidocaine. Can J Anaesth 41:486–491, 1994.

27. Virachit K, Girard M: The utilization of 2-chloroprocaine for blocks of the lumbar plexus and sciatic nerve (French). Can J Anaesth 41:919–924, 1994.

28. Kirchmair L, Entner T, Wissel J, et al: A study of the paravertebral anatomy for ultrasound-guided posterior lumbar plexus block. Anesth Analg 93:477–481, 2001.

29. Tokat O, Turker Y, Uckunkaya N, Yilmazlar A: A clinical comparison of psoas compartment and inguinal paravascular blocks combined with sciatic nerve block. J Int Med Res 30:161–167, 2002.

30. De Biasi P, Lupescu R, Burgun G, et al: Continuous lumbar plexus block: Use of radiography to determine catheter tip location. Reg Anesth Pain Med 28:135–139, 2003.

31. Breslin D, Martin G, Macleod D, et al: Central nervous system toxicity following the administration of levobupivacaine for lumbar plexus block: A report of two cases. Reg Anesth Pain Med 28:144–147, 2003.

32. Weller R, Gerancher J, Crews J, Wade K: Extensive retroperitoneal hematoma without neurologic deficit in two patients who underwent lumbar plexus block and were later anticoagulated. Anesthesiology 98:581–585, 2003.

33. Winnie AP, Ramamurthy S, Durrani Z: The inguinal paravascular technic of lumbar plexus anesthesia. Anesth Analg; 52:989–996, 1973.

34. Marhofer P, Schrogendorfer K, Koinig H, et al: Ultrasonic guidance improves sensory block and onset time of three-in-one block. Anesth Analg 85:854–857, 1997.

35. Marhofer P, Schrogendorfer K, Wallner T, et al: Ultrasonic guidance reduces the amount of local anesthetic for 3-in-1 blocks. Reg Anesth Pain Med 23:584–588, 1998.

36. Winnie AP: An immobile needle for nerve blocks. Anesthesiology 31:557–558, 1969.

37. Winnie AP, Ramamurthy S, Durrani Z, Radonjic R: Plexus blocks for lower extremity surgery. Anesth Rev 1:11–16, 1974.

38. Urbanek B, Duma A, Kimberger O, et al: Onset time, quality of blockade, and duration of three-in-one blocks with levobupivacaine and bupivacaine. Anesth Analg 97:888–892, 2003.

39. Seeberger M, Urwyler A: Paravascular lumbar plexus block: Block extension after femoral nerve stimulation and injection of 20 vs. 40 ml mepivacaine 10 mg/ml. Acta Anaesthesiol Scand 39:769–773, 1995.

40. Ng H, Cheong K, Lim A, et al: Intraoperative single-shot "3-in-1" femoral nerve block with ropivacaine 0.25%, ropivacaine 0.5% or bupivacaine 0.25% provides comparable 48-hr analgesia after unilateral total hip replacement. Can J Anaesth 48:1102–1108, 2001.

41. Weber A, Fournier R, Van Gessel E, et al: Epinephrine does not prolong the analgesia of 20 mL ropivacaine 0.5% or 0.2% in a femoral three-in-one block. Anesth Analg 93:1327–1331, 2001.

42. Snoeck M, Vree T, Gielen J, Lagerwert J: Steady state bupivacaine plasma concentrations and safety of a femoral "3-in-1" nerve block with bupivacaine in patients over 80 years of age. Int J Clin Pharmacol Ther 41:107–113, 2003.

43. Schwarz S, Franciosi L, Ries C, et al: Addition of femoral 3-in-1 blockade to intraarticular ropivacaine 0.2% does not reduce analgesic requirements following arthroscopic knee surgery. Can J Anaesth 46:741–747, 1999.

44. Bonicalzi V, Gallino M: Comparison of two regional anesthetic techniques for knee arthroscopy. Arthroscopy 11:207–212, 1995.

45. Winnie AP, Candido KD, Torres M: Continuous peripheral nerve blocks for the management of trauma to the extremities. In Rosenberg A, Grande C, Bernstein R (eds): Pain Management and Regional Anesthesia in Trauma. WB Saunders, New York, 1999, pp 224–238.

46. Rosenblatt R: Continuous femoral anesthesia for lower extremity surgery. Anesth Analg 59:631–632, 1980.

47. Postel J, Marz P: Continuous block of the lumbar plexus ("3-in-1 Block") in pre- and post-operative pain therapy (German). Reg Anaesth 7:140–143, 1984.

48. Nebler R, Schwippel U: Continuous plexus blockade with the "3-in-1" block catheter technique in pain therapy (German). Reg Anaesth 11:54–57, 1988.

49. Anker-Möller E, Spangsberg N, Dahl J, et al: Continuous blockade of the lumbar plexus after knee surgery: A comparison of the plasma concentration and analgesic effect of bupivacaine 0.25% and 0.125%. Acta Anaesthesiol Scand 34:468–472, 1990.

50. Singelyn F, Van Roy C, Goosens F, et al: A high position of the catheter increases the success rate of continuous "3-in-1" block. Anesthesiology 85:A723, 1996 (abstract).

51. Capdevila X, Biboulet P, Morau D, et al: Continuous three-in-one block for postoperative pain after lower limb orthopedic surgery: Where do the catheters go? Anesth Analg 94:1001–1006, 2002.

52. Serpell M, Millar F, Thomson M: Comparison of lumbar plexus block versus conventional opioid analgesia after total knee replacement. Anaesthesia 46:275–277, 1991.

53. Eriksson E, Haggmark T, Saartok T, et al: Knee arthroscopy with local anesthesia in ambulatory patients. Methods, results and patient compliance. Orthopedics 9:186–188, 1986.

54. De Andres J, Bellver J, Febre E, et al: A comparative study of analgesia after knee surgery with intraarticular bupivacaine, intraarticular morphine, and lumbar plexus block. Anesth Analg 77:727–730, 1993.

55. Hord A, Roberson J, Thompson W, et al: Evaluation of continuous femoral nerve analgesia after primary total knee arthroplasty. Anesth Analg 70:S164, 1990 (abstract).

56. Dahl J, Christiansen C, Daugaard J, et al: Continuous blockade of the lumbar plexus after knee surgery – Postoperative analgesia and bupivacaine plasma concentrations. Anaesthesia 43:1015–1018, 1988.

57. Shultz P, Christensen E, Anker-Möller E, et al: Postoperative pain treatment after open knee surgery: Continuous lumbar plexus block with bupivacaine versus epidural morphine. Reg Anesth 16:34–37, 1991.

58. Uhrbrand A, Jensen T: Iatrogenic femoral neuropathy after blockade of the lumbar plexus (3-in-1 block) (German). Ugeskrift for Laeger 150:428–429, 1988.

59. Johr M: A complication of continuous femoral nerve block (German). Reg Anaesth 10:37–38, 1987.

60. Lynch J, Trojan S, Arhelger S, Krings-Ernst I: Intermittent femoral nerve blockade for anterior cruciate ligament repair. Use of a catheter technique in 208 patients. Acta Anaesth Belg 42:297–312, 1991.

61. Candido KD, Sukhani R, Kendall MC, et al: Neurostimulation assisted femoral nerve block (FNB): Anatomical indicators for seeking the optimal motor response. A-1115. Presented at the American Society of Anesthesiologists Annual Meeting, San Francisco, CA, 14 October 2003.

62. Allen H, Liu S, Ware P, et al: Peripheral nerve blocks improve analgesia after total knee replacement surgery. Anesth Analg 87:93–97, 1998.

63. Hirst G, Lang S, Dust W: Femoral nerve block. Single injection versus continuous infusion for total knee arthroplasty. Reg Anesth 21:292–297, 1996.

64. Wang H, Boctor B, Verner: The effect of single-injection femoral nerve block on rehabilitation and length of hospital stay after total knee replacement. Reg Anesth Pain Med 27:139–144, 2002.

65. Dauri M, Polzoni M, Fabbi E, et al: Comparison of epidural, continuous femoral block and intraarticular analgesia after anterior cruciate ligament reconstruction. Acta Anaesthesiol Scand 47:20–25, 2003.

66. Tetzlaff J, Andrish J, O'Hara J Jr, et al: Effectiveness of bupivacaine administered via femoral nerve catheter for pain control after anterior cruciate ligament repair. J Clin Anesth 9:542–545, 1997.

67. Frost S, Gossfeld S, Kirkley A, et al: The efficacy of femoral nerve block in pain reduction for outpatient hamstring anterior cruciate ligament reconstruction: A double-blind, prospective, randomized trial. Arthroscopy 16:243–248, 2000.

68. Albert T, Yelnik A, Bonan I, et al: Effectiveness of femoral nerve selective block in patients with spasticity: preliminary results. Arch Phys Med Rehabil 83:692–696, 2002.

69. Singelyn F, Vanderelst P, Gouverneur J: Extended femoral nerve sheath block after total hip arthroplasty: Continuous versus patient-controlled techniques. Anesth Analg 92:455–459, 2001.

70. Edwards N, Wright E: Continuous low-dose 3-in-1 nerve blockade for postoperative pain relief after total knee replacement. Anesth Analg 75:265–267, 1992.

71. Vloka J, Hadzic A, Mulcare R, et al: Femoral and genitofemoral nerve blocks versus spinal anesthesia for outpatients undergoing long saphenous vein stripping surgery. Anesth Analg 84:749–752, 1997.

72. Williams B, Kentor M, Vogt M, et al: Femoral-sciatic nerve blocks for complex outpatient knee surgery are associated with less postoperative pain before same-day discharge: A review of 1,200 consecutive cases from the period 1996–1999. Anesthesiology 98:1206–1213, 2003.

73. Vloka J, Hadzic A, Drobnik L, et al: Anatomical landmarks for femoral nerve block: A comparison of four needle insertion sites. Anesth Analg 89:1467–1470, 1999.

74. Vloka J, Hadzic A, Drobnik L, et al: Anatomical landmarks for femoral nerve block: A comparison of four needle insertion sites. Anesth Analg 89:1467–1470, 1999.

75. Casati A, Fanelli G, Magistris L, et al: Minimum local anesthetic volume blocking the femoral nerve in 50% of cases: A double-blind comparison between 0.5% ropivacaine and 0.5% bupivacaine. Anesth Analg 92:205–208, 2001.

76. Mulroy M, Larkin K, Batra M, et al: Femoral nerve block with 0.25% bupivacaine improves postoperative analgesia following outpatient arthroscopic anterior cruciate ligament repair. Reg Anesth Pain Med 26:24–29, 2001.

77. Eledjam J, Cuvillon P, Capdevila X, et al: Postoperative analgesia by femoral nerve block with ropivacaine 0.2% after major knee surgery: Continuous versus patient-controlled techniques. Reg Anesth Pain Med 27:604–611, 2002.

78. Cuvillon P, Ripart J, Lalourcey L, et al: The continuous femoral nerve block catheter for postoperative analgesia: bacterial colonization, infectious rate and adverse effects. Anesth Analg 93:1045–1049, 2001.

79. Jones SF, White A: Analgesia following femoral neck surgery. Lateral cutaneous nerve block as an alternative to narcotics in the elderly. Anaesthesia 40:682–685, 1985.

80. Shannon J, Lang S, Yip R, Gerard M: Lateral femoral cutaneous nerve block revisited: A nerve stimulator technique. Reg Anesth 20:100–104, 1995.

81. Bridenbaugh P, Wedel D: The lower extremity: Somatic blockade. *In* Cousins MJ, Bridenbaugh PO (eds): Neural Blockade in Clinical Anesthesia and Management of Pain, ed 3. Lippincott-Raven, Philadelphia, 1998, pp 373–394.

82. Sunderland S: Obturator nerve. *In* Sunderland S (ed): Nerves and Nerve Injuries. E & S Livingstone, Edinburgh, 1968, pp 1096–1109.

83. Kawaguchi M, Hashizume K, Iwata T, Furuya H: Percutaneous radiofrequency lesioning of sensory branches of the obturator and femoral nerves for the treatment of hip joint pain. Reg Anesth Pain Med 26:576–581, 2001.

84. McNamee DA, Parks L, Milligan KR: Post-operative analgesia following total knee replacement: An evaluation of the addition of an obturator nerve block to combined femoral and sciatic nerve block. Acta Anaesthesiol Scand 46:95–99, 2002.

85. Atanasoff P, Weiss B, Horst A, et al: Electroneurographic study on the obturator nerve. Anesthesiology 81:A1043, 1994 (abstract).

86. Atanasoff P, Weiss B, Brull S, et al: Compound motor action potential recording distinguishes different onset of motor block of the obturator nerve in response to etidocaine or bupivacaine. Anesth Analg 82:317–320, 1996.

87. Atanassoff PG, Weiss BM, Brull SJ, et al: Electromyographic comparison of obturator nerve block to three-in-one block. Anesth Analg 81:529–533, 1995.

88. Atanassoff PG, Weiss BM, Brull SJ: Lidocaine plasma levels following two techniques of obturator nerve block. J Clin Anesth 8:535–539, 1996.

89. Bouaziz H, Vial F, Jochum D, et al: An evaluation of the cutaneous distribution after obturator nerve block. Anesth Analg 94:445–449, 2002.

90. Fujita Y, Kimura K, Furukawa Y, Takaori M: Plasma concentrations of lignocaine after obturator nerve block combined with spinal anaesthesia in patients undergoing transurethral resection procedures. Br J Anaesth 68:596–598, 1992.

91. Wassef M: Interadductor approach to obturator nerve blockade for spastic conditions of adductor thigh muscles. Reg Anesth 18:13–17, 1993.

92. Akata T, Murakami J, Yoshinaga A: Life-threatening haemorrhage following obturator artery injury during transurethral bladder surgery: A sequel of an unsuccessful obturator nerve block. Acta Anaesthesiol Scand 43:784–788, 1999.

93. Ellis H, Feldman S: Anatomy for Anaesthetists, ed 3. Blackwell Scientific, Oxford, 1977, pp 221–224.

94. Romanoff ME, Cory PC, Kalenak A, et al: Saphenous nerve entrapment at the adductor canal. Am J Sport Med 17:478–481, 1989.

95. Mansour NY: Sub-sartorial saphenous nerve block with the aid of a nerve stimulator. Reg Anesth 18:266–268, 1993.

96. Bouaziz H, Benhamou D, Narchi P: A new approach for saphenous nerve block. Reg Anesth 21:490, 1996.

97. Bouaziz H, Narchi P, Zetlaoui PJ, et al: Lateral approach to the sciatic nerve at the popliteal fossa combined with saphenous nerve block. Tech Reg Anesth Pain Manage 3:19–22, 1999.

98. Van der Wal M, Lang SA, Yip RW: Transsartorial approach for saphenous nerve block. Can J Anaesth 40:542–546, 1993.

99. Bonica JJ: The Management of Pain, ed 2. Lea Febiger, Philadelphia, 1990, p 1928.

100. Katz J: Atlas of Regional Anesthesia. Appleton-Century Crofts, Prentice-Hall, Norwalk, CT, 1985, pp156–157.

101. Comfort VK, Lang SA, Yip RW: Saphenous nerve anaesthesia – A nerve stimulator technique. Can J Anaesth 43:852–857, 1996.

102. Bridenbaugh PO: The lower extremity: Somatic blockade. *In* Cousins MJ, Bridenbaugh PO (eds): Neural Blockade in Clinical Anesthesia and Management of Pain, ed 2. JB Lippincott, New York, 1988, pp 417–441.

103. Brown DL: Regional Anesthesia and Analgesia. WB Saunders, Philadelphia, 1996, pp 288–289.

104. De May JJ, Deruyck LJ, Cammu G, et al: A paravenous approach for the saphenous nerve block. Reg Anesth Pain Med 26:504–506, 2001.

105. Benzon HT, Calimaran AL, Hausman J: Saphenous nerve blockade. ASA Annual Meeting, New Orleans, LA, 16 October 2001.

106. Kofoed H: Peripheral nerve blocks at the knee and ankle in operations for common foot disorders. Clin Orthop Rel Res 168:97–101, 1982.

107. Ericksson E: Illustrated Handbook in Regional Anesthesia. AB Astra, Copenhagen, 1969, p 110.

108. Capdevila X, Biboulet PH, Bourgeba M, et al: Comparison of the 3 in 1 and fascia iliaca compartment block in adults: Clinical and radiographic analysis. Anesth Analg 86:1039–1044, 1998.

109. Lopez S, Gros T, Bernard N, et al: Fascia iliaca compartment block for femoral bone fractures in prehospital care. Reg Anesth Pain Med 28:203–207, 2003.

110. Longo S, Williams D: Bilateral fascia iliaca catheters for postoperative pain control after bilateral total knee arthroplasty: A case report and description of a catheter technique. Reg Anesth 22:372–377, 1997.

111. Ganapathy S, Wasserman R, Watson J, et al: Modified continuous three-in-one block for postoperative pain after total knee arthroplasty. Anesth Analg 89:1197–1202, 1999.

112. Dalens B, Vanneuville G, Tanguy A: Comparison of the fascia iliaca compartment block with the 3-in-1 block in children. Anesth Analg 69:705–713, 1989.

113. Doyle E, Morton N, McNicol L: Plasma bupivacaine levels after fascia iliaca compartment block with and without adrenaline. Paediatr Anaesth 7:121–124, 1997.

114. Morau D, Lopez S, Biboulet P, et al: Comparison of continuous 3-in-1 and fascia iliaca compartment blocks for postoperative analgesia: feasibility, catheter migration, distribution of sensory block, and analgesic efficacy. Reg Anesth Pain Med 28:309–314, 2003.

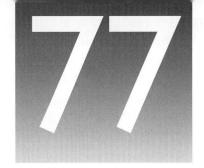

Sciatic Nerve Block

**Radha Sukhani, M.D., and
Honorio T. Benzon, M.D.**

The sciatic nerve provides sensory innervations to the entire leg below the knee except for its medial aspect, which is innervated by the saphenous nerve. Sciatic nerve block in conjunction with lumbar plexus block, femoral nerve block, or saphenous nerve block can be used to provide perioperative analgesia for surgical procedures of the lower extremity. Lower extremity peripheral nerve blocks provide cost-effective anesthesia and postoperative analgesia with a favorable postoperative recovery profile. In this regard peripheral nerve blocks have the following distinct advantages over general or central neuraxial anesthesia: (1) no autonomic blockade with no risk of hemodynamic instability and urinary retention; (2) unilateral block with no risk of spinal hematoma in an anticoagulated patient; (3) prolonged postoperative analgesia when extended block is provided either by injecting a long-acting local anesthetic or by a continuous infusion of local anesthetic via an indwelling catheter and infusion pump; (4) minimal need for postoperative nursing due to minimal side effects such as uncontrolled pain, emesis, sedation (airway), and respiratory depression; and (5) early ambulation and discharge: patients with unilateral blocks for lower extremity surgery can be ambulated on crutches and discharged early with minimal or no risk of the aforementioned side effects. Increasing demands for peripheral nerve block techniques by orthopedic surgeons can be attributed to the rapid growth of ambulatory surgery over the last decade. A single-shot and continuous sciatic (popliteal) blocks for patients undergoing reconstructive foot and ankle surgery and varicose vein stripping have been recognized as safe and effective techniques for perioperative analgesia with high ratings for patient satisfaction.[1-7]

Despite the potential advantages, lower extremity nerve blocks are infrequently used in clinical practice. The primary reason for this clinical trend is a general perception amongst clinical anesthesiologists that sciatic nerve block is technically demanding with a variable success rate.[8-10] This perception may stem from unfamiliarity with the technique because most residency training programs are deficient in the teaching of peripheral nerve blocks, specifically, the lower extremity nerve blocks.[11-13] There has been an explosion in the description of new techniques of sciatic nerve blockade over the last decade as practitioners of regional anesthesia continue to explore for a simple approach to block this nerve. These techniques block the sciatic nerve at varying anatomical sites along the course of nerve from the pelvis to the popliteal fossa (Table 77-1).[8-10,14-23] Additionally a significant amount of research is being done to define strategies to reduce latency and improve the success of a complete block of the two neural components of sciatic nerve, the tibial and peroneal nerves.[20,24,25]

REGIONAL ANATOMY PERTINENT TO SCIATIC NERVE BLOCK

The sciatic nerve is the largest nerve in the body measuring 0.8 to 1.5 cm in width. It is the continuation of the sacral plexus arising from L4, L5 and S1, S2, S3 nerve roots. The roots that form the sciatic nerve exit from the pelvis through the greater sciatic foramen and travel on the anterior surface of the piriformis muscle. From its origin to its termination, the two divisions of the sciatic nerve—tibial nerve (medial position) and peroneal nerve (lateral position)—are distinctly separate. The two divisions, however, are combined into one large single nerve trunk by a connective tissue sheath. Proximally the nerve lies over the posterior surface of the ischium between the ischial tuberosity and greater trochanter of the femur. In this location the sciatic nerve is accompanied by the posterior cutaneous nerve of the thigh and the inferior gluteal artery. Distal to piriformis muscle the nerve lies sandwiched between the gemelli, quadratus femoris, and adductor magnus muscles anteriorly and gluteus maximus muscle posteriorly. In the infragluteal location the sciatic nerve lies over adductor magnus muscle and is crossed obliquely in the mediolateral direction by the long head of the biceps femoris. The sciatic nerve, therefore, lies at first lateral and subsequently deep to the long head of the biceps femoris muscle in the upper thigh. In its entire course, from its origin to its termination in the distal thigh, the sciatic nerve lies deep and covered by large muscle mass except in the infragluteal region. For a brief 3 to 4 cm distance in this location the nerve lies lateral to long head

TABLE 77-1. **PUBLISHED APPROACHES TO SCIATIC NERVE AND POPLITEAL NERVE BLOCKS**

Approach by Investigation	Year	Site	Patient Position	Additional Blocked Nerves
Labat (Paucet); posterior	1922	Distal to piriformis in proximity of greater sciatic foramen	Lateral (Sim's)	PCN
Winnie modification of Labat; posterior	1975	Distal to piriformis in proximity of greater sciatic foramen	Lateral (Sim's)	PCN
Ichiyanagi et al.; supine lateral	1959	Subgluteal space	Supine	PCN
Guardini et al.; supine lateral	1985	Subgluteal space	Supine	PCN
Raj; supine posterior	1975	Between greater trochanter and ischial tuberosity	Supine	PCN
Mansour; parasacral	1993	Level of greater sciatic foramen	Lateral (Sim's)	PCN, obturator pudendal
Beck's anterior approach	1962	Upper thigh; level of greater trochanter	Supine	–
Chelly's modification of Beck's approach	1999	Upper thigh; level of greater trochanter		–
Benedetto et al.; posterior	2002	Subgluteal space	Lateral (Sim's)	–
Sukhani et al.; posterior	2003	Infragluteal parabiceps	Prone or lateral (Sim's)	–
Ronie et al.; posterior	1980	Popliteal fossa	Prone	–
Vloka et al.; lateral	1996	Popliteal fossa	Supine	–
Hadzic et al.		Popliteal fossa; intertendinous	Prone	–

PCN, posterior cutaneous nerve of thigh.

of the biceps femoris muscle covered only by subcutaneous tissue and skin with no overlying musculature.[20] In the infragluteal region the nerve lies posteromedial to the femur in the close proximity of the lesser trochanter. The sciatic nerve continues distally in the thigh along the posteromedial aspect of femur under the biceps femoris muscle. At the cephalad portion of popliteal fossa or distal third of thigh, the sciatic nerve divides into its two terminal branches, the posterior tibial and common peroneal nerves. The division may occur higher in the thigh. The two divisions of the sciatic nerve are distinctly separate for the entire length of the nerve, but are combined into one large trunk by a common connective tissue sheath. The need for two separate injections to achieve surgical anesthesia of the tibial and common peroneal divisions of the sciatic nerve has been attributed to this anatomical feature.[26–28]

TECHNIQUES OF SCIATIC NERVE BLOCK

To be widely accepted in clinical anesthesia practice, a nerve block technique must be technically simple, use easily identifiable landmarks, produce minimal patient discomfort, and provide prompt onset of surgical anesthesia. Although several approaches to sciatic nerve block have been described, the block has not achieved wide acceptance amongst clinicians because of limitations with respect to identifying bony landmarks (particularly in overweight patients), substantial patient discomfort (needle passage through dense musculature), unpredictable success, and latency of the block. Recently published reports on sciatic nerve block have addressed some of these limitations with respect to the technique latency and success of the block.[19,20]

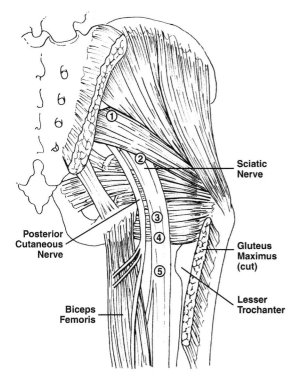

FIGURE 77-1. Sites for the various posterior approaches to sciatic nerve block. (1) Parasacral approach of Mansour—at the point where the nerve exits from greater sciatic foramen. (2) Labat approach—at the lower border of the piriformis fossa. (3) Raj's approach—midway between the greater trochanter and ischial tuberosity. (4) Subgluteal approach (di Benedetto et al.)—over the adductor magnus, 4 cm caudal to the midpoint of a line joining the greater trochanter and the ischial tuberosity. (5) Infragluteal parabiceps (Sukhani et al.)—between the lesser trochanter and lateral border of the biceps femoris as the nerve overlies the adductor magnus.

The sciatic nerve can be blocked at different levels along its entire length as it exits the pelvis at the greater sciatic foramen to its termination in the lower thigh. The following describes the different approaches to sciatic nerve block in the order from its origin to its termination (Table 77-1; Fig. 77-1). To the description of each technique is added its advantages and limitations.

Parasacral Approach of Mansour: Mansour described the parasacral approach to sciatic nerve block in 1993.[16] The approach is the most proximal of all the described approaches to sciatic nerve block. It aims at depositing the local anesthetic solution within the fascial plane enclosing the nerve roots of sacral plexus before they unite to form the main trunk of the sciatic nerve under the piriformis muscle. The sacral plexus consists of fibers from L4 to S3 nerve roots. In addition to blocking the components of the sciatic nerve, the parasacral approach additionally blocks the posterior cutaneous nerve of the thigh, pudendal nerve, and obturator nerve, which runs in close proximity of the sacral plexus. Using a single-injection technique the overall success rate of surgical anesthesia in the distribution of the sciatic nerve was noted to be 97% and 93% in the distribution of obturator nerve.[29]

SURFACE ANATOMY AND TECHNIQUE: The patient is placed in the lateral (Sim's) position with the limb to be operated on uppermost. The posterior superior iliac spine (PSIS) and ischial tuberosity are identified and marked. A line is constructed between these two points. The point of needle entry is approximately three finger widths (6 cm) from the PSIS. In the average-sized patient the bony rim of the greater sciatic foramen can be palpated in the close vicinity of the marked needle entry site. A 100 mm 22-gauge insulated block needle is inserted at the anesthetized marked site and advanced in a sagittal plane. The needle is walked off the contour of the greater sciatic foramen into the pelvis. The advancing needle usually contacts the nerve roots of the sacral plexus at 5 to 8 cm depth from the marked entry site at the skin. The contact with the nerve roots produces an evoked motor response (EMR) at the ankle. An appropriate volume (20 to 30 mL) of local anesthetic is injected when an appropriate EMR at ankle/foot is obtained at <0.5 mA (see Table 77-2 for appropriate EMR).

TABLE 77-2. MAJOR MUSCLES SUPPLIED BY BRANCHES OF THE SCIATIC NERVE AND THEIR ACTION WITH REGARD TO MOVEMENT OF THE FOOT AND TOES

Muscle Supplied	Action
I. Tibial nerve	
A. Wide part of sciatic nerve	
1. Gastrocnemius	Plantar flexion
2. Soleus	Plantar flexion
B. After division of sciatic nerve	
1. Tibialis posterior	Inversion; assist in plantar flexion
2. Flexor digitorum longus	Plantar flexion (toes)
3. Flexor hallucis longus	Plantar flexion (toes)
4. Soleus	Plantar flexion (toes)
II. Deep peroneal (anterior tibial) nerve	
1. Tibialis anterior	Inversion; dorsiflexion
2. Extensor hallucis longus	Dorsiflexion
3. Extensor digitorum longus	Dorsiflexion
4. Peronius tertius	Dorsiflexion
5. Extensor digitorum brevis	Extension (toes)
III. Superficial peroneal nerve	
1. Peroneus longus	Eversion; assist in plantar flexion
2. Peroneus brevis	Eversion; assist in plantar flexion

The sural nerve has no muscular branch.
Data compiled and reproduced from Calilet R: Foot and Ankle Pain. FA Davis, Philadelphia, 1983, pp 1–46; Mayo Clinic and Mayo Foundation: Clinical Examinations in Neurology. WB Saunders, Philadelphia, 1981, pp 168–188.

ADVANTAGES AND LIMITATIONS: The approach has been claimed to be technically easy and provides a high success rate of the block of the two components of the sciatic nerve. The needle does not traverse the bulk of glutei muscles so the approach causes less discomfort to the patient. The posterior femoral cutaneous nerve and the obturator nerve are blocked. The associated block of the obturator nerve is an advantage because obturator nerve anesthesia is a necessary component of regional anesthesia for major surgery of the knee (total knee arthroplasty).

The parasacral approach is a block of the sacral plexus within the pelvis. The needle, therefore, lies in the close proximity of vascular and visceral structures within the pelvis. There are no reports of visceral puncture with the parasacral approach; however, experience with the technique is still limited. The parasacral approach blocks the pudendal nerve with resultant anesthesia of the perineum. Almost 100% of patients who receive this block will report unilateral perineal anesthesia. Despite the close proximity of somatic and sympathetic nerve supply of the bladder to the injection site and resultant blockade of these nerves, voiding difficulties requiring bladder catheterizations are uncommon.[29]

Classic Posterior Approach to Sciatic Block: The classic posterior approach blocks the sciatic nerve at the level of the greater sciatic notch distal to the piriformis muscle (Fig. 77-1).[8,14] The approach is expected to block the two components of the sciatic nerve, posterior cutaneous nerve of the thigh, and pudendal nerve.

SURFACE ANATOMY AND TECHNIQUE: The patient is placed in the lateral (Sim's position) with the side to be blocked uppermost and rotated forwards. The upper thigh and knee are flexed 90° and the dependent lower extremity is extended. A line (line 1) is constructed between the tip of greater trochanter and the PSIS. Line 1 is bisected and a perpendicular line is drawn inferiorly from the midpoint of the bisected first line (line 2). A third line (line 3) is constructed between the tip of the greater trochanter and the sacral hiatus. The point of intersection between lines 2 and 3 is the needle entry site. A 100 to 150 mm (depending on the size of the patient) insulated 22-gauge block needle is inserted perpendicular to the skin and advanced until an appropriate EMR (see Table 77-2) is obtained at ankle/foot at <0.5 mA. If an EMR is not obtained the needle is redirected laterally or medially until an EMR is elicited. The depth of the nerve from the skin usually ranges from 70 to 150 mm. An appropriate volume (20 to 30 mL) of local anesthetic is injected after ensuring negative aspiration and absence of paresthesia.

ADVANTAGES AND LIMITATIONS: The sciatic nerve is blocked at the point of its origin distal to the piriformis so there is greater likelihood of blocking the two components of the sciatic nerve as well as the posterior cutaneous nerve of the thigh. The approach requires the needle to traverse the bulky gluteal musculature to reach the sciatic nerve producing significant pain and discomfort. It has been claimed that dysesthesias associated with the block are more common after this approach.[30]

Supine Lithomy Approach: This approach blocks the sciatic nerve at a more distal level between the ischial tuberosity

and the greater trochanter.[9] The approach is expected to block the two components of the sciatic nerve. The posterior cutaneous nerve of the thigh may not be blocked because the nerve descends, distal to the piriformis muscle, medially into the thigh over the posterior surface of the biceps femoris muscle.

SURFACE ANATOMY AND TECHNIQUE: The patient is in the supine position with the extremity to be blocked supported in a position of the hip in maximal flexion and knee flexion at 90°. This can be achieved by an assistant holding the leg to be blocked, which is cumbersome, or by supporting the flexed leg (90° flexion at hip and knee) on a picket fence frame. Maximal flexion at the hip thins out the gluteus maximus muscle and decreases redundant tissue at the buttock. A line is constructed between the tip of the greater trochanter and ischial tuberosity. The midpoint of the line is the point of the needle entry. A 100 mm insulated 22-gauge needle is inserted through the marked site in a direction perpendicular to the skin. The elicitation of appropriate EMR at <0.5 mA and guidelines of local anesthetic injection are similar to the techniques described above. If sciatic nerve stimulation is not achieved the needle is directed in the lateral or medical direction until EMR of sciatic nerve stimulation is achieved.

ADVANTAGES AND LIMITATIONS: The sciatic nerve in this approach is more superficial than for any of the other gluteal approaches. The approach is expected to produce less discomfort (less musculature to traverse) and the patient is in the supine position for the block which can be useful in obese patients and patients with painful traumatic injuries to the extremity. Positioning of the lower extremity in this approach is cumbersome and may require an assistant.

Anterior Approach to Sciatic Block: The anterior approach to sciatic block was first described by Beck in 1962 and subsequently modified by Chelly and Delauney in 1999.[10,17] The approach requires the needle to traverse the muscles of the anterior compartment of the leg to block the sciatic nerve as it lies in the proximity of the lesser trochanter of the femur. The two components of the sciatic nerve lie in close proximity but the posterior cutaneous nerve of the thigh, which overlies the posterior surface of biceps femoris muscle, may not be close enough to be blocked.

SURFACE ANATOMY AND TECHNIQUE: The patient is placed supine with the lower extremities in neutral position. A line is constructed between the anterior superior iliac spine and the pubic tubercle. This line marks the reflection of the inguinal ligament. The second line is constructed parallel to the first line, i.e., along the inguinal ligament, at the level of the greater trochanter. In Beck's approach a perpendicular line is drawn at the junction of the lateral two-thirds and medial one-third of the first line (inguinal ligament). The needle entry site for Beck's approach is the junction of the perpendicular and the second line. In Chelly's modification the inguinal ligament line is bisected and a perpendicular line is extended down from the bisected point by 8 cm. Chelly's modification does not require palpation of the greater trochanter.

The block is performed with a 150 mm, 22-gauge insulated block needle because the nerve lies deep under the muscles of the anterior thigh. The needle in its passage through the anterior thigh may encounter the femoral nerve (indicated by patellar snap by electrostimulation). If femoral nerve stimulation persists the needle should be oriented laterally to bypass the femoral nerve. The sciatic nerve may not be encountered until a depth of 12 to 15 cm. Local anesthetic is injected when appropriate EMR is obtained at <0.5 mA.

ADVANTAGES AND LIMITATIONS: The anterior approach is unique in that it can be performed with the patient supine without limb flexion or additional patient positioning. Furthermore, the time required for a combination of blocks (femoral nerve block, perifemoral saphenous nerve block) is reduced because only one area of skin preparation is required.

The accessibility of the sciatic nerve using an anterior approach at the level of the lesser trochanter has been questioned recently. Vloka et al.[31] reported that the sciatic nerve at this site lies posterior to the lesser trochanter and is not accessible to the needle using the direct anterior approach. Cadaver dissections and magnetic resonance imaging have demonstrated that in the majority of the subjects the position of the sciatic nerve relative to the lesser trochanter made it inaccessible from the anterior approach at this level.[31,32] Two strategies to overcome this limitation include the insertion of the needle at a more distal level (4 cm distal to the lesser trochanter) and internal rotation of the foot (femur) so the sciatic nerve moves medial to the lesser trochanter.[31,32]

Lateral Approach to Sciatic Block (Ichiyanagi, 1959; Guardini et al., 1985): Ichiyanagi described the technique of blocking the sciatic nerve via a lateral approach, with the patient in the supine position.[15] The technique did not become popular because of technical difficulties in performing the block. Guardini et al. in 1985 described a new lateral approach and claimed it to be technically easier.[18] In this technique the sciatic nerve is blocked in the subgluteal space where the nerve lies just dorsal to the plane of the quadratus femoris muscle between the femur and ischial tuberosity (Fig. 77-1). The other structures besides the sciatic nerve that lie in the subgluteal space are the posterior cutaneous nerve of the thigh, the interior gluteal nerve and vessels, and the ascending branch of the circumflex femoral artery. The sciatic nerve is blocked as it lies along the lower border of the quadratus femoris muscle in the subgluteal space.

SURFACE ANATOMY AND TECHNIQUE: The block is performed with the patient in the supine position and the hip in neutral position. The site of needle insertion is 3 cm distal to the point of maximum lateral prominence of the greater trochanter along the posterior profile of the femur. The correct location of the needle insertion site can be verified by feeling the ischial tuberosity with the nondominant hand. The ischial tuberosity serves as the medial reference point for advancing the needle.

The needle is inserted through the anesthetized marked site perpendicular to the skin and the major axis of the limb and advanced towards the femur. Once the needle contacts the femur it is withdrawn slightly, redirected 20° under the femur, and advanced toward the ischial tuberosity. The sciatic nerve is usually contacted at a depth of 8 to 12 cm. Local anesthetic solution is injected after appropriate EMR of the sciatic nerve stimulation is obtained.

ADVANTAGES AND LIMITATIONS: The block can be performed with the patient in the supine position. Despite the authors' claims of simplicity, the approach has not received wide acceptance. The approach can produce significant patient discomfort because: (1) the needle has to travel through substantial tissue planes to reach the nerve; (2) the advancing needle can stimulate other motor nerves including the inferior gluteal nerve and the nerves to the biceps femoris muscle causing patient discomfort; and (3) multiple redirection attempts may be needed to contact the nerve which lies in a plane posterior to the femur.

Posterior Subgluteus Approach (di Benedetto et al.): The subgluteus posterior approach is one of several proximal approaches to sciatic nerve block. This approach blocks the nerve at a point more distal to that of the classic posterior approach described by Labat.[14,19] The nerve in the subgluteus location overlies the adducor magnus, posterior to the lesser trochanter, and is approximately 3 cm above the lower limit of the gluteus maximus muscle.

SURFACE ANATOMY AND TECHNIQUE: The patient is placed in the lateral position with the extremity to be blocked uppermost and rolled forward with the knee in the flexed position. A line is drawn from the greater trochanter to the ischial tuberosity and a second line is drawn from the midpoint of this line extending caudally for 4 cm. The needle insertion site is the distal point of the second line. The stimulating 100 mm, 22-gauge insulated needle is inserted through the anesthetized needle entry site with a 90° angle to the skin and advanced until sciatic nerve stimulation is observed. An appropriate volume of local anesthetic is injected when an appropriate motor response is obtained at <0.5 mA.

ADVANTAGES AND LIMITATIONS: Compared to the classic posterior approach, the posterior subgluteus approach is easy and reliable. It produces less patient discomfort because the nerve is located at a shallower depth and the needle traverses less muscle tissue (the average depth from the skin is 4.5 cm with the subgluteus approach and 6.7 cm for the classic posterior approach). The nerve is located in a relatively superficial plane with minimal overlying muscle tissue and the placement of catheter for an extended sciatic block is relatively easy. A limitation is that the approach is distal and may not block the posterior cutaneous nerve of the thigh.

Infragluteal Parabiceps Approach: As in the posterior subgluteus approach, described by Benedetto et al., the infragluteal parabiceps approach blocks the sciatic nerve at a site more distal to the classic posterior approach described by Labat.[20] Distal to the gluteus maximus the sciatic nerve lies over the adductor magnus and is crossed obliquely in the mediolateral direction by the long head of the biceps femoris muscle. The sciatic nerve therefore lies further lateral and subsequently deep to the long head of the biceps femoris. For a short distance of 3 to 4 cm, where the nerve is lateral to the long head of the biceps femoris, there is no overlying musculature and the nerve is covered only by skin and subcutaneous tissue (Fig. 77-2). The approach to the nerve in this area is determined by using two easily identifiable soft tissue landmarks: the lateral border of the biceps femoris muscle and the lower border of the gluteus maximus muscle (gluteal crease) (Fig. 77-3).

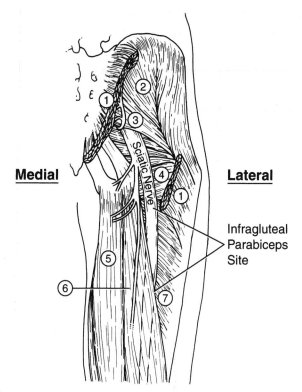

FIGURE 77-2. Schematic representation of muscular relationship of sciatic nerve in the proximity of the block site for the infragluteal parabiceps approach. 1, Gluteus maximus; 2, gluteus medius; 3, piriformis; 4, quadratus femoris; 5, semitendinosus; 6, biceps femoris; 7, adductor magnus.

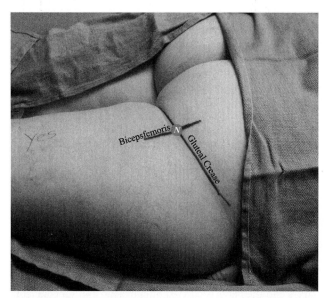

FIGURE 77-3. Surface anatomy for infragluteal parabiceps approach. The needle insertion site (N) lies at the point where gluteal crease line and lateral border of the biceps femoris muscle cross each other.

SURFACE ANATOMY AND TECHNIQUE: The surface landmarks for this approach are the lateral border of the biceps femoris and the gluteal crease. The lateral border of the biceps femoris muscle is identified by asking the patient to flex the knee while resistance is applied to the calf muscles. The gluteal crease is a consistent landmark. When more than one gluteal crease is present, the proximal crease is accepted as the landmark. The site of needle insertion is along the lateral border of the biceps femoris 0 to 1 cm caudal to the gluteal crease. After anesthetizing the skin a 100 mm, 22-gauge insulated block needle is inserted at an angle of 70° to 80° to the skin with a cephalad and anterior orientation within the parasagittal plane. To seek the sciatic nerve the needle is moved only in one plane from the lateral to medial direction. The femur lies lateral to the nerve and the biceps femoris is medial to the nerve (Fig. 77-4). If the needle contacts the femur, it is withdrawn to the superficial tissue plane, the skin is retracted medially in 2 to 3 mm increments, and the needle reintroduced. If biceps contraction is encountered with the needle advancement it indicates that the needle is inserted too far medially. If this occurs the needle is withdrawn to the superficial tissue plane, the skin is retracted laterally in 2 to 3 mm increments, and the needle is reintroduced until the nerve is stimulated.

The type of EMR, whether plantar flexion, inversion, eversion, or dorsiflexion, affects the latency and success of complete block of the sciatic nerve using the neurostimulation technique of nerve identification. EMR inversion is associated with complete block of the two components of the sciatic

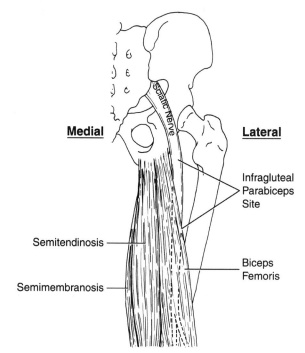

FIGURE 77-4. The sciatic nerve at the infragluteal parabiceps site lies between the lesser traochanter of the femur laterally and biceps femoris medially. Needle contact with bone indicates that the needle is lateral to the sciatic nerve and should be redirected medially while stimulation of the biceps femoris indicates that the needle tip is medial to the sciatic nerve and should be redirected laterally.

nerve in 100% cases with the shortest latency to sensory and motor block of both components of the sciatic nerve.[20,24]

ADVANTAGES AND LIMITATIONS: The infragluteal approach is easy, reliable, and produces less patient discomfort because the needle traverses minimal or no muscle tissue. To seek the nerve the needle adjustments have to be made only in the lateral (femur) to medial (biceps femoris) direction (Fig. 77-4). Since the sciatic nerve is blocked at a distal site in the upper thigh, the posterior cutaneous nerve of the thigh is not blocked by this approach.

SCIATIC NERVE BLOCK AT THE POPLITEAL FOSSA

Anatomy: The popliteal fossa is a diamond-shaped area bounded by the semitendinosus and semimembranosus muscles medially, the biceps femoris muscle laterally, and by the two heads of the gastrocnemius muscle inferiorly (Fig. 77-5).[21,24] The popliteal vessels are located medial to the sciatic nerve. Although the sciatic nerve is usually one nerve, the tibial and common peroneal nerves can be visualized within the sciatic nerve. Occasionally, the tibial and common peroneal nerves are two separate nerves as soon as they descend from the sacrosciatic foramen, the tibial nerve medially and the common peroneal nerve laterally. If the sciatic nerve is one nerve, it divides into its tibial and common peroneal branches at the apex of the popliteal fossa, between 4 and 13 cm above the popliteal crease (Fig. 77-5).[24] The tibial nerve immediately gives off the sural nerve and, at the level just above the sole of the foot, gives off the medial calcaneal nerve. The tibial nerve then continues as the posterior tibial nerve that terminates into the medial plantar and lateral plantar nerves. The common peroneal nerve gives off a sural communicating branch and, once it is below the head of the fibula, divides into the deep peroneal and superficial peroneal nerves. While the major branches of the sciatic nerve have muscular branches, the sural nerve has no motor function.

The sensory innervation of the foot is supplied by branches of the tibial nerve, the common peroneal nerve, and the saphenous nerve. The posterior tibial nerve supplies the sole of the foot, the deep peroneal nerve the web between the big toe and the second toe, the superficial peroneal the dorsum of the foot, and the sural nerve the lateral aspect of the heel and foot and fifth toe. The saphenous nerve, which is the terminal branch of the femoral nerve, supplies the medial aspect of the foot, from the medial malleoli to midway between the malleoli and the big toe. There are several variations in the sensory innervation of the foot.[33] The sural nerve may innervate the lateral aspect of the foot up to the second toe while the medial cutaneous branch of the superficial peroneal nerve may cross-innervate the medial aspect of the foot.[33,34] These variations in sensory innervations ought to be taken into consideration when a specific area on the foot is partially numb after a specific peripheral nerve block.

The sural nerve has no motor functions while the branches of the sciatic nerve have muscular branches (Table 77-1). Dorsiflexion of the foot is secondary to action of the muscles supplied by the deep peroneal nerve, whereas eversion is due to action of the muscles supplied by the superficial peroneal nerve. Plantar flexion results from the action of the muscles supplied by the tibial nerve, with some assistance from the peroneus muscles that are supplied by the superficial peroneal nerve. Inversion of the foot is due to action of both the tibialis posterior muscle which is innervated by the tibial nerve, and the tibialis anterior muscle which is supplied by the deep peroneal nerve.[24,35,36]

The use of a nerve stimulator is recommended in the performance of sciatic block at the popliteal fossa. Elicitation of foot inversion is the best response since it signifies stimulation of both branches of the sciatic nerve (Fig. 77-6).[24] Either the sciatic nerve is stimulated before it gives off its tibial and peroneal branches or the tip of the needle is located between the two nerves. Elicitation of foot dorsiflexion signifies stimulation of the deep peroneal nerve while plantar flexion signifies stimulation of the tibial nerve.[24] Elicitation of one of these responses implies that the needle has to be redirected medially or laterally to elicit the other response to block both branches of the sciatic nerve.

Indications: Popliteal nerve blocks are indicated for sensory and motor blockade of the foot, either for anesthesia for surgery of the foot or for diagnostic/therapeutic blockade for pain management. The block is especially useful when ankle blocks are contraindicated because of the presence of swelling or infection in the ankle. In contrast to ankle blocks wherein up to four injections may be given, one or two injections are adequate for popliteal nerve block. Popliteal sciatic nerve blocks are also performed for postoperative pain management.

Technique:
POSTERIOR APPROACH: The patient is usually prone, although the block can be performed with the patient in the slightly lateral decubitus position. The popliteal fossa is aseptically prepared and draped. An insulated needle is inserted 5 to 7 cm above the popliteal crease and 1 cm lateral to a line that bisects the superior part of the fossa. The needle is advanced at a 45° angle to the skin and inserted to a depth of 2 to 5 cm until a motor response is elicited with a nerve stimulator.[21,24,37] The stimulating current of the nerve stimulator is initially set between 1 and 1.5 mA and the needle is advanced until the desired motor response is visible. The needle is advanced slowly until maximum motor response of the foot is elicited.

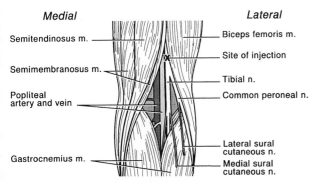

Medial   Lateral

Semitendinosus m. — Biceps femoris m.
— Site of injection
Semimembranosus m. — Tibial n.
Popliteal artery and vein — Common peroneal n.
Gastrocnemius m. — Lateral sural cutaneous n.
— Medial sural cutaneous n.

FIGURE 77-5. Anatomy of the popliteal fossa and technique of sciatic nerve blockade (see text for the technique of nerve blockade). (Reproduced with permission from Benzon HT, Kim C, Benzon HP, et al: Correlation between evoked motor response of the sciatic nerve and sensory blockade. Anesthesiology 87:547–552, 1997.)

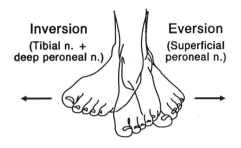

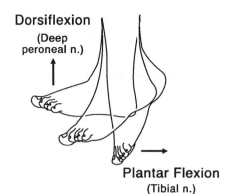

FIGURE 77-6. Elicited motor response of the foot in response to stimulation of the major branches of the sciatic nerve. The nerve responsible for each elicited motor response is indicated; note that the superficial peroneal nerve assists in the elicitation of plantar flexion.

The stimulus intensity is decreased and visible motor response is elicited with the smallest possible current. The needle is considered close to the nerve when the stimulating current is between 0.3 and 0.8 mA, preferably <0.5 mA.[38] The proximity of the insulated needle to the nerve is confirmed when an injection of 1 or 2 mL of local anesthetic results in an immediate cessation of the EMR.[39] While several motor responses can be elicited, including eversion, inversion, dorsiflexion, or plantar flexion, elicited inversion or combined inversion/plantar flexion is the preferred response.[1] A volume of 30 mL of local anesthetic is adequate to block the sciatic nerve.

Sciatic nerve block at the popliteal fossa may result in patchy sensory blockade of the foot. This is probably secondary to the considerable size of the sciatic nerve (between 0.9 and 1.5 cm), the thickness of its epineurium, the presence of fat in the popliteal fossa, and the variable level at which the sciatic nerve divides into the tibial and common peroneal nerves.[24,40] The mean distance above the popliteal crease at which the sciatic nerve divides into its major branches is 6.5 ± 2.7 cm with a range of 1 to 11 cm.[41] To eliminate the variations in the site of bifurcation of the sciatic nerve as a factor, a nerve stimulator is recommended to identify the nerve being stimulated and to use a double-injection technique. As stated, elicited inversion of the foot or combined inversion/plantar flexion is recommended. Our clinical experience is that inversion or combined foot inversion/plantar flexion is difficult to elicit. To facilitate the performance of the block, we advocate the double-injection technique wherein two 15 mL injections are made after the tibial (elicited plantar flexion) and peroneal (elicited foot dorsiflexion or eversion) nerves are stimulated. If the peroneal response (dorsiflexion or eversion) is elicited first, then the needle is moved medially a few millimeters to elicit the tibial response (plantar flexion) since the tibial nerve is medial to the peroneal nerve.[42] If the tibial response is elicited first, then the needle is moved laterally to stimulate the peroneal nerve. Although slightly higher stimulating intensities are needed, there is no difficulty identifying the second response after 15 mL of local anesthetic are injected.[42] More rapid onset of block and increased efficacy of the block have been noted with the double-injection technique.[43]

One disadvantage of the posterior approach is the prone position of the patient. The approach can be done with the patient in the lateral decubitus position and supine positions, although it is harder to perform and if performed in the supine position, an assistant is required to hold the patient's leg up (with the knee bent).

LATERAL APPROACH TO POPLITEAL SCIATIC NERVE BLOCK: The lateral approach to popliteal sciatic nerve block was first described by Collum and Courtney.[44] In this approach the patient is supine. The upper edge of the patella and the groove between the tendon of the biceps femoris and the iliotibial tract are palpated. Identification of the groove is made easier by flexion followed by extension of the patient's knee. The site of needle insertion is at the intersection of a line drawn from the upper edge of the patella and the intermuscular groove. The insulated needle is inserted 20° to 30° posteriorly in relation to the horizontal plane and directed slightly caudad.[45] The 30° angle relative to the horizontal plane results in close location of the needle tip to the nerves and the injection of the solution lateral and posterior to the popliteal vessels.[46] Since the common peroneal nerve is located laterally, it is stimulated first followed by the tibial nerve. As stated previously, the common peroneal nerve is identified by elicitation of dorsiflexion or eversion and the tibial nerve by plantar flexion. Local anesthetic (10 to 15 mL) is injected each time after the nerve is stimulated at <0.5 mA. As in the posterior approach, a double stimulation technique is recommended.

It should be noted that other authors insert their needle at a higher level. Vloka et al.[47] insert their needle 7 cm cephalad to the lateral femoral epicondyle, in the groove between the biceps femoris and the vastus lateralis muscles. At 7 cm above the femoral condyle, the sciatic nerve runs in a sheath which allows the cephalad spread of injected solutions. Vloka et al. advance their needle until they contact the shaft of the femur. They then withdraw their needle and redirect it posteriorly at a 30° angle to the horizontal plane. The needle is slowly advanced until dorsiflexion of the foot is elicited. After injection of local anesthetic, the needle is directed medially and slightly posterior to identify the tibial nerve.

The posterior and lateral approaches are equally effective. More attempts were necessary in the lateral approach and stimulation of the common peroneal nerve was more frequent in the lateral approach,[48] not a surprising finding in view of the lateral position of the nerve. One advantage of the lateral approach is that the patient is supine. There may be a slight discomfort with the lateral approach because of passage of the needle through the vastus lateralis or biceps femoris muscle.

Postoperative pain is a common reason for unplanned hospital admissions after surgery. Popliteal sciatic nerve block has been used in the management of postoperative pain. Rongstad et al.[4] reported the efficacy of popliteal sciatic nerve blocks. Their patients took an average of three hydrocodone tablets within the first 24 hours after their operation. In comparison to ankle blocks, popliteal sciatic blocks resulted in a longer duration of analgesia.[3]

SCIATIC NERVE BLOCK IN CHILDREN

Dalens el al.[49] compared the posterior, anterior, and lateral approaches to the sciatic nerve block in 180 pediatric patients, aged between 3 months and 18 years and weighing between 5.5 and 70 kg. The sciatic nerve was located by electrical stimulation. The depth of the sciatic nerve from the skin was significantly less with the posterior approach than with either the lateral or anterior approach. The overall success rate was 90% in the three groups with significantly fewer difficulties encountered in the posterior versus the anterior approach. No neurological sequelae were observed. The authors concluded that the posterior and lateral approaches are the most suitable approaches to sciatic nerve block in children.

CONTINUOUS SCIATIC NERVE BLOCK

Single-injection techniques of peripheral nerve blocks provide only a finite length of postoperative analgesia. Using a long-acting local anesthetic such as 0.625% chirocaine with epinephrine 1:200,000 for sciatic nerve block, the duration of postoperative analgesia following reconstructive ankle surgery was noted to be 19 ± 6 hours.[20] Continuous peripheral nerve blocks are optimal for providing prolonged postoperative analgesia.[50,51] However, issues such as complexity of the technique with respect to the placement and maintenance of the catheter, potential for nerve injury, and risk of systemic toxicity with continuous infusions of potent long-acting local anesthetic limit the applicability and acceptance of continuous catheter technology in a busy ambulatory or community hospital setting.[52,53] In a recent survey 228 patients undergoing upper and lower extremity outpatient procedures were treated with continuous peripheral nerve block catheters for 24 hours in an ambulatory surgery center. In this group 90% of catheters were functional after 24 hours and there were no complications at 1 and 7 days follow-up. Despite functional catheters, 59% to 80% of patients required supplemental oral or intravenous opioids during the 24-hour observation period.[54] The role of continuous peripheral nerve catheters continues to evolve both in inpatient and outpatient settings.[52,53]

CHOICE OF LOCAL ANESTHETICS AND ADJUNCTS

A single injection of 20 to 30 mL of a long-acting local anesthetic such as bupivacaine provides 12 to 24 hours (19 ± 6 hours) of postoperative analgesia.[20] This long duration favors the use of a single-injection technique for postoperative analgesia for the vast majority of orthopedic surgical procedures below the knee. The use of a continuous catheter technique is indicated primarily when postoperative analgesia greater than 24 hours is desired.

Historically, the sciatic nerve block has been considered as that with the longest latency to onset of surgical anesthesia. The delay in the onset of block can be minimized by observing the appropriate technique (see section on the methods of nerve localization) and by using higher concentrations of local anesthetic.[29,54,55] A quick onset of block with prolonged

postoperative analgesia is an important goal in peripheral nerve blocks. Although intermediate-acting local anesthetics such as mepivacaine and lidocaine have a faster onset time to surgical anesthesia compared to bupivacaine, the duration of the postoperative analgesia is limited to 4 to 6 hours. Ropivacaine 0.75% for sciatic block was found to have an onset time similar to 2% mepivacaine and duration of postoperative analgesia between 0.5% bupivacaine and 2% mepivacaine (ropivocaine 670 ± 227 minutes, bupivacaine 880 ± 312 minutes, and mepivacaine 251 ± 47 minutes).[56] Levobupivacaine is the most recently introduced long-acting local anesthetic. In a double-blind randomized comparison of 0.5% levobupivacaine versus 0.5% bupivacaine, the two local anesthetics were comparable with respect to onset of surgical anesthesia (5 to 60 minutes) and duration of postoperative analgesia (8 to 24 hours).[57]

For a continuous infusion technique of lower extremity nerve blocks, a dilute solution of a long-acting local anesthetic such as bupivacaine 0.1% to 0.25% or ropivacaine 0.2% is appropriate.[5,6,51,58–60] The administration of these concentrations at 8 to 10 mL/hour for 48 to 72 hours does not result in toxic blood levels of local anesthetics. The published data support that a patient-controlled infusion with or without a baseline continuous infusion is superior over a continuous infusion; the amount of local anesthetic can be reduced without affecting the quality of pain relief and patient satisfaction.[60,61]

LOCAL ANESTHETIC ADJUNCTS

Local anesthetic adjuncts such as epinephrine, clonidine, and opioids are added for the purposes of prolonging analgesia and anesthesia and minimizing blood levels of a local anesthetic.

Epinephrine: The addition of epinephrine to local anesthetics for peripheral nerve blocks has beneficial as well as adverse effects. The beneficial effects include the prolongation of the duration and intensity of the block for most of the local anesthetics. This has been attributed to local vasoconstriction with prolongation of nerve exposure to the local anesthetics. Epinephrine acts as a marker for intravascular injection. It minimizes systemic blood levels of the local anesthetic and reduces systemic toxicity by decreasing the absorption of the local anesthetic. The adverse effects of adding epinephrine to the local anesthetic include hemodynamic side effects such as tachycardia, a 10% to 15% increase in heart rate that lasts up to 90 minutes. There is a potential risk of perioperative neural injury through reduction of nerve blood flow. A decrease in blood flow of 20% to 30% has been reported with the addition of 5 μg/mL of epinephrine to lidocaine.[62,63] The risk of nerve injury with epinephrine-induced vasoconstriction may be increased in patients with compromised neural blood flow such as diabetic neuropathy and in normal patients with inadvertent intraneural injection. It is, therefore, prudent to use weaker concentrations of epinephrine (1:300,000 or 1:400,000) or avoid its use in patients with compromised neural blood flow from diabetes or atherosclerotic disease.

Clonidine: Clonidine is a peripheral alpha-2 adrenergic agonist. It potentiates conduction blockade of the local anesthetic by blocking conduction of the A-alpha and C fibers.[64] The clinical effects of clonidine are dependent on the type of local anesthetic with which it is used and the total dose used. The side effects (hypotension, bradycardia, sedation) with clonidine are unlikely when a total dose of up to 1.5 μg/kg is used (the maximum dose is ≤150 μg). Whereas the prolongation of analgesia with clonidine is well documented when it is added to the intermediate-acting local anesthetics, its ability to do the same when it is added to long-acting local anesthetics such as bupivacaine is less clear.[64,65]

Opioids: The data on the beneficial effect of opioids as an adjunct to local anesthetics in prolonging analgesia following peripheral nerve blocks are conflicting and not substantiated.[66,67]

METHODS OF NERVE LOCALIZATION

Two methods of peripheral nerve localization have been used in clinical practice: elicitation of paresthesia and a neurostimulation technique using electrical stimulation of the targeted neural elements with a low-intensity electrical current. Since the technique allows a more objective evaluation of the targeted neural elements being stimulated, neurostimulation technology has replaced the paresthesia approach especially for lower extremity blocks. Because of the size of the sciatic nerve and because of the two distinct components within the epineurial sheath, a single-injection technique may result in incomplete block of the sciatic nerve.[28,29] The use of the nerve stimulator allows for a precise identification of the two components of the sciatic nerve.[20,24] Using a nerve stimulator and a single-injection technique, two strategies have been proposed to improve the latency and success of a complete block of the sciatic nerve:

1. The proximity of the stimulating needle tip to both components of the sciatic nerve is ensured prior to local anesthetic injection. The EMR to neurostimulation determines the sciatic nerve component being stimulated (see Table 77-2 for nerve component, muscles supplied, and the foot movement for each muscle).[24,36] There are four possible foot movements in response to sciatic nerve stimulation: (1) plantar flexion—represents the action of muscles supplied by the tibial nerve, with some assistance from the peroneus muscles which are supplied by the superficial peroneal nerve; (2) dorsiflexion—represents the action of muscles supplied by the deep peroneal nerve; (3) inversion—represents the stimulation of both deep peroneal nerve which supplies the tibialis anterior muscle, and the tibial nerve which supplies the tibialis posterior muscle; and (4) eversion—represents the action of muscles supplied by superficial peroneal nerve. Elicitation of EMR inversion to neurostimulation therefore implies that the stimulating needle is lying in the middle of the sciatic nerve resulting in stimulation of both tibial and deep peroneal nerves. The deep peroneal nerve is located medially within the common peroneal nerve closer to the tibial nerve compared to superifical peroneal nerve.[24] The clinical studies correlating the four EMRs to the latency and success of a complete block of the sciatic nerve support this hypothesis.[20,24]

2. A close proximity of the stimulating needle tip to the sciatic nerve is ensured by eliciting an evoked motor response of either of the two components of the sciatic nerve at a current strength ≤0.4 mA. Using this endpoint Vloka et al. reported 100% success in achieving complete block of the sciatic nerve at the popliteal fossa, regardless of the type of EMR obtained.[25] The authors, however, have not been able to achieve 100% block of sciatic nerve using this strategy.

Historically, sciatic nerve block has been known to have variable success rate ranging from 33% to 95% and long latency requiring 30 minutes for a complete block.[10,18,29] By applying the two strategies outlined above, i.e., aiming for EMR inversion at ≤0.4 mA, one can achieve 100% success with a latency of <10 minutes for sciatic nerve block.[20]

COMPLICATIONS OF SCIATIC NERVE BLOCK

The sciatic nerve unlike the brachial plexus above the clavicle does not lie in the close vicinity of other nerves, sympathetic chain, or central neuraxis. Therefore, there are no complications related to the spread of local anesthetics to the adjacent structures. The exception, however, is the parasacral approach of Mansour[16] where the local anesthetic is deposited on the sacral plexus within the pelvis in the close vicinity of pelvic vasculature and viscera. The complications of sciatic nerve can be categorized into:

- Systemic toxicity due to high blood concentration of local anesthetics secondary to intravascular injection or local anesthetic overdose.
- Neurologic complication.

Systemic Toxicity: Providing anesthesia and analgesia for lower extremity surgery requires blockade of other nerves or the lumbar plexus to provide complete coverage of the surgical site. This translates to the administration of relatively larger doses of local anesthetics and, therefore, a finite risk of systemic toxicity from high blood level from absorption of the local anesthetic. Several studies have examined the blood levels of local anesthetics following combined blocks of lower extremity utilizing higher than recommended doses of local anesthetics.[68,69] Mepivacaine, lidocaine, and bupivacaine in doses exceeding 150% of the recommended doses did not produce systemic toxicity or excessive plasma levels. This may be related to the slower absorption of local anesthetics from the relatively avascular injected sites in lower extremity blocks. The addition of epinephrine to the local anesthetics in the combined blocks also minimizes the blood levels of the local anesthetics by slowing absorption.[63]

Neurologic Injury: Neurologic injury secondary to sciatic nerve block is infrequent. In a recent report on major complications of regional anesthesia in France peripheral neuropathy following sciatic nerve block occurred in 2.4 per 10,000 cases (2 cases amongst 8507 sciatic blocks performed).[70] In comparison, the frequency of peripheral neuropathy following popliteal block was much higher at 31.5 per 10,000 cases (3 cases amongst 952 popliteal blocks performed). The use of nerve stimulation for peripheral nerve blocks in the series did not prevent occurrence of neurologic injury. Strategies one can adopt to minimize the risk of neurologic injury following peripheral nerve block include the following:

- Moderate doses of sedation should be used, ensuring that the patient is coherent and conversant during the entire procedure and is able to report paresthesia if it occurs.

- EMR elicited at currents ≤0.5 mA ensures that the needle is close enough to the nerve to obtain a successful block. The EMR at currents lower than 0.2 mA, however, may suggest that the needle is too close to nerve with a risk of nerve damage from intraneural injection of local anesthetic. When using neurostimulation technology for nerve location, therefore, one must be certain that there is no brisk motor response at currents ≤0.2 mA and there is no discernible motor response at currents <0.1 mA.[55]
- Epinephrine in the local anesthetic solution has an impact on nerve blood flow and has been implicated in the neurologic injury following peripheral nerve blocks.[63] The theoretical risk of epinephrine-induced ischemic nerve injury is increased in patients with compromised blood flow from diabetes and atherosclerotic disease. It is preferable to use weaker concentrations (1:300,000 to 1:400,000) of epinephrine with local anesthetic solutions in patients at potential risk for ischemic nerve injury.

SUMMARY

Lower extremity nerve blocks are rapidly gaining in popularity for surgical anesthesia and postoperative analgesia. In patients undergoing painful orthopedic procedures of the lower extremity these blocks provide distinct advantages over general and central neuraxial anesthesia in inpatient and outpatient settings. Extended sciatic and femoral nerve blocks using long-acting local anesthetics or continuous catheter techniques permit superior postoperative analgesia with minimal side effects. Several new techniques have been described which are easy and practical and produce minimal patient discomfort. Neurostimulation technology has allowed precise identification of the larger neural elements to be blocked with minimal risk of nerve injury and discomfort to the patient. Neurostimulation technology is evolving with new research studies that are directed at improving the latency and success of lower extremity blocks. The risk of neurologic injury is minimal with lower extremity blocks. The judicious selection of local anesthetic drugs and adjuncts and the observance of appropriate precautions when locating the nerve by neurostimulation further reduce this risk.

KEY POINTS

- The sciatic nerve is the largest nerve in the body and innervates the entire leg below the knee and the foot except for its medial aspect which is innervated by the saphenous nerve. Its two divisions, the tibial nerve and the peroneal nerve, are separate but are covered by a continuous connective tissue sheath.
- The sciatic nerve can be blocked at different levels along its entire length as it exits the pelvis at the greater sciatic foramen to its termination in the popliteal fossa. Of the different approaches, the posterior subgluteus and the infragluteal parabiceps approaches are associated with less patient discomfort since the sciatic nerve is blocked at shallower depths compared to the other approaches.
- The use of the nerve stimulator facilitates easy identification of the sciatic nerve. The EMR should be obtained at stimulation intensities ≤0.4 mA. The appropriate EMR is inversion because it signifies stimulation of both divisions of the sciatic nerve (see Table 77-2). With inversion, blockade of

both components of the sciatic nerve is ensured and the latency of the block is shortened.

- Sciatic nerve block in the popliteal fossa can be performed through the posterior approach or lateral approach. The two approaches are equally effective. The lateral approach can be performed with the patient in the supine position while the posterior approach is usually done with the patient in the prone position.
- Evoked inversion may not be easy to elicit in the popliteal nerve block. The block can be facilitated by the two-stimulation technique. The first response is accepted and the other response is elicited after injection of the local anesthetic.
- The two-stimulation technique takes advantage of the anatomical relationship of the tibial and common peroneal nerves: the tibial nerve is located medially and the common peroneal nerve laterally. The needle is redirected after the initial evoked foot response is elicited. After plantar flexion is elicited (signifying stimulation of the tibial nerve) and the local anesthetic injected, the needle is moved laterally to block the common peroneal nerve. Either dorsiflexion (stimulation of the deep peroneal nerve) or eversion is elicited (stimulation of the superficial peroneal nerve) and the remaining local anesthetic injected. Conversely, the needle is moved medially after stimulation of the peroneal nerve and the tibial nerve blocked.
- The two-stimulation technique can be performed with the sciatic nerve block at the popliteal fossa because there is some distance between the tibial and peroneal nerves. The technique is difficult to perform with the other approaches to sciatic nerve blockade because of the close proximity of the tibial and peroneal nerves.

REFERENCES

1. Singelyn FJ, Gouverneur JA, Gribomont BF: Popliteal sciatic nerve block aided by a nerve stimulator. A reliable technique for foot and ankle surgery. Reg Anesth 16:278–281, 1991.
2. Hansen E, Eshelmon MR, Cracchiolo A: Popliteal fossa neural blockade as the sole anesthetic technique for outpatient foot and ankle surgery. Foot Ankle Int 21:38–44, 2000.
3. Mcleod DH, Wong DHW, Claridge RJ: Lateral popliteal sciatic nerve block compared with subcutaneous infiltration for analgesia following foot surgery. Can J Anaesth 41:673–676, 1994.
4. Rongstad K, Mann RA, Prieskorn DP, et al: Popliteal sciatic nerve block for postoperative analgesia. Foot Ankle Int 17:378–382, 1996.
5. Singelyn F, Aye F, Governeur JM: Continuous popliteal sciatic block: An origin technique to provide postoperative analgesia after foot surgery. Anesth Analg 84:383–386, 1997.
6. Ilfield BM, Money TE, Wang RD, Enneking FK: Continuous popliteal sciatic nerve block for postoperative pain control at home. A randomized, double blind, placebo controlled study. Anesthesiology 97:959–965, 2002.
7. Vloka JD, Hadzic A, Mulcare R, et al: Combined popliteal and posterior cutaneous nerve of the thigh for short saphenous vein stripping in outpatients: An alternative to spinal anesthetisia. J Clin Anesth 9:618–622, 1997.
8. Winnie AP: Regional anesthesia. Surg Clin North Am 54: 861–892, 1975.
9. Raj PP, Parks RI, Watson TD, et al: A new single supine approach to sciatic/femoral nerve block. Anesth Analg 54:489–494, 1975.
10. Beck GP: Anterior sciatic nerve block. Anesthesiology 24: 222–224, 1963.

11. Hadzic A, Vloka JD, Kuroda MM, et al: The practice of peripheral nerve blocks in the United States: A national survey. Reg Anesth Pain Med 23:241–246, 1998.

12. Smith MP, Juray Sprung MED, Zura A, et al: A survey of exposure to regional anesthesia technique in American anesthesia residency training program. Reg Anesth Pain Med 24:11–16, 1999.

13. Kopacz DJ, Neal JM: Regional anesthesia and pain medicine: Residency training – The year 2000. Reg Anesth Pain Med 24:9–14, 2002.

14. Labat G: Regional Anesthesia. Its Technique and Clinical Applications, ed 2. WB Saunders, Philadelphia, 1930, p 33.

15. Ichiyanagi K: Sciatic nerve block: Lateral approach with patient supine. Anesthesiology 20:601–604, 1959.

16. Mansour NY: Reevaluating the sciatic nerve block: Another landmark for consideration. Reg. Anesth 18:322–323, 1993.

17. Chelly JE, Delauney L: A new approach to the sciatic nerve block. Anesthesiology 91:1655–1660, 1999.

18. Guardini R, Waldron BA, Wallace WA: Sciatic nerve block: A new lateral approach. Acta Anesthesiol Scand 29:515–519, 1985.

19. Benedetto P, Bertini L, Casati A, et al: A new posterior approach to the sciatic nerve block: A prospective, randomized comparison with the classic posterior approach. Anesth Analg 93:1040–1044, 2001.

20. Sukhani R, Candido KD, Doty R, et al. Infragluteal–parabiceps scatic nerve block: An evaluation of a novel approach using a single injection technique. Anesth Analg 96:868–873, 2003.

21. Rorie DK, Byer D, Nelson DO, et al: Assessment of the block of the sciatic nerve in the popliteal fossa. Anesth Analg 59:371–376, 1980.

22. Vloka JD, Hadzic A, Koorn R, et al: Supine approach to the sciatic nerve in the popliteal fossa. Can J Anaesth 43:964–997, 1996.

23. Hadzic A, Vloka J, Singson R, et al: A comparison of intertendinous and classical approaches to popliteal nerve block using magnetic resonance imaging simulation. Anesth Analg 94:1321–1324, 2002.

24. Benzon HT, Kim C, Benzon HP, et al: Correlation between evoked motor response of the sciatic nerve and sensory blockade. Anesthesiology 87:548–552, 1997.

25. Vloka JD, Hadzic A: The intensity of current at which sciatic nerve stimulation is achieved is more important factor in determining the quality of nerve block than the type of motor response obtained [letter to the editor]. Anesthesiology 88:148–50, 1998.

26. Bailey SL, Parkinson SK, Little WL, et al: Sciatic nerve block: A comparison of single versus double injection technique. Reg Anesth 19:9–13, 1994.

27. Davies MJ, McGlode DP: One hundred sciatic nerve blocks: A comparison of single versus double injection technique. Reg Anesth 19:9–13, 1994.

28. Bouaziz H, Paqueron X, Macalou D, et al: The lateral approach block of sciatic nerve at the popliteal level: One or two stimulations. Anesthesiology 89:A838, 1998.

29. Morris GF, Lang SA, Dust WM, et al: The parasacral sciatic nerve block. Reg Anesth 22:223–228, 1997.

30. Brown DL: Sciatic block. In Atlas of Regional anesthesia, ed 2. WB Saunders, Philadelphia, 1999, pp 95–101.

31. Vloka JD, Hadzic A, April E, et al: Anterior approach to the sciatic nerve block: The effects of leg rotation. Anesth Analg 92:460–462, 2001.

32. Ericksen ML, Swenson JD, Pace NL: The anatomic relationship of the sciatic nerve to the lesser trochanter: Implications for anterior sciatic nerve block. Anesth Analg 95:1971–1974, 2002.

33. Sarrafian SK. Anatomy of the Foot and Ankle. JB Lippincott, Philadelphia, 1983, pp 313–332.

34. Benzon HT, Calimaran AL, Hausman J: Saphenous nerve blockade. Presented at the ASA Annual Meeting, New Orleans, LA, 16 October 2001.

35. Calilet R: Foot and Ankle Pain. FA Davis, Philadelphia, 1983, pp 1–46.

36. Mayo Clinic and Mayo Foundation: Clinical Examinations in Neurology. WB Saunders, Philadelphia, 1981, pp 168–188.

37. Singelyn FJ, Gouverneur JA, Gribomont BF: Popliteal sciatic nerve block aided by a nerve stimulator: A reliable technique for foot and ankle surgery. Reg Anesth 16:178–281, 1991.

38. Benzon HT. In reply – The intensity of the current at which sciatic nerve stimulation is achieved is more important factor in determining the quality of nerve block than the type of motor response obtained. Anesthesiology 88:1410–1411, 1998.

39. Sims JK: A modification of landmarks for infraclavicular approach to brachial plexus block. Anesth Analg 56:554, 1977.

40. Vloka JD, Hadzic A, Lesser JB, et al: A common epineural sheath for the nerves in the popliteal fossa and its possible implications for sciatic nerve block. Anesth Analg 84:387–390, 1997.

41. Vloka JD, Hadzic A, April E, Thys DM: The division of the sciatic nerve in the popliteal fossa: Anatomical implications for popliteal nerve blockade. Anesth Analg 92:215–217, 2001.

42. Benzon HT: Popliteal sciatic nerve block. Posterior approach. Tech Reg Anesth Pain Manage 3:23–27, 1999.

43. Bailey SL, Parkinson SK, Little WL, Simmerman SR: Sciatic nerve block. A comparison of single versus double injection technique. Reg Anesth 19:9, 1994.

44. Collum CR, Courtney PG: Sciatic nerve blockade by the lateral approach to the popliteal fossa. Anaesth Intens Care 21:236–237, 1993.

45. Bouaziz H, Narchi P, Zetlaoui PJ, et al: Lateral approach to sciatic nerve at the popliteal fossa combined with saphenous nerve block. Tech Reg Anesth Pain Manage 3:19–22, 1999.

46. Zetlaoui PJ, Bouaziz H: Lateral approach to the sciatic nerve in the popliteal fossa. Anesth Analg 87:79–82, 1998.

47. Vloka JD, Hadzic A, Kitain E, et al: Anatomic considerations for sciatic nerve block in the popliteal fossa through the lateral approach. Reg Anesth 21:414, 1996.

48. Hadzic A, Vloka J: A comparison of the posterior versus lateral approaches to the block of the sciatic nerve in the popliteal fossa. Anesthesiology 88:1480–1486, 1998.

49. Dalens B, Tanguy A, Vanneuville G: Sciatic nerve blocks in children: Comparison of the posterior, anterior, and lateral approaches in 180 pediatric patients. Anesth Analg 70:131–137, 1990.

50. Ilfeld BM, Money TE, Wang RD, et al: Continuous popliteal sciatic nerve blocks for postoperative pain control at home: A randomized, double blinded, placebo controlled study. Anesthesiology 97:959–965, 2002.

51. di Benedetto P, Casati A, Bertini L, et al: Postoperative analgesia with continuous sciatic nerve block after foot surgery: A prospective randomized comparison between the popliteal and subgluteal approaches. Anesth Analg 94:996–1000, 2002.

52. Klein SM: Beyond the hospital: Continuous peripheral nerve blocks at home [editorial]. Anesthesiology 96:1283–1284, 2002.

53. Liu SS, Salinas FU: Continuous plexus and peripheral nerve blocks for postoperative analgesia. Anesth Analg 96:263–272, 2003.

54. Grant SA, Nielsen KC, Greengrass RA, et al. Continuous peripheral nerve blocks for ambulatory surgery. Reg Anesth Pain Med 26:209–214, 2001.

55. Hadzic A, Vloka J, Hadzic N, et al. Nerve stimulations used for peripheral nerve blocks vary in their electrical characteristics. Anesthesiology 98:969–974, 2003.

56. Smith BE, Siggins D: Low volume, high concentration block of the sciatic nerve. Anesthesia 43:8–11, 1988.

57. Fanelli G, Casati A, Beccaria P, et al: A double bind comparison of ropivacaine, bupivacaine and mepivacaine during sciatic and femoral nerve blockade. Anesth Analg 87:597–600, 1998.

58. Chelly JE, Greger J, Gebhand R, et al: Continuous femoral nerve blocks improve recovery and outcome of patients undergoing total knee arthroplasty. J Anthroplasty 16:436–445, 2001.

59. Chudinov A, Bercenstadt H, Salai M, et al: Continuous psoas compartment block for anesthesia and perioperative analgesia in patients with hip fractures. Reg Anesth Pain Med 24:563–568, 1999.

60. Singelyn F, Gouverneur JM: Extended "three-in-one" block after total knee arthroplasty: Continuous versus patient controlled analgesia techniques. Aneth Analg 91:176–180, 2000.

61. Singelyn F, Seguy S, Gouverneur JM: Interscalene brachial plexus analgesia after open shoulder surgery: Continuous versus patient controlled analgesia infusion. Anesth Analg 89:1216–1220, 1999.

62. Bernards CM, Kopacz DJ: Effect of epinephrine on lidocaine clearance in vivo: A microdialysis study in humans. Anesthesiology 91:962–968, 1999.

63. Neal JM: Effect of epinephrine in local anesthetics on the central and peripheral nervous systems: Neurotoxicity and neural blood flow. Reg Anesth Pain Med 28:124–134, 2003.

64. Eisenach JC, de Kock M, Klimscha W: α-2-adrenergic agonists for regional anesthesia: A clinical review of clonidine (1984–1995). Anesthesiology 85:655–674, 1996.

65. Culebras X, Van Gessel E, Hoffmeyer P, et al: Clonidine combined with a long acting local anesthetic does not prolong postoperative analgesia after brachial plexus block but does induce hemodynamic changes. Anesth Analg 92:199–204, 2001.

66. Murphy DB, McCartney CJ, Chen VW: Novel analgesic adjuncts for brachial plexus block: A systematic review. Anesth Analg 90:1122–1128, 2000.

67. Reuben SS, Rueben JP: Brachial plexus anesthesia with verapamil and/or morphine. Anesth Analg 91:379–383, 2000.

68. Elmos C, Etanassoff PG: Combined inguinal paravascular (3-in-1) and sciatic nerve blocks for lower limb surgery. Reg Anesth 18:88, 1993.

69. Misna G, Pridie AK, McClymont C, et al: Plasma concentration of bupivacaine following combined sciatic and femoral 3-in-1 nerve blocks in open knee surgery. Br J Anaesth 66:310, 1991.

70. Auroy Y, Benhamou D, Bargues L, et al: Major complications of regional anesthesia in France. The SOS regional anesthesia hotline service. Anesthesiology 97:1274–1280, 2002.

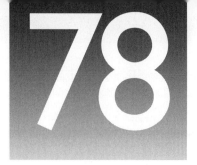

Ankle Block

**Robert Doty, Jr., M.D., and
Radha Sukhani, M.D.**

Ankle block is a common and successful means of providing surgical anesthesia and postoperative analgesia for midfoot and forefoot surgery. Depending on the technique utilized it can also provide anesthesia for surgery on the hind foot. Familiarity with the anatomy and innervation of the foot allows more precise location of the five nerves involved in performing an ankle block and a higher success of complete block.

The nerve supply to the foot and ankle is provided by four terminal branches of the sciatic nerve and the saphenous nerve (a terminal branch of the femoral nerve). The cutaneous innervation of these five branches supplying the foot is as follows[1] (Fig. 78-1):

1. *Posterior tibial nerve*—plantar surface of the foot and toes by its three divisions: medial plantar nerve, lateral plantar nerve, and medial calcaneal nerve.
2. *Deep peroneal nerve*—the dorsal surface of the foot between the great and second toe.
3. *Sural nerve*—the lateral surface of the foot (dorsolateral cutaneous nerve), and the heel (lateral calcaneal nerve). A medial branch unites with the intermediate cutaneous nerve of the superficial peroneal nerve innervating the web spaces of the third and fourth toes.
4. *Superficial peroneal nerve*—the dorsal surface of the foot and toes, except the web space between the first and second toes and the lateral aspect of the foot including the fifth toe and lateral half of the fourth toe.
5. *Saphenous nerve*—the skin over the medial malleolus, medial surface of the foot up to the medial arch and to the medial side of the great toe.

Thus, complete ankle block involves anesthesia of all five nerves—the posterior tibial nerve being the major component nerve as it innervates all five toes.

POSTERIOR TIBIAL NERVE (PTN)

Anatomy:[1] The PTN is one of the two terminal divisions of the sciatic nerve and consists of muscular, cutaneous, and articular branches. It extends from the arch of the soleus muscle to the tibiotalocalcaneal canal. In the upper two-thirds of the leg the nerve is located deep in the posterior compartment. In the lower one-third of the leg the nerve assumes a superficial location as the soleus and gastrocnemius muscles converge to form the Achilles tendon. At this level the PTN courses along the medial border of the Achilles tendon between the flexor digitorum longus, which lies anteromedially, and the musculotendinous flexor hallucis longus, which lies posterolateral to the nerve (Fig. 78-2). In this location the PTN lies lateral and posterior (thus more superficial) to the posterior tibial artery and vein (Fig. 78-3). In the talocalcaneal canal the PTN divides into its two terminal branches: the medial and lateral plantar nerves. In 93% of cases this division occurs in the talocalcaneal canal within 2 cm of the tip of medial malleolus. In 7% of cases this division occurs at a more proximal level. Therefore, blocking the PTN at a distal site in these patients may result in partial block of the nerve.

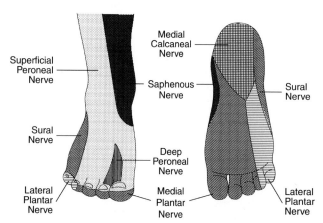

FIGURE 78-1. Cutaneous innervation of the foot: The medial plantar nerve, lateral plantar nerve, and medial calcaneal nerve are branches of the posterior tibial nerve.

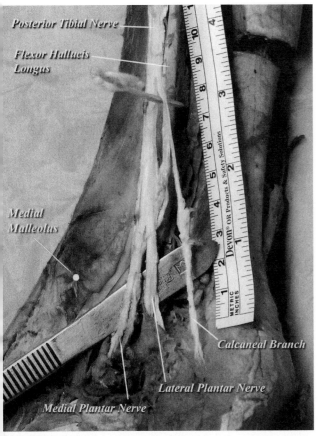

Posterior Tibial Nerve

Flexor Hallucis Longus

Medial Malleolus

Calcaneal Branch

Lateral Plantar Nerve

Medial Plantar Nerve

FIGURE 78-2. Terminal branches of the posterior tibial nerve. The medial calcaneal nerve can originate as high as 8 to 10 cm above the tip of the medial malleolus. The medial and lateral plantar nerves usually divide in the talocalcaneal canal within 2 cm of the tip of the medial malleolus, sometimes higher.

The PTN also gives off a medial calcaneal branch that has a variable origin. In 40% of cases the medial calcaneal branch originates high above the talocalcaneal canal (Fig. 78-2). The cutaneous branches of the medial calcaneal nerve supply the medial side of the heel.

The medial plantar nerve (MPN) is longer than the lateral plantar nerve (LPN). The MPN supplies the muscular branches to the abductor hallucis, flexor digitorum brevis, flexor hallucis brevis, and lumbricals. Neurostimulation of the MPN produces flexion of all toes except the great toe and abduction of the great toe. The LPN supplies muscular branches to the abductor digiti minimi, adductor hallucis, quadratus plantae, short flexors, and opponens of the fifth and fourth toes (sometimes the third toe), lumbricals, and interossei. Neurostimulation of the LPN produces adduction of the great toe, abduction of the fifth toe, and contraction of the musculotendinous arch of the foot (contraction of the quadratus plantae).

Posterior Tibial Nerve Block: The PTN can be blocked by two approaches: the distal (traditional) approach and the proximal approach.

DISTAL APPROACH (TRADITIONAL SITE): The PTN can be blocked at the level of the medial malleolus within 2 to 3 cm of its tip, and thus within the tibiocalcaneal canal. The nerve in this location lies under the flexor reticulum, posterior to the tibial artery and vein. The limitations of the PTN block at the distal traditional site are:

- The diffusion barrier imposed by the flexor reticulum.
- A partial and incomplete block because the calcaneal branch may have taken off at higher level (40%) and the two terminal divisions of the nerve—medial and lateral plantar nerves—may have separated (7% to 13% of cases).
- In patients with an altered and/or distorted ankle anatomy (inflammation, edema, poor vascular anatomy) the block may be technically difficult and the results may be disappointing.

The technique of traditional distal PTN block[2,3] is as follows. After appropriate sedation, the patient is placed either in the prone position, or in the supine position with the foot elevated high by blankets under the calf, or the knee flexed to allow access to the back of the ankle. The needle entry site is marked 2 to 3 cm proximal to the tip of the medial malleolus (or at the superior border of the medial malleolus) approximately 1 cm from the medial border of the Achilles tendon, posterior to the tibial artery pulsation (if palpable). After appropriate aseptic precautions and superficial local anesthetic infiltration of the marked site, a 22-gauge, 1.5-inch B bevel needle or a 50 mm, 22-gauge insulated needle (if a neurostimulation technique is used) is directed toward the posterior aspect of the tibia, posterior to the tibial artery pulsation, until a paresthesia or appropriate motor response is obtained or bone is contacted (Fig. 78-3). If neurostimulation is not being used, after bone contact is obtained and the needle withdrawn 1 to 2 mm off the bone, 5 to 7 mL of local anesthetic is injected incrementally checking for negative aspiration of blood. If a neurostimulation technique is used, the needle is redirected medially or laterally until an appropriate evoked motor response is obtained at <0.5 mA (see below).

PROXIMAL APPROACH TO PTN BLOCK: In the proximal approach to PTN block the posterior tibial nerve is blocked before it has given off its medial calcaneal branch and before it divides into its two terminal branches: the MPN and LPN. This approach is practiced extensively at the authors' institution and is associated with a high success of complete block. A consistent location of the posterior tibial nerve in the lower third of the leg is 7 cm above the medial malleolus in line with, and slightly anterior to, the medial border of the Achilles tendon (Fig. 78-4). The nerve at this location lies between the tendon of the flexor digitorum and the musculotendinous flexor hallucis longus.

The needle entry site is marked 7 cm from the superior border of the medial malleolus and approximately 1 cm anterior to the medial border of the Achilles tendon in the groove between the flexor digitorum and flexor hallucis longus. After appropriate aseptic precautions and superficial local anesthetic infiltration of the marked site, a 50 mm, 22-gauge insulated needle is introduced in a direction that is anterior and slightly caudad 60° to the sagittal plane until an appropriate evoked motor response (see below) is obtained at <0.5 mA. A loss of resistance or a "pop" may be felt as the needle penetrates the intermuscular fascia septa between the flexor digitorum and flexor hallucis muscles. Isolated flexion of the great toe represents direct stimulation of the musculotendinous flexor hallucis tendon indicating that the needle tip is too deep and

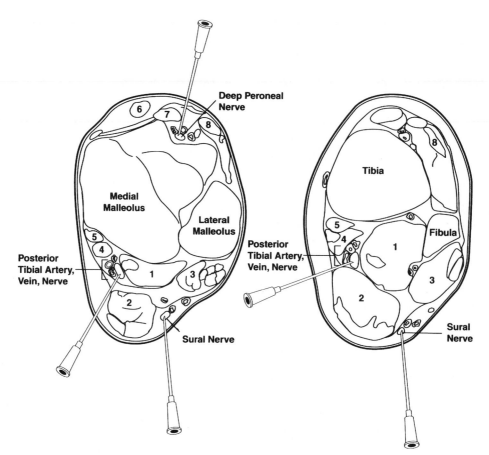

FIGURE 78-3. Cross-sections of the lower extremity. The needle is inserted 2 cm proximal to the tip of the medial malleolus in the figure on the left and inserted 7 to 8 cm proximal to the tip of the medial malleolus in the figure on the right. 1, Musculotendinous flexor hallucis longus tendon; 2, Achilles tendon; 3, peroneal tendon; 4, flexor digitorum longus tendon; 5, tibialis posterior tendon; 6, tibialis anterior tendon; 7, extensor hallucis longus tendon; 8, extensor digitorum longus tendon.

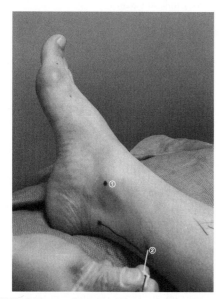

FIGURE 78-4. Proximal approach to posterior tibial nerve block. The site of block is measured 7 cm proximal from the tip of the medial malleolus (1) and approximately 1 cm anterior to the medial border of the Achilles tendon in the groove between the flexor digitorum longus and flexor hallucis tendons (2). The block needle is directed anterior and slightly caudad 60° to the sagittal plane of the Achilles tendon.

posterior and should be withdrawn and directed anteriorly. Aspiration of blood during needle advancement indicates the needle tip is too anterior and medial to the PTN. The needle should then be withdrawn and directed posteriolaterally until the appropriate motor response is obtained. A volume of 7 to 10 mL of local anesthetic is injected incrementally checking for negative aspiration of blood.

Anatomical Indicators for Neurostimulation of the PTN: The PTN has two neural components: the MPN and the LPN. The MPN is the longer anterior component. Neurostimulation of each component produces distinct evoked motor response as outlined below.

NEUROSTIMULATION OF THE MEDIAL PLANTAR NERVE

- Plantar flexion of all toes except the great toe. A very important point to note, as mentioned previously, is isolated plantar flexion of the great toe represents direct stimulation of the musculotendinous flexor hallucis longus. Using plantar flexion of the great toe as an endpoint for local anesthetic injection, therefore, will result in a failed block. If plantar flexion of the great toe is encountered, the needle is posterior and should be withdrawn and redirected more anterior to the Achilles tendon.
- Abduction of the great toe.

NEUROSTIMULATION OF THE LATERAL PLANTAR NERVE
- Contraction of the tendinous plantar arch of the midfoot.
- Abduction of the fifth toe.
- Adduction of the great toe.

NEUROSTIMULATION OF THE MAIN TRUNK OF THE PTN
- Plantar flexion of all the toes except the great toe.
- Adduction of the great toe (adduction is dominant compared to abduction).
- Contraction of the tendinous arch of the midfoot.
- Abduction of the fifth toe.

Other Approaches to PTN Block
MIDTARSAL APPROACH:[4] The PTN can be blocked distal to the flexor reticulum where it is relatively superficial. The posterior tibial artery is palpated distal to the medial malleolus. The needle is inserted on either side of the posterior tibial artery and advanced towards the calcaneus. After bony contact is made, the needle is withdrawn 2 to 3 mm and 5 to 7 mL of local anesthetic is injected. This a more distal block of the PTN for mid- or forefoot surgery and the calcaneal branch may be missed.

SUBCALCANEAL APPROACH:[5] Distal to the medial malleolus the bony ridge on the calcaneus can normally be palpated. The PTN is in close and consistent relation to this bony ridge. The needle is inserted posteroinferiorly to the bony ridge until a bony contact is made. The needle is withdrawn and 5 to 7 mL of local anesthetic is injected. This is also a more distal block for mid- or forefoot surgery and the calcaneal branch may be missed.

DEEP PERONEAL NERVE (DPN) BLOCK

Anatomy:[1] In the distal third of the leg the DPN passes behind the extensor hallucis longus tendon. Approximately 2.5 to 5 cm above the ankle the DPN is located between the tendons of the extensor digitorum and extensor hallucis longus tendons. In the majority of cases the DPN lies laterally to the anterior tibial artery proximally. The nerve then becomes more medial, just lateral to the extensor hallicus longus tendon at the level of the malleoli. The DPN divides into lateral and medial terminal branches 1 cm above the ankle joint in 98% of cases. In 1.2% of cases the branching occurs higher. The lateral branch supplies the extensor digitorum brevis and divides to become the second, third, and fourth interosseous nerves. The medial branch is the longer of the two branches and divides to supply dorsal cutaneous branches to the great toe and the second toe.

Technique: The most consistent location of the DPN is 2.5 cm above the level of the ankle joint at the upper border of extensor hallucis longus (EHL) laterally and extensor digitorum longus (EDL) medially. Dorsiflexion of the great toe (EHL) and small toes (EDL) allows identification of these two tendons. The needle is advanced perpendicular to the ankle joint (lower anterior tibia) until bone is contacted, the needle is withdrawn 1 to 2 mm, and 5 mL of local anesthetic is injected. If a nerve stimulator is being used (2 to 3 mA current is often needed at 0.1 ms), the evoked motor response obtained is a muscle twitch of the extensor digitorum brevis: extension of the lateral four toes.

SUPERFICIAL PERONEAL NERVE (SPN) BLOCK

Anatomy:[1] The SPN is a sensory branch of the common peroneal nerve. After coursing in the anterolateral compartment of the leg, the nerve pierces the deep fascia 10 to 15 cm from the tip of lateral malleolus. From this point the SPN lies subcutaneously and divides into branches that supply the dorsum of the foot and toes.

Technique: The SPN can be blocked by subcutaneous infiltration of 5 to 7 mL of local anesthetic between the lateral border of the tibia to the superior aspect of the lateral malleolus.

SURAL NERVE BLOCK

Anatomy:[1] The sural nerve is formed by the union of the medial sural nerve—a branch of the tibial nerve—and the lateral sural nerve—a branch of the common peroneal nerve. The sural nerve courses along the lateral border of the Achilles tendon and is posteromedial to the short saphenous vein. The sural nerve turns around the posterior border of the lateral malleolus and passes 1 to 1.5 cm from the tip of the lateral malleolus from which it is separated by peroneal tendons. At the level of the base of the fifth metatarsal, the nerve divides into its two terminal branches: medial and lateral. The lateral branch (dorsolateral cutaneous nerve) supplies sensory innervation to the lateral border of the foot, and the fourth and fifth toes. The medial branch unites with the intermediate cutaneous nerve of the superficial peroneal nerve innervating the web spaces of the third and fourth toes.

The sural nerve also gives off two lateral calcaneal branches above the tip of the lateral malleolus. A very consistent superficial anatomical location of the sural nerve is 7 to 10 cm above the tip of the lateral malleolus just at the lateral border of the Achilles tendon. The short saphenous vein may be visible and courses in close vicinity (anterolaterally) to the nerve at this point.

Technique: The patient may lie in the prone position or in the supine position with the knee flexed, to expose the back of the lower leg and ankle. The needle entry site is anterolateral to the Achilles tendon at the level of the lateral malleolus. The needle is introduced through the skin aiming for the lateral border of the lateral malleolus and fibula. Local anesthetic solution (up to 5 mL) is infiltrated just anterolateral (approximately 1 to 2 cm) to the lateral border of the Achilles tendon. The nerve may be blocked 7 to 10 cm above the superior border of the lateral malleolus just at the lateral border of Achilles tendon posteromedially to the short saphenous vein. The nerve is very superficial at this site and block of the lateral calcaneal nerves is also accomplished (Fig. 78-3).

For surgery on the midfoot or third and fourth toes, a full sural nerve block may not be needed if the lateral aspect of the foot is to be avoided. However, the medial branch of the sural nerve, which unites with the intermediate cutaneous nerve of the superficial peroneal nerve, can be blocked with 3 to 5 mL of local anesthetic superficially infiltrated at the anterior border of the lateral malleolus.

TABLE 78-1. APPROXIMATE DURATIONS OF SURGICAL ANESTHESIA AND POSTOPERATIVE ANALGESIA FOR DIFFERENT LOCAL ANESTHETIC DRUGS

Local Anesthetic Drug	Duration of Surgical Anesthesia (hours)	Duration of Postoperative Analgesia (hours)
Lidocaine 1.5–2%	2–2.5	3–5
Mepivacaine 1.5–2%	3–4	5–6
Bupivacaine 0.25%	–	5–6
Bupivacaine 0.5% and 0.625%	5–6	12–24
Lidocaine/mepivacaine plus bupivacaine	3–4	8–12

Epinephrine should not be added to local anesthetic solution for ankle block as this may impair the vascular supply distally in the foot.

SAPHENOUS NERVE BLOCK

Anatomy:[1] The saphenous nerve is the terminal branch of the femoral nerve. The nerve becomes superficial at the medial border of the knee joint as it pierces the fascia between the gracilis and sartorius muscles. It runs distally in the cleft behind the medial border of the tibia just posterior to the great saphenous vein. It divides into branches, one branch ending at the ankle. The second branch passes in front of the medial malleolus, close to the long saphenous vein. It provides cutaneous innervation to the medial site of the foot extending up to the medial side of the big toe.

Technique: The saphenous nerve is blocked by subcutaneous infiltration of 3 to 5 mL of local anesthetic along the upper border of the medial malleolus near the greater saphenous vein.

LOCAL ANESTHETIC CHOICE AND DOSE FOR ANKLE BLOCK

The PTN is a fairly large nerve and is the major component nerve involved in performing an ankle block for surgical procedures of the midfoot, forefoot, and hind foot. If the needle tip is in the close vicinity to the nerve as indicated by paresthesia or an appropriate evoked motor response, as mentioned above, at a stimulating current of <0.5 mA, a smaller volume of local anesthetic (5 to 7 mL) may suffice. If such definite endpoints are not present, it is preferable to use a higher (10 to 12 mL) local anesthetic volume to ensure adequate diffusion of the local anesthetic.

Duration of surgery, and, most importantly, duration of postoperative analgesia is an important consideration in the selection of local anesthetic agent for ankle block (Table 78-1).

REFERENCES

1. Sarrafian SK: Anatomy of the Foot and Ankle, Descriptive, Topographic, Functional, ed 2. JB Lippincott, Philadelphia, 1993.
2. Brown D: Regional Anesthesia, ed 2. WB Saunders, Philadelphia, 1999, pp 289–290.
3. Sarrafian SK, Ibrahim IN, Breihan JH: Ankle foot peripheral nerve block for midfoot and forefoot surgery. Foot and Ankle 4:86–90, 1983.
4. Sharrock ME, Waller JF, Fierro LE: Midtarsal block for surgery of the forefoot Br J Anesth 58:37–40, 1986.
5. Wassef MR: Posterior tibial nerve block. A new approach using bony landmark of the sustentaculum tali. Anaesthesia 46:841–844, 1991.

Issues in Peripheral Nerve Blocks: Use of Nerve Stimulators, Multiple- versus Single-Injection Techniques, and Use of Adjuvants

Kenneth D. Candido, M.D.,
Jeffrey A. Katz, M.D., and
Honorio T. Benzon, M.D.

USE OF NERVE STIMULATORS

Overview: Although much has been written on the use of nerve stimulators in peripheral nerve blockade, there remains controversy about the role relative to other approaches, such as the elicitation of paresthesia or the use of transarterial methods.[1] Nonetheless, it has particular advantage in those situations where the surrounding anatomy is not consistent relative to the target nerve's location (e.g., obturator or popliteal nerve block) or where patient cooperation may not be present. With the development of equipment specially suited for peripheral nerve stimulation for regional anesthesia and the ready availability of associated equipment such as insulated needles and stimulating catheter sets, it would appear that the use of nerve stimulation in regional anesthesia is likely to continue to increase.

History: In 1912, about one year after Kulenkampff's description of brachial plexus blockade via the axillary approach, Perthes used electrical stimulation to locate the brachial plexus.[2,3] However, since his equipment was cumbersome, inconvenient, and required the use of needles insulated with lacquer, it was largely disregarded. In 1955 Pearson demonstrated how motor nerve stimulation could be used to locate peripheral nerves, but it was the introduction in 1962 by

Greenblatt and Denson of a convenient transistorized unit that the method became practical.[1] They demonstrated how motor nerves could be stimulated using voltages (later demonstrated to be a crude parameter relative to current) without eliciting pain and how the voltage required reflected the distance of the needle from the target nerve.[2]

Later issues addressed the concern that insulated needles of that time (using modified needles or plastic catheters) altered the tactile sensitivity during the procedure, so studies on uninsulated needles were performed. It was found that standard, unsheathed needles could be used successfully for nerve localization for regional anesthesia.[4]

Technical Issues: Excellent reviews have been published on the technical aspects of nerve stimulator design and application.[5] To appreciate the design and application of nerve stimulators for regional anesthesia, it is useful to understand the electrophysiology of stimulation.

PULSE CHARACTER AND POLARITY: The ability to stimulate a nerve depends upon both the current applied (pulse amplitude) and the duration of current application (pulse width). Smaller nerve fibers (A-delta or C) require longer current durations than larger fibers (A-alpha motor) to be stimulated for a

TABLE 79-1. **NERVE TYPE AND DURATION OF STIMULUS**

Nerve Site from Cat	Nerve Type	Chronaxis (µs)
Sural nerve	A-alpha A-delta	50–100 170
Saphenous	C	400

The chronaxes (duration of stimulus) needed to stimulate various types of mammalian nerves for a given current. Note that large motor fibers in a mixed-fiber peripheral nerve may be stimulated with short stimulation durations while pain fibers are not affected, allowing motor twitch to be elicited in the absence of pain or paresthesia.

Modified from Raj P, Banister R: Aids to localization of peripheral nerves. In Raj PP (ed): Textbook of Regional Anesthesia. Churchill-Livingstone, New York, 2002, pp 251–283.

given current. Hence in mixed peripheral nerves, by limiting the duration of the pulse width it is possible to stimulate only motor fibers without triggering pain. A short pulse width of 50 to 100 microseconds is optimal (Table 79-1). Furthermore, shorter pulse widths provide better discrimination of the distance of the needle tip from the nerve (i.e., longer pulse widths are more likely to stimulate a nerve when the tip is too far away, whereas with short pulse widths it takes much more current to stimulate distant nerves).[5]

Another important consideration in the design and use of nerve stimulators is in the assignment of the (negative) cathode to the exploring needle and the (positive) anode to the ground lead. Less current is required to stimulate a nerve in this configuration, since when the needle is the cathode current flows toward it, causing depolarization of nerve tissue near the needle; if the needle is the anode then hyperpolarization of the nerve occurs.[6,7] This has been shown to have clinical relevance during brachial plexus blockade, with the current required for stimulation being tripled when the positive lead is connected to the needle.[8]

STIMULATING DISTANCE AND CURRENT REQUIRED:
The basis of nerve stimulation for regional anesthesia is the concept that the current required to stimulate the nerve is directly related to the distance of the needle tip from the nerve. Current density diminishes quickly as one moves further from the stimulating needle tip. For example, if a stimulus of 0.1 mA is needed to depolarize a nerve when the needle is touching the nerve, at 0.5 cm from the nerve 2.5 mA will be needed and at 1 cm 10 mA will be needed.[5] Based on these theoretical calculations, it is very unlikely that a nerve will be stimulated until the needle tip is within a centimeter of it.

An early study of obturator nerve blocks demonstrated that 0.5 mA was needed for direct stimulation of the obturator nerve, and when 1 to 3 mA was needed to elicit motor response the subsequent block was usually unsuccessful.[9] Another study examining interscalene, supraclavicular, and axillary approaches to the brachial plexus found that currents ranging from 0.2 to 1.5 mA were "readily obtainable and sufficient for localization" of the plexus in all locations.[10]

The concept of minimum current required for stimulation is reviewed further in the Clinical Issues section below.

INSULATED VS. UNINSULATED NEEDLES:
A debated issue relating to accuracy of needle placement concerns the use of insulated vs. uninsulated needles for stimulating. Uninsulated needles are effective despite the fact that current may escape along their entire length, because the greatest current density is at the tip (Fig. 79-1). Some even take the position that the pattern of current spread from uninsulated needles allows more precise positioning of the needle tip next to the nerve than insulated needles.[11] However, uninsulated needles can mislead needle placement by stimulating a nerve even though the tip of the needle has passed the nerve. Furthermore, higher currents are needed to stimulate nerves using uninsulated vs. insulated needles.[12] Using the saphenous nerve of an in vivo cat model, it was found that on average a minimally stimulating current of 0.5 mA (range 0.2 to 0.9 mA) located the tip of an insulated needle an average of 0 cm from the nerve (range 0 to 0.2 cm past the nerve). This is in comparison to an average minimally stimulating current of 1.2 mA (range 0.7 to 1.5 mA) and a distance of 0.4 cm past the nerve (0 to 0.8 cm past the nerve) using uninsulated needles.[12]

Despite these advantages of insulated needles, some hold that their expense and the altered resistance to insertion through tissues do not justify their exclusive use.

CURRENT OUTPUT OF THE STIMULATOR:
The stimulator should provide a reliable and constant current in the face of changing resistance as the needle passes through various tissues. This predictability greatly facilitates the use of current strength as an indicator of needle proximity to the nerve. The resistance to current flow may vary during a procedure by as much as a factor of 20 according some sources,[5] although a resistance load of 1 to 2 kΩ is most often what is clinically encountered.[13]

Constant current in the face of changing resistance can be provided through the use of current multipliers in the stimulator.[14] Most units monitor the current set by the user compared to the current actually delivered to the patient

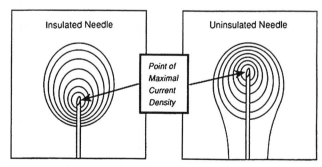

FIGURE 79-1. The differences between the current densities for insulated and uninsulated needles. The lines represent points of equal current density. Note that for the uninsulated needle the center is proximal to the needle tip and the pattern extends up the shaft. (From Pither C: Nerve stimulation. In Raj PP (ed): Clinical Practice of Regional Anesthesia. Churchill Livingstone, New York, 1991, p 164.)

(which should be clearly shown on a digital display on the unit); when there is a difference due to high resistance, an increased voltage is automatically applied to maintain a constant current at the user set amount.[15] However, while most units in fact provided reasonably accurate current outputs in the range >1 mA set by the manufacturers, a study demonstrated highly variable output in current ranges that are currently being used clinically, namely 0.1 to 0.5 mA.[15] As a result, when using these lower currents, the practitioner must employ clinical judgment in order to ensure that an underestimation of delivered current (i.e., more current being delivered than operator thinks) does not result in missed blocks and perhaps more importantly that an overestimation of delivered current (less current being delivered than operator thinks) does not result in an intraneural injection.

OTHER DESIGN ISSUES: Other considerations in the design of a nerve stimulator are a low-battery indicator, a current output range of at least 0.1 to 5 mA, and a linear scale current controller (i.e., half of a dial turn provides half the current of a full dial turn). While some maintain that the option for a high output of up to 10 mA has value, such an option may pose a hazard to the patient with the potential for an inadvertent delivery of a large current directly to a peripheral nerve.[16]

Clinical Issues
KNOWLEDGE OF ANATOMY AND BLOCK SUCCESS:
Nerve stimulation may have its greatest advantage in those situations where there are no clear anatomic landmarks indicating nerve location precisely (e.g., popliteal nerve,[17] lateral femoral cutaneous nerve,[18] sciatic nerve, lumbar plexus) or in those situations where production of paresthesia might be unreliable (in the recovery room or following opioid administration). It may also provide benefit in those situations where a transarterial technique (specifically axillary block) might result in hematoma or interfere with distal vascular surgery (e.g., A-V fistula creation). However, it should be emphasized that use of a nerve stimulator for regional anesthesia still necessitates knowledge of the anatomy involved and of the pharmacology of the agents being used. Simply demonstrating nerve stimulation at a low current is not enough to ensure that subsequent injection of local anesthetic will provide adequate block.[19]

For example, injection into the brachial plexus sheath may be accomplished using a nerve stimulator; however, should the injection be performed too distally in the axilla despite evidence of appropriate stimulation, the local anesthetic will not bathe the more proximal plexus thereby missing those nerves supplying the wrist, forearm, and elbow. In a study of blockade of the sciatic nerve, stimulation producing inversion of the foot resulted in more complete anesthesia than with other evoked motor responses, reflecting stimulation of a part of the sciatic nerve most relevant to lower extremity anesthesia for foot and ankle surgery: injection in response to any movement of the foot might not produce the desired anesthesia.[20]

The literature is replete with case series of successful application of nerve stimulators for regional anesthesia.[16] More notable, therefore, are the few that reflect the view that nerve stimulation offers no advantage over other (paresthesia, transarterial) methods. One study comparing three techniques of axillary block (transarterial, paresthesia, and nerve stimulation) found use of the nerve stimulator to provide no greater

success than the other two methods; in fact, it appeared that a trend toward nerve stimulation being least effective existed.[21] Studies conducted even by strong proponents of the technique have found that in axillary block nerve stimulation does not offer higher success rates than other methods, yet still requires the additional equipment and preparation.[22] Others using nerve stimulation to facilitate interscalene blocks (compared to paresthesia technique) also found it to provide no greater likelihood of success.[19,23] All of these studies serve to underline the concept that it is the application of the technique and knowledge behind the methodology that results in successful regional anesthesia, so that no one methodology is always superior.

CURRENT NEEDED FOR NERVE LOCALIZATION AND PARESTHESIAS:
The amount of current producing muscle stimulation that indicates proper placement of the needle prior to injection is subject to some debate, despite the animal data noted previously. For example, some would maintain that the initial current to be used after skin entry should be 1 mA, and the successful placement would be noted with stimulation at 0.2 mA.[24] Others, however, note that levels of stimulation using currents of 0.2 mA (and in some cases merely less than 1 mA) pose a risk of intraneural injection.[25]

A prospective database of regional anesthesia complications in France over a 10-month period involving 487 anesthesiologists and 158,083 regional anesthetics noted 56 major complications, including 12 cases of nerve injury following peripheral neural blockade. While the incidence of complications was low and factors such as specific operator technique and experience could not be evaluated, it is sobering to note that of the 12 cases (7 of whom still had symptoms more than 6 months following the blocks), 9 were performed using nerve stimulators. Of those 9, 2 reported paresthesia during the procedure and 3 reported specifically using final stimulating currents of <0.5 mA.[26]

The relationship of paresthesia to motor stimulation is another area of controversy and some puzzlement. In a study of 30 patients undergoing interscalene block for shoulder surgery all patients had successful blocks performed and all successfully had the brachial plexus identified by use of paresthesia. However, once paresthesia was obtained in all patients, motor stimulation was then performed and it was found that only 30% were able to demonstrate any motor response at currents <1.0 mA, despite the subsequent successful block.[27] The authors suggested that this might be due to the anatomic separation of motor from sensory fascicles in peripheral nerves, with the probing needle encountering sensory nerves while being too far away to stimulate motor nerves. They further propose that the likelihood of a stimulating needle to produce either motor or sensory stimulation first would depend upon the ratio of motor to sensory nerves plus the topographic organization in the mixed nerve being blocked. However, in our experience using primarily nerve stimulation for interscalene blocks, paresthesia is rarely obtained before motor stimulation, and others also note this pattern.[28] Additionally, it seems unlikely that fascicles are so far removed from each other that a needle on a sensory fascicle would not be within the immediate vicinity of a motor fascicle. Perhaps more notable is that no clear evidence of the mechanism of paresthesia by a probing needle has ever been published to date, and the assumption that a paresthesia involves actual contact with the nerve may or may not be correct.[28]

The above relationship of paresthesia to motor stimulation provides a warning: that lack of motor response does not mean that sensory fibers have not been violated. It would be possible therefore to continue probing with a stimulating needle in an overly sedated patient with the operator oblivious to sensory nerves being approached. Further, paresthesias have repeatedly been targeted as a possible cause of persistent dysesthesia following plexus blockade.[29–31] Although patient cooperation is not required with the use of a nerve stimulator, the ability to monitor for paresthesia and intraneural injection (with subsequent nerve injury) is critical. Some maintain that with a nerve stimulator, once minimal current stimulation has been established, one should confirm that a reduction of current (e.g., to <0.3 mA) results in cessation of muscle twitching, thereby confirming that the needle is not intraneural.[32] Cases of paresthesia and nerve injury occurring while using nerve stimulators have been reported,[33] and other more disturbing case reports in the literature emphasize the need for clinical judgment in the use of neural stimulation for regional anesthesia.[34]

USE IN SENSORY NERVE BLOCKADE: Although designed primarily to stimulate motor nerves, studies show that nerve stimulators can be used to locate purely sensory nerves for neural blockade. In one study examining blockade of the lateral femoral cutaneous nerve the procedure took significantly longer using the nerve stimulator, but successful block rates were much higher and onset of block began within 1 minute vs. 7 minutes for infiltration techniques. The endpoint used was a paresthesia referred to the lateral aspect of the knee at 0.6 mA.[18]

Method: Preparation for regional anesthesia using a nerve stimulator should be no different from that of other techniques except for the stimulator equipment. Following preparation of medications and airway materials, placement of appropriate monitors, and preparation of the injection site, a ground electrode (positive) from the stimulator should be placed on the patient at a site distant from the block site and away from superficial peripheral nerves. The needle can be attached to the negative electrode of the stimulator either through connections in specially designed needles or using an alligator clip attached to the proximal end of the needle. Many patients may find the motor twitching of the stimulator unpleasant. Since total alertness is not a requirement for this technique, sedation should be considered.

Once the needle has entered the skin, the nerve stimulator should be turned on and set to stimulate at 1 to 2 Hz with an initial current of 1 to 2 mA or less (although both higher and lower initial currents have been proposed). As the needle is advanced, motor response to the nerve stimulator in the distribution of the target nerve should be monitored. When any motor response occurs, whether to local stimulation from the needle passing through a muscle or from the target muscles, the current output should be decreased immediately to limit the twitching to the minimum amount needed to confirm motor response. Excessive motor twitching can be extremely unpleasant and should be minimized, as one study noted a 53% incidence of patients reporting the stimulation as being painful.[35]

As the needle approaches the target nerve, the current output should be decreased. Optimally, currents of 0.5 mA with target motor response are desired, but some report consistent success with currents less than 1 mA. It should be noted that uninsulated needles will require higher currents compared to insulated needles.

Another marker sometimes used to indicate appropriate needle placement is the sudden reduction in motor response following the injection of only 2 mL of solution.[36] This rapid response is not the result of neural blockade, but rather the result of the nerve being displaced away from the needle tip. This has been confirmed in studies where air produced the same sudden response as local anesthetic.[2] In theory, if the needle is past the nerve or lying just lateral to the nerve and the shaft of the needle is causing stimulation, then injection will not change the motor response and the needle should be slightly withdrawn and the test repeated. This test is not commonly mentioned in published reports describing nerve stimulation for regional anesthesia and is used infrequently.

Conclusion: While nerve stimulation as a method of facilitating regional anesthesia offers several advantages over other methods including the avoidance of hematoma and possible nerve damage through paresthesia, it also requires costly equipment. These costs are further increased if specially purchased insulated needles are used. It also requires the use of an assistant to manipulate the stimulator (although there are reports of various work-arounds for this obstacle, including foot-pedal controllers and using makeshift sterile attachments to the stimulator control dials) and may require additional time to locate the nerve. However, it offers an additional option toward approaching blocks that might otherwise be difficult due to anatomic or patient considerations and should be available in any institution wanting to offer regional anesthesia.

MULTIPLE- VS. SINGLE-INJECTION TECHNIQUES

Axillary Brachial Plexus Block: Single-injection techniques of axillary blockade often result in incomplete sensory anesthesia. This may be related to insufficient proximal spread of the local anesthetic[37] or to inadequate circumferential spread of the local anesthetic to the various nerves of the brachial plexus.[38,39] The spread of local anesthetic may be hindered by septa within the axillary sheath,[40] although a later study showed the velamentous septa to be incomplete and not a significant barrier to the spread of the local anesthetic.[41] Increasing the volume may improve the quality of the sensory blockade[42] while increasing the concentration of the local anesthetic tends to improve the motor blockade.[43] Studies showed that the musculocutaneous and radial nerves are particularly more difficult to block.[43,44] Multiple-injection techniques have been proposed to improve the quality and shorten the latency of peripheral nerve blocks.

In axillary brachial plexus blocks it was shown that increasing the number of nerve stimulations or nerve paresthesias increased the success rate of the block.[45] A double-injection technique was noted to be superior to a single-injection technique.[46] To better improve the success rate of axillary blocks, Lavoie et al.[47] looked at the efficacy of stimulating the four nerves of the brachial plexus. In a prospective, randomized, double-blind study they showed that the stimulation of the musculocutaneous, radial, median, and ulnar nerves or stimulation of the musculocutaneous and one of the three nerves resulted in a higher success rate compared to stimulation of either the radial, median, or ulnar nerve alone.[47]

Stimulation of just one nerve resulted in a 50% success rate and there was no difference in the quality of blockade when single injection of the three nerves was compared. The four-nerve stimulation technique has been shown to have a high success rate and rapid onset of blockade.[48,49] Compared to elicitation of paresthesias involving the four nerves, nerve stimulation resulted in an overall higher success rate (91% vs. 76%) with improved chance of anesthetizing the radial and musculocutaneous nerves.[50] The paresthesia technique was also related to a higher incidence of venous puncture and poor acceptance by the patient secondary to discomfort during the block.[50] The four-nerve stimulation technique is time consuming and stimulation of all four nerves may be difficult in view of the injected local anesthetic permeating the adjacent nerves. In an effort to decrease the number of injections Sia et al.[51] compared the double- (radial and median nerves) and triple-injection (radial, median, and musculocutaneous nerves) techniques and found that the success rate was better (90% vs. 76%) and the time to perform the block was shorter (5 vs. 6 minutes) in the three-nerve stimulation technique. They did not stimulate the ulnar nerve because they found in an earlier study that ulnar nerve stimulation is not essential in axillary brachial plexus block.[52]

The specific evoked motor activities for stimulation of the nerves are as follows. Musculocutaneous: arm flexion; radial: forearm supination, extension of wrist and fingers; median: pronation of forearm, wrist flexion, flexion of lateral three fingers; ulnar: wrist flexion, adduction of all fingers, flexion of lateral two fingers toward thumb.[50]

Femoral Nerve Block: Multiple-injection techniques in femoral nerve block involve stimulation of the nerve to the vastus medialis (evidenced by contraction of the vastus medialis muscle), of the nerve to the vastus intermedius (contraction of the vastus intermedius muscle with movement of the patella), and of the nerve to the vastus lateralis (contraction of the vastus lateralis muscle). As little as 4 mL of local anesthetic has been injected for each nerve for a total of 12 mL. Compared to a single-injection technique, the multiple-injection technique decreased the onset sensory block (10 ± 4 minutes vs. 30 ± 11 minutes).[53] Although it took longer to perform the block (4 minutes vs 3 minutes), the multiple-injection technique decreased the total preoperative time because of the shorter time it took for the block to take effect.[53] The volume required to block the branches of the femoral nerve is smaller (14 mL vs. 23 mL) with the multiple-injection technique.[54]

Sciatic Nerve Block: A double-stimulation technique in sciatic nerve blocks involves the stimulation of the tibial and common peroneal nerves and injection of 10 mL of local anesthetic each time. Compared to a single-stimulation technique, where 20 mL of the local anesthetic is injected after stimulation of either the tibial or peroneal nerve, the onset of the block is more rapid and the sensory block more complete.[55]

In popliteal sciatic nerve block the tibial and common peroneal branches of the sciatic nerve can also be individually stimulated and injected. A volume of 10 to 15 mL of local anesthetic is injected per nerve. If the tibial nerve is stimulated then the needle is moved laterally to stimulate the common peroneal nerve.[56] Conversely, the needle is moved medially after stimulation of the peroneal nerve. Stimulation of the tibial nerve is evidenced by evoked plantar flexion while dorsiflexion

and eversion signifies stimulation of the deep peroneal and superficial peroneal nerves, respectively.[20]

In the lateral approach to popliteal sciatic nerve block the two-injection technique involves the injection of 10 mL of local anesthetic after stimulation of the tibial and peroneal components.[57] The two-stimulation technique has been shown to increase the success rate of the block (88% vs. 54%) compared to a single-injection technique, specifically inversion.[57] The results of the study were a little surprising in view of the study by Benzon et al. that showed 100% success rate when inversion was used as the endpoint in the posterior approach to sciatic nerve block.[20] The discrepancy of the results may be due to the 40 mL volume used by Benzon and the more posterior location of the tibial nerve in relation to the common peroneal nerve. The posterior approach to popliteal sciatic nerve block may have favored a posterior spread of the local anesthetic compared to the lateral approach resulting in a complete block.

Clinicians are hesitant to adopt the multiple-stimulation technique because of possible increased neural injury from the nerve stimulations. A prospective study of 3,996 patients who underwent multiple-injection techniques of sciatic–femoral blocks, axillary blocks, and interscalene blocks showed an incidence of neurologic dysfunction of 1.7%.[58] Complete recovery occurred within 4 to 12 weeks in all the patients except one who took 25 weeks to recover. The risk of permanent neurologic injury is similar to that reported after regional anesthesia.[59]

ADJUVANTS TO LOCAL ANESTHETICS IN PERIPHERAL NERVE BLOCKS

Adjuvant drugs for peripheral nerve blocks include medications added to the primary local anesthetic agent to shorten the latency of onset or augment the duration of neural blockade. Adjuvants may also signify agents added to improve the analgesic potency, or the quality of resultant analgesia. Probably the most commonly used adjuvant in clinical practice for peripheral nerve blockade is the addition of dilute concentrations of epinephrine to the local anesthetic solution. The chief vascular action of epinephrine is exerted upon smaller arterioles and precapillary sphincters, although large veins and even arteries also respond to epinephrine. Epinephrine diminishes cutaneous blood flow by constricting precapillary vessels and small venules. This effect is largely mediated by alpha-1-adrenergic receptor agonism. Braun, in 1903, characterized epinephrine as a "chemical tourniquet."[60] Braun also coined the term "conduction anesthesia" and proposed that the adjuvant use of epinephrine might be important to produce conduction anesthesia in regions of the body distinct from the extremities.[61] Local anesthetic solutions may be packaged with dilute epinephrine concentrations added, or the epinephrine may be freshly added to the local anesthetic solution immediately prior to use. Epinephrine ampules contain a 1:1000 concentration, or 1.0 mg epinephrine in 1 mL solution, from which epinephrine is freshly drawn up to be added to local anesthetic solutions. In ampule form epinephrine, as the hydrochloride, is dissolved in water, and sodium chloride is added for tonicity. Sodium bisulfite (not exceeding 0.1%) is added as an antioxidant. Prepackaged local anesthetic solutions containing epinephrine usually have a lower pH as compared to plain solutions. This may delay the onset of local anesthetic neural blockade activity, since onset is largely a function of pKa.

The vasoconstrictive effect of epinephrine is pH dependent. As long ago as 1924 Alpern[62] found that the vasoconstrictive effect of adrenalin (epinephrine) was totally abolished below a pH of 5.6, that it became effective at a pH of 6.6, and that its effect was markedly enhanced at a pH of 7.8 or above. It appears that the hydrogen ion concentration of the blood actually regulates the response of vascular smooth muscle to (intravenously administered) adrenalin, and this may be extrapolated to the microvascular millieu of the vaso nervorum surrounding a peripheral nerve. This finding has significant implication for understanding the ability (or lack thereof) of alkalinization of local anesthetics to exert a clinically significant change in the onset or duration of conduction anesthesia, as is discussed below. Adding epinephrine to local anesthetic solutions immediately prior to their administration to produce a final epinephrine concentration of 1:200,000 to 1:400,000 (5 to 2.5 µg/mL) is recommended for several reasons. The addition of epinephrine to local anesthetic solutions produces vasoconstriction in the tissues at the site of local anesthetic injection. This vasoconstriction of the local milieu may reduce the peak serum levels of local anesthetic by limiting its absorption from the site of administration into the systemic circulation.[63] The higher the vascularity of a region, the greater the proportional effect on duration of neural blockade with the addition of epinephrine. Additionally, by decreasing the "local" vascular flow in the region of the injection, the local anesthetic may have a longer "residence time" at the site of the peripheral nerve due to decreased local anesthetic clearance from the injection site.[64] More local anesthetic molecules reaching the peripheral nerve membrane may improve both the depth and duration of anesthesia. In a well-conducted study on the effect of epinephrine on lidocaine clearance in vivo using perineural microdialysis catheters, Bernards and Kopacz demonstrated that epinephrine prolongs the sensory block produced by lidocaine by decreasing local blood flow and by slowing the lidocaine clearance.[64] A prolonged neural blockade effect with the addition of epinephrine to solutions of lidocaine, mepivacaine, and bupivacaine for peripheral neural blockade is well demonstrated.[63,65,66] This effect appears less significant for the highly lipophilic etidocaine and especially for ropivacaine, however, possibly due to the intrinsic vasoconstrictor activity of ropivacaine alone.[67] Other vasoconstrictor agents such as phenylephrine and norepinephrine have also been used as additives to local anesthetics. However, neither agent has demonstrated any consistent advantage as compared to epinephrine. Adding epinephrine to local anesthetic for peripheral nerve block, then, prolongs the duration of anesthesia and analgesia; increases the intensity, extent, and success rate of most local anesthetic blocks; reduces and delays peak levels of local anesthetics in the blood; produces a "bloodless field"; delays the onset of tachyphylaxis (acute tolerance); and may obviate the need for continuous techniques. Epinephrine has also proved to be a valuable marker or "test dose" to rule out unintended vascular injection of local anesthetic (or rapid systemic uptake) during the performance of techniques requiring the intermittent injection of relatively larger volumes of local anesthetic. Moore and Batra[68] suggested using a test dose of a local anesthetic solution containing 15 µg of epinephrine (i.e., 3 mL of a solution containing epinephrine in a 1:200,000 concentration). They noted that the dose reliably ascertains whether an intravascular injection has occurred, particularly during epidural block, since this dose of epinephrine rapidly (within 20 to 30 seconds) and

reproducibly produces an elevation in systolic blood pressure and heart rate.

The addition of epinephrine to local anesthetic solutions is generally contraindicated in cases of severe hypertension (especially during pregnancy), presence of tachydysrhythmias, unstable angina, patients on medications such as MAO that modify the metabolism or action of catecholamines, and for use in peripheral nerve blocks of the digits, wrist, ankle, and penis, especially in atherosclerotic patients. In atherosclerotic or diabetic patients adding epinephrine to local anesthetic solutions may theoretically contribute to perioperative neural injury by reducing blood flow to an already compromised nerve.

The carbonization of local anesthetic agents (addition of carbon dioxide) has been demonstrated in vitro to produce a reduction in time to onset of various local anesthetic agents. The mechanism is believed to be due to the rapid diffusion of carbon dioxide across the nerve membrane, lowering the intracellular pH, and trapping the cationic form (active form binding to receptors in the sodium channel) of the local anesthetic in the intracellular phase.[69,70] In vivo studies of the clinical effectiveness of carbonation of local anesthetic agents in significantly reducing latency to onset of local anesthetics have produced variable results.[71] While not available in the USA, carbonated solutions of lidocaine are clinically available in Canada.[63]

Attempts have been made to reduce the latency of onset or prolong the duration of local anesthetic neural blockade by adding sodium bicarbonate 8.4% to local anesthetic solutions immediately prior to injection. Increasing the pH of the acidic solution closer to the pKa of the local anesthetic makes relatively more of the local anesthetic available in the nonionized, lipid-soluble base form that crosses the nerve membrane.[63] Thus, the rate of diffusion across the nerve sheath and nerve membrane should theoretically be enhanced, resulting in a more rapid onset of anesthesia. The effect of this alkalinization of the local anesthetic solution is greatest for commercially prepared local anesthetics containing epinephrine due to the lower pH required to maintain the stability of the epinephrine-containing solution. The time to onset of plain local anesthetic solutions with epinephrine added immediately prior to local anesthetic injection is shorter than commercially prepared local anesthetic solutions containing epinephrine due to the higher pH (i.e., closer to pKa) of the plain solutions. Indeed, Candido et al. demonstrated that the addition of bicarbonate to plain bupivacaine for lower extremity plexus block did not alter the onset or duration of anesthesia.[69] They suggested that increasing the pH of a local anesthetic towards its pKa increases the amount of local anesthetic existing in the uncharged (base) form. The alkalinization of the local anesthetic should provide more free base, and provide a more rapid onset of anesthesia. In addition, since more of the free base is available, a greater number of local anesthetic molecules should reach the anesthetic receptors within the nerve membrane, resulting in a more intense block and a prolonged duration of action. The resultant increase in pH in this study, however, produced a clinically insignificant increase in the amount of free base in the solution, and therefore the onset and duration of action of bupivacaine was not significantly affected. Similar findings were noted by the same investigators using plain (no added epinephrine) mepivacaine for upper extremity plexus anesthesia, whereby added bicarbonate had little or no effect on onset or duration of anesthesia.[70] The shortened latency of onset and prolonged duration of action experienced by alkalinization of local anesthetic solutions containing epinephrine may be due to a reactivation of the vasoconstrictor activity of the epinephrine itself, which is inactivated at a low pH as described above, and may not be the result of an increase in the relative amount of free base (which tends to be modest in most cases).[69,71]

Another study showed that the addition of sodium bicarbonate to lidocaine in epidural anesthesia resulted in a shorter onset and a more intense blockade of the L5 and S1 nerve roots.[72] In this study[72] the effect of sodium bicarbonate was demonstrated by dermatomal somatosensory evoked potential monitoring. The addition of sodium bicarbonate to the local anesthetic solution immediately prior to injection or in volumes greater than that recommended (distinct for each particular local anesthetic agent) may result in precipitation of the base form of the local anesthetic.[63] In summary, clinical evidence supports the addition of bicarbonate immediately prior to injection of local anesthetic solutions containing epinephrine, but does not support the routine addition of sodium bicarbonate to improve the block onset time induced by plain local anesthetic (without added epinephrine).

The alpha-2$_A$-specific adrenergic agonist clonidine has been studied as an adjuvant to local anesthetics for peripheral nerve block. Clonidine, an imidazoline, was synthesized in the 1960s and was found to produce transiently vasoconstriction, followed by a more prolonged activation of central alpha-2-receptors with reduction in sympathetic nervous system impulses. More readily available and more extensively used in Europe, clonidine has demonstrated a significant benefit in terms of prolonging the duration of local anesthetic sensory neural blockade without effecting motor blockade.[71] Clonidine is suspected of enhancing the local anesthetic effects on peripheral nerves through a direct neuronal, pharmacodynamic effect. Kopacz and Bernards utilized their peripherally placed microdialysis catheter methodology to attempt to differentiate the potential for a pharmacodynamic vs. a pharmacokinetic effect of clonidine. They found that clonidine had a pharmacokinetic effect on decreasing the clearance of lidocaine at the peripheral nerve during the first 60 minutes following injection. Thereafter, clonidine appeared to have a predominant pharmacodynamic effect potentiating the sensory neural blockade effects of the lidocaine.[73] Iskander and colleagues demonstrated that the effect of peripherally injected clonidine as an adjuvant to local anesthetic neural blockade is indeed a peripheral rather than a systemic, generalized response.[74] They used a solution of mepivacaine and clonidine to block selectively the median and musculocutaneous nerves using a mid-humeral block technique. The radial and ulnar nerves were blocked using a plain solution of mepivacaine without clonidine. The addition of clonidine to mepivacaine in this study significantly prolonged the duration of sensory block only in the median and musculocutaneous distributions with no effect on motor block. On the other hand, Erlacher and colleagues showed that the addition of clonidine to 0.75% concentrations of ropivacaine for axillary brachial plexus block was ineffective in shortening latency to onset, prolonging duration of analgesia, or improving on the quality of the block.[75] Culebras et al., using a systemic control group, also demonstrated that interscalene brachial plexus blocks incorporating clonidine were not different from bupivacaine blocks in regards onset of action, duration of anesthesia, or duration of analgesia.[76] Additionally, there were hemodynamic changes experienced by the group receiving clonidine, but not in the bupivacaine group. It appears that the choice of local anesthetic and type of peripheral nerve block affect the efficacy of adding clonidine, as does the dose of clonidine. Nevertheless, the addition of clonidine to local anesthetic solutions has shown significant analgesic potential with minimal adverse systemic side effects at doses up to 150 µg in adult patients,[65,66,74,77–86] with one study demonstrating hemodynamic changes at 150 µg.[76] At doses exceeding 150 µg, systemic side effects including hypotension, bradycardia, and sedation become more frequent and clinically significant. As systemic administration of clonidine exhibits a long half-life (12 ± 7 hours), these side effects might be of prolonged duration, possibly limiting consideration of using larger doses in clinical practice.

Several opioid analgesics have been used as adjuncts to local anesthetic peripheral neural blockade including the mu-agonists morphine,[87–90] fentanyl,[91–94] sufentanil,[95,96] and alfentanil;[97] the partial mu-agonist and kappa-agonist butorphanol;[98,99] and the partial mu-agonist buprenorphine.[88,100,101] The ability of the opioids to produce an analgesic benefit through a peripheral mechanism has been somewhat variable. Many of the clinical studies examining the analgesic benefit of opioid analgesics added to local anesthetic peripheral neural blockade have generally not had adequate systemic control groups to clearly define a peripheral mechanism of action.[71] Morphine has been shown to improve postoperative analgesia when added to lidocaine for peripheral nerve block as compared to systemic control in one study,[102] while it failed to do so in another.[89] Sufentanil added to a combination of lidocaine and bupivacaine doubled analgesic duration following brachial plexus block vs. a control group.[95] In another study using the same opioid mixed with plain mepivacaine 1.5% for axillary block, however, analgesia was not only not prolonged vs. placebo, but patients receiving sufentanil also experienced more nausea and somnolence.[96] Butorphanol without local anesthetic administered as a perineural infusion near the axillary perivascular brachial plexus decreased pain as compared to a systemic infusion.[99] Buprenorphine, a partial mu-agonist, has demonstrated significant prolongation of postoperative analgesia when added to local anesthetics for perivascular brachial plexus blocks, both via the subclavian as well as by the axillary routes.[88,100,101] Buprenorphine is structurally more similar to the mu-antagonists naltrexone and nalmefene as well as to the partial mu-agonists butorphanol and nalbuphine than it is to morphine. It is a semisynthetic, highly lipophilic agent derived from thebaine that is 25 to 50 times more potent than morphine. In two recent studies Candido et al. demonstrated that the addition of 0.3 mg buprenorphine to 40 mL of a local anesthetic mixture provided 3 times the duration of postoperative analgesia vs. a saline placebo control. Importantly, buprenorphine mixed with the local anesthetic solution also resulted in a doubling of duration of postoperative analgesia when compared to an IM control group receiving the same dose of buprenorphine systemically. Their work supports the work of Fields[103] and Stein[104] in animals who suggested that there exist peripheral opiate receptors on the central processes of primary afferent nerves that are migratory in response to inflammatory states (i.e., postsurgical trauma). Since buprenorphine dissociates very slowly from the mu-receptor (half-life = 166 minutes, vs. 7 minutes for fentanyl) it may prove to be an ideal choice when considering an adjuvant for prolonging postoperative analgesia.

A variety of other drugs used as adjuvants to local anesthetic peripheral blockade have been reported in the literature including tramadol,[105] verapamil,[87] and neostigmine.[106,107] Tramadol is an analgesic that is antagonized by alpha-2 and opioid antagonists. It appears to have a peripheral analgesic effect somewhat similar to clonidine. Verapamil, in doses of 2.5 mg added to lidocaine for axillary brachial plexus block, increased the duration of surgical anesthesia in one study.[87] Neostigmine, an anticholinesterase agent, is theorized to affect peripheral cholinergic stimulation, which modifies pain transmission. Unfortunately, neostigmine is associated with significant side effects including nausea, bradycardia, and bronchoconstriction. The utility of each of these agents as adjuvants to local anesthetic peripheral neural blockade requires additional studies.

In summary, the literature supports the safety and efficacy of epinephrine and clonidine as additions to local anesthetic for peripheral neural blockade. Both agents have demonstrated the ability to increase the duration of intensity of local anesthetic neural blockade. Dexmedetomidine and tizanidine, other alpha-2-adrenergic agonists, may have the potential to act like clonidine as adjuncts to local anesthetics for peripheral nerve block, but this remains to be seen. The addition of bicarbonate to local anesthetic is somewhat time consuming and the clinical benefit is questionable as related to its ability to hasten the onset of local anesthetic neural blockade, particularly for plain, nonepinephrine-containing solutions of local anesthetic. Opioids, particularly buprenorphine, with activity via peripheral opioid receptors or other, yet undetermined mechanisms may be of benefit in extending the duration of postoperative analgesia following local anesthetic peripheral neural blockade, but the evidence at this point does not support their widespread use in this application. Opioids with activity for peripheral non-mu-opioid receptors (i.e., kappa-agonist activity) await additional study.[103,104] Adenosine added to local anesthetics may hold promise for future applications. Adenosine receptors are located in the superficial layers of the dorsal horn of the spinal cord, and antinociceptive effects of adenosine have been noted following its administration systemically and intrathecally. Whether or not adenosine has a role in peripheral nerve block analgesia remains to be seen. The application of other agents with peripheral effects at Na^+, K^+, Ca^{2+}, and other ion channels or peripheral neural membrane receptors represents the future with respect to the study of other agents as additives to local anesthetics for peripheral neural blockade.

REFERENCES

1. Winnie A: Plexus Anesthesia, WB Saunders, Philadelphia, 1983, pp 215–217.
2. Raj P: Adjuvant techniques in regional anesthesia. In Raj P (ed): Handbook of Regional Anesthesia. Churchill Livingstone, New York, 1985, pp 250–258.
3. Perthes von G: Uker leitungsanasthesia unter zuhilfenahme elektrischer reizung. Medizinische Monatsschrift 47:2545–2548, 1912.
4. Raj P, Montgomery S, Nettles D, et al.: Infraclavicular brachial plexus block: A new approach. Anesth Analg (Cleve) 52:897, 1973.
5. Pither C, Raj P, Ford D: The use of peripheral nerve stimulators for regional anesthesia: A review of experimental characteristics, technique, and clinical applications. Reg Anesth 10:49–58, 1985.
6. Ford D, Pither C, Raj P: Electrical characteristics of peripheral nerve stimulators: Implications for nerve localization. Reg Anesth 9:73–77, 1984.
7. Rosenberg H, Greenhow D: Peripheral nerve stimulator performance: The influence of output polarity and electrode placement. Canad Anaesth Soc J 25:424–426, 1978.
8. Tulchinsky A, Weller R, Rosenblum M, Gross J: Nerve stimulator polarity and brachial plexus block. Anesth Analg 77:100, 1993.
9. Magora E, Rozin R, Ben-Menachem Y, et al.: Obturator nerve block: An evaluation of technique. Br J Anaesth 41:695, 1969.
10. Riegler F: Brachial plexus block with the nerve stimulator: Motor response characteristics at three sites. Reg Anesth 17:295–299, 1992.
11. Jones R, De Jonge M, Smith B: Voltage fields surrounding needles used in regional anaesthesia. Br J Anaesth 68:515–518, 1992.
12. Ford D, Pither C, Raj P: Comparison of insulated and uninsulated needles for locating peripheral nerves with a peripheral nerve stimulator. Anesth Analg 63:925–928, 1984.
13. Valentinuzzi E: Bioelectrical impedance techniques in medicine: I. Bioimpedance measurement. Crit Rev Biomed Eng 24:223–255, 1996.
14. Technical Data Sheet provided by Braun Medical, Inc.
15. Hadzic A, Vloka J, Hadzic N, et al: Nerve stimulators used for peripheral nerve blocks vary in their electrical characteristic. Anesthesiology 98:969–974, 2003.
16. Raj P, Banister R: Aids to localization of peripheral nerves. In Raj P (ed): Textbook of Regional Anesthesia. Churchill-Livingstone, New York, 2002, pp 251–283.
17. Singelyn F, Gouverneur J, Gribomont B: Popliteal sciatic nerve block aided by a nerve stimulator. Reg Anesth 16:278–281, 1991.
18. Shannon J, Lang S, Yip R, Gerard M: Lateral femoral cutaneous nerve block revisited. Reg Anesth 20:100–104, 1995.
19. Smith B: Efficacy of a nerve stimulator in regional anaesthesia: Experience in a resident training programme. Anaesthesia 31: 778, 1976.
20. Benzon H, Kim C, Silverstein M, et al: Correlation between evoked motor response of the sciatic nerve and sensory blockade. Anesthesiology 87:547–552, 1997.
21. Goldberg M, Gregg C, Larijani G, Norris M, et al.: A comparison of three methods of axillary approach to brachial plexus blockade for upper extremity surgery. Anesthesiology 66:814–816, 1987.
22. Baranowski A, Pither C: A comparison of three methods of axillary brachial plexus anaesthesia. Anaesthesia 45:362, 1990.
23. McClain D, Finucane B: Interscalene approach to the brachial plexus. Paresthesia vs. nerve stimulator [abstract]. Reg Anesth 8:39, 1983.
24. Vloka J, Hadzic A: The intensity of the current at which sciatic nerve stimulation is achieved is more important factor in determining the quality of nerve block than the type of motor response obtained [letter]. Anesthesiology 88:1408–1410, 1998.
25. Benzon H: The intensity of the current at which sciatic nerve stimulation is achieved is more important factor in determining the quality of nerve block than the type of motor response obtained – Reply [letter]. Anesthesiology 88:1410–1411, 1998.
26. Auroy Y, Benhamou D, Bargues L, et al: Major complications of regional anesthesia in France. Anesthesiology 97:1274–1280, 2002.
27. Urmey W, Stanton J: Inability to consistently elicit a motor response following sensory paresthesia during interscalene block administration. Anesthesiology 96:552–554, 2002.
28. Carter C, Sandberg W: What happened to the paresthesia [letter]? Anesthesiology 98:588, 2003.
29. Selander D, Edshage S, Wolff T: Paresthesiae or no paresthesiae – Nerve lesions after axillary blocks. Acta Anaesth Scand 23:27–33, 1979.
30. Plevak D, Linstromberg J, Danielson D: Paresthesia vs. nonparesthesia, the axillary block [abstract]. Anesthesiology 59: A216, 1983.
31. Selander D: Axillary plexus block: Paresthetic or perivascular. Anesthesiology 66:726–728, 1987.

32. Choquet O, Jochum D, Estebe J, et al: Motor response following paresthesia during interscalene block: Methodological problems may lead to inappropriate conclusions. Anesthesiology 98:587–588, 2003.

33. Moore D, Mulroy M, Thompson G: Peripheral nerve damage and regional anaesthesia [editorial]. Br J Anaesth 73:435, 1994.

34. Benumof JL: Permanent loss of cervical spinal cord function associated with interscalene block performed under general anesthesia. Anesthesiology 93:1541–1544, 2000.

35. Nielsen Z, Rotboll-Nielsen P, Rassmussen H: Patients' experiences with multiple stimulation axillary block for fast-track ambulatory hand surgery. Acta Anaesthesiol Scand 46:789–793, 2002.

36. Montgomery S, Raj P, Nettles D, et al: The use of the nerve stimulator with standard unsheathed needles in nerve blockade. Anesth Analg (Cleve) 52:827, 1973.

37. Winnie AP, Radonjic R, Akkineni SR, Durrani Z: Factors influencing distribution of local anesthetic injected into the brachial plexus sheath. Anesth Analg 58:225–234, 1979.

38. Koscielniak-Nielsen ZJ, Christensen LQ, Stens-Pedersen HL, Brushoj J: Effect of digital pressure on the neurovascular sheath during perivascular axillary block. Br J Anaesth 75:702–706, 1995.

39. Yamamoto K, Tsunehisa T, Ohmura S, Kobayashi T: The effects of arm position on central spread of local anesthetics and on quality of the block with axillary brachial plexus block. Reg Anesth Pain Med 24:36–42, 1999.

40. Thompson GE, Rorie DK: Functional anatomy of the brachial plexus sheaths. Anesthesiology 59:117–122, 1983.

41. Partridge BL, Katz J, Bernirschke K: Functional anatomy of the brachial plexus sheath: Implications for anesthesia. Anesthesiology 66:743–747, 1987.

42. Vester-Andersen T, Husum B, Lindenburg T, et al: Perivascular axillary block: IV. Blockade following 40, 50, or 60 ml of mepivacaine 1% with adrenaline. Acta Anaesthesiol Scand 28:99–105, 1984.

43. Vester-Andersen T, Eriksen C, Christiansen C: Perivascular axillary block: III. Blockade following 40 ml of 0.5%, 1%, and 1.5% mepivacaine with adrenaline. Acta Anaesthesiol Scand 28:95–98, 1984.

44. Lanz E, Theiss D, Jankovic D: The extent of blockade following various techniques of brachial plexus block. Anesth Analg 62:55–58, 1983.

45. Baranowski AP, Piuther CE: Comparison of three methods of axillary brachial plexus anaesthesia. Anaesthesia 45:362–365, 1990.

46. Inberg P, Annila I, Annila P: Double-injection method using peripheral nerve stimulator is superior to single injection in axillary brachial plexus block. Reg Anesth Pain Med 24:509–513, 1999.

47. Lavoie J, Martin R, Tetrault JP, et al: Axillary brachial plexus block using a peripheral nerve stimulator: Single or multiple injections. Can J Anaesth 39:583–586, 1992.

48. Koscielnak-Nielsen ZJ, Stens-Pedersen HL, Knudsen Lippert F: Readiness for surgery after axillary block: Single or multiple injection techniques. Eur J Anaesthesiol 14:164–171, 1997.

49. Koscielnak-Nielsen ZJ, Hesselberg L, Fejberg V: Comparison of transarterial and multiple nerve stimulation techniques for an initial axillary block by 45 ml of mepivacaine with 1% adrenaline. Acta Anaesthesiol Scand 42:570–575, 1998.

50. Sia S, Bartolli M, Lepri A, et al: Multiple-injection axillary brachial plexus block: A comparison of two methods of nerve localization-nerve stimulation versus paresthesia. Anesth Analg 91:647–651, 2000.

51. Sia S, Lepri A, Ponzecchi P: Axillary brachial plexus block using peripheral nerve stimulator: A comparison between double- and triple-injection techniques. Reg Anesth Pain Med 26:499–503, 2001.

52. Sia S, Bartoli M: Selective ulnar nerve localization is not essential for axillary brachial plexus using a multiple nerve stimulation technique. Reg Anesth Pain Med 26:12–16, 2001.

53. Casati A, Fanelli G, Beccaria P, et al: The effects of the single or multiple injection technique on the onset time of femoral nerve blocks with 0.75% ropivacaine. Anesth Analg 91:181–184, 2000.

54. Casati A, Fanelli G, Beccaria P, et al: The effects of the single or multiple injections on the volume of 0.5% ropivacaine required for femoral nerve blockade. Anesth Analg 93:183–186, 2001.

55. Bailey SL, Parkinson SK, Little WL, Simmerman SR: Sciatic nerve block. A comparison of single versus double injection technique. Reg Anesth 19:9, 1994.

56. Benzon HT. Popliteal sciatic nerve block: Posterior approach. Tech Reg Anesth Pain Manage 3:23–27, 1999.

57. Paqueron X, Bouaziz H, Macalou D, et al: The lateral approach to the sciatic nerve at the popliteal fossa: one or two injections? Anesth Analg 89:1221–1225, 1999.

58. Fanelli G, Casati A, Garancini P, Torri G: Nerve stimulator and multiple injection technique for upper and lower limb blockade: Failure rate, patient acceptance, and neurologic complications. Anesth Analg 88:847–852, 1999.

59. Auroy Y, Narchi P, Messiah A, et al: Serious complications related to regional anesthesia. Anesthesiology 87:479–486, 1997.

60. Braun H: Local Anesthesia. Its Scientific Basis and Practical Use, ed 3. Lea & Febiger, Philadelphia, 1914.

61. Braun H: Ueber den Einfluss der Vitalitat der Gewebe auf die ortlichen und allgemeinen Giftwirkungen localanasthesirender Mittel und uber die Bedeutung des Adrenalins fur die Localanasthesie. Arch Klin Chir 9:541, 1903.

62. Alpern D: The dependence of the contractility of peripheral vessels on the H-ion concentration in the perfusing fluid [German]. Pflugers Arch 205:578–589, 1924.

63. Covino BG, Wildsmith JAW: Clinical pharmacology of local anesthetic agents. In Cousins MJ, Bridenbaugh PO (eds): Neural Blockade in Clinical Anesthesia and Management of Pain, ed 3. Lippincott-Raven, Philadelphia, 1998, pp 97–128.

64. Bernards CM, Kopacz DJ: Effect of epinephrine on lidocaine clearance in vivo: A microdialysis study in humans. Anesthesiology 91:962–968, 1999.

65. Eledjam JJ, Deschodt J, Viel EJ, et al: Brachial plexus block with bupivacaine: Effects of added alpha-adrenergic agonists: Comparison between clonidine and epinephrine. Can J Anaesth 38:870–875, 1991.

66. Gaumann D, Forster A, Griessen M, et al: Comparison between clonidine and epinephrine admixture to lidocaine in brachial plexus block. Anesth Analg 75:69–74, 1992.

67. McClure JH: Ropivacaine. Br J Anaesth 76:300–307, 1996.

68. Moore DC, Batra MS: The components of an effective test dose prior to epidural block. Anesthesiology 55:693–696, 1981.

69. Candido KD, Winnie AP, Covino BG, et al: Addition of bicarbonate to plain bupivacaine does not significantly alter the onset or duration of plexus anesthesia. Reg Anesth 20:133–138, 1995.

70. Candido KD, Raza SM, Vasireddy AP: pH adjusted mepivacaine for upper extremity conduction anesthesia [abstract]. Reg Anesth 14(Suppl 2):93, 1989.

71. Crews JC: Adjuvants in peripheral neural blockade. ASRA Annual Meeting Syllabus. 28th Annual Spring Meeting, 3–6 April 2003.

72. Benzon HT, Toleikis JR, Dixit P, et al: Onset, intensity of blockade and somatosensory evoked potential changes of the lumbosacral dermatomes after epidural anesthesia with alkalinized lidocaine. Anesth Analg 7:515–516, 1993.

73. Kopacz DJ, Bernards CM: Effects of clonidine on lidocaine clearance in vivo: A microdialysis study in humans. Anesthesiology 95:1371–1376, 2001.

74. Iskandar H, Guillaume E, Dixmerias F, et al: The enhancement of sensory blockade by clonidine selectively added to mepivacaine after midhumeral block. Anesth Analg 93:771–775, 2001.

75. Erlacher W, Schuschnig C, Orlicek F, et al: The effects of clonidine on ropivacaine 0.75% in axillary perivascular plexus block. Acta Anaesthesiol Scand 44:53–57, 2000.

76. Culebras X, Van Gessel E, Hoffmeyer P, Gamulin Z: Clonidine combined with a long acting local anesthetic does not prolong postoperative analgesia after brachial plexus block but does induce hemodynamic changes. Anesth Analg 92:199–204, 2001.

77. Gaumann DM, Brunet PC, Jirounek P: Clonidine enhances the effects of lidocaine on C-fiber action potential. Anesth Analg 74:719–725, 1992.

78. Erlacher W, Schuschnig C, Koinig H, et al: Clonidine as adjuvant for mepivacaine, ropivacaine and bupivacaine in axillary perivascular brachial plexus block. Can J Anaesth 48:522–525, 2001.

79. Murphy DB, McCartney CJ, Chan VW: Novel analgesic adjuncts for brachial plexus block: A systematic review. Anesth Analg 90:1122–1128, 2000.

80. Madan R, Bharti N, Shende D, et al: A dose response study of clonidine with local anesthetic mixture for peribulbar block: A comparison of three doses. Anesth Analg 93:1593–1597, 2001.

81. Ivani G, Conio A, De Negri P, et al: Spinal versus peripheral effects of adjunct clonidine: Comparison of the analgesic effect of a ropivacaine–clonidine mixture when administered as a caudal or ilioinguinal-iliohypogastric nerve blockade for inguinal surgery in children. Paediatr Anaesth 12:680–684.

82. El Saied AH, Steyn MP, Ansermino JM: Clonidine prolongs the effect of ropivacaine for axillary brachial plexus blockade. Can J Anaesth 47:962–967, 2000.

83. Mjahed K, el Harrar N, Hamdani M, et al: Lidocaine–clonidine retrobulbar block for cataract surgery in the elderly. Reg Anesth 21:569–575, 1996.

84. Singelyn FJ, Dangoisse M, Bartholomee S, Gouverneur JM: Adding clonidine to mepivacaine prolongs the duration of anesthesia and analgesia after axillary brachial plexus block. Reg Anesth 17:148–150, 1992.

85. Bernard JM, Macaire P: Dose-range effects of clonidine added to lodocaine for brachial plexus block. Anesthesiology 87:277–284, 1997.

86. Singelyn FJ, Gouverneur JM, Robert A: A minimum dose of clonidine added to mepivacaine prolongs the duration of anesthesia and analgesia after axillary brachial plexus block. Anesth Analg 83:1046–1050, 1996.

87. Reuben SS, Reuben JP: Brachial plexus anesthesia with verapamil and/or morphine. Anesth Analg 91:379–383, 2000.

88. Viel EJ, Eledjam JJ, De La Coussaye JE, d'Athis F: Brachial plexus block with opioids for postoperative pain relief: Comparison between buprenorphine and morphine. Reg Anesth 14:274–278, 1989.

89. Racz H, Gunning K, Della Santa D, Forster A: Evaluation of the effect of perineural morphine on the quality of postoperative analgesia after axillary plexus block: A randomized double-blind study. Anesth Analg 72:769–772, 1991.

90. Flory N, Van Gessel E, Donald F, et al: Does the addition of morphine to brachial plexus block improve analgesia after shoulder surgery? Br J Anaesth 75:23–26, 1995.

91. Gobeauz D, Landais A, Bexon G, et al: Addition of fentanyl to adrenalinized lidocaine for the brachial plexus block [French]. Cah Anesthesiol 35:195–199, 1987.

92. Gobeaux D, Landais A: Use of 2 opioids in blocks of the brachial plexus [French]. Cah Anesthesiol 36:437–440, 1988.

93. Fletcher D, Kuhlman G, Samii K: Addition of fentanyl to 1.5% lidocaine does not increase the success of axillary plexus block. Reg Anesth 19:183–188, 1994.

94. Kardash K, Schools A, Concepcion M: Effects of brachial plexus fentanyl on supraclavicular block. A randomized double-blind study. Reg Anesth 20:311–315, 1995.

95. Bazin JE, Massoni C, Bruelle P, et al: The addition of opioids to local anesthetics in brachial plexus block: The comparative effects of morphine, buprenorphine and sufentanil. Anaesthesia 52:858–862, 1997.

96. Bouaziz H, Kinirons BP, Macalou D, et al: Sufentanil does not prolong the duration of analgesia in a mepivacaine brachial plexus block: A dose response study. Anesth Analg 90:383–387, 2000.

97. Gormley WP, Murray JM, Fee JPH, Bower S: Effect of the addition of alfentanil to lignocaine during axillary brachial plexus anaesthesia. Br J Anaesth 76:802–805, 1996.

98. Wajima Z, Shitara T, Nakajima Y, et al: Comparison of continuous brachial plexus infusion of butorphanol, mepivacaine and mepivacaine–butorphanol mixtures for postoperative analgesia. Br J Anaesth 75:548–551, 1995.

99. Wajima Z, Nakajima Y, Kim C, et al: IV compared with brachial plexus infusion of butorphanol for postoperative analgesia. Br J Anaesth 74:392–395, 1995.

100. Candido KD, Winnie AP, Ghaleb AH, et al: Burprenorphine added to the local anesthetic for axillary brachial plexus block prolongs postoperative analgesia. Reg Anesth Pain Med 27:162–167, 2002.

101. Candido KD, Franco CD, Khan MA, et al: Buprenorphine added to the local anesthetic for brachial plexus block to provide postoperative analgesia in outpatients. Reg Anesth Pain Med 26:352–356, 2001.

102. Bourke DL, Furman WR: Improved postoperative analgesia with morphine added to axillary block solution. J Clin Anesth 5:114–117, 1993.

103. Fields HL, Emson PC, Leigh BK, et al: Multiple opiate receptor sites on primary afferent fibres. Nature 284:351–353, 1980.

104. Stein C: Peripheral mechanisms of opioid analgesia. Anesth Analg 76:182–191, 1993.

105. Kapral S, Gollmann G, Waltl B, et al: Tramadol added to mepivacaine prolongs the duration of an axillary brachial plexus blockade. Anesth Analg 88:853–856, 1999.

106. Bouaziz H, Paqueron X, Bur ML, et al: No enhancement of sensory and motor blockade by neostigmine added to mepivacaine axillary plexus block. Anesthesiology 91:78–83, 1999.

107. Bone HG, Van Aken H, Booke M, Burkle H: Enhancement of axillary brachial plexus block anesthesia by coadministration of neostigmine. Reg Anesth Pain Med 24:405–410, 1999.

Peripheral Sympathetic Blocks

Antoun Nader, M.D., and
Honorio T. Benzon, M.D.

STELLATE GANGLION BLOCK

Anatomy: The cervical sympathetic trunk contains three interconnected ganglia: the superior, middle, and inferior cervical ganglia. In 80% of people the lowest cervical ganglion is fused with the first thoracic ganglion to form the cervicothoracic (stellate) ganglion.[1] If not connected, the first thoracic ganglion is labeled as the stellate ganglion. The cervical ganglia receive preganglionic fibers from the lateral gray column of the spinal cord; the myelinated preganglionic cell axons originate from the anterolateral horn of the spinal cord. The nerve fibers emerge from the upper thoracic spinal cord through the ventral spinal root, joining the spinal nerves at the start of the ventral rami. They leave the spinal nerve through the white rami communicantes, which enter the corresponding thoracic ganglia, through which they ascend into the neck. The preganglionic fibers for the head and neck emerge from the upper five thoracic spinal nerves (mainly the upper three), ascending in the sympathetic trunk to synapse in the cervical ganglia. The preganglionic fibers supplying the upper limb originate from the upper thoracic segment, probably T2–T6, ascend via the sympathetic trunk to synapse in the cervicothoracic ganglion, where postganglionic fibers pass to the brachial plexus. The white ramus to the cervicothoracic ganglion contains most of the preganglionic fibers for the head and neck; these ascend the trunk to the superior cervical ganglion from which postganglionic branches supply vasoconstrictor and sudomotor nerves to the face and neck, secretory fibers to the salivary glands, dilator pupillae, and nonstriated muscle in the eyelid and orbitalis. Blockade of this ramus leads to ptosis, miosis, enophthalmos, and loss of sweating of the face and neck (Horner's syndrome). The cervicothoracic ganglion sends gray ramus communicantes to the seventh and eighth cervical and first thoracic nerves and gives off a cardiac branch, branches to nearby vessels, and sometimes a branch to the vagus nerve. To achieve successful sympathetic denervation of the head and neck, one should block the stellate ganglion because all preganglionic nerves either synapse or pass through the ganglion on their way to the more cephalad ganglia. Blood vessels of the upper limb beyond the first part of the axillary artery receive their sympathetic supply via branches of the adjacent brachial plexus. The first and second (and occasionally the third) intercostal nerves may be interconnected by postganglionic fibers from their gray rami; these fibers provide another pathway by which postganglionic nerves pass from the upper thoracic ganglia to the brachial plexus. These anomalous pathways have been termed Kuntz's nerves and are implicated in cases of inadequate relief of sympathetic mediated pain despite evidences of cervical ganglia block.

The cervical sympathetic chain lies anterior to the prevertebral fascia which is the fascia enclosing the prevertebral muscle. It is enclosed within the lateral aspect of the alar fascia (the thin layer of fascia immediately anterior to the prevertebral fascia which separates the cervical sympathetic chain from the retropharyngeal space). It is medial to the carotid space. The carotid sheath is connected to the alar fascia by a variable mesothelium-like fascia. The fascial plane enclosing the cervical sympathetic chain may be in direct communication with several spaces including the space in front of the scalenus anterior muscle, the brachial plexus, spinal nerve roots, the prevertebral portion of the vertebral artery, and between the endothoracic fascia and the thoracic wall muscle at the T1–T2 level. These communications may explain some of the side effects of stellate ganglion block. In the upper thorax the thoracic sympathetic chain lies lateral to the longus colli muscle and posterior to the endothoracic fascia, which is the inferior continuation of the prevertebral fascia.

The cervicothoracic ganglion lies on or just lateral to the longus colli muscle between the base of the seventh cervical transverse process and the neck of the first rib (which are posterior to the ganglion), the vertebral vessels are anterior, and the nerve roots that contribute to the inferior portion of the brachial plexus are posterior to the ganglion. The vertebral artery, which originates from the subclavian artery, passes over the ganglion and enters the vertebral foramen, posterior to the anterior tubercle of C6.

Effects of Stellate Ganglion Block: The effects of stellate ganglion block are secondary to neural inhibition in its sphere of innervation, including increased blood flow as a result of peripheral vasodilatation. Brain blood volume may increase.[2] The increase in blood flow can be reversed by prostaglandin (PGE1) infusion.[3] Left stellate ganglion block has been shown to increase heart rate and blood pressure and to activate the sympathetic neural outflow to the skeletal muscle with no deleterious effect on the left ventricular function.[4] In left-sided block the QTc interval and the QTc dispersion interval is decreased.[5] Although the autonomic innervation of sinus node is mainly through the right stellate ganglion, blockade of the right stellate ganglion may attenuate both sympathetic and parasympathetic activities resulting in inconsistent changes in the RR interval and corrected QT interval.[6] Stellate ganglion block may increase the retinal venous blood velocity without changing the retinal vessel diameter.[7] The intraocular pressure on the blocked side may decrease[8] and the ocular oxygen tension and ocular temperature may increase.[9] The tympanic temperature may drop significantly 5 minutes after a stellate ganglion block and the decrease in temperature may persist for more than 30 minutes.[10] Stellate ganglion block may modulate the immune system,[11] although neural blockade alone cannot completely explain the effects of the block on the immune and endocrine systems. Other mechanisms of action besides vasodilatation have been suggested including the regulation of melatonin secretion by the pineal gland. Plasma melatonin levels are suppressed triggering the recovery of a physiological melatonin rhythm. Since the rhythm of melatonin secretion influences many organs, recovery of its rhythm restores various physiological biorhythms.[12]

Clinical Indications for Cervicothoracic Ganglion Block:

The therapeutic efficacy of stellate ganglion block has not been tested by randomized, controlled clinical trials and some of its clinical indications are based largely on anecdotal cases. The clinical indications for stellate ganglion block in Japan are broader than in the USA or Europe. It is not only used for diseases of the head, neck, and upper extremity, but also in systemic diseases. Although there may be grounds for the extensive clinical indications, the evidences have been insufficient to support the routine use of stellate ganglion blocks in these conditions. Moreover, there are other alternatives that are efficacious and yield immediate results.

The common indications of stellate ganglion block include complex regional pain syndrome (CRPS), acute pain of herpes zoster, postherpetic neuralgia, and acute and chronic vasculopathies of the head, neck, and upper extremity.

Other reported clinical indications include the following:[12]

- Head: migraine, tension headache, cluster headache, temporal arteritis, cerebral angiospasm, cerebral thrombosis.
- Face: Bell's palsy, Hunt's syndrome, atypical facial hair, masticatory muscle syndrome, temporomandibular arthrosis.
- Eye: retinal vascular occlusion, retinal pigment degeneration, uveitis, optic neuritis, macular edema, corneal herpes, corneal ulcer, allergic conjunctivitis.
- Ear, nose, throat: allergic rhinitis, nasal polyps, acute or chronic sinusitis, sudden deafness, Meniere's disease, benign paroxysmal position vertigo.
- Neck, shoulder: Raynaud's disease, Raynaud's syndrome, acute arterial occlusion, and upper Buerger disease, neck-shoulder-arm syndrome, traumatic cervical extremity syndrome, thoracic outlet syndrome, scapulohumeral periarthritis, postoperative edema, tennis elbow, hyperhidrosis, frostbite, shoulder stiffness, phantom limb pain, stump pain.
- Circulatory system: myocardial infarction, angina pectoris, sinus tachycardia, neurocirculatory asthenia.

Technique: An intravenous line is started and standard resuscitative equipment must be readily accessible. The patient is placed in the supine position with the head slightly lifted forward and tilted backwards to straighten the esophagus and move it away from the transverse processes. The mouth is slightly opened to relax the neck muscles. The cricoid cartilage is palpated to discern the level of the C6 transverse process. Identification of the skin crease just caudal to thyroid level may be helpful as it is found to cross the C6 transverse process level in 71% of cases.[13] The Chassaignac's tubercle at C6 is identified. In most individuals the tubercle is located approximately 3 cm cephalad to the sternoclavicular joint at the medial border of the sternocleidomastoid muscle. The trachea and carotid pulse are palpated by the insertion of two fingers between the sternocleidomastoid muscle and the trachea (Fig. 80-1). The carotid artery is retracted laterally away from the needle entry site. A 22-gauge, short-beveled 4 to 5 cm needle is advanced downward, perpendicular to the table plane, until it touches bone and then withdrawn approximately 2 mm to avoid injection into the periosteum. The needle is in contact with either the C6 tubercle or the junction between the C6 vertebral body and the tubercle. The C6 tubercle is covered by the prevertebral fascia whereas the longus colli muscle is located at the lateral aspect of the body of the vertebra and the medial aspect of the transverse process. Injection into the substance of the longus colli muscle may result in a spread pattern that is often localized to the course of the muscle. Injection anterior to the C6 tubercle places the majority of solution anterior to the stellate ganglion. The solution may reach the ganglion especially when the drug travels in a caudad direction to the thoracic level. Therefore, sympathetic denervation of the upper extremity after C6 paratracheal injection is a complex phenomenon not entirely explained by bulk contact of local anesthetic with the stellate ganglion.[14] This has led many investigators to refer to this type of block as a cervicothoracic sympathetic block.

Careful aspiration must be performed prior to any injection. An initial test dose of 0.5 to 1 mL must be injected slowly since intravascular injection of less than 1 mL of local anesthetic results in loss of consciousness and seizure activity.[1] Computed tomography, magnetic resonance imaging, ultrasound, radionuclide tracers, and fluoroscopy may be used to confirm correct needle placement. Fluoroscopy is the most practical method. After 1 to 2 mL of contrast material is injected, spread of the contrast is characteristically seen. If contrast medium is not easily visualized, improper placement including intravascular, intrathecal, epidural, or intrapleural should be suspected.

The choice of medication and the volume of the solution vary according to the preference of the physician. Volumes of 5 to 20 mL have been used.[1] A larger volume is suggested when a sympathetic block to the arm is required. However, larger volumes (20 mL) are associated with an increased incidence of recurrent laryngeal nerve block.[1] Due to the high vascularity at the injection site, the plasma local anesthetic levels may

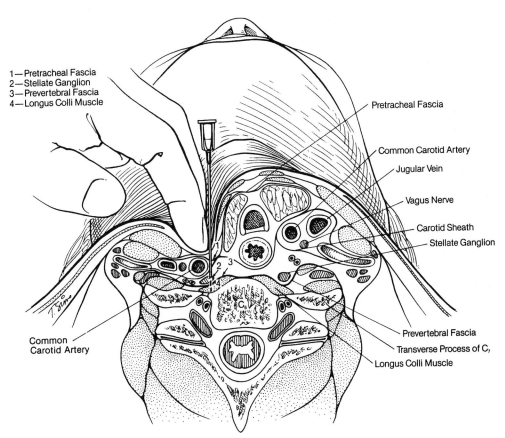

1—Pretracheal Fascia
2—Stellate Ganglion
3—Prevertebral Fascia
4—Longus Colli Muscle

Pretracheal Fascia

Common Carotid Artery

Jugular Vein

Vagus Nerve

Carotid Sheath

Stellate Ganglion

Prevertebral Fascia

Transverse Process of C$_7$

Longus Colli Muscle

Common
Carotid Artery

FIGURE 80-1. Cross-sectional anatomy of the technique of paratracheal approach to stellate ganglion block at the level of C6. (From Raj PP: Chronic pain. *In* Raj PP (ed): Clinical Practice of Regional Anesthesia. Churchill Livingtone, New York, 1991, p 489.)

be higher than after other types of nerve blocks.[15] Opioids, including fentanyl and morphine, and clonidine have been used alone or in combination with local anesthetics.[1]

Alternative Approaches

C7 ANTERIOR APPROACH: This approach is similar to the C6 anterior approach. However, C7 has a vestigial tubercle so the C6 tubercle should be identified first and the C7 transverse process can be located one fingerbreadth caudally. In this approach less volume is needed to achieve a sympathetic blockade. The approach has some disadvantages including increased incidence of vertebral artery puncture since the artery lies anterior to the C7 transverse process and increased risk of pneumothorax since the dome of the lung lies in close proximity to the injection site.

POSTERIOR THORACIC APPROACH: A posterior approach to the thoracic sympathetic chain has been described. It is most frequently done with imaging guidance such as fluoroscopy or computed tomography. The needle is inserted 2 to 4 cm lateral to the upper thoracic (T1, T2, or T3) spinous process adjacent to the body of the vertebra. A 22-gauge, 8 to 10 cm needle is used. The lamina is contacted then the needle is moved laterally off the lamina, parallel to the sagittal plane, until it passes through the costotransverse ligament at a depth of 2 cm beyond the lamina. The block can be done with the loss-of-resistance technique or a contrast material is injected to document spread in the area.

Side Effects and Complications: Cervical ganglion block causes ptosis, miosis, nasal congestion, and warmth of the face. Recurrent laryngeal nerve block results in hoarseness, subjective feeling of lump in the throat, or subjective shortness of breath. Phrenic nerve block may lead to respiratory difficulty in patients with preexisting lung disease.

Intravascular injection of the local anesthetic may lead to loss of consciousness, apnea, hypotension, and seizures. Intravascular injection of air may result in cerebral air embolism. A transient locked-in syndrome with hemodynamic stability, eyelid movements, apnea, and motor paralysis has been reported.[1] Brachial plexus block is secondary to the needle being inserted too posterior or from the spread of the medication along the prevertebral fascia. Intrathecal, subdural, or epidural injection may require respiratory assistance. Puncture of the pleura results in pneumothorax. The risk of pneumothorax is increased with the C7 approach. Myoclonus of the hand and arm, persistent cough, sinus arrest, intercostal neuralgia, and migraine have all been reported.[1] Contralateral spread of the drug may occur from the injection of large volumes of the local anesthetic. Bleeding and hematoma formation cause tracheal compression and airway compromise and may require emergency tracheostomy. Properly performed, stellate ganglion block is a safe and easy procedure. Complications are rare, with an incidence of 0.17%;[1] these occur early and are of short duration. Full resuscitative equipment should always be available when stellate ganglion block is performed.

LUMBAR PARAVERTEBRAL SYMPATHETIC BLOCK

Anatomy: The sympathetic chain lies along the anterolateral surface of the lumbar vertebral bodies, the psoas muscle and fascia separating the sympathetic nerves from the somatic nerves. The lumbar sympathetic chain contains pre- and post-ganglionic fibers to the pelvis and lower extremities. The location of the sympathetic ganglia on the vertebra at the level of the second and third lumbar vertebral bodies, where the sympathetic innervation of the lower extremities mostly originates from, was studied in cadavers. The ganglia were most frequently found at the level of the lower third of the second lumbar vertebra, at the L2–L3 interspace, and at the upper third of the third lumbar vertebra.[16] Therefore, the best site for placement of the tip of the needle is the anterolateral surface of the lower third of the second vertebral body or at the upper third of the third vertebral body.[16] The segmental artery and vein pass along the midportion of the lumbar vertebral body in a tunnel under the dense fascia. Solutions injected at the mid-vertebral level may pass posteriorly in this tunnel to the epidural space. Crossover of the sympathetic fibers to the other side has been described.

Indications: Lumbar sympathetic blocks are performed to determine the degree of sympathetic-mediated pain in a patient with acute or chronic pain, as prognostic or therapeutic blocks in patients with sympathetic mediated pain, for the improvement of blood flow in patients with vascular insufficiency of their lower extremities, and for the management of neuralgic pain associated with peripheral nerve injuries such as those following trauma or limb amputation.

Technique: The patient is placed prone with a pillow underneath the lower abdomen to reduce lumbar lordosis. Blind insertion of the needle has been described. However, radiologic confirmation is preferable because of variability of the body habitus, the uncertainty of the vertebral level of insertion, and to confirm correct placement of the needle tip. The earlier techniques involve injections at the L2, L3, and L4 vertebrae. More recent techniques described the use of a single needle.[17,18] In the technique of Hatangdi and Boas the midline is marked and the tip of the twelfth rib palpated on the side to be injected. The site of insertion of the needle is 2 to 3 cm below and medial to the tip of the twelfth rib, opposite the body of L3 (Fig. 80-2).[18] A 5- to 7-inch, 22-gauge needle is inserted 8 to 10 cm from the midline, at a 30° to 45° angle, lateral to the spinous process, to reach the anterolateral aspect of the vertebra. Correct placement of the needle is confirmed by the injection of 2 to 3 mL of nonionic contrast that shows a linear spread of the dye along the anterolateral aspect of the vertebral bodies (Fig. 80-3). A volume of 15 to 20 mL of local anesthetic is then injected. Some authors first identify the psoas muscle by injecting 0.5 to 1 mL of dye, visualizing the "psoas stripe," then advancing the needle until it is anterior to the psoas muscle.[19] For neurolytic blocks, a two-needle technique is recommended, one needle at L2 and the other needle at L3.[18] The injection of 2 to 4 mL of 6% phenol at each site allows better control of the spread of the neurolytic agent, in contrast to an injection of 6 to 10 mL of phenol at one site. Some investigators recommend confirmation of correct needle placement by demonstration of a temperature increase after

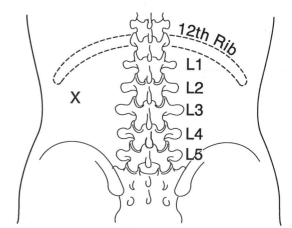

FIGURE 80-2. Single-needle technique of lumbar sympathetic blockade.[18] X is the site of the needle insertion.

injection of a small volume of local anesthetic, before the phenol is injected. A volume of 1 mL of air or local anesthetic is injected before the needle is removed to prevent depositing the neurolytic solution on the somatic nerves during removal of the needle. The patient is kept on the side for 15 to 30 minutes to prevent the phenol from spreading laterally toward the genitofemoral nerve or posteriorly between the slips of origin of the psoas major muscle and along the fibrous tunnel occupied by the rami communicantes, toward the somatic nerve roots.[20] The patient is then turned supine and instructed not to raise his/her head for at least 1 hour.

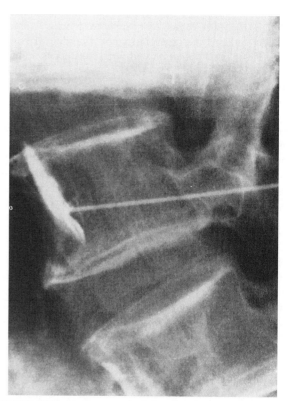

FIGURE 80-3. Linear spread of the dye along the anterolateral aspect of the vertebral body.

Insertion of the needle at 10 cm from the midline is the preferred site by some investigators.[21] Insertion of the needle closer to the midline take the needle path close to the somatic nerve roots. The more lateral the needle insertion the closer is the tip of the needle to the sympathetic chain. There is also less risk of piercing the roots of the lumbar plexus or encountering the transverse process.

Complications of lumbar paravertebral sympathetic block include bleeding from puncture of the lumbar vessels or the aorta, hematuria, infection, orthostatic hypotension, perforation of the abdominal viscera, transient backache and stiffness, epidural or subarachnoid blockade, lumbar plexus block, and segmental nerve injury. There is a 5% to 40% incidence of postblock neuralgia but this is usually of limited duration. The genitofemoral nerve passes below L3 so injection at L4 is not advisable.

Radiofrequency Lumbar Sympathectomy: Rocco described the use of radiofrequency (RF) sympathectomy to relieve the pain of sympathetic maintained pain, i.e., CRPS type I.[22] The site of RF sympatholysis was slightly cephalad to the middle of the L3 vertebra; contrast material was injected to confirm the correct placement of the needle. Reproduction of the pain, spread of the dye, rapidity of temperature rise in the legs, and increase in the pulse amplitude were useful guides to appropriate placement of the needle tip. The needle tip was heated to 80°C and the temperature maintained for 90 seconds. Of the 20 patients who had RF sympathectomy, 5 continued to have pain relief 5 months to 3 years after the last RF procedure while 15 had temporary relief or no relief at all. Rocco concluded that despite the early sympathetic blockade, as confirmed by a warm foot, long-lasting relief with RF sympathectomy was difficult to obtain.[22]

MONITORING THE ADEQUACY OF SYMPATHETIC BLOCKADE

Successful stellate ganglion block denervates the upper cervical segments to produce Horner's syndrome that includes ptosis, miosis, and anhydrosis. Other signs include unilateral nasal stuffiness (Guttman's sign), hyperemia of the tympanic membrane, and warmth of the face. The presence of Horner's syndrome signifies cephalic sympathetic blockade and does not imply sympathetic denervation of the arm.[23] If the block is used to treat the shoulder or upper limb, additional signs are needed to determine sympathetic blockade in the area. Complete block is reliably detected when a test of adrenergic fiber activity (thermography, plethysmography, laser Doppler flowmetry) is combined with a test of sympathetic cholinergic (sudomotor) fiber activity (sweat test, sympathogalvanic response).

Increase in skin temperature is the most commonly used clinical sign of sympathetic blockade. Commonly, skin temperature is measured by using adhesive thermocouple probes that are placed distally to the extremity being monitored. For continuous skin temperature measurements, thermocouple devices are placed bilaterally. It is important to allow the patient some time to accommodate to the room temperature before the first temperature measurements are taken. If an infrared thermography unit is used, an average sensitivity to skin temperature changes is about 0.1°C. Another qualitative thermography technique is liquid crystal thermography, with a

reported sensitivity of about 0.8°C. Different investigators considered different increases in skin temperature as signifying effective sympathetic blockade. After a stellate ganglion block, skin temperature increases of 1.5°C,[24] 3.8°C,[25] and 7.5°C[26] have been considered as signifying successful sympathetic blockade. A mean increase of 3°C was noted after a lumbar paravertebral sympathetic block.[27] Hogan et al. recommended that the ipsilateral temperature increase should exceed that of the contralateral side to indicate successful sympathetic blockade.[23] Stevens et al. found that a temperature increase that was 2°C higher than the contralateral extremity signified complete sympathetic blockade in most patients but it was not sufficient to guarantee a complete sympathetic block in all their patients.[28] The magnitude of temperature increases after complete sympathetic blockade depends on the baseline values; greater increases are noted in patients with lower preblock temperatures.[29] With vasodilation, the skin temperature will approximate core body temperature. Since the upper limit of skin temperature in the fingers and toes is 35 to 36°C,[30] patients other than those with organic peripheral vascular disease can approach 35 to 36°C as a limit of complete sympathetic blockade.[29] Patients whose baseline skin temperatures are low because of vasoconstriction (those with late-stage CRPS) will have large increases after complete sympathetic blockade. A patient who has vasodilation of the involved extremity, someone with early-stage CRPS, cannot be expected to have a large temperature increase. The absolute change in temperature of the affected extremity is greater if temperature is measured more distally (e.g., index finger rather than upper arm).

Laser Doppler flowmetry is a sensitive method to evaluate skin blood flow and to detect the presence of sympathetic blockade. Most of the devices available today have a low-power laser source and flexible fiberoptic light guides, which deliver laser light to the skin. When light is reflected from the moving red blood cells, the device has a shift in frequency that can then be analyzed in real time. Some investigators consider a 50% or greater increase in the skin blood flow to signify successful sympathetic block.[31]

Blood flow can be determined accurately by using plethysmographic methods such as venous-occlusion plethysmography. A transducer is placed on the finger to measure the change of the finger volume over time, or the whole foot or hand is placed in a water bath that is attached to the transducer. Rapid inflation of the venous tourniquet around the finger allows arterial blood to enter the finger but prevents venous blood to leave. The finger's rate of volume increase is measured using the volume transducer and typical plethysmographic trace is produced. The slope first rapidly increases then reaches a plateau phase when enough blood has entered the finger to equalize the venous and tourniquet pressures. After successful sympathetic block of the extremity, there is a marked increase of the upward slope because of a significant increase in the pulse wave. Investigators found a better correlation of the blood flow measured by volume plethysmography with skin surface temperature gradients than blood flow measurements by laser Doppler flowmetry.[31]

Abolition of sweating and of the sympathogalvanic response (SGR) are among the standard tests of complete sympathetic blockade.[23–34] The older starch iodine test is messy and cumbersome while the newer sweat tests, the cobalt blue and the ninhydrin sweat tests, are easier to perform. Benzon et al. have modified the preparation of the two sweat tests.[34] For the cobalt

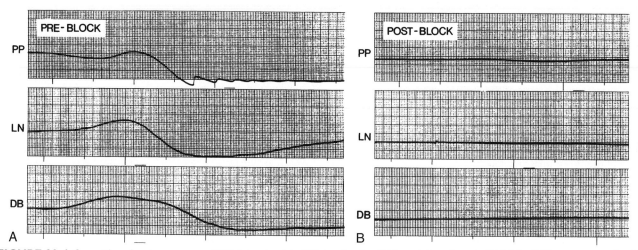

FIGURE 80-4. Sympathogalvanic responses (SGRs) to pinprick (PP), loud noise (LN), and deep breath (DB). The SGRs were completely abolished after the sympathetic block.

blue filter paper, 0.5 M CoCl₂ in 70% ethanol is used while 2% ninhydrin in 70% ethanol with 1 mL of 4 M acetate buffer (pH 5.5) per 100 mL solution is utilized for the ninhydrin filter paper. Seventy percent ethanol is used because it dries up rapidly and does not require heating of the filter paper. The solutions (cobalt blue or ninhydrin) are applied evenly on a Whatman No. 1 filter paper at 2 mL/100 cm². The papers are dried at room temperature and stored in a desiccator. The sweat tests are performed in the following manner. The patient's fingers or toes are wiped dry and the cobalt blue- or ninhydrin-impregnated filter paper is taped on them. A transparent tape is used so the change in color of the cobalt blue paper secondary to sweating can be seen. Sweating is signified by a change in color of the cobalt blue filter paper from blue to pink and the appearance of purple dots in the ninhydrin filter paper. Unfortunately, the cobalt blue and ninhydrin sweat tests are not available commercially.

The SGR can be recorded using a regular ECG machine. The right arm and left arm leads of the ECG are placed on the dorsum and palm of the hand (or dorsum and sole of the foot), the other leads are placed on the contralateral extremity, and the lead selector switch turned to lead I. The stimulus can be a deep breath, pinprick, or loud noise. The response consists of an upward or downward deflection of the ECG tracing; it can be monophasic or biphasic. Partial sympathetic block reduces the response while complete block abolishes it, i.e., the tracing is a straight line (Fig. 80-4). The SGR has several shortcomings including marked variations in the responses of patients to the different stimuli and difficulty in obtaining a satisfactory recording under clinical conditions. There is also a rapid habituation to the stimuli used, i.e., the patient has no SGR in the absence of a sympathetic block after several SGR recordings with the same stimulus.

The two sweat tests are more reliable than the SGR in predicting complete sympathetic blockade.[34] The sensitivities of the sweat tests and the SGR were found to be 90%. The specificity of the SGR was 56% compared to 100% for the sweat tests; their accuracy was 74% and 95%, respectively.[34] Since these tests are rarely used clinically, temperature increases to 35 or 36°C can be considered as signifying complete sympathetic blockade.

Relief of pain does not imply complete sympathetic blockade since patients with chronic pain may exhibit complete pain relief after partial sympathetic blockade. Partial pain relief, on the other hand, signifies one of two things. The patient's pain may be due to causes other than sympathetic-mediated pain (e.g., combined somatic sensory- and sympathetic-mediated pain or combined sympathetic-mediated and central pain) or the sympathetic blockade may be partial. A sign of complete sympathetic blockade is therefore necessary in these instances. It is also valuable after surgical or chemical sympathectomy to demonstrate complete sympathetic interruption and to correlate recurrence of pain with sympathetic recovery.[35]

KEY POINTS

- The cervicothoracic ganglion lies on or just lateral to the longus colli muscle between the base of the seventh cervical transverse process and the neck of the first rib. The vertebral vessels are anterior and the nerve roots that contribute to the inferior portion of the brachial plexus are posterior to the ganglion.
- The intravascular injection of a small volume (1 mL) of local anesthetic may result in convulsion. This is secondary to injection of the local anesthetic into the vertebral artery.
- The appearance of Horner's syndrome does not signify sympathetic blockade of the upper extremity. Signs of sympathetic blockade of the arm must be documented.
- The lumbar sympathetic ganglia are most frequently found at the lower third of the L2, the L2–L3 interspace, and at the upper third of L3. Therefore, the best site for placement of the needle is at the anterolateral surface of the lower third of L2 or at the upper third L3. The genitofemoral nerve passes below L3 so injection at L4 is not advisable when chemical neurolytic block is performed.
- Increase in skin temperature is the most commonly used clinical sign of sympathetic blockade. The magnitude of temperature increases after complete sympathetic blockade depends on the baseline values. Greater increases are noted in patients with lower preblock temperatures. Since the upper limit of skin temperature in the fingers and toes is 35 to 36°C, patients without organic peripheral vascular

disease can approach 35 to 36°C as a sign of complete sympathetic blockade.

- Abolition of sweating and of the SGR are the standard tests of complete sympathetic blockade. The two sweat tests are more reliable than the SGR in predicting complete sympathetic blockade. Since these tests are rarely used clinically, temperature increases to 35 or 36°C can be considered as signifying complete sympathetic blockade.

REFERENCES

1. Marples IL, Atkin RE: Stellate ganglion block. Pain Rev 8:3–11, 2001.

2. Okubo Y, Ogata H: Brain blood volume measured with near infrared spectroscopy increased after stellate ganglion block. Masui – Japanese J Anesthesiol 44:423–427, 1995.

3. Okuda Y, Kitajima T: Imbalance of blood flow induced by sympathetic blood flow was corrected by prostaglandin E1. Masui – Japanese J Anesthesiol 45:27–29, 1996.

4. Ikeda T, Iwase S, Sugiyama Y, et al: Stellate ganglion block is associated with increased tibial nerve muscle activity in humans. Anesthesiology 84:843–850, 1996.

5. Egawa H, Okuda Y, Kitajima T, Minami J: Assessment of QT interval and QT dispersion following stellate ganglion block using computerized measurements. Reg Anesth Pain Med 26:539–544, 2001.

6. Fujiki A, Masuda A, Inoue H: Effects of unilateral stellate ganglion block on the spectral characteristics of heart rate variability. Japanese Circulat J 63:854–858, 1999.

7. Kiuchi Y, Hirota A, Takamatsu M, et al: Effects of stellate ganglion block on human retinal blood flow. Nippon GanKa Gakkai Zasshi – Acta Societatis Ophthalmologicae Japonicae 104:29–33, 2000.

8. Nagahara M, Tamaki Y, Araie M, et al: The acute effects of stellate ganglion block on circulation in human ocular fundus. Acta Ophthalmol Scand 79:45–48, 2001.

9. Masuda R, Yokoyoma K, Kajiwara K, et al: The effects of stellate ganglion block on conjunctival oxygen tension and intraocular pressure in patients with retinal vein occlusion. Masui – Japanese J Anesthesiol 44: 828–833, 1995.

10. Murakuwa K, Noma K, Ishida K, et al: Changes of tympanic temperature by stellate ganglion block. Masui – Japanese J Anesthesiol 44:824–827, 1995.

11. Yokoyama M, Nakatsuka H, Itano Y, et al: Stellate ganglion block modifies the distribution of lymphocytes subsets and natural-killer cell activity. Anesthesiology 92:109–115, 2000.

12. Uchida K, Tateda T, Hino H: Novel mechanism of action hypothesized for stellate ganglion block related to melatonin. Med Hypoth 59:446–449, 2002.

13. Cha YD, Lee SK, Kim TJ, et al: The neck crease as a landmark of Chasaignac's tubercle in stellate ganglion block: Anatomical and radiological evaluation. Acta Anaesthesiol Scand 46:100–102, 2002.

14. Christie JM, Martinez CR: Computerized axial tomography to define the distribution of solution after stellate ganglion nerve block. J Clin Anesth 7:306–311, 1995.

15. Yokoyama M, Mizobuchi S, Nakatuska H, et al: Comparison of plasma lidocaine concentrations after injection of a fixed small volume in the stellate ganglion, the lumbar epidural space, or a single intercostal nerve. Anesth Analg 87:112–115, 1998.

16. Umeda S, Arai T, Hatano Y, et al: Cadaver anatomic analysis of the best site for chemical lumbar sympathectomy. Anesth Analg 66:643, 1987.

17. Brown EM, Kunjappan V: Single-needle lateral approach for lumbar sympathetic block. Anesth Analg 4:725, 1975.

18. Hatangdi VS, Boas RA: Lumbar sympathectomy: A single-needle technique. Br J Anaesth 57:285, 1985.

19. Sprague RS, Ramamurthy S: Identification of the anterior psoas sheath as a landmark for lumbar sympathetic block. Reg Anesth 15:253, 1990.

20. Breivik H, Cousins MJ, Lofstrom JB: Sympathetic neural blockade of upper and lower extremity. In Cousins MJ, Bridenbaugh PO (eds): Neural Blockade in Clinical Anesthesia and Management of Pain, ed 3. JB Lippincott, Philadelphia, 1998, pp 435–437.

21. Cherry DA, Rao DM: Lumbar sympathetic and coeliac plexus blocks – An anatomical study in cadavers. Br J Anaesth 54:1037, 1982.

22. Rocco AG: Radiofrequency lumbar sympatholysis: The evolution of a technique for managing sympathetically maintained pain. Reg Anesth 20:3, 1995.

23. Hogan QH, Taylor ML, Goldstein M, et al: Success rates in producing sympathetic blockade by paratracheal injection. Clin J Pain 10:139, 1994.

24. Carron H, Litwiller R: Stellate ganglion block. Anesth Analg 54:567, 1975.

25. Ready LB, Kozody R, Barsa JE, Murphy TM: Side-port needles for stellate ganglion block. Reg Anesth 7:160, 1982.

26. Erickson SJ, Hogan QH: CT-guided injection of the stellate ganglion: Description of technique and efficacy of sympathetic blockade. Radiology 188:707, 1993.

27. Hatangdi VS, Boas RA: Lumbar sympathectomy: A single-needle technique. Br J Anaesth 57:285, 1985.

28. Stevens RA, Stotz A, Kao TC, et al: The relative increase in skin temperature after stellate ganglion block is predictive of a complete sympathectomy of the hand. Reg Anesth Pain Med 23:266–270, 1998.

29. Benzon HT, Avram MJ: Temperature increases after complete sympathetic blockade. Reg Anesth 11:27, 1986.

30. Coller FA, Maddock WG: The differentiation of spastic from organic vascular occlusion by the skin temperature response to high environmental temperature. Ann Surg 96:719, 1932.

31. Kapural L, Mekhail N: Assessment of sympathetic blocks. Tech Reg Anesth Pain Manage 5:82–87, 2001.

32. Malmqvist EL, Bengstsson M, Sorensen J: Efficacy of stellate ganglion block: A clinical study with bupivacaine. Reg Anesth 17:340, 1992.

33. Dhuner KG, Edshage S, Wihelm A: Ninhydrin test – An objective method for testing local anaesthetic drugs. Acta Anaesthesiol Scand 4:189, 1960.

34. Benzon HT, Cheng SC, Avram MJ, et al: Sign of complete sympathetic blockade: Sweat test or sympathogalvanic response? Anesth Analg 64:415, 1985.

35. Benzon HT: Importance of documenting complete sympathetic denervation after sympathectomy. Anesth Analg 74:599, 1992.

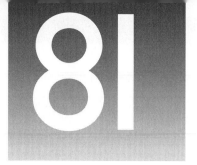

Complications After Peripheral Nerve Block

**Joseph M. Neal, M.D., and
James R. Hebl, M.D.**

Peripheral nerve blocks are subject to a unique set of potential complications that will likely become increasingly relevant as anesthesiologists predictably expand their practice of peripheral regional anesthesia.[1] The generally held opinion that peripheral nerve blocks are safer than neuraxial blocks is an oversimplification. In surveys of French anesthesiologists Auroy et al.[2,3] reported that death, cardiac arrest, respiratory arrest, and permanent neurologic injury were significantly more likely to occur with neuraxial blocks. Although these complications are reported after peripheral nerve block, they are decidedly rare (Table 81-1).[2,3] Most serious peripheral nerve block complications are related to unintended intravascular injection of local anesthetic or peripheral nerve injury. Seizures are twice as likely to occur during peripheral nerve block as compared with all regional anesthetics (1.2 versus 0.6/10,000 patients, respectively), and four to five times more frequent than the rate associated with epidural anesthesia. Presumably, this is secondary to the large volume of local anesthetics commonly used during peripheral nerve blockade. Conversely, neurologic injury occurs less frequently after peripheral nerve block than subarachnoid block (2.4 versus 3.4/10,000 patients, respectively).[3] Complication profiles for specific peripheral blocks are less well studied, but in the case of interscalene block, the overall incidence of short- and long-term complications is about 0.4%.[4] Peripheral catheter techniques do not increase the risk of serious nerve injury or infection.[4,5] Overall, the practice of peripheral nerve block is remarkably safe, yet retains the potential for life-altering complications. This chapter addresses the vascular, neurologic, pulmonary, anesthetic toxicity, and infectious complications of peripheral nerve block (Table 81-2).

VASCULAR COMPLICATIONS

Intravascular Injection: Common use of vascular landmarks during the performance of peripheral blocks raises the potential for unintentional intravascular injection of local anesthetic. Intravascular injection without subsequent seizure activity happens in 0.2% of transarterial axillary blocks, even after careful aspiration and test dosing.[6] Whether the local

TABLE 81-1. MAJOR COMPLICATIONS RELATED TO REGIONAL ANESTHESIA

Technique	Death	Cardiac Arrest	Respiratory Failure	Seizure	Neurologic Injury
All regional anesthetics	0.3	0.7	0.4	0.6	1.6
Spinal	0.7	2.4	0.5	0.2	3.4
Epidural	0	0	0.8	0.8	0
Peripheral nerve blocks	0.2	0.2	0.4	1.2	2.4

Data represent estimated number per 10,000 patients.
Modified from Auroy Y, Benhamou D, Bargues L, et al: Major complications of regional anesthesia in France. The SOS regional anesthesia hotline service. Anesthesiology 97:1274–1280, 2002.

TABLE 81-2. PERIPHERAL NERVE BLOCKS: COMPLICATIONS AND ESTIMATED FREQUENCY

Complication	Estimated Occurrence
Vascular complications	
Intravascular injection	0.2%*
Seizure: all peripheral blocks	1.2/10,000 patients
Seizure: axillary, interscalene, supraclavicular	1.3, 7.6, 7.9/1,000 patients
Bruising	20%*
Vasospasm	1%*
Permanent anesthesia-related nerve injury	0.02–0.4%
Pulmonary complications	
Hemidiaphragmatic paresis	100%†
Pneumothorax	<0.01 to 6.1%‡
Unintended local anesthetic destinations	
Subarachnoid/epidural	Rare† to ~5%§
Cervical sympathetic chain	20–90%
Recurrent laryngeal nerve	1–20%
Hypotensive/bradycardic events (awake interscalene)	13–24%
Infectious complications	Very rare

* Transarterial axillary block.
† Interscalene block.
‡ Supraclavicular block.
§ Psoas block.

anesthetic is injected intra-arterially or intravenously is critically important. Direct intra-arterial injection during brachial plexus block can result in immediate seizure activity after small volumes of local anesthetic. Direct injection into the vertebral or carotid arteries, or retrograde injection via the subclavian artery, can cause seizures with as little as 3 mg bupivacaine or 14 mg lidocaine.[7] Indeed, seizure frequency is significantly greater with interscalene or supraclavicular block (7.6 and 7.9/1,000 patients, respectively), as compared with the axillary approach (1.3/1,000).[8] In contradistinction to injection into arteries supplying the brain, similar-volume intravenous injection is less likely to result in seizure because local anesthetic is partially cleared by the lung and then distributed throughout the body. However, large-volume intravascular injection can still result in serious cardiotoxicity, particularly when local anesthetics with cardiotoxic profiles are used. Peak plasma levels subsequent to local anesthetic uptake from subcutaneous or interstitial tissues can be delayed 30 to 60 minutes, and are influenced by total local anesthetic dose, vasoconstrictors, and block site. In these cases peak plasma levels may be sufficient to cause systemic local anesthetic toxicity, including seizures. The risk of delayed toxicity is highest with intercostal nerve block, less with plexus blocks, and least with local subcutaneous infiltration.

Avoidance of intravascular injection is paramount for preventing systemic local anesthetic toxicity. Meticulous technique includes frequent aspiration, incremental dosing, and epinephrine-containing intravascular test doses. Basing local anesthetic dosing on body weight has minimal value, because peak plasma local anesthetic concentrations correlate poorly with patient mass (weight or body surface area) (Fig. 81-1).[9] For large-volume perivascular blocks (femoral, popliteal fossa, brachial plexus), consideration should be given to avoiding local anesthetics with high cardiotoxicity profiles: bupivacaine, etidocaine > ropivacaine, l-bupivacaine >> lidocaine, mepivacaine. Lower extremity peripheral blocks represent a particularly high risk of systemic toxicity because multiple, moderate-volume individual nerve blocks are often necessary for full anesthetic effect.

Systemic local anesthetic toxicity is the most serious complication of intravenous regional anesthesia. Large volumes of local anesthetic can breach a pneumatic tourniquet and enter the systemic circulation after rapid, high-pressure injection, particularly into a proximal vein. Slow (90 seconds) injection into a distal vein greatly reduces the likelihood of this complication. Local anesthetic can also enter the circulation during tourniquet deflation. To avoid high postblock plasma levels of local anesthetic, it is recommended that tourniquets not be deflated until at least 30 minutes following the initial injection sequence. The efficacy of tourniquet cycling (deflation/reinflation) to attenuate peak plasma levels is unclear, but the practice is generally unnecessary if more than 45 minutes have passed since local anesthetic injection.

Vascular Injury: Minor hematoma and bruising is exceedingly common after perivascular nerve blocks, particularly using the

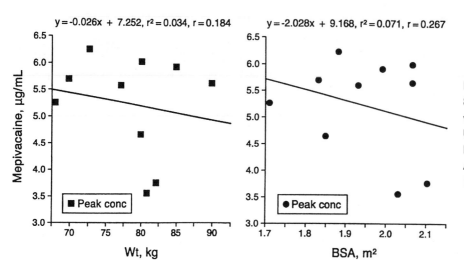

FIGURE 81-1. Peak plasma levels after 800 mg mepivacaine do not correlate with weight or body surface area. (From Urmey WF: Upper extremity blocks. *In* Brown DL (ed): Regional Anesthesia and Analgesia. WB Saunders, Philadelphia, 1996, p 272, Fig. 16–20.)

axillary approach, where bruising is apparent in ~20% of patients.[10] When evidence of vascular compromise, such as absent distal pulse or extremity pallor, is temporally related to peripheral block placement, vascular injury should be part of the differential diagnosis. Local anesthetic- or needle-induced vasospasm, which occurs in 1% of transarterial axillary blocks,[6] typically resolves within 10 to 15 minutes. However, in cases of persistent arterial vasospasm interventions such as intra-arterial lidocaine, topical warming, or nitroglycerine paste has been suggested.[11] Conversely, prolonged vascular insufficiency may indicate direct arterial compression secondary to hematoma formation or needle-induced arterial wall injury, dissection, or pseudoaneurysm.[7] In rare cases surgical exploration may be necessary to restore distal perfusion. Surgical indications include: (1) hematoma expansion, (2) neurologic deterioration, (3) unchanged neurologic examination despite a resolving hematoma, and (4) documented vascular or lymphatic obstruction.[6,12]

When compared to neuraxial hemorrhagic complications associated with the concurrent use of anticoagulants our knowledge of how abnormal coagulation affects peripheral nerve blocks is sparse.[13] Careful consideration should be given before placing blocks in the proximity of noncompressible vascular structures in patients with prolonged coagulation parameters or abnormal platelet function. Psoas compartment block may represent a particularly increased risk, as hemorrhagic complications have been reported in patients given low molecular weight heparin or other anticoagulants after block placement.[14]

NEUROLOGIC COMPLICATIONS

Permanent anesthesia-related nerve injury (ARNI) lasting over 9 months is relatively rare (<0.02% to 0.4%).[7] In a large survey of complications the frequency of neurologic injury was generally 0 to 3/10,000 patients across a wide spectrum of peripheral blocks, except for an inexplicably large rate (32/10,000) in patients undergoing popliteal fossa block.[3] Regional anesthetic techniques are more likely to be associated with ARNI medicolegal claims as compared with general anesthesia.[15] Neither regional anesthesia in patients with pre-existing neuropathology[16] nor continuous axillary catheter techniques increase the risk of neurologic injury.[5]

Peripheral nerve injury usually becomes evident within 48 to 72 hours of surgery. Injuries secondary to hematoma formation, postoperative edema, or intraoperative traction or transection typically manifest themselves immediately, while injury secondary to reactive tissue or scarring can be delayed for up to 3 weeks. The vast majority of perioperative peripheral nerve injuries resolve within 6 weeks, with less than 0.4% resulting in permanent sequelae.[7] Because most injuries resolve quickly, it is acceptable to delay formal neurologic evaluation for 6 to 8 weeks. However, some experts recommend more immediate consultation to help localize injury site, document pre-existing occult or subclinical neurologic pathology (such as pre-existing subclinical diabetic neuropathy or carpal tunnel syndrome), and/or to ensure appropriate rehabilitation prescription.

When faced with evidence of a neurologic deficit following peripheral nerve block, it is imperative that the anesthesiologist considers a complete differential diagnosis (Table 81-3). In addition to ARNI, surgical factors that may cause or worsen nerve injury include improper positioning, direct nerve trauma, traction injury, or ischemic insult secondary to hematoma, edema, or constrictive tourniquets or dressings. Certain surgeries, most notably shoulder[17] and elbow procedures, are particularly prone to peripheral nerve injury. Patient factors such as advanced age, diabetes mellitus, male gender, or pre-existing neuropathy may also predict or further exacerbate perioperative nerve injury.[7]

The mechanisms of peripheral nerve injury can be arbitrarily categorized as mechanical, chemical, or a combination of the two.

Mechanical Injury: Direct neural trauma secondary to needle injury has been postulated to play a significant role in perioperative peripheral nerve injury. The significance of paresthesia elicitation is most controversial, because some studies link injury to documented paresthesia within a particular nerve's distribution,[2,18] while others have been unable to link consistently paresthesia to subsequent injury.[15] Indeed, the very definition of what a paresthesia represents varies among experts: indirect pressure transmitted from perineural tissues, direct needle-to-nerve contact, or needle within the nerve. Consensus opinion appears to accept paresthesia per se as not indicating nerve injury, but rather representing information

TABLE 81-3. DIFFERENTIAL DIAGNOSIS OF PERIOPERATIVE NERVE INJURY

Anesthesia-related factors
Mechanical injury
    Direct needle injury
    Ischemia: hematoma, edema
Chemical injury
    Local anesthetic toxicity
    Vasoconstrictors or preservatives

Surgery-related factors
Improper positioning
Ischemia: tourniquet, dressing, edema, hematoma
Direct nerve injury
Traction injury

Patient-related factors
Advanced age
Male gender
Diabetes mellitus
Chemotherapy-induced neuropathy

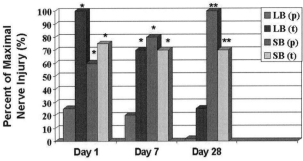

FIGURE 81-2. Rat sciatic nerve injury as a function of time and needle bevel orientation. LB, long bevel; SB, short bevel; p, parallel to nerve fibers; t, transverse to nerve fibers. (Modified by permission of Oxford University Press from Rice ASC, McMahon SB: Peripheral nerve injury caused by injection needles used in regional anaesthesia: Influence of bevel configuration, studied in a rat model. Br J Anaesth 9:433–438, 1992.)

Whether patients with compromised PNBF, such as those with diabetes mellitus or chemotherapy-induced neuropathy, are at higher risk of peripheral nerve injury from chemical insult is not known.[7]

Double Insult: As alluded to, perioperative nerve injury is poorly understood. In the vast majority of patients needle-to-nerve contact (paresthesia) and the use of common clinical concentrations of local anesthetic/epinephrine solutions appears to be exceedingly safe. Some experts suggest that ARNI may require a dual insult or "double crush" injury.[7] Animal experiments also suggest that duality may be important,[23,24] although confirmatory human studies are absent. In the absence of complete or near-complete nerve transection, needle-induced injury appears to be quite rare. Indeed, needles are routinely introduced into nerves in the course of microneurography[25] or surgical repair, albeit in these cases anesthetic solution is not injected. However, when the blood–nerve barrier is compromised by needle trauma or surgical injury, the application of local anesthetics, with or without epinephrine, has produced neurotoxicity in animal models.[7]

Prevention: The dual insult theory suggests that attention to technique may significantly reduce the likelihood of perioperative peripheral nerve injury. There is no clinical evidence to suggest that the incidence of ARNI is higher with any specific regional anesthetic technique: transarterial, paresthesia, or peripheral nerve stimulation.[7] Complete avoidance of paresthesias may be impossible;[18] and paresthesias per se appear to be neither causative nor predictive of nerve injury. Furthermore, the use of a peripheral nerve stimulator does not guarantee avoidance of intraneural injection or peripheral nerve injury.[3] Thus, vigilant awareness of the signs of intraneural injection is paramount to prevention, because it causes disruption of the nerve–blood barrier, which in turn elevates the potential for chemical-induced nerve injury. Initial injection of local anesthetic near a nerve should be performed slowly and with very small volumes. Patient complaint of pain should prompt immediate cessation of injection and withdrawal or repositioning of the needle.

that the needle and nerve are sufficiently close to warrant interpretation as either endpoint or warning sign.[19] More significant is the patient's ability to appreciate pain during local anesthetic injection, which likely is indicative of intraneural injection and should halt further injection.[7] Masking the patient's ability to appreciate this unpleasant sensation, as by provision of general anesthesia or deep sedation, has been linked to significant neurologic injury in anesthetized patients undergoing femoral and interscalene block.[20] The risks of placing other peripheral blocks in patients undergoing general anesthesia are undefined.

Smaller-gauge needles cause less nerve damage, but the role of needle bevel design is controversial. In animals nerve penetration is more difficult to accomplish with a blunt needle as compared with a sharp needle. However, if nerve penetration does occur, blunt needles are associated with significantly greater structural damage that takes longer to heal. Furthermore, a needle penetrating a nerve with the bevel parallel to its fibers causes less structural damage that recovers faster than when the bevel is placed in a transverse orientation (Fig. 81-2).[7] In humans no randomized clinical trials exist to clarify the relative safety of one needle design over another.

Chemical Injury: Direct peripheral nerve injury can theoretically be caused or worsened by chemical toxicity from local anesthetics, vasoconstrictors, and/or preservatives and excipients.[21] When applied to peripheral nerves in a time- and concentration-dependent manner, all local anesthetics are potentially neurotoxic and/or decrease peripheral nerve blood flow (PNBF). Animal studies demonstrate that commonly used agents, such as lidocaine 2%, reduce PNBF by 40%, and the addition of epinephrine further reduces flow to 20% of baseline.[22] However, vast experience suggests that such reductions, if indeed they occur in humans, are well tolerated.

PULMONARY COMPLICATIONS

Pneumothorax: Proximity of the brachial plexus to the lung cupula, particularly on the right side, risks violation of the pleural space and resultant pneumothorax. While this complication is particularly associated with the supraclavicular approach, it has also been reported after the interscalene, intersternocleidomastoid, suprascapular, and infraclavicular approaches. The incidence of pneumothorax following the classic Kulenkampff supraclavicular approach (needle directed caudad towards the first rib) is reported to be as high as 6.1%.[7] Contemporary supraclavicular techniques such as the "plumb bob" and first rib palpation were designed in part to reduce the risk of pneumothorax, and while reports of pneumothorax concurrent with their use appears to be less frequent, controlled trials are lacking. Because symptoms are typically delayed 6 to 12 hours after block placement, selection of supraclavicular block in ambulatory patients should be made with caution. Patient complaint of pleuritic chest pain or dyspnea should prompt the obtaining of a chest radiograph in full expiration to rule out pneumothorax.

Phrenic Nerve Paresis: The phrenic nerve (C3–C5) is intimately associated with the brachial plexus and as such hemidiaphragmatic paresis is common after approaches above, but typically not below, the clavicle (Fig. 81-3). When assessed with ultrasonography, 100% of patients undergoing interscalene block will exhibit hemidiaphragmatic paresis that may be associated with up to 37% reduction in pulmonary spirometric values.[26] Reduced concentrations of ropivacaine,[27] digital pressure applied to the interscalene groove cephalad to the point of injection,[28] or smaller volumes of local anesthetic do not reduce the occurrence of phrenic nerve blockade. Hemidiaphragmatic paresis persists in some patients with a continuous local anesthetic infusion via an interscalene catheter,[29] although respiratory function with patient-controlled interscalene analgesia does not differ significantly from patients who receive patient-controlled intravenous opioid analgesia.[30] The risk of phrenic nerve involvement following supraclavicular block (about 50%) is less than that reported with the interscalene approach, but its occurrence is unpredictable.[31] Thus, above the clavicle brachial plexus blocks are relatively contraindicated in patients with moderate to severe respiratory disease who are unable to withstand an approximate 30% decrement in pulmonary function. Similar concerns apply to patients with vocal cord paralysis or preexisting phrenic nerve dysfunction. Alternatively, the infraclavicular and axillary approaches have no significant effect on respiratory function.[32]

UNINTENDED LOCAL ANESTHETIC DESTINATIONS

The vast network of neural structures that reside within the neck predicts an ease of exposure to local anesthetic solutions originally intended for the brachial plexus. The most serious of these unintended destinations are the subarachnoid and epidural spaces, and the underlying spinal cord (Fig. 81-4). In normal-sized patients the vertebral column is <4 cm from the skin overlying the interscalene groove. Practitioners should thus be prepared for potential rapid development of symptoms consistent with high spinal anesthesia or cervical epidural block. Of greater concern, particularly in anesthetized or heavily sedated patients, is needle placement into the spinal cord with subsequent intramedullary injection and permanent spinal cord injury.[20] Unintended epidural injection can also occur in at least 1.8% of lumbar plexus blocks,[33] but the mechanism

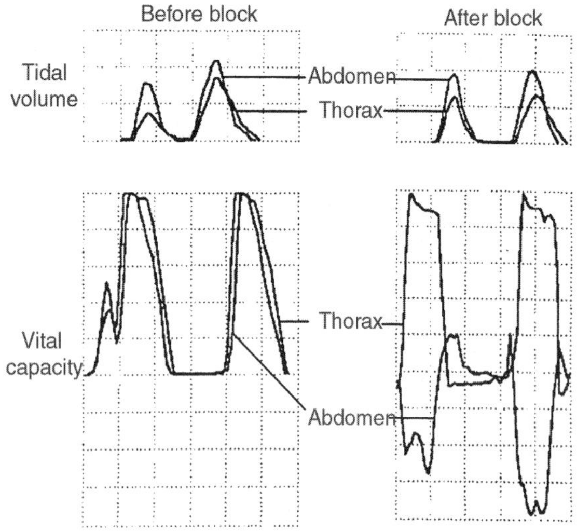

FIGURE 81-3. Plethysmogram before and after supraclavicular block. Negative abdominal excursion represents paradoxical diaphragm motion indicative of hemidiaphragmatic paresis. (From Neal JM, Moore JM, Kopacz DJ, et al: Quantitative analysis of respiratory, motor, and sensory function after supraclavicular block. Anesth Analg 86:1241, 1998, Fig. 2.)

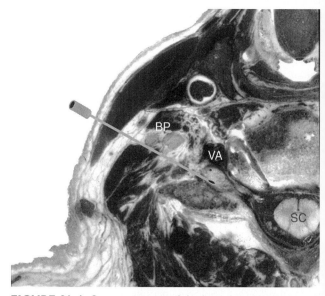

FIGURE 81-4. Cryomicrotome of the human neck demonstrating the proximity of the spinal cord, subarachnoid and epidural spaces, and spinal nerve root cuff (needle point) to the brachial plexus. Top of the figure is anterior. BP, brachial plexus; VA, vertebral artery; SC, spinal cord. (From Neal JM, Hebl JR, Gerancher JC, Hogan QH: Brachial plexus anesthesia: Essentials of our current understanding. Reg Anesth Pain Med 27:417, 2002, Fig. 15.)

involves translocation of local anesthetic in a retrograde fashion through the intervertebral foramen.

Other cervical neural structures unintentionally anesthetized during brachial plexus block placement include the recurrent laryngeal nerve (RLN) and cervical sympathetic nerves. The RLN is commonly anesthetized after interscalene block and less so after supraclavicular block (1%); this presents as hoarseness and/or the sensation of inability to clear one's throat. Horner's syndrome (ipsilateral miosis, anhydrosis, and ptosis) occurs as a result of cervical sympathetic chain anesthesia and is associated with either the interscalene or supraclavicular approach (20% to 90%). These unintended side effects of local anesthetic spread dissipate as the local anesthetic block resolves, and therefore require only patient reassurance.[7]

HYPOTENSIVE/BRADYCARDIC EVENTS

Sudden-onset hypotensive/bradycardic events (HBE) may occur in about 20% of awake, sitting patients undergoing shoulder surgery with interscalene block.[34] The purported mechanism for these events, still unproven, involves the Bezold–Jarisch reflex. Cardiac preload, which is reduced by preoperative volume restriction and the beach-chair position, and exogenous epinephrine[35] combine to create the scenario of a vigorously contracting empty ventricle. Resultant stimulation of mechanoreceptors in the ventricular wall initiates reflex bradycardia and hypotension. Somewhat analogous to the well-described HBE associated with spinal anesthesia, this complication typically occurs 30 to 60 minutes after block placement. Beta blockade with metoprolol (titrated to a heart rate <60 beats/minute or a maximum 10 mg dose) decreases its frequency, but glycopyrrolate has no beneficial effects.[34] For reasons unclear, HBE are infrequent in sitting shoulder surgery patients in whom general anesthesia is administered, with or without supplemental interscalene block.

MUSCLE INJURY

Direct muscle injury consequent to local anesthetic toxicity has been reported following retrobulbar and interscalene block, and presumably is possible with other blocks placed near muscle masses. The risk of this complication is particularly high when relatively large volumes of local anesthetic are placed into or around small muscles (retrobulbar blocks), or when muscles are exposed to local anesthetics over a prolonged time (continuous interscalene blocks). Interference with calcium metabolism is the proposed etiology of myonecrosis, which has been associated with all local anesthetics, particularly bupivacaine. Recovery occurs as myocytes replenish themselves.[7]

INFECTION

Infection can complicate any regional technique. The infectious source can be exogenous due to contaminated equipment or medication, or endogenous secondary to a bacterial source residing in the patient that seeds to the remote site of needle or catheter insertion. Although infection at the site of needle insertion is an absolute contraindication to regional anesthesia, common sense dictates that encroaching cellulitis, lymphangitis, or erythema would also preclude a regional technique.

Indwelling catheters may theoretically increase the risk of infectious complications. Gaumann et al.[36] reported a 27%

colonization rate for indwelling axillary catheters that had remained in situ an average of 3.7 ± 0.7 days. However, no signs of local or systemic infection were noted in any patient. Similarly, Bergman et al.[5] reported a single (0.2%) superficial axillary infection in 405 consecutive continuous axillary catheters. Continuous femoral nerve catheters in patients receiving standardized antibiotic therapy have a reported 57% colonization rate after 48 hours, with *Staphylococcus epidermidis* being the most frequent organism. Neither cellulitis nor abscess occurred in this series, but three (1.4%) transitory bacteremias were likely related to catheter use. Patients presented with increased temperatures and symptoms of bacteremia at both 24 and 48 hours, which dissipated upon removal of the catheter, and without the addition of antibiotic therapy.[37]

There are no definitive recommendations regarding continuous catheter use and routine antibiotic prophylaxis. Signs and symptoms of local or systemic infections should be treated with catheter removal and appropriate antibiotic therapy. In rare circumstances retained catheter fragments may also be a source of infection, requiring surgical intervention and debridement.

HOLLOW VISCUS PENETRATION

Unintended penetration of hollow organs is a potential complication of lower extremity peripheral nerve blocks. The classic Labat approach to the sciatic nerve risks penetration of intraperitoneal organs if the block needle is allowed to pass beyond the rim of the sciatic foramen. Likewise, unintentionally deep placement of a block needle through the obturator foramen risks penetration of the rectum, bladder, or vagina. Penetration of these organs is typically a benign event, but potentially may cause bleeding or infection. Avoidance is best assured by knowledge of the technique, and awareness of needle depth and the location of key bony landmarks, most notably the rims of the sciatic and obturator foramina.

CONCLUSION

Complications related to peripheral nerve block range from merely nuisance to life altering. The most common side effects of peripheral blocks are limited to the duration of local anesthetic effect and rarely have significant physiologic impact. Two complications hold particular importance because of their potential for significant harm. Intravascular injection associated with peripheral nerve block is much more common than generally recognized and can lead to significant systemic local anesthetic toxicity. Meticulous aspiration and incremental injection will reduce the likelihood of this complication in most patients. While permanent neurologic injury is exceedingly rare, it can occur even when standard of care is followed. Adherence to simple principles such as avoiding intraneural injection should reduce its frequency to an acceptable level of risk versus benefit.

KEY POINTS

- Intravascular injection leading to seizure is significantly more common after peripheral nerve blocks than neuraxial techniques.
- Long-term postoperative nerve injury is rare (~2.4/10,000 patients).

- The patient's ability to recognize, and the anesthesiologist's ability to respond to, an intraneural injection of local anesthetic is significantly more important for the prevention of anesthesia-related nerve injury than whether or not a paresthesia is elicited, or a block needle is sharp or dull.
- Ideal management of postoperative nerve injury mandates the consideration of surgical and patient-related etiologies, as well as those related to the provision of anesthesia.
- All above-the-clavicle brachial plexus blocks have the potential to affect respiration by causing hemidiaphragmatic paresis.
- Although reported in up to 24% of awake patients with interscalene block undergoing shoulder surgery in the sitting position, hypotensive/bradycardic events are decidedly rare in the setting of general anesthesia with or without supplemental interscalene block.
- Infectious complications associated with peripheral nerve block are extremely rare.

REFERENCES

1. Hadzic A, Vloka JD, Kuroda MM, et al: The practice of peripheral nerve blocks in the United States: A national survey. Reg Anesth Pain Med 23:241–246, 1998.
2. Auroy Y, Narchi P, Messiah A, et al: Serious complications related to regional anesthesia. Results of a prospective survey in France. Anesthesiology 87:479–486, 1997.
3. Auroy Y, Benhamou D, Bargues L, et al: Major complications of regional anesthesia in France. The SOS regional anesthesia hotline service. Anesthesiology 97:1274–1280, 2002.
4. Borgeat A, Ekatodramis G, Kalberer F, et al: Acute and nonacute complications associated with interscalene block and shoulder surgery. A prospective study. Anesth Analg 95:875–880, 2001.
5. Bergman BD, Hebl JR, Ken J, et al: Neurologic complications of 405 consecutive continuous axillary catheters. Anesth Analg 96:247–252, 2003.
6. Stan TC, Krantz MA, Solomon DL, et al: The incidence of neurovascular complications following axillary brachial plexus block using a transarterial approach. Reg Anesth 20:486–492, 1995.
7. Neal JM, Hebl JR, Gerancher JC, et al: Brachial plexus anesthesia: Essentials of our current understanding. Reg Anesth Pain Med 27:402–428, 2002.
8. Brown DL, Ransom DM, Hall JA, et al: Regional anesthesia and local anesthetic-induced systemic toxicity: Seizure frequency and accompanying cardiovascular changes. Anesth Analg 81:321–328, 1995.
9. Urmey WF: Upper extremity blocks. In Brown DL (ed): Regional Anesthesia and Analgesia, ed 1. WB Saunders, Philadelphia, 1996, pp 254–278.
10. Cooper K, Kelley H, Carrithers J: Perceptions of side effects following axillary block used for outpatient surgery. Reg Anesth 20:212–216, 1995.
11. Merrill DG, Brodskey JB, Hentz RV: Vascular insufficiency following axillary block of the brachial plexus. Anesth Analg 60:162–164, 1981.
12. Pearce H, Lindsay D, Leslie K: Axillary brachial plexus block in two hundred consecutive patients. Anaesth Intens Care 24:453–458, 1996.
13. Horlocker TT, Wedel DJ, Benzon H, et al: Regional anesthesia in the anticoagulated patient: Defining the risks (the second ASRA consensus conference on neuraxial anesthesia and anticoagulation). Reg Anesth Pain Med 28:172–197, 2003.
14. Weller RS, Gerancher JC, Crews JC, et al: Extensive retroperitoneal hematoma without neurologic deficit in two patients who underwent lumbar plexus block and were later anticoagulated. Anesthesiology 93:581–585, 2003.
15. Cheney FW, Domino KB, Caplan RA, et al: Nerve injury associated with anesthesia: A closed claims analysis. Anesthesiology 90:1062–1069, 1999.
16. Hebl JR, Horlocker TT, Sorenson EJ, et al: Regional anesthesia does not increase the risk of postoperative neuropathy in patients undergoing ulnar nerve transposition. Anesth Analg 93:1606–1611, 2001.
17. Lynch NM, Cofield RH, Silbert PL, et al: Neurologic complications after total shoulder arthroplasty. J Shoulder Elbow Surg 5:53–61, 1996.
18. Selander D, Edshage S, Wolff T: Paresthesiae or no paresthesiae? Nerve lesions after axillary blocks. Acta Anaesth Scand 23:27–33, 1979.
19. Neal JM: How close is close enough? Defining the "paresthesia chad" [editorial]. Reg Anesth Pain 26:97–99, 2001.
20. Benumof JL: Permanent loss of cervical spinal cord function associated with interscalene block performed under general anesthesia. Anesthesiology 93:1541–1544, 2000.
21. Hodgson PS, Neal JM, Pollock JE, et al: The neurotoxicity of drugs given intrathecally (spinal). Anesth Analg 88:797–809, 1999.
22. Myers RR, Kalichman MW, Reisner LS, et al: Neurotoxicity of local anesthetics: Altered perineural permeability, edema, and nerve fiber injury. Anesthesiology 64:29–35, 1986.
23. Gentili F, Hudson AR, Hunter D, et al: Nerve injection injury with local anesthetic agents: A light and electron microscopic, fluorescent microscopic, and horseradish peroxidase study. Neurosurg 6:263–272, 1980.
24. Selander D, Brattsand R, Lundborg G, et al: Local anesthetics: Importance of mode of application, concentration and adrenaline for the appearance of nerve lesions. Acta Anaesthesiol Scand 23:127–136, 1979.
25. Eckberg DL, Wallin BG, Fagius J, et al: Prospective study of symptoms after human microneurography. Acta Physiol Scand 137:567–569, 1989.
26. Urmey WF, McDonald M: Hemidiaphragmatic paresis during interscalene brachial plexus block: Effects on pulmonary function and chest wall mechanics. Anesth Analg 74:352–357, 1992.
27. Casati A, Fanelli G, Cedrati V, et al: Pulmonary function changes after interscalene brachial plexus anesthesia with 0.5% and 0.75% ropivacaine: A double blind comparison with 2% mepivacaine. Anesth Analg 88:587–592, 1999.
28. Urmey WF, Grossi P, Sharrock NE, et al: Digital pressure during interscalene block is clinically ineffective in preventing anesthetic spread to the cervical plexus. Anesth Analg 83:366–370, 1996.
29. Pere P, Pitkanen M, Rosenberg PH, et al: Effect of continuous interscalene brachial plexus block on diaphragm motion and on ventilatory function. Acta Anaesthesiol Scand 36:53–57, 1992.
30. Borgeat A, Perschak H, Bird P, et al: Patient-controlled interscalene analgesia with ropivacaine 0.2% versus patient-controlled intravenous analgesia after major shoulder surgery. Effects on diaphragmatic and respiratory function. Anesthesiology 92:102–108, 2000.
31. Neal JM, Moore JM, Kopacz DJ, et al: Quantitative analysis of respiratory, motor, and sensory function after supraclavicular block. Anesth Analg 86:1239–1244, 1998.
32. Rodriguez J, Barcena M, Rodriguez V, et al: Infraclavicular brachial plexus block effects on respiratory function and extent of block. Reg Anesth Pain Med 23:564–568, 1998.
33. De Biasi P, Lupescu R, Burgun G, et al: Continuous lumbar plexus block: Use of radiography to determine catheter tip location. Reg Anesth Pain Med 28:135–139, 2003.
34. Liguori GA, Kahn RL, Gordon J, et al: The use of metoprolol and glycopyrrolate to prevent hypotension/bradycardic events during shoulder arthroscopy in the sitting position under interscalene block. Anesth Analg 87:1320–1325, 1998.

35. Sia S, Sarro F, Lepri A, et al: The effect of exogenous epinephrine on the incidence of hypotensive/bradycardic events during shoulder surgery in the sitting position during interscalene block. Anesth Analg 97:583–588, 2003.

36. Gaumann DM, Lennon RL, Wedel DJ: Continuous axillary block for postoperative pain management. Reg Anesth 13:77–82, 1988.

37. Cuvillon P, Ripart J, Lalourcey L, et al: The continuous femoral nerve block catheter for postoperative analgesia: Bacterial colonization, infectious rate, and adverse effects. Anesth Analg 93:1045–1949, 2001.

Complications After Neuraxial Blockade

Lila A. Sueda, M.D.

Centroneuraxial blockade still accounts for more than 70% of regional anesthesia procedures and there is no doubt that it is the mainstay of regional anesthesia.[1] While permanent neurologic injuries are rare (0.02% to 0.07%), transient injuries occur and are more common (0.01% to 0.8%).[1,2] This chapter addresses some of the complications following centroneuraxial blockade including transient neurologic symptoms, back pain following chloroprocaine epidural, epidural hematoma, epidural abscess, adhesive arachnoiditis, and cauda equina syndrome.

TRANSIENT NEUROLOGIC SYMPTOMS

Intrathecal lidocaine has enjoyed a long clinical history of success since its introduction in 1948. It has been used for millions of spinal anesthetics and has proven itself to be safe and reliable for spinal anesthesia. The first prospective safety study of intrathecal lidocaine concluded that lidocaine was safe for spinal anesthesia.[3] However, in 1993 Schneider et al.[4] were the first to publish a case report of 4 patients with transient radiating pain without neurologic deficits following the injection of hyperbaric 5% lidocaine in the subarachnoid space for surgery in the lithotomy position. Initially the term transient radicular irritation (TRI) was used to describe this syndrome. The terminology was later changed to transient neurologic syndrome (TNS) to more accurately reflect the symptomatology as well as the clear-cut lack of an etiology. Since 1993, several case series[5,6] as well several prospective, randomized controlled studies[7–10] have examined this syndrome.

Definition: Transient neurologic symptoms have been defined as pain or dysesthesia or both occurring in the legs or buttocks. Symptoms typically appear within the first 24 hours after a full recovery from spinal anesthesia and resolve completely within 72 hours.[11] Despite the transient nature of symptoms, a recent prospective, randomized clinical trial comparing the incidence and functional impact of TNS between 1% and 5% intrathecal lidocaine showed that patients with

TNS experienced functional impairment with walking and sitting during the first 48-hour postoperative period.[12]

Incidence: The risk of developing TNS is significantly higher after spinal anesthesia with lidocaine than with the other local anesthetics. Prospective, randomized trials reveal an incidence of TNS with intrathecal lidocaine between 0% and 40%.[7–11,13–24] In studies that have compared lidocaine and mepivacaine the incidence of TNS with mepivacaine has approached that of lidocaine.[10,16,21] However, it is difficult to draw definitive conclusions because of the small sample size. Bupivacaine, prilocaine, and procaine, on the other hand, were associated with a lower frequency of TNS than lidocaine.[7–9,13–15,19,20,24] (Table 82-1).

Etiology: While the etiology of TNS remains largely unknown, possible causes of TNS have been speculated upon in the clinical literature. These possibilities include direct neurotoxicity of local anesthetics, needle trauma, patient positioning, pooling of local anesthetic, muscle spasm, early mobilization, and neural ischemia secondary to stretching of the sciatic nerve.[25] However, there has been no connection to neurologic pathology in the literature. Electromyography, nerve conduction studies, and somatosensory-evoked potential testing

TABLE 82-1. INCIDENCE OF TRANSIENT NEUROLOGIC SYMPTOMS (TNS) BY LOCAL ANESTHETIC

Local Anesthetic	Incidence of TNS (%)
Bupivacaine	0 to 7
Lidocaine	0 to 40
Mepivacaine	0 to 37
Prilocaine	1 to 3
Procaine	6

revealed no abnormalities in human volunteers with TNS after lidocaine spinal anesthesia.[26]

Risk Factors: As mentioned previously, the use of intrathecal lidocaine has been shown in prospective, randomized trials to be a risk factor for the development of TNS. In particular, the use of intrathecal lidocaine in patients undergoing surgery in the lithotomy position has been associated with a 30% to 35% incidence of TNS[13] whereas the incidence is lower (i.e., 4% to 8%)[14] in surgery performed in the supine position. However, it has been shown that changing the concentration of lidocaine from 5% to 1% or 0.5% does not decrease the incidence of TNS.[12,18]

Other risk factors identified in clinical studies to be important predictors for the development of TNS include ambulatory surgery (i.e., outpatient status)[27] as well as the type of surgery performed (knee arthroscopy and lithotomy positions). For example, surgery in the lithotomy position has an incidence of TNS of 30% to 36%, knee arthroscopy an incidence of 18% to 22%, and surgery in the supine position an incidence of 4% to 8%.[3]

Treatment: Despite the transient nature of this syndrome, TNS is associated with a significant amount of discomfort as well as functional impairment and treatment can be difficult. Therefore, the prevention of TNS is paramount by the selective use of intrathecal lidocaine. Treatment is usually symptomatic and options include opioids, nonsteroidal anti-inflammatory drugs (NSAIDs), muscle relaxants, and symptomatic therapy, such as the use of heating pads or leg elevation.[28] NSAIDs, by far, have been the most successful class of drugs used in the treatment of this syndrome.

BACK PAIN AFTER CHLOROPROCAINE

Reports of minor localized backache after regional anesthesia are quite common with a higher incidence of backache following epidural rather than spinal anesthesia. While the needles used may contribute, there are other causes of backache following regional anesthesia that should be considered.[1] For example, the use of local anesthetic agents may be a factor.

Definition: In 1987 a revised formulation of 2-chloroprocaine was marketed by Astra and was named Nesacaine-MPF (methylparaben-free) and contained disodium EDTA (ethylenediaminetetraacetic acid) as a preservative.

In 1988 several cases of severe backache following epidural anesthesia with Nesacaine-MPF were reported to Astra and the US Food and Drug Administration (FDA).[29] The lumbar back pain following epidural anesthesia with Nesacaine-MPF occurs immediately after regression of epidural anesthesia (i.e., within 30 minutes of dissipation of epidural anesthesia). The back pain is characterized as a diffuse burning sensation confined to the lower back, but sometimes can be severe, requiring opioid analgesia to relieve the pain. It usually resolves within 24 hours.[30]

Incidence: Stevens et al.[30] reported a 50% incidence of backache following EDTA-containing chloroprocaine epidural anesthesia. In a more recent study Na and Mulroy[31] found that the incidence of back pain after 2-chloroprocaine without preservative was low and mild.

Etiology: Animal models have demonstrated tetanic contraction followed by paralysis of hindlimbs as well as moderate to severe focal degeneration of spinal nerve roots with subarachnoid injection of disodium EDTA. Pretreatment with calcium prevented the tetanic contractions and hindlimb paralysis. Based on this, it has been suggested that chelation of Ca^{2+} ions by disodium EDTA in lumbar muscles is responsible for the back pain observed in patients. Hypocalcemic tetany of the psoas or quadratus lumborum muscles may occur as a result of leakage of EDTA-containing solutions out of the epidural space after a high-volume injection.[32] However, the exact mechanism of back pain following chloroprocaine epidural anesthesia remains unknown.

Risk Factors: Factors proposed to contribute to back pain following chloroprocaine epidural anesthesia include the preservative EDTA, injection of large volumes of chloroprocaine, and local infiltration with chloroprocaine. Of all the factors listed, total volume and concentration of chloroprocaine administered correlate with the incidence and severity of back pain.[30]

Treatment: Back pain following chloroprocaine epidural anesthesia is self-limiting and usually resolves within 24 hours. However, severe cases of back pain have been treated effectively with epidural fentanyl or systemic opioid analgesia. Prevention is also important by keeping the total volume of chloroprocaine low or the using the preservative-free form of the drug.[30]

EPIDURAL HEMATOMA

Definition: Epidural hematoma, defined as symptomatic bleeding within the spinal neuraxis, is a rare, but potentially catastrophic complication of centroneuraxial blocks.[33] Hemorrhage most commonly occurs in the epidural space because of the prominent epidural venous plexus and a spinal/epidural needle or catheter can traumatize these vessels. It is a medical emergency and if unrecognized can lead to spinal cord compression with permanent neurologic sequelae. Epidural hematomas can occur in the face of coagulopathies (i.e., disease states, administration of anticoagulants) and traumatic needle insertion, but can also occur in the absence of obvious risk factors. Epidural hematomas usually present within 0 to 2 days and are characterized by back pain, sensory deficit, and changes in bowel and bladder function.

Incidence: The actual incidence of neurologic dysfunction from epidural hematomas associated with centroneuraxial blocks is unknown. The incidence of epidural hematoma cited in the literature is estimated to be less than 1 in 220,000 spinal and less than 1 in 150,000 epidural anesthetics.[34]

Risk Factors: In a literature review Vandermeulen et al.[35] reported 61 cases of spinal hematoma between 1906 and 1994. These cases of spinal hematoma were associated with centroneuraxial blocks and in 68% of the patients the spinal hematomas were associated with a hemostatic abnormality (i.e., heparin use, coagulopathy, thrombocytopenia, antiplatelet use, oral anticoagulants, thrombolytics, and dextran). In 87% of the patients either a clotting abnormality or difficulty with needle placement was present. Neurologic compromise

TABLE 82-2. DIFFERENTIAL DIAGNOSIS OF BACK PAIN

Syndrome	Onset	Duration	Symptoms	Treatment
TNS	24 hours	72 hours	Pain/dysesthesia in legs or buttocks	Selective use of intrathecal lidocaine, NSAIDs, muscle relaxants, symptomatic treatment
Chloroprocaine	Within 30 minutes after regression of anesthesia	24 hours	Diffuse, burning sensation in lower back	Epidural fentanyl, systemic opioids
Epidural hematoma	0 to 2 days		Back pain, sensory deficit, changes in bowel and bladder function	MRI, neurosurgical consultation, surgical evacuation of hematoma

MRI, magnetic resonance imaging; NSAID, nonsteroidal anti-inflammatory drug; TNS, transient neurologic syndrome.

presented as progression of sensory or motor block in 68% of the patients and bowel/bladder dysfunction in 8% of the patients.

The use of anticoagulants in the surgical population for the prevention of perioperative deep vein thrombosis is a common practice. This practice reduces the morbidity and mortality associated with thromboembolic complications related to surgery. However, this creates challenges for the anesthesiologist in the management of patients undergoing centroneuraxial blocks, as concern exists for the potential of spinal bleeding. It is generally agreed that regional anesthesia is contraindicated in the anticoagulated patient.

Treatment: The avoidance of centroneuraxial blocks in the presence of anticoagulation is paramount. The reader is referred to the second ASRA consensus conference on neuraxial anesthesia and anticoagulation for guidelines.[36] Early diagnosis of epidural hematoma and intervention is paramount to prevent permanent neurologic injury. Immediate neurologic imaging (i.e., magnetic resonance imaging (MRI)) is warranted when epidural hematoma is suspected to ensure timely surgical evacuation of the hematoma. Vandermeulen et al.[35] demonstrated that prognosis was good if patients underwent laminectomy within 8 hours of the onset of neurologic symptoms. However, only 38% of patients had partial or good neurologic recovery (Table 82-2).

EPIDURAL ABSCESS

Infections can complicate centroneuraxial anesthetic techniques and are particularly concerning when they occur around the spinal cord or within the spinal canal. Infections of the central neural axis, such as arachnoiditis, meningitis, and cord compression secondary to epidural abscess, can occur after spinal or epidural anesthesia, are rare, and appear as individual case reports in the literature.

Definition: Abscess formation after epidural or spinal anesthesia can be superficial involving only the skin and soft tissue, or can occur within the epidural space with associated spinal cord compression. Superficial infections typically present as

local tissue edema, erythema, drainage, and fever. They rarely result in neurologic impairment. Epidural abscesses, on the other hand, present days to weeks after centroneuraxial block as severe localized back pain, neurologic disturbances (i.e., lower-limb paraplegia, urinary or fecal incontinence, or radiating pain), and fever with associated leukocytosis. Most epidural abscesses are not related to the placement of epidural catheters, but rather related to infections of the skin, soft tissue, spine, or to hematogenous spread to the epidural space.[37]

Incidence: Epidural abscesses may occur spontaneously in approximately 1:10,000 hospital admissions in the USA.[38] Epidural abscesses, however, may also occur in patients receiving epidural anesthesia and/or analgesia. The actual incidence of epidural abscess following epidural anesthesia is unknown and is thought to vary widely. A prospective 1-year study conducted in Denmark revealed an incidence of epidural abscess after epidural analgesia of 1:1,930 catheters.[38]

Etiology: The pathogenesis of an epidural abscess typically involves 1 of 5 mechanisms: (1) direct inoculation of bacteria either at time of epidural catheter insertion or by contaminated injection/infusion; (2) contiguous spread from a nearby site of infection; (3) spinal instrumentation/neurosurgery; (4) lymphatic spread from a paraspinous lesion; or (5) hematogenous spread, which is thought to be the most common mechanism.[39]

A colonization rate of 6% to 22% of epidural catheters has been shown. However, very few appear to be clinically significant, leading to infection. The rate of epidural catheter-associated infection is reported as 0.8% to 3.7% and 5.3%. Local infection rates of 4.3%, 5.3%, and 12% have been reported.[39] *Staphylococcus aureus* is the most common causative organism in epidural abscess, accounting for more than 60% of cases; however, in recent years the spectrum of causative organisms is broadening to include streptococci, Gram-negative aerobes and anaerobes, mycobacteria, fungi, and parasites.[39]

Not only does the epidural abscess cause direct spinal cord compression by spreading axially, but it is thought that the inflammatory abscess is also responsible for causing ischemia by compromising vascular supply to the spinal cord or by causing a hypercoagulable state (i.e., thrombosis).[39]

Risk Factors: Predisposing factors to the development of epidural abscess include diabetes mellitus, intravenous drug abuse, long-term renal failure, alcoholism, malignancy, trauma (i.e., presence of hematoma), corticosteroid use, or any other cause of an altered immune status.[39]

Treatment: Prompt diagnosis of an epidural abscess with blood cultures and MRI is crucial as the prognosis depends on rapid diagnosis and treatment. Current recommended treatment of an epidural abscess consists of urgent laminectomy, decompression, and evacuation of pus with appropriate high-dose parenteral antimicrobial therapy for 1 month, followed by oral therapy for 2 months. In selective cases, such as poor surgical risk or absence of neurological deficits, conservative treatment may be warranted.[39]

Recommendations to minimize epidural catheter-related infections such as the use of strict aseptic technique, filter, closed delivery system, preparation of epidural infusate under sterile conditions, minimal drug changes, and inspection of the epidural site every 8 hours should be followed to minimize this risk of epidural abscess.

ADHESIVE ARACHNOIDITIS

Definition: Arachnoiditis has been defined as an acute, local inflammatory response followed by a proliferative phase characterized by fibrosis, adhesion, and scarring that involves the arachnoid layer of the meningeal sac.[40]

Arachnoiditis begins days, weeks, or months following spinal anesthesia and typically presents as a gradual, progressive weakness with sensory loss in the lower extremities that can progress to complete paraplegia.[40]

Incidence: As with other neurologic complications, the exact incidence of arachnoiditis is unknown. However, the incidence of adhesive arachnoiditis is extremely rare.

Etiology: Arachnoiditis has resulted from infections, epidural abscesses, myelograms, blood in the intrathecal space, neuro-irritants, neurotoxic and/or neurolytic substances, surgical interventions in the spine, intrathecal corticosteroids, and trauma.[40]

Adhesive arachnoiditis occurs in response to the injection of chemical substances (i.e., local anesthetics, radiographic materials) in the intrathecal space. When progressive, the subarachnoid space becomes obliterated by adhesions. Blood vessels can get entrapped in the adhesions thereby resulting in ischemia of the spinal cord.[40]

This process is dependent on the dose of medication injected, its concentration, the number of attempts, as well as the immune responsiveness of the patient and the neural tissue.[40]

Risk Factors: Traumatic taps, blood in the cerebrospinal fluid, paresthesias, and injection of neurotoxic or neuroirritant substances into the subarachnoid space have been identified as potential risk factors for adhesive arachnoiditis. The presence of these may necessitate deferment of the procedure rather than attempting centroneuraxial blockade at a different level.[40]

Treatment: The presence of blood in the cerebrospinal fluid, traumatic tap, or paresthesias may require deferment of the surgical procedure to allow for adequate neurological monitoring of the patient. Should neurologic symptoms occur, a complete neurologic examination is indicated. This should be followed by a MRI study of the affected area to determine the presence of a pathologic lesion (i.e., medullary lesion, cauda equina, or radicular lesion).[40]

Because adhesive arachnoiditis represents an inflammatory process, therapy with intravenous methylprednisolone and NSAIDs may reduce the evolution into a more permanent proliferative phase.[40]

CAUDA EQUINA SYNDROME

Definition: Cauda equina syndrome is a complex syndrome involving the terminal portion of the spinal cord. The small autonomic fibers are primarily affected; therefore, presenting symptoms often include autonomic insufficiency, changes in bowel and bladder function, paraplegia, alterations in temperature regulation and sweating, as well as alterations in sensation to pinprick, temperature, and proprioception in the distribution of the lumbar and sacral nerve roots.[41–43]

Incidence: Cauda equina syndrome is an extremely rare and devastating complication of spinal anesthesia. Auroy et al.[44] in a prospective survey of French anesthesiologists reported 5 cases of cauda equina syndrome out of a total of 41,251 spinal anesthetics. Loo and Irested[42] reported 6 cases of cauda equina syndrome during the period 1993–1997.

Etiology: The potential causes of cauda equina syndrome include direct or indirect trauma to the nerve roots, spinal cord ischemia, infection, and neurotoxic reaction of locally injected drugs.[41–43] Because the nerves in the cauda equina lack any protective sheath, they are particularly vulnerable to injury from high concentrations of local anesthetics. Repeated injections of local anesthetics through spinal micocathethers or by a repeat spinal injection to improve inadequate spinal anesthesia have been associated with cauda equina syndrome.[41–43] Case reports also demonstrate that it can occur after a single spinal injection of local anesthetic.[41] It is thought that maldistribution and pooling of toxic concentrations of hyperbaric local anesthetic in the area of the cauda equina nerve roots may be responsible for this syndrome. This led to the recall of exemption by the FDA of spinal microcatheters in 1992.[41–43]

Treatment: Unfortunately, there is no treatment for cauda equina syndrome. Rather treatment is expectant and supportive. Frequent bladder scans to determine the volume of residual urine and repeated catherization may help patients regain bladder function by preventing overdistention of the detrusor muscle. Additionally, active rehabilitation should play an important role in patients affected by cauda equina syndrome. Finally, prevention of this syndrome is important by avoiding the use of spinal microcatheters, high concentrations and total doses of local anesthetics, waiting 10 minutes in the case of failed spinal anesthesia to repeat the spinal anesthesia with the same dose, and choosing L2–L3 if a hyperbaric solution is to be used to enhance cephalad spread[45] (Table 82-3).

TABLE 82-3. DIFFERENTIAL DIAGNOSIS OF EPIDURAL ABSCESS, ADHESIVE ARACHNOIDITIS, AND CAUDA EQUINA SYNDROME

Syndrome	Onset	Characteristics	Treatment
Epidural abscess	2–7 days	Backache, progressive neurologic symptoms, fever	Antibiotics, possible surgical decompression
Adhesive arachnoiditis	Days, weeks, or months after spinal anesthesia	Progressive weakness, sensory loss, progressing to complete paraplegia	No effective treatment, consider intravenous corticosteroids, NSAIDs
Cauda equina syndrome	Variable	Loss of bowel/bladder function, paraplegia, sensory deficits	No effective treatment

NSAID, nonsteroidal anti-inflammatory drug.

REFERENCES

1. Faccenda KA, Finucane: Complications of regional anesthesia: Incidence and prevention. Drug Safety 24:413–442, 2001.
2. Horlocker TT, McGregor D, Matsushige DK, et al: A retrospective review of 4767 consecutive spinal anesthetics: Central nervous system complications. Anesth Analg 84:578–584, 1997.
3. Pollock JE: Transient neurologic symptoms: Etiology, risk factors, and management. Reg Anesth Pain Med 27:581–586, 2002.
4. Schneider M, Ettlin T, Kaufmann M, et al: Transient neurologic toxicity after hyperbaric subarachnoid anesthesia with 5% lidocaine. Anesth Analg 76:1154–1157, 1993.
5. Beardsley D, Holman S, Gantt R, et al: Transient neurologic deficits after spinal anesthesia: Local anesthetic maldistribution with pencil point needles? Anesth Analg 81:314–320, 1995.
6. Rodriquez-Chinchilla R, Rodriquez-Pont A, Pintanel T, et al: Bilateral severe pain at L3–4 after spinal anaesthesia with hyperbaric 5% lignocaine. Br J Anaesth 76:328–329, 1996.
7. de Weert T, Traksel M, Gielen M, et al: The incidence of transient neurological symptoms after spinal anesthesia with lidocaine compared with prilocaine. Anaesthesia 55:1020–1024, 2000.
8. Hampl KF, Heinzmann-Wiedmer S, Luginbuehl MC, et al: Transient neurologic symptoms after spinal anesthesia. Anesthesiology 88:629–633, 1988.
9. Hodgson PS, Liu SS, Batra MS, et al: Procaine compared with lidocaine for incidence of transient neurologic symptoms. Reg Anesth Pain Med 25:218–222, 2000.
10. Liguori GA, Zayas VM, Chisholm MF: Transient neurologic symptoms after spinal anesthesia with mepivacaine and lidocaine. Anesthesiology 88:619–623, 1998.
11. Hampl KF, Schneider MC, Pargger H, et al: A similar incidence of transient neurologic symptoms after spinal anesthesia with 2% and 5% lidocaine. Anesth Analg 83:1051–1054, 1996.
12. Tong D, Wong J, Chung F, et al: Prospective study on incidence and functional impact of transient neurologic symptoms associated with 1% versus 5% hyperbaric lidocaine in short urologic procedures. Anesthesiology 98:485–494, 2003.
13. Hampl KF, Schneider MC, Thorin D, et al: Hyperosmolarity does not contribute to transient radicular irritation after spinal anesthesia with hyperbaric 5% lidocaine. Reg Anesth 20:363–368, 1995.
14. Pollock JE, Neal JM, Stephenson CA, et al: Prospective study of the incidence of transient radicular irritation in patients undergoing spinal anesthesia. Anesthesiology 84:1361–1367, 1996.
15. Martinez-Bourio R, Arzuaga M, Quintana JM, et al: Incidence of transient neurologic symptoms after hyperbaric subarachnoid anesthesia with 5% lidocaine and 5% prilocaine. Anesthesiology 88:624–628, 1998.
16. Salmela L, Aromma U: Transient radicular irritation after spinal anesthesia induced with hyperbaric solutions of cerebrospinal fluid-diluted lidocaine 50 mg/ml or mepivacaine 40 mg/ml or bupivacaine 5 mg/ml. Acta Anaesthesiol Scand 42:765–769, 1998.
17. Hiller A, Karjalainen K, Balk M, et al: Transient neurologic symptoms after spinal anesthesia with hyperbaric 5% lidocaine or general anesthesia. Br J Anaesth 82:575–579, 1999.
18. Pollock J, Liu S, Neal J, et al: Dilution of spinal lidocaine does not alter the incidence of transient neurologic symptoms. Anesthesiology 90:445–449, 1999.
19. Keld DB, Hein L, Dalgaard M, et al: The incidence of transient neurologic symptoms after spinal anesthesia in patients undergoing surgery in the supine position. Hyperbaric lidocaine 5% versus hyperbaric bupivacine 0.5%. Acta Anaesthesiol Scand 44:285–290, 2000.
20. Ostgaard G, Hallaraker O, Ulveseth OK, et al: A randomized study of lidocaine and prilocaine for spinal anesthesia. Acta Anaesthesiol Scand 44:436–440, 2000.
21. Salazar F, Bogdanovich A, Adalia R, et al: Transient neurologic symptoms after spinal anesthesia using isobaric 2% mepivacaine and isobaric 2% lidocaine. Acta Anaesthesiol Scand 45:24–45, 2001.
22. Lindh A, Andersson AS, Westman L: Is transient lumbar pain after spinal anesthesia with lidocaine influenced by early mobilization? Acta Anaesthesiol Scand 45:290–293, 2001.
23. Philip J, Sharma S, Gottumukkla V, et al: Transient neurologic symptoms after spinal anesthesia with lidocaine in obstetric patients. Anesth Analg 92:401–404, 2001.
24. Aouad M, Siddik S, Jalbout M, et al: Does pregnancy protect against intrathecal lidocaine-induced transient neurologic symptoms? Anesth Analg 92:405–409, 2001.
25. Pollock JE: Neurotoxicity of intrathecal local anaesthetics and transient neurological symptoms. Best Pract Res Clin Anaesthesiol 17:471–484, 2003.
26. Pollock JE, Burkhead D, Neal JM, et al: Spinal nerve function in five volunteers experiencing transient neurologic symptoms after lidocaine subarachnoid anesthesia. Anesth Analg 90:658–665, 2000.
27. Freedman JM, Li D, Drasner K, et al: Transient neurologic symptoms after spinal anesthesia: An epidemiologic study of 1,863 patients. Anesthesiology 89:633–641, 1998.
28. Pollock JE: Transient neurologic symptoms: Etiology, risk factors, and management. Reg Anesth Pain Med 27:581–586, 2002.

29. Munnur U, Suresh MS: Backache, headache, and neurologic deficit after regional anesthesia. Anesthesiol Clin North Am 21:71–86, 2003.

30. Stevens RA, Urmey WF, Urquhart BL, et al: Back pain after epidural anesthesia with chloroprocaine. Anesthesiology 78: 492–497, 2000.

31. Na KB, Mulroy MF: Back pain after epidural 2-chloroprocaine. Reg Anesth Pain Med 28:A53, 2003.

32. Stevens RA: Back pain following epidural anesthesia with 2-chloroprocaine. Reg Anesth 22:299–302, 1997.

33. Horlocker TT, Wedel DJ, Benzon H, et al: Regional anesthesia in the anticoagulated patient: Defining the risks (the second ASRA consensus conference on neuraxial anesthesia and anticoagulation). Reg Anesth Pain Med 28:172–197, 2003.

34. Horlocker TT, Wedel DJ: Neurologic complications of spinal and epidural anesthesia. Reg Anesth Pain Med 25:83–98, 2000.

35. Vandermeulen EP, Van Aken H, Vermylen J, et al: Anticoagulants and spinal-epidural anesthesia. Anesth Analg 79:1165–1177, 1994.

36. Horlocker TT, Wedel DJ, Benzon H, et al: Regional anesthesia in the anticoagulated patient: Defining the risks (the second ASRA consensus conference on neuraxial anesthesia and anticoatulation). Reg Anesth Pain Med 28:172–197, 2003.

37. Horlocker TT, Wedel DJ: Neurologic complications of spinal and epidural anesthesia. Reg Anesth Pain Med 25:83–98, 2000.

38. Wang LP, Hauerberg J, Schmidt JF: Incidence of spinal epidural abscess after epidural analgesia. Anesthesiology 91:1928–1936, 1999.

39. Brookman CA, Rutledge MLC: Epidural abscess: Case report and literature review. Reg Anesth Pain Med 25:428–431, 2000.

40. Aldrete JA: Neurologic deficits and arachnoiditis following neuroaxial anesthesia. Acta Anaesthesiol Scand 47:3–12, 2003.

41. Gerancher JC: Cauda equina syndrome following a single spinal administration of 5% hyperbaric lidocaine through a 25-gauge Whitacre needle. Anesthesiology 87:687–689, 1997.

42. Loo CC, Irested L: Cauda equina syndrome after spinal anaesthesia with hyperbaric 5% lignocaine: A review of six cases of cauda equina syndrome reported to the Swedish pharmaceutical insurance 1993–1997. Acta Anaesthesiol Scand 43:371–379, 1999.

43. Kubina P, Gupta A, Oscarsson A, et al: Two cases of cauda equina syndrome following spinal-epidural anesthesia. Reg Anesth 22: 447–450, 1997.

44. Auroy Y, Benhamou D, Bargues L, et al: Major complications of regional anesthesia in France. Anesthesiology 97:1274–1280, 2002.

45. Abouleish E: Cauda equina syndrome, continuous spinal anesthesia and repeated spinal block is there a relationship? Reg Anesth 17:356–357, 1992.

Anticoagulants and Neuraxial Anesthesia

Honorio T. Benzon, M.D.

The issue of anticoagulant use during neuraxial injection came to the fore in 1997 when the American Society of Regional Anesthesia and Pain Medicine (ASRAPM) convened a panel of experts to discuss the increased number of reports of epidural hematoma. The reports coincided with the introduction of low-molecular-weight heparin and the lack of definite guidelines on its use in patients who had neuraxial procedure. The panel published their guidelines in a supplemental issue of the ASRAPM journal, *Regional Anesthesia and Pain Medicine*, in 1998.[1] The guidelines, which set standards for patient safety, were widely adhered to by the different medical specialties. A new set of antiplaletet drugs, not covered by the guidelines, was later introduced. The ASRAPM reconvened the panel and published their revised guidelines in 2003 (Table 83-1).[2] This chapter covers the problem of deep vein thrombosis and neuraxial injections in the presence of anticoagulants. The necessity of the anticoagulants in the perioperative setting and in cardiac events is reviewed so the anesthesiologist will gain a better perspective on the indications and usage of these anticoagulants.

PERIOPERATIVE DEEP VENOUS THROMBOSIS

In this chapter the discussion on postoperative deep vein thrombosis (DVT) is focused on its occurrence in total joint replacement surgery because of the high incidence of DVTs in patients who undergo this type of surgery. It is also in these patients that neuraxial anesthesia is frequently performed.

Approximately 50% of DVTs after total joint surgery begin intraoperatively, with the highest incidence occurring during the surgery and the first postoperative day.[3] Almost 75% of DVTs develop within the first 48 hours after surgery. Other investigators identified the fourth postoperative day as the peak occurrence of DVT and another smaller peak incidence on day 13. The risk of DVT is minimal after postoperative day 17.[3]

The predisposing factors to the development of DVTs during surgery include stasis, intimal injury, and hypercoagulability.[4] Some of the risk factors for the development of DVTs are previous history of DVT or pulmonary embolism, major surgery (operations involving the abdomen, pelvis, and lower extremities), age over 60, obesity, malignancy, increased duration of surgery, prolonged immobilization, presence of varicose veins, and the use of estrogen.[4] The problem is most pronounced in total joint operations where intraoperative factors predispose to the development of DVTs. During total hip replacement (THR), the lower extremity is placed into positions of flexion, rotation, and adduction. These manipulations may damage the femoral vein and produce severe venous stasis.[5] Intraoperative venograms performed during total hip arthroplasty revealed significant occlusion and twisting of the femoral vein causing stagnation of the limb blood flow.[6] In total knee replacements (TKR), the knee is flexed, causing compression of the blood vessels, to ensure alignment of the prosthesis and a tourniquet is used. The tourniquet compresses the underlying venous structures causing intimal injury to the vessel. The increased coagulability of the blood is aggravated by decreases in antithrombin III and tissue plasminogen activator (t-PA).[7,8]

The incidences of DVT in patients without prophylaxis are 54% to 57% for total hip arthroplasty and 40% to 84% for TKR.[4,9–11] Most of the DVTs after TKR are located in the calf veins (24% to 60% of DVTs) compared to the more proximal veins (3% to 20% of DVTs).[6] In contrast, a higher incidence of DVTs after THR develop in the more proximal veins. Some 46% of DVTs after THR develop in the posterior tibial or peroneal veins compared to 12% to 35% in the proximal veins of the thigh or popliteal fossa.[3] There is a greater tendency of proximal veins to embolize to the lung; hence the reason for the higher incidence of pulmonary embolism in THR surgery. Although calf vein thromboses do not embolize to the lung as much, 24% of these thromboses propagate to the more proximal veins.[12] Fatal pulmonary embolism occurs in 0.34% to 6% for THR and 0.2% to 0.7% for TKR.[4]

Ascending venous contrast venography is considered the most reliable diagnostic test for DVT,[13] its sensitivity approaching 100%.[14] It is invasive, requires a radiology suite, and is more expensive than the other tests. There is also a risk of contrast nephropathy and allergic reactions.[13] B-mode compression

TABLE 83-1. **SUMMARY OF GUIDELINES ON ANTICOAGULANTS AND NEURAXIAL BLOCKS**[1,2]

I. Antiplatelet medications

1. Aspirin, NSAIDs, COX-2 inhibitors

   May continue

   Pain clinic patients: aspirin preferably stopped 2 to 3 days in thoracic and cervical epidurals (author's preference: see text)

2. Thienopyridine derivatives

   (a) Clopidogrel (Plavix): discontinue for 7 days

   (b) Ticlopidine (Ticlid): discontinue for 14 days

   Do not perform a neuraxial block in patients on more than one antiplatelet drug

3. Glycoprotein IIb/IIIa inhibitors: time to normal platelet aggregation

   (a) Abciximab (Reopro) = 24 to 48 hours

   (b) Eptifibatide (Integrilin) = 4 to 8 hours

   (c) Tirofiban (Aggrastat) = 4 to 8 hours

   Antiplatelet medications (ASA, Plavix) are usually given after glycoprotein IIb/IIIa inhibitors. The above guidelines on aspirin and Plavix should be adhered to.

II. Warfarin

Check INR

INR ≤1.5 before neuraxial block or epidural catheter removal

III. Heparin

1. Subcutaneous heparin (5,000 u SC q 12 hours)

   Subcutaneous heparin is not a contraindication against a neuraxial block

   Neuraxial block should preferably be performed before SC heparin is given

   Risk of decreased platelet count with SC heparin therapy >5 days

2. Intravenous heparin

   Neuraxial block: 2 to 4 hours after the last intravenous heparin dose

   Wait ≥1 hour after neuraxial block before giving intravenous heparin

IV. Low-molecular-weight heparin (LMWH)

No concomitant antiplatelet medication, heparin, or dextran

A. LMWH preoperative

   (a) Wait 12 hours before a neuraxial block:

   Enoxaparin (Lovenox) 0.5 mg/kg BID (prophylactic dose)

   (b) Wait 24 hours before a neuraxial block:

   Enoxaparin (Lovenox), 1 mg/kg BID (therapeutic dose)

   Enoxaparin (Lovenox), 1.5 mg/kg QD

   Dalteparin (Fragmin), 120 u/kg BID

   Dalteparin (Fragmin), 200 u/kg QD

   Tinzaparin (Innohep), 175 u/kg QD

B. LMWH postoperative

   LMWH should not be started until after 24 hours after surgery

   LMWH should not be given until ≥2 hours after epidural catheter removal

C. Patients with epidural catheter who are given LMWH

   The catheter should be removed at the earliest opportunity

   Enoxaparin (0.5 mg/kg): remove the epidural catheter ≥12 hours after last dose

   Enoxaparin (1 to 1.5 mg/kg), dalteparin, tinzaparin: remove the epidural catheter ≥24 hours after last dose

   Restart the LMWH ≥2 hours after the catheter removal

   Summary recommendations for LMWH (preoperative and postoperative):

   Wait 24 hours except for patients on low-dose enoxaparin (0.5 mg/kg) in which case a 12-hour interval is adequate.

   Wait 2 hours after the catheter is removed before starting LMWH

Continued

TABLE 83-1. SUMMARY OF GUIDELINES ON ANTICOAGULANTS AND NEURAXIAL BLOCKS[1,2]—CONT'D

V. Specific Xa inhibitor: fondaparinux (Arixtra)
Short onset, long duration (plasma half-life: 21 hours)
ASRA: no definite recommendation
If neuraxial procedure *has to be performed*, recommend single-needle atraumatic placement, avoid indwelling catheter

VI. Fibrinolytic/thrombolytic drugs
No data on safety interval for performance of neuraxial procedure
Follow fibrinogen levels
ASRA: no definite recommendation

VII. Thrombin inhibitors
Desirudin (Revasc)
Lepirudin (Refludan)
Bivalirudin (Angiomax)
Argatroban (Acova)
Anticoagulant effect lasts 3 hours
Monitored by aPTT
ASRA: no recommendation at this time because of paucity of data

VIII. Herbal therapy
Mechanism of anticoagulant effect and time to normal hemostasis:
   Garlic: inhibits platelet aggregation, increased fibrinolysis; 7 days
   Ginko: inhibits platelet-activating factor; 36 hours
   Ginseng: increased PT and PTT; 24 hours
ASRA: neuraxial block not contraindicated for single herbal medication use
No data on combined herbal therapy

The guidelines are the same for the placement and removal of epidural catheters.
aPTT, activated partial thromboplastin time; ASRA, American Society of Regional Anesthesia; COX, cyclooxygenase; INR, international normalized ratio; NSAID, nonsteroidal anti-inflammatory drug; SC, subcutaneous.

ultrasonography ± Doppler is the first-line modality for confirming diagnosis in symptomatic patients.[13] It is portable and the most accurate noninvasive study of DVTs.[14] Failure of the vein to compress is indirect evidence that a thrombus is present.[14]

PERIOPERATIVE PROPHYLAXIS OF DEEP VEIN THROMBOSIS

The prevention of DVT after total joint surgery includes intraoperative, mechanical, and pharmacologic measures. The use of epidural hypotensive anesthesia is associated with improved visualization of the operative field, less intraoperative blood loss, and shorter duration of surgery.[5] All of these factors lead to a lower incidence of DVT formation. Mechanical devices decrease stasis by augmenting venous flow in the lower legs,[12] and appear to have a fibrinolytic effect through a reduction in plasminogen activator inhibitor.[5] Various types of mechanical devices include calf-length sleeve, thigh-length stockings, and foot pump devices.[12] In patients who underwent TKR the use of intermittent pulsatile compression of the plantar venous plexus and aspirin was found to be superior to aspirin alone in preventing DVTs (27% to 59%).[15] A combination of mechanical

and pharmacologic measures is probably the most efficacious way of preventing DVT.

The pharmacologic management of DVTs includes the use of aspirin, warfarin, low-molecular-weight heparin (LMWH), and the thrombin inhibitors. Aspirin irreversibly blocks the platelet cyclooxygenase (COX) enzyme inhibiting the formation of thromboxane A_2 that causes platelet aggregation. Most regimens use doses of 325 to 650 mg twice a day. The risks of aspirin use are gastritis and gastric erosions or ulcers. While there were early reports of the efficacy of aspirin in DVT prophylaxis in total joint surgery, later evaluations showed it not to be very effective. The incidence of DVT when aspirin alone is used in TKR ranges from 41% to 78%.[12]

Heparin, LMWH, and warfarin are used perioperatively to prevent DVTs after surgery. For warfarin, the usual dosing regimen is 5 mg given the night of surgery, followed by adjustment of the dose to maintain an international normalized ratio (INR) of 2.0 to 2.5. Higher INRs may result in hemarthromas. The incidence of DVT with warfarin is 25% to 59%.[12] The therapy is maintained for 1 month after surgery. Because of warfarin's delayed effect and the early development of postoperative thrombus (most postoperative DVTs occur intraoperatively or in the first 2 days), some surgeons add a LMWH as a "bridge therapy" while the effect of warfarin is commencing. For patients who are on chronic warfarin intake, the drug is stopped 4 to 6 days before the surgery. Heparin or LMWH are administered during the time the warfarin is discontinued then stopped the day before surgery.

The prophylactic dose of heparin is 3,500 units subcutaneously (SC) every 8 hours, 2 days before the surgery. The other dosing regimen is 3,500 units of heparin SC 2 hours before surgery, followed by 3,500 units SC every 8 hours beginning the evening of surgery. The dose is then adjusted to maintain the activated partial thromboplastin time (aPTT) at the top of the normal value of the laboratory. Heparin is prescribed for 7 to 10 days after the surgery after which warfarin is started. Heparin is not widely used for postoperative prophylaxis after total joint surgery probably because of the better bioavailability and predictability of LMWH. However, heparin is commonly used in general surgery for postoperative DVT prophylaxis.

LMWH is an effective prophylaxis against DVT after total joint surgery.[16–19] It appears to be more effective than warfarin. The incidences of DVT in patients who had total hip surgery are 5% with enoxaparin and 12% with warfarin.[17,18] Dalteparin is also associated with lower incidence of DVTs after total hip arthroplasty when compared to warfarin (13% versus 24%).[19] Compared to mechanical prophylaxis, LMWH is more effective in reducing the incidence of DVTs (27% versus 65%).[20] The LMWH therapy is continued for 1 to 2 weeks after the surgery. With this extended, out-of-hospital prophylaxis, the incidence of DVTs has been shown to decline from 22% with placebo to 8% with either enoxaparin or dalteparin. Fondaparinux, a specific Xa inhibitor, is given for 5 to 9 days after surgery at a daily dose of 2.5 mg. The drug reduces the incidence of venous thromboembolism by 57%, comparable to enoxaparin.[21]

The oral antithrombin agents are undergoing clinical trials and show some promise. A recent study showed ximelagatran, in doses of 36 mg twice a day, is superior to warfarin for the prevention of deep venous thromboembolism after TKR surgery.[22] The efficacy was primarily related to a decreased incidence of distal DVT, although there was also decreased incidence of proximal DVT (note that proximal DVTs are more associated with pulmonary embolism than distal DVTs).

VENOUS THROMBOEMBOLISM: PHARMACOLOGIC PROPHYLAXIS AND TREATMENT

Venous thromboembolism includes DVT and pulmonary embolism and has been considered to be a chronic disease.[23] Most patients with venous thromboembolism have a systemic disorder including a hereditary hypercoagulable state. Almost one-third of patients with a history of DVT have a recurrence within 8 years of the initial event.[24] Recurrences of DVTs involve the contralateral leg in half of the patients supporting the role of systemic hypercoagulability in the pathogenesis of DVT.[23,25]

There are two phases in the treatment of symptomatic DVT: the initial treatment and secondary prophylaxis.[23,26] The initial treatment consists of either intravenous unfractionated heparin or subcutaneous LMWH while oral anticoagulants such as warfarin are used for secondary prophylaxis. The efficacy of an initial therapy of 5- to 10-day course of heparin was shown by clinical trials. The first trial, done in patients with symptomatic pulmonary embolism, was stopped prematurely after 35 patients were studied because 25% died and another 25% had nonfatal recurrence in the no treatment group compared to no recurrences or death in the patients treated with a combination of heparin and warfarin.[27] Another trial that was stopped prematurely compared a combination of heparin and vitamin antagonists with vitamin K antagonists alone. The study showed the incidence of recurrence was three times as high in the patients who did not have the initial treatment with heparin.[28]

The risk of recurrent thromboembolism requires the need for secondary prophylaxis. This need was shown by studies by Lagerstedt et al. and Hull et al. The patients in the two studies had initial treatment with heparin then randomized to vitamin K antagonists versus no treatment in the study by Lagerstedt et al.[29] or to low-dose subcutaneous unfractionated heparin versus vitamin K antagonist in the study of Hull et al.[30] The studies showed the risk of recurrent venous thromboembolism was significantly higher in the patients with no or inadequate prophylaxis.

Based on the classic studies mentioned above,[27–30] heparin has been used as the initial treatment and warfarin for the long-term prevention of recurrence of venous thromboembolism.[23,26] It has been recommended that the dose of warfarin be adjusted to maintain an INR between 2.0 and 3.0.[31–34] The absence of recurrent venous thrombosis during treatment at these INR levels suggested that an INR of 2 may be greater than is necessary for the long-term prevention of venous thrombosis. This led investigators to compare the efficacy and safety of low-intensity warfarin therapy (target INR of 1.5 to 1.9) with the conventional-intensity warfarin therapy (target INR of 2.0 to 3.0).[35,36] The results of the studies done so far have not been uniform. One study, the PREVENT (Prevention of Recurrent Venous Thromboembolism) study,[35] compared low-intensity warfarin therapy with placebo and found that the warfarin treatment resulted in 48% reduction of venous thromboembolism, major hemorrhage, or death and 76% to 81% reduction in the risk of recurrent venous thromboembolism. The study concluded that long-term, low-intensity warfarin therapy is highly effective in preventing recurrent venous thromboembolism. The other study compared low-intensity warfarin therapy with conventional-intensity warfarin therapy and found that the conventional therapy was more effective: 6 of 369 patients had recurrent venous thromboembolism compared to 16 of 369 patients in the low-intensity warfarin group.[36] The investigators also found that the low-intensity warfarin treatment did not reduce the risk of clinically important bleeding: there were 9 major bleeding episodes in the low-intensity warfarin group compared to 8 in the conventional-intensity therapy group.[36] It appears therefore that the target INR should be between 2.0 and 3.0 since lower INRs result in more recurrence and no advantage with regards the risk of bleeding.[26] INRs above 3.0 result in more bleeding with no added benefit in the prevention of recurrent venous thrombosis.[37,38]

The duration of warfarin treatment is based on the history of recurrence and the presence of predisposing factors. When venous thromboembolism develops in a patient with reversible or time-limited risk factors, the patient should be treated with an oral anticoagulant for at least 3 months. The treatment is extended to 6 months in patients with a first episode of idiopathic venous thromboembolism while patients with recurrent idiopathic venous thromboembolism or a long-term risk factor such as cancer, antithrombin deficiency, or antiphospholipid-antibody syndrome are treated for 12 months or longer.[39] Patients with venous thromboembolism who undergo treatment with vitamin K antagonists go through three different phases. The first period occurs during treatment, the second period is the first 6 to 12 months after treatment, and the third phase is the subsequent years.[26] The risk of recurrence is reduced by 90% during treatment; a catch-up phenomenon occurs during the second phase when the incidence of recurrence is 5% to 10%, then the risk of recurrence stabilizes at 1% to 2% during the subsequent years. There appears to be no added benefit by continuing therapy beyond 12 months, and treatment beyond this period depends on the preference of the individual patient.[26]

ANTICOAGULANTS FOR ACUTE MYOCARDIAL INFARCTION, STROKE PROPHYLAXIS, AND PATIENTS WITH HYPERCOAGULABLE CONDITIONS

Anticoagulants are used in acute myocardial infarction, stroke prophylaxis, and in patients with hypercoagulable conditions such as systemic lupus erythematosus. In 1999 a task force of the American College of Cardiology and the American Heart Association issued practice guidelines for the management of patients with acute myocardial infarction.[40] They recommended a combination of (1) aspirin, or ticlopidine or clopidogrel for patients with aspirin intolerance; (2) therapeutic anticoagulation with heparin or LMWH; and (3) administration of platelet glycoprotein (GP) IIb/IIIa receptor antagonist. For patients whose symptoms are less than 6 hours, intravenous thrombolytic therapy is recommended.

There is increased use of clopidogrel in patients with acute coronary syndrome. In these patients the administration of aspirin and clopidogrel for up to 9 months was more effective than aspirin alone in reducing the combined incidence of death from cardiovascular causes, myocardial infarction, or stroke.[41] This combined therapy, however, resulted in increased risk of bleeding. It is for this reason that some physicians delay prescribing clopidogrel until the results of coronary angiography are known and confirm that bypass grafting is not necessary.[42] In patients who undergo percutaneous coronary intervention the administration of clopidogrel and aspirin reduces the risk of vessel thrombosis when compared to aspirin alone.[43] The continuation of these drugs for 9 to 12 months after a coronary procedure (such as balloon angioplasty, bare-metal placement, drug-eluting stent, and brachytherapy) further reduces the incidence of major adverse cardiovascular events (death, myocardial infarction, or stroke) compared to aspirin alone.[43,44] A higher dose of clopidogrel, 300 mg, given 6 hours before the procedure made the combination effective.[44] In patients undergoing percutaneous coronary intervention a loading dose of clopidogrel, 300 to 600 mg, is given 4 to 6 hours before the procedure followed by a maintenance dose of 75 mg daily for 9 to 12 months.[42]

The glycoprotein IIb/IIIa inhibitors abciximab, eptifibatide, and tirofiban have been shown to reduce subsequent myocardial infarction and the need for coronary revascularization.[45,46] Patients who are at high risk (patients with ongoing ischemia, elevated serum troponin concentrations, or ischemic ST-segment abnormalities) are given infusions of tirofiban or eptifibatide

for 48 to 72 hours or until 12 to 24 hours after the coronary intervention. The antiplatelet effect of these drugs is maximal within minutes of administration. These drugs are administered concomitantly with aspirin. The role of these drugs in patients with unstable angina who undergo diagnostic coronary angiography has not been established.[42] It appears that patients who undergo percutaneous coronary intervention and those with acute coronary syndromes who are at low risk for ischemic complication may receive aspirin and clopidogrel only.[42] Additional studies will establish the role of additional glycoprotein IIb/IIIa inhibitors in coronary interventions.[42,47]

Anticoagulants, specifically clopidogrel or dipyridamole, are used in patients who are at high risk for having a stroke. This is because a study of 6,602 patients showed that the development of stroke decreased from 37% with placebo to 18% with aspirin and to 16% with dypiridamole.[48]

RELEVANT PHARMACOLOGY OF ANTICOAGULANTS AND IMPLICATIONS FOR NEURAXIAL BLOCKADE

Antiplatelet Drugs: Aspirin irreversibly binds to the platelet COX enzyme inhibiting the formation of thromboxane A_2 that causes platelet aggregation resulting in the formation of an adequate but fragile clot. Most regimens use doses of 325 to 650 mg twice a day. Lower doses of aspirin are more effective in preventing clot formation since higher doses may have a paradoxical effect. Lower doses block the platelet COX enzyme decreasing the formation of thromboxane A_2 which causes platelet aggregation. Higher doses of aspirin inhibit the COX enzyme in the platelets and in the vascular endothelium; this inhibition results in decreased levels of PGI2 which inhibits platelet aggregation. The ultimate effect of higher dosages is therefore a reflection of the antagonistic effects of reduced levels of thromboxane A_2 and PGI2. Benzon et al. compared the bleeding times of patients who were on daily low-dose aspirin (1 to 2 tablets of 325 mg aspirin), medium-dose aspirin (3 to 10 tablets), and high-dose aspirin (more than 10 tablets) and found that the mean bleeding times and the incidences of prolonged bleeding times were the same in the three groups.[49] Nonsteroidal anti-inflammatory drugs (NSAIDs) also bind to the platelet COX enzyme but the binding is reversible.

The bleeding time has been used as a screening test for platelet or capillary function. It is not a good indicator of platelet function, recent antiplatelet therapy, or surgical blood loss.[50] It has been shown to be a poor predictor of operative hemorrhage in a patient with negative history of bleeding diathesis. There is large intra- and interpatient variability in the results of the test. The platelet function analyzer (PFA) is a test of in vitro platelet function. It is a good screening test for von Willebrand disease, monitoring the effect of DDAVP administration, and is abnormal after antiplatelet therapy.[51,52] The test simulates the process of primary hemostasis (platelet adhesion and aggregation) by measuring the ability of platelets to occlude a microscopic aperture in a membrane coated with collagen and epinephrine (C-EPI) or collagen and adenosine diphosphate (C-ADP) under controlled high shear rates. The time required to obtain a complete platelet plug is the closure time in seconds. The normal closure times are 60 to 160 seconds for C-EPI and 50 to 124 seconds for C-ADP. Aspirin and NSAIDs intakes prolong the closure time of C-EPI while von

Willebrand disease, low platelet count (<100,000/UL), low hematocrit (<30%), and renal failure prolong the closure time for C-ADP.

There have been several studies that looked into the incidence of intraspinal hematoma in patients who were on aspirin or NSAIDs.[49,53–56] Some of these studies looked at large number of patients, including 1,422[55] and 1,214[56] patients and found no incidence of intraspinal hematoma.[55,56] Although there have been case reports of intraspinal hematoma in patients on aspirin and NSAIDs, there were complicating factors in these case reports.[57] These included concomitant heparin administration,[58] epidural venous angioma,[58] and technical difficulty in performing the procedure.[59–61] Technical difficulties in performing the injection has been identified as a major risk factor in the development of intraspinal hematoma after neuraxial injections.[57,59–61]

The COX enzyme catalyzes the synthesis of prostaglandins from arachidonic acid. COX activity is associated with distinct isoenzymes, COX-1, COX-2, and COX-3.[62–66] COX-1 is expressed constitutively throughout the body and plays an essential role in homeostatic processes such as platelet aggregation, gastrointestinal protections, and renal function. COX-2 is expressed in inflammatory cells and is involved in the synthesis of prostaglandin-mediating pathologic processes such as pain, fever, inflammation, and carcinogenesis.[62–64] Both COX-1 and COX-2 messenger RNA are expressed in the lung, heart, and kidney; only COX-1 mRNA is present in the liver. While COX-1 prostaglandins are responsible for physiologic functions, COX-2 prostaglandins mediate pathophysiologic and inflammatory processes including pain. The COX-3 enzyme is selectively inhibited by analgesic/antipyretic drugs such as acetaminophen, phenacetin, and antipyrine and inhibited by some NSAIDs. Inhibition of COX-3 may represent a central mechanism by which drugs such as acetaminophen decrease pain and fever.[65]

The COX-2 inhibitors have analgesic effects with minimal side effects. Several studies showed the perioperative analgesic property in different surgical settings.[67–74] They have less gastrointestinal toxicity[64,75,76] and were recommended by the American College of Rheumatology to patients who are at increased risk for serious upper gastrointestinal adverse events.[77] Compared to aspirin or NSAIDS, the effects of the COX-2 inhibitors on platelet aggregation and bleeding times were not different from a placebo.[78–80] The amount of blood loss was not increased during spinal fusion surgery when COX-2 inhibitors were given preoperatively.[81] These effects make these drugs ideal for perioperative use when neuraxial injections are planned.

The thienopyridine drugs ticlopidine and clopidogrel have no direct effect on arachidonic acid metabolism. They inhibit platelet aggregation by inhibiting ADP receptor-mediated platelet activation.[42,82] These drugs also modulate vascular smooth muscle reducing vascular contraction.[83] Clopidogrel is 40 to 100 times more potent than ticlopidine.[84] The doses employed are 75 mg daily for clopidogrel and 250 mg twice a day for ticlopidine. Ticlopidine is rarely used because it causes hypercholesterolemia, neutropenia, and thrombocytopenic purpura. There is also a possible delayed antithrombotic effect of ticlopidine and may not offer protection in the cardiac patient for the first 2 weeks of ticlopidine therapy. Clopidogrel is preferred because it has a better safety profile. It appears to have a better effect than aspirin in patients with peripheral vascular disease and is increasingly used in these patients.[85] The maximal inhibition of ADP-induced platelet aggregation with clopidogrel occurs 3 to 5 days after initiation of a standard dose (75 mg), but within 4 to 6 hours after the administration of a large loading dose (300 to 600 mg).[86] The large loading dose is given to patients before they undergo percutaneous coronary intervention.[42,44] There has been a case report of spinal hematoma in a patient on ticlopidine.[61] While there has been no case of intraspinal hematoma in a patient on clopidogrel alone, there has been a case of quadriplegia in a patient on clopidogrel, diclofenac, and possible aspirin.[57]

ASRA RECOMMENDATIONS FOR ANTIPLATELET THERAPY AND NEURAXIAL BLOCK

The ASRA concluded that neuraxial blocks may be performed in patients on aspirin or NSAIDs.[87] This recommendation is supported by numerous studies that showed the safety of neuraxial injections in patients who were on these medications. The safety of neuraxial blocks in patients on COX-2 inhibitors is obvious. For clopidogrel, it is recommended that the drug be discontinued for 7 days before a neuraxial injection. In contrast, a delay of 10 to 14 days is recommended with ticlopidine. This is because the half-life of ticlopidine increases from 12 hours after a single dose to 4 to 5 days after a steady state is reached.

Aspirin and NSAIDs alone do not significantly increase the risk of spinal hematoma. The combination of these drugs, however, increases the risk of spontaneous hemorrhagic complications, bleeding at puncture sites, and spinal hematoma.[2] Spinal hematomas have been reported in patients on LMWH and antiplatelet medications and in patients on combined clopidogrel and aspirin therapy.[2,57] The society cautioned the performance of intraspinal injections in patients who are on combined antiplatelet medications. This recommendation should be borne in mind in view of the increased use of combined clopidogrel and aspirin therapy in cardiac patients.

The above recommendations apply to patients having neuraxial injections for surgery and for pain clinic interventions. In the pain clinic the interventional physician has to decide whether it is prudent to continue the aspirin or NSAIDs before a neuraxial injection. If the indication for the aspirin is not strong, e.g., routine daily aspirin in an elderly but healthy patient, then the physician may choose to stop the medication especially in cervical and thoracic injections. This is because in these patients it is difficult to differentiate between new or old symptoms (numbness and weakness) or between real and imagined pathology. Greater caution is advised in cervical and thoracic injections since the epidural space is narrower in these levels, the presence of the spinal cord in the area (lumbar injections are performed below the level of the conus medullaris), and the fact that the studies on neuraxial injections in the presence of antiplatelet therapy were done in patients who had lumbar injections only.

For patients on clopidogrel, the present author stops the clopidogrel for 7 days and puts the patients on aspirin therapy. This change is made after discussion with the managing physician. The aspirin is then continued up to the time of injection, after which the patient is switched back on clopidogrel after the block. For patients on combined clopidogrel and aspirin therapy, the clopidogrel is stopped and the aspirin continued. It is very important that the managing physician is informed about these changes and a mutual decision arrived at. In the surgical setting, these drugs are usually stopped by the surgeons before the surgery.

WARFARIN: PHARMACOLOGY AND ASRA RECOMMENDATIONS

Warfarin is an oral anticoagulant that inhibits the vitamin K-dependent, post-translational carboxylation of certain N-terminal glutamic acid residues in prothrombin and factors II, VII, IX, and X—a modification that endows these proteins with the ability to bind calcium ions strongly and to function normally.[88–90] It also inhibits the anticoagulant proteins C and S. Both factor VII and protein C have short half-lives (6 to 7 hours) and increase in the INR is the result of the competing effects of reduced factor VII and protein C and the washout of existing clotting factors. The unpredictability of the INR values during the initial stage of warfarin therapy was shown by a study in which 2 of 24 patients had INRs greater than 2.0 at 36 hours after warfarin intake.[91] It was found that the incidence of INRs ≤ 1.5 was 3% on postoperative day (POD) 1 or 36 hours after warfarin intake, 38% on POD2, 52% on POD3, and 59% on POD4 (Table 83-2).[92] Prophylactic anticoagulation (INRs of 2.0 to 2.5) is reached 48 to 72 hours after the initial dose. The anticoagulant effect of warfarin is primarily dependent on the levels of factor II that has a half-life of 50 hours. Maximal anticoagulation is reached in 4 to 5 days when factor II is sufficiently reduced. The most common dosing regimen is 5 mg given the night of surgery followed by adjustment of the dose to maintain an INR of 2.0 to 2.5. Higher INRs may result in hemarthromas. Because of warfarin's delayed effect and the early development of postoperative thrombus, some surgeons add LMWH as a "bridge therapy" while the effect of warfarin is commencing. This is done in patients who are at high risk for thromboembolism;

some physicians add heparin during the initial stage of warfarin therapy to hasten the anticoagulation. The risks of warfarin usage are bleeding and the rare occurrence of skin necrosis. Its drawbacks include the necessity of monitoring its effect with serial INR monitoring, its interaction with a host of other drugs, and the fact that it has to be stopped a few days before surgery.[88,89]

The ASRA recommended an INR of 1.5 for safe placement and removal of the epidural catheter.[89] This value was based on studies that showed excellent hemostasis during surgery when the INR value was ≤ 1.5.[90] Several studies on the levels of clotting factors at different INR values showed that the decline of these factors may not be significant at an INR of 1.5. At INR values of 1.5 to 2.0, the concentrations of factor II were found to be 74% to 82% of baseline while factor VII levels were 27% to 54% of baseline values.[91] Levels of 20% of normal are considered adequate for normal hemostasis at the time of major surgery. A study[93] found that during the initial phase of warfarin administration and at an INR of 2.1 ± 1, factors II and VII were 65% ± 28% and 25% ± 20% of control values. Another study found that under stable anticoagulation with warfarin, at INRs of 1.3 to 2, the concentrations of the clotting factors were 0.65 IU/mL for factor VII (reference interval: 0.6 to 1.6), 0.75 IU/mL for factor IX (reference interval: 0.7 to 1.3), and 0.47 IU/mL for factor X (reference interval: 0.7 to 1.26).[94]

The same INR value was recommended for removal of the epidural catheter.[89] It should be noted that the same laboratory values apply to placement and removal of the epidural catheter[95] since intraspinal hematomas have occurred after removal of the catheter.[96] The safety of removing the epidural catheters at these values was shown by Horlocker et al.[97] and Wu and Perkins.[98] A question that remains is the rate of decline of the INR after the warfarin is discontinued. It was found that, in general, the INR decreases exponentially after the discontinuation of warfarin, the onset of maximal decrease occurring at 24 to 36 hours after the last dose of warfarin.[99]

TABLE 83-2. INTERNATIONAL NORMALIZED RATIOS (INRs) AFTER WARFARIN INTAKE

Postoperative Day	Warfarin Dose (mg)	Cumulative Warfarin Dose (mg)	INR	Patients with INR > 1.5
0	4.98 ± 0.1 (4–5)	4.98 ± 0.1 (4–5)	0.9 ± 0.1 (0.8–1.1)	0/24 (0%)*
1	4 ± 1.2 (0†–6)	9 ± 1.1 (5–11)	1.1 ± 0.2 (0.8–1.7)	2/60 (3%)
2	3.2 ± 1.8 (0†–7.5)	12.2 ± 2.3 (5–18.5)	1.4 ± 0.5 (0.9–3.9)	23/60 (38%)
3	3.4 ± 2.2 (0†–9)	15.8 ± 4 (5–27.5)	1.6 ± 0.6 (1.0–4.1)	31/59‡ (52%)
4	3.3 ± 2 (0†–7.5)	18.8 ± 5.2 (7–28.5)	1.6 ± 0.5 (1.1–3.8)	29/49‡ (59%)

Data shown are mean ± standard deviation (range). Postoperative day 0 = operative day. Warfarin was administered in the evening of surgery while PTs and INRs were measured in the morning.
* Only 24 of 60 patients had preoperative PT/INR.
† Some patients had their warfarin discontinued because of prolonged PT/INR.
‡ Some patients were discharged on the third and fourth postoperative days, accounting for the smaller number of patients.
From Benzon HT, Esposito P: Timing of removal of epidural catheters in anticoagulated patients. ASA annual meeting, San Diego, CA, 21 October 1997. Anesthesiology 87(3A):A798, 1997.

White et al.[99] showed that at a baseline mean INR of 2.6, the INR decreased to 1.6 at 65 hours (2.7 days) and 1.1 at 115 hours (4.7 days) after the last dose of warfarin. It should be noted, however, that those patients had wide variabilities in their INRs[99] and that several variables affect the clearance of warfarin. There is a 10% increase per year decrease in clearance in patients over the age of 20 to 70 years.[100] Smoking results in a 10% increase in clearance while the coadministration of other drugs (inducers of phenytoin or phenobarbital) results in increased clearance.[100]

HEPARIN AND LMWH: PHARMACOLOGY AND ASRA RECOMMENDATIONS

Heparins are glycosaminoglycans that consist of chains of alternating residues of D-glucosamine and uronic acid, either glucoronic acid or iduronic acid. Unfractionated heparin is a heterogeneous mixture of polysaccharide chains ranging in molecular weight from 3,000 to 30,000.[89] A unique pentasaccharide sequence, randomly distributed along the heparin chains, binds to antithrombin (AT).[101] The binding of the heparin pentasaccharide to AT causes a conformational change in AT that accelerates its ability to inactivate thrombin, factor Xa, and factor IXa. In addition, unfractionated heparin releases tissue factor pathway inhibitor from endothelium, enhancing its activity against factor Xa.[102] The anticoagulant effect of heparin is not linear but increases disproportionately with increasing dosages. The anticoagulant effect of subcutaneous heparin takes 1 to 2 hours but the effect of intravenous heparin is immediate. The aPTT is used to monitor the effect of heparin; therapeutic anticoagulation is achieved with a prolongation of the aPTT to greater than 1.5 times the baseline value or a heparin level of 0.2 to 0.4 U/mL.[103] The aPTT is usually not prolonged by the subcutaneous administration of low doses of heparin and is not monitored.

Heparin is either administered as an intravenous injection or as subcutaneous injection for DVT prophylaxis. The risk factors in the development of intraspinal hematoma in patients who are given heparin were identified by Ruff and Dougherty as follows:[104] (1) an interval of less than 1 hour between the lumbar puncture and heparin administration; (2) concomitant use of other anticoagulants such as aspirin; and (3) traumatic needle placements. For patients who are scheduled for vascular procedures and given intravenous heparin during the surgery, it was noted that it was safe to perform preoperative neuraxial blocks if some precautions are observed.[105] The cancellation of the proposed surgery has been recommended in cases of bloody or traumatic taps but there appears to be no data to support this recommendation. In summary, the ASRA guidelines on the performance of neuraxial procedures in patients who are anticoagulated with heparin are as follows:[2,106] (1) the neuraxial technique should be avoided in patients with other coagulopathies; (2) although the occurrence of bloody or difficult needle placement increases the risk of hematoma, discussion with the surgeon of the risk/benefit ratio should determine cancellation or noncancellation of the case; (3) the heparin administration should be delayed for 1 hour after needle placement; (4) indwelling neuraxial catheters should be removed 2 to 4 hours after the last heparin dose, and the patient's coagulation status is evaluated and reheparinization occurs 1 hour after catheter removal; and (5) minimal concentrations of local anesthetics should be used for early detection of signs of spinal hematoma and the patient is monitored postoperatively for signs of hematoma.

In general surgery and urology patients who undergo major procedures, the heparin is continued in the postoperative period for DVT prophylaxis. Heparin, 5,000 U, is given subcutaneously every 12 hours. The changes in the aPTT appear to be barely detectable; the very few patients have prolongations of their aPTT do not exceed 1.5 times the normal levels. Liu and Mulroy noted the relative safety of performing neuraxial procedures and continuing the epidural catheters in these patients.[2,106] The case report of spinal hematoma after the ASRA guidelines came out occurred in a patient who had other risk factors and in whom the ASRA guidelines were not followed.[2] The continued use of subcutaneous heparin for more than 4 days warrants the determination of the patient's platelet count to detect the development of heparin-induced thrombocytopenia.

There appears to be a continuing debate as to whether neuraxial procedures should be performed in patients who undergo cardiopulmonary bypass. In these patients the following precautions have been recommended: (1) neuraxial procedures should be avoided in patients with a known coagulopathy; (2) surgery should be delayed 24 hours in the patient with a traumatic tap; (3) the time from the neuraxial procedure to the systemic heparinization should exceed 1 hour; (4) heparinization and reversal should be monitored and controlled tightly; and (5) the epidural catheter should be removed when normal coagulation is restored and the patient should be monitored closely for signs of spinal hematoma after the catheter is removed.[107]

Heparin is not the ideal anticoagulant: it is a mixture of molecules of which only a fraction has anticoagulant activity. It binds to platelet factor IV which is released from activated platelets, to a number of plasma proteins, and to high-molecular-weight multimers of von Willebrand factor that is released from platelets and endothelial cells.[88,108] The heparin–antithrombin complex is also not very effective in neutralizing clot-bound thrombin. These factors result in an unpredictable anticoagulant effect of heparin necessitating careful laboratory monitoring when it is used in therapeutic dosages. Finally, heparin causes immunologic thrombocytopenia and immune-mediated thrombosis.[88] These drawbacks of heparin led to increased use of the LMWHs.

LOW-MOLECULAR-WEIGHT HEPARIN

LMWHs are the fractionated forms of heparin with a mean molecular weight of 5,000.[108,109] Similar to unfractionated heparin, LMWH activates antithrombin accelerating antithrombin's interaction with thrombin and factor Xa. LMWH, like unfractionated heparin, also releases tissue factor pathway from the endothelium. While unfractionated heparin has equivalent activity against thrombin and factor Xa, LMWH has a greater activity against factor Xa. The plasma half-life of the LMWHs ranges from 2 to 4 hours after an intravenous injection and 3 to 6 hours after a subcutaneous injection. The LMWHs have a longer half-life, and dose-independent clearance compared to heparin resulting in a more predictable anticoagulant response. The reduced binding with plasma proteins and endothelium results in the LMWHs' better bioavailability and predictability than unfractionated heparin. The recovery of anti-factor Xa activity after a subcutaneous injection of

LMWH approaches 100% compared to approximately 30% for unfractionated heparin.[110] Laboratory monitoring is not necessary except in patients with renal insufficiency or those with body weight less than 50 kg or more than 80 kg.[108] The r time from the thrombelastogram, a test that is easily available, was found to correlate with the serum anti-Xa concentration.[111]

Clinical studies showed the efficacy and safety of LMWHs in the prevention and treatment of venous thrombosis. They have been used a prophylaxis against thromboembolism in surgical settings such as general surgery,[112] total hip and knee replacements,[16–20,113–117] surgery for hip fractures,[118] and multiple trauma.[119] Also, LMWHs have been used in unstable angina,[120–122] acute myocardial infarction,[123] and ischemic stroke.[124]

There are three commercially available LMWHs in the USA: enoxaparin (Lovenox), dalteparin (Fragmin), and tinzaparin (Innohep). Enoxaparin is either given once daily or every 12 hours while the two other drugs are given once a day. There are very few studies that directly compared the different LMWHs. A review of the literature showed the three drugs to have comparable efficacy in the treatment and prevention of venous thromboembolism.[125] Enoxaparin and dalteparin have similar efficacy in the prevention of venous thrombosis after general surgery and after total hip replacement. The two drugs also have comparable efficacy in the prevention of death or myocardial infarction among patients with unstable angina. For all remaining indications, the literature supports the use of enoxaparin.[125]

The recommendations of the ASRA for patients receiving LMWH and neuraxial anesthesia are as follows:[2,126]

- Monitoring of anti-Xa level is not recommended.
- The administration of antiplatelet or oral anticoagulant medications with LMWHs may increase the risk of spinal hematoma.
- The presence of blood during needle placement and catheter placement does not necessitate postponement of surgery. However, the initiation of LMWH therapy should be delayed for 24 hours postoperatively.
- The first dose of LMWH prophylaxis should be given no earlier than 24 hours postoperatively and only in the presence of adequate hemostasis.
- In patients who are on LMWH needle/catheter placement should occur at least 12 hours after the last prophylactic dose of enoxaparin or 24 hours after dalteparin (120 U/kg every 12 hours or 200 U/kg every 12 hours), tinzaparin (175 U/kg daily), or after higher doses of enoxaparin (1 mg/kg every 12 hours).
- There should be a 12-hour interval between the last prophylactic dose of enoxaparin and removal of the epidural catheter. For higher doses of enoxaparin, a 24-hour delay is recommended.
- The LMWH may be administered 2 hours after the epidural catheter is removed.

FONDAPARINUX

Fondaparinux is a synthetic anticoagulant that is a selective Xa inhibitor.[127] Studies showed the incidence of DVT following major hip and knee surgery to be lower with fondaparinux compared to enoxaparin.[128] It was also found to be as effective as unfractionated heparin in the initial treatment of hemodynamically stable patients with pulmonary embolism.[129] Because it is synthesized chemically, it exhibits batch-to-batch consistency. The drug is rapidly absorbed, reaching a maximum concentration within 1.7 hours of dosing and has a half-life of 17 hours.[127] It has a 100% bioavailability. A dose of 2.5 mg is given subcutaneously 6 hours after surgery then once a day. The risk of spinal hematoma in patients on fondaparinux is not known at this time. The ASRA recommended that neuraxial injections should involve single-needle pass, atraumatic needle placements, and avoidance of intraspinal catheters.[126]

THROMBIN INHIBITORS

Hirudo medicinalis, the medicinal leech, produces hirudin, a direct thrombin inhibitor.[88] Hirudin acts independently of antithrombin and other plasma proteins.[130] The commercially available thrombin inhibitors include the recombinant hirudin derivatives desirudin (Revasc), lepirudin (Refludan), and bivalirudin (Angiomax), and the synthetic L-arginine derivative argatroban (Acova). These drugs can neutralize free and clot-bound thrombin and are used in the treatment of thrombosis in patients with heparin-induced thrombocytopenia and in the prevention of thromboembolic complications after total hip replacement.[131,132] Their anticoagulant effect is present for 1 to 3 hours and is monitored by the aPTT.[2] There has been no case report of spinal hematoma in patients who had thrombin inhibitors and had neuraxial anesthesia. This is most probably related to anesthesiologists waiting at least 3 to 4 hours after the thrombin inhibitor was given.

A new oral thrombin inhibitor, ximelagatran, is undergoing clinical trials in the prevention of venous thromboembolism after total joint replacements and in the secondary prevention of venous thromboembolism.[22,133] Ximelagatran is the first new oral anticoagulant since warfarin. It is converted to melagatran, the mean bioavailability of which is 20% after a single dose of ximagalatran. Melagatran has predictable and reproducible pharmacokinetic and pharmacodynamic properties, with a low binding affinity to plasma proteins. The maximum plasma concentration of melagatran is achieved within 2 hours of oral administration of ximelagatran and its half-life is 3 hours.[134] Ximelagatran is administered at a fixed dose of 24 mg twice daily without monitoring of blood coagulation.[133] The ease of administration and the lack of monitoring for this drug will probably result in its greater use in the future.

HERBAL THERAPIES

The use of herbal medications in the USA has increased tremendously. The most commonly used herbal medications are garlic, ginkgo, and ginseng. Garlic inhibits platelet aggregation and its effect on hemostasis appears to last 7 days. Ginkgo inhibits platelet-activating factor and its effect lasts 36 hours. Ginseng has heterogeneous effects. It inhibits platelet aggregation in vitro and prolongs both thrombin time and activated partial thromboplastin time in laboratory animals. Its effect lasts 24 hours.[2]

SUMMARY

The problems of perioperative DVT and venous thromboembolism have been discussed in this chapter. The perioperative prophylaxis against the development of DVTs and the prophylaxis and management of venous thromboembolism have also been discussed. A knowledge of the interaction between the anticoagulants and neuraxial anesthesia and epidural postoperative analgesia will lead to the safe use of the neuraxial procedures and better safety of the patients.

KEY POINTS

- Some 50% of DVTs after total joint surgery begin intraoperatively; the highest incidence occurs during surgery and the first postoperative day. Almost 75% of DVTs develop within the first 48 hours after surgery.
- Recent studies showed that conventional-intensity warfarin therapy (target INR of 2.0 to 3.0) was more effective than low-intensity warfarin therapy (target INR of 1.5 to 1.9) in reducing recurrent venous thromboembolism. In addition, low-intensity-warfarin therapy did not reduce the risk of clinically important bleeding. Anesthesiologists will therefore continue to see target INRs of 2.0 to 3.0 when warfarin is used for venous thromboemnbolism. This INR value conflicts with the INR of 1.5 that was deemed safe by the ASRA for neuraxial procedures.
- The maximal inhibition of ADP-induced platelet aggregation with clopidogrel occurs 3 to 5 days after initiation of treatment with standard doses of 75 mg but within 4 to 6 hours after the administration of 300 to 600 mg. These large loading doses are given to patients who undergo percutaneous coronary interventions.
- The PFA is a test that simulates platelet adhesion and aggregation by measuring the ability of the platelets to occlude a microscopic aperture in a membrane coated with collagen and epinephrine (C-EPI) or collagen and ADP (C-ADP). Aspirin and platelets prolong the closure time of C-EPI (normal: 60 to 160 seconds) while von Willebrand disease, low platelet count, low hematocrit, and renal failure prolong the closure time for C-ADP (normal: 50 to 124 seconds).
- Case reports of intraspinal hematoma after aspirin and NSAIDs had complicating factors such as concomitant administration of other anticoagulant, epidural vascular abnormalities, and technical difficulties. The intake of different antiplatelet medications has been identified as a major risk factor in the development of spinal hematoma after neuraxial injections.
- Heparin binds to platelet factor IV, to plasma proteins, and to the von Willebrand factor released from platelets and endothelial cells. The heparin–antithrombin complex is not very effective in neutralizing clot-bound thrombin.

REFERENCES

1. Heit JA, Horlocker TT (eds): Neuraxial anesthesia and anticoagulation. Reg Anesth Pain Med 23:S129–S193, 1998.
2. Horlocker TT, Wedel DJ, Benzon HT: Regional anesthesia in the anticoagulated patient: Defining the risks (the second ASRA consensus conference on neuraxial anesthesia and anticoagulation). Reg Anesth Paain Med 28:171–197, 2003.
3. O'Meara PM, Kaufman EE: Prophylaxis for venous thromboembolism in total hip arthroplasty: A review. Orthopedics 13:173–178, 1990.
4. Merli GJ: Deep vein thrombosis and pulmonary embolism prophylaxis in joint replacement surgery. Rheum Dis Clin North Am 25:639–656, 1999.
5. Miric A, Lombardi P, Sculco TP: Deep vein thrombosis prophylaxis: A comprehensive approach for total hip and total knee arthroplasty patient populations. Am J Orthop 29:269–274, 2000.
6. Kim YH, Kim JS: Incidence and natural history of deep-vein thrombosis after total knee arthroplasty. JBJS 84B:566–670, 2002.
7. Gitel S, Salvanti E, Wessler S, et al: The effect of total hip replacement and general surgery on antithrombin III in relation to venous thrombosis. JBJS 1979;61–A:653–656
8. Ericksson B, Ericksson E, Erika G, et al: Thrombosis after hip replacement: Relationship to the fibrinolytic system. Acta Orthop Scand 60:159–163, 1989.
9. Cohen S, Ehrlich G, Kauffamn M, et al: Thrombophlebitis following knee surgery. JBJS 55A:106–112, 1973.
10. Stulberg B, Insall J, William G, et al: Deep vein thrombosis following total knee replacement: An analysis of six hundred and thirty-eight arthroplasties. JBJS 66A:194–201, 1984.
11. Stringer M, Steadman C, Hedges A, et al: Deep vein thrombosis after elective knee surgery: An incidence study in 312 patients. JBJS 71B:492–497, 1989.
12. Westrich GH, Haas SB, Mosca P, Peterson M: Meta-analysis of thromboembolic prophylaxis after total knee arthroplasty. JBJS 82B:795–800, 2000.
13. De Wet CJ, Pearl RG: Postoperative thrombotic complications. Venous thromboembolism: Deep vein thrombosis and pulmonary embolism. Anesth Clin North Am 17:895–922, 1999.
14. Rosen CL, Tracy JA: The diagnosis of lower extremity deep venous thrombosis. Emerg Clin North Am 19:895–923, 2001.
15. Westrich GH, Sculco TP: Prophylaxis against deep venous thrombosis after total knee arthroplasty. Pneumatic plantar compression and aspirin compared to aspirin alone. JBJS 78A:826–834, 1996.
16. Leclerc JR, Geerts W, Desjardins L, et al: Prevention of deep vein thrombosis after major knee surgery. A randomized double-blind trial comparing a low molecular weight heparin fragment to placebo. Thromb Haemost 67:417–423, 1992.
17. Colwell C, Spiro T, Trombridge A, et al: Use of enoxaparin, a low molecular weight heparin and unfractionated heparin for the prevention of deep venous thrombosis after elective hip replacement. JBJS 76A:3–114, 1994.
18. RD Heparin Arthroplasty Group: RD heparin compared with warfarin in prevention of venous thromboembolic disease following total hip or knee arthroplasty. JBJS 76A:1174–1185, 1994.
19. Hull RD, Pineo GF, Francis C, et al: Low-molecular-weight heparin prophylaxis using dalteparin in close proximity to surgery versus warfarin in hip arthroplasty patients: A double-blind, randomized comparison. The North American Fragmin Trial investigators. Arch Intern Med 160:2199–2207, 2000.
20. Blanchard J, Meuwly JY, Leyvraz PF, et al: Prevention of deep-vein thrombosis after total knee replacement. Randomized comparison between a low-molecular weight heparin (nadroparin) and mechanical prophylaxis with foot-pump system. JBJS 81B: 654–659, 1999.
21. Cannavo D: Use of neuraxial anesthesia with selective factor Xa inhibitors. Am J Orthop 31(Suppl 11):21–23, 2002.
22. Francis CW, Berkowitz SD, Comp PC, et al: Comparison of ximelagatran with warfarin for the prevention of venous thromboembolism after total knee replacement. N Engl J Med 349: 1703–1712, 2003.
23. Schafer AI: Warfarin for venous thromboembolism – Walking the dosing tightrope. N Engl J Med 348:1478–1480, 2002.
24. Prandoni P, Lensing AW, Cogo A, et al: The long-term clinical course of acute deep vein thrombosis. Ann Intern Med 125:1–7, 1996.
25. Schulman S, Rhedin A-S, Lindmarker P, et al: A comparison of six weeks with six months of oral anticoagulant therapy after a first episode of venous thromboembolism. N Engl J Med 332: 1661–1665, 1995.

26. Buller HR, Prins MH: Secondary prophylaxis with warfarin for venous thromboembolism. N Engl J Med 349:702–704, 2003.

27. Barritt DW, Jordan SC: Anticoagulant drugs in the treatment of pulmonary embolism: A controlled trial. Lancet 1:1309–1312, 1960.

28. Brandjes DPM, Heijboer H, Buller HR, et al: Acenocoumarol and heparin compared with acenocoumarol alone in the initial treatment of proximal-vein thrombosis. N Engl J Med 327:1485–1489, 1992.

29. Lagerstedt CI, Olsson CG, Fagher BO, et al: Need for long-term anticoagulant treatment in symptomatic calf-vein thrombosis. Lancet 2:515–518, 1985.

30. Hull R, Delmore T, Genton E, et al: Warfarin sodium versus low-dose heparin in the long-term treatment of venous thrombosis. N Engl J Med 301:855–858, 1979.

31. Schulman S, Rhedin A-S, Lindmarker P, et al: A comparison of six weeks with six months of oral anticoagulant therapy after a first episode of venous thromboembolism. N Engl J Med 332:1661–1665, 1995.

32. Schulman S, Granqvist S, Holmstrom M, et al: The duration of oral anticoagulant therapy after a second episode of venous thromboembolism. N Engl J Med 336:393–398, 1997.

33. Kearon C, Gent M, Hirsh J, et al: A comparison of three months of anticoagulation with extended anticoagulation for a first episode of idiopathic venous thromboembolism. N Engl J Med 340:901–907, 1999.

34. Agnelliu G, Prandoni P, Santamaria MG, et al: Three months versus one year of oral anticoagulant therapy for idiopathic deep venous thrombosis. N Engl J Med 345:165–169, 2001.

35. Ridker PM, Goldhaber SZ, Danielson E, et al: Long-term, low-intensity warfarin therapy for the prevention of recurrent venous thromboembolism. N Engl J Med 348:1425–1434, 2003.

36. Kearon C, Ginsberg JS, Kovacs MJ, et al: Comparison of low-intensity warfarin therapy with conventional-intensity warfarin therapy for long-term prevention of recurrent venous thromboembolism. N Engl J Med 349:631–639, 2003.

37. Prins MH, Hutten BA, Koopman MM, Buller HR: Long-term treatment of venous thromboembolic disease. Thromb Haemost 82:892–898, 1999.

38. Hull R, Hirsh J, Jay R, et al: Different intensities of oral anticoagulant therapy in the treatment of proximal-vein thrombosis. N Engl J Med 307:1676–1681, 1982.

39. Hyers TM, Agnelli G, Hull RD, et al: Antithrombotic therapy for venous thromboembolic disease. Chest 119(Suppl):176S–193S, 2001.

40. Ryan TJ, Antman EM, Brooks NH, et al: ACC/AHA guidelines for the management of patients with acute myocardial infarction. J Am Coll Cardiol 34:890–909, 1999.

41. The Clopidogrel in Unstable Angina to Prevent Recurrent Events Trial investigators: Effects of clopidogrel in addition to aspirin in patients with acute coronary syndromes without ST-segment elevation. N Engl J Med 345:494–502, 2001.

42. Lange RA, Hillis LD: Antiplatelet therapy for ischemic heart disease. N Engl J Med 350:277–280, 2004.

43. Mehta SR, Yusuf S, Peters RJ, et al: Effects of pretreatment with clopidogrel and aspirin followed by long-term therapy in patients undergoing percutaneous coronary intervention: the PCI-CURE study. Lancet 358:527–533, 2001.

44. Steinhubl SR, Berger PB, Mann JT, et al: Early and sustained dual oral antiplatelet therapy following percutaneous coronary intervention: A randomized controlled trial. JAMA 288:2411–2420, 2002.

45. The PURSUIT trial investigators: Inhibition of platelet glycoprotein IIb/IIIa with eptifibatide in patients with acute coronary syndromes. N Engl J Med 339:436–443, 1998.

46. The Platelet Receptor Inhibition in Ischemic Syndrome Management in Patients Limited by Unstable Signs and Symptoms (PRISM-PLUS) Study investigators: Inhibition of the platelet glycoprotein IIb/IIIa receptor with tirofiban in unstable angina and non-Q-wave myocardial infarction. N Engl J Med 338:1488–1497, 1998.

47. Kasatrati A, Mehili J, Schuhlen H, et al: A clinical trial of abciximab in elective percutaneous coronary intervention after pretreatment with clopidogrel. N Engl J Med 350:232–238, 2004.

48. Diener HC, Cunha L, Farber C, et al: European Stroke Prevention Study 2. Dipyridamole and acetylsalicylic acid in the secondary prevention of stroke. J Neurol Sci 143:1–13, 1996.

49. Benzon HT, Brunner EA, Vaisrub N: Bleeding time and nerve blocks after aspirin. Reg Anesth 9:86–90, 1984.

50. Rodgers RPC, Levin J: A critical reappraisal of the bleeding time. Sem Thromb Hemost 16:1–20, 1990.

51. Fressinaud E, et al: Screening for von Willebrand disease with a new analyzer using high shear stress: A study of 60 cases. Blood 91:1325–1331, 1998.

52. Mammen EF, et al: PFA-100 system: A new method for assessment of platelet dysfunction. Sem Thromb Hemost 24:195–202, 1998.

53. Horlocker TT, Wedel DJ, Offord KP: Does preoperative antiplatelet therapy increase the risk of hemorrhagic complications associated with regional anesthesia? Anesth Analg 70:631–634, 1990.

54. Horlocker TT, Wedel DJ, Schroeder DR, et al: Preoperative antiplatelet therapy does not increase the risk of spinal hematoma associated with regional anesthesia. Anesth Analg 80:303–309, 1995.

55. CLASP (Collaborative Low-Dose Aspirin Study in Pregnancy) Collaborative Group: CLASP: a randomized trial of low-dose aspirin for the prevention and treatment of pre-eclampsia among 9364 pregnant women. Lancet 343:619–629, 1994.

56. Horlocker TT, Bajwa ZH, Ashraft Z, et al: Risk assessment of hemorrhagic complications associated with nonsteroidal anti-inflammatory medications in ambulatory pain clinic patients undergoing epidural steroid injection. Anesth Analg 95:1691–1697, 2002.

57. Benzon HT, Wong HY, Siddiqui T, Ondra S: Caution in performing epidural injections in patients on several antiplatelet drugs. Anesthesiology 91:1558–1559, 1999.

58. Eastwood DW: Hematoma after epidural anesthesia: Relation of skin and spinal angiomas. Anesth Analg 73:352–354, 1991.

59. Greensite F, Katz J: Spinal subdural hematoma associated with attempted epidural anesthesia and subsequent spinal anesthesia. Anesth Analg 59:72–73, 1980.

60. Gerancher JC, Waterer R, Middleton J: Transient paraparesis after postdural puncture spinal hematoma in a patient receiving ketorolac. Anesthesiology 86:490–494, 1997.

61. Mayumi T, Dohi S: Spinal subarachnoid hematoma after lumbar puncture in a patient receiving antiplatelet therapy. Anesth Analg 62:777–779, 1983.

62. Fitzgerald GA, Patrono C: The coxibs, selective inhibitors of cyclooxygenase-2. N Engl J Med 345:433–442, 2001.

63. McCrory CR, Lindahl SGE: Cyclooxygenase inhibition for postoperative analgesia. Anesth Analg 95:169–176, 2002.

64. Gajraj NM: Cyclooxygenase-2 inhibitors. Anesth Analg 96:1720–1738, 2003.

65. Chandrasekharan NV, Dai H, Roos KLT, et al: COX-3, a cyclooxygenase-1 variant inhibited by acetaminophen and other analgesic/antipyretic drugs: Cloning, structure, and expression. PNAS 99:13926–13931, 2002.

66. Warner TD, Mitchell JA: Cyclooxygenase-3 (COX-3): Filling in the gaps toward a COX continuum? PNAS 99:13371–13373, 2002.

67. Reuben SS, Connelly NR: Postoperative analgesic effects of celecoxib or rofecoxib after spinal fusion surgery. Anesth Analg 91:1221–1225, 2000.

68. Daniels SE, Desjardins PJ, Talewaker S, et al: The analgesic efficacy of valdecoxib vs. oxycodone/acetaminophen after oral surgery. JADA 133:611–621, 2002.

69. Camu F, Beecher T, Recker DP, et al: Valdecoxib, a COX-2-specific inhibitor, is an efficacious, opioid-sparing analgesic in patients undergoing hip arthroplasty. Am J Ther 9:43–51, 2002.

70. Malan TP, Marsh G, Hakki SI, et al: Parecoxib sodium, a parenteral cyclooxygenasae 2 selective inhibitor, improves morphine analgesia and is opioid-sparing following total hip arthroplasty. Anesthesiology 98:950–956, 2003.

71. Barton SF, Langeland FF, Snabes MC, et al: Efficacy and safety of intravenous parecoxib sodium in relieving acute postoperative pain following gynecologic laparotomy surgery. Anesthesiology 97:306–314, 2002.

72. Desjardins PJ, Shu VS, Recker DP, et al: A single preoperative dose of valdecoxib, a new cyclooxygenase-2 specific inhibitor, relieves post-oral surgery or bunionectomy pain. Anesthesiology 97:565–573, 2002.

73. Buvanendran A, Kroin JS, Tuman KJ, et al: Effects of perioperative administration of a selective cycloxygenase 2 inhibitor on pain management and recovery of function after knee replacement: A randomized controlled trial. JAMA 290:2411–2418, 2003.

74. Sinatra RS, Shen Q J, Halaszynski T, et al: Preoperative rofecoxib oral suspension as an analgesic adjunct after lower abdominal surgery: The effects of an effort-dependent pain and pulmonary function. Anesth Analg 98:135–140, 2003.

75. Silverstein F, Faich G, Goldstein J, et al: Gastrointestinal toxicity with celecoxib vs nonsteroidal anti-inflammatory drugs for osteoarthritis and rheumatoid arthritis: The CLASS study – A randomized controlled trial. JAMA 284:1247–1255, 2000.

76. Bombardier C, Laine L, Reicin A, et al: Comparison of upper gastrointestinal toxicity of rofecoxib and naproxen in patients with rheumatoid arthritis. N Engl J Med 343:1520–1528, 2000.

77. Recommendations for the medical management of osteoarthritis of the hip and knee: 2000 update. American College of Rheumatology Subcommittee on Osteoarthritis Guidelines. Arthritis Rheum 43:1905–1915, 2000.

78. Lessee PT, Hubbard RC, Karim A, et al: Effects of celecoxib, a novel, cyclooxygenase-2-inhibitor, on platelet function in healthy adults: A randomized, clinical trial. J Clin Pharmacol 40:124–132, 2000.

79. van Heeken H, Schwartz JI, Depre M, et al: Comparative inhibitory activity of rofecoxib, meloxicam, diclofenac, ibuprofen and naproxen on COX-2 versus COX-1 in healthy volunteers. J Clin Pharmacol 40:1109–1120, 2000.

80. Greenberg H, Gottesdiener K, Huntington M, et al: A new cyclooxygenase-2-inhibitor, rofecoxib (VIOXX) did not alter the antiplatelet effects of low-does aspirin in healthy volunteers. J Clin Pharmacol 40:1509–1515, 2000.

81. Reuben SS, Connelly NR: Postoperative analgesic effects of celecoxib or rofecoxib after spinal fusion surgery. Anesth Analg 91:1221–1225, 2000.

82. Schror K: Antiplatelet drugs: A comparative review. Drugs 50:7–28, 1995.

83. Yang LH, Fareed J: Vasomodulatory action of clopidogrel and ticlopidine. Thromb Res 86:479–491, 1997.

84. Boneu B, Destelle G, on behalf of the study group: Platelet antiaggregating activity and tolerance of clopidogrel in atherosclerotic patients. Thromb Haemost 76:939–943, 1996.

85. CAPRIE Steering Committee: A randomized blind trial of clopidogrel versus aspirin in patients at risk of ischaemic stroke (CAPRIE). Lancet 348:1329–1339, 1996.

86. Helft G, Osende JI, Worthley SG, et al: Acute antithrombotic effect of a front-loaded regimen of clopidogrel in patients with atherosclerosis on aspirin. Arterioscler Thromb Vasc Biol 29:2316–2321, 2000.

87. Urmey WF, Rowlingson JC: Do antiplatelet agents contribute to the development of perioperative spinal hematoma? Reg Anesth Pain Med 23:146–151, 1998.

88. Shapiro SS: Treating thrombosis in the 21st century. N Engl J Med 349:1762–1764, 2003.

89. Enneking FK, Benzon HT: Oral anticoagulants and regional anesthesia: A perspective. Reg Anesth Pain Med 23:140–145, 1998.

90. Kearon C, Hirsh J: Management of anticoagulation before and after elective surgery. N Engl J Med 336:1506–1511, 1997.

91. Harrison L, Johnston M, Massicote MP, et al: Comparison of 5-mg and 10-mg doses in initiation of warfarin therapy. Ann Intern Med 126:133–136, 1997.

92. Benzon HT, Esposito P: Timing of removal of epidural catheters in anticoagulated patients. ASA annual meeting, San Diego, CA, 21 October 1997. Anesthesiology 87(3A):A798, 1997.

93. Weinstock DM, Chang P, Aronson DL, Kessler CM: Comparison of plasma prothrombin and factor VII and urine prothrombin F1 concentrations in patients on long-term warfarin therapy and those in initial phase. Am J Hematol 57:193–199, 1998.

94. Jerkeman A, Astermark J, Hedner U, et al: Correlation between different intensities of anti-Vitamin K treatment and coagulation parameters. Thromb Res 98:467–471, 2000.

95. Horlocker TT: When to remove a spinal or epidural catheter in an anticoagulated patient. Reg Anesth 18:264–265, 1993.

96. Vandermeulen EP, Van Aken H, Vermylen J: Anticoagulants and spinal-epidural anesthesia. Anesth Analg 79:1165–1177, 1994.

97. Horlocker TT, Wedel DJ, Schlichting JL: Postoperative epidural analgesia and oral anticoagulant therapy. Anesth Analg 79:89–93, 1994.

98. Wu CL, Perkins FM: Oral anticoagulant prophylaxis and epidural catheter removal. Reg Anesth 21:517–524, 1996.

99. White RH, McKittrick T, Hutchinson R, Twitchell J: Temporary discontinuation of warfarin therapy: Changes in the international normalized ratio. Ann Intern Med 122:40–42, 1995.

100. Mungall DR, Ludden TM, Marshall J, et al: Population pharmacokinetics of racemic warfarin in adult patients. Pharmacokinet Biopharm 13:213–227, 1985.

101. Rosenberg RD, Bauer KA: The heparin–antithrombin system: A natural anticoagulant mechanism. In Colma RW, Hirsch J, Marder VJ, Salzman EW (eds): Hemostasis and Thrombosis: Basic Principles and Clinical Practice, ed 3. JB Lippincott, Philadelphia, 1994, pp 837–860.

102. Abildgaard U, Lindahl AK, Sandset PM: Heparin requires both antithrombin and extrinsic pathway inhibitor for its anticoagulant effect in human blood. Haemostasis 21:254–257, 1991.

103. Murray DJ, Brodsnahan WJ, Pennell B, et al: Heparin detection by the activated coagulation time: A comparison of the sensitivity of coagulation tests and heparin assays. J Cardiothorac Vasc Anesth 11:24–28, 1997.

104. Ruff DL, Dougherty JH: Complications of anticoagulation followed by anticoagulation. Stroke 12:879–881, 1981.

105. Rao TL, El-Etr AA: Anticoagulation following placement of epidural and subarachnoid catheters: An evaluation of neurologic sequelae. Anesthesiology 55:618–620, 1981.

106. Liu SS, Mulroy MF: Neuraxial anesthesia and analgesia in the presence of standard heparin. Reg Anesth Pain Med 23:157–163, 1998.

107. Chaney MA: Intrathecal and epidural anesthesia and analgesia for cardiac surgery. Anesth Analg 84:1211–1221, 1997.

108. Weitz JI: Drug therapy: Low-molecular-weight heparins. N Engl J Med 337:688–698, 1997.

109. Horlocker TT, Heit JA: Low molecular weight heparin: Biochemistry, pharmacology, perioperative prophylaxis regimens, and guidelines for regional anesthetic management. Anesth Analg 85:874–885, 1997.

110. Bara L, Billaud E, Gramond G, et al: Comparative pharmacokinetics of a low molecular weight heparin (PK 10 169) and unfractionated heparin after intravenous and subcutaneous administration. Thromb Res 39:631–636, 1985.

111. Klein S, Slaughter T, Vail PT, et al: Thrombelastography as a perioperative measure of anticoagulation resulting from low molecular weight heparin: A comparison with anti-Xa concentrations. Anesth Analg 91:1091–1095, 2000.

112. Kakkar W, Cohen AT, Edmonson RA, et al: Low molecular weight versus standard heparin for prevention of venous thromboembolism after major abdominal surgery. Lancet 341: 259–265, 1993.

113. Nurmohamed MT, Rosendaal FR, Buller HR, et al: Low-molecular weight heparin versus standard heparin in general and orthopedic surgery: A meta-analysis. Lancet 340:152–156, 1992.

114. German Hip Arthroplasty Trial (GHAT) Group: Prevention of deep vein thrombosis with low molecular weight heparin in patients undergoing total hip replacement: A randomized trial. Arch Orthop Trauma Surg 111:110–120, 1992.

115. Hull R, Raskob G, Pineo G, et al: A comparison of subcutaneous low-molecular weight heparin with warfarin sodium for prophylaxis against deep-vein thrombosis after hip or knee implantation. N Engl J Med 329:1370–1376, 1993.

116. Leclerc JR, Geerts WH, Desjardins L, et al: Prevention of venous thromboembolism after knee arthroplasty: A randomized, double-blind trial comparing enoxaparin with warfarin. Ann Intern Med 124:619–626, 1996.

117. Heit JA, Berkowitz SD, Bona R, et al: Efficacy and safety of low molecular weight heparin (ardeparin sodium) compared to warfarin for the prevention of venous thromboembolism after total knee surgery: A double-blind, dose-ranging study. Thromb Haemost 77:32–38, 1997.

118. Barsotti J, Gruel Y, Rosset P, et al: Comparative double-blind study of two dosage regimens of low-molecular weight heparin in elderly patients with a fracture of the neck of the femur. J Orthop Trauma 4:371–375, 1990.

119. Geerts WH, Jay RM, Code KI, et al: A comparison of low-dose heparin with low-molecular weight heparin as prophylaxis against venous thromboembolism after major trauma. N Engl J Med 335:701–707, 1996.

120. Gurfinkel EP, Manos EJ, Mejail RI, et al: Low-molecular weight heparin versus regular heparin or aspirin in the treatment of unstable angina and silent ischemia. J Am Coll Cardiol 26:313–318, 1995.

121. Fragmin During Instability in Coronary Artery Disease (FRISC) Study Group: Low-molecular weight heparin during instability in coronary artery disease. Lancet 347:561–568, 1996.

122. Cohen M, Demers C, Gurfinkel EP, et al: A comparison of low-molecular-weight heparin with unfractionated heparin for unstable coronary artery disease. N Engl J Med 337:447–452, 1997.

123. Cohen M: The role of low-molecular weight heparin in the management of acute coronary syndromes. J Am Coll Cardiol 41:S55–S61, 2003.

124. Kay R, Wong KS, Yu, et al: Low-molecular-weight-heparin for the treatment of acute ischemic stroke. N Engl J Med 333: 1588–1593, 1995.

125. White RH: Low-molecular-weight heparins: Are they all the same? Br J Haematol 121:12–20, 2003.

126. Horlocker TT, Wedel DJ: Neuraxial block and low molecular weight heparin: Balancing perioperative analgesia and thromboprophylaxis. Reg Anesth Pain Med 23:164–177, 1998.

127. Bauer KA: Fondaparinux: Basic properties and efficacy and safety in venous thromboembolism prophylaxis. Am J Orthop 31:4–10, 2002.

128. Turpie AG, Bauer KA, Eriksson BL, Lassen MR: Fondaparinux vs enoxaparin for the prevention of venous thromboembolism in major orthopedic surgery: A meta-analysis of 4 randomized double-blind studies. Arch Intern Med 162:1833–1840, 2002.

129. The Matisse Investigators: Subcutaneous fondaparinux versus intravenous unfractionated heparin in the initial treatment of pulmonary embolism. N Engl J Med 349:1695–1702, 2003.

130. Verstraete M: Direct thrombin inhibitors: Appraisal of the antithrombin/hemorrhagic balance. Thromb Haemost 78: 357–363, 1997.

131. Greinacher A, Eichler P, Lubenow N, Luz M: Heparin-induced thrombocytopenia with thromboembolic complications: Meta-analysis of 2 prospective trials to assess the value of parenteral treatment with lepirudin and its therapeutic aPTT range. Blood 96:846–851, 2000.

132. Eriksson BI, Wille-Jorgense P, Kalebo P, et al: A comparison of recombinant hirudin with a low-molecular weight heparin to prevent thromboembolic complications after total hip replacement. N Engl J Med 337:1329–1335, 1997.

133. Schulman S, Wahlander K, Lundstrom T, et al: Secondary prevention of venous thromboembolism with the oral direct thrombin inhibitor ximelagatran. N Engl J Med 349:1713–7121, 2003.

134. Erickson UG, Bredberg U, Gislen K, et al: Pharmacokinetics and pharmacodynamics of ximelagatran, a novel oral direct thrombin inhibitor, in young healthy male subjects. Eur J Pharmacol 59:35–43, 2003.

Index

Note: page numbers in *italics* indicate illustrations; page numbers with suffix 't' indicate tables

ELSEVIER
CHURCHILL
LIVINGSTONE

The Curtis Center
170 S Independence Mall W 300E
Philadelphia, Pennsylvania 19106

ESSENTIALS OF PAIN MEDICINE AND REGIONAL ANESTHESIA
Second Edition

ISBN: 0-443-06651-5

NOTICE

Anesthesiology is an ever-changing field. Standard safety precautions must be followed, but as new research and clinical experience broaden our knowledge, changes in treatment and drug therapy may become necessary or appropriate. Readers are advised to check the most current product information provided by the manufacturer of each drug to be administered to verify the recommended dose, the method and duration of administration, and contraindications. It is the responsibility of the licensed prescriber, relying on experience and knowledge of the patient, to determine dosages and the best treatment for each individual patient. Neither the publisher nor the author assumes any liability for any injury and/or damage to persons or property arising from this publication.

Previous edition copyrighted 1999.

International Standardized Book Number 0-443-06651-5

Acquisitions Editor: Natasha Andjelkovic
Developmental Editors: Melissa Fisch and Katie Miller
Publishing Services Manager: Joan Sinclair
Project Manager: Cecelia Bayruns

Printed in the United States of America.

Last digit is the print number: 9   8   7   6   5   4   3   2   1

Essentials of Pain Medicine and Regional Anesthesia

Second Edition

Honorio T. Benzon, MD
Professor of Anesthesiology
Senior Associate Chair, Academic Affairs
Chief, Division of Pain Medicine
Director, Pain Medicine Fellowship Program
Northwestern University Feinberg School of Medicine
Chicago, Illinois

Srinivasa N. Raja, MD
Professor of Anesthesiology and Critical Care
Director of Pain Research
Division of Pain Medicine
Johns Hopkins University School of Medicine
Baltimore, Maryland

Robert E. Molloy, MD
Assistant Professor of Anesthesiology
Associate Chair, Residency Program
Northwestern University Feinberg School of Medicine
Chicago, Illinois

Spencer S. Liu, MD
Staff Anesthesiologist
Virginia Mason Medical Center
Clinical Professor of Anesthesiology
University of Washington School of Medicine
Seattle, Washington

Scott M. Fishman, MD
Chief, Division of Pain Medicine
Professor of Anesthesiology
Department of Anesthesiology and Pain Medicine
University of California, Davis
Sacramento, California

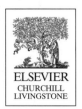

ELSEVIER
CHURCHILL
LIVINGSTONE